S0-AZR-738

PREPARATION FOR EXAMINATION

examination step-by-step

sample documentation & diagnoses

CRITICAL THINKING

HEALTH HISTORY AND REVIEW OF SYSTEMS

HEALTH HISTORY

Biographical information
Chief complaint
Present health/present illness
  Introduction
  Investigation of symptoms—chronological story
  Negative information
  Relevant family information
  Disability assessment
Past health history
  Past general health
  Childhood illnesses
  Accidents and disabling injuries
  Hospitalizations
  Operations
  Major acute and chronic illnesses
  Immunizations
  Medications and transfusions
  Allergies
Current health information
  Allergies
  Habits
  Medications
  Exercise patterns
  Sleep patterns
  Family health history
REVIEW OF SYSTEMS (for each system: usual health, health maintenance practices, health screenings and results, common symptoms, and common problems)
  Physical systems
    General
    Skin
    Hair
    Nails

SKIN, HAIR, AND NAILS

SKIN

Inspection of Each Area of Body
  Color
  Symmetry
  Uniformity
  Thickness
  Pigmentation
  Lesions
Palpation of Each Area of Body
  Moisture (dry, sweaty, oily, scaly)
  Temperature
  Thickness
  Mobility/turgor
Inspection and Palpation of Lesions
  Size
  Color
  Surface texture (flat, raised, indurated)
  Pattern
  Location and distribution
  Exudates

HAIR

Inspection
  Quantity
  Distribution
  Pattern of loss
  Color
Palpation
  Texture

SCALP

Inspection
  Condition

FACE, HEAD, AND NECK

FACE
Expression
Symmetry
Periorbital edema
HEAD
Inspection
Position
Involuntary movements
Skull
Size
Shape
Symmetry
Nose
External
Shape
Size
Color
Vascular markings
Lesions
Skin condition
Septum in midline
Symmetry
Deformity
Internal
Nasal mucosa
Color
Swelling
Exudate
Bleeding
Nasal septum
Bleeding
Perforation
Deviation
Inferior and middle turbinates
Color
Swelling
Exudate
Polyps
Lips
Color
Moisture
Lesions (blisters and ulcers)
Cracks at corners
Mouth
Denture(s)
Fit
Mucosa
Color
Lesions (ulcerations)
Lumps, thickening
Teeth
General condition
Caries
Coloration

EYES

Visual Acuity
Snellen chart
Rosenbaum chart or newspaper
Visual Fields
Confrontation test
Extraocular Movements
Six cardinal positions
Corneal light reflex
Cover-uncover test
Inspection
Symmetry, alignment
Shape
Position
Lids and lashes
Position
Palpebral fissures
Redness, swelling, lumps
Conjunctiva and sclera
Clarity
Eversion of lid, if indicated
Redness, discharge
Cornea
Clarity
Light reflex
Arcus senilis
Anterior chamber
Clarity
Depth
Lacrimal apparatus
Puncta
Swelling, redness
Lacrimal sac
Iris
Color
Shape
Flutter movements

Face, Head, and Neck *cont'd*

Missing teeth
Gums
  Condition
  Sensitivity to pressure
  Retraction
  Color
  Lesions (blisters and ulcers)
Tongue and sublingual area
  Color
  Symmetry
  Coating
  Texture
  Lesions (blisters and ulcers)
Palate (hard and soft)
  Irritation
  Lesions (blisters and ulcers)
  Malformation
Oropharynx (including tonsils)
  Color
  Presence and condition of tonsils
  Swelling
  Lesions
  Uvula

Palpation
  Scalp
  Temporal artery pulses
  Temporomandibular joint
  Sinuses
    Frontal
    Maxillary

NECK
Inspection
  Distended veins
  Swelling
  Masses
  Scars

Palpation
  Lymph nodes
  Trachea
    Position
    Deviation
  Thyroid
    Size
    Shape
    Configuration
    Nodules, cysts
    Symmetry

Auscultation
  Carotid arteries
  Thyroid (bruits)

Eyes *cont'd*

Pupils
  Equal
  Size
  Shape
  Reaction to light and accommodation
    Each eye separately
    Both eyes simultaneously

Ophthalmoscopic Examination
Lens clarity
Red reflex
Optic disc
  Size, shape
  Color
  Margins
Physiologic cup
Retinal vessels
  Color
  Arteriolar light reflex
  Arteriole/vein ratio
  Arteriovenous crossing characteristics
Retinal background
  Regularity
  Color
  Microaneurysms
  Hemorrhages
  Exudates
Macula and fovea centralis
  Regularity
  Color

Health History and Review of Systems *cont'd*

Head and face
Eyes
Ears
Nose and sinuses
Mouth and throat
Neck and nodes
Breasts
Respiratory system
Cardiovascular system
Gastrointestinal system
Urinary system
Genital system and reproductive history
Sexual history
Musculoskeletal system and extremities
Central nervous system
Endocrine system
Hematopoietic system
Functional status
Sociological system
  Relationships with family and significant others
  Environment
  Occupational history
  Economic status and resources
  Educational level
  Daily profile
  Patterns of health care
  Relevant cultural information
Psychological system
  Cognitive abilities
  Responses to illness and health
  Response to care
  Cultural implications for care
  Developmental data
  Nutritional data

Skin, Hair, and Nails *cont'd*

Palpation
  Lumps, lesions

NAILS
Inspection
  Angle
  Contour
  Color
  Ridges
  Lesions
  Infection
  Cleanliness

Palpation
  Texture
  Consistency
  Thickness
  Adherence to nail bed

EARS, NOSE, MOUTH, AND THROAT

EXTERNAL EAR

Inspection
Position
Shape
Symmetry

Preauricular and postauricular nodes

INTERNAL EAR

Inspection Using Otoscope
Condition of auditory canal
Tympanic membrane
  Color
  Cone of light
  Landmarks

NOSE, MOUTH, AND THROAT

Inspection
Nose
External nose and paranasal sinuses
  Shape
  Symmetry
Internal nose
  Nasal mucosa

Evaluation of Hearing
Hears spoken voice
Repeats whispered words
Rinne—vibrating tuning fork to mastoid process to forehead
Weber—tuning fork to mastoid process to compare AC:BC ratio

Palpation
Pinna
Tragus
Mastoid process

Musculoskeletal System   *cont'd*

Extend arms and try flexing against resistance (biceps muscle)
Flex arms and extend against resistance (triceps muscle)
Shrug shoulders against resistance (trapezius muscle)

ELBOWS

Inspection (in both flexed and extended positions)
Carrying angle
Contour

Palpation
Ulna extensor surface
Nodules
Olecranon process
Olecranon grooves

Contour
Equality
Acromioclavicular joint
Contour
Equality

Palpation
Shoulders
Bursal sites

Range of Motion
Extend both arms forward (flexion)
Extend both arms backward (hyperextension)
Put hands behind back (internal rotation)
Put hands behind head (external rotation)

Muscle Strength
Hold arms upward against resistance (deltoid muscle)

MUSCULOSKELETAL SYSTEM

Evaluate skeletal integrity while evaluating range of motion. Range-of-motion deviation or limitation to be observed includes:

1. Joint swelling, tenderness, or deformity
2. Crepitation
3. Movement symmetry
4. Strength
5. Condition of surrounding tissue, muscle, etc.

GENERAL

Posture
Body size

Inspection
Gait
Movement
Ability to change positions
Discomfort
Alignment and stature
Deformities
Spinal curvatures
Atrophied or hypertrophied limbs

HEAD

Inspection
Musculature
Facial symmetry
Skinfolds
Muscles
Wrinkles

Musculoskeletal System   *cont'd*

Extend fingers against resistance
Flex fingers against resistance
Spread fingers apart against resistance
Push fingers together against resistance

HIPS

Inspection
Iliac crest
  Height
  Symmetry
Gluteal folds

Palpation
Hips and pelvis
Stability
Tenderness
Crepitus

Range of Motion
While supine:
Raise leg above body with knee extended
Bring knee to chest while keeping other leg straight
Swing leg laterally and medially while keeping knee straight
Foot on opposite patella
Move flexed knee down (external rotation)
Flex knee and rotate leg (internal rotation)
Swing straightened leg behind body (prone or standing)

Muscle Strength
While supine:
Raise extended leg against resistance
Bring both legs together against resistance

Musculoskeletal System *cont'd*

Lateral epicondyles
Tenderness

Range of Motion
Bend and straighten elbow
Palm up (supination)
Palm down (pronation)

HANDS AND WRISTS

Inspection
Hands (dorsal and palmar)
Position
Shape
Contour
Fingers
Position
Shape
Contour
Number
Wrists

Palpation
Hands
Wrist joints

Range of Motion
Spread fingers apart and back
Make fists
Touch thumb to fingertips
Touch thumb to base of little finger
Bend fingers up and down at metacarpophalangeal joint
Bend hand up and down at wrist
Turn hand to right and left with palm facing down

Muscle Strength
Maintain wrist flexion against resistance
Extend wrist against resistance
Squeeze first two fingers as hard as possible

Musculoskeletal System *cont'd*

Perform alternate leg crossing
Hamstring muscles
Gluteal muscles
Abductor muscles
Adductor muscles

KNEES

Inspection
Natural concavities
Swelling

Palpation
Joint space
Popliteal space

Range of Motion
Bend knee
Straighten and stretch leg

Muscle Strength
Extend leg against resistance (quadriceps muscle strength)
Bend knee against resistance (hamstring muscle strength)

ANKLES AND FEET

Inspection
Weight-bearing and non-weight-bearing positions
Position
Size
Contour
Number of toes

Palpation
Ankle joint
Achilles tendon
Metatarsophalangeal joints

Ears, Nose, Mouth, and Throat *cont'd*

Color, swelling, exudate
Septum
Symmetry
Perforation
Bleeding
Inferior and middle turbinates
Color, swelling
Exudate, polyps

Mouth and Throat
Lips
Teeth
Gums
Tongue
Buccal mucosa
Parotid ducts
Hard and soft palates
Sublingual areas
Presence and condition of tonsils

Uvula rises midline when saying "ah"
Pharynx

Palpation

Nose
External nose and paranasal sinuses
Occlude each nostril to assess patency
Check nose for tenderness
Apply pressure over frontal and maxillary sinuses

Mouth
With gloved hand, palpate gums, mucosa, and sublingual area

Percussion
Direct percussion over frontal and maxillary sinuses

Musculoskeletal System *cont'd*

Palpation
Temporomandibular joint

Range of Motion
Open and close mouth
Project lower jaw
Move jaw from side to side

Muscle Strength
Bite down hard (masseter muscles)
Clench teeth, pressing down on chin

CERVICAL SPINE

Inspection
Skinfolds
Alignment
Symmetry
Muscles
Alignment
Symmetry

Palpation
Cervical spine

Range of Motion
Touch chin to chest
Extend head backward
Bend head laterally to each shoulder
Rotate head from side to side

Muscle Strength
Push cheek against hand (right and left sides)
Push forehead against hand
Push head back against hand

SHOULDERS

Inspection
Muscles

BREASTS AND REGIONAL LYMPHATICS

Inspection
Positions
  At rest
  Arms over head
  Sitting with hands pressed into hips
  Leaning forward
Skin
  Color
  Lesions
  Surface characteristics
Breasts and areolae
  Size
  Configuration
  Symmetry at rest and with motion
  Dimpling
  Retraction
  Surface characteristics
Nipples
  Surface characteristics
  Color
  Plane

Palpation
Supraclavicular nodes
Infraclavicular nodes
Axillary nodes
Breasts
  Consistency
  Masses
Areolar areas
  Masses
Nipples
  Discharge

Musculoskeletal System *cont'd*

Range of Motion
Point foot up
Point foot down
Inversion
Eversion
Rotation

Muscle Strength
Flex foot upward against resistance
Push foot down against resistance

THORACIC AND LUMBAR SPINE

Inspection
Alignment

Palpation
Spinous processes
  Tenderness
  Spasm
Paravertebral muscles
  Tenderness
  Spasm

Range of Motion
Bend back as far as possible (hyperextension)
Bend sideways (lateral bending)
Twist shoulders bilaterally (stabilize pelvis)
Slowly bend forward to touch toes

ABDOMEN

Inspection
Skin color
Scars
  Presence
  Location
Striae
  Color
  Distribution
  Amount
Dilated veins
Lesions (rashes)
Umbilicus
  Contour
  Location
  Inflammation
  Hernia
Contour
  General shape
  Local bulges

Auscultation (do before percussion and palpation in all four quadrants)
Bowel sounds
  Frequency
  Character
  Timing
  Quality
Bruits
Friction rub over liver and spleen

Percussion
Tympany in all four quadrants
Liver
  Size
Identify gastric bubble

HEART AND BLOOD VESSELS

HEART

Inspection
Apical impulse
Retractions, lifts, heaves

Palpation
Apical impulse
Pulsation, thrill, vibration
Aortic
Pulmonary
Third left interspace
Right ventricular
Apical
Epigastric

Auscultation
Apical rate and rhythm
Identify first and second heart sounds
  Location
  Intensity
  Timing
  Splitting
Precordial areas
  Aortic
  Pulmonic
  Tricuspid
  Mitral
Listen with diaphragm, then bell
  Location
  Rate
  Rhythm
  Intensity
  Splitting
  Extra sounds
Murmurs
  Timing
  Pitch
  Location
  Radiation
  Intensity
  Pitch
  Quality

BLOOD VESSELS

Inspection
Venous peripheral vascular pulse
Jugular
  Highest point pulsation seen
  Angle client lying
  Amplitude and timing of pulses

Heart and Blood Vessels *cont'd*

Arms
  Color
  Symmetry
Legs
  Color
  Symmetry
  Venous pattern
  Varicosities
  Edema
  Pigmentation
  Rashes
  Scars, ulcers
Palpation
Arterial peripheral vascular
  pulses
    Carotid
    Radial
    Brachial
    Femoral
    Popliteal
    Posterior tibial
    Dorsalis pedis
  Assess arterial peripheral
    pulses
    Rate
    Rhythm/pattern
    Amplitude
    Variations
    Contour
    Symmetry
  Arms
    Edema
    Compare radial pulses
      Volume
    Skin
      Temperature
      Texture
  Legs
    Skin
      Temperature
      Texture
    Edema
    Phlebitis
  Inguinal lymph nodes
  Femoral artery tenderness
  Phlebitis
  Capillary refill time

Abdomen *cont'd*

Spleen
  Size
Light Palpation (in all four quadrants)
Identify organ locations
Masses
Tenderness
Increased resistance
Hernia
Deep Palpation (in all four quadrants)
Masses
  Location
  Size
  Shape
  Consistency
  Mobility
Tenderness
Pulsation
Liver (deep breath and hold)
  Tenderness
  Size
  Contour of edge
Spleen (deep breath and hold)
  Tenderness
Kidney
  Tenderness
Aorta
  Pulsation
Umbilicus
  Bulges
  Nodules
  Umbilical ring

THORAX AND LUNGS

Inspect all four general thoracic areas—apical, anterior, posterior, and lateral.

Inspection
Respiration
  Rate
  Pattern
  Inspiratory/expiratory ratio
  Audible adventitious sounds
Use of accessory muscles of respiration
Skin
  Condition
  Color
  Superficial venous patterns
Thorax
  Size
  Shape
  Symmetry
  Contour
  Muscle development

Palpation
General assessment
  Skin tone
  Temperature
  Tenderness
  Unusual sensations
Thoracic expansion
Tactile fremitus

Percussion
Survey
Diaphragmatic excursion

Auscultation
Survey
Adventitious sounds
Vocal resonance

NEUROLOGICAL SYSTEM

MENTAL STATUS

General Appearance
Grooming
Manner of dress
Posture
Coordination

Cognitive Functions
Orientation
Attention span
Memory
  Immediate—digit recall
  Recent—What did you eat for lunch today?
  Remote—Where were you born?

Intellectual Functions
Abstraction ability—proverbs
  A bird in the hand is worth two in the bush.
  A rolling stone gathers no moss.
Comprehension—give client information to be recalled at a later time
Computation
  Subtract 7 from 100.
Ability to read
Insight and judgment
  What do you feel is causing your problem?
  What would you do if you were in a theater when a fire broke out?

Behavior
Mood
Characteristics of speech
  Pattern
  Quality

Neurological System *cont'd*

VIII Acoustic
Hearing acuity—whispered voice
Weber—tuning fork on center of forehead
Rinne—tuning fork on mastoid process
Otoscopic examination
Balance standing with eyes closed (Romberg)

IX Glossopharyngeal
Say "ah"
Gag reflex
Sensory—taste on posterior one third of tongue

X Vagus
Say "ah"
Listen to spoken voice
Observe ability to swallow

XI Spinal Accessory
Turn head side to side and shrug shoulders against resistance

XII Hypoglossal
Tongue strength and symmetry of movement

CEREBELLAR FUNCTION
Finger-to-nose movements
Finger-nose-finger movements
Rapid alternating movements
Heel to shin
Romberg (see Cranial Nerves)

MOTOR COORDINATION
Observe gait
Balance
  Walk heel to toe
  Walk on toes

GENITALIA AND INGUINAL AREA
Gloves must be worn during this examination.

FEMALE EXTERNAL
Palpation of external inguinal area

Inspection
Skin
  Color
  Condition
  Integrity
Hair
  Characteristics and distribution
Labia majora and minora
  Symmetry
  Color
  Inflammation
Clitoris
  Length

Urethral opening
  Discharge
  Inflammation
Vaginal opening
  Size
  Condition
Perineum
  Condition
  Inflammation
  Lesions
Anus
  Condition

Palpation
Labia
Skene's glands
Bartholin's glands

Support of pelvic musculature
Perineum
Vaginal introitus musculature
Assessment for rectocele, cystocele, enterocele, and uterine prolapse

FEMALE INTERNAL

Speculum Examination
Inspection of cervix and os
  Color
  Position
  Size
  Surface characteristics

Genitalia and Inguinal Area *cont'd*

  Tenderness or induration
Scrotum
  Surface characteristics
    Size
    Tenderness
    Consistency
    Masses
  Spermatic cords
    Consistency
    Size
    Tenderness
    Masses
  Testes
    Size
    Unusual tenderness
    Shape
    Masses
    Mobility
    Consistency
  Epididymis
    Location
    Masses
    Consistency

ANUS, RECTUM, AND PROSTATE

Inspection
Sacrococcygeal area
Perineal area
Inflammation
Lesions
Hemorrhoids
Fissures

Palpation
Anal sphincter tone
Internal sphincter tone

Rectal wall
Surface characteristics
Lesions
Masses
Prostate and seminal vesicles (males)
Size
Shape
Surface characteristics
Consistency
Tenderness

Genitalia and Inguinal Area *cont'd*

Discharge
Shape
Specimens for cervical and
  vaginal smears and
  cultures
Inspection of vaginal wall
Color
Surface characteristics
Discharge

Bimanual Palpation
Vaginal wall
Smoothness, lesions
Cervix and fornices
Size
Shape
Position
Mobility
Patency of os
Surface characteristics

Tenderness
Uterus
Size
Position
Shape
Mobility
Tenderness
Adnexal
Masses
Tenderness
Cul-de-sac
Masses
Tenderness

MALE
Inspection
Skin
Color
Lesions
Swelling

Hair
Distribution
Penis
Surface characteristics
Foreskin
Inflammation
Urethral meatus
Position
Inflammation
Discharge

Palpation
Inguinal area
Nodes
Swelling
Bulging
Penis
Inflammation
Discharge

Neurological System *cont'd*

Rate
Organization
Volume
Diction
Facial expressions

CRANIAL NERVES
I Olfactory
Simple odors
II Optic
Snellen chart (distant)
Read print (near)
Visual fields by confrontation
Ophthalmoscopic examination
III Oculomotor
Pupil constriction
Extraocular movements
Lid position

IV Trochlear
Downward and medial EOMs
V Trigeminal
Sensory (pain and touch) to three divisions
  on face with sharp object and cotton
  wisp
Motor—clench jaw and palpate masseter
  muscles
Corneal reflex—cotton wisp over cornea
VI Abducens
EOMs (lateral movements)
VII Facial
Sensory—taste on anterior two thirds of
  tongue
Motor—wrinkle forehead, close eyes, smile,
  puff cheeks

Neurological System *cont'd*

Walk on heels
Stand on one foot
Hop on one foot
Deep knee bend

SENSORY FUNCTION
Light touch (dull) sensation to face,
  extremities
Pain (sharp) sensation to face, extremities
Temperature (hot, cold) sensation
Vibration sense to extremities
Tactile discrimination
Point localization
Stereognosis/graphesthesia
Two-point discrimination—palms,
  thighs, back
Extinction—touch perceived bilaterally
Position sense—fingers, toes

REFLEXES
Deep tendon
Biceps
Triceps
Brachioradialis
Patellar
Ankle (Achilles)
Superficial
Plantar
Abdominal
Cremasteric
Gluteal

SPECIAL TESTS
Mini-Mental Status Examination
Pain assessment scale
Glasgow Coma Scale

HEALTH & PHYSICAL ASSESSMENT

HEALTH & PHYSICAL ASSESSMENT

second edition

Violet H. Barkauskas, PhD, RN, FAAN
Associate Professor
School of Nursing
University of Michigan
Ann Arbor, Michigan

Kathryn Stoltenberg-Allen, MSN, RN
Formerly Assistant Professor
Department of Public Health Nursing
College of Nursing
University of Illinois at the Medical Center
Chicago, Illinois

Linda Ciofu Baumann, PhD, RN, CS-ANP
Professor
School of Nursing
University of Wisconsin–Madison
Madison, Wisconsin

Cynthia Darling-Fisher, PhD, RN, FNC
Assistant Professor and Coordinator
Family Nurse Practitioner Program
School of Nursing
University of Michigan
Ann Arbor, Michigan

 Mosby

St. Louis Baltimore Boston Carlsbad Chicago Minneapolis New York Philadelphia Portland
London Milan Sydney Tokyo Toronto

Dedicated to Publishing Excellence

A Times Mirror
Company

Vice President and Publisher: Nancy L. Coon
Executive Editor: Sally Schrefer
Associate Developmental Editor: Rae L. Robertson
Project Manager: Deborah L. Vogel
Senior Production Editor: Judith Bange
Layout Artist: Jeanne Genz
Designer: Pati Pye
Manufacturing Manager: Linda Ierardi

SECOND EDITION
Copyright © 1998 by Mosby–Year Book, Inc.

Previous edition copyrighted 1994

Printed in the United States of America
Composition by Clarinda Company
Lithography/color film by Clarinda Company
Printing/binding by Von Hoffmann Press, Inc.

Mosby–Yearbook, Inc.
11830 Westline Industrial Drive
St. Louis, Missouri 63146

Library of Congress Cataloging in Publication Data

Health & physical assessment / Violet H. Barkauskas . . . [et al.]. —
    2nd ed.
        p.   cm.
    Includes bibliographical references and index.
    ISBN 0–8151–2776–6
    1. Nursing assessment.   2.   Medical history taking.   3.   Physical
diagnosis.   I.   Barkauskas, Violet.
    [DNLM: 1.   Physical Examination—nurses' instruction.   2.   Nursing
Assessment.   WB 200 H434 1997]
    RT48.H38   1997
    616.07′5—dc21
    DNLM/DLC
    for Library of Congress
                                                    97-14864
                                                        CIP

97 98 99 00 01/9 8 7 6 5 4 3 2 1

contributors & reviewers

CONTRIBUTORS

Beverly A. Priefer, PhD, RN
Geriatrics Research, Education, and Clinical Center
William S. Middleton Memorial Veterans Hospital;
Assistant Clinical Professor
School of Nursing
University of Wisconsin–Madison
Madison, Wisconsin
Chapter 26: Aging Clients

Gail Underbakke, MS, RD
Nutrition Coordinator
Preventive Cardiology Program and Department of Family
    Medicine
University of Wisconsin Medical School
Madison, Wisconsin
Chapter 5: Nutritional Assessment

REVIEWERS FOR FIRST AND SECOND EDITIONS

Cheryl Anderson, PhD, RN
Department of Obstetrics
University of Texas at Arlington
Arlington, Texas

Gary Arnold, MD, FACS
Assistant Professor
College of Nursing
University of Southwestern Louisiana
Lafayette, Louisiana

Eileen K. Baldwin, MSN, RN
Department of Nursing
Allentown College of St. Francis de Sales
Center Valley, Pennsylvania

Donna H. Bedsole, EdD, RN
School of Nursing
Troy State University
Montgomery, Alabama

Charlotte Breithaupt, MN, RN
School of Nursing
Baylor University
Dallas, Texas

Mary Ann Broda, PhD, RN, CPNP
Assistant Professor, Parent-Child Nursing
University of Michigan
Ann Arbor, Michigan

Pamela S. Brown, MS, RN
Blessing-Rieman College of Nursing
Quincy, Illinois

Brenda Leigh Cameron, MScN, RN
Assistant Professor
Faculty of Nursing
University of Alberta
Edmonton, Alberta

Linda S. Dillion, MS, RN
School of Nursing
Baylor University
Dallas, Texas

Marty Downey, BSN, RN, CCRN
Boise, Idaho

Linda A. Eastham, MSN, RN, FNP
Charlottesville, Virginia

Helen Hansen, MS, RN
Instructor
College of Nursing
University of Tulsa
Tulsa, Oklahoma

Janice Hausauer, MS, RN, CCRN
Adjunct Assistant Professor
Department of Nursing
Montana State University
Bozeman, Montana

Anne Hummer, PhD, RN
University of Detroit
Detroit, Michigan

Mary C. Kavoosi, PhD, RN
Clarion University
Oil City, Pennsylvania

Nancy Lospinoso, MS, RN, ONC
Orange, New Jersey

Meredith A. McCord, MS, RN
Assistant Professor
Adult Health and Illness Nursing
Oregon Health Sciences University
Portland, Oregon

Graham McDougall, PhD, RN, CS
Assistant Professor
Gerontological Nursing
Frances Payne Bolton School of Nursing
Case Western Reserve University
Cleveland, Ohio

Jolyne McGregor, PhD, RN
ADN Instructor
Trinity Valley Community College
Health Science Center
Kaufman, Texas

Donna T. Mitchell, PhD, RN, CS
Associate Professor
Department of Nursing
University of Rio Grande
Rio Grande, Ohio

Joan C. Murphy, MS, RN
Director, College of Nursing
Utica College
Utica, New York

Yvonne G. Newberry, MSN, RN, FNP
Department of Obstetrics and Gynecology
University of Virginia Health Sciences Center;
Clinical Faculty, School of Nursing
University of Virginia
Charlottesville, Virginia;
Clinical Faculty
Medical College of Virginia–Virginia Commonwealth
    University
Richmond, Virginia

Alice Palmer, MS, RN, OCN
Program Chair/Assistant Director
Nursing Technology
Health Technologies Division
Cincinnati State Technical and Community College
Cincinnati, Ohio

Marybeth Paradowski, MPH, MSN, RN
Assistant Professor, Nursing
Allentown College of St. Francis de Sales
Center Valley, Pennsylvania

Charlene Pope, MPH, RN, CNM
Clinical Associate Faculty
Women's Health Care/School of Nursing
University of Rochester
Rochester, New York

Deborah A. Raines, PhD, RNC
Maternal Child Nursing Department
School of Nursing
Virginia Commonwealth University
Richmond, Virginia

Patricia K. Reed, MA, RN, CNAA
Albany Medical Center
Project Learn
Albany, New York

Cindy Roach, DSN, RN
Associate Professor
Beth-El College of Nursing and Health Sciences
University of Colorado at Colorado Springs
Colorado Springs, Colorado

Julie Sanford, MSN, RN, CCRN
Clinical Assistant Professor
Department of Adult Health Nursing
College of Nursing
University of South Alabama
Mobile, Alabama

Susan D. Schaffer, MS, RN, CFNP
Assistant Professor of Nursing
Old Dominion University
Norfolk, Virginia

Anita Singleton, MSN, EdS, RN
Assistant Professor
School of Nursing
Missouri Southern State College
Joplin, Missouri

Elaine Steinke, PhD, RN
Department of Nursing
Wichita State University
Wichita, Kansas

dedications

To family, friends, colleagues, and students who have extended their love, support, wisdom, encouragement, and perspective during our professional lives and during the development of this book, especially:

Sally Dymek and Sally Ann Dymek
V.H.B.

Lawrence, Laurel, Matthew, and Douglas Allen
Jim and Sadye Stoltenberg
Drs. Mara and Alexandru Nitu
Carolyn Piatek
The women of Hersong
K.S-A.

Alice Simonds, mentor and teacher
L.C.B.

Daniel C., Cara, and Noah Fisher
Elaine C. and R. Clement Darling
Clem and Julie Darling
Wendy and Doug Nickerson
Elisabeth and Michael Botelho
C.D-F.

preface

Health and Physical Assessment reflects recent changes in the practice of health assessment by nurses. This new edition represents our beliefs in holistic health assessment as the basis for nursing intervention and practice. Health assessment is presented as the systematic collection of data that health professionals can use to make decisions about how they will intervene to promote, maintain, or restore health. Our goal for this text is to provide an innovative product that reflects and anticipates the ways in which nursing practice and health care are changing.

Health and Physical Assessment is designed for students and beginning practitioners. It contains the theory and skills necessary to collect a comprehensive health history and to perform a complete physical examination. These skills can be most effectively mastered when the text is used within a structured learning environment, which includes supervised student practice in skills laboratories or clinical settings. Because *Health and Physical Assessment* contains a great deal of substantive detail on examination techniques and findings, the student is not expected to outgrow the text but to continue to use it as a valuable reference in clinical practice.

Throughout this text, the consumer of health care is referred to as the *client* because the term implies the ability of a person, whether well or sick, to contract for health care as a responsible participant, along with the providers, in the health care process. Health care providers cannot expect consumers to accept assessment or intervention unless they have been actively included in the process.

■ ORGANIZATION

The content in *Health and Physical Assessment* is organized in four units. Unit I, *Taking the Health History*, introduces the linkages from health assessment to subsequent steps of the client care process—diagnosis, care planning, and implementation. It also consists of thorough discussions of the art and science of effectively taking and recording a comprehensive health history for purposes of health or illness assessment and management. Unit II, *Holistic Assessment*, assists the reader in understanding and assessing a client holistically, with chapters on developmental, nutritional, and sleep assessment and cultural considerations in health assessment.

Unit III, *Physical Assessment*, follows the traditional body-system approach and contains detailed, richly illustrated discussions of the physical examination of body systems or regions. The chapters in Unit III are consistently organized and include the following headings and content:

Anatomy and Physiology
Health History
Preparation for Examination
Technique for Examination and Normal Findings
Variations from Health
Sample Documentation and Diagnoses

The last chapter in this unit assists the reader in bringing together all physical assessment components into a logical system for performing the comprehensive physical examination.

Although this book focuses on the assessment of the healthy adult client, no comprehensive text on health assessment can ignore the special assessment techniques required by clients of other age groups and with special health needs. Thus Unit IV, *Assessing Special Populations*, includes chapters that present assessment techniques unique to pregnant women, children, older adults, and individuals with functional limitations. These client groups are frequently served by nurse practitioners.

■ FEATURES

- **Color photographs** of physical examination techniques are extensively used to enhance learning, and carefully crafted illustrations clarify significant aspects of the discussion, especially anatomy and physiology.

- **Preparation for Examination** boxes quickly present needed equipment and special considerations for preparing the client and setting for an examination.
- **Helpful Hint** boxes provide tips from experienced practitioners for performing a thorough and accurate assessment.
- **Examination Step-by-Step** boxes provide a quick overview of the physical examination discussed in a chapter.
- **Teaching Self-Assessment** is included in all applicable chapters and provides information on health promotion.
- **Cultural Considerations** boxes provide information on variations in findings that may represent cultural anomalies.
- **Sample Documentation and Diagnoses** boxes highlight the importance of documenting assessment findings and formulating nursing diagnoses, and can serve as models for documentation in the clinical setting.
- A **Glossary** is included as a reference at the end of the book and provides definitions of key terms that appear in the text.

▌ SUPPLEMENTS

An *Instructor's Manual and Test Bank to accompany Health and Physical Assessment* is available. The *Instructor's Manual* includes, for every chapter in the text, learning objectives and detailed lecture outlines, and the *Test Bank* includes approximately 1000 questions with answers.

A *Student Workbook and Laboratory Manual* is available that includes helpful learning exercises to aid the student in obtaining a thorough understanding of the material covered in *Health and Physical Assessment*. Laboratory checklists and skills checklists are also included to guide the student through learning the components of physical assessment.

▌ ACKNOWLEDGMENTS

It is our pleasure to express gratitude to a number of individuals who helped us prepare this publication. Without their support and assistance it would not have been possible. The beautiful color photographs are the products of Don Price, Tim Ford, Joe Welch, and Lin Goings of BMC Photographics, University of Michigan. Illustrations were prepared by Holly Fischer and Valorie Loomis of Biomedical Communications, University of Michigan, and Barbara Cousins. Youngshook Han, of the University of Wisconsin-Madison, greatly facilitated the library research for Dr. Baumann. Ms. Stoltenberg-Allen especially thanks Jean Gittings and Mary Spawn for their assistance with library research and computer searches.

We wish to especially acknowledge the assistance of Rae Robertson and Sally Schrefer from Mosby for making this hard work an enjoyable and rewarding experience.

Violet H. Barkauskas
Kathryn Stoltenberg-Allen
Linda Ciofu Baumann
Cynthia Darling-Fisher

contents

Unit III
PHYSICAL ASSESSMENT

Unit IV
ASSESSING SPECIAL POPULATIONS

HEALTH *&* PHYSICAL ASSESSMENT

chapter **1**

Clinical Reasoning in Determining Health Status

The chapters that follow present methods to collect data when performing a general health assessment. The examiner uses these data to formulate conclusions about the client's health status. To reach a conclusion, or diagnosis, the practitioner uses a process known as clinical reasoning, or decision making. This chapter discusses the process of clinical reasoning and its relationship to the nursing process and nursing diagnosis. In addition, it presents some methods for facilitating decision making.

■ CLINICAL REASONING PROCESS

Process of Gathering Information

The first step in clinical reasoning is gathering information. The general health assessment provides the data or information needed to formulate a diagnosis and eventually a plan of treatment and evaluation. The data-gathering process includes:

1. Data collection
2. Data validation
3. Data organization
4. Pattern identification

Data collection

Data include information gathered from the first encounter with the client and during the health interview and physical examination. Laboratory data, if applicable, are also considered. These components of a database are part of a general health assessment. In later follow-up with a client, the practitioner focuses the assessment by collecting data on a specific problem or concern.

Data are collected using a system or framework. In the physical examination, the examiner can collect data using several organizing principles: head-to-toe, regional areas of the body (e.g., pelvic examination), or body systems (e.g., cardiovascular or neurological). Each of these methods provides a logical, organized framework for collecting physical assessment data. The practitioner's decision about which method to use is influenced by both priority needs of the client and personal preference. For example, if you see a client for a periodic health examination, you would use a head-to-toe approach. However, if a client who appears in acute distress stated she had just injured her hand, you would begin the assessment by focusing on the body region affected.

As you develop expertise as a practitioner, you will

develop your own approach to data collection that is appropriate to the circumstances, such as the client's age, sex, emotional state, and acuity of the health problem or concern. Whatever approach is used, you must think about the range of possibilities and develop a sensitivity to the possible meaning of all signs and symptoms.

Data validation

Validation is the process of making sure the data collected are accurate. Data obtained using an instrument with a measurement scale can be validated by repeating the measure. For example, if a weight on the clinic scale indicates a 10-pound weight loss since the last visit, you can repeat the weight to validate this measure. Verify information with the client by direct observation or interview. Preferably, validate information yourself, rather than relying on information obtained by others, especially if it involves subjective data open to interpretation. Strategies to validate data include the following:

1. Recheck your own data. Go back to an area of the physical examination that you need to palpate or observe again.
2. Be sure other factors did not influence the accuracy of the data (e.g., while in a hurry to obtain a blood pressure, you used the wrong-size blood pressure cuff).
3. Always recheck information that is grossly abnormal. For example, repeat a systolic blood pressure reading of 260 mm Hg.
4. Ask someone, preferably more experienced, to collect the same data. If you hear a grade III systolic heart murmur on physical examination, have another clinician also listen to the heart.
5. Recheck previous documentation yourself or with other clinicians to see if abnormal findings were previously recorded.

Data organization

Data are organized by clustering. The ability to do this efficiently depends on the examiner's knowledge, skill, and preference. Theoretical frameworks help to organize data and are discussed in more detail later in this chapter. The different chapters in this book present various frameworks for health assessment. For example, Chapter 16 presents a systems approach (cardiovascular). Chapters 4 and 26 present a developmental approach that modifies the health history and physical examination for the client's age.

Pattern identification

The examiner analyzes the data to determine if gaps exist or if more data are needed to make a diagnosis. For example, if a client states he has a loss of appetite, obtaining a weight is critical to determine if weight loss has occurred. You would compare the current weight with previous weights to determine if a pattern of weight change is evident. If no previous weights were recorded, you and the client would plan to obtain weight data at a designated frequency over the next month. You would then assess these data to detect any pattern of weight change.

Medical Diagnostic Reasoning Process

Many investigators have studied how physicians diagnose illness. By comparison, few studies concern nursing decision making. However, some of the research that has been done suggests that physicians and nurses use similar clinical reasoning processes. This conclusion seems reasonable, since researchers have suggested that both tradition and necessity require nurses to make both medical and nursing judgments.

The medical diagnostic reasoning process includes four major steps (Table 1.1).

Cue recognition

In the first phase of diagnostic reasoning, the practitioner must recognize that a cue is significant. A cue is a piece of information. It can consist of either subjective or objective data. For example, a subjective cue might be the client's statement, "I feel nervous." In contrast, an objective cue might be observing a client's hand tremor.

Whether a cue is considered significant depends on the practitioner's ability to distinguish between normal and abnormal behavior, physical characteristics, and diagnostic findings. This ability, in turn, depends on the

table **1.1** Stages of Diagnostic Reasoning	
Stage	**Example**
Cue recognition	Look at client's face— notice cyanosis as abnormal
Hypothesis formulation	Client is experiencing impaired gas exchange
Hypothesis testing	Arterial blood gas result: pH 7.32, PCO_2 55 m, PO_2 65. The client appears restless and confused. Weak cough effort
Hypothesis evaluation	Do enough data exist to confirm the diagnosis of impaired gas exchange? If yes, then diagnosis is made. "Impaired gas exchange related to . . ."

examiner's knowledge base and expertise. You must stay attuned to even slight variations of normal findings, since they may have a significance that is not at first obvious. A knowledgeable and experienced practitioner, for example, might note the slight pallor of a client's nail beds and consider the diagnosis of anemia. In contrast, an inexperienced student might not even notice the subtle change in nail bed color.

In summary, during the first phase of diagnostic reasoning, cue recognition, the practitioner receives thousands of pieces of information. Next, he or she begins to sort the data, keeping some pieces of information and ignoring others. This process of sorting information is called clinical judgment. The remaining data or cues serve as a more efficient resource for the next step in the process: hypothesis formulation.

Hypothesis formulation

During the second phase of diagnostic reasoning, the practitioner decides on possible explanations for the cues recognized in the previous step. This phase is often referred to as hypothesis formulation. Inference is the process of perceiving and interpreting a cue. The examiner must be a critical observer to pick up all cues available. Before making any conclusions, the examiner first clusters or links the cues to determine any patterns. One cue, in isolation, is rarely enough to suggest a particular hypothesis or diagnosis. Rather, the presence of several cues that are usually or always associated with a specific problem helps indicate what other further information is necessary before arriving at a conclusion.

As in the first phase, an examiner's knowledge and expertise strongly influence the diagnostic reasoning process. The practitioner's knowledge influences the interpretation and relative importance of the remaining cues. Often the novice jumps to early and erroneous conclusions because he or she misinterprets cues, focuses on only one cue, or fails to eliminate irrelevant cues from the cues considered. As a practitioner gains knowledge and experience, he or she builds associations between cues and clinical situations. These associations enable the examiner to cluster cues into meaningful groups and formulate hypotheses.

The formulation of hypotheses or tentative conclusions helps focus further data collection efforts on a manageable group of possibilities. However, the examiner must be careful not to limit further investigation to only one hypothesis, since the likelihood of an accurate final diagnosis increases when several explanations are considered. The examiner must think about the more likely problems, since common problems occur with more frequency, while at the same time entertaining the probability that a rare problem might be presenting itself.

Hypothesis testing

During the third stage of diagnostic reasoning, the practitioner focuses on gathering data to support or reject the previously generated hypotheses. This phase is called hypothesis testing. Examiners use many different data collection strategies during this stage. Tables 1.2 and 1.3 list methods of continued inquiry. One or more of these techniques may be appropriate for a given clinical situation. In addition, the practitioner may be more comfortable using some methods rather than others.

Throughout the hypothesis testing phase, the practitioner needs to guard against having biases about hypotheses. Some of these biases may lead to prematurely accepting a possible explanation or prematurely rejecting an explanation (Table 1.4).

table 1.2	*General Strategies for Hypothesis Testing*	
Approach	**Explanation**	**Example**
Cue based	Explore each aspect of initial cues until all facets are covered	Facial cyanosis—mucous membranes, ears, skin color
Hypothesis driven	Investigate the defining characteristics to confirm their presence or absence	Hypoxia? Hypercapnia? Restlessness? Confusion? Irritability? Inability to move secretions?
Systematic	Review body systems	Start with respiratory system, then move to cardiovascular system, etc.
Hit or miss	No recognizable strategy	Ask client when last bowel movement took place

table **1.3**	*Hypothesis Testing Strategies Used by Experts*
Strategy	**Explanation**
Confirmation	Seek data to confirm hypothesis
Elimination	Eliminate hypothesis based on absence of key signs and symptoms (defining characteristics)
Discrimination	Investigate defining characteristics that separate diagnoses with similar signs and symptoms (i.e., look for those characteristics that are different)
Exploration	Consider investigation of diagnoses with similar manifestations

table **1.4**	*Biases Affecting Diagnosis*
Bias	**Explanation**
Frequency of occurrence	If the diagnosis being considered has been made frequently, it has a higher probability of being chosen.
Recency of experience	If the clinician has made the considered diagnosis in the recent past, the clinician may be more familiar with this diagnosis than with other related diagnoses.
Profoundness of memory	Vivid impressions of cases in which a certain diagnosis was made can influence decision making in favor of this diagnosis.

HELPFUL HINT *To minimize bias in hypothesis testing:*
- *Don't maintain a narrow focus.*
- *Don't jump to conclusions.*
- *Do explore alternative explanations.*
- *Do keep an open mind.*
- *Do take your time.*

Hypothesis evaluation

After the practitioner has investigated all reasonable explanations for the initial set of cues, he or she must evaluate each hypothesis in light of the new evidence collected and reach a final diagnosis or conclusion. Hypothesis evaluation requires synthesis of all data that have been collected, since information obtained to refute one hypothesis may support another. You might also find that the data suggest that more than one problem exists.

Careful recording of data collected is crucial. Failure to document data fully increases the chance that information necessary to evaluate the hypothesis will be lost or forgotten. Missing data, in turn, can lead to erroneous conclusions. Chapter 23 contains an example of one form that can be used to record data during the assessment process.

During this phase of diagnostic reasoning, the practitioner determines which explanation has the most sup-

porting data and chooses this hypothesis as the diagnosis. In some cases, however, the examiner can merely eliminate hypotheses until only the one with the highest probability remains.

▪ INFLUENCE OF THEORETICAL FRAMEWORKS ON CLINICAL REASONING

Although nurses and physicians seem to use the same general clinical reasoning process, these two groups of professionals reach conclusions that are quite different. The reason for this difference stems from each profession's focus of concern.

Medical and Nursing Concerns

The focus of medicine is the diagnosis and treatment of disease. The knowledge base physicians use is derived, in part, from cell and germ theories. The organizing framework for the biomedical model is biochemical or biophysical systems. As a result, physicians concentrate their investigations on biological abnormalities and on identifying the cause of such disorders. Traditionally, how human psychosocial and socioeconomic factors have an impact on health has not been a focus of medicine.

In contrast, nursing's primary focus is the diagnosis of human responses to actual or potential health problems. These responses may result in health problems but

may not be disease states. Nursing assessment focuses on the client's physical, psychological, and spiritual reactions to illness and the environment. Nurses use many theoretical frameworks to explain these phenomena. Some examples are Roy's adaptation model, Orem's self-care model, and the unitary person framework proposed by the North American Nursing Diagnosis Association (NANDA).

Theory-Based Clinical Reasoning: The Unitary Person Framework

Using a framework to guide assessment and decision making is beneficial because it helps organize knowledge and provides direction for further investigation of initial cues. A framework also provides practitioners with specific terminology, which facilitates more effective communication between members of the same discipline. NANDA has been instrumental in providing a common language to communicate nursing findings and a common framework to explain the phenomena nurses observe. The language provided by NANDA consists of nursing diagnoses arranged in a taxonomy, or meaningful pattern, based on the unitary person framework.

NANDA Taxonomy: A Nursing Classification System

The NANDA taxonomy is a nursing diagnosis classification system arranged in a hierarchy from the general to the specific based on the unitary person framework. The unitary person framework suggests that a person's health status is manifested by observable phenomena that can be classified into nine human response patterns. The most general concept of the system is the unitary person. A slightly more specific concept is health. Health, in turn, is determined by functioning within the nine human response patterns. The nine response patterns have subcategories that identify specific human patterns and behaviors within each particular response pattern. These nine human response patterns act as the major categories for the NANDA taxonomy of approved nursing diagnoses (see box above, right).

The next level of this system consists of nursing diagnoses and other subcategory headings that NANDA's Taxonomy Committee has determined to be related to a particular pattern. The boxed material on pp. 6-7 shows diagnoses arranged according to the nine human response patterns of the unitary person framework.

The NANDA taxonomy can be used to guide clinical decision making. A practitioner can select the general response pattern and assess for signs and symptoms associated with that response pattern. Response patterns are broad and can be further defined.

For example, the examiner wishing to evaluate the

Nine Human Response Patterns of the Unitary Person Framework

1. Exchanging: Mutual giving and receiving
2. Communicating: Sending messages
3. Relating: Establishing bonds
4. Valuing: Assigning worth
5. Choosing: Selection of alternatives
6. Moving: Activity
7. Perceiving: Reception of information
8. Knowing: Meaning associated with information
9. Feeling: Subjective awareness of information

From Sparks SM, Taylor CM: *Nursing diagnosis reference manual,* Springhouse, Pa, 1991, Springhouse Corp.

exchanging pattern might start by assessing the client's elimination, since "altered elimination" is one diagnosis found in this pattern.

The examiner then decides which type of elimination to evaluate first—bowel or urinary. He or she chooses bowel elimination.

Next, the examiner looks for signs and symptoms of diarrhea, constipation, or incontinence. Nursing diagnoses have been defined and determined to have certain signs and symptoms, called defining characteristics. These defining characteristics are cues for diagnostic reasoning.

Occasionally, the examiner can make even more specific diagnoses (e.g., "colonic constipation" [see box on p. 6]).

A practitioner can also use the NANDA taxonomy to investigate a specific finding, such as an abdomen that is firm to palpation. Other cues may be associated with this finding (e.g., the client's complaint of a feeling of abdominal fullness). Based on these cues, the examiner makes a tentative diagnosis of constipation. The practitioner then tests this diagnosis by searching for the presence of its other defining characteristics, such as client reports of no bowel movement for 3 days. If several of these signs and symptoms are present, the examiner can make the diagnosis of "constipation."

The predictive relationships between defining characteristics and nursing diagnoses are not perfect. These relationships are initially based on the observations of experienced clinicians who propose new nursing diagnoses. Much research is currently being conducted to validate the defining characteristics of the diagnoses accepted by NANDA. Although the association of a cluster of signs and symptoms with a nursing diagnosis may be strong, no single group of characteristics ever absolutely indicates a particular nursing diagnosis.

NANDA-Approved Nursing Diagnoses

PATTERN 1: EXCHANGE
Altered nutrition: more than body requirements
Altered nutrition: less than body requirements
Altered nutrition: potential for more than body requirements
Risk for infection
Risk for altered body temperature
Hypothermia
Hyperthermia
Ineffective thermoregulation
Dysreflexia
Constipation
Perceived constipation
Colonic constipation
Diarrhea
Bowel incontinence
Altered urinary elimination
Stress incontinence
Reflex incontinence
Urge incontinence
Functional incontinence
Total incontinence
Urinary retention
Altered (specify type) tissue perfusion (renal, cerebral, cardiopulmonary, gastrointestinal, peripheral)
Fluid volume excess
Fluid volume deficit
Risk for fluid volume deficit
Decreased cardiac output
Impaired gas exchange
Ineffective airway clearance
Ineffective breathing pattern
Inability to sustain spontaneous ventilation
Dysfunctional ventilatory weaning response (DVWR)
Risk for injury
Risk for suffocation
Risk for poisoning
Risk for trauma
Risk for aspiration
Risk for disuse syndrome
Altered protection
Impaired tissue integrity
Altered oral mucous membrane
Impaired skin integrity
Risk for impaired skin integrity
Decreased adaptive capacity: intracranial
Energy field disturbance

PATTERN 2: COMMUNICATING
Impaired verbal communication

PATTERN 3: RELATING
Impaired social interaction
Social isolation
Risk for loneliness
Altered role performance
Altered parenting
Risk for altered parenting
Risk for altered parent/infant/child attachment
Sexual dysfunction
Altered family processes
Caregiver role strain
Risk for caregiver role strain
Altered family process: alcoholism
Parental role conflict
Altered sexuality patterns

PATTERN 4: VALUING
Spiritual distress (distress of the human spirit)
Potential for enhanced spiritual well-being

PATTERN 5: CHOOSING
Ineffective individual coping
Impaired adjustment
Defensive coping
Ineffective denial
Ineffective family coping: disabling
Ineffective family coping: compromised
Family coping: potential for growth
Potential for enhanced community coping
Ineffective community coping
Ineffective management of therapeutic regimen (individuals)
Noncompliance (specify)
Ineffective management of therapeutic regimen: families
Ineffective management of therapeutic regimen: community
Ineffective management of therapeutic regimen: individual
Decisional conflict (specify)
Health-seeking behaviors (specify)

PATTERN 6: MOVING
Impaired physical mobility
Risk for peripheral neurovascular dysfunction
Risk for perioperative positioning injury
Activity intolerance
Fatigue
Risk for activity intolerance
Sleep pattern disturbance
Diversional activity deficit

NANDA-Approved Nursing Diagnoses—cont'd

PATTERN 6: MOVING—cont'd
Impaired home maintenance management
Altered health maintenance
Feeding self-care deficit
Impaired swallowing
Ineffective breastfeeding
Interrupted breastfeeding
Effective breastfeeding
Ineffective infant feeding pattern
Bathing/hygiene self-care deficit
Dressing/grooming self-care deficit
Toileting self-care deficit
Altered growth and development
Relocation stress syndrome
Risk for disorganized infant behavior
Disorganized infant behavior
Potential for enhanced organized infant behavior
PATTERN 7: PERCEIVING
Body image disturbance
Self-esteem disturbance
Chronic low self-esteem
Situational low self-esteem
Personal identity disturbance
Sensory/perceptual alterations (specify) (visual, auditory, kinesthetic, gustatory, tactile, olfactory)

Unilateral neglect
Hopelessness
Powerlessness
PATTERN 8: KNOWING
Knowledge deficit (specify)
Impaired environmental interpretation syndrome
Acute confusion
Chronic confusion
Altered thought processes
Impaired memory
PATTERN 9: FEELING
Pain
Chronic pain
Dysfunctional grieving
Anticipatory grieving
Risk for violence: self-directed or directed at others
Risk for self-mutilation
Post-trauma response
Rape-trauma syndrome
Rape-trauma syndrome: compound reaction
Rape-trauma syndrome: silent reaction
Anxiety
Fear

Using the NANDA taxonomy method of assessment and decision making may be difficult at first, since nurses traditionally have not been taught to organize their thinking in this manner. As more nursing diagnoses are developed, defined, and verified, the taxonomy will continue to be refined. This, in turn, will make the nursing diagnosis process easier.

■ USING A CLASSIFICATION SYSTEM TO FACILITATE CLINICAL REASONING

Classification systems such as the NANDA taxonomy serve as road maps for diagnostic reasoning. From any given location in the classification scheme, a practitioner can investigate in the direction of either a more general or a more specific conclusion, whichever is appropriate for the situation.

Body Systems Approach

One classification system frequently used in physical assessment is the body systems approach. Using a body systems approach, an examiner might choose to evaluate the gastrointestinal system. This is a general category that consists of several organs and tissues. After choosing the system to assess, the practitioner focuses on evaluating the functioning of the various organs and tissues. With an abnormal finding, the examiner then searches for additional signs and symptoms known to be associated with this finding to make a diagnosis.

Examiners can also use the body systems approach to move from a specific complaint or finding to an evaluation of the functioning of one or more systems. For example, a practitioner investigating tachycardia might first search for other cardiac-related signs and symptoms. However, during this search, the practitioner observes that the client has abdominal distress, has difficulty concentrating, and describes a smothering sensation. The diagnostic process might then involve assessing environmental variables for other data to confirm the tentative nursing diagnosis of anxiety related to situational crisis.

Theoretical Frameworks

Nurses, as well as physicians, have traditionally used the body systems approach to assessment. However, this approach does not always facilitate the formulation of

nursing diagnoses. To ease the process of making nursing diagnoses, nurses must use a theory-based approach to assessment and decision making.

Maslow's hierarchy of needs

Maslow's hierarchy of needs is a system of classifying human needs based on the idea that lower-level physiological needs must be met before higher-level abstract needs can be met. By considering categories of needs, the nurse can provide more holistic care. Nursing diagnoses can be related to each of the categories in Maslow's hierarchy:

1. Physiological needs—oxygen, food, elimination, temperature control, sex, movement, rest, comfort
2. Safety and security—safety from physical or psychological threat; protection, continuity, stability, lack of danger
3. Love and belonging—affiliation, affection, intimacy, support, reassurance
4. Self-esteem—sense of self-worth, self-respect, independence, dignity, privacy, self-reliance
5. Self-actualization—recognition and realization of one's potential, growth, health, autonomy

Orem's universal self-care demands

For humans to function, they must be able to meet universal self-care demands. If a person is not able to meet these demands, a self-care deficit occurs. In Orem's theory, the goals of nursing include helping the client to overcome circumstances that interfere with or cause self-care deficits.

Gordon's functional health patterns

The most widely used organizing framework for nursing diagnoses is based on functional health patterns described by Marjory Gordon. The 11 health patterns allow for easy organization of basic nursing information obtained during an initial health assessment (see also Chapter 3: The Health History). Gordon's functional health patterns are as follows:

1. Health-perception–health-management pattern
2. Nutritional-metabolic pattern
3. Elimination pattern
4. Activity-exercise pattern
5. Sleep-rest pattern
6. Cognitive-perceptual pattern
7. Self-perception–self-concept pattern
8. Role relationship pattern
9. Sexuality-reproductive pattern
10. Coping-stress-tolerance pattern
11. Value-belief pattern

■ CLINICAL REASONING AND THE NURSING PROCESS

Assessment

The nursing process consists of five phases: assessment, diagnosing, planning, implementation, and evaluation. The assessment phase includes history taking and physical examination and ends with the determination of actual or potential nursing diagnoses. This definition implies that some form of clinical reasoning has occurred.

During the initial phase of clinical reasoning, the practitioner performs a cursory initial assessment for significant cues. This initial assessment can be as simple as eliciting the client's presenting complaint and making general observations concerning the client's appearance. After clustering the initial cues and formulating tentative hypotheses, the examiner performs a second, more focused assessment. Thus assessment and clinical reasoning are intertwined.

Nursing Diagnoses

Nursing diagnoses are actual or potential problems that can be prevented, resolved, or reduced through independent nursing interventions. The nursing focus is holistic and includes comfort as well as cure. The culmination of nursing assessment and clinical reasoning is the formulation of nursing diagnoses.

According to NANDA's recommendations, a nursing diagnosis should be stated in a problem–etiology–signs and symptoms (P-E-S) format. This format also conveniently summarizes the key defining characteristics leading to the final diagnosis. Following is a sample nursing diagnosis:

Problem (P)—Impaired physical mobility

Etiology (E)—"related to" a fractured tibia; status after cast application

Signs and symptoms (S)—"as manifested by"; client states, "I can't walk without help. I feel clumsy using crutches." The client requires standby assistance when ambulating to the bathroom; is observed to position crutches correctly during ambulation.

Diagnostic statement: Impaired physical mobility related to a fractured tibia after cast application manifested by statements that she cannot walk without help and feels clumsy, and observation that she needs standby assistance when using crutches correctly.

When nursing diagnoses are recorded in this manner, any nurse reading the diagnostic statement is able to determine how the diagnosis was reached. In addition, nursing diagnoses written in P-E-S format provide clues about possible nursing interventions by indicating which defining characteristics are present and therefore

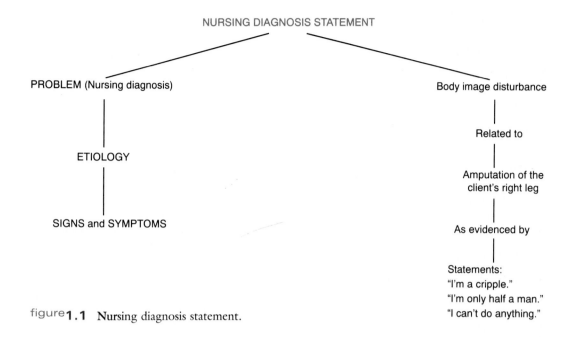

NURSING DIAGNOSIS STATEMENT

PROBLEM (Nursing diagnosis)

ETIOLOGY

SIGNS and SYMPTOMS

Body image disturbance

Related to

Amputation of the client's right leg

As evidenced by

Statements:
"I'm a cripple."
"I'm only half a man."
"I can't do anything."

figure**1.1** Nursing diagnosis statement.

require intervention. In this way, nursing diagnoses can also assist in the planning phase of the nursing process. For example, the diagnosis in Figure 1.1 suggests planning interventions that would allow the client to ventilate feelings regarding the loss of a leg. Another suggested intervention would be fostering the client's independence by encouraging self-care and personal decision making.

> **HELPFUL HINT** *A nursing diagnosis is* not:
> - *A diagnostic test (schedule for mammogram)*
> - *A nursing problem (difficulty visualizing cervix)*
> - *A medical diagnosis (fractured tibia)*
> - *A nursing goal (teach breast self-examination)*

Planning and Clinical Management
Prioritize diagnoses

Whenever you develop more than one diagnosis, assign priority to each diagnosis to plan care. In your plan, first address the diagnoses with the highest priority. Some needs may be emergency needs such as:

> *High risk for violence: self-directed* related to suicide attempt manifested by repeated statements: "I want to shoot myself" and possession of a handgun.

You may prioritize other needs as intermediate. Low-priority needs do not directly relate to a specific, current problem. An organizing framework, such as Maslow's hierarchy of needs, will help you assign priorities.

Establish outcomes or goals

Establish goals to let others know what is to be accomplished and when. The examiner must also assess the client's preferences and expectations before establishing goals. Short-term goals are those that can be met relatively quickly (days or weeks), and long-term goals can be met over months or years. For example, a short-term goal for a client would be "Increase skill in breast self-examination." The long-term goal would be "Client incorporates monthly breast self-examination into lifestyle habits."

Outcomes are the specific measurable events associated with each goal, including a time frame by which the expected outcomes should be accomplished. The client outcome is a statement of behavior that demonstrates an improvement in, or resolution of, the problem.

To continue with the previous example, the client outcome related to the short-term goal would be "The client will be able to perform a breast self-examination after observing a demonstration." The outcome related to the long-term goal would be "At 1-year follow-up the client will report performing monthly breast self-examination." Each of these outcomes is stated in measurable terms, one verified by practitioner observation and one by data obtained in an interview.

Intervention

Once you have prioritized and identified client outcomes, record a plan of action and specific nursing strategies for meeting the goals. The etiology of a prob-

lem or response pattern guides selection of the specific interventions. When listing nursing interventions, include when the action should be done; who should be involved; and the frequency, quantity, and method to be used. For example, "The employee health nurse will offer on-site 1-hour classes twice yearly on breast self-examination technique to all female employees." Methods of intervention include assessing, teaching, counseling, consulting, and referring.

When implementing nursing interventions, determine the difference between nursing diagnoses and collaborative problems. Nursing diagnoses relate to health problems or potential problems that nurses can independently treat. Independent nursing interventions are within the legal scope of nursing practice and require no supervision or direction by others.

On the other hand, collaborative interventions involve direction from, or collaboration with, an appropriate and legally designated health care professional. Collaborative problems can be prevented, resolved, or reduced through collaborative or interdependent nursing interventions.

Each time you identify a problem or potential problem, ask yourself "Can I initiate the treatment independently?" If the answer is no, another licensed health care professional, usually a physician, must provide collaboration or direction.

Evaluation

The criteria for evaluation are the same as the goals or outcomes identified during planning. To evaluate goal achievement, compare the documented outcome criteria with the client's actions or behaviors. Once you have determined whether the client has achieved the outcomes, gather data to analyze what factors contributed to success or failure. Factors that may contribute to unsuccessful outcomes might be:

New problems developed.
The original problem changed.
The interventions were not appropriate.
The goals were unrealistic.
The intervention did not fit the client.

After you have evaluated the goals and outcomes, develop a revised plan of care with new goals, outcomes, and interventions. Work with the client on all phases of this process, including how to revise the care plan. This evaluation process is ongoing as long as the practitioner has a role in caring for the client.

■ SUMMARY

Clinical reasoning is an integral part of the nursing process. All five phases of the clinical reasoning process occur during nursing assessment. The end products are nursing diagnoses. The NANDA taxonomy provides a classification system and a language for communicating. Nursing diagnoses written in the P-E-S format contribute useful information to the rest of the nursing process. Nursing diagnoses are used to organize assessment data, as a basis for care planning and evaluation, and as a focus for nursing documentation.

This book introduces the student practitioner to skills and techniques for obtaining and organizing data from clients. Examples in each chapter demonstrate beginning steps in clinical and diagnostic reasoning.

chapter **2**

Interviewing Skills and Techniques

■ PURPOSE OF THE INTERVIEW

Developing Relationships

The major purpose of interviewing a client before performing the physical examination is to obtain a health history. Practitioners must be skillful in communication techniques to enable a client to fully share life experiences relevant to his or her health status. When the initial interview is problem focused, the practitioner also asks about the signs and symptoms associated with the client's problems or concerns.

Beginning with introductions, the practitioner observes and analyzes the client's reactions to the interview. The examiner must establish a climate of trust to promote interaction necessary for a therapeutic relationship, or an interaction that maintains a focus on the client's needs. As a practitioner, you can create a climate of trust by the way you introduce yourself, by how you conduct the interview, and through the environment you arrange for the interview. To create a respectful and warm environment, introduce yourself, including your full name and your role in the agency; describe your understanding of the purpose of the interview; and address the client by his or her full name or surname (Figure 2.1).

Another way to promote trust and acknowledge the client as an active participant in the interview is to ask about the client's primary concerns and goals for the visit. Use communication skills that create a climate in which the client feels free to talk about his or her health condition. These strategies are necessary for obtaining the most reliable data about both the client's physical and mental status (see Chapter 19: Neurological System, Including Mental Status).

Contracting

The initial interview is the basis for establishing a client-provider contract. Contracting is an agreement between the provider and client that makes explicit the expectations of each party. For example, the provider might state that for the client to receive appropriate preventive care, the client will agree to make an appointment at least yearly. The client is then encouraged to respond. It is not necessary to label this agreement a

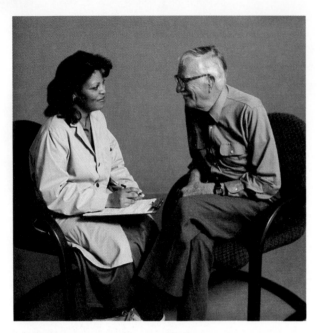

figure**2.1** Establishing a climate that is comfortable and respectful to the client promotes communication.

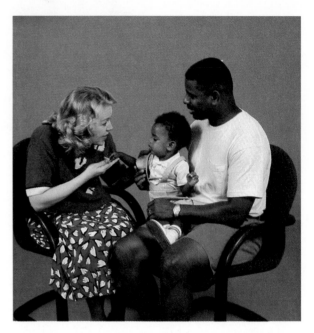

figure**2.2** The practitioner modifies the interview by the client's age and the presence of other family members.

"contract," but it is important for the client and provider to agree on the plan and modify it as needed.

Sometimes contracts are written, but most often they are verbal agreements. Written contracts are often useful when using behavior modification techniques for dealing with behavior changes, such as smoking cessation or medication taking.

Timing is important when the examiner introduces discussion of a contract. Allow enough time so that you and the client have exchanged introductions and you have some awareness of the client's needs and the purpose of the visit. However, it is important not to wait until the very end of the visit to discuss a plan of care or treatment. Adequate time should be available for negotiating any modifications to the course of action or plan based on the client's response.

Modifications in the Interview

The interview will be modified by the age of the client, the reason for the visit, and the existing relationship between you and the client. A young child will be accompanied by a parent or adult who will be the major source of information. It is important to remember that although the adult may be providing the verbal information, the child needs to feel included in the interview. Introduce yourself to the child, ask the child questions, and let the child touch equipment. Adults may also prefer to have a family member or significant other with them during a health visit. Confirm with the client that he or she chooses to have another person present and

acknowledge the presence and concerns of the family member or significant other (Figure 2.2).

On the first visit with a client who is being seen for a general health assessment, allocate adequate time to obtain baseline data and develop a relationship with the client. When you see a client who has an acute problem, focus less time on past history and put greater emphasis on understanding the immediate problem. A practitioner who has known a client and/or the family members over many years may be quite familiar with many aspects of the client's health status and may need a shorter amount of time for a visit. However, a provider in this situation will need to periodically and systematically update history information.

Guide for Focusing the Physical Examination

Always ask for basic information, such as the client's reason for seeking care, his or her current health status, information about allergies, medications taken, levels of stress, and support available to cope with health concerns (see Chapter 3: The Health History). The focus and types of questions you ask will vary according to the client's presenting problem or concerns. Chapters 10 through 27 include history questions related to a specific body system or to the health concerns of special populations (such as children, the elderly, and the functionally limited).

From information obtained in the history, you will

I.D. #: _____

NAME: _____

PHONE: _____

GYNECOLOGY CLINIC
Confidential To be completed by patient

ELIGIBILITY: E P F O M C
                          O

DATE: _____

Reason for Visit

First Day of Last   Drug Allergies   Present Medications
Menstrual Period

REPRODUCTIVE HISTORY: Age at 1st period _____ Date of Last Pap _____

Number of: Live births _____   Pregnancies _____   Abortions _____   Miscarriages _____

Have you ever had: Breast _____   Uterus/Tube_____   Sexually_____   Abnormal Pap _____
                      Abnormality   Infection   Transmitted
                                                               Disease

Other OB/Gyn Problems:_____

Did your mother take DES (a hormone) while pregnant with you? ❏ Yes ❏ No ❏ Unsure

Do you have: **Flow:** ❏ excessively heavy   ❏ missed periods
                                    ❏ excessively light

❏ painful periods
❏ spotting between periods
❏ unusual discharge/infection
❏ sexual concerns

Are you sexually active? ❏ Yes ❏ No

Current contraception? (Specify) _____

List any problems you are experiencing: _____

FAMILY HISTORY:

Have any members of your immediate family i.e., Grandparent(s) Parent(s) Sibling(s) ever had

❏ high blood pressure   ❏ heart attack or stroke
❏ diabetes   ❏ cancer, type _____

MEDICAL HISTORY: please check any condition(s) that applies to you

❏ heart disease   ❏ anemia   ❏ gallbladder disease   ❏ kidney or bladder infections
❏ high blood pressure   ❏ asthma   ❏ cancer   ❏ thyroid disease
❏ migraine headaches   ❏ epilepsy   ❏ high cholesterol   ❏ liver disease/jaundice
❏ blood clots (leg or lungs) ❏ diabetes   ❏ sickle cell disease   ❏ surgery, type _____
❏ eating disorder   ❏ depression   ❏ other _____

HEALTH BEHAVIORS: (Please refer to pamphlet (p) or video (v) for more information)

Do you: (Please check all that apply to you)

❏ smoke (p)   ❏ eat a well balanced diet (p)
❏ have a weight problem (p)   ❏ exercise regularly (p)
❏ have a history of alcohol or other drug use (p)   ❏ perform monthly self breast examinations (p) (v)
❏ more than 2 sexual partners in the past six months (p) (v)   ❏ have Rubella immunization (p)

figure**2.3** Self-administered history form.

determine what to explore in more depth during the physical examination. For example, if a client's major reason for a visit is a cough, nasal congestion, and fullness in the head, focus on examining the head, eyes, ears, nose, and throat (HEENT), as well as the lungs. A neurological or musculoskeletal examination, for example, may not be necessary during that visit.

HELPFUL HINT *A self-administered history form helps the practitioner to focus the interview and can save time (Figure 2.3).*

Therapeutic Use of Self

The use of certain personal qualities of the interviewer to support the client's perspective or feelings is called therapeutic use of self. For example, an interviewer might say, "As a woman I have also experienced . . ." or "As a mother I can understand how difficult this can be . . ." This technique can be especially helpful when the client's background, such as ethnicity, race, or socioeconomic status, appears to be very different from the examiner's background. It helps to find a common connection that can facilitate communication.

■ CONDUCTING THE INTERVIEW

Health History

Begin by finding out the client's chief complaint, or major reason for seeking care. It is also important to find out why the client came at this point in time. It may be that it was simply a convenient time or that an acute problem started to get worse and the client felt the need for treatment. Other underlying concerns related to a chief complaint may exist. An individual may have had a "blue-black" mole for a number of years and now wants it evaluated "immediately." By asking what triggered the visit now, you may find that a friend or relative recently died of malignant melanoma and the client is now concerned about having cancer. Because you are aware of the concern, you can provide the appropriate evaluation, reassurance (if appropriate), and education about the warning signs of melanoma.

A client may also have a specific agenda that is not obvious from the stated reason for a visit. By asking a question such as "How did you hope I could help you today?" toward the end of the visit, you can identify the client's underlying concerns, as well as address the health issues obvious to a clinician (Molde, 1986).

You may also obtain data from secondary sources, such as parents, guardians, family members, significant others, written records, and interpreters. However, the client must sign a written consent for a provider to obtain information from other existing health records. The use of interpreters is discussed in more detail later in this chapter under Cultural Variation.

Client explanatory models

You can ask the client a series of questions to uncover his or her explanatory model (Kleinman, Eisenberg, and Good, 1978). Answers to these questions provide a meaningful explanation of the events surrounding an illness and suggest the appropriate course of action. The questions also help to uncover the client's level of understanding about a health problem. These questions include:

What do you think caused your problem?
Why do you think it started when it did?
What do you think your illness does to you?
What are the symptoms?
How long do you think it will last?

Based on information you obtain, you can develop a plan that will be sensitive to the client's needs and level of understanding.

Dimensions of a symptom

Symptoms are the perceived changes in body sensations or functions. During an interview, obtain a thorough understanding of the dimensions of a symptom. This understanding will help guide the focus of the physical examination. Seven criteria can be used to describe a symptom: location, quality, quantity, timing, setting in which it occurs, aggravating or alleviating factors, and associated symptoms.

Dimensions of a symptom	Questions to ask
1. Location	"Where do you feel it? Does it move around? Does it radiate? Show me where it hurts."
2. Quality or character	"What does it feel like?"
3. Quantity or severity	"On a scale of 1 to 10, with 10 being the worst pain you could have, how would you rate the discomfort you have now?" "How does this interfere with your usual activities?" "How bad is it?"
4. Timing	"When did you first notice it? How long does it last? How often does it happen?"
5. Setting	"Does this occur in a particular place or under certain circumstances? Is it associated with any specific activity?"
6. Aggravating or alleviating factors	"What makes it better? What makes it worse?"
7. Associated symptoms	"Have you noticed other changes that occur with this symptom?"

Preparation for the Interview: Client and Environment

A comfortable, private, and quiet environment is essential for conducting an interview. Meet the client before he or she has undressed for the physical examination. In some clinics, clients are asked to undress before they meet the clinician. If you are in such a situation, try to at least introduce yourself before the client undresses. Address the client using his or her full name or surname. Identify yourself using your full name and title. This greeting respectfully acknowledges the client and conveys your personal accountability as part of the health care team.

You and the client should both be comfortably seated during the interview. To put the client at ease, directly state that the information you obtain will be confidential, recorded in the medical record, and shared only with those individuals directly involved in the care and treatment plan.

During the interview you will need to take some notes regarding dates, events, or short phrases related to specific aspects of the history. It is not desirable to complete the final report during the interview because doing so diverts attention from the client. You will need practice to determine what relevant information to document during the interview and what data can be later written or dictated into the permanent record. History forms that are partially completed by the client before the interview and flow sheets are useful devices for facilitating documentation of history information (see Figure 2.3).

Techniques for Conducting the Interview

Start with the concerns the client stated in the chief complaint. Be aware of the pace of your questions and the tone of your voice. You do not want to appear rushed or abrupt.

Types of questions

Open-ended questions. Open the interview with a broad opening statement, such as "Tell me what brings you here today." You can prompt the client to explain details using minimal verbal activity. For example, you might say, "You feel . . . ?"

The aim of an open-ended question is to elicit a response that is more than one or two words. A client will answer this type of question by describing signs or symptoms in his or her own words and at his or her own pace. Examples of open-ended questions are "Can you tell me a little about yourself?" or "How have you been feeling since your last visit?" A risk of asking an open-ended question is that the client may be unable to focus on the topic being asked or may take an excessive

amount of time to tell his or her story. In such cases you will need to focus the interview.

Closed-ended questions. A closed-ended question requires a response of one or two words, such as "yes" or "no," or a brief statement regarding marital status, age, or a list of medications the client may be taking. An examiner asks closed-ended questions when specific information is required, such as the client's age or the possible presence of a specific health risk (e.g., smoking), or when the client has a limited ability to respond (e.g., because of anxiety, lack of verbal skill, or physical discomfort). If a practitioner is rushed, he or she may ask more closed-ended questions to speed up the process of obtaining a history of the problem. A word of caution: Failure to allow clients to express in their own words the nature of their problem may lead to inaccurate conclusions and in the long run waste time.

Directive questions. Directive questions lead the client to focus on one set of thoughts. This type of question is most often used in reviewing systems or in evaluating functional status. Allow the client time for reflection, at least 5 to 10 seconds, before you ask the next question. For example, you might ask, "Have you experienced any problems with urination in the past, such as infections or unusual frequency, urgency, or difficulty urinating?"

> **HELPFUL HINT** *To ask the clearest questions, use simple words. For example, it is better to ask, "Does Quan have pain?" than to ask, "Is Quan experiencing any discomfort?" when obtaining information from a secondary source.*

Permission-giving questions. Frequently you will need to ask clients questions about sensitive areas or concerns. One way to deal with such questions is to ask clients in a way that lets them know that it is all right to speak of such things to you. For example, you might tell a male client, "Many young men I see have questions or concerns about sexually transmitted diseases; what questions do you have?"

Use of silence

Periods of silence during the interview can be helpful for both you and the client. Short periods of silence allow the client to organize his or her thoughts. During silent periods, you can observe the client's emotional state and note nonverbal cues. Silence may also indicate that either you or the client may need time to reflect on what was just said.

Validating information from the interview

Clarification. Use clarification to obtain more information about conflicting, vague, or ambiguous statements. By asking the client to elaborate on, or clarify, the thoughts and feelings he or she has expressed, you will communicate understanding. An example of clarification is "You say you feel out of sorts. Tell me what you mean."

Restatement. Restatement involves repeating what the client has said using different words. It is a way to acknowledge that you are listening to the client and to validate your interpretation of what the client has said. An example is "I'd like to review the timing of your symptoms with you. You said that first you experienced a headache; then nausea and vomiting followed an hour later. Is that correct?"

Reflection. Reflection is repeating a phrase or sentence the client just said. This suggests to the client that you are still interested in the topic being discussed and you would like further elaboration on the facts or feelings involved. An example of reflection follows:

Client: I love my children, but sometimes they are so misbehaved that I am afraid I'll hurt them.

Interviewer: You are afraid you might hurt them?

Use reflection to describe nonverbal behavior and ask the client what it means. For example, "I notice that you haven't taken your sunglasses off. Is there a reason?" Verbalizing that you perceive what the client feels communicates empathy. For example, "I see you have tears in your eyes. You must feel quite sad about this."

Confrontation. In confrontation, you make the client aware that what you observe is not consistent with what he or she said. An example is "You are telling me how depressed you feel, but I notice you are smiling a lot." Another example is "You said you were so sick this morning you stayed home from work, yet you show no distress now. Can you help me understand what is going on?"

Interpretation. During interpretation, you share with the client the conclusion you have drawn from the information you obtained in the interview. Sharing your interpretation or the meaning of the facts provides the client with an opportunity to confirm, deny, or offer an alternative interpretation.

Summary. The use of summary is a technique that orders and condenses the information obtained during an interview to help clarify the situation being discussed. This is particularly useful when you obtain information from a client who has difficulty conveying the sequence of events.

When you terminate the interview, it may be helpful to summarize the information you obtained to highlight the main areas discussed. A summary also allows the client to assess whether information pertinent to his or her health problem was completely obtained and can help demonstrate to both the client and the examiner what was accomplished during the interview.

Focusing/refocusing

Focusing or refocusing involves guiding the direction of the interview. During focusing or refocusing, you attempt to help the client expand on a particular topic of concern. It is particularly useful if the client comes in for an acute complaint but has multiple health problems. It is also useful if the client begins to ramble or avoids a particular topic. When attempting to focus the interview, acknowledge the value of the information being given but redirect the discussion to the problem at hand. An example is "I would like to hear about your past history shortly; for the moment I need more information about your headaches."

Nonverbal communication

Body posture. Body language is the conveyance of messages by movements or gestures of the body or limbs, facial expressions, and eye contact. Body posture may convey anxiety, boredom, attention, or indifference. Both the examiner and the client communicate nonverbally. In a closed-body posture, one holds limbs in a defensive position, close to the body as though hugging oneself. This often conveys mistrust or anxiety. An open-body posture is one that is more relaxed, with arms extended or hanging loosely at sides. An examiner who remains standing during an interview conveys a message of time urgency. An examiner who is seated comfortably during the interview conveys to the client that they will take some time to conduct the interview.

Facial expressions such as frowns or smiles are indi-

CULTURAL CONSIDERATIONS

NONVERBAL BEHAVIOR VARIATIONS

Appropriate nonverbal behavior is subject to considerable cultural variation. In the dominant culture of the United States, it is important to look directly at the person with whom you are speaking. In other cultures (Asian, Native American, Indochinese, Arab, Appalachian), looking directly at another person may be a sign of disrespect or aggression. In many cultures it is not acceptable for a younger person or woman to have direct eye contact with a male. In many Asian cultures it is considered inappropriate to openly express pain or sadness to a stranger.

cators of emotional states such as anxiety, fear, surprise, or joy.

Eye contact. Use eye contact and eye movement to engage or remove yourself from a situation. You may convey the message that the interview is over by looking at a watch or clock. A client who looks around the room while answering questions or talking and avoids eye contact with the examiner may have anxiety about the situation being discussed. Prolonged direct gaze into the examiner's eyes or an excess or absence of blinking might be cues to the client's mental status.

Mirroring activity. Mirroring involves awareness of nonverbal aspects of the client's communication to you (e.g., speed and volume of speech, and body position). Imitate or mirror these characteristics in an unobtrusive way. For example, if a client is sitting forward with her arms folded across her chest, you can also fold your arms across your chest and lean forward in the client's direction. This is an action that individuals who are engrossed in a conversation frequently do without thinking. Mirroring has been shown to increase the client's comfort level and sense of rapport. It is also a nonverbal way to evaluate how comfortable the client is with the discussion. If in the course of the interview, the client suddenly changes from an open-body posture that had been similar to your own posture to a closed-body posture, the discussion may have raised a sensitive topic or the client may have lost interest in the discussion.

Interpersonal distance. Interpersonal distance is the distance between two individuals interacting. This may vary by the nature of the relationship or cultural practices. The distance most acceptable in the dominant culture of the United States is to be close enough to be able to extend one's arm to shake hands, to hear a moderate- to low-volume voice, and to clearly observe the client. Trust is best developed from this distance.

Cultural variation

If you work with a particular cultural group, it is necessary to obtain some understanding of the group's health beliefs and practices, as well as some language skills to facilitate communication. The use of interpreters may be critical (see box at right). A useful guide for overcoming barriers in cross-cultural communication is the LEARN model (Berlin and Fowkes, 1983):

L   Listen with sympathy and understanding to the client's perception of the problem.
E   Explain your perceptions of the problem.
A   Acknowledge and discuss the differences and similarities.
R   Recommend a course of action.
N   Negotiate an agreement.

Given current projections about the number of cultural groups who will receive health care in the United

---

Guidelines for the Use of Interpreters

1. Unless you are fluent in the client's language, use an interpreter.
2. Allow extra time when using an interpreter. The interview becomes a discussion among people.
3. Avoid using family members as interpreters. They may respond to your questions based on their own knowledge without asking the client.
4. Make sure the interpreter has a basic understanding of medical terminology. Become familiar with the meaning of special words or phrases that connote practices or traditions of a particular cultural group.
5. Make sure the interpreter understands the confidential nature of the information obtained in the interview.
6. Direct questions to the client. The client may then direct responses to you directly or to the interpreter.
7. Some cultures are unfamiliar with direct questions. If necessary, adjust the type and tone of your questions to a style that is more conversational. Use short questions with minimal jargon.
8. Using repetition, validate information you heard; summarize what you heard at the end of the interview.
9. Instructions to the client may need to be in writing in the client's language to ensure clear understanding.
10. Get feedback from the interpreter about the client's emotional state and comprehension.

States in the next 50 years, it is unrealistic to assume that health care providers can have in-depth knowledge of the health practices and beliefs of multiple cultural groups. It is unwise to assume that because a client is a member of a particular cultural or ethnic group, he or she holds a certain belief. Beliefs within a cultural or ethnic group vary as much as they do among different groups.

Therefore the ability to uncover health care beliefs in each client is an essential skill for any health care provider. Questions to elicit a client's explanatory model of an illness (Kleinman, Eisenberg, and Good, 1978) is one approach to gathering this information. (See also Chapter 7: Cultural Considerations in Health Assessment.)

CULTURAL CONSIDERATIONS

DEVELOPING CULTURAL SENSITIVITY

1. Recognize that cultural diversity exists.
2. Demonstrate respect for people as unique individuals, with culture as one factor that contributes to their uniqueness.
3. Respect the unfamiliar.
4. Identify and examine your own cultural beliefs.
5. Recognize that some cultural groups have definitions of health and illness as well as practices that attempt to promote health and cure illness, which may differ from your own.
6. Be willing to modify health care delivery in keeping with the client's cultural background.
7. Do not expect all members of one cultural group to behave in exactly the same way.
8. Appreciate that each person's cultural values are ingrained and therefore very difficult to change.

From Stulc DM: The family as a bearer of culture. In Cookfair JN: *Nursing process and practice in the community*, St Louis, 1991, Mosby.

Listening

Listening is probably the most effective communication technique available. Active listening is concentrating on what the client is saying so that subtle cues may be detected. Active listening gives the client the nonverbal message that he or she is "a person of worth" whose opinions, ideas, and concerns are valued. Active listening involves blocking out environmental noise and distractions, as well as intrusive thoughts you may have about what to do next.

Providing support

Acceptance. Never discount what the person says. Acceptance is recognition of what is said without necessarily agreeing. An example is "You say you fear this pain could mean that you have cancer."

Touch. The art of touching is one of the most intimate forms of nonverbal communication. It precedes speech in every person's life. Cultural traditions prescribe the ritual of touch or define the taboos. For example, in North American middle-class culture, touch (when used by health care providers) conveys a message of closeness, encouragement, and caring. A warm handshake can be a familiar comfort to a client who is concerned about a health problem and who is fearful of unfamiliar surroundings. Clients may also express appreciation and trust in the health care provider by hugging

or initiating touch. Other cultural groups see touch as an invasion of privacy.

Many Asian cultures believe that the head is the most sacred part of the body. The clinician should therefore obtain permission before touching an Asian client's head. Many Asians believe that the feet are the lowest part of the body, and it is therefore disrespectful to show the bottom of your shoe to the client or point your toe at him or her.

Openness to more information. It is important not to appear too rushed or impatient, because the client may hesitate to share concerns that could be crucial to identifying and treating a problem. Before concluding an interview, ask, "Do you have any additional concerns you want to discuss?" This question encourages the client to bring up important issues, which may save a great deal of time in the long run.

■ COMMON ERRORS IN INTERVIEWING

Giving Advice

By giving advice or telling clients what to do, you communicate that they may not be capable of handling the problem. You also accept responsibility for the outcomes. A health care provider should provide sufficient information about risks, side effects, and benefits of available treatment and management options so that clients can decide what is right for themselves.

Changing the Subject

Changing the subject introduces a new topic inappropriately. A client may be expressing concern about the discomfort of the examination, and the practitioner asks what medication he is taking. Practitioners may do this unintentionally when feeling, for example, both pressured for time and anxious about ensuring that they obtain specific information.

Social Versus Therapeutic Response

A social response focuses attention on the practitioner instead of the client. An example is a client stating that she just returned from a trip to South America and the practitioner responding by talking about her own vacation. The sharing of this story by the practitioner becomes the focus of the interchange. A therapeutic response focuses attention on the client. In the above example, after the client states that she just returned from a trip to South America, a therapeutic response by the practitioner would be "Tell me about your trip."

False Reassurance

In an attempt to reassure the client, statements may be made that are not true, such as "It will be all right," "You'll be just fine," or "You'll get over it."

CULTURAL CONSIDERATIONS

COMMUNICATION VARIATIONS

1. Assess your personal beliefs about persons from different cultures.
   - Review your personal beliefs and past experiences.
   - Set aside any values, biases, ideas, or attitudes that are judgmental and may negatively affect care.
2. Assess communication variables from a cultural perspective.
   - Determine the ethnic identity of a client, including generation in America.
   - Use the client as a source of information when possible.
   - Assess cultural factors that may affect your relationship with the client and respond appropriately.
3. Plan care based on communicated needs and cultural background.
   - Learn about the client's cultural customs and beliefs.
   - Encourage the client to reveal his or her cultural interpretation of health, illness, and health care.
   - Be sensitive to the uniqueness of the client.
   - Identify sources of discrepancy between the client's and your own conceptions of health and illness.
4. Modify communication approaches to meet cultural needs.
   - Be attentive to signs of fear, anxiety, and confusion in the client.
   - Learn how listening is communicated in the client's culture.
   - Use appropriate active listening techniques.
   - Adopt an attitude of flexibility, respect, and interest to help bridge barriers imposed by culture.
5. Communicate in a nonthreatening manner.
   - Conduct the interview in an unhurried manner.
   - Follow acceptable social and cultural amenities.
   - Ask general questions during the information-gathering stage.
   - Be patient with a respondent who gives information that may seem unrelated to the client's health problem.
   - Develop a trusting relationship by listening carefully, allowing time, and giving the client your full attention.
6. Use validating techniques in communication.
   - Be alert for feedback that the client is not understanding you.
   - Do not assume meaning is interpreted without distortion.
7. Be considerate of reluctance to talk when the subject involves sexual matters.
   - Be aware that in some cultures sexual matters are not discussed freely with members of the opposite sex.
8. Adopt special approaches when the client speaks a different language.
   - Use a caring tone of voice and facial expression to help alleviate the client's fears.
   - Speak slowly and distinctly, but not loudly.
   - Use gestures, pictures, and playacting to help the client understand.
   - Repeat the message in different ways if necessary.
   - Be alert to words the client seems to understand, and use them frequently.
   - Keep messages simple and repeat them frequently.
   - Avoid using medical terms and abbreviations that the client may not understand.
   - Use an appropriate language dictionary.
9. Use interpreters to improve communication.
   - Ask the interpretor to translate the message, not just the words.
   - Use an interpreter who is culturally sensitive.

Modified from Giger J, Davidhizar R: *Transcultural nursing,* ed 2, St Louis, 1995, Mosby.

Overloading or Underloading the Client with Questions

Overloading is continuing to ask a client questions before he or she has a chance to answer the first one. Underloading is failing to answer when a client asks a question or failing to respond to cues. An example might be:

Client: "This is going to hurt." Client is wincing, teeth clenched.

Nurse: Smiles and prepares the injection.

Jumping to Conclusions

The following is an example of jumping to conclusions, or making assumptions without verifying information: A client who is sexually active states that she does not use a birth control method and the practitioner responds, "How long have you been trying to get pregnant?" The client might lack knowledge of birth control methods or may be in a homosexual relationship where pregnancy is not a risk.

Halo Effect

Because of the "halo effect," the practitioner may neglect to ask about potential problem areas because the client appears to be happy, prosperous, and coping well. In fact, the client may have serious financial or psychosocial problems that she does not feel comfortable discussing. For example, although the practitioner might say, "Oh, I never asked Mrs. Smith about her alcohol intake; she seems like such a well-adjusted person and has such a nice family," Mrs. Smith may in fact have a serious problem with alcohol.

Biased Questions

Biased questions make assumptions about the client's feelings or behavior and may lead the examiner to make false conclusions. An example is "You practice safe sex, don't you?" This question not only assumes that the client is sexually active and knows what "safer sex" means, but also conveys a certain negative judgment on the part of the practitioner toward someone who does not practice safer sex.

Interview Vignettes

The following is an example of an appropriate sequence of questions. Can you identify the techniques of interviewing used?

Provider: Hello, Mr. Chang, my name is Linda Jones, the nurse practitioner at the clinic. What brings you here today?

Mr. Chang: I'm worried about my heart.

Ms. Jones: Worried?

Mr. Chang: Yes. I was gardening last week and noticed that it became very hard for me to catch my breath after raking only 10 or 15 minutes. I know this is a sign of a heart problem.

Ms. Jones: Yes, shortness of breath can be a sign of a heart problem. But there can be other reasons someone becomes short of breath. I need to get more information from you before coming to any conclusions. I'm going to ask you some questions about the symptoms you experience that cause you concern . . .

The following is an example of an inappropriate sequence of questions. (Can you identify the common errors discussed in the chapter?

Provider: Hello, my name is Linda. I'm a special kind of a nurse. What's your name?

Mr. Chang: George Chang.

Provider: Well, George, what's wrong with you today?

Mr. Chang: I'm not sure, but I'm worried about my heart.

Provider: Oh, at your age it's unlikely you have a heart problem. And, anyway, it's my job to diagnose the problem. I just need for you to tell me what your symptoms are. Do you have chest pain?

Mr. Chang: No.

Provider: Do you have trouble breathing?

Mr. Chang: Well, yes, as a matter of fact, that was my biggest worry

Provider: (Interrupts.) You don't look like you're having trouble breathing to me. By the way, exactly how old are you?

chapter

The Health History

■ PURPOSE

The health history is an extremely important part of
the health assessment. It serves as the primary vehicle by
which the practitioner establishes rapport with the
client. The history-taking interview helps the practition-
er assess and diagnose the client's health needs and
problems and obtain knowledge of these matters within
the context of that particular client's life. The health his-
tory not only documents the client's needs and prob-
lems, but also provides a picture of the client as a whole
person, in relation to his or her social and physical envi-
ronment. Thus it registers both the deficits and abnor-
malities and the strengths that will support health inter-
ventions and care.

Other important components of the history database
are the client's perceptions regarding health, illness,
therapies, and experiences with health care providers
and delivery systems. Understanding these beliefs, per-
ceptions, and responses is necessary to providing future
care that is relevant and, consequently, effective.

The practitioner implements the health history in
two phases: (1) the client interview phase, which elicits
the information, and (2) the documentation of data
phase. The sequence for obtaining a history, as present-
ed in this chapter, follows a systematic method for
recording the history. The client interview itself may not
proceed in the same sequence because of the nature of
the client's health need or problem, the condition of the
client, or other contextual variables. The interviewer
needs to understand the essential components of a
health history fully, develop a personal scheme for tak-
ing a health history, and be ready to alter the sequence
and nature of data obtained according to the conditions
of a particular encounter.

The health history usually is done in the examiner's
office or in the client's home or hospital room. If the in-
terview takes place in the examiner's space, the examin-
er can control the environment to facilitate privacy,
comfort, and quiet. However, if the interview is done in
the client's space, the examiner must assess the environ-

ment and, in some instances, alter it to facilitate an adequate interview. For example, closing the curtains in a multibed hospital room or requesting that the television be turned off in the home will make the environment more conducive to the interview situation.

Whether the examiner or the client initiates the encounter, the client will have certain ideas about its purpose and content. Clarification of the client's purpose and expectations and orientation of the client to the examiner's goals and methods early in the encounter will minimize the potential for misunderstanding and frustration. Often the client's priorities are different from those of the examiner, or the examiner may have an inaccurate perception of the client's goals. The interviewer must clarify any discrepancies and negotiate priorities if the encounter is to be productive.

The various types of health histories include the following:

1. A *complete health history*, as described in this chapter, is taken on the initial visit to a health care facility when the health care providers within that facility will be providing comprehensive and/or continuous care.
2. An *interval health history* is used to collect information during visits subsequent to the one in which the initial database was collected. Depending on the time since the last entry to the history and the purpose of the encounter, selected information about current needs and problems and updates of health history information are obtained.
3. A *problem-focused* or *chief complaint–focused health history* is used to collect data about a specific problem system or region. Examples of such health histories are included in the systems and region examination chapters in this book.

The interviewer should strive for balance between allowing clients to talk freely and tell their story in their own way and using time efficiently. Clients must be able to provide information that they consider relevant. However, the examiner must probe, clarify, and quantify client information in structured ways. Because the examiner is the "expert" in history taking, he or she must take the lead in managing the interview to obtain appropriate information as efficiently as possible. Also, time is not an unlimited resource. Often other clients are waiting for services, and the examiner must control the costs of encounters.

Because it is usually not possible to write the entire health history during the interview, the interviewer takes notes. Forms are useful in structuring note taking and are appropriate for many data components. The interviewer records as much of the health history as possible during the interview, and the remainder is added as soon as possible after the interview has been completed.

■ PREPARATION: CLIENT AND ENVIRONMENT

Organize the environment for the history in a manner that will increase the physical and psychological comfort of the client (see box below). At the first encounter, introduce yourself to the client with a formal greeting and use the client's full name. In a clinic setting, seat yourself facing the client. Allow the client to remain in street clothes until the history portion of the assessment has been completed.

Make sure that you and the client understand each other's expectations for the encounter. Brief the client about the purposes and structure of a health history, and ask the client about his or her expectations early in the interaction.

■ FORMAT

The health history described in this chapter is extremely detailed and complete. In many actual client care situations, it may not be possible, or even appropriate, to obtain the complete history at the first encounter or at all. For clients who are receiving continuous care, the history can be done in portions during several encounters. For clients who require episodic care, deci-

---

Preparation for the Health History

1. Establish an environment that is conducive to effective communication—private, comfortable, and quiet.
2. Introduce yourself to the client.
3. Address the client formally by his or her full name.
4. If children or others are in attendance, determine the client's wishes about the presence of the additional person(s) during the interview and examination.
5. Allow the client to state the problems and his or her expectations for the encounter.
6. Orient the client to the purposes, structure, and components of the health history.
7. If this is not the client's first encounter with the health system and a record exists of past data and care for the client, review this record with the client.
8. Make some judgment early in the interview about the priorities for the encounter, given your and the client's constraints. Communicate and negotiate priorities with the client.

sions regarding the data that are essential for immediate therapy will guide the content of the history.

The beginning health historian should practice obtaining the complete health history to develop skill in interviewing and in recording data and to establish priorities for focused interviews. During this practice process, the learner will gain an appreciation for the information obtained from each portion of the health history.

The recommended format for the complete health history is as follows (see box below for suggested scripts for the introduction of each component):

1. Biographical information
2. Client's reason for seeking care (chief complaint)
3. Present health and present illness status
4. Past health history
5. Current health information
6. Family health history
7. Review of systems
   a. Physical systems
   b. Functional status
   c. Sociological system
   d. Psychological system
8. Developmental data
9. Nutritional data

Biographical Information

At the beginning of any health record, list commonly used, and sometimes critical, biographical information. Obtain this information early during the client's first visit or at admission. Otherwise, the information may be omitted and later needed in an emergency or at a time when the client is unavailable or unable to respond.

In the introductory biographical section of the history, record the information listed in the box on p. 24. Sometimes this information is recorded by an assistant in the health care setting, or it may be on the record from a previous encounter. If the information is already recorded, review it with the client to verify that it is complete, accurate, and up-to-date.

First, record the client's name. Since persons who live in an ethnically homogenous geographical area often have similar names, it is important that this key information be exact. Precise identification, including first, middle, and last names, assists in ensuring accurate information retrieval and coordination. If additional identifying information is needed, record the parents' names, including the mother's maiden name.

Next, record the client's full mailing address and telephone numbers. Also include the name, address, and telephone number of one of the client's friends or rela-

---

Suggested Script for Introducing Components of the Health History

BIOGRAPHICAL INFORMATION

"I will start the history by asking you some general questions about yourself. First, could you please give me the correct spelling of your full name?"

CLIENT'S REASON FOR SEEKING CARE

"Please tell me why you came to see me today."

PAST HEALTH HISTORY

"Because some of the health problems you had in the past may have some implications for what we do today, I will now be asking you about your past illnesses, health problems, and immunizations."

CURRENT HEALTH INFORMATION

"Because my advice must take into account your current health habits and practices, I will now ask you various questions about your current habits and medications."

FAMILY HEALTH HISTORY

For ill client: "Because others in your family may have health problems that relate to your problems or affect your treatment, I will ask you some questions about their health."

For well client: "Because others in your family may have health problems that relate to your current health risks and future health, I will ask you some questions about their health."

REVIEW OF SYSTEMS

Physical Systems and Functional Status

"Up to now in the interview, we have concentrated on certain parts of your body. To have a complete picture of your physical health, I will now ask you a number of questions about the other parts of your body."

Sociological Systems and Psychological Systems

"Because I want to know more about you as a total person, I will now ask you some questions about you, your family, and your relationships with others."

DEVELOPMENTAL DATA

(Usually the interview up to this point in the history will provide information for this section.)

NUTRITIONAL DATA

"Because nutrition is important to health, I will next ask you some questions about your diet."

Client Biographical Information

Full name
Address and telephone numbers
   Client's permanent
   Contact of client (person to contact in case of
    emergency)
Birth date
Sex
Race
Ethnicity
Religion
Marital status
Social Security number
Occupation
   Usual
   Present
Birthplace
Source of referral
Usual source of health care
Source and reliability of information
Date of interview

tives. This person should be someone with whom the client is in frequent contact and who would be willing and able to relay a message to the client in an emergency or if the client cannot be located.

The birth date, sex, race, ethnicity, religion, marital status, and birthplace entries are self-explanatory. Many health problems and needs are related to age, sex, race, or social situation. This information provides initial insight into the client as a unique person and can be correlated with the client's needs and problems discovered later in the history.

Justifiable reasons for recording the client's Social Security number include the precise identification of each client and potential access to a large pool of health-related information. The potential for violation of client confidentiality is a disadvantage.

A significant difference may exist between the client's current and usual occupations. The nature of the difference may indicate the severity of the client's health problems and the level of disability resulting from them. In addition, knowledge of past occupations might provide clues to past or present environmental hazards contributing to the present illness. A mine worker with a respiratory system complaint is an example.

Knowledge of the client's birthplace provides geographical information associated with the origin of problems and cultural implications for therapy and health maintenance.

If the current caregiver is not the usual and primary source of the client's care, record the name and address of the individual or institution so identified by the client. In addition, document the reason that the client is entering a new health care system. The client may be in crisis, may be dissatisfied with past care, or may be "shopping." If the past source of care possesses significant data about the client's health and if the client intends to continue in the current health care system, ask the client to sign a permission for the transfer of information. Later in the health history, you will have the opportunity to record, in some detail, past patterns of health care.

The source of client payment for care is usually included on administrative records. However, noting this information in the health history might be useful in guiding choices of interventions.

Next, make a statement about the source of the information to follow. In most instances the source is the client, but do not assume that this is so unless the source is specifically identified. If the information is given by someone other than the client, describe the nature of the informant's contact with the client. For example, in the case of a child, a history given by a grandmother who resides with the child should be viewed differently from one given by a grandmother who visits the child once a week.

Along with the statement of the informant, give an evaluation of that person's reliability. For example, you could describe the informant as "inconsistent," "unclear about recent events," "evasive," or "cooperative and reliable." Such statements serve as simple criteria by which the remainder of the information in the history is judged by other health care providers. In addition, this type of information may indicate a need to retake or supplement the history at a future date or to consult with other informants to verify the data.

HELPFUL HINT   *For effective interviewing:*
- *Make judgments about the balance between allowing the client to talk in an unstructured way and the need to control the interview.*
- *Avoid questions that can be answered with yes or no if details are needed.*
- *Clarify the client's diagnostic statements and conclusions.*
- *Be alert to concerns that the client is having difficulty in presenting.*
- *Avoid the formulation of premature conclusions about the nature of the client's problem.*
- *Avoid judgmental statements.*

In some cases a translator will be needed to assist with the interview. The translator may be a stranger to the client or a friend or family member. If such a person has been involved, note this information on the record along with the relationship to the client (e.g., stranger, family member, friend). Note also any effect the use of a translator may have had on the reliability of the information obtained. See Chapter 2 for guidelines regarding the use of interpreters.

HELPFUL HINT *When taking a history through an interpreter:*
- *Ask the interpreter to translate as close to verbatim as possible.*
- *Advise the interpreter to clarify the meaning of a message if it is unclear and to avoid translating literally if the message does not seem to make sense*
- *Advise the interpreter not to engage in side conversations, especially those that include the provision of advice, with the client*

It is important to date the history. In a situation in which the client's condition changes rapidly, events can be correlated only if their temporal relationships are known.

For suggestions about how to conduct an effective health history interview, see the Helpful Hint on p. 24.

Client's Reason for Seeking Care (Chief Complaint)

Record the reason for seeking care as a short statement in the client's own words and in quotation marks, indicating the client's purpose for requesting health care at this time. In the case of a well client, the statement of the reason for seeking care may be the client's request for a health examination for health screening or health promotion.

With an ill client, the statement is sometimes called a chief complaint (CC), defined as the acute or chronic problem that is the client's priority for treatment. Whenever relevant, include a notation of the duration of the problem. The duration stated by the client may not be the actual time span of the symptoms. However, it indicates the time during which the complaint was important enough to motivate the client to seek help.

Keep in mind that the reason for seeking care is not a diagnostic statement. In fact, formulating this statement in diagnostic terms can be hazardous. For example, a client who has frequent asthmatic attacks may ap-pear for treatment with respiratory system complaints and state that he or she is having an "asthmatic attack." However, this may not be the actual situation. In this early portion of the history, care must be taken to avoid client and interviewer bias. Otherwise, the interview and the problem solving may be set in one, potentially incorrect, direction.

The following are examples of good statements of reasons for seeking care:

Chest pain for 3 days.

Swollen ankles for 2 weeks.

Fever and headache for 24 hours.

Pap smear needed. Last Pap 9/8/96.

Physical examination needed for camp.

In contrast, the following are examples of inadequately stated chief complaints:

Thinks she might be pregnant.

Sick.

Nausea and vomiting.

Hypertension.

The client's reason for seeking care may seem superfluous, especially since the next section of the history involves a description of the health need or problem in detail. However, this entry is one of the few places in the recorded histories of encounters with the health care system where clients are given the opportunity to have their needs recorded in their own words. Too often, practitioners lose sight of the clients' priorities for care. The consistent documentation of clients' reasons for seeking care assists in keeping the system responsive to their perceived needs.

In some instances a client presents several complaints. However, do not state more than three in this portion of the history, and note the client's priorities as stated. All the client's problems can be addressed in the present health/present illness (PH/PI) portion of the health history.

Be alert to the possibility that some clients may be reluctant to state their priority for seeking health care and may provide the interviewer with a reason perceived to be more acceptable than the actual reason. Watch for clues to any underlying and unstated concerns throughout the interview.

Present Health/Present Illness Status

The present health/present illness section describes the information relevant to the client's reasons for seeking care. For a well client, the interviewer commonly describes the client's usual health and briefly summarizes his or her health maintenance needs and activities.

When the client has a health problem, this portion of the health history challenges the practitioner's interviewing, clinical knowledge, and written communication skills. The practitioner must learn the minute details of the chief complaint and its associated phenomena. First,

the information must be comprehensive. Second, it must be recorded logically and concisely. Third, it must provide the practitioner with enough information to initiate additional assessment and the intervention measures.

The interviewing and recording for the present illness portion of the health history is especially difficult for beginning practitioners because the processes involved require both skill in interviewing and history taking and clinical knowledge. Outlining the progression of the present illness before writing the narrative discussion is sometimes helpful. Although the student who is learning health assessment has probably not yet studied client care management, the student may find that the use of clinical management references for the system(s) discussed with the client will often provide valuable learning by highlighting important omissions, which can be incorporated in future interviews.

The following are the components of the present health/present illness section of the health history:

A. Introduction
  1. Client summary
  2. Usual health
B. Investigation of symptoms: chronological story
  1. Onset
    a. Date
    b. Manner (gradual or sudden)
    c. Duration
    d. Precipitating factors
  2. Course since onset
    a. Incidence (frequency)
    b. Manner
    c. Duration (longest, shortest, and average times)
    d. Patterns of remissions and exacerbations
  3. Location
  4. Quality
  5. Quantity
  6. Setting
  7. Associated phenomena
  8. Alleviating or aggravating factors
C. Negative information
D. Relevant family information
E. Disability assessment

Introduction

The introduction to the present illness section should be succinct. Its major purpose is to provide the reader with a general orientation to the client.

State the client's previous visits or admissions, if any, to the institution or service. Next, briefly summarize the client's biographical data (usually age, race, marital status, employment status, and occupation). If the client is being hospitalized and also has been hospitalized in the past, note the client's total number of hospitalizations and the number of hospitalizations for complaints related to the present illness.

Next, describe the client's usual health; record any significant past diagnoses and past and current health problems.

Investigation of symptoms: chronological story

Initiate the exploration of symptoms by saying to the client: "Tell me about it [the problem mentioned in the chief complaint statement]," or "How did it [the problem] start, and what has happened since it started?" The client usually will respond to this inquiry with a long but diagnostically incomplete discourse about health problems and needs. Exercise skill in determining when to interrupt the client—specifically, when to direct the responses by asking additional, clarifying questions and when to allow the client to continue the narration of events perceived as significant by that individual.

Create a mental or written list of the areas of symptom investigation, based on the body systems on regions affected, to be explored as an aid in attaining comprehensive information. Regardless of the nature of the problem, each of the dimensions of symptom analysis is relevant, and any health problem analysis would be incomplete without the description of all areas (see box on p. 27).

Determine the onset and chronological sequence of the client's problem. The client is apt to remember best the most recent episode of illness. When a prolonged illness is being discussed, the client will need direction in tracing the problem to its first symptomatic event. Once this first event has been identified, investigate it in detail and specify its date, manner of onset, duration, and precipitating factors.

Determine the usual manner of onset for the illness episodes. Note specifically any change in onset. When many episodes have occurred, specify the longest, shortest, and average durations of the episodes. If there have been only several episodes, identify the length of each one.

Describe each symptom's course since onset. Determine its frequency as a specific time interval. Clients may state vaguely that they have a symptom "all the time." Such a statement may mean once a month to one client or 10 times a day to another. To obtain specific information, ask, "How many times a day [or a week or a month] does it occur?" Although suggesting answers with questions is to be avoided, occasionally it may be necessary to pursue the issue of frequency by asking leading questions (e.g., "Does it occur more often than five times a day?").

For prolonged illnesses, describe the patterns of remission and exacerbation according to their duration

Symptom Analysis

ONSET

When the symptoms started—as specific a date as possible

Manner in which the symptoms started—sudden or gradual

Duration of symptoms in the initial occurrence

Factors that seemed to precipitate or be associated with the initial event

COURSE SINCE ONSET

Frequency—in a specific time interval (e.g., per day/per month) logical to the situation

Manner of onset for subsequent events

Duration—longest, shortest, and average times

Patterns of improvement and exacerbation, including condition between episodes of the symptom(s)

Previous episodes and treatment

LOCATION

Specific location

Radiation

QUALITY

Unique properties of the complaint (e.g., if pain— dull, aching, sharp, nagging, throbbing, stabbing, squeezing)

If discharge—color, consistency, composition

QUANTITY

Severity, size, extent, number, amount

Amount in a common measure (e.g., tablespoons)

Severity measured in estimated amount of, for example, pain on a scale of 1 to 10, or general response (e.g., is the client able to continue what he had been doing or does he need to lie down?)

Exact size of lesions (e.g., pinhead, dime)

SETTING

Environment—place, air quality, people, activity, etc., when symptom occurs

ASSOCIATED PHENOMENA

Occur with the chief complaint—can be precipitating, concurrent, or ensuing

Effect of chief complaint on the same or related body systems

ALLEVIATING AND AGGRAVATING FACTORS

Initial response—nature and effect

Remedies tried—nature and effect

What makes the symptom worse

What makes the symptom better

Effects of movement, position, diet, medications

CLIENT'S UNDERLYING CONCERN

Meaning/attribution of the symptom to the client (e.g., fear of heart attack, [cancer])

Why concerned at this time (e.g., new symptom, worse episode than in the past, feeling stressed)

---

and frequency. Be watchful for environmental or other clues that might be precipitating factors for the illness events.

For recording the symptoms, several methods can be used to assist readers in identifying temporal relationships easily. Describe the initial event first, then the subsequent events. A chronological story can be indexed in the left-hand column of the history sheet, with *prior to admission (PTA)* or *visit (PTV)* used as a reference. For example, the chronological index can be listed as follows: "6 years PTA," "3 years PTA," "6 months PTA," or "1 day PTA," with the corresponding narrative alongside it and continuing below the temporal index heading.

One method of demonstrating the progression of an illness is to use a diagram illustrating the disease process (Figure 3.1). This type of diagram is especially helpful with multisymptomatic illnesses.

As the chronological story evolves, integrate the other areas of symptom investigation into the text of the narrative. Whenever appropriate, describe the sign's or symptom's location, quality, quantity, setting, associated phenomena, and alleviating and aggravating factors, especially when a change in pattern occurs.

Determine the exact site of the sign or symptom. Subjective events, such as pain, pose certain problems. Having a client point to the exact location of pain and trace its radiation with a finger assists in determining the site. Use body hemispheres and anatomical landmarks in recording the location.

Quality refers to the unique properties of the complaint. Signs such as discharge are described according to their color, texture, composition, appearance, and odor. Sound and temperature may be descriptive attributes of other phenomena. Subjective events such as pain challenge the descriptive skills of the practitioner. The quality of pain is frequently characterized as dull, aching, sharp, nagging, throbbing, stabbing, or squeez-

figure**3.1** Example of a graph to illustrate symptomatic progression of an illness.

ing. Whenever appropriate, use the client's descriptions with quotation marks.

Quantity refers to the size, extent, number, or amount (e.g., of pain, rash, discharge, or lesion). With objective events reported by the client, ask the client to refer to common measurements, such as centimeters, cups, or tablespoons in describing approximate amounts. In describing subjective events (e.g., pain), remember that evaluations such as "a little" or "a lot" have different meanings for different persons. The quality of subjective phenomena can be more accurately conveyed by describing the client's response to the symptom. For example, when the pain occurs, does the client stop and sit or continue with activities? Another commonly understood method of quantification is a scale of 1 to 10 to assess pain.

Whenever illness occurs, the client is in a particular environment, either with someone or alone. It may be useful to ask about the setting in which certain symptoms occur because, physically or psychologically, the setting may have an effect on the client. This information can provide the practitioner with clues to the cause of the problem and implications for treatment.

Associated phenomena are those symptoms, such as nausea and vomiting, that occur with the chief complaint. They may be related to the chief complaint or may be part of a totally different syndrome. Often the client will spontaneously identify these events. Always ask if there is anything else occurring with the chief complaint, or inquire about the presence or absence of certain specific events. Review the system or systems associated with the chief complaint or the purpose of the visit. Record the client's positive responses and com-

pletely describe all reported symptoms. Document the negative responses in the negative information section.

When an illness occurs, initially the affected person often adapts to it or attempts self-treatment. The individual may decrease activity, eat more or less, wait, or actively medicate and treat himself or herself. Often cultural responses to illness and treatment influence this self-care. The client's actions in response to the problem and the effect of these actions should be addressed in a nonjudgmental way. If there has been professional intervention, the nature, source, and effect of each intervention need to be recorded. The client, through treatment or accommodation, may have discovered something that alleviates the symptom. Therefore the client should be asked what makes the situation better. The client's solution may provide valuable therapeutic data and may reflect the individual's adaptation to illness.

If the client has not already suggested a cause for the problem(s), ask whether the client has any thoughts about why he or she is having the problem(s) at this time. Also ask the client about what makes the chief complaint worse. Usually the client has noticed aggravating factors but may need assistance in recalling them. Inquire about the effect of movement, positioning, or eating, for example. Again, this information may offer valuable therapeutic data.

Negative information

In the analysis of a problem, negative information is as significant as positive information for determining the diagnosis. Thoroughly review each system implicated in the present illness section. Record the client's positive replies in the text of the chronological story. Document

all negative information in this separate category of the present illness section.

Relevant family history

Ask the client whether any problem similar to the chief complaint is known to exist among blood relatives. Record positive replies, specifically identifying the relative and the problem. Document negative replies in general terms (e.g., "None of the client's blood relatives has diabetes"). In the case of a client who is adopted, the family history of the biological family (if known) must be differentiated from that of the adoptive family, in which bloodlines are not shared.

Disability assessment

The purpose of the disability assessment is to determine the extent to which the symptoms identified in the present illness section have affected the client's total life. Note physiological effects, as well as sociological, psychological, and financial consequences of the problem.

Past Health History

The purpose of the past health history (PH) section of the health history is to identify all of the client's major past health problems. Past illnesses may have some effect on the client's current health needs and problems. In addition, information about the management of and response to past problems provides some indication of the client's possible response to current and future health issues.

The following information is obtained and recorded in the past history section of the health history:

1. Past general health
2. Childhood illnesses
3. Accidents and disabling injuries
4. Hospitalizations
5. Operations
6. Major acute and chronic illnesses
7. Immunizations
8. Medications and transfusions
9. Allergies

Ask about the client's usual health status. Try to elicit a sense of the client's perception of, and feelings about, his or her usual health status.

The recording of childhood illnesses is probably more relevant to, and more easily obtained for, a child's history than it is for an adult's. At minimum, however, ask all adults if they have had rheumatic fever. Whenever a positive reply is given, determine the age of the client at occurrence, the fact or absence of a medically confirmed diagnosis, and the short-term and long-term effects of the disease.

Ask the client to recall all accidents and disabling injuries, regardless of whether hospitalization occurred or treatment was handled on an outpatient basis. Determine and record the precipitating event, extent of injury, fact or absence of medical care, names of the practitioner and institution, and sequelae. Be alert to the possibility of patterns of injury or the presence of consistent environmental hazards.

Determine whether any hospitalizations have occurred, and record descriptions of them, including all the times that the client was admitted to an inpatient unit. Include the dates of stay, primary practitioner, name and address of the hospital, admitting complaint, discharge diagnosis, and follow-up care and sequelae. Record any obstetrical hospitalizations in this section or in the review-of-systems portion of the health history (review of female genital system).

Record all operations together, under the specific operations category. Include a description of the nature of the repair or removal, making it as complete as possible. Frequently, clients are unaware of the exact nature of their operations. It may be necessary to consult past records for accurate and complete information.

If the client has had major acute illnesses or chronic illnesses that have not required hospitalization, note the course of treatment, the person making the diagnosis, and the follow-up care and sequelae.

Information under the categories of hospitalizations, operations, and other major illnesses may, in some instances, be redundant. Do not record detailed information more than once. Instead, state the presence of a past problem and refer the reader to the section where the original notation was made.

Information regarding medications currently being taken is covered in the next section of the health history. At this point, ask about previous medications that may have been taken for a long time and/or those that might have an effect on the current health need or problem. Given current concerns about blood transfusions and AIDS, be sure to record information about blood transfusions in this section.

Record all immunizations according to type and date. Accurate immunization records are commonly kept for children but not usually for adults. For adults, obtain the exact (or at least approximate) date of the last tetanus immunization, as well as flu and pneumonia immunization in the elderly.

Current Health Information

The purpose of the current health information section is to record major, current, health-related information. A recommended outline for the information is as follows:

1. Allergies
   a. Environmental
   b. Ingestion
   c. Drug
   d. Other

2. Habits
   a. Alcohol
   b. Tobacco
   c. Drugs
   d. Caffeine
3. Medications taken regularly (names, dosages, frequency, intended effect, and compliance)
   a. By health care provider prescription
   b. By self-prescription
4. Exercise patterns
5. Sleep patterns

Ask specifically about allergies to food, environmental factors, animals, and drugs. If the client reports an allergy, obtain specific information about the causative factor, reaction, diagnosis of the causative factor, therapy, and sequelae. Exercise caution in assessing drug allergies. A drug reaction may not always be an allergic response. It may be an interaction with a concurrently administered drug, a misdose, a side effect, or an adverse effect.

Habits relevant to the health of an individual are excessive alcohol or caffeine ingestion, smoking, and the addictive use of legal or illegal mood-altering substances. In recording habits, note the number of cigarettes, ounces, or tablets per day, along with the duration of the habit. Determine and record both past and current use of these substances.

If therapy is to be planned by informed practitioners logically, all medications currently being used by the client must be known and recorded. Clients usually admit to vague patterns, such as taking "a white pill once a day for water," but they may forget to tell the practitioner about the aspirin or antacid they take several times a day unless they are specifically asked about nonprescription items. This portion of the health history presents the opportunity to educate clients about the

names, doses, and uses of their medications and the necessity of knowing such information.

Explore the pattern of physical and sedentary activities in the client's usual routine. Include a weekly or daily profile of the individual's usual activities.

Describe the client's sleep pattern. Record the daily routine for a typical week. Determine the client's assessment of the adequacy of his or her sleep and satisfaction with the pattern.

Family Health History

The purpose of the family health history (FH) section is to learn about the general health of the client's blood relatives, spouse, and children and to identify any illnesses of a genetic, familial, or environmental nature that might have implications for the client's current or future health problems and needs, or their solution or resolution. Genetic problems are those that are directly inherited through the genes. Familial problems are ones that have not yet been demonstrated to be genetic exclusively but appear more often in family clusters for various reasons. An example of a familial problem is alcoholism. Environmental problems (e.g., exposure to toxic substances) may be shared by families.

The health status of the client's family is significant for several reasons. First, the client's health status affects, and is affected by, health conditions in other family members. Communicable disease is an example of this situation. Second, heredity and constitutional factors are associated with the causation of many diseases. A strong family history of certain problems might offer important clues in assessment and diagnosis.

Inquire about the health of the client's relatives, including maternal and paternal grandparents, parents, siblings, aunts, uncles, spouse, and children. In certain situations information regarding roommates, sexual

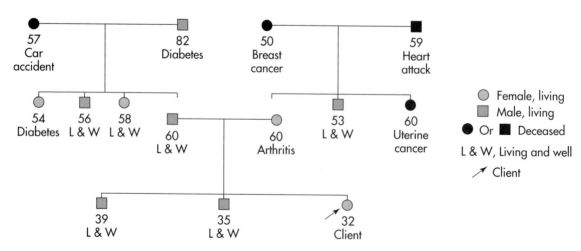

figure**3.2**   Example of a family tree to illustrate family health.

partners, and significant others might be relevant to a family history. Information also needs to be obtained about the current health status of, presence of disease in, and current age or age at death of each family member. If a member is deceased, record the cause of death.

If the client's established or possible illnesses have known or suspected familial tendencies, question the client again about similar problems of family members.

Inquire about the presence of the following diseases because of their genetic, familial, or environmental tendencies: alcoholism, allergies, epilepsy, diabetes, hematological disorders (e.g., hemophilia, sickle cell anemia, thalassemia, hemolytic jaundice, or severe anemia), Huntington's chorea, cancer, hypertension, arteriosclerosis, gout, obesity, coronary artery disease, tuberculosis, and kidney disease. Often printed history forms list these diseases. Check whether or not the client or a family member has the diagnosis. Inquire about selected additional health problems because of the client's family history, occupation, socioeconomic status, ethnic origins, or environment.

The information in the family history section can be outlined in the record or put in the form of a family tree chart. Figure 3.2 is an example of such a chart. This type of chart is especially useful in situations in which genetically transmitted diseases are present or suspected or if the understanding of family composition is an important factor in management. The traditionally used symbols for genogram notations are included in the box on p. 31. For an adopted individual, two genograms may be useful if the information is available. The genogram for the biological family would indicate genetic health issues and familial ones that may be genetically linked. The genogram for the adoptive family would include familial health issues and those affected by environment.

Certain health problems are linked to specific population or ethnic groups. Table 3.1 contains information about health problems that have been noted in relatively high frequencies in particular groups.

Review of Systems

The review-of-systems (ROS) portion of the history includes a collection of data about the past and present health of each of the client's systems. This review of the client's physical, functional, sociological, and psychological health status may identify problems not uncovered previously in the history. It also provides an opportunity to indicate the client's strengths and weaknesses.

Generally, this portion of the history is organized from a cephalad-to-caudad body direction and from physical to psychosocial factors. The client is told that he or she will be asked a number of questions. For both beginning and experienced interviewers, a checklist or written reminder of the routine is useful.

Physical systems

In the review of physical systems, ask a question about the client's symptoms, then pause to allow the client to think and respond. If the client responds positively, analyze the symptoms according to the characteristics of symptoms discussed in the present health/present illness section of the history. Ask questions quickly enough to be efficient, yet slowly enough to allow the client time to think. In general, emphasize the presence of past or current common anatomical or functional problems of the system and the health functioning and maintenance of the system.

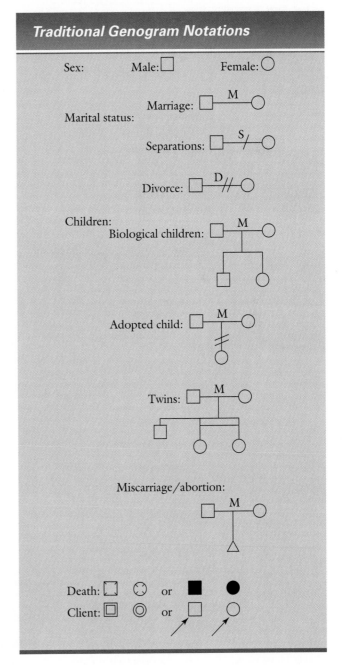

table 3.1   *Distribution of Selected Genetic Traits and Disorders by Population or Ethnic Group*

Ethnic or population group	Genetic or multifactorial disorder present in relatively high frequency	Ethnic or population group	Genetic or multifactorial disorder present in relatively high frequency
Africans	Sickle cell disease Hereditary persistence of hemoglobin F G-6-PD deficiency, African type Lactase deficiency, adult β-Thalassemia	Jews— Ashkenazi	Tay-Sachs disease (infantile) Niemann-Pick disease (infantile) Gaucher disease (adult type) Familial dysautonomia (Riley-Day syndrome) Bloom syndrome Torsion dystonia Factor XI (PTA) deficiency
Amish	Limb-girdle muscular dystrophy Pyruvate kinase deficiency Hemophilia	Jews— Sephardi	Familial Mediterranean fever Ataxia-telangiectasia Cystinuria Glycogen storage disease III
Armenians	Familial Mediterranean fever Familial paroxysmal polyserositis	Lapps	Congenital dislocation of the hip
Burmese	Hemoglobin E disease	Lebanese	Dyggve-Melchoir-Clausen syndrome
Chinese	Alpha thalassemia G-6-PD deficiency, Chinese type Lactase deficiency, adult	Mediterranean peoples	G-6-PD deficiency, Mediterranean type β-Thalassemia Familial Mediterranean fever
Costa Ricans	Malignant osteopetrosis		
English	Cystic fibrosis Hereditary amyloidosis, type III	Middle Eastern peoples	Dubin-Johnson syndrome Ichthyosis vulgaris Werdnig-Hoffman disease G-6-PD deficiency, Mediterranean type Phenylketonuria Metachromatic leukodystrophy
Eskimos	Congenital adrenal hyperplasia Pseudocholinesterase deficiency Methemoglobinemia		
Finns	Congenital nephrosis Generalized amyloidosis syndrome, V Polycystic liver disease Retinoschisis Aspartyglycosaminuria Diastrophic dwarfism	Nova Scotia Acadians	Niemann-Pick disease
		Polish	Phenylketonuria
French Canadians	Tyrosinemia Morquio syndrome	Polynesians	Clubfoot
		Portuguese	Joseph disease
Gypsies	Cogenital glaucoma	Scandinavians	Cholestasis-lymphedema Sjögren-Larsson syndrome Krabbe disease Phenylketonuria
Hopi Indians	Tyrosinase-positive albinism		
Iceland	Phenylketonuria		
Indians (American)	Ear anomalies	Scots	Phenylketonuria Cystic fibrosis Hereditary amyloidosis, type III
Irish	Phenylketonuria Neural tube defects	Thai	Lactase deficiency, adult Hemoglobin E disease
Japanese	Acatalasemia Cleft lip/palate Oguchi disease	Zuni Indians	Tyrosinase-positive albinism

Modified from Wong DL: *Whaley and Wong's nursing care of infants and children,* ed 5, St Louis, 1995, Mosby.

It is important to translate the signs and symptoms into questions and terms that the client can understand. For example, questions concerning a symptom such as intermittent claudication need to be presented in descriptive lay terms. Examples of questions related to intermittent claudication follow:

"Do you ever have any cramplike pains in your legs?"

"When do these cramps occur?"

"What happens to the pain if you rest your legs?"

In documenting the health history, record the presence or absence of all signs or symptoms included in the inquiry. Using the general description "negative" for a total system is meaningless. If such a broad notation is made, the reader will not know which questions were asked and consequently will not understand the context of "negative." If the reader is also the recorder, he or she probably will not, at a later time, remember which specific questions were asked. An exception might exist in a health care system where the review of physical systems section is routinized and where "negative" indicates an inquiry into, and a negative response to, predetermined, universally known, and always reviewed items of exploration.

In the present health/present illness section of the health history, a body region or system may have already been reviewed, along with exploration of a health problem. In this situation, in the review of physical systems section, a notation is made that refers the reader to the present health/present illness section for information about that system.

Systems and body regions to review and areas of exploration about the health status, functional and anatomical problems, and health maintenance of those systems are presented in the following list. The purpose of the encounter, plans for care continuity, time, and the condition of the client will affect the detail with which the review of systems is executed. The listing of areas for exploration in this chapter is very comprehensive. In actual client care situations, the practitioner would choose areas of review appropriate to the particular situation.

GENERAL

Usual state of health
Episodes of chills
Episodes of weakness or malaise
Fatigue
Fever
Odors
Recent and significant gain or loss of weight (if present, amount, time interval, and possible causes are recorded)
Sweats
Usual, maximum, and minimum weight

SKIN

Usual condition
Care habits, including use of sunscreen
Previously diagnosed and treated disease
Color changes
Dryness
Ecchymosis
Lesions
Masses
Petechiae
Pruritus
Temperature changes
Texture changes

HAIR

Usual state of health
Alopecia, or hair loss
Excessive growth or change in distribution
Texture changes
Use of dyes

NAILS

Usual state of health
Changes in appearance
Texture changes

HEAD AND FACE

Usual state of health
Dizziness
History of trauma
Injuries
Pain
Syncope
Unusual or frequent headaches

EYES

Usual state of health
Pattern of eye examinations
Visual acuity, without and with corrective lenses, if applicable
Date of last ophthalmological examination and results
Cataracts
Changes in visual fields or vision
Diplopia
Excessive tearing
Glaucoma
Infections
Pain
Photophobia
Pruritus
Redness
Unusual discharge or sensations
Visual disturbances, such as "rainbows" around lights, flashing lights, or blind spots

EARS

Usual state of health
Care habits, especially cleaning
Use of prosthetic devices
Discharge
Hearing ability
Infections
Otalgia
Presence of excessive environmental noise
Tinnitus, buzzing, or ringing
Vertigo (subjective or objective)

NOSE AND SINUSES

Usual state of health
Olfactory ability
Discharge (seasonal associations)
Epistaxis
Frequency of colds
Obstruction
Pain in infraorbital or sinus areas
Postnasal drip
Sinus infection
Sneezing (frequent or prolonged)

MOUTH AND THROAT

Usual state of health
Pattern of dental care
Pattern of dental hygiene
Use of prosthetic devices
Abscesses
Bleeding or swelling of gums
Change in taste
Dryness
Dysphagia
Excessive salivation
Hoarseness
Lesions
Odors
Pain
Sore throats
Voice changes

NECK AND NODES

Usual state of health
Masses
Node enlargement
Pain with movement or palpation
Swelling
Tenderness

BREASTS

Usual state of health
Self-examination pattern
Dimpling
Discharge

Masses
Pain
Tenderness

RESPIRATORY AND CARDIOVASCULAR SYSTEMS

Usual state of health
Past diagnosis of respiratory or cardiovascular system disease
Date of last roentgenogram and electrocardiogram and results
Cough
Cyanosis
Dyspnea (if present, amount of exertion precipitating it is recorded)
Edema
Hemoptysis
High blood pressure
Orthopnea (number of pillows needed to sleep comfortably is recorded)
Pain (intensity [e.g., scale of 1 to 10], exact location, radiation, and effect of respiration are recorded)
Palpitations
Paroxysmal nocturnal dyspnea
Sputum (if present, amount, color, and characteristics are described)
Stridor
Wheezing

GASTROINTESTINAL SYSTEM

Usual state of health
Previous roentgenograms or x-ray results; endoscopic results (e.g., sigmoidoscopy)
Abdominal pain
Appetite
Ascites
Bowel habits
Change in stool color
Constipation
Diarrhea
Dyschezia
Dyspepsia
Dysphagia
Flatulence
Food idiosyncrasies
Hematemesis
Hemorrhoids
Hernia
Indigestion
Infections
Jaundice
Melena
Nausea
Previously diagnosed problems
Pyrosis
Recent changes in habits

Rectal bleeding
Rectal discomfort
Thirst
Vomiting

URINARY SYSTEM

Usual state of health
Past diagnosed problems and infections
Usual pattern of urination
Change in stream
Dysuria
Enuresis
Flank pain
Frequency
Hematuria
Hesitancy of stream
Incontinence
Nocturia
Oliguria
Polyuria
Retention
Stress incontinence
Suprapubic pain
Urgency
Urine color change
Urine odor change

GENITAL SYSTEM (MALE)

Usual state of health
Impotence
Lesions
Masses (testicular)
Pain
Prostate problems
Swelling
Urethral discharge

GENITAL SYSTEM (FEMALE)

Usual state of health
Frequency of Pap smear and results
Care habits
Diagnosed problems
Dyspareunia
Lesions
Menstrual history
  Age at menarche
  Amenorrhea
  Amount of flow
  Date of last menstrual period (LMP)
  Date of last normal menstrual period (LNMP)
  Duration of flow
  Dysmenorrhea
  Frequency of menses
  Menorrhagia
  Metrorrhagia

Polymenorrhea
Pruritus
Vaginal discharge
Obstetrical history (for each pregnancy)
  Complications of pregnancy
  Condition, sex, and weight of baby
  Date of delivery
  Description of labor
  Duration of pregnancy
  Place of prenatal care and hospitalization
  Postpartum course
  Prenatal course
  Type of delivery (vaginal, cesarean section)

SEXUAL HISTORY (BOTH SEXES)

Ability to perform and enjoy satisfactory sexual
  intercourse
Age of onset of sexual activity
Health of sexual partners
Infertility
Problems with sexual function or sexuality
Satisfaction with sexual activity
Sexual practices
Sexual preference
Sexually transmitted diseases
Sterility
Use of condoms and other contraceptives

EXTREMITIES AND MUSCULOSKELETAL SYSTEM

Usual state of health
Past diagnosis of disease
Extremities
  Coldness
  Deformities
  Discoloration
  Edema
  Intermittent claudication
  Pain
  Thrombophlebitis
Muscles
  Cramping
  Pain
  Weakness
Bones and joints
  Back pain
  Deformities
  Fractures
  Heat
  Limitation of movement
  Pain
  Redness
  Stiffness
  Swelling

CENTRAL NERVOUS SYSTEM

Usual state of health
Past diagnosis of disease
Anxiety
General behavior change
Loss of consciousness
Mood change
Nervousness
Seizures
Speech
　Aphasia
　Dysarthria
Cognitive ability
　Changes in memory
　Disorientation
　Hallucinations
Motor
　Ataxia
　Imbalance
　Paralysis
　Paresis
　Tic
　Tremor
　Spasm
Sensory
　Pain
　Paresthesia (hyperesthesia, anesthesia)

ENDOCRINE SYSTEM

History of physical growth and development
Adult changes in size of head, hands, or feet
Diagnosis of diabetes or thyroid disease
Dryness of skin or hair
Exophthalmos
Goiter
Hair distribution
Hormone therapy
Hypoglycemia
Intolerance of heat or cold
Polydipsia
Polyphagia
Polyuria
Postural hypotension
Presence of secondary sex characteristics
Weakness

HEMATOPOIETIC SYSTEM

Past diagnosis of hematopoietic disease
Anemia
Bleeding tendencies
Blood transfusion
Blood type
Bruising
Exposure to radiation
Lymphadenopathy

Functional status

If the client has functional limitations, measure the extent of abilities. Chapter 27 contains approaches and tools for the specific assessment of functional abilities. If this area of assessment is included, choose tools appropriate to the client group being assessed.

Sociological system

Diagnosis and treatment cannot be effectively done by knowing the client's physical status only. Since the client is a unique and whole person, diagnosis and treatment must be addressed within the context of that person. Therefore it is necessary to gather, in some organized way, information about the client's sociological, psychological, developmental, and nutritional status.

The following is a suggested organization of sociological data:

1. Relationships with family and significant others
   a. Client's position in the family
   b. Persons with whom client lives
   c. Persons with whom client relates
   d. Recent family crisis or changes
2. Environment
   a. Home
   b. Community
   c. Work
   d. Recent changes in environment
   e. Residence/travel outside of home country
3. Occupational history
   a. Jobs held
   b. Satisfaction with present and past employment
   c. Current place of employment
4. Economic status and resources
   a. Source of income
   b. Perception of adequacy or inadequacy of income
   c. Effect of illness on economic status
5. Educational level
   a. Highest degree or grade attained
   b. Judgment of intellect relative to age
6. Daily profile
   a. Rest-activity patterns
   b. Social activities
   c. Special weekend activities
   d. Recent changes in daily activities
7. Patterns of health care
   a. Private and public primary care agencies
   b. Dental care
   c. Preventive care
   d. Emergency care
8. Relevant cultural information
   a. Where client was born—if an immigrant, length of residence in current country
   b. Ethnic affiliation and strength of ethnic affiliation

c. Primary language and other languages spoken and read

d. Cultural beliefs and practices as they relate to health, illness, and health care

This outline is useful for gathering the sociological data for the majority of adult clients; however, it may be necessary to make adaptations for some individuals. Many clients may be unaccustomed to extensive questioning about nonphysical matters during the taking of a health history. Therefore the use of such data may need to be explained to the client, by stating, for example, "To treat you most effectively, it is important that I know something about you as a person."

First, ask about the client's role or roles in the family and household. A member may have a societally assigned role relating to birth (e.g., that of son, father, or grandfather). In addition, the client may have a circumstantially defined role (e.g., that of provider, "black sheep," or child). Identify all roles if possible.

Next, inquire about the people whom the client lives with and relates to on a regular basis. This information can be useful in hypothesizing, for example, the effect that a long illness of the care provider may have on the family. Also, identify strengths by the presence of strong family or friend relationships. Ask the client about the closeness and compatibility of these relationships. Sometimes unsatisfactory social relationships produce stress, which can be a factor in exacerbating or causing illness.

Ask the client if any recent event has had a significant impact on his or her health. Resultant positive data might provide clues of causation or implications for prevention of illness.

Physical and psychological environments can have a profound effect on an individual's health status and potential. Ask about the client's satisfaction with the appearance and general comfort of house, community, and work situations. Also, inquire whether the client considers the environment healthy or unhealthy. The pursuit of "why" when clients identify problems will provide some insight into the client's value system, possible information regarding significant health hazards, clues to the cause of the present illness, and a validation of the dissatisfaction. Again, ask about recent change or loss. Record positive responses.

Residence and travel outside of one's own country can affect health because of changes in water, food, and environmental conditions as well as response to indigenous health problems. Ask about time spent outside of the home country and recent travel.

Occupational history information can be used to specify past environmental hazards, determine the fit between personal ability and productivity, and plan rehabilitation. Inquire about jobs held, satisfaction with those jobs, and place of current employment.

Although it is usually not necessary to know the client's exact annual income, find out the source of that income and his or her assessment of its adequacy. Identify clients whose resources are insufficient to enable them to follow therapy, and make appropriate referral for financial assistance. For a probable prolonged illness, discuss and record financial reserves. If the client is covered by any health insurance, note the type of insurance, name of the insurer, and policy number.

Determine the educational level of the client and record the highest degree or grade completed. In addition, make a judgment about the client's intellectual ability relative to age. Interviewing up to this point in the history has provided the opportunity for extensive observation of the client's understanding, response, and judgment.

> **HELPFUL HINT** *Assess the client's ability to read before providing written materials. For bilingual clients, provide written materials in the preferred language if possible.*

Knowing the client's daily pattern helps in understanding the client as a person, with habits that encourage or impede health. Ask the client to describe a typical 24-hour day and to indicate weekend differences. Specifically, identify work, activity, sleep, rest, and recreational pursuits in the recording.

Part of the client's past social interaction has been with the health care system, and past responses may predict future patterns. Ask about health agencies used for acute, preventive, and maintenance health care. Determine whether the client is a health facility "shopper" or whether his or her care has had continuity.

For detailed information regarding cultural assessment, see Chapter 7.

Psychological system

The following information needs to be obtained during the psychological assessment of the client:

1. Cognitive abilities
   a. Comprehension
   b. Learning patterns
   c. Memory
2. Responses to illness and health
   a. Reaction to illness
   b. Coping patterns
   c. Value of health
3. Response to care
   a. Perceptions of the caregivers
   b. Compliance
4. Cultural implications for care
   a. Patterns of therapy
   b. Patterns of illness response

table 3.2   *Religious Beliefs Influencing Health and Health Care*

Religious Affiliation	Beliefs
Adventist	Some believe in divine healing and practice anointing with oil and use of prayer May desire Communion or baptism when ill Believe in man's choice and God's sovereignty Saturday is Sabbath for many
Baptist	"Laying on of hands" May encounter some resistance to some therapies, such as abortion Believe God functions through physician Some believe in predestination; may respond passively to care
Black Muslim	Faith healing unacceptable Maintenance of personal habits of cleanliness
Buddhist Churches of America	Illness believed to be a trial to aid development of soul; illness due to Karmic causes May be reluctant to have surgery or certain treatments on holy days Cleanliness believed to be of great importance Family may request Buddhist priest for counseling Optimistic outlook; teach ways to overcome fears, anxieties, apprehension
Church of Christ Scientist	Deny existence of health crisis; see illness and sin as errors of mind that can be altered by prayer Oppose human intervention with drugs or other therapies; however, accept legally required immunizations Many adhere to belief that disease is a human mental concept that can be dispelled by "spiritual truth" to the extent that they refuse all medical treatment May desire services of practitioner or reader; will sometimes refuse even emergency treatment until a reader has been consulted
Church of Jesus Christ of Latter Day Saints (Mormons)	Devout adherents believe in divine healing through anointment with oil and "laying on of hands" by church officials (elders) Medical therapy not prohibited Financial support for the sick available through well-funded welfare system Discourage use of tobacco
Eastern Orthodox	Anointment of the sick No conflict with medical science
Episcopal (Anglican)	Some believe in spiritual healing Rite for anointing the sick available but not mandatory
Friends (Quakers)	No special rites or restrictions
Greek Orthodox	Health crisis handled by ordained priests; deacon may also serve in some cases Holy Communion administered in hospital Some may desire the Sacrament of Holy Unction performed by a priest Believe every reasonable effort should be made to preserve life until termination by God

Modified from Wong DL: *Whaley and Wong's nursing care of infants and children,* ed 5, St Louis, 1995, Mosby.
*NOTE: Not all members of any religious affiliation believe in all formal and informal tenets across religions. The beliefs listed have been noted to be characteristic of substantial numbers of the members of the listed religions.

table 3.2 *Religious Beliefs Influencing Health and Health Care—cont'd*	
Religious Affiliation	**Beliefs**
Hindu	Illness or injury believed to represent sins committed in previous life Accept most modern medical practices
Islam (Muslim/Moslem)	Faith healing not acceptable unless psychological condition of patient is deteriorating; performed for morale Ritual washing after prayer; prayer takes place 5 times daily (on rising, midday, afternoon, early evening, and before bed); during prayer, face Mecca and kneel on prayer rug Older Muslims often have a fatalistic view that may interfere with compliance with therapy
Jehovah's Witness	Adherents are generally absolutely opposed to blood transfusions, including banking of own blood; individuals can sometimes be persuaded in emergencies May be opposed to use of albumin, globulin, factor replacement, and vaccines Not opposed to giving blood sample
Judaism (Orthodox and Conservative)	May resist surgical procedures during Sabbath, which extends from sundown Friday until sundown Sunday Seriously ill and pregnant women are exempt from fasting Illness is grounds for violating dietary laws
Mennonite	Deep concern for dignity and self-determination of individual that would conflict with shock treatment or medical treatment affecting personality or will
Nazarene	Believe in divine healing but not exclusive of medical treatment
Pentecostal (Assembly of God)	No restrictions regarding medical care Deliverance from sickness is provided for in atonement; may pray for divine intervention in health matters and seek God in prayer for themselves and others when ill Some insist illness is divine punishment; most consider it an intrusion of Satan
Orthodox Presbyterian	Blood transfusion accepted when advisable Believe science should be used for relief of suffering
Roman Catholic	Encourage anointing of sick, although this may be interpreted by older members of church as equivalent to old terminology "extreme unction" or "last rites"; they may require careful explanation if reluctance is associated with fear of imminent death Traditional church teaching does not approve of contraceptives or abortion
Russian Orthodox	Adherents believe in divine healing, but not exclusive of medical treatment
Unitarian Universalist	Most believe in the general goodness of their fellow humans and appreciate the expression of that goodness by visits from their clergy and fellow parishioners during times of illness

Selected Cultural Beliefs Related to Health and Health Care

ASIAN-AMERICANS

Chinese

A healthy body is viewed as a gift from parents and ancestors and must be cared for.

Health is one of the results of balance between the forces of yin (cold) and yang (hot), the energy forces that rule the world; illness is caused by imbalance.

Chi is innate energy.

Blood is the source of life and is not regenerated; lack of chi and blood results in deficiency that produces fatigue, poor constitution, and long illness.

There is wide use of medicinal herbs that are applied in prescribed ways.

The goal of therapy is to restore the balance of yin and yang.

Folk healers are herbalists, spiritual healers, temple healers, or fortune healers.

Japanese

Three major belief systems are (1) Shinto (religious influence stating that humans are inherently good, evil is caused by outside spirits, and illness is caused by contact with polluting agents (e.g., blood, corpses, skin diseases); (2) Chinese and Korean influence (health is achieved through harmony and balance between self and society, with disease caused by disharmony with society and not caring for one's body); and (3) Portuguese influence (upholds the germ theory of disease).

Believe evil is removed by purification.

Energy is restored by acupuncture, acupressure, massage, and moxibustion along affected meridians.

Use natural herbs.

Believe in the removal of diseased parts.

Trend is to use both Western and Oriental healing methods.

Care for disabled is viewed as the family's responsibility; take pride in their children's good health; seek preventive care and medical care for illnesses.

Vietnamese

Good health is a balance between yin (cold) and yang (hot).

Health results from harmony with existing universal order; attained by pleasing good spirits and avoiding evil ones.

Practice some restrictions to prevent incurring wrath of evil spirits.

Many use rituals to prevent illness.

Believe a person's life is predisposed toward certain phenomena by cosmic forces; belief in am duc, the amount of good deeds accumulated by ancestors.

Family uses all means possible before consulting outside agencies for health care.

Fortune-tellers determine event that caused disturbance.

May visit temple to procure divine instruction; use astrologer to calculate cyclical changes and forces; seek generalist health healers.

Certain illnesses, such as pustules or open wounds, are considered only temporary and should be ignored.

Filipinos

Believe God's will and supernatural forces govern the universe.

Illness, accidents, and other misfortunes are God's punishment for violations of His will.

Some use amulets as a shield from witchcraft or as a good luck piece; Catholics substitute religious medals and other items.

AFRICAN-AMERICANS

Illness is either natural (due to forces of nature when not adequately protected [e.g., cold air, pollution, food and water]) or unnatural (due to evil influences [e.g., witchcraft, voodoo, hoodoo, hex, fix, rootwork]); symptoms are often associated with eating.

Serious illness is sent by God as punishment (e.g., parents punished by illness or death of a child; can be avoided; may resist health care because illness is the "will of God").

Self-care and folk medicine are very prevalent; folk therapies are usually religious in origin; attempt home remedies first.

Poorer people do not seek help until illness occurs; usually seek help from an "old lady" (woman with common knowledge of herbs; specializes in pediatric care); a spiritualist (received gift from God for healing incurable diseases or solving personal problems; strongly based in Christianity); a priest or priestess (most powerful leader and involved in voodoo); or a root doctor (supplies herbs, oils, candles, and ointments).

Prayer is common means for prevention and treatment of illness.

Modified from Wong DL: *Whaley and Wong's nursing care of infants and children,* ed 5, St Louis, 1995, Mosby.

Selected Cultural Beliefs Related to Health and Health Care—cont'd

HAITIANS

Illness is either natural or supernatural. Supernatural illness is caused by angry voodoo spirits, enemies, or the dead, especially deceased relatives. Natural illness is due to irregularities of blood volume, flow, purity, viscosity, color, and/or temperature (hot/cold); gas; movement and consistency of mother's milk; hot/cold imbalance of the body; bone displacement; or movement of diseases. Natural illnesses are based on conceptions of natural causation.

Health is a personal responsibility.

Health is maintained by good dietary and hygienic practices.

Natural illnesses are treated by home remedies first; supernatural illness is treated by healers: voodoo priest or priestess, midwife, or herbalist or leaf doctor.

Amulets and prayer are used to protect against illness due to curses or willed by evil people.

HISPANICS

Mexican-Americans (Latinos, Chicanos, Raza-Latinos)

Health belief is strongly associated with religion; some maintain good health is a result of good luck and a reward for good behavior and that illness is punishment from God for wrongdoing or is caused by forces of nature or the supernatural.

Some believe in body imbalance causing illness, especially imbalance between caliente (hot) and frio (cold), or "wet" and "dry."

Illness is prevented by behaving properly, eating proper foods, working a proper amount of time, praying, wearing religious medals or amulets, and sleeping with relics in the home.

Seek help from curandero or curandera, especially in rural areas; this person receives his or her position by birth, apprenticeship, or a "calling" via a dream or vision; treatments involve use of herbs, rituals, and religious artifacts; for severe illnesses, make promises, visit shrines, offer medals and candles, and pray.

Puerto Ricans

Subscribe to the "hot-cold" theory of disease causation.

Some illness is caused by evil spirits and forces.

Use the health care system infrequently.

Seek a folk healer who uses herbs and rituals; consult a spiritualist medium for mental disorders. Santeria is the system, and practitioners are called santeros.

Cuban-Americans

Prevention and good nutrition are related to good health.

Are diligent users of the medical model.

Have eclectic health-seeking practices, including preventive measures, extensive use of the health care system, and sometimes medicine of both religious and nonreligious origin; home remedies are used; in many instances seek assistance from santeros (Afro-Cuban healers) and spiritualists to complement medical treatment.

NATIVE AMERICANS

Believe health is a state of harmony with nature and the universe.

All disorders are believed to have aspects of the supernatural.

Show respect of the body through proper management.

Theology and medicine are strongly interwoven.

Seek care from medicine persons: altruistic persons who must use powers in purely positive ways; persons capable of both good and evil—perform negative acts against enemies; diviner-diagnosticians who diagnose but do not have powers or skill to implement medical treatment; specialists who use herbs as curative but nonsacred medical procedures; medicine persons who use herbs and rituals; and singers who cure by the power of their song.

In assessing cognitive abilities, determine the client's comprehension ability. Usually, comprehension can be assessed well indirectly rather than directly. Up to this point in the history-taking process, the client has demonstrated his or her ability to respond to rather complex questions. With this background in mind, record your judgment summary regarding the client's general comprehension ability.

Because education should be an essential component of all therapy, determine the client's health-learning patterns. Some clients need personal instructions. Others learn best through reading or group discussion. Knowing the client's preference can enable efficient use of provider effort and also involve the client in decision making concerning the process of therapy.

Discuss the client's behavior in past illnesses and in

health to help predict future responses. Ask questions such as the following: "What does health mean to you, and what do you do to keep yourself healthy?" "How do you feel, and what do you do when you become slightly ill? When you become very ill?" "Who do you go to for help if you are ill?" Most clients will be able to answer these questions easily. Record a concise summary of the client's responses. This information can indicate the client's strengths and weaknesses and possible problems in therapy.

Skill may be required in learning the client's real responses to care, since people are often placed in a position of subjugation by the health care system. Ask the client how comfortable he or she feels in asking questions of health care providers and whether he or she feels like a partner in care with them. You may record answers verbatim or summarize them.

Ask about the client's degree of compliance with past courses of therapy. If compliance has been minimal, determine the reasons for noncompliance. Problems resulting from lack of understanding and financial constraints are more easily solved than problems relating to distrust, indifference, or denial.

If the client is of a cultural group that is different from yours and that of the majority of the care providers, ask the client what he or she expects of care and therapy and if his or her culture has particular traditions regarding persons with similar needs. If the chief complaint is an illness, ask about the feelings and responses of the client and significant others to the fact of the illness. The responses may help to guide the care provider in a more efficient direction and to avoid unacceptable routes of intervention. (For more information on the collection of culturally relevant information, see Chapter 7, Table 3.2, and the box on pp. 40-41.)

Developmental Data

A detailed description of the developmental assessment is presented in Chapter 4. At minimum, the recording of these data includes a summary of the client's development to date and a statement of current developmental functioning.

Nutritional Data

A detailed description of nutritional assessment is presented in Chapter 5. The recording of data minimally includes a description of an average day's food intake; an assessment of adequacy, inadequacy, or excess of the components of the basic four food groups; and the presence of any past nutritional problems.

Concluding the Health History

At the completion of the history, it is often useful to verbally summarize the key points of the history with the client. Also, this is a good time to ask the client if

Screening for Problem Drinking

The U.S. Preventive Services Task Force (1996) recommends screening to detect problem drinking for all adult and adolescent clients. The screening method endorsed is a careful history of alcohol use or the use of standard screening questionnaires. Routine measurement of biochemical markers was not recommended in asymptomatic persons. The AUDIT Structured Interview was highlighted as a clinical tool for screening (U.S. Preventive Services Task Force, 1996, p. 577). The tool's key questions are:

1. How often do you have a drink containing alcohol?
2. How many drinks do you have on a typical day when you are drinking?
3. How often do you have six or more drinks on one occasion?
4. How often during the last year have you found that you were unable to stop drinking once you had started?
5. How often during the last year have you failed to do what was normally expected of you because of drinking?
6. How often during the last year have you needed a first drink in the morning to get yourself going after a heavy drinking session?
7. How often during the last year have you had a feeling of guilt or remorse after drinking?
8. How often during the last year have you been unable to remember what happened the night before because you had been drinking?
9. Have you or someone else been injured as a result of your drinking?
10. Has a relative, doctor, or other health care worker been concerned about your drinking or suggested you cut down?

there is any additional pertinent information that has not yet been shared.

■ ORGANIZATION BY FUNCTIONAL HEALTH PATTERNS

The format for the health history presented in this chapter is based on the traditional approaches in health care delivery systems. Within nursing, alternate systems of health assessment are being developed around the organizing framework of functional health patterns (Gordon, 1994). Functional health patterns are defined as

sequences of health behavior across time. Following is the currently used taxonomy of functional health patterns. Listed under each pattern are areas of specific assessment relevant to that health pattern.

Health Perception–Health Management Pattern

This category describes the client's perceived pattern of health and well-being and how health is managed. It includes the relevance of health perception to current activities and future planning. Also included is the individual's health risk management and general health care behavior, such as adherence to mental and physical health promotion activities, medical or nursing prescriptions, and follow-up care.

Reason for seeking health care
Current and usual health status
Perception of individual's own health
Health management and adherence behavior
Risk factors—family, health habits, environment
Preventive health screening activities

Nutritional-Metabolic Pattern

This area describes the pattern of food and fluid consumption relative to metabolic need and pattern indicators of local nutrient supply. It includes daily eating times, types and quantity of food and fluids consumed, particular food preferences, and use of nutrient or vitamin supplements. This area also describes breast-feeding and infant-feeding patterns. It includes reports of any skin lesions and general ability to heal; the condition of skin, hair, nails, mucous membranes, and teeth; and measurements of body temperature, height, and weight.

General information—height, weight, appetite
Food and fluid intake
Weight patterns
Activity level
Psychosocial/cultural/personal influences
Nutrition information
Pertinent physiological alterations
Drug history
Skin and dental problems

Elimination Pattern

This category describes the patterns of excretory function (bowel, bladder, and skin). It includes the individual's perceived regularity of excretory function, use of routines or laxatives for bowel elimination, and any changes or disturbances in time pattern, mode of excretion, quality, or quantity. Also included are any devices used to control excretion.

Bladder elimination
    Usual pattern of voiding
    Self-care practices
    Symptoms of altered bladder elimination
    Pertinent physiological alterations
Bowel elimination
    Usual pattern of defecation
    Self-care practices
    Symptoms of altered bowel elimination
    Pertinent physiological alterations
Skin problems

Activity-Exercise Pattern

This area describes the pattern of exercise, activity, leisure, and recreation. It includes activities of daily living requiring energy expenditure, such as hygiene, cooking, shopping, eating, working, and home maintenance. Also included are the type, quantity, and quality of exercise, including sports, that describe the typical pattern for the individual. Factors that interfere with the desired or expected pattern for the individual (e.g., neuromuscular deficits and compensations, dyspnea, angina, or muscle cramping on exertion, and cardiac/pulmonary classification, if appropriate) are noted. Leisure patterns are also included and describe the activities that the individual undertakes as recreation either with a group or as an individual. Emphasis is on the activities of high importance or significance to the individual.

Usual activities
Self-care activities
Adequacy of energy for requirements
Symptoms related to activity and exercise
Pertinent physiological alterations
Functional status

Sleep-Rest Pattern

This category describes the patterns of sleep, rest, and relaxation during the 24-hour day. It includes the individual's perception of the quality and quantity of sleep and rest, and perception of energy level. Also noted are aids to sleep, such as medications or nighttime routines that the individual employs.

Usual sleep pattern
Sleep/bedtime rituals
Sleep environment
Sleep position
Psychophysiological influences
Sleep-pattern disturbance symptoms

Cognitive-Perceptual Pattern

This class describes the sensory-perceptual and cognitive pattern. It includes the adequacy of sensory modes, such as vision, hearing, taste, touch, or smell, and the compensation or prosthetics used for disturbances. Reports of pain perception and how pain is managed are also noted when appropriate. In addition, the cognitive functional abilities, such as language, memory, and decision making, are included.

Special senses
   Eyes and vision
   Ears and hearing
Other special senses
Symptoms of neurological dysfunction
Pertinent physiological alterations and medications
Learning styles
Comfort

Self-Perception–Self-Concept Pattern

This area describes the self-concept pattern and the perceptions of self. It includes the individual's attitudes about himself or herself, perception of abilities (cognitive, affective, or physical), body image, identity, general sense of worth, and general emotional pattern. Patterns of body posture and movement, eye contact, voice, and speech are noted.
   Social identity
   Personal identity
   Physical self
   Self-esteem
   Self-concept threats

Role-Relationship Pattern

This class describes the pattern of role engagements and relationships. It includes the individual's perception of the major roles and responsibilities in current life situations. Satisfaction or disturbances in family, work, or social relationships and responsibilities related to these roles are noted.
   Roles
   Family relationships
   Family problems
   Family functioning
   Work environment
   Neighborhood environment

Sexuality-Reproductive Pattern

This category describes the patterns of satisfaction or dissatisfaction with sexuality and delineates the reproductive pattern. It includes the individual's perceived satisfaction or disturbances in his or her sexuality. The female's reproductive stage, premenopausal or postmenopausal, and any perceived problems are also noted.
   Sex roles and gender identification
   Knowledge about sexuality and reproduction
   Concerns about sexual performance and satisfaction
   Reproductive history
   Use of contraception

Coping–Stress Tolerance Pattern

This area describes the general coping pattern and the effectiveness of the pattern in terms of stress tolerance. It includes the individual's reserve or capacity to resist challenge to self-integrity, modes of handling stress, family or other support systems, and perceived ability to control and manage situations.
   Nature of stresses
   Perception of stresses/roles
   Coping strategies
   Resolution of stress

Value-Belief Pattern

This class describes the pattern of values, goals, or beliefs (including spiritual) that guide choices or decisions. It includes what is perceived as important in life, the quality of life, and any perceived conflicts in values, beliefs, or expectations that are health related.
   Culture
   Spirituality
   Values

■ COMPUTER-ASSISTED HISTORY

Computer science is an important and permanent component of health care technology, and the computer can be an important tool in obtaining the client health history. Studies have demonstrated that the use of the computer in history taking can save the practitioner time and yield a reliable, comprehensive, and readable printout. In addition, this approach is acceptable to clients. In situations where personnel is in short supply and time allocated to history taking is routinely inadequate, the computer-assisted history can be superior to a verbal history.

Computer systems for history taking can be either client- or practitioner-interactive systems. The client-interactive systems are more commonly used because they can save the practitioner time. A number of client-interactive, computerized history-taking systems are available. Self-administered histories involve the client's either completing a paper-and-pencil questionnaire or interacting with a computer. With the paper-and-pencil questionnaire, the client's responses are computerized in a variety of ways, and the practitioner receives a printout of those responses. In the client-interactive systems, the client responds to inquiries from a computer terminal. In general, clients have viewed computer-assisted interviews favorably, and printouts from such systems have been complete, accurate, and legible.

In any client self-administered system, the practitioner's time is needed to review the client's history. Usually this review involves only a small amount of time. However, the amount of time spent by the client in the history-taking process is not shortened by the computer-assisted methods. The client's age, the number of client problems, and the time required by the client to complete the instructional portion of the computer pro-

gram are positively correlated with the overall time needed to complete a computer-assisted history. The number of the client's years of formal education is negatively correlated with the overall time.

The computer-assisted history is more appropriate for the ambulatory client than for the hospitalized client. The ambulatory client can be scheduled for a computer interview or can complete a form for computerization that will yield a printout for the practitioner within several days. For hospitalized clients, information is generally needed immediately, and client access to terminals becomes problematic. Also, the hospitalized client often is too ill to complete a questionnaire or to use a computer terminal.

Practitioner-based computer systems for history taking involve either the practitioner's direct interaction with a computer, which is programmed for questions related to the history and into which answers are placed, or the practitioner's completion of a form that is computer processed at a later time. The practitioner-interactive systems require a terminal for each practitioner, a situation that may not be cost-effective in ambulatory care situations. A more common approach is to perform computer processing of questionnaires. The advantage of this method is that it produces a legible printout, an improvement over most handwritten documents.

The computer-assisted history can be as effective as the verbal history. In fact, it may be more effective because remembering items for review is not a problem. Any question that can be asked verbally can be programmed into a computer system, and computer technology allows for additional, branching questions if the client gives certain significant responses. Before additional assessment is done and therapy is begun, it is important for the practitioner to discuss, review, and verify the information to determine the validity of significant responses. The client may have misunderstood instructions, or mechanical errors may be reflected in the information.

As computers become more prevalent in health care systems, especially microcomputers, the use of computer-assisted histories is likely to increase. However, there will always exist situations in which the computer-assisted history is not feasible and a verbal history is necessary. Therefore skill in history taking is, and will continue to be, an important ability of the health care practitioner.

■ WRITTEN RECORD

The written record is the permanent, legal, and working documentation of what the practitioner sees, hears, and feels during the examination. It serves as the baseline for evaluation of subsequent changes and decisions related to therapy. This record is used by readers who do not have access to the recorder and is consequently subject to interpretation.

The recorded history must be accurate, objective, clear, complete, and concise. It should be free of recorder bias. In particular, the history is not the place for the recorder to include his or her opinions of possible diagnoses. Other portions of a client's record allow for the recorder to elaborate on hypotheses and plans.

In addition, the practitioner should integrate the client's responses in an accurate but objective way. This can be accomplished in one of two ways: (1) by paraphrasing the client, using statements such as "States he had the same symptoms 4 years ago" or "Denies chest pain," or (2) by quoting the client directly (e.g., "The pain was so severe, I fell back into the chair I had just gotten up from").

Because most health histories are read by many health care providers over time, the clarity and organization of the presentation are important. A clear presentation is often difficult for the beginning health historian to achieve, but feedback about written histories from colleagues and instructors can assist in identifying strengths and deficits in this area. Most beginners must pay specific attention to chronology and to the quality and quantity of symptoms.

The written record should be a complete history of the practitioner-client encounter. It should be specific enough for the reader to determine clearly what questions were asked, what areas of examination were covered, and the results of the interview and examination. An entry such as "Eyes—negative" or "Eyes—normal" does not supply any information regarding what questions were asked about the eyes. The range of "normal" is wide, and any change in condition, even within the range of normal, may be significant for an individual client.

Although the written record must be complete, it should also be concise. A reader should be able to locate and read regional entries easily. A verbose and disorganized record may be even less effective than an incomplete one because its appearance may frustrate the busy reader, who simply will not read it. The record does not need to be composed of complete sentences. In fact, the use of clear phrases can save both time and space.

Two examples of documented health histories are presented in the boxed material on pp. 46-56. One is an example of a history taken from a well client. The other is an example of a history taken from an ill client being admitted to a hospital. An example of a documented physical examination is included in Chapter 23.

Example of Health History Documentation: Well Client

CLIENT: Mary Rose Doe

ADDRESS: 1056 N. East St.
          St. Louis, MO 63047

TELEPHONE: 278-9274

CONTACT: Mrs. Elsa Smith (mother)

ADDRESS: 3496 Oak St.
          St. Louis, MO 63047

TELEPHONE: 926-8711

BIRTH DATE: Feb. 6, 1959   SEX: Female   RACE: Black

RELIGION: Methodist (active)   MARITAL STATUS: Married

SOCIAL SECURITY NUMBER: 396-47-8911

USUAL OCCUPATION: Grade school teacher

PRESENT OCCUPATION: Same—Greenwich School

BIRTHPLACE: Greenwood, Mississippi

SOURCE OF REFERRAL: Self

USUAL SOURCE OF HEALTH CARE: St. Louis Health Maintenance Organization
                              4693 C. Division St.
                              St. Louis, MO 63044

SOURCE AND RELIABILITY OF INFORMATION: Client; cooperative, apparently reliable

DATE OF INTERVIEW: Dec. 12, 1996

REASON FOR VISIT: Annual physical examination; last examination, 11/95

PRESENT HEALTH STATUS

Usual Health

This is the third St. Louis HMO visit for this 37-year-old black, married, female schoolteacher who has been in good health for all of her life. Client has been hospitalized twice for the purposes of normal childbirth only. Has no major chronic diseases.

Summary

Client is presently well and requests a physical examination for health maintenance and screening purposes. Is concerned about a strong family history of hypertension and believes that monitoring of her blood pressure status is important. Also requests a Pap smear and evaluation for continuance of oral contraceptives. Has been taking oral contraceptives since the birth of her last child in 1983. Client enrolled in the health plan a year ago.

PAST HEALTH HISTORY

Childhood Illnesses

Had rubella, chickenpox—not diagnosed by a physician. Has not had rheumatic fever.

Injuries

None.

Hospitalizations

See obstetrical data in Review of Physical Systems.
1. Age 20 (1979). Childbirth.
2. Age 24 (1983). Childbirth.

Operations

None.

Major Illnesses

None.

Example of Health History Documentation: Well Client—cont'd

CURRENT HEALTH INFORMATION

Allergies

None known. Denies allergy to penicillin, other drugs, foods, or environmental components. Has had a course of penicillin (10 days, oral).

Immunizations

Had full DPT series when a preschooler. Had oral polio when an adolescent. No others.

Habits

Cigarettes—smoked 15 cigarettes a day for 5 years (age 20 to 25). No smoking since age 25.
Illicit drugs—none.
Alcohol—drinks 3 to 4 mixed drinks a weekend.
Coffee, tea—drinks approximately 10 cups of coffee a day. Drinks tea rarely.

Medications

Norinyl 1/35 taken currently. Oral contraceptive used since 1983.
Aspirin (ASA) for headache—takes approximately 10 gr twice a month.
Milk of magnesia for constipation—takes 1 tablespoon about once a month.
One-a-Day multiple vitamins—takes 1 a day.

Exercise Patterns

Attends aerobics classes 2 to 3 times a week during the winter. In summer, walks 3 to 4 times a week.

Sleep Patterns

Sleeps 7 to 8 hours a night regularly with occasional naps on weekends.

FAMILY HEALTH HISTORY

Denies family history of diabetes, blood disorder, gout, obesity, tuberculosis, epilepsy, kidney disease, or gastrointestinal disease.

continued

Example of Health History Documentation: Well Client—cont'd

REVIEW OF PHYSICAL SYSTEMS

General
Usually well. Usual-minimum-maximum weight: 135-125-160 lb. No recent increase or decrease in weight. Denies fatigue, malaise, chills, sweats, fever, seizures, or fainting. Reports height as 5 ft 6 in.

Skin, Hair, and Nails
Denies lesions, color change, ecchymoses, masses, petechiae, texture changes, pruritus, sweating, or unusual odors. No alopecia or brittle hair. Denies brittle, cracking, or peeling nails. No birthmarks. Washes hair once a week; does not use dyes.

Head and Face
Denies pain, dizziness, vertigo, or history of injury or loss of consciousness.

Eyes
Has worn corrective lenses since age 7; currently wears contact lenses all day. Denies recent change in visual acuity, pain, infection, watery or itching eyes, diplopia, blurred vision, glaucoma, cataracts, or decreased peripheral vision. Last ophthalmoscopic examination, 2 years ago.

Ears
Denies hearing loss, discharge, pain, irritation, or ringing in ears. Cleans ears with cotton-tipped applicator.

Nose and Sinuses
States she has sinus pain, congestion, and subsequent nasal discharge several times each winter. Takes Contac prn (approximately 1 q 12 hours × 3 days) for each episode of rhinitis; gets relief. Denies epistaxis, soreness, excessive sneezing, obstructed breathing, or injuries. States olfaction is good.

Oral Cavity
Visits a dentist every 6 months for cleaning and examination. Brushes teeth twice a day. Denies toothache, lesions, soreness, bleeding of gums, coated tongue, disturbance of taste, hoarseness, or frequent sore throat.

Neck
Denies pain, stiffness, limitation of movement, or masses.

Nodes
Denies enlarged or tender nodes in neck, axillary, or inguinal area.

Breasts
Denies masses, pain, tenderness, or discharge. Examines breasts monthly, right after menses.

Chest and Respiratory System
Denies pain, wheezing, shortness of breath, dyspnea, hemoptysis, or cough. Denies history of asthma, pneumonia, or bronchitis. Obtains annual PPD tests—have been negative.

Cardiovascular System
Denies precordial pain, palpitations, cyanosis, edema, or intermittent claudication. Denies diagnosis of heart murmur, hypertension, coronary artery disease, or rheumatic fever.

Gastrointestinal System
Denies history of GI disease. Appetite good. Daily bowel movements; stools are always brown. Denies pain, constipation, diarrhea, flatulence, vomiting, hemorrhoids, hernias, jaundice, pyrosis, or bleeding. Has never had GI x-rays.

Genitourinary System
Denies history of bladder or kidney infections, hematuria, urgency, frequency, dysuria, incontinence, nocturia, polyuria, or VD. Menses—onset 13 years; frequency, every 26 to 30 days; duration, 5 days; flow, heavy for 3 days, light for 2 days; last menstrual period (LMP), 12/1/96. Denies dysmenorrhea, menorrhagia, menorrhagia discharge, or pruritus. Last Pap smear, 12/95.

Example of Health History Documentation: Well Client—cont'd

Obstetrical History

1. Sept. 12, 1979. Girl, 6 lb, 8 oz. Vaginal delivery at St. Francis Hospital, St. Louis. Prenatal, intrapartum, and postpartum course normal for mother and baby.
2. Oct. 9, 1983. Boy 7 lb, 2 oz. Vaginal delivery at St. Francis Hospital, St. Louis. Prenatal, intrapartum, and postpartum course normal for mother and baby.

Sexual History

Age at first intercourse was 17 years. Enjoys intercourse with husband—no dyspareunia and able to achieve satisfactory orgasm most of the time. Using oral birth control medication. Not sure yet if she will have another child. Will consider sterilization when family is complete.

Extremities

No past problems. Denies deformities, varicose veins, thrombophlebitis, joint pain, stiffness, swelling, gout, arthritis, limitation of movement, color changes, or temperature changes.

Back

No past problems. Denies pain, stiffness, or limitation of movement; no history of disk disease.

Central Nervous System

No past problems. Denies loss of consciousness, clumsiness of movement, difficulty with balance, weakness, paralysis, tremor, neuralgia, paresthesia, history of emotional disorders, drug or alcohol dependency, disorientation, memory lapses, or seizures. Speech articulate.

Hematopoietic System

No past problems. Denies excessive bleeding and bruising, blood transfusions, or excessive exposure to x-rays or toxic agents. Blood type A, Rh positive.

Endocrine System

Denies history of diabetes or thyroid disease, polyuria, polydipsia, polydysplasia, intolerance to heat or cold, or hirsutism.

REVIEW OF SOCIOLOGICAL SYSTEM

Family Relationships

Lives in own home with husband and 2 children. Husband is a schoolteacher also; couple shares finances, child-rearing, and housekeeping responsibilities. Client's parents live 1/2 mile away, and relationships are described as "good." Couple has several close friends; also, siblings are in frequent contact. No recent family crisis or change.

Occupational History

Has been a grade school teacher for 5 years. No other jobs. Holds bachelor's and master's degrees and feels secure that she can retain her job as long as she wants it. Enjoys children and states job is very satisfying.

Economic Status

Client and husband achieve a combined gross income of over $90,000 a year. Feels this is very adequate. Belongs to an HMO. Assesses coverage as "good."

Daily Profile

During the week, works 8 AM to 3 PM. Returns home around 3:30 and works until 5 PM on school work. Then cooks dinner and interacts with family. Has meetings 1 or 2 evenings a week. Weekends, client and husband usually have 1 evening out with friends, to movie or concert. Family attends church each Sunday. Client is involved with photography as a hobby. Frequently bicycles in summer and downhill skis in winter. Walks 2 miles a day.

Educational Level

Highest degree attained is the master's degree. Obtains most of health knowledge by reading.

Patterns of Health Care

Has always had a primary care provider. Cared for by Dr. Richard Smith, a family practitioner until first pregnancy. Then seen regularly by Dr. Janice Lawson for obstetric and gynecologic care. Family enrolled in HMO a year ago. Receives regular dental care through the HMO.

continued

Example of Health History Documentation: Well Client—cont'd

Environmental Data

Birthplace—Greenwood, Miss. Grew up in Trenton, N.J.

Home—family lives in their own 8-room home in a residential St. Louis neighborhood. Client describes home as comfortable. Has lived there for 10 years.

Community—community is middle income, integrated, consisting primarily of young, professional families.

Work—teaches fourth grade in a community school. States that the work situation is fairly good. School is in good condition, and classes are small. A recent stress is a new assistant principal with whom client does not get along. May consider transfer to another school.

REVIEW OF PSYCHOLOGICAL SYSTEM

Cognitive Abilities

Oriented to time, place, and person (×3). Is articulate, asks questions, has a good memory. Able to understand directions.

Response to Illness

States she has never been seriously ill, so does not know what personal response would be. Feels she is "too busy" to be ill for any length of time. Uses resources of the HMO for preventive and therapeutic needs of self and family.

Response to Care

States she enjoys encounters with health care providers. States she usually follows through on the advice that is given. Feels that the services of the HMO are adequate to meet her family care needs and she has been very satisfied with the care to date.

Cultural Implications

Client states she and her family are involved in a racially integrated community. She grew up in a predominantly black northern community. Cannot identify any way in which her black culture would especially affect her response to illness or therapy in the case of illness. Active Methodist; believes that religious concerns would influence her response to illness and treatment.

DEVELOPMENTAL DATA

Adult female; wife, mother, and career teacher.

NUTRITIONAL DATA

Diet adequate; high in fats and carbohydrates. Has no food intolerances.

Usual breakfast—toast with butter, fried egg, orange juice, and coffee with cream.

Usual lunch—eats with schoolchildren; consists of meat, 1 vegetable, 1 carbohydrate, dessert, and beverage.

Dinner—meat (beef, chicken, or pork), salad, 1 vegetable, potato or bread, dessert, and coffee with cream.

Snacks—may have cheese and crackers or peanuts in the evening.

Example of Health History Documentation: Ill Client

CLIENT: John Donald Doe
ADDRESS: 9037 N. Sheridan St.
St. Louis, MO 63125
TELEPHONE: 735-1946
CONTACT: Mrs. Clara Doe (mother)
ADDRESS: Same address as above; client will move in with mother after discharge from hospital
TELEPHONE: Same telephone number as above
BIRTH DATE: March 3, 1960   SEX: Male   RACE: White
RELIGION: Presbyterian (inactive)   MARITAL STATUS: Separated
SOCIAL SECURITY NUMBER: 097-32-7259
USUAL OCCUPATION: Offset printer
PRESENT OCCUPATION: None; on disability for 1 year
BIRTHPLACE: New York, N.Y.
SOURCE OF REFERRAL: Self
USUAL SOURCE OF HEALTH CARE: Dr. Christopher Ryan
1346 W. North Ave.
St. Louis, MO 63122
SOURCE AND RELIABILITY OF INFORMATION: Client; attempted to be cooperative; however, was frequently vague about the nature and time of events
DATE OF INTERVIEW: Jan. 9, 1996
CHIEF COMPLAINT: "Pain in the left side of stomach for 2 days."
PRESENT ILLNESS

Usual Health

This is the fifth Healer's Hospital admission for this 35-year-old white, separated, unemployed male who has been drinking an average of 2 to 3 fifths of hard liquor daily. Total past admissions number 8; one of these has been for a hemorrhoidectomy. Client is presently on disability income as a result of a diagnosis of tuberculosis (11/94). Also has a history of drug abuse and gastric ulcer.

CHRONOLOGICAL STORY

18 Years PTA*

Began drinking heavily and regularly.

7 Years PTA

Diagnosed as having a gastric ulcer by Dr. Ryan. Treated by him on an outpatient basis with Maalox and Xanax prn. Had x-rays at that time. Has complained of slight to moderate gastric discomfort and food intolerance intermittently since then. Unable to relate the specific frequency or specific characteristics of episodes of illness. States that they are usually accompanied by "hangovers." Generally experiences left upper quadrant discomfort, feelings of hunger, nausea, and vomiting of mucous material 6 to 8 hours after drinking heavily. Drinks heavily 3 to 4 days a week and states symptoms occur approximately 2 times a week. Appetite generally has been good. Meal patterns are erratic. Takes Xanax for sleep each night. Drinks 2 to 3 8-oz bottles of Maalox per week. No pattern of follow-up care with Dr. Ryan. Symptoms relieved somewhat with Maalox. Bowel movements have been regular, formed, and brown.

1 Day PTA

Had not been drinking the night before. Awoke at approximately 7:00 AM and took several alcoholic drinks (amount approximately 1 cup). An hour after an attempt to drink orange juice at 9:00 AM, experienced nausea and vomiting.

---

*PTA, Prior to admission.

continued

Example of Health History Documentation: Ill Client—cont'd

At 10:00 AM walked to his mother's home (2 blocks). On arriving, experienced a sharp, continuous, nonradiating pain in his upper left abdominal area. The intensity required him to lie down. Position changes provided no relief. A whole bottle of Maalox did not affect the pain, which built in intensity over the next 2 hours. After 2 hours the pain remained constant but was more nagging than sharp. Tried to take some soup and orange juice but immediately vomited it. At 2:00 pm vomited approximately 1 cup of green-colored matter again, and this time there were red streaks in the vomitus, which was a green, thick material. (Exact amount of vomitus or blood streaks unknown.)

Throughout the remainder of the afternoon and early evening, took 5 mg Xanax for a total of 4 times. Obtained no relief; pain remained nagging and continuous. Was able to walk with no increase in discomfort but felt most comfortable lying down.

At bedtime took a sleeping pill but states it did not really help him sleep. Spent a fitful night, and the pain persisted with increased intensity. States he took his temperature at midnight and had a fever of 102° F.

Date of Admission

Rose at 9:00 AM and was driven to Dr. Ryan's office but found it closed. Then came directly to Healer's urgent care clinic, where he was seen and admitted.

NEGATIVE INFORMATION

Denies unusual weakness, chills, or fever before the onset of symptoms. Denies injury to the abdomen, unusual activity or exercise, pain in other locations, diarrhea, constipation, change in stools, jaundice, ascites, flatulence, hemorrhoids, rectal bleeding, or dysphagia.

RELEVANT FAMILY HISTORY

The only significant family history for a serious, persistent gastrointestinal disorder was a maternal uncle who was a heavy drinker and who died of stomach cancer at age 40.

DISABILITY ASSESSMENT

Client states that he has not felt really well in the past 7 years. Has not spent a great deal of time in bed but has not worked regularly and has been either drinking or "hung over" most of the time. Was diagnosed as having tuberculosis, 11/94, and was placed on a disability income plan at that time. This insurance will cover medical expenses.

PAST HEALTH HISTORY

Childhood Illnesses

Exact illnesses or dates unknown. Assumes he had all childhood illnesses (measles, mumps, chickenpox); denies history of rheumatic fever.

Injuries

Client unable to provide exact dates for any of the following:

1. Age 9 (1969). Hit in the eye by rock. States has had a permanent decrease in vision in left eye. No medical care.
2. Age 14 (1974). In an automobile accident. Was hospitalized at Lakeside Hospital, Chicago, for 1 week. Physician unknown. Discharged from hospital with no follow-up required.
3. Age 15 or 16 (1975 or 1976). Fractured right ankle while playing football. Cast applied at Johnson Hospital, Chicago, and was followed in their orthopedic clinic. Apparently healed.
4. Age 18 (1978). Head injury from blow with blunt object, which was thrown. Was unconscious for approximately 30 minutes. Head sutured in emergency room (ER) of Healer's Hospital, St. Louis. No follow-up except for removal of sutures. No sequelae.
5. Age 21 (1981). Stab wound in left shoulder; was attacked and robbed. Sutured in ER of Lakeside Hospital, Chicago. No follow-up except for removal of sutures. No sequelae.

Hospitalizations

1. Age 10 (1970). Hernia repair at Lakeside Hospital, Chicago. Dates and events of hospitalization unclear.
2. Age 14 (1974). Automobile accident. See item 2 under Injuries.
3. Age 20 (1980). Pneumonia. Under the care of Dr. Warner at St. Peter's Hospital, Chicago. Hospitalized for 2 weeks during December. No follow-up.

Example of Health History Documentation: Ill Client—cont'd

4. Age 23 (1983). Surgery for priapism at Lakeside Hospital. Under the care of Dr. Meyer. Follow-up for 1 year after surgery because was unable to obtain an erection. No other complications or current disability.
5. Age 24 (1984). Heroin drug overdose. Under the care of Dr. Ryan, Healer's Hospital, St. Louis. Hospitalized for 2 weeks; was to start methadone maintenance; did not. Dates of stay not known.
6. Age 26 (1986). Heroin drug overdose. Under the care of Dr. Ryan, Healer's Hospital. In the hospital for 1 week. Discharged against medical advice.
7. Age 28 (1988). Heroin drug overdose. Under the care of Dr. Ryan. Hospitalized at Healer's Hospital for 2 weeks (1/83). Discharged on methadone maintenance.
8. Age 28 (1988). Hemorrhoidectomy. Under the care of Dr. Ryan and Dr. Jones, Healer's Hospital. Hospitalized 1 week. No complications; 1 follow-up visit.

Operations
See Hospitalizations for details.
1. Age 10 (1970). Hernia repair.
2. Age 23 (1983). Correction of priapism.
3. Age 28 (1988). Hemorrhoidectomy.

Other Major Illnesses
1. Age 23 (1983). Diagnosed as having gastric ulcer by Dr. Ryan after an outpatient evaluation including x-rays. See Present Illness section for follow-up and sequelae.
2. Age 34 (1994). Tuberculosis diagnosed and treated by staff of the St. Louis Health Department as an outpatient. Medications for 1 year. Off medications for the past 3 months. Followed with yearly x-rays and evaluation.

CURRENT HEALTH INFORMATION

Allergies
None known. Denies allergies to penicillin, other drugs, foods, or environmental components; has had at least 3 courses of penicillin.

Immunizations
Unknown.

Habits
Cigarettes—smokes 1 pack a day. Habit regular since age 12.
Hard drugs—all types, including heroin. 1984-1988 had a "$90-a-day-habit." No recent history.
Alcohol—started to drink heavily at age 16. Drinking decreased during period of drug addiction. Has been drinking 2 to 3 fifths of hard liquor a day for the past 2 years.
Coffee—drinks 6 to 7 cups a day.

Medications
Xanax 5 mg prn for gastric distress.
Maalox—for ulcer prn with varied dosage since 1983. Prescribed by Dr. Ryan. Client states he uses 2 to 3 8-oz bottles a week.
Valium—10 mg prn for ulcer and nervousness since 1983. Client states he uses at least 1 to 2 tablets a day.
Methadone—40 mg daily for 6 months, 1988. Given through drug abuse program.
Streptomycin—IM daily, dose? For TB, 11/94 to 9/95.
INH—tid for TB, 11/94 to 9/95.
Salve—name unknown, a nonprescription drug; topically every day for scaling skin on soles of feet; since approximately 8/89.
Magnesium citrate—for constipation approximately once (×1) monthly or less frequently; prescribed by self. Uses 1 tbsp prn.
Sleeping pill—prn. Name and dose unknown. Prescribed by Dr. Ryan; 1 every night.

Exercise Patterns
Largely sedentary due to lifestyle and low energy. No regularly scheduled exercise.

Sleep Patterns
Sleeps about 7 to 8 hours during a 24-hour period. Often patterns are irregular because of alcohol consumption.

continued

Example of Health History Documentation: Ill Client—cont'd

FAMILY HEALTH HISTORY

Maternal and paternal grandparents deceased. Ages at death and causes of death unknown. Denies family history of diabetes, blood disorders, arteriosclerosis, gout, obesity, coronary artery disease, tuberculosis, cancer, hypertension, epilepsy, kidney disease, or allergic disorders. Uncertain about health history of aunts and uncles.

Mother—age 56; alive and well.

Father—deceased, age 50, 1975; cause unknown.

Siblings—no maternal miscarriages.

    1. ♀ Age 31; alive and well.

    2. ♂ Age 20; deceased 1988; drug overdose.

    3. ♀ Age 25; alive and well.

    4. ♂ Age 23; alive and well.

Children

    1. ♂ Age 10; alive and well.

    2. ♂ Age 7; alive and well.

Wife—age 31; obese, otherwise well.

REVIEW OF PHYSICAL SYSTEMS

General

Chronically ill, white male adult; usual weight about 176 lb. Reports approximately 10-lb weight loss over the past 3- to 4-month period. Feels this is a result of not eating when drinking heavily. States he has felt a generalized fatigue and malaise for over 1 year, since onset of TB, but denies requiring daily naps or extra sleep. States he cannot exercise because of fatigue. Denies chills (other than those associated with present illness), sweats, and seizures.

Skin, Hair, and Nails

Denies lesions, color changes, ecchymoses, petechiae, texture changes, unusual odors, or infections. Pruritus; soles of feet dry and scaling for 6 months; condition stable (using nonprescription salve, name unknown). States he has had small cracks at corners of mouth for 1 month. Denies cold sores. States hair breaks off and falls out but denies patchy alopecia. Denies brittle, cracking, or peeling nails. States bites nails. Has 1 birthmark on upper back but is not aware of any change in size or color.

Head and Face

Denies pain, headache, dizziness, or vertigo. History of injury with blow to forehead. Reports frequent losses of consciousness after drinking; duration unknown, probably 1 to 8 hours.

Eyes

Has worn corrective lenses since 1970, age 10. States right eye 20/20, left eye 20/50. History of 1 eye injury, age 9. States visual acuity decreased after injury. Denies pain, infection, watery or itching eyes, diplopia, blurred vision, glaucoma, cataracts, decreased peripheral vision. Last ophthalmological examination 2 years ago.

Ears

Denies hearing loss. Denies discharge, pain, irritation, or ringing in ears. States he was "cut in a fight" on right auricle. Cleans ears with a toothpick.

Nose and Sinuses

Denies sinus pain, postnasal drip, discharge, epistaxis, soreness, excessive sneezing, or obstructed breathing. Denies injuries. States he has approximately 2 colds a year. Reports decreased sense of smell; attributes this to smoking.

Oral Cavity

Complains of frequent dryness in mouth and cracking of lips and tongue. No false teeth. Central incisors and lateral incisors missing in upper arch. Left bicuspids missing in lower arch. Gums bleed frequently. Denies hoarseness, pain, odor, frequent sore throats, voice change. Dental care infrequent. Brushes teeth "occasionally."

Neck

Denies pain, stiffness, or limitation of range of motion. Denies masses.

Example of Health History Documentation: Ill Client—cont'd

Nodes
Denies enlarged or tender nodes in neck, axillary, or inguinal area.

Breasts
Denies surgery, pain, masses, or discharge.

Chest and Respiratory System
Denies pain, wheezing, asthma, or bronchitis. History of pneumonia, age 20 (see Hospitalizations). Denies shortness of breath or dyspnea. Sleeps on 2 pillows but is not dependent on them for breathing. History of TB, 1994-1995. Last chest x-ray on present admission, negative. States he had 1 episode of hemoptysis, 1983, associated with his ulcer. Details of this unclear. States he has "smoker's cough" (dry cough in the morning) but denies sputum.

Cardiovascular System
Denies chest pain, coronary artery disease, rheumatic fever, or heart murmur. Denies hypertension, palpitations, cyanosis, or diagnosis of cardiac disorder. States he has occasional slight edema in right ankle.

Gastrointestinal System
See Present Illness. Also see Hospitalizations re: hemorrhoidectomy. Appetite good. Denies melena, clay-colored stools, or diarrhea. Takes laxative, magnesium citrate, approximately ×1 monthly or less for constipation. Denies jaundice. Reports decreased appetite with alcohol intake but denies specific intolerance to any food.

Genitourinary System
Denies bladder or kidney infections, urgency, frequency, hesitancy, painful micturition, incontinence, nocturia, or polyuria, history of VD. Denies testicular pain. History of surgery for priapism with inability to have erection for 1 year following surgery. No dysfunction at present. States sex life is "fair." Alcohol decreases "urge." Heterosexual. No homosexual encounters. Has had 5 sexual partners in the last 5 years. Has not used condoms.

Extremities
See Past Health History. Reports swelling of ankle without pain. Denies varicose veins, thrombophlebitis, joint pain, stiffness, swelling, gout, arthritis, limitation of movement, or color changes.

Back
Denies pain, stiffness, limitation of movement, or disk disease.

Central Nervous System
Reports loss of consciousness (1978) following blow to head; duration approximately 30 minutes. Denies clumsiness of movement, weakness, paralysis, tremor, neuralgia, or paresthesia. States he is a "nervous" person but denies history of nervous breakdown. History of drug and alcohol abuse. States he will periodically (every 2 to 3 weeks) have spontaneous jerky movement of legs during rest. There are 4 to 5 movements in each episode. This has never occurred while legs were bearing weight. Denies disorientation or memory disorders. Denies seizures or epilepsy. "Passes out" frequently after heavy alcohol ingestion and sleeps for 5 to 6 hours. Wakes with headache and nausea.

Hematopoietic System
Denies bleeding, bruising, blood transfusion, or exposure to x-rays or toxic agents.

Endocrine System
Denies diabetes, thyroid disease, or intolerance to heat or cold. Growth has been within normal range.

REVIEW OF SOCIOLOGICAL SYSTEM

Family Relationships
Has been separated from wife for 6 to 7 months and is in the process of being divorced. States his marital problems do not interfere with seeing his children. Plans to move to his mother's home when discharged from hospital. States relationships with his family of origin are good.

continued

Example of Health History Documentation: Ill Client—cont'd

Occupational History

Offset printer since 1986. Presently unemployed. Was advised not to work for 6 months when TB was diagnosed and has not been "able to get back to work." States he liked that occupation but expresses no urgency to return to work.

Economic Status

On disability income because of TB and need to rest. States he does not have trouble making ends meet on present income. Expresses no concern for financial status of wife and children who are on "welfare" and being assisted by wife's family.

Daily Profile

Lives alone in a room. States he spends time during the day at home or with friends, drinking. Has no special hobbies or activities to occupy time. Has habit of heavy daily drinking. States "I just hang around all day." Does do some spur-of-the-moment traveling. Weekdays are no different than weekends. States he dropped out of college because of disinterest.

Educational Level

States he is "smart enough." Dropped out of college after 2 years because of disinterest. States he has no aspiration except to "get by in life."

Patterns of Health Care

Has maintained relationship with same physician for episodic care for the last 10 years. Does return for periodic examinations and follow-up when symptoms "scare him."

Environmental Data

Birthplace—New York, N.Y. No travel outside of USA; no armed forces duty.

Home—Plans to move to his mother's home. Will share the 5-bedroom residence with his mother and 2 siblings.

Neighborhood is residential; describes it as "beautiful."

REVIEW OF PSYCHOLOGICAL SYSTEM

Cognitive Abilities

Oriented to present events. Has fairly adequate vocabulary. Has a fair to poor memory. Cannot recall details of some important events. No history of psychiatric treatment.

Response to Illness

States he "quit" drinking when he entered the hospital and plans to abstain in the future. Verbalizes that his health problems are his own fault and that he will die soon if he does not resolve them. States illness does not bother him except when "it gets out of control." Definition of health entails being able to play baseball again.

Response to Care

States he has sometimes not followed medical advice because of fear or because drugs or alcohol did not allow him to think "straight." "People have been nice to me." States all care has been "OK."

Cultural Implications

Inactive Presbyterian at present but is concerned about conflict with religious beliefs and lifestyle. Fourth-generation American.

DEVELOPMENTAL DATA

Adult male who has had problems with interpersonal relationships in his marriage. Has demonstrated drug and alcohol abuse since entering adulthood. Does not express concern regarding his inability to work; has abandoned his college attendance. Immediate plans for the future involve moving in with his mother and trying to stop drinking. Speaks of his children as playmates; expresses few fathering needs or activities.

NUTRITIONAL DATA

States he does not eat or has erratic meal patterns when drinking heavily and must build his tolerance to food by taking liquids such as soup or juices after drinking. States he does eat 3 complete meals daily when not drinking. Includes foods from the four basic food groups.

chapter

4

Developmental Assessment Across the Life Span

◼ PURPOSE OF DEVELOPMENTAL ASSESSMENT

Birth is the first of numerous developmental stages over the life span. From infancy through old age, individuals continue to develop some aspect of who they are. Each person is unique, but his or her individuality occurs within some broadly shared patterns.

The family is a powerful influence on human development. How each person develops through each phase of life and how he or she comes to view the world and interact with the people in it are largely learned within the family. While the focus of this chapter is on the individual, it is always with the acknowledgment that all individuals are part of family units, or substitutes for family units, for at least some significant portion of their lives.

Humans are dynamic, complex, changing beings. They interact continuously with the environment, and their responses to life are highly individualized. Personal growth and development patterns along with social, cultural, economic, and historical forces affect each person's responses to life.

While you are learning to obtain a health history and perform a physical examination, you are focusing on assimilating new skills, handling new tools, performing new techniques, remembering lists of questions for the health history, and performing the many components of the physical examination. However, from the onset of this learning process, you need to remember to include a perspective on the individual client as a whole person. The whole person includes the mind, body, and spirit. You cannot assess parts of the person in isolation from the other parts or from the whole. You must take into account the client's life developmental processes and the phases of growth and maturation through which that person is progressing. Take time to observe the client as a person and to discuss and discover the client's world— her or his interaction and growth within the self, with significant others, and with society at large.

Discussing developmental phases, stages, or crises with the client can provide both of you with a perspective of greater breadth and depth on the client's life situation and its relationship to health or illness. As a health care practitioner, you are in a position to help in-

dividuals and families look at the developmental aspects of their lives. Your openness in discussing the life tasks of individuals can help them appreciate the appropriateness and normalcy of their own or their children's growth patterns, changes, behaviors, and feelings. With anticipatory guidance parents can gain a greater appreciation of ways to support their child's development. Your guidance may also assist those who are blocked in their growth to understand and deal with the problem area more effectively. Help clients review their past, compare it with the present, look at progressive phases and intervals, and plan for the future in whatever ways are appropriate and necessary.

You should not expect to learn everything about a client's developmental accomplishments in one or even several interviews. It is a personal story that requires time and trust. Determining the presence of a developmental deficit is sometimes difficult in a busy clinical setting. You may need additional time to focus attention on assessing development, or you may need to seek the assistance of others who specialize in the field.

You can perform some developmental assessment during each encounter with a client of any age. With children, have a parent or primary caregiver present, since this person will be the main source of information. This person's descriptions are essential because limited opportunities exist to observe a child's behavior and responses in the clinical setting. In addition, keep in mind that the behavior demonstrated may not be typical because of stress from the unfamiliar environment or the particular problems related to the child's illness.

Record developmental assessment data in the health history.

For further information on the developmental changes of children and older adults, see Chapter 25: Pediatric Clients and Chapter 26: Aging Clients.

STAGES OF DEVELOPMENT

Developmental stages and categories are used for purposes of organization. In life, such stages are not totally distinct or exclusive. During particular phases, certain aspects of growth may be more prominent, but many overlap. Some of the early work done on the development of children by Jean Piaget and of children and adults by Erik Erikson was based on a "stage" approach. One stage and its accomplishments was followed by another, and moving from one to the other was premised on the completion of tasks at the earlier level. Piaget asserted that biological growth combines with children's interaction with the environment to take them up a development staircase, step-by-step, with each step signaling an increase in complexity of the child's thinking. He believed that changes in memory, perceptual skills, learning ability, and other aspects of

---

Some General Characteristics of Growth and Development

1. Growth and development are cyclical. Children tend to grow in spurts, then level off for periods. Adolescents tend to have cycles of outward activity and then inner reflection. Adults also experience periods of greater outward involvement and inner orientation.
2. Growth and development continue throughout the life cycle. From birth until death, some aspect of the complex human being is changing. This process of growth and development is both universal and unique and includes physical, emotional, psychological, social, and cognitive components. It ranges from changes that are slow, subtle, and often elusive to those that occur with astonishing rapidity.
3. All aspects of the growth and development of an individual are interrelated. The physical, mental, social, emotional, sexual, moral, and spiritual components of the self are all a part of the complex matrix that is the whole person.
4. There are periods of readiness for certain developmental tasks. During these periods a degree of maturation is necessary for the behavior to occur. If the appropriate environment or stimulus is not present, the behavior may not develop, may be delayed, or may occur in a defective way.

---

mental development all occurred in this fashion. More recently, it has been argued that more variations in children's growth can be observed and that some children develop in one area much more quickly than in others. General characteristics of growth and development are presented in the box above.

SELECTED THEORIES OF HUMAN DEVELOPMENT

There are numerous theorists in the field of human development. Only a brief description of a few of them is included here. (You need to refer to other texts in the field for a comprehensive overview of this broad subject.) The approach in this chapter is to provide a beginning framework for assessing the personhood of each individual.

The developmental aspect of infancy and childhood has received much attention and study since the late 1800s. A considerable amount of literature has surfaced

on these phases, although much still remains to be studied and understood. Of more recent vintage are the studies and theories about adolescence and old age. The most recent literature on human development is material on the age span between youth and old age: middle adulthood.

This chapter organizes developmental assessment around eight major life phases based on age:

Infancy: Birth to 12 months
Toddler years: 1 to 3
Preschool years: 3 to 6
School-age years: 6 to 12
Adolescence: approximately 11-13 to 20
Young adulthood: approximately 20 to 30-35
Middle adulthood: approximately 30-35 to 65-70
Late adulthood: approximately 65-70 to 95+

Characteristics of each stage are described. The length of the chronological divisions increases with each division, ranging from months for infants to decades for adults.

Erik Erikson—Psychosocial Development

Erikson is one of the theorists who suggested a developmental framework for the entire life span (Erikson, 1963). His framework is outlined here and is incorporated into the discussion at the various stages of growth used in this chapter. Erikson believed that individuals view the self in a social context. He suggested eight developmental stages and for each stage identified a central task and a threat to the accomplishment of that task. These central tasks are called developmental "crises," not in the sense of an emergency but rather to designate a necessary turning point when development must move one way or another. Each crisis is marked by a pair of opposite qualities that the person must resolve and integrate in order to proceed with ego development. Dealing with each task at a particular stage of development provides the basis for progress to the next stage. As a person faces each challenge, she or he assumes both increased vulnerability and increased potential. A new strength emerges that contributes to further development. Erikson viewed the task of identity as the major task of life. These stages and tasks are shown in Table 4.1.

Jean Piaget—Intellectual Development

Piaget's theory concerns intellectual, or cognitive, development. He believed that intellectual acts are the act of adaptation to, and organization of, the perceived environment. He noted certain signposts of development that indicate maturation and growth. The newborn perceives the world as a vague mass but gradually integrates the various sensory inputs from sight, sound, touch, taste, and smell. The young child does not understand that objects continue to exist even though they cannot be seen, but the child gradually learns that objects have constancy—they are there even when they cannot be seen. The use of symbols and language to represent reality is another developmental milestone in childhood. A young schoolchild gains the cognitive ability to focus on more than one aspect of a situation and to realize that although things may change superficially, they remain basically the same. Piaget described four major stages of intellectual development. These stages are listed in the box below.

table 4.1	Erikson's Eight Stages of Development	
Stage	**Task**	**Threat**
Infancy	Trust	Mistrust
Toddler years	Autonomy	Shame and doubt
Preschool years	Initiative	Guilt
School-age years	Industry	Inferiority
Adolescence	Identity	Identity diffusion
Early adulthood	Intimacy	Isolation
Middle adulthood	Generativity	Self-absorption
Late adulthood	Integrity	Despair

Piaget's Stages of Cognitive Development

1. Sensorimotor stage—ages 0 to 2. Primary concern is learning about physical objects.
2. Preoperational stage—ages 2 to 7. Primary concern is with symbols in language, dreams, and fantasy.
3. Concrete operational stage—ages 7 to 11. Primary concern is the ability to use thinking to represent objects and events. The child is increasingly able to use numbers and words to classify, serialize, and understand principles of conservation.
4. Formal operational stage—ages 11 to 15. Primary concern is logical thought, thinking about one's own thoughts as well as those of others.

Sigmund Freud—Development of Sexuality

The sex of a child is genetically determined, but the development of human sexuality is influenced by many aspects of life: physical, mental, emotional, and sociocultural. Sexuality is a large dimension of life related to many aspects of total personality functioning. It is expressed through cultural beliefs, attitudes, stereotypes, feelings, self-image, and body image.

Freud thought that sexual feelings were present from infancy, changing from one form to another into adulthood. Freud's four stages of psychosexual development center on the early years of life. At each stage, instinctual sexual energy (libido) is invested in different areas of the body. He believed that at each stage a conflict exists that must be resolved satisfactorily before the individual can progress to the next stage and that a person can become fixated at any stage. These resolutions or fixations determine how an individual interacts with others. The box below lists Freud's stages of sexual development.

Freud's Stages of Sexual Development

1. Oral stage—infancy through 18 months. During this period the oral region (the sensory area of the mouth, lips, and tongue) provides the greatest sensual satisfaction. Sucking and swallowing reduce tension and provide pleasure.
2. Anal stage—ages 18 months to 3 years. During this period the greatest amount of sensual pleasure is obtained from the anal and urethral areas. Toilet training is a source of tension between child and parent.
3. Phallic stage—ages 3 to 5 years. The region of greatest sensual pleasure is the genital region. The Oedipal/Electra complex occurs in the later part of the phallic stage. During this stage the child "loves" the parent of the opposite sex. The parent of the same sex is considered a rival.
4. Latency stage—ages 6 to 12 years. At the beginning of the latency stage, the child is resolving the Oedipal/Electra conflict, so this is a phase of sexual latency. During this period children form close relationships with others of their own age and sex. They direct energy to physical and intellectual quests.
5. Genital stage—puberty to adulthood. Increased hormones stimulate sexual development. Sexual urges reawaken but are now directed outside the family.

Freud's theory has had a strong and lasting impact in the field of psychology. Many now feel, however, that while his focus on the sexual aspect of development was important, it was also narrow and limited and that human psychological and sexual development need to be considered in the broader context of the whole person.

Carl Jung

Jung focused his extensive psychoanalytic work on the adult years of life. Jung's first developmental stage, extending from about 18 to 35 or 40, was called "youth." He saw this stage as being marked by individual development, involvement in the outside world, and investment in a family. During this period the individual's task is to give up the world of childhood while broadening one's horizons and engaging in the task-oriented and achievement-oriented work of the world. Jung saw the second half of life as beginning at age 35 or 40, with the change in orientation occurring slowly, developing largely through the unconscious. During this time many individuals become increasingly oriented to the inner life through reflection. Throughout life there is a drive toward individuation of the self and an effort to develop those aspects of the personality that have been underdeveloped, such as the qualities of extroversion, introversion, intuition, sensing, feeling, or thinking.

Carol Gilligan

Recent studies focusing on men's or women's development across the life span have provoked controversy over the applicability of previous theories to both sexes. Many of the theories on human growth and development were developed based on research or observations of males only, or with only a small sample of females. In her study of the psychosocial processes by which women develop, Carol Gilligan takes the position that women's development does not match men's development because women's identity formation takes place in a context of an ongoing relationship with the mother rather than separation from the mother. The female child experiences attachment to the mother that does not require separation for self and sexual identity that the male child requires. Masculine identity becomes defined through separation and is threatened by intimacy, whereas feminine identity is defined through attachment and is threatened by separation. This leads to life experiences where males tend to have greater difficulty with relationships, whereas females have greater difficulty with individuation. Gilligan notes that when maturity is equated with personal autonomy, a focus on relationships appears to be a weakness rather than a human strength, and she suggests that both forces must be in balance as the person moves toward maturity.

■ TOOLS FOR DEVELOPMENTAL ASSESSMENT

Numerous tools are available to assess child development, and a few are available to assess certain aspects of adult development. Some of the more commonly used ones are presented here. These tools assess various components, including gross motor skills, fine motor skills, personal-social behaviors, and language abilities. As a health care practitioner, you will not be administering intelligence tests. Special training in the administration of each tool and careful adherence to standardized procedures are necessary to obtain valid results.

For adolescents through adults, you can accomplish much assessment by talking with the client in an accepting, unrushed manner. Use nonthreatening questions about thoughts, feelings, work, family, and other activities, accompanied by an attitude of active listening to encourage clients to share significant information about themselves regarding their own development tasks and accomplishments.

Screening Tools Used with Infants and Children

Screening tools assist in determining an infant's or child's progress in accomplishing age-appropriate developmental tasks. For further information on childhood assessment tools, see Chapter 25.

Denver II

The Denver II (the 1989 revision of the Denver Developmental Screening Test [DDST] (Figure 4.1) is a screening tool commonly used to assess the developmental level from 1 month to 6 years of age. It is easy to administer, useful for determining developmental level, and helpful in providing guidance to parents. A series of developmental tasks are used to determine whether a child's development is within the normal range. The Denver II provides a developmental profile of the individual child in four areas: personal-social, fine motor–adaptive, language, and gross motor skills. If development in any of these four areas is questionable when compared with normal standards, refer the child for an in-depth evaluation. Children who have questionable or abnormal scores on the Denver II are at risk for developing later problems in school regardless of their intelligence. The Denver II is a *screening* tool; it is *not* a *diagnostic* tool, nor is it an intelligence test.

Denver Prescreening Developmental Questionnaire

The Denver Prescreening Developmental Questionnaire (PDQ) (Figure 4.2) is a brief test answered by the parent. It identifies those children who will need a more thorough screening with the Denver II (or the DDST). It assesses the same four categories as the Denver II, and it can be administered quickly and easily. The questionnaire consists of 97 questions, divided according to the child's age. The parent is asked to answer the questions from the appropriate age grouping.

Denver Articulation Screening Examination

The Denver Articulation Screening Examination (DASE) (see box on pp. 66-67) is used to detect articulation disorders in children ages 2½ to 7 years. It assesses a child's ability to imitate word sounds, which provides information on a child's speech development. The child is asked to repeat 30 different sound elements: the tester listens for errors in articulation.*

Goodenough-Harris Drawing Test

The Goodenough-Harris Drawing Test is used to screen children between the ages of 3 and 12 years. Children are requested to draw a man, a woman, and a representation of the self. The interpretation is based on a gradual increase in the complexity of the figures as the child becomes older.

Adult Assessment Tools

Although few tools are available to assess life changes and their effects on adults, two that have been developed are the Recent Life Changes Questionnaire and the Life Experiences Survey. Both attempt to assess life stresses and to indicate a possible relationship between life stresses and susceptibility to physical and psychological problems or illnesses.

Recent Life Changes Questionnaire

The Recent Life Changes Questionnaire (Rahe, 1975) is a self-administered questionnaire containing a list of events that subjects respond to by checking those events that they have experienced in the previous 6 months to 1 year (Table 4.2). To determine the scores for these events, the researchers had a large group of subjects rate each of the items with regard to the amount of social readjustment each event required. Mean values for each item were taken to represent the average amount of social readjustment required. The values, called Life Change Units, were added to yield a life stress score. Studies using this tool have shown correlations between high recent life change scores and the

Text continued on p. 66

*Further information on the Denver II, PDQ, DASE, and other developmental screening and training materials can be obtained from Denver Developmental Materials, Inc.
P.O. Box 6919
Denver, CO 80206-0919
(303) 355-4729

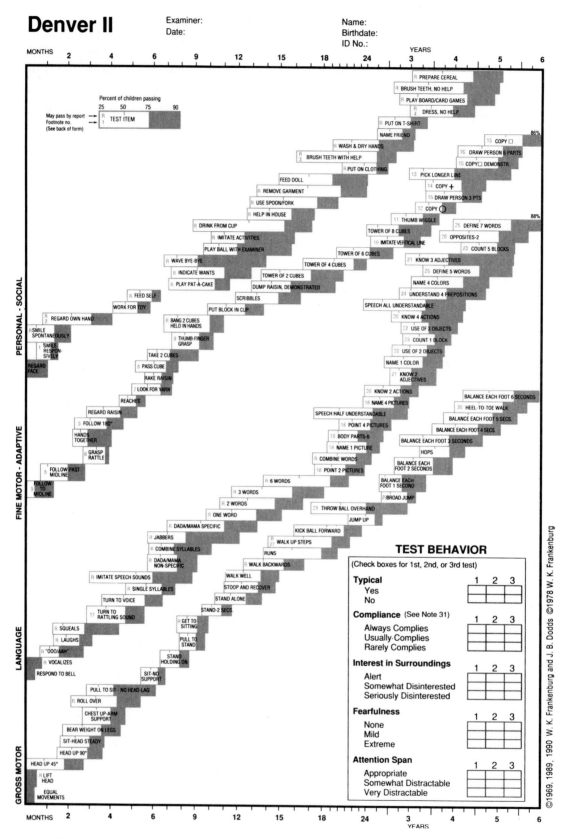

figure **4.1**   Denver II Developmental Screening Test. *(From WK Frankenburg and JB Dodds, 1990.)*

DIRECTIONS FOR ADMINISTRATION

1. Try to get child to smile by smiling, talking or waving. Do not touch him/her.
2. Child must stare at hand several seconds.
3. Parent may help guide toothbrush and put toothpaste on brush.
4. Child does not have to be able to tie shoes or button/zip in the back.
5. Move yarn slowly in an arc from one side to the other, about 8" above child's face.
6. Pass if child grasps rattle when it is touched to the backs or tips of fingers.
7. Pass if child tries to see where yarn went. Yarn should be dropped quickly from sight from tester's hand without arm movement.
8. Child must transfer cube from hand to hand without help of body, mouth, or table.
9. Pass if child picks up raisin with any part of thumb and finger.
10. Line can vary only 30 degrees or less from tester's line. $\sqrt{}$
11. Make a fist with thumb pointing upward and wiggle only the thumb. Pass if child imitates and does not move any fingers other than the thumb.

12. Pass any enclosed form. Fail continuous round motions.
13. Which line is longer? (Not bigger.) Turn paper upside down and repeat. (pass 3 of 3 or 5 of 6)
14. Pass any lines crossing near midpoint.
15. Have child copy first. If failed, demonstrate.

When giving items 12, 14, and 15, do not name the forms. Do not demonstrate 12 and 14.

16. When scoring, each pair (2 arms, 2 legs, etc.) counts as one part.
17. Place one cube in cup and shake gently near child's ear, but out of sight. Repeat for other ear.
18. Point to picture and have child name it. (No credit is given for sounds only.)
    If less than 4 pictures are named correctly, have child point to picture as each is named by tester.

19. Using doll, tell child: Show me the nose, eyes, ears, mouth, hands, feet, tummy, hair. Pass 6 of 8.
20. Using pictures, ask child: Which one flies?... says meow?... talks?... barks?... gallops? Pass 2 of 5, 4 of 5.
21. Ask child: What do you do when you are cold?... tired?... hungry? Pass 2 of 3, 3 of 3.
22. Ask child: What do you do with a cup? What is a chair used for? What is a pencil used for?
    Action words must be included in answers.
23. Pass if child correctly places <u>and</u> says how many blocks are on paper. (1, 5).
24. Tell child: Put block **on** table; **under** table; **in front of** me, **behind** me. Pass 4 of 4.
    (Do not help child by pointing, moving head or eyes.)
25. Ask child: What is a ball?... lake?... desk?... house?... banana?... curtain?... fence?... ceiling? Pass if defined in terms of use, shape, what it is made of, or general category (such as banana is fruit, not just yellow). Pass 5 of 8, 7 of 8.
26. Ask child: If a horse is big, a mouse is __? If fire is hot, ice is __? If the sun shines during the day, the moon shines during the __? Pass 2 of 3.
27. Child may use wall or rail only, not person. May not crawl.
28. Child must throw ball overhand 3 feet to within arm's reach of tester.
29. Child must perform standing broad jump over width of test sheet (8 1/2 inches).
30. Tell child to walk forward, ⟨⟨⟨⟩⟩⟩→ heel within 1 inch of toe. Tester may demonstrate.
    Child must walk 4 consecutive steps.
31. In the second year, half of normal children are non-compliant.

OBSERVATIONS:

figure**4.1, cont'd** Denver II Developmental Screening Test.

REVISED DENVER PRESCREENING DEVELOPMENTAL QUESTIONNAIRE (R-PDQ)

0-9 MONTHS

Child's Name _____

Person Completing R-PDQ: _____

Relation to Child: _____

For Office Use		
Today's Date:	____ yr ____ mo ____ day	
Child's Birthdate:	____ yr ____ mo ____ day	
Subtract to get Child's Exact Age:	____ yr ____ mo ____ day	
R-PDQ Age: (____ yr ____ mo ____ completed wks)		

CONTINUE ANSWERING UNTIL 3 "NOs" ARE CIRCLED

		For Office Use

1. Equal Movements
When your baby is lying on his/her back, can (s)he move each of his/her arms as easily as the other and each of the legs as easily as the other? Answer **No** if your child makes jerky or uncoordinated movements with one or both of his/her arms or legs.

Yes   No   (0) FMA

2. Stomach Lifts Head
When your baby is on his/her stomach on a flat surface, can (s)he lift his/her head off the surface?

Yes   No   (0-3) GM

3. Regards Face
When your baby is lying on his/her back, can (s)he look at you and watch your face?

Yes   No   (1) PS

4. Follows To Midline
When your child is on his/her back, can (s)he follow your movement by turning his/her head from one side to facing directly forward?

Yes   No   (1-1) FMA

5. Responds To Bell
Does your child respond with eye movements, change in breathing or other change in activity to a bell or rattle sounded outside his/her line of vision?

Yes   No   (1-2) L

6. Vocalizes Not Crying
Does your child make sounds other than crying, such as gurgling, cooing, or babbling?

Yes   No   (1-3) L

7. Smiles Responsively
When you smile and talk to your baby, does (s)he smile back at you?

Yes   No   (1-3) PS

		For Office Use

8. Follows Past Midline
When your child is on his/her back, does (s)he follow your movement by turning his/her head from one side *almost all the way to the other side?*

Yes   No   (2-2) FMA

9. Stomach, Head Up 45°
When your baby is on his/her stomach on a flat surface, can (s)he lift his/her head 45°?

Yes   No   (2-2) GM

10. Stomach, Head Up 90°
When your baby is on his/her stomach on a flat surface, can (s)he lift his/her head 90°?

Yes   No   (3) GM

11. Laughs
Does your baby laugh out loud without being tickled or touched?

Yes   No   (3-1) L

12. Hands Together
Does your baby play with his/her hands by touching them together?

Yes   No   (3-3) FMA

13. Follows 180°
When your child is on his/her back, does (s)he follow your movement from one side *all the way* to the other side?

Yes   No   (4) FMA

14. Grasps Rattle
It is important that you follow instructions carefully. Do *not* place the pencil in the palm of your child's hand. When you touch the pencil to the back or tips of your baby's fingers, does your baby grasp the pencil for a few seconds?

Yes   No   (4) FMA

TRY THIS   NOT THIS

(Please turn page)

0-9 MONTHS (R-PDQ)

CONTINUE ANSWERING UNTIL 3 "NOs" ARE CIRCLED

	For Office Use

15. Sits, Head Steady
When sitting, can your child hold his/her head upright and steady? Answer **No** if his/her head falls to either side or upon his/her chest.   Yes   No   (4) GM

16. Stomach Chest Up-Arm Support
When your baby is on his/her stomach on a flat surface, can (s)he lift his/her chest using his/her arms for support?   Yes   No   (4-1) GM

17. Squeals
Does your baby make happy high-pitched squealing sounds which are not crying?   Yes   No   (4-2) L

18. Rolls Over
Has your baby rolled over at least 2 times, from stomach to back, or back to stomach?   Yes   No   (4-3) GM

19. Regards Raisin
Can your child focus his/her eyes on small objects the size of a pea, a raisin, or a penny?   Yes   No   (5) FMA

20. Reaches For Object
Can your child pick up a toy if it is placed within his/her reach?   Yes   No   (5) FMA

21. Smiles Spontaneously
Does your child smile at crib toys, pictures, or pets when (s)he is playing by himself/herself?   Yes   No   (5) PS

22. Pull To Sit, No Headlag
With your baby on his/her back, gently pull him/her up to a sitting position by his/her wrists. Does your baby hold his/her neck stiffly like the baby in the picture below left? Answer **No** if his/her head falls back like the baby in the picture below right.   Yes   No   (6-1) GM

Yes   No

Side #2

	For Office Use

23. Sits, Looks For Yarn
Please follow directions carefully. Get your baby's attention with a scarf, handkerchief, or a tissue and then drop it *out of sight.* Did your baby try to find it? For example, did (s)he look for it under the table or continue to watch where it disappeared?   Yes   No   (7-2) FMA

24. Passes Cube Hand To Hand
Can your baby pass something, such as a small block or a small cookie, from one hand to the other? Long objects like a spoon or rattle do not count.   Yes   No   (7-2) FMA

25. Sits, Takes 2 Cubes
Can your baby pick up 2 things, such as toys or cookies, and hold one in each hand at the same time?   Yes   No   (7-2) FMA

26. Bears Some Weight On Legs
When you hold your baby under his/her arms, can (s)he bear some weight on his/her legs? Answer **Yes** only if (s)he tries to stand on his/her feet and supports some of his/her own weight.   Yes   No   (7-3) GM

27. Rakes Raisin, Attains
Can your baby pick up small objects, such as raisins or pieces of food with his/her hand using a raking or grabbing motion?   Yes   No   (7-3) FMA

28. Sits Without Support
Without being propped by pillows, a chair, or wall, can your child sit by himself/herself for 60 seconds?   Yes   No   (7-3) GM

29. Feed Self Crackers
Can your baby feed himself/herself a cracker or cookie? Answer **No** if (s)he has never been given one.   Yes   No   (8) PS

30. Turns To Voice
When your child is playing and you come up *quietly* behind him/her, does (s)he sometimes turn his/her head as though (s)he heard you? *Loud sounds do not count.*   Yes   No   (8-1) L

figure **4.2**   Denver Prescreening Developmental Questionnaire (PDQ). *(From WK Frankenburg, 1986.)*

Denver Articulation Screening Examination (DASE)

DENVER ARTICULATION SCREENING EXAMINATION

(For Children 2.5 to 6 Years of Age)

Instructions: Have child repeat each word after you. Circle the underlined sounds that he or she pronounces correctly. Total number of correct sounds is the raw score. Use charts below to score results.

NAME
HOSPITAL NO.
ADDRESS

Date: _____ Child's age: _____ Examiner: _____ Raw score: _____
Percentile: _____ Intelligibility: _____ Result: _____

1. table	6. zipper	11. sock	16. wagon	21. leaf
2. shirt	7. grapes	12. vacuum	17. gum	22. carrot
3. door	8. flag	13. yarn	18. house	
4. trunk	9. thumb	14. mother	19. pencil	
5. jumping	10. toothbrush	15. twinkle	20. fish	

Intelligibility (circle one):   1. Easy to understand   3. Not understandable
                                2. Understandable half of the time   4. Cannot evaluate

Comments:

From AF Drumwright and WK Frankenburg, 1971-1973.

development of health problems. This tool combines a life stress score based on both desirable and undesirable events; health care professionals should take these differences into account in assessing an individual's life changes and their impact on health. They also should consider the client's own assessment of both the intensity of the life changes and the strength of his or her coping abilities.

Life Experiences Survey

The Life Experiences Survey (Sarason, Johnson, and Siegel, 1978) is a self-report tool that allows respondents to indicate events they have experienced over the past year (Table 4.3). It includes events that occur fairly frequently and allows respondents to weigh the desirability or undesirability of events. Ratings are on a seven-point scale from extremely negative (−3) to extremely positive (+3). A positive change score is obtained by adding those events rated as positive, a negative change score is obtained by adding the negatively rated events, and a total change score is obtained by combining those two values.

As the integrated nature of the human organism becomes more fully understood, we will likely gain a better understanding of the relationship between life changes and problems of a psychological nature. The cause-effect relationship is often unclear between life changes and health status, and the effect of life changes or stresses differs from person to person depending on unique characteristics, including the degree of perceived control over events and the degree of psychosocial assets.

Text continued on p. 72

Denver Articulation Screening Examination (DASE)—cont'd

To score DASE words: Note raw score for child's performance. Match raw score line (extreme left of chart) with column representing child's age (to the closest *previous* age group). Where raw score line and age column meet denotes percentile rank of child's performance when compared with other children that age. Percentiles above heavy line are *abnormal,* below heavy line are *normal.*

Percentile rank

Raw score	2.5 yr	3.0 yr	3.5 yr	4.0 yr	4.5 yr	5.0 yr	5.5 yr	6 yr
2	1							
3	2							
4	5							
5	9							
6	16							
7	23							
8	31	2						
9	37	4	1					
10	42	6	2					
11	48	7	4					
12	54	9	6	1	1			
13	58	12	9	2	3	1	1	
14	62	17	11	5	4	2	2	
15	68	23	15	9	5	3	2	
16	75	31	19	12	5	4	3	
17	79	38	25	15	6	6	4	
18	83	46	31	19	8	7	4	
19	86	51	38	24	10	9	5	1
20	89	58	45	30	12	11	7	3
21	92	65	52	36	15	15	9	4
22	94	72	58	43	18	19	12	5
23	96	77	63	50	22	24	15	7
24	97	82	70	58	29	29	20	15
25	99	87	78	66	36	34	26	17
26	99	91	84	75	46	43	34	24
27		94	89	82	57	54	44	34
28		96	94	88	70	68	59	47
29		98	98	94	84	84	77	68
30		100	100	100	100	100	100	100

To score intelligibility:

		NORMAL	ABNORMAL
	2.5 years	Understandable half of the time or easy to understand	Not understandable
	3 years and older	Easy to understand	Understandable half of the time or not understandable

Test result: 1. Normal on DASE and intelligibility = *normal*
  2. Abnormal on DASE or intelligibility = *abnormal**

*If abnormal on initial screening, rescreen within 2 weeks. If abnormal again, child should be referred for complete speech evaluation.

table 4.2　*Recent Life Changes Questionnaire*

Life Change Unit (LCU) Weights for Life Change Events		Life Change Unit (LCU) Weights for Life Change Events	
	HEALTH		**HOME AND FAMILY**
	Within the Time Periods Listed, Have You Experienced:		***Within the Time Periods Listed, Have You Experienced:***
	1. An illness or injury that:		14. A change in residence:
42	(a) Kept you in bed a week or more, or took you to the hospital?	28	(a) A move within the same town or city?
25	(b) Was less serious than described above?	38	(b) A move to a different town, city, or state?
29	2. A major change in eating habits?	26	15. A change in family "get-togethers"?
31	3. A major change in sleeping habits?	52	16. A major change in the health or behavior of a family member (illness, accidents, drug, or disciplinary problems, etc.)?
30	4. A change in your usual type or amount of recreation?		
40	5. Major dental work?	39	17. A major change in your living conditions (home improvements or a decline in your home or neighborhood)?
	WORK		
	Within the Time Periods Listed, Have You:		
38	6. Changed to a new type of work?	105	18. The death of a spouse?
33	7. Changed your work hours or conditions?		19. The death of a:
	8. Had a change in your responsibilities at work:	105	(a) Child?
		64	(b) Brother or sister?
31	(a) More responsibilities?	66	(c) Parent?
29	(b) Less responsibilities?		(d) Other close family member?
31	(c) Promotion?	46	20. The death of a close friend?
51	(d) Demotion?		21. A change in marital status of your parents:
38	(e) Transfer?		
	9. Experienced troubles at work:	38	(a) Divorce?
39	(a) With your boss?	33	(b) Remarriage?
35	(b) With co-workers?	50	22. Marriage?
30	(c) With persons under your supervision?		(NOTE: Questions 23-33 concern marriage. For persons never married go to item 34.)
31	(d) Other work troubles?		
38	10. Experienced a major business readjustment?	34	23. A change in arguments with your spouse?
49	11. Retired?	29	24. In-law problems?
	12. Experienced being:		25. A separation from spouse:
64	(a) Fired from work?	49	(a) Due to work?
57	(b) Laid off from work?	56	(b) Due to marital problems?
29	13. Taken courses by mail or studied at home to help you in your work?	45	26. A reconciliation with spouse?
		62	27. A divorce?
			28. A gain of a new family member?
		49	(a) Birth of a child?
		45	(b) Adoption of a child?
		57	(c) A relative moving in with you?

From Rahe RH: Epidemiological studies of life change and illness, *Int J Psychiatry Med* 6(1-2):133-146, 1975.

table 4.2	*Recent Life Changes Questionnaire—cont'd*

Life Change Unit (LCU) Weights for Life Change Events		Life Change Unit (LCU) Weights for Life Change Events	
37	29. Wife beginning or ceasing work outside the home?		**FINANCIAL**
60	30. Wife becoming pregnant?		***Within the Time Periods Listed, Have You:***
29	31. A child leaving home:	26	52. Taken on a moderate purchase, such as a television, car, freezer, etc.?
28	(a) Due to marriage?	39	53. Taken on a major purchase or a mortgage loan, such as a home, business, property, etc.?
30	(b) To attend college?		
29	(c) For other reasons?	57	54. Experienced a foreclosure on a mortgage or loan?
53	32. Wife having a miscarriage or abortion?		55. Experienced a major change in finances:
31	33. Birth of a grandchild?	27	(a) Increased income?
	PERSONAL AND SOCIAL	60	(b) Decreased income?
	Within the Time Periods Listed, Have You Experienced:	43	(c) Credit rating difficulties?
33	34. A major personal achievement?		**SUBJECTIVE LIFE CHANGE UNIT (SLCU) INSTRUCTIONS**
31	35. A change in your personal habits (your dress, friends, lifestyle, etc.)?		***Instructions for Scoring Your Adjustment to Your Recent Life Changes***

FINANCIAL

Within the Time Periods Listed, Have You:

SUBJECTIVE LIFE CHANGE UNIT (SLCU) INSTRUCTIONS

Instructions for Scoring Your Adjustment to Your Recent Life Changes

LCU	Event
49	36. Sexual difficulties?
32	37. Beginning or ceasing school or college?
28	38. A change of school or college?
29	39. A vacation?
29	40. A change in your religious beliefs?
28	41. A change in your social activities (clubs, movies, visiting)?
32	42. A minor violation of the law?
57	43. Legal troubles resulting in your being held in jail?
25	44. A change in your political beliefs?
32	45. A new, close, personal relationship?
39	46. An engagement to marry?
35	47. A "falling out" of a close personal relationship?
30	48. Girlfriend (or boyfriend) problems?
40	49. A loss or damage of personal property?
44	50. An accident?
45	51. A major decision regarding your immediate future?

Persons adapt to their recent life changes in different ways. Some people find the adjustment to a residential move, for example, to be enormous, while others find very little life adjustment necessary. You are now requested to "score" each of the recent life changes that you marked with an "X" as to the amount of adjustment you needed to handle the event.

Your scores can range from 1 to 100 "points." If, for example, you experienced a recent residential move but felt it required very little life adjustment, you would choose a low number and place it in the blank to the right of the question boxes. On the other hand, if you recently changed residence and felt it required a near maximal life adjustment, you would place a high number, toward 100, in the blank to the right of that question's boxes. For immediate life adjustment scores you would choose intermediate numbers between 1 and 100.

Please go back through your questionnaire and for each recent life change you indicated with an "X," choose your personal life adjustment score (between 1 and 100), which reflects what you saw to be the amount of life adjustment necessary to cope with or handle the event. Use both your estimates of the intensity of the life change and its duration to arrive at your scores.

table 4.3 *The Life Experiences Survey*

Listed below are a number of events which sometimes bring about change in the lives of those who experience them and which necessitate social readjustment. *Please check those events which you have experienced in the recent past and indicate the time period during which you have experienced each event.* Be sure that all check marks are directly across from the items they correspond to.

Also, for each item checked below, *please indicate the extent to which you viewed the event as having either a positive or negative impact on your life* at the time the event occurred. That is, *indicate the type and extent of impact that the event had.* A rating of −3 would indicate an extremely negative impact. A rating of 0 suggests no impact either positive or negative. A rating of +3 would indicate an extremely positive impact.

	0 to 6 mo	7 mo to 1 yr	Extremely negative	Moderately negative	Somewhat negative	No impact	Slightly positive	Moderately positive	Extremely positive
1. Marriage			−3	−2	−1	0	+1	+2	+3
2. Detention in jail or comparable institution			−3	−2	−1	0	+1	+2	+3
3. Death of spouse			−3	−2	−1	0	+1	+2	+3
4. Major change in sleeping habits (much more or much less sleep)			−3	−2	−1	0	+1	+2	+3
5. Death of close family member:									
a. Mother			−3	−2	−1	0	+1	+2	+3
b. Father			−3	−2	−1	0	+1	+2	+3
c. Brother			−3	−2	−1	0	+1	+2	+3
d. Sister			−3	−2	−1	0	+1	+2	+3
e. Grandmother			−3	−2	−1	0	+1	+2	+3
f. Grandfather			−3	−2	−1	0	+1	+2	+3
g. Other (specify)			−3	−2	−1	0	+1	+2	+3
6. Major change in eating habits (much more or much less food intake)			−3	−2	−1	0	+1	+2	+3
7. Foreclosure on mortgage or loan			−3	−2	−1	0	+1	+2	+3
8. Death of close friend			−3	−2	−1	0	+1	+2	+3
9. Outstanding personal achievement			−3	−2	−1	0	+1	+2	+3
10. Minor law violations (traffic tickets, disturbing the peace, etc.)			−3	−2	−1	0	+1	+2	+3
11. *Male:* Wife/girlfriend's pregnancy			−3	−2	−1	0	+1	+2	+3
12. *Female:* Pregnancy			−3	−2	−1	0	+1	+2	+3
13. Changed work situation (different work responsibility, major change in working conditions, working hours, etc.)			−3	−2	−1	0	+1	+2	+3
14. New job			−3	−2	−1	0	+1	+2	+3
15. Serious illness or injury of close family member:									
a. Father			−3	−2	−1	0	+1	+2	+3
b. Mother			−3	−2	−1	0	+1	+2	+3
c. Sister			−3	−2	−1	0	+1	+2	+3
d. Brother			−3	−2	−1	0	+1	+2	+3

From Sarason IG, Johnson JH, Siegal JM: Assessing the impact of life changes: development of life experiences survey, *J Consult Clin Psychol* 46(5):932-946, 1978.

| table **4.3** | **The Life Experiences Survey—cont'd** | | | | | | | | |

	0 to 6 mo	7 mo to 1 yr	Extremely negative	Moderately negative	Somewhat negative	No impact	Slightly positive	Moderately positive	Extremely positive
e. Grandmother			−3	−2	−1	0	+1	+2	+3
f. Grandfather			−3	−2	−1	0	+1	+2	+3
g. Spouse			−3	−2	−1	0	+1	+2	+3
h. Other (specify)			−3	−2	−1	0	+1	+2	+3
16. Sexual difficulties			−3	−2	−1	0	+1	+2	+3
17. Trouble with employer (in danger of losing job, being suspended, demoted, etc.)			−3	−2	−1	0	+1	+2	+3
18. Trouble with in-laws			−3	−2	−1	0	+1	+2	+3
19. Major change in financial status (a lot better off or a lot worse off)			−3	−2	−1	0	+1	+2	+3
20. Major change in closeness of family members (increased or decreased closeness)			−3	−2	−1	0	+1	+2	+3
21. Gaining a new family member (through birth, adoption, family member moving in, etc.)			−3	−2	−1	0	+1	+2	+3
22. Change of residence			−3	−2	−1	0	+1	+2	+3
23. Marital separation from mate (due to conflict)			−3	−2	−1	0	+1	+2	+3
24. Major change in church activities (increased or decreased attendance)			−3	−2	−1	0	+1	+2	+3
25. Marital reconciliation with mate			−3	−2	−1	0	+1	+2	+3
26. Major change in number of arguments with spouse (a lot more or a lot less arguments)			−3	−2	−1	0	+1	+2	+3
27. *Married male:* Change in wife's work outside the home (beginning work, ceasing work, changing to a new job, etc.)			−3	−2	−1	0	+1	+2	+3
28. *Married female:* Change in husband's work (loss of job, beginning new job, retirement, etc.)			−3	−2	−1	0	+1	+2	+3
29. Major change in usual type and/or amount of recreation			−3	−2	−1	0	+1	+2	+3
30. Borrowing more than $10,000 (buying home, business, etc.)			−3	−2	−1	0	+1	+2	+3
31. Borrowing less than $10,000 (buying car, TV, getting school loan, etc.)			−3	−2	−1	0	+1	+2	+3
32. Being fired from job			−3	−2	−1	0	+1	+2	+3
33. *Male:* Wife/girlfriend having abortion			−3	−2	−1	0	+1	+2	+3

continued

| table 4.3 | *The Life Experiences Survey—cont'd* | | | | | | | |

	0 to 6 mo	7 mo to 1 yr	Extremely negative	Moderately negative	Somewhat negative	No impact	Slightly positive	Moderately positive	Extremely positive
34. *Female:* Having abortion			−3	−2	−1	0	+1	+2	+3
35. Major personal illness or injury			−3	−2	−1	0	+1	+2	+3
36. Major change in social activities, e.g., parties, movies, visiting (increased or decreased participation)			−3	−2	−1	0	+1	+2	+3
37. Major change in living conditions of family (building new home, remodeling, deterioration of home, neighborhood, etc.)			−3	−2	−1	0	+1	+2	+3
38. Divorce			−3	−2	−1	0	+1	+2	+3
39. Serious injury or illness of close friend			−3	−2	−1	0	+1	+2	+3
40. Retirement from work			−3	−2	−1	0	+1	+2	+3
41. Son or daughter leaving home (due to marriage, college, etc.)			−3	−2	−1	0	+1	+2	+3
42. Ending of formal schooling			−3	−2	−1	0	+1	+2	+3
43. Separation from spouse (due to work, travel, etc.)			−3	−2	−1	0	+1	+2	+3
44. Engagement			−3	−2	−1	0	+1	+2	+3
45. Breaking up with boyfriend/ girlfriend			−3	−2	−1	0	+1	+2	+3
46. Leaving home for the first time			−3	−2	−1	0	+1	+2	+3
47. Reconciliation with boyfriend/girlfriend			−3	−2	−1	0	+1	+2	+3
Other recent experiences that have had an impact on your life. List and rate.									
48. _____			−3	−2	−1	0	+1	+2	+3
49. _____			−3	−2	−1	0	+1	+2	+3
50. _____			−3	−2	−1	0	+1	+2	+3

■ INFANCY: BIRTH TO 12 MONTHS

More dramatic changes occur within the brief period of infancy than during any other time of life. During the period from birth to 12 months, the child develops from a dependent, helpless newborn to a busy little person who is mobile and communicative and relates to people in terms of their importance in her or his life. Infants enter the world with all sensory systems functioning in at least a rudimentary fashion. They begin to interact with and influence their environment from the moment of birth. As the neuromuscular system becomes more integrated, they are intent on taking in everything in the environment within their reach. Soon they can display a wide range of primary, unselfconscious emotions: interest, distress, disgust, joy, anger, surprise, sadness, and fear. They are responsive to the caregivers' mood: sadness or happiness affects their behavior.

The boxed material on pp. 74-78 summarizes child development using the categories of motor development, language development, and personal-social-adaptive development. (These categories are slightly different from, but complementary to, the categories used in the text.)

figure**4.3**   Infancy.

Physical Development

The rate of growth during the first few months and years of life is greater than at any other time. The average full-term infant weighs about 7 to 7½ pounds (3.4 kg) and is about 20 inches (50 cm) long. An infant typically loses up to 10% of that weight during the first few days, then regains it within 10 days and continues to gain steadily. Although infants vary, most double their birth weight by 4 to 6 months and triple it by 1 year. Length increases by about 50% during the first year.

Marked changes occur in body contour during infancy. The head grows at a rapid rate during the first year, and the head circumference is greater than the chest circumference. Growth in head circumference reflects brain growth, most of which occurs during the first 2 years of life. The thickness of the subcutaneous fat increases during the first year, reaching a peak around 9 months, then decreasing during the second year. Teeth begin to erupt, and the infant advances from a liquid diet to table food.

The newborn makes many rapid adjustments necessary to sustain life outside the uterus, which are actually a continuum of the development during fetal life. At birth, respirations are initiated and changes in the circulatory system occur, the digestive system begins to assimilate the food obtained from an external source, body wastes are excreted, and maintenance of body heat depends on the infant's own resources. Behavior includes many reflex actions that reflect the immaturity of the newborn's nervous system but also assist in adaptation with the new environment. One of the most strik-

ing physiological changes is the continuing maturation and increasing function of the nervous system. Myelination continues at a rapid rate during the first months of life but is not completed for several years. The functional development of various body structures probably corresponds to the order of myelination and occurs in a cephalocaudal direction, from head to foot. The development of head control precedes sitting, standing, and walking. As the brain and central nervous system continue to develop, an increasingly sophisticated range of cognitive and behavioral skills follows.

The first 3 months of life can be called a period of adjustment. Reflexes become more regulated during the first month, and the infant learns how to search, to suck, and to let needs be known. Sleeping and feeding patterns become more regular. The tonic neck reflex becomes more prominent at the end of the first month. (The tonic neck reflex is a normal response in newborns. It consists of extending the arm and the leg on the side of the body to which the head is quickly turned while the infant is supine and flexing the limbs of the opposite side.) During the second and third months, new behaviors appear that are not reflexes. The infant begins to follow objects with the eyes, allowing exploration of the environment. There is coordination of hand and mouth movement, such as sucking the thumb at will. The grasp reflex gradually lessens as more purposeful movements begin. The infant begins to prolong interesting events that occur more or less by accident. The little wails that precede crying may be continued for their own sake. The squeals of the 2- to 3-month-old baby are loud, repeated, and joyful. The infant begins to smile in response to environmental stimuli and to vocalize. Most responses are generalized and frequently involve movements of the whole body. The infant during this period has social responses but does not discriminate; any person who can satisfy the infant's needs is accepted.

By 3 months of age, the baby becomes more discriminating and begins to differentiate his or her mother from others and produces special types of smiles and crying for her. This is the beginning of attachment behavior and the development of awareness of the self as separate from the mother. Between 3 and 6 months, or even earlier, the infant repeats some actions that are interesting and prolongs those that occur accidentally, such as repeated hitting of suspended toys to produce movement. There is more imitation of facial movements and beginning imitation of sounds. The infant attempts somewhat of a search for a displaced object, but not a true search. Infantile reflexes are replaced by purposeful movements, especially those seen in the development of eye-hand coordination. The infant begins to reach for and grasp objects with a raking motion. The tonic neck reflex and Moro reflex disappear during the fifth or sixth month. (The Moro reflex is a normal mass reflex in a

Text continued on p. 79

Child Development from 1 Month to 5 Years

1 MONTH

Motor

1. Moro reflex present.
2. Vigorous sucking reflex present.
3. Lying prone (face down): lifts head briefly so chin is off table.
4. Lying prone: makes crawling movements with legs.
5. Held in sitting position: back is rounded, head held up momentarily only.
6. Hands tightly fisted.
7. Reflex grasp of object with palm.

Language

8. Startled by sound; quieted by voice.
9. Small throaty noises or vocalizations.

Personal-Social-Adaptive

10. Ringing bell produces decrease of activity.
11. May follow dangling object with eyes to midline.
12. Lying on back: will briefly look at examiner or change activity.
13. Reacts with generalized body movements when tissue paper is placed on face.

2 MONTHS

Motor

1. Kicks vigorously.
2. Energetic arm movements.
3. Vigorous head turning.
4. Held in ventral suspension (prone): no head droop.
5. Lying prone: lifts head so face makes an approximate 45° angle with table.
6. Held in sitting position: head erect but bobs.
7. Hand goes to mouth.
8. Hands often open (not clenched).

Language

9. Is cooing.
10. Vocalizes single vowel sounds, such as: ah-eh-uh.

Personal-Social-Adaptive

11. Head and eyes search for sound.
12. Listens to bell ringing.
13. Follows dangling object past midline.
14. Alert expression.
15. Follows moving person with eyes.
16. Smiles back when talked to.

3 MONTHS

Motor

1. Lying prone: lifts head to 90° angle.
2. Lifts head when lying on back (supine).
3. Moro reflex begins to disappear.
4. Grasp reflex nearly gone.
5. Rolls side to back (3-4 months).

Language

6. Chuckling, squealing, grunting, especially when talked to.
7. Listens to music.
8. Vocalizes with two different syllables, such as: a-a, la-la (not distinct), oo-oo.

Personal-Social-Adaptive

9. Reaches for but misses objects.
10. Holds toy with active grasp when put into hand.
11. Sucks and inspects fingers.
12. Pulls at clothes.
13. Follows object (toy) side to side (and 180°).
14. Looks predominately at examiner.
15. Glances at toy when put into hand.
16. Recognizes mother and bottle.
17. Smiles spontaneously.

4 MONTHS

Motor

1. Sits when well supported.
2. No head lag when pulled to sitting position.
3. Turns head at sound of voice.
4. Lifts head (in supine position) in effort to sit.
5. Lifts head and chest when prone, using hands and forearms.
6. Held erect: pushes feet against table.

Language

7. Laughs aloud (4-5 months).
8. Uses sounds, such as: m-p-b.
9. Repeats series of same sounds.

Personal-Social-Adaptive

10. Grasps rattle.
11. Plays with own fingers.
12. Reaches for object in front with both hands.
13. Transfers object from hand to hand.
14. Pulls dress over face.
15. Smiles spontaneously at people.
16. Regards raisin (or pellet).

Child Development from 1 Month to 5 Years—cont'd

5 MONTHS

Motor
1. Moro reflex gone.
2. Rolls side to side.
3. Rolls back to front.
4. Full head control when pulled to or held in sitting position.
5. Briefly supports most of weight on legs.
6. Scratches on tabletop.

Language
7. Squeals with high voice.
8. Recognizes familiar voices.
9. Coos or stops crying on hearing music.

Personal-Social-Adaptive
10. Grasps dangling object.
11. Reaches for toy with both hands.
12. Smiles at mirror image.
13. Turns head deliberately to bell.
14. Obviously enjoys being played with.

6 MONTHS

Motor
1. Supine: lifts head spontaneously.
2. Bounces on feet when held standing.
3. Sits briefly (tripod fashion).
4. Rolls front to back (6-7 months).
5. Grasps foot and plays with toes.
6. Grasps cube with palms.

Language
7. Vocalizes at mirror image.
8. Makes four or more different sounds.
9. Localizes source of sound (bell, voice).
10. Vague, formless babble (especially with family members).

Personal-Social-Adaptive
11. Holds one cube in each hand.
12. Puts cube into mouth.
13. Resecures dropped cube.
14. Transfers cube from hand to hand.
15. Conscious of strange sights and persons.
16. Consistent regard of object or person (6-7 months).
17. Uses raking movement to secure raisin or pellet.
18. Resists having toy taken away.
19. Stretches out arms to be taken up (6-8 months).

8 MONTHS

Motor
1. Sits alone (6-8 months).
2. Early stepping movements.
3. Tries to crawl.
4. Stands few seconds, holding on to object.
5. Leans forward to get an object.
6. Held in sitting position: head erect but bobs.

Language
7. Two-syllable babble, such as a-la, ba-ba, oo-goo, a-ma, mama, dada (8-10 months).
8. Listens to conversation (8-10 months).
9. "Shouts" for attention (8-10 months).

Personal-Social-Adaptive
10. Works to get toy out of reach.
11. Scoops pellet.
12. Rings bell purposely (8-10 months).
13. Drinks from cup.
14. Plays peek-a-boo.
15. Looks for dropped object.
16. Bites and chews toys.
17. Pats mirror image.
18. Bangs spoon on table.
19. Manipulates paper or string.
20. Secures ring by pulling on the string.
21. Feeds self crackers.

10 MONTHS

Motor
1. Gets self into sitting position.
2. Sits steadily (long time).
3. Pulls self to standing position (on bed railing).
4. Crawls on hands and knees.
5. Walks when held or around furniture.
6. Turns around when left on floor.

Language
7. Imitates speech sounds.
8. Shakes head for "no."
9. Waves "bye-bye."
10. Responds to name.
11. Vocalizes in varied jargon-patterns (10-12 months).

Personal-Social-Adaptive
12. Plays "pat-a-cake."
13. Picks up pellet with finger and thumb.
14. Bangs toys together.

continued

Child Development from 1 Month to 5 Years—cont'd

15. Extends toy to a person.
16. Holds own bottle.
17. Removes cube from cup.
18. Drops one cube to get another.
19. Uses handle to lift cup.
20. Initially shy with strangers.

1 YEAR

Motor

1. Walks with one hand held.
2. Stands alone (or with support).
3. Secures small object with good pincer grasp.
4. Pivots in sitting position.
5. Grasps two cubes in one hand.

Language

6. Uses "mama" or "dada" with specific meaning.
7. "Talks" to toys and people, using fairly long verbal patterns.
8. Has vocabulary of two words besides "mama" and "dada."
9. Babbles to self when alone.
10. Obeys simple requests, such as: "Give me the cup."
11. Reacts to music.

Personal-Social-Adaptive

12. Cooperates with dressing.
13. Plays with cup, spoon, saucer.
14. Points with index finger.
15. Pokes finger (into stethoscope) to explore.
16. Releases toy into your hand.
17. Tries to take cube out of box.
18. Upwraps a cube.
19. Holds cup to drink.
20. Holds crayon.
21. Tries to imitate scribble.
22. Imitates beating two cubes together.
23. Gives affection.

15 MONTHS

Motor

1. Stands alone.
2. Creeps upstairs.
3. Kneels on floor or chair.
4. Gets off floor and walks alone with good balance.
5. Bends over to pick up toy without holding on to furniture.

Language

6. May speak four to six words (15-18 months).
7. Uses jargon.
8. Indicates wants by vocalizing.
9. Knows own name.
10. Enjoys rhymes or jingles.

Personal-Social-Adaptive

11. Tilts cup to drink.
12. Uses spoon but spills.
13. Builds tower of two cubes.
14. Drops cubes into cup.
15. Helps turn page in book, pats picture.
16. Shows or offers toy.
17. Helps pull off clothes.
18. Puts pellet into bottle without demonstration.
19. Opens lid of box.
20. Likes to push wheeled toys.

18 MONTHS

Motor

1. Runs (stiffly).
2. Walks upstairs—one hand held.
3. Walks backward.
4. Climbs into chair.
5. Hurls ball.

Language

6. May say 6 to 10 words (18-21 months).
7. Points to at least one body part.
8. Can say "hello" and "thank you."
9. Carries out two directions (one at a time), for instance: "Get ball from table."—"Give ball to mother."
10. Identifies two objects by pointing (or picking up), such as: cup, spoon, dog, car, chair.

Personal-Social-Adaptive

11. Turns pages.
12. Builds tower of three to four cubes.
13. Puts 10 cubes into cup.
14. Carries or hugs a doll.
15. Takes off shoes and socks.
16. Pulls string toy.
17. Scribbles spontaneously.
18. Dumps raisin from bottle after demonstration.
19. Uses spoon with little spilling.

Child Development from 1 Month to 5 Years—cont'd

21 MONTHS

Motor

1. Runs well.
2. Walks downstairs—one hand held.
3. Walks upstairs alone or holding on to rail.
4. Kicks large ball (when demonstrated).

Language

5. May speak 15 to 20 words (21-24 months).
6. May combine two to three words.
7. Asks for food, drink.
8. Echoes two or more words.
9. Takes three directions (one at a time), for instance: "Take ball from table."—"Give ball to Mommy."—"Put ball on floor."
10. Points to three or more body parts.

Personal-Social-Adaptive

11. Builds tower of five to six cubes.
12. Folds paper once when shown.
13. Helps with simple household tasks (21-24 months).
14. Removes some clothing purposefully (besides hat or socks).
15. Pulls person to show something.

2 YEARS

Motor

1. Runs without falling.
2. Walks up and down stairs.
3. Kicks large ball (without demonstration).
4. Throws ball overhand.
5. Claps hands.
6. Opens door.
7. Turns pages in book, singly.

Language

8. Says simple phrases.
9. Says at least one sentence or phrase of four or more syllables.
10. Can repeat four to five syllables.
11. May reproduce about five or six consonant sounds. (Typically: m-p-b-h-w.)
12. Points to four parts of body on command.
13. Asks for things at table by name.
14. Refers to self by name.
15. May use personal pronouns, such as: I-me-you (2-2½ years).

Personal-Social-Adaptive

16. Builds five- to seven-cube tower.
17. May cut with scissors.

18. Spontaneously dumps raisin from bottle (without demonstration).
19. Throws ball into box.
20. Imitates drawing vertical line from demonstration.
21. Parallel play predominant.

2½ YEARS

Motor

1. Jumps in place with both feet.
2. Tries standing on one foot (may not be successful).
3. Holds crayon by fingers.
4. Imitates walking on tiptoe.

Language

5. Refers to self by pronoun (rather than name).
6. Names common objects when asked (key, penny, shoe, box, book).
7. Repeats two digits (one of three trials).
8. Answers simple questions, such as: "What is this?"—"What does the kitty say?"

Personal-Social-Adaptive

9. Builds tower of eight cubes.
10. Pushes toy with good steering.
11. Helps put things away.
12. Can carry breakable objects.
13. Puts on clothing.
14. Washes and dries hands.
15. Eats with fork.
16. Imitates drawing a horizontal line from demonstration.
17. May imitate drawing a circle from demonstration.

3 YEARS

Motor

1. Stands on one foot for at least 1 second.
2. Jumps from bottom stair.
3. Alternates feet going upstairs.
4. Pours from a pitcher.
5. Can undo two buttons.
6. Pedals a tricycle.

Language

7. Repeats six syllables, for instance: "I have a little dog."
8. Names three or more objects in a picture.
9. Gives sex. ("Are you a boy or a girl?")
10. Gives full name.
11. Repeats three digits (one of three trials).

continued

Child Development from 1 Month to 5 Years—cont'd

12. Knows a few rhymes.
13. Gives appropriate answers to: "What: swims-flies-shoots-boils-bites-melts?"
14. Uses plurals.
15. Knows at least one color.
16. Can reply to questions in at least three-word sentences.
17. May have vocabulary of 750 to 1000 words (3-3½ years).

Personal-Social-Adaptive
18. Understands taking turns.
19. Copies a circle (from model, without demonstration).
20. Builds three-block pyramid.
21. Dresses with supervision.
22. Puts 10 pellets into bottle in 30 seconds.
23. Separates easily from mother.
24. Feeds self well.
25. Plays interactive games, such as "tag."

4 YEARS

Motor
1. Stands on one foot for at least 5 seconds (two of three trials).
2. Hops at least twice on one foot.
3. Can walk heel-to-toe four or more steps (with heel 1 inch or less in front of toe).
4. Can button coat or dress; may lace shoes.

Language
5. Repeats ten-word sentences without errors.
6. Counts three objects, pointing correctly.
7. Repeats three to four digits (4-5 years).
8. Comprehends: "What do you do if: you are hungry, sleepy, cold?"
9. Spontaneous sentences, four to five words long.
10. Likes to ask questions.
11. Understands prepositions, such as: on-under-behind, etc. ("Put the block *on* the table.")
12. Can point to three out of four colors (red, blue, green, yellow).
13. Speech is now an effective communication tool.

Personal-Social-Adaptive
14. Copies cross (+) without demonstration.

15. Imitates oblique cross (×).
16. Draws a man with four parts.
17. Cooperates with other children in play.
18. Dresses and undresses self (mostly without supervision).
19. Brushes teeth, washes face.
20. Compares lines: "Which is longer?"
21. Folds paper two to three times.
22. Can select heavier from lighter object.
23. Cares for self at toilet.

5 YEARS

Motor
1. Balances on one foot for 8 to 10 seconds.
2. Skips, using feet alternately.
3. May be able to tie a knot.
4. Catches bounced ball with hands (not arms) in two of three trials.

Language
5. Knows age ("How old are you?")
6. Performs three tasks (with one command), for instance: "Put pen on table—close door—bring me the ball."
7. Knows four colors.
8. Defines use for: fork-horse-key-pencil, etc.
9. Identifies by name: nickel-dime-penny.
10. Asks meaning of words.
11. Asks many "why" questions.
12. Relatively few speech errors remain—90% of consonant sounds are made correctly.
13. Counts number of fingers correctly.
14. Counts by rote to 10.
15. Comments on pictures (descriptions and interpretations).

Personal-Social-Adaptive
16. Copies a square.
17. Copies oblique cross (×) without demonstration.
18. May print a few letters (5-5½ years).
19. Draws man with at least six identifiable parts.
20. Builds a six-block pyramid from demonstration.
21. Transports things in a wagon.
22. Plays with coloring set, construction toys, puzzles.
23. Participates well in group play.

young infant elicited by a sudden loud noise resulting in flexion of the legs, an embracing posture of the arms, and usually a brief cry.) At 3 months the infant, while prone, can raise the head and chest from a surface with arms extended, and at 4 months the head can be held steadily while the infant is supported in the sitting position. At 6 to 7 months the infant can sit without support. Crawling typically begins at about 9 months. At about the same time, the baby will begin to pull up to a standing position while holding onto something for support. At 10 to 11 months the child starts to "cruise," walking while holding onto the furniture. Walking alone usually begins at about 12 months, though it may be several months earlier or later.

Fine motor skill development includes using the hands and fingers for grasping. The infant is born with a grasp reflex, which disappears by about 3 months. At 4 months the infant seems to discover his or her hands and inspects them. By 5 months the baby is able to grasp with two hands. By 10 months the pincer grasp, with the index finger in apposition to the thumb, is present. The child can pick up finger foods and small toys.

Cognitive Development

Piaget defined the infancy stage of cognitive development as the sensorimotor period. Mental development during this period begins with reflexes and ends with the early appearance of language and other symbolic ways of representing the world. The infant is egocentric, and sensorimotor learning is related to the self. The infant changes from response through reflexes (crying, grasping, rooting, and sucking) to organization of sensorimotor activities in relation to the environment. Even the very young infant is a cognitive being capable of rather sophisticated mental operations. For example, infants are more responsive to a new stimulus than to one that has been repeated several times, showing discrimination known as habituation. They are also able to imitate certain facial gestures, such as sticking out the tongue or opening the mouth, which are indications of early cognitive abilities and integrative function.

During the first 7 to 9 months of life, the infant's learning is focused on bodily actions. At around 8 to 9 months the concept Piaget called "object permanence" can be observed. The infant learns that objects and people continue to exist even when she or he cannot see them. The 5-month-old infant will not reach for an object after it is hidden, but the 8-month-old infant will. Through this sequence of mental and physical actions and the gradual development of memory, the child begins to have a sense of self as separate from, and yet a part of, the environment. It is the beginning of the child's construction of reality.

The first mode of communication is crying. Although all the cries may sound the same initially, by about 1 month of age, the parents are usually able to differentiate the meaning of cries of varying pitch and intensity. For example, the infant has different cries for discomfort and hunger. Vocalization during this period changes from babbling and cooing to the use of several words that can be understood. Generally, the baby laughs at about 3 months, babbles at about 4 months, and by 9 or 10 months can imitate the sounds of others. By 12 months several words besides "mama" and "dada" are acquired.

Psychosocial Development

During the first year of life, great strides in behavioral development occur. The infant develops social skills that bond the baby with others in the environment. Socially, the infant progresses from staring at faces and crying to smiling, demanding company, vocalizing, and actively participating in games.

The period between 6 and 12 months is dominated by the social modality of "taking and holding on" as described by Erikson. It is a period of attachment behavior. The infant at 8 to 9 months of age has a beginning concept of permanence and becomes fearful that the mother or other primary caregiver will disappear. The infant actively initiates contact with the caregiver and seeks to maintain that contact. There is true searching for a vanished object, although the search may be in several inappropriate places. Behavior becomes more complex and aggressive. The infant coordinates earlier repetitive actions into behaviors with a purposeful aim. Now the child explores objects more fully by rubbing, banging, and chewing and by discovering the correct procedures for manipulating them. Motor development is dramatic as coordination increases. The pincer grasp, using thumb and forefinger, develops.

Erikson described this first stage of ego development as one of trust versus mistrust. During this critical period of personality development, the child develops a sense of trust based on consistent nurturing in terms of food, warmth, comfort, and the presence of the mother. Successful growth during this period means that the child comes to trust both the self and the people in the environment. The threat at this stage is mistrust of the environment and self. According to Erikson (1963), a sense of trust develops when there is a mutual regulation of the baby's pattern of accepting things and the mother's way of giving them that changes as the baby develops. The social modality of the baby's development during the first 6 months is to satisfy needs by getting, receiving, and accepting. This is not passive behavior, since the infant influences people in the environment from birth. The first reflexive behaviors of looking, rooting, sucking, and crying elicit responses in the mother or other caretaking adults that cause them to act in ways that will meet the infant's needs. Parental bond-

ing is influenced by these behaviors. The infant's social modality during the second half of the first year is taking and holding on, which begins with the eruption of teeth and the ability to sit upright and voluntarily reach out. The infant begins to be aware of being separate from the mother. The infant may become more demanding of the mother and is faced with the frustrations that result when the pleasure experienced in biting or grasping and holding on to things is met with interference. The infant displays helpless rage when strong desires are thwarted. When this behavior is understood and the infant continues to receive loving attention, trust in self and others can be maintained and strengthened. Some of the infant's early emotional expressions, such as timidity and shyness or boldness and sociability, may indicate enduring personality characteristics. Temperament, or basic behavioral style, is inborn. Aspects of temperament include activity level; regularity in biological functioning (hunger, sleep, elimination); readiness to accept new people and situations; adaptability to change; sensitivity to noise, light, and other sensory stimuli; mood (cheerfulness or unhappiness); intensity of responses; distractibility; and persistence. Infants vary in these characteristics from birth and have a tendency to continue in one style, although parental handling and experiences may cause change.

Freud described infancy as the oral stage. The pleasure zone is the mouth; the child seeks to take in everything for sensory exploration and takes great pleasure in sucking and eating. Weaning and teething are challenges at this stage.

■ TODDLER YEARS: 1 TO 3

The child enters the toddler years well equipped to continue learning about the self and the world. Autonomy blossoms as the child begins to recognize self as separate from others. Toddlers have a sense of hope and trust and are developing intellectual and motor skills. A basic competence develops with the expansion of language, memory, and self-control. The toddler years are characterized by energetic exploration and intense inquisitiveness, and also by some obstinate and ritualistic behaviors. Ego growth is rapid during the second and third years of life as the child learns about people and objects in the environment and gradually gains increasing mastery over impulses and bodily functions.

Physical Development

The rate of growth in height and weight decreases during the second year of life. The toddler gains an average of 5½ pounds (2.5 kg) in weight and 4 to 5 inches (10 to 13 cm) in height. The child's adult height will be roughly twice what it is at age 2. As the growth rate in height and weight decreases, it becomes less consistent month by month.

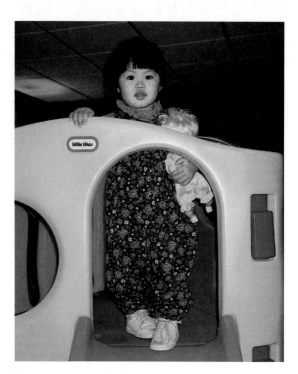

figure**4.4**   Toddler years.

The changes in the child's physical appearance are dramatic. The toddler who is beginning to walk looks top-heavy, with short legs and a potbelly. Fat pads fill the arch of the foot, and most young children appear to be flat-footed until 3 or 4 years of age. There is also a tendency for the legs to bow outward and for lordosis to be apparent. Gradually the child becomes less chubby, the abdomen becomes flatter, and the face loses its baby look. The posture and body proportions change as the chest becomes larger in proportion to the head and abdomen. After 2 years of age, the extremities continue to grow faster than the trunk, and the jaw and lower face grow more rapidly than the cranium. The subcutaneous fat decreases rapidly in thickness during the second year.

Visual acuity improves: at 2 years of age, it is about 20/40. The brain reaches 75% of its adult weight by 3 years of age. Myelination in the spinal cord is almost complete by age 2. The skin changes after the first year, becoming firmer with less water content. The primary teeth continue to erupt, and the child will have the full complement of 20 primary teeth early during the third year, when the second molars erupt.

Gross and fine motor skills increase during the toddler years as a result of the myelination of nerve fibers. Neuromuscular maturation contributes to gross motor abilities, such as sitting, crawling, standing, and walking, and to fine motor skills, such as scribbling and using a pincer grasp. The child usually walks by about 12 months, though it may be as early as 9 months or as late

as 18 months. By age 2 the toddler can run and can walk up and down stairs. Toilet training, a major developmental milestone, is also dependent on neuromuscular maturation and generally occurs around age 3.

As the toddler learns to perform self-care skills such as drinking, eating, dressing, toothbrushing, and bathing, her or his sense of independence and competence is enhanced. Initially, the child's efforts are clumsy and incomplete, but by about 3 years of age, the child displays a fair degree of competence in these areas. Competence increases with physical maturation and is enhanced by parents who give their child the opportunity to practice these skills.

On average, during the toddler years, girls' development tends to be a bit ahead of boys' development. Girls talk, walk, and are toilet trained a month or two earlier than boys.

Cognitive Development

During the second year of life, the child is in the sensorimotor stage as described by Piaget. The toddler, increasingly ready for independence, experiments with new ways to achieve a goal. During the last half of the second year, the child reaches a cognitive milestone: he or she becomes capable of the mental representation of external events. The toddler can think through plans to achieve a goal, rather than performing and watching what happens. The concept of object permanence is developed: the toddler searches for an object even when it is not visible.

Language skills increase dramatically during the toddler years. The use of language reflects the child's cognitive development. Speech enables the child to become more independent, as well as to better make needs known. Most children begin to use a few words at about 14 months, though some do not begin until around age 2. By age 2 most children have an effective vocabulary (words that can be spoken and/or understood) of 250 to 300 words. The first words a child learns are nouns of one syllable; subsequently the noun is connected with an action verb. During the second year, the child moves from having personal, nonverbal mental images of objects and events and the use of words and gestures invested with personal meaning, to having the capacity for thought and communicative language. A burst of vocabulary occurs toward the end of the second year. This is a period of symbolic thought, a time when the toddler can use mental symbols and words to refer to objects and people, seen and unseen, and to anticipate future events. Language develops sequentially, with adjectives and adverbs following the use of nouns and verbs. The toddler gradually learns other grammatical components of the language from 18 months on. By the third birthday the child has an effective vocabulary of about 900 words. The greater the child's vocabulary and comprehension, the more the cognitive processes can advance.

As children share speech and communication with adults, they also learn ideas, attitudes, and values.

The toddler's thinking is characterized by centering, which means that only one aspect of an object or event is perceived by the child, and by egocentrism, the notion that there is only one point of view—the child's own. Toddlers are unaware of how other people think.

Psychosocial Development

Autonomy and independence are major goals for a toddler. The core task for this stage of ego development as described by Erikson is autonomy versus shame. Each child is developing a sense of individuality and separateness from other people. The toddler experiences autonomy in many ways, including the ability to gain a new level of control over motor abilities, bodily functions, and self-care skills; making and acting on decisions; coping with problems or getting the necessary help; and giving generously or holding on. Neuromuscular and cognitive development make it possible for the toddler to explore and experiment, which lead to a sense of autonomy. Failure to establish autonomy results in a sense of shame and of doubt in one's ability to function effectively.

Freud described the period from 18 months to 3 years as the anal stage of psychosexual development. The focus of this stage is on the buildup and release of tension at the orifices. The child experiences pleasure from expelling urine and feces. However, the parents begin to insist that these actions occur only at the proper time and in the proper location. Toilet training is part of socializing the child. Self-control and delayed gratification are necessary skills for socialized behavior. Freud believed that the parent's approach to toilet training and the child's response greatly influence the personality of the individual.

Socialization is an important aspect of the child's development during the toddler years. Socialization is the process by which an individual becomes a member of a social group by acquiring the group's values and behaviors. In our society, socialization during this period focuses on numerous issues, including bowel and bladder habits, cleanliness, control of anger and aggressive behaviors, acquisition of language skills, and control of excessive motor activities, egocentric behavior, and antisocial behavior.

During infancy the child had few restrictions or responsibilities. The toddler must develop new roles and relationships with the world and the people in it. The rules for acceptable behavior are changing, and the growing child must adapt.

Social relationships during this period continue to revolve mainly around the parents or other primary caregivers, but the toddler is increasingly equipped to expand her or his social world to include siblings, other children, relatives, and neighbors. Through social relationships the

toddler learns about socially approved behaviors, such as cooperation, sharing, waiting one's turn, and respecting the feelings and possessions of others.

Socialization as a male or female begins during infancy. From 1 to 3 years of age, the child has a beginning awareness of sexual differences and sexual roles. Children begin exploring their own bodies and those of others. This is normal and is an important means for the toddler to learn about physical differences between males and females. Parents generally interact differently with boys and girls and have different expectations regarding behaviors and attitudes such as dependence/independence, achievement, vigor, cooperation/competition, and assertiveness. The attributes that are affirmed or negated by the parents greatly influence the child's sex role development. Observation and imitation of the same-sex parent also contribute to gender identity.

The toddler is uninhibited in the pursuit of personal goals. She or he wants to explore everything in the environment. Since the toddler has not yet acquired any sense of judgment or discrimination, parents are constantly balancing the child's drive to explore and experience with the need to protect the child from situations that could be harmful or are beyond the child's ability level. This leads to conflict with the parents when the child encounters restrictions that the parent must set to protect the child or help her or him adapt to socially acceptable behaviors. Displays of the toddler's temper are common, especially when the child is also fatigued. While temper tantrums are expressions of frustration, they may provoke fear in the child because he or she also wants to please the parent and desires the parent's love and approval. An environment that is safe for exploration and allows the child to make choices is beneficial. It is also important for the parents to maintain control of their own emotions in situations where the toddler is not yet prepared to do so. As the toddler matures and gains greater control over self and environment, many situations become less stressful.

Play is important developmental work for the toddler. It is a process of exploration and discovery. Gradually, as the child begins to form mental images, play becomes more imaginative and imitative. The child thoroughly enjoys newly acquired abilities and manipulates objects with persistence and enthusiasm. Play provides practice for newly acquired motor skills. The toddler exhibits repetitive play and enjoys putting things in and out of containers. Children who are given the freedom to explore and make reasonable choices develop a sense of self-assurance and spontaneity. If the toddler is not allowed to play in a safe and interesting environment or if play activities are stopped by constant limit setting, the child may begin to doubt his or her ability to accomplish tasks or to meet new challenges.

Young toddlers engage in parallel play, where they play beside, but not with, each other. Initially they treat other children like objects; toddlers may push, pinch, bite, or poke others because they have no inner sense that this may hurt. Gradually the toddler moves into interactive play with peers.

The toddler gradually becomes able to play alone for longer periods of time, but attachment behavior continues. Periodically, the toddler seeks out the parent or caregiver, particularly if there is a problem or perceived threat. When faced with a new person or situation, most toddlers have more assurance if the parent is present, and they return to the parent quickly if things become too difficult.

The toddler is sensitive to changes in the environment. If one alteration occurs in the toddler's world, it is as if everything changes and becomes strange and unmanageable. Consistent routines for daily activities are helpful. They allow the child to anticipate what will happen, learn the behaviors that are expected, and gain a sense of control. Routines, habits, or rituals may be particularly important around mealtime or at bedtime, when the child must deal with separation and darkness. If parents do everything the same way each night, the child is reassured that the world will not change while he or she sleeps.

During the toddler years the child learns to cope with separation from the parents or caregivers. Fear of separation begins at about 7 months. Between the ages of 1 and 3 years, long separations are not well tolerated and may damage the child emotionally. Although unable to express or understand the feelings, the child is able to sense loss. Learning to tolerate brief separations is an important developmental task. As children learn that parents return, they become more accepting and adaptable.

Closely related to separation anxiety are the fears and fantasies commonly expressed by toddlers. The child may experience nightmares or behavioral changes, such as anxiety about taking a bath or about flushing the toilet for fear of disappearing. The toddler's feeling of power may contribute to these fears because the child believes that by wishing something, it can be made to happen. For example, the child fears that by wishing harm toward someone, it may occur. Imaginary beings and animals, some of them ferocious, are common in the imaginations of toddlers. Some of the child's own aggressive feelings may be projected onto the imaginary being. Sympathetic understanding of these fears and fantasies by the parents helps them deal with the child's concern about separation.

Emotional feelings and reactions vary in toddlers depending on age and temperament and on how others in their environment react to them. A toddler cannot express or explain personal emotions, so they are expressed in behaviors. These behaviors may include

showing affection, sharing, playing cooperatively, timidity, contrariness, selfish or aggressive behavior, temper tantrums, or dawdling. A degree of self-awareness, and emotions such as pride, sympathy, jealousy, guilt, and shame begin to emerge during the second year. Parents need to be sensitive to the acting out of the toddler's emotions, and the need to be supportive and loving in helping the toddler as he or she learns to deal with various emotions.

The word "no" is spoken with increasing frequency during the toddler years. This is often labeled "negativism," but it is essential to the child's efforts to gain self-control and a sense of mastery over the environment. The child may be saying "no" and at the same time complying with the parent's request.

Children begin to develop a self-concept at a very young age. By the time a child enters the toddler years, and certainly during these years, the child has positive or negative perceptions of the self and a personal sense of worth. Adults in the child's world are very influential in determining the direction of the child's inner sense of self. Supportive reinforcement of positive feelings is essential for nurturing an emotionally healthy human being.

■ PRESCHOOL YEARS: 3 TO 6

The preschool years are marked by physical, social, emotional, and intellectual development. While the child still has many dependent needs and behaviors, she or he is also beginning to exhibit more independence in

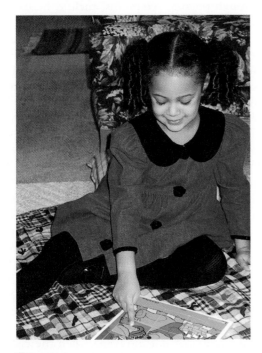

figure**4.5** Preschool years.

actions and thoughts. The child is developing a sense of self as a social person in relation to other people and is also learning a great deal about the physical world. Preschool children are emerging from their toddler years and becoming social beings. Expanded language and gross motor skills enable them to explore further in the environment. Preschoolers are involved in increasing independence, developing basic motor and language skills, and adding to their social skills.

Physical Development

Physical growth continues at a slow rate. On average, the preschooler gains about 1.5 to 2.5 kg (3 to 5 pounds) in weight, and 5 to 7 cm (2 to 2¾ inches) per year. The face and body become more slender as the baby fat disappears. The musculoskeletal system continues to develop, with muscles growing and cartilage changing to bone. Most of the bone growth is in the long bones. At about age 5 the child begins to lose the first set of teeth. Visual acuity reaches 20/20 between 4 and 5 years of age.

Preschoolers have an increased sense of balance and enjoy both gross and fine motor skills. Their ability to run, jump, hop, swim, skate, and ride tricycles and bicycles demonstrates their increasing gross motor abilities. Their use of building toys and art materials exhibits their increase in coordination and fine motor skills.

The preschooler is dependent on parents and other caregivers for nutritious foods and good eating habits. Family food preferences, culture, and lifestyle also influence food selections. Appetite fluctuates, and many preschoolers go for several months without gaining weight. However, for some preschoolers excessive eating may be a problem and is a cause for concern, since lifetime habits are beginning during these years. During the preschool years the child learns to eat with the family and to enjoy many of the foods that the family eats. The child should be able to feed himself or herself early in the preschool years, and should be using eating utensils with little difficulty toward the end of the preschool years.

The preschooler shows increasing skills in dressing and other personal care skills. Toilet training is usually completed before or during the early preschool years.

Cognitive Development

Piaget described the child from 2 to 7 years of age as being in the preoperational stage of cognitive functioning. The child is increasingly able to use mental symbols to represent people, objects, and events. This means that the child is able to think about people, for example, without seeing or hearing them. This is liberating for the child, making it possible to act out thoughts during play. The preschooler's thinking is still limited by the inability to focus on more than one aspect of a situation at

a time. At times, preschoolers will group unrelated characteristics of a person or event together into a confusing whole. A major characteristic of this period is egocentric thinking: children in this stage cannot see another's point of view and assume that their own viewpoint is shared by everyone. This affects the preschooler's language, thought, and reasoning. The older preschooler begins to be able to consider more aspects of a situation, another person's viewpoint, and the intent and outcome of behavior. Cognitive growth of the preschooler includes increasing memory ability.

Language development includes use of an increasing number of words, improved articulation, use of correct grammatical structure, and a growing ability to categorize objects in the environment using words. The early preschooler uses both communicative and noncommunicative speech. When using communicative speech, the child tries to communicate a message to a listener. Noncommunicative speech consists of monologues during which the child converses out loud to herself or himself, although others may be present. The child may repeat and elaborate on statements made by parents and other adults. These monologues are often a source of great amusement to other people.

Interactions with parents, siblings, relatives, other adults, and peers all contribute to the child's educational process. In addition, many preschoolers begin structured educational programs, such as Headstart, nursery school, or preschool, when they are 3 or 4 years of age. An environment at home or away from home that stimulates and affirms discovery and learning is necessary for the child to practice new skills and extend earlier experiences.

Psychosocial Development

The child identifies with the parents and is motivated to try to be what they want and to be like them. The child becomes more socially responsive and able to give love and affection. The development of initiative is characterized by the wish to "become," in which the child wants to find out what kind of person he or she can be. During the earlier years, the child undergoes a growth of the sense of self as a separate person with some power to influence the environment and to control impulses and his or her own body. These accomplishments make it possible to approach new tasks with feelings of confidence and an abundance of energy. The child becomes intrusive in a desire to attack new situations. Preschool children are noisy, active, and on the move. They thrust themselves into each situation, driven by curiosity and imagination. Erikson described this stage of ego development, particularly around 4 to 5 years of age, as one of initiative versus guilt. The child now has adequate energy, motor skills, and mental ability to attack new tasks with gusto and determination. When the parent provides encouragement and enthusiasm, while also protecting the child from harm, the child learns self-sufficiency, direction, and purpose. If the parent prevents the child from doing tasks she or he is capable of trying, or ridicules or punishes the child, the child learns guilt and shame and a sense of inadequacy. The child may then experience these negative feelings when he or she tries to do the same thing, or even when the child thinks about trying it again. This can have long-term effects on the child's psychological makeup.

The preschooler's social environment increasingly extends beyond the family and other primary caregivers to include other adult and peer encounters. The child learns to interact more easily with unfamiliar people. Temperament enables some children to do this with great ease; other children require more encouragement. Experiencing a variety of interactions with people of all ages is important for preschoolers to help them develop a range of personal-social behaviors.

The preschooler is able to experience many feelings, including happiness, joy, affection, excitement, wonder, anger, frustration, jealousy, sadness, loneliness, and fear, all of which are normal emotions. Emotional feelings and reactions are determined by both innate temperament and the pattern of emotional expression of adults around the child. Children need to be able to express the range of their emotions in a supportive and loving environment, and to begin to name and understand their own emotional reactions. Preschool children who experience a death, loss, separation, significant change in lifestyle, or illness require support and help in dealing with their feelings. Preschoolers may express their feelings through physical symptoms, such as headaches or stomachaches, or they may become irritable or withdrawn. The finality of death is not well understood by a child at this age. She or he may ask many questions and continue to search for the lost person. The most important aspect of dealing with a loss or death is for the parents to be gentle and honest with the child.

The behaviors of a preschool child are a composite of many interacting factors, including heredity, culture, the environment, and developmental level. The child continually experiments with old and new behaviors. As the child's experience moves beyond the home, she or he encounters a vast number of experiences that affect behavior. As the behavioral repertoire enlarges, the preschooler tries many new behaviors. Many of these are useful and help the child develop. However, some are negative, harmful, or dangerous and must be curtailed. Some of the common negative behaviors of the preschooler are negative use of language, negative facial gestures, aggressive or hostile behavior, excessively dependent behavior, and noncompliance. If the parent or other caregiver does not intervene when the child displays negative behaviors, behavioral problems may de-

velop. Some discipline is necessary, but it must be delivered within the context of love and concern for the child's present and future well-being. The preschooler is developing concepts of "good" and "bad." If a child behaves in an unacceptable manner and is told repeatedly that he or she is "bad," this affects self-image. The situation is similar with a child who is repeatedly told that he or she is "good" and then becomes limited in self-expression and self-development to someone else's definition of "good." Adults should identify the behavior rather than labeling the child. Children become restricted by labels and may find it difficult to move beyond them to enlarge their field of experience.

Play during the preschool years becomes increasingly more social, imaginative, and complex. While playing together, children develop concepts, imagination, neuromuscular coordination, and language. "Let's pretend" is a favorite phrase and activity. Through imaginative play the child tries out the roles of different people in a variety of situations. In play the child can take on any role and master fears. The child can have feelings of strength and adequacy instead of smallness and vulnerability.

Imaginary playmates are important to some preschoolers. They may include these "playmates" in dreams, fantasies, and certain daily rituals, such as eating, as well as including them in their play. Rituals continue to be a significant part of the preschooler's daily pattern.

By internalizing the parents' standards and ideals, the child gradually develops a sense of moral responsibility and a conscience, which makes resisting temptation possible even though the parents are not present. The child can feel guilt for misbehavior, and at about 5 years of age he or she even has some feelings of guilt for wanting to misbehave. This early conscience is modified through the years of childhood as intellectual abilities increase and the ability to identify reasons for moral action becomes more mature.

Sexuality Patterns

Love and admiration for the parents and other significant adults intensify during the preschool years, although they may be mixed with defiance at times; identification with the parents increases. Sexual identification began at an earlier age when the child learned that he was a boy or that she was a girl, but during the preschool years it is heightened. It becomes evident as the child begins to imitate the parent of the same sex, learns more of a sex role identity, and becomes acutely aware of sexual differences. The interest in the parent of the opposite sex is somewhat romantic, which results in conflict when the child learns that he or she cannot replace the parent of the same sex, whom the child also loves. These feelings of intense love and the wish to be rid of one parent can cause anxiety, guilt, and fear because the child believes that wishes are as real as the actual deed. Because the child cannot compete with this larger and more powerful rival, she or he resolves the tension by identifying with the parent of the same sex. Freud called this the Oedipal complex for boys and the Electra complex for girls, named after characters in Greek mythology. Parents and other significant adults influence early sex role development.

The preschooler is very interested in his or her own body and its intactness and how it compares with that of other children. This sexual curiosity is an important developmental phase and helps the child gain an understanding of sexual identity. The child's curiosity may be manifested in direct questions to parents about sex. Such questions are an attempt to understand how the body functions and why girls and boys are different. Curiosity may also be evident in overt behaviors such as actual visual exploration of oneself or of the opposite sex. The sexual development of the preschooler also centers around resolution of the Oedipal complex for boys and the Electra complex for girls. According to Freud's psychoanalytical theory, a boy wishes to possess his mother solely and thus competes with his father to win affection from his mother. The child imitates the behaviors of the same-sex parent closely in an attempt to replace that parent, thus taking on characteristics of masculinity or femininity and resolving the complex. By the end of the preschool period, the child begins to realize that such a sexual relationship is not possible and instead expresses interest in the same-sex peer group. Nevertheless, child-rearing practices and imitation of the same-sex parent influence the specific sex typing of the child. One activity related to sexuality that tends to confuse or disturb parents is the preschooler's interest in masturbation, or self-stimulation of the genitals. If this behavior is not excessive, it is both normal and healthy, since it is part of a child's bodily exploration and helps satisfy sexual curiosity.

When assessing sex and sexuality, it is important to also determine the parents' perceptions of both male and female sex roles, their understanding of sexual development in the preschooler, and any biases they may have as a result of certain attitudes or beliefs.

■ SCHOOL-AGE YEARS: 6 TO 12

During the middle years of childhood, from ages 6 to 10, the child moves from the close ties of family and home to the larger world of peers, school, and neighborhood. The family "romance" is less intense, and the child is able to go out into the world. This is the period of latency during which the child is free from earlier concentration on sexuality and strong basic drives. The child can now direct energy toward learning the skills

figure**4.6**   School-age years.

and competencies of the mind and body that lead to practical achievements and accomplishment in the world. Tremendous intellectual growth occurs during this lull before the "storm" of adolescence, and the child is introduced to experiences that help in learning the fundamentals of society and culture.

Physical Development

Physical growth during the middle years of childhood is relatively slow and smooth. The most pronounced period of growth usually comes toward the end of this stage, at 10 to 12 years of age. Some children begin the growth spurt as early as age 8 or 9. The increments in weight are less regular than those in the young infant and child, and weight may remain stationary for weeks at a time. The approximate annual increase in weight is about 5 to 7 pounds. The average annual increase in height is approximately 2 to 3 inches. Boys on average are taller and heavier than girls until the adolescent growth spurt, which occurs earlier in girls.

The physical changes that occur make school-age children more agile and graceful. They become slimmer, with longer legs and a lower center of gravity than the younger child. They are stronger and better coordinated and are able to fit into the adult physical environment more easily. The size of the cranium increases only slightly, because nearly 90% of the growth of the brain is accomplished by age 7. The lower parts of the face continue to grow, giving the child a more mature appearance and making room for the larger teeth to erupt. The first permanent teeth, which usually erupt at 6 to 6½ years of age, are usually the mandibular central incisors. The eruption of the large permanent teeth contributes to the temporarily less attractive appearance of the school-age child.

The eyeball continues to grow until 10 or 12 years of age. Visual acuity is usually 20/20 to 20/30 between 4 and 5 years of age, but depth perception is not very accurate until 6 to 7 years of age. Hearing is well established at a much earlier age. Growth of lymphoid tissue increases steadily until puberty and then decreases. This accounts for the abundance of lymphoid tissues such as adenoids and tonsils. The skeleton continues to ossify, with cartilage being replaced by bone. The child acquires the basic neuromuscular mechanisms by age 6 or 7 and spends the school years refining physical skills, resulting in an increase in motor skills and coordination. Thus the school-age child engages in repetitive practice in all areas of neuromuscular activities from the fine motor skills of writing, drawing, and playing instruments to the large motor skills used in baseball, biking, running, and swimming, depending on individual interests.

The appetite fluctuates, and eating nutritiously may become a problem. Problems with excessive weight may also begin to occur. Although taste preferences continue to influence what the child eats, the ongoing establishment of good eating habits is important.

Cognitive Development

The cognitive development of the school-age child, according to Piaget, is characterized by the ability to begin to do mentally what the child would have had to do with real action at an earlier age. Piaget termed this the stage of concrete operations, meaning that the child can now use mental representations or symbols of objects and events. What had to be done physically before, the child can now experience mentally. This enables the child to use numbers, read, order objects on an increasing or decreasing scale, and classify objects by a common characteristic. The stage of concrete operations begins at about age 8. The school-age child also begins to see the multiple characteristics of objects rather than centering on any one aspect. Piaget also found that during these years the child masters the concept of conservation. Piaget's classic test illustrating the principle of conservation is to give the child two jars of equal size containing equal amounts of liquid. The contents of one jar are then poured into two smaller containers of equal size, and the child is asked whether the amount of liquid poured into the two smaller jars is still the same as that remaining in the other container. Younger children cannot comprehend that the liquid has been conserved when placed in smaller containers. The older child comprehends that the quantity remains the same. She or he is beginning to distinguish the difference between how things seem and how they really are.

Throughout the school years, memory and language skills increase. This enhances the child's ability to share experiences and observations and to articulate questions and new understandings. Older children can think more logically because they can now make mental compar-

isons rather than actually manipulating objects, can see the whole as well as the parts, and have mastered the concept of conservation.

As school-age children develop, thinking gradually becomes more logical. Egocentric thinking and behavior progressively diminish and are replaced by a larger view of self and others. Children begin to realize that their own is not the only point of view and that others see things differently. This new ability to reason and to carry out mental operations in solving problems is limited in an important respect. They cannot yet differentiate clearly between their own assumptions and the facts. In other words, they treat their own hypotheses as if they were facts and reject facts that do not agree with that position.

Creativity continues to develop in the young school-age child. Frequently, however, children appear more reluctant to express creativity while they are in school, perhaps because of the responses of adults who are more interested in the "right" answers. This attitude can suppress the child's creative impulses, because adult approval is so important.

As children internalize the standards and ideals of the significant adults around them, they begin to develop a conscience and sense of moral behavior. They have greater knowledge of what is right and wrong, although they may break the rules made by adults. They begin to have feelings of guilt about misbehavior. The younger child may follow certain rules somewhat rigidly and be quick to condemn the supposed wrongs of others. This early sense of morality is expanded and modified during the years of middle childhood as intellectual skills increase and the ability to understand reasons for moral thought and action matures. Parents can enhance their child's moral growth by modeling their own values, such as honesty and fairness, at every opportunity, and by helping the child understand punishment as the result of a deed and not as a judgment of the child's worth.

School is an exciting adventure, and most children anticipate it eagerly. Mixed in with the excitement are often some fears and anxieties. The child needs to separate from home and parents, adjust to new authority figures, accept restrictions on previously acceptable activities, learn new routines, and participate in large groups. These situations can create tension within the child. This transition can be facilitated by parents and teachers who express understanding and encouragement.

Certain characteristics are indicators of readiness to enter the world of school. Of course, one child is unlikely to possess all of these. Some of these characteristics include the ability to communicate, ability to participate in social interactions, capacity to make friends, ongoing attainment of a basic body of knowledge, and independence in basic self-care activities.

Psychosocial Development

Erikson described the ego development stage of middle childhood as a period focused on industry versus inferiority. This is a stage when ideally the child develops a sense of industriousness and accomplishment rather than a sense of inadequacy. During this period the child leaves home for school, where the views, esteem, and approval of people outside the family become important. The child becomes a worker, one who is required to develop intellectual, physical, and social skills that contribute to a sense of adequacy. The child's attainments in cognitive, interpersonal, and social development are significant. The child is now able to see a higher organization of behavior in which to participate. The child wants to operate in socially accepted ways of thinking and behaving, can understand another person's point of view, and is able to take what she or he hears and sees and compare it with what is already known of reality. The child learns to reason and act according to rules, which allows for benefit from the school experience and for participation in organized sports or other activities. Participation in activities that develop skills both in cooperation and competition is beneficial.

Achievement at this stage enhances feelings of competence, confidence, and industry. The child who achieves in some areas begins to feel rewarded both from outside sources, such as teachers and parents, and from within, by feelings of satisfaction. The child who does not achieve in some way begins to develop feelings of inferiority, low self-esteem, loss of confidence, and a sense of incompetence. These feelings may haunt the developing individual for many years, even when success and achievement come later. Children experience success during this stage of industry as they participate in many productive activities. School-age children's great desire to win at games and willingness to work to achieve a variety of skills demonstrate their need to be adequate in their own eyes, as well as in the eyes of others. Parents, teachers, and other adult figures should encourage school-age children even when performance is incomplete or imperfect. And adults must realize that success comes sooner for some children than for others.

Freud described the period of relative sexual quiet as a time of latency. In terms of sexual development, middle childhood is a span of time between the sexual struggles and resolutions of earlier childhood and the sexual turbulence of adolescence. Awareness of sexuality is not absent; curiosity, questions, and jokes remain a part of the child's growing sexual identity.

By 6 years of age, the child's personality has become structured. Through accomplishment of earlier developmental tasks, the child has achieved a concept of the self, acquired a sense of trust, developed autonomy with some power over impulses and the environment, and in-

corporated standards of the culture as interpreted by the parents.

During these school years the peer group becomes increasingly important, and the child needs to find a place in a group of peers. The child is ready to be involved in the private world of children, where adults are not always welcome. At ages 6 and 7, peers are partners in play, with boys and girls participating together much of the time. During ages 8 and 9 the child usually selects a best friend and moves toward group activities with friends of the same sex. Feelings of group solidarity and belonging are promoted by secret languages, codes, and clubs, as well as a common culture. Together, children explore ideas and values, learn fair play, practice leadership roles, and experience cooperation and compromise. Children who show difficulty with peer relationships may have problems in developing future relationships.

As these children move into the larger world of school and peers, they continue to need their parent(s). Demands for conformity are placed on them by people outside the family, such as teachers, scout leaders, and peers. The family should be children's source of strength and support. They continue to need the approval of parents, teachers, and other important adults for their uniqueness and any special talents. As children approach adolescence, they view their parents in a more critical light. This puts a strain on the parent-child relationship and can lead to tension and arguments. Parents need to understand the changing viewpoint of the child and reassure him or her of their continuing love, even when this is difficult. Parents also need to allow greater independence and responsibility for the child in appropriate areas. This reinforces the child's sense of self and prepares the child for future developmental stages.

■ ADOLESCENCE: 11-13 TO 20

Adolescence is the period of life beginning with puberty and extending for about 7 to 10 years to the onset of adulthood. The age boundaries of adolescence vary but range from 11-13 to 19-22, and sometimes longer. Adolescence generally extends to the time when the person is physically and psychologically mature, ready to assume adult responsibilities and to be self-sufficient. Throughout the adolescent years the individual struggles with the transition from the role of a child to the role of an adult and struggles to develop a personal identity. The adolescent moves toward greater independence and personal freedom to make decisions.

Developmental Tasks

The adolescent faces the following developmental tasks:

1. Searching for self-identity and a sense of self-worth

2. Achieving a gradual independence from parents
3. Establishing relationships with peers
4. Developing academic and vocational skills
5. Adjusting to rapid physical and sexual changes
6. Developing an internalized set of values
7. Considering choices for a career
8. Developing the ability to think logically and analytically

According to Erikson, the task of adolescence is the development of ego identity versus role confusion. The formation of a self-identity separate from others is a process that begins in infancy and continues throughout adulthood, but it has a very distinct focus during adolescence. Without the emerging understanding of self-identity as expressed through interests, preferences, and personality temperament, individuals feel confused about who they are in comparison with the group. Part of the need to identify the self as a separate person is the need to establish independence from the parents.

The word *conflict* is often associated with the words *teenager* and *adolescent,* and adolescence is truly a stage of conflict and turmoil, as well as one of high growth potential in the physical, sexual, and social areas. The adolescent must learn to cope with increasingly intense impulses, developing sexuality, and an altering body form. Spurts of growth occur, along with increased muscular energy and strength. The reproductive system matures; the individual develops secondary sexual characteristics and becomes capable of reproduction. The social world broadens in adolescence, and the individual develops a growing sensitivity to the perceived judgments of others.

Stages of Adolescence

Adolescence may be divided into four phases or stages:

1. Preadolescence
2. Early adolescence
3. Middle adolescence
4. Late adolescence

Preadolescence

Preadolescence is a stage covering the years of 10 through 12 for girls and 10 to 11 through 13 for boys. It is characterized by increases in physical activity, energy, and restlessness. Running is more natural than walking, and sitting still even for a short time may be nearly impossible. Muscular strength, skill, and agility are very important to the individual and among peers. Adolescents may have quiet moments during which they seem to be simply staring into space. They may have fears, worries, and concerns but are generally not interested in talking about them. Signs of earlier childhood problems such as nervous habits, childish antics, or bed-wetting may reappear temporarily.

Preadolescence is a continuation of the change in primary affiliation with parents and their codes to primary affiliation with peers. These years are often trying times for parents because the parent-child bonds appear to be loosening and breaking. Although preadolescents love and feel loyalty toward their parents, they may frequently treat them with surprising suspicion, distrust, and irritability. They are easily offended and respond to seemingly minor incidents with the ready accusation that adults do not understand them and treat them unfairly. Other adults in the neighborhood may receive more admiration than the parents receive. Parental recommendations regarding use of language and matters of appearance and cleanliness are often met with indignation and conflict. Preadolescents are increasingly sensitive about having a parent see their bodies and about public displays of affection toward parents. They are often seemingly unaware of the effect of their own inconsiderateness on the feelings of others and appear surprised when it is pointed out to them that their behavior has caused some hurt.

At this stage boys and girls typically have little to do with each other socially. Girls may move through this phase more quickly than boys. Clique and secret club formation is a prominent characteristic. If peer codes do not meet with parental approval, they are all the more desirable. The changes of preadolescence are not easy for the parents, nor are they easy for the preadolescent. Conflicting and painful situations are common, but the preadolescent must experience these to move on in establishing an individual identity.

Early adolescence

Early adolescence begins with puberty and lasts for several years (11 to 12 through 13 to 14 for females and 12 to 14 through 15 to 16 for males). The growth spurt focuses attention on the self and on the task of becoming comfortable with body changes and appearance. The teen tries to separate from the parents; the dependency-independency struggle is apparent by less involvement in family activities, criticism of parents, and rebellion against parental and other adult discipline and authority. Conformity to, and acceptance of, peer group standards and peer friendships gain importance. The peer group usually consists of same-sex friends; however, the early adolescent shows an increased interest in the opposite sex. Early adolescence usually coincides with menarche in females and active spermatogenesis in males.

Middle adolescence

Middle adolescence begins when physical growth is completed and usually extends from age 13 to 14 through age 16 for females and from age 14 to 16 through age 18 to 20 for males. The major tasks during

figure**4.7**   Early adolescence.

figure**4.8**   Middle adolescence.

this period are an increased sense of ego identity, attainment of greater independence, interest in the future and career possibilities, and establishment of heterosexual relationships. The individual is working to overcome feelings of insecurity and inadequacy and to move toward self-assurance and independence. Peer group allegiance, at a peak in 15- to 16-year-olds, is manifested by clothing, food, fads, musical preference, and common jargon. Most teenagers relate increasingly with the opposite sex, whereas some begin to be aware of their homosexual orientation. The middle adolescent gradually becomes more self-assured and able to make some independent decisions. For these reasons, the youth at this stage has particular difficulty in adjusting to controlling or confining situations. Some societal privileges and responsibilities increase during middle adolescence, such as driving a car. Experimentation with adultlike behavior and risk taking is common in an attempt to prove oneself to peers. Sexual experimentation often begins now as a result of social exploration and physical maturation. Family relationships and communication may be disrupted as the adolescent's activity outside the home is increased. Changes in cognitive functioning may first be evident in that the adolescent moves to abstract thinking, returning to more concrete thinking during times of stress.

Late adolescence

Late adolescence may occur from about age 17 to 18 until 20 to 25 years of age. The person has usually finished adolescent rebellion, formed some significant views, and established a fairly stable sense of self. Many youths are not yet committed to one occupation, and they often question relationships to existing social, vocational, and emotional roles and lifestyles. The late adolescent may be a student or an apprentice. Lack of economic freedom may be a concern and can lead to prolonged dependence on parents. Continued dependence may lead to delayed maturity. The late adolescent is clarifying his or her value system and examining issues of philosophy, religion, life and death, and ethical decisions. The peer group has lost its primary importance, and a relationship with a particular person may become the focal point for social activity. There is more individual dating and fewer group activities with friends; often the first emotionally intimate relationship develops. The late adolescent may take a major step in establishing independence from parents by moving away from home. Activities with family members tend to decrease, and more adultlike friendships begin between late adolescents and their parents as the earlier family turbulence subsides. At that point, the person is developmentally a young adult, having made the transition from adolescence. He or she is more realistically aware of strengths and self-limitations, as well as the limitations of others.

Thought processes become more logical, and the ability to use abstract ideas increases. The end of late adolescence is marked by planning for the future in the form of higher education, occupation, and committed relationships.

Some fluctuation in this progression may continue to some degree for several years in the direction of greater maturation. The task of finding an acceptable career that is personally satisfying and potentially economically adequate assumes a more central position during the later high school years and subsequent period of college, vocational training, or apprenticeship. This is a time of becoming ready to leave the parents' home both physically and emotionally.

At age 18, people may marry without parental consent and may vote. At age 21, individuals attain most adult privileges and responsibilities conferred by society. At this time an individual is allowed to drink alcoholic beverages, sign a binding financial document, and accept full legal penalties for crimes.

The end of adolescence is more difficult to define than the beginning. Our society observes no specific ritual of passage into adulthood. The adolescent may remain dependent on the parents because of economic need or educational endeavors. In general, the adolescent moves into adulthood when she or he can prepare realistic plans for the future, including plans for education, occupation, and a shared or single lifestyle. The status of young adulthood is reached when the adolescent begins to adjust to societal responsibilities and moves toward achieving personal life goals.

Physical Development

Puberty marks the beginning of adolescence. It is characterized by dramatic physical and physiological changes, including the beginning of the ability to reproduce. There is a spurt of rapid growth in height, weight, and muscular development. Secondary sex characteristics appear, and the reproductive organs mature. In girls puberty lasts about 3 years, from age 10 or 11 to 14. Menarche, the onset of menses, usually occurs at 12 to 13 years, though it may begin about a year earlier or several years later. It often begins just after the peak of the physical growth spurt. In boys puberty lasts about 4 years, from ages 12 to 16.

Girls between the ages of 10 and 12 experience a spurt in height; by age 14 or 15 their growth is nearly complete. During these years, girls grow 2.5 to 5 inches (6 to 12.5 cm) and gain 8 to 10 pounds (3.5 to 4.5 kg). Boys have their rapid growth spurt between ages 12 and 14. By age 16, their growth is nearly complete. Boys grow an average of 3 to 6 inches (7.5 to 15 cm) and gain 12 to 14 pounds (5.5 to 6.5 kg). An adolescent's self-concept is continually readjusting as the body changes.

Sexual development and sexuality

Adolescents struggle with notions of body image and what is normal growth and development. At this stage teenagers begin to develop curiosity and interest in sexual relationships. They are very aware of the development of secondary sex characteristics and continually compare how their body looks with the appearance of their peers and to some ideal standard of attractiveness.

Frequently, formerly supportive adults are confused or uncomfortable with the teenager's sexual curiosity. In addition, the changing roles of males and females leave many teenagers with little idea of what is expected from them.

Females. Menarche may occur anywhere between 10 and 16 years of age. In the United States, the average age of onset is at about 12½ years of age. Ovulation usually begins 12 to 24 months after menarche. The onset of menarche varies among population groups and is influenced by heredity, nutrition, health care, and other environmental factors. Most adolescent girls view the menarche as a normal developmental milestone separating them from childhood. They may view it with curiosity or pride. Others view the onset of menstruation with fear or anxiety. A wide variety of attitudes exist among different groups in society. The presence of physical discomfort during and/or around the time of menstruation may also lead to a negative reaction, with some females experiencing headaches, backaches, cramps, and abdominal pain. They may also experience mood changes before menstruation, such as depression, irritability, anxiety, and a sense of low self-esteem.

Secondary sex characteristics in the female begin to develop at puberty and may take 2 to 8 years for completion. Breast development, often the earliest sign of puberty in girls, occurs between the ages of 8 and 18. Pubic hair develops between years 11 and 14.

Males. Spermatogenesis (sperm production) and seminal emissions mark puberty and sexual maturity in the male. The first ejaculate of seminal fluid occurs about 1 year after the penis has begun its adolescent growth, and nocturnal emissions (loss of seminal fluid during sleep) occur at about age 14. Just as the onset of menstruation produces a new set of feelings in girls, nocturnal emissions may produce new feelings, including pride, fear, or shame. Erotic dreams may accompany the nocturnal emissions.

Secondary sex characteristics in the male also begin before puberty and may take 2 to 5 years for completion. Changes in body shape, growth of body hair, and muscle development may continue until 19 or 20, or even until the late 20s. Testicular enlargement is usually the first pubescent change, starting between ages 10 and 13 and ending between ages 13 and 17. The penis and scrotum enlarge; the scrotum reddens, and scrotal skin changes texture. Hair grows at the axilla and pubic area between ages 12 and 16. The growth of facial and chest hair usually occurs somewhat later, around age 16. The voice begins to deepen at age 13 or 14.

Sexual role development

Maturation of an individual's sexual identity involves more than development of primary and secondary sexual characteristics and strong sexual impulses. It also involves the ability and desire to give and receive love, respect, and affection. The development of a sexual identity begins very early in life, but it is particularly strong during adolescence because of the physical changes and the search for self-identity. Conflict with parents over issues of sexual identity and behavior is common. This conflict is due in part to the changes between childhood and adolescence in what parents find acceptable, such as kissing others, and in part because of the differences between what different generations believe is acceptable.

Intellectual curiosity about sexuality and the act of sexual intercourse is a major component in adolescent sexual development. Frustration at this age results from a general lack of sufficient information about sex.

Traditional attitudes and values regarding sexuality are changing. Because of the dichotomy of American values relating to sexual behavior and rules for sexual identity, present-day adolescents are left to search for their own sexual identity and moral code with very few parental or societal guidelines. Understandably, many teenagers have difficulty establishing a consistent sexual identity.

Adolescent pregnancy

Teen pregnancies occur within all cultural and socioeconomic groups. Teenagers may find it difficult to deal with the tension between their emotional needs and their developing sexuality. During this time of sexual development and exploration of a sexual role, pregnancy may occur. Babies born to teen mothers are at risk for low birth weight and related problems. If both parents are not committed to caring for the child, this complicates the already-difficult situation. Frequently the teen mother is left with little support to take on the enormous burden of raising a child while she is still developing herself.

Educating adolescents about sexuality, birth control, and the realities of parenting is very important in avoiding unwanted pregnancy and helping teens learn about the responsibilities of parenthood.

Skin

Skin texture changes during adolescence. Sebaceous glands become more active and increase in size. Acne may develop. The sweat glands are fully developed and begin to secrete in response to emotional stimuli.

Health risks

Physical health is generally good. Risks to the health of adolescents include poor judgment resulting in accidents, drug or alcohol abuse, unwanted pregnancy, or sexually transmitted diseases. Emotional stress due to unmet or unrealistic expectations may show up as depression, anorexia nervosa, or suicide attempts. Accidents and suicide are the leading causes of death in the adolescent population.

Cognitive Development

During adolescence the mind has a great ability to acquire and use knowledge. The thought process of the adolescent becomes more logical, and the ability to use abstract ideas increases. The adolescent is working on the beginning structure of a philosophy of life. This process requires the use of abstract thinking. Piaget described this level of cognitive process as the period of formal operations. This thinking moves beyond the concrete into the area of abstract thought where reasoning occurs and symbolic and logical processes are used. Abstract thinking is a new and deeper level of consciousness. It allows for greater creativity and inner awareness. The individual can contemplate the past and future, as well as the present, can develop theories, and can consider scientific hypotheses. Abstract thinking liberates the person for mental processes of greater depth and breadth. This can be a period of academic and creative achievement for the adolescent.

The conscious development of a personal value system also occurs during this period. This is another component of the search for self-identity. Part of the questioning of the values of parents and institutions is the process of developing a set of values that works for the person. The adolescent becomes more aware of inconsistencies, hypocrisy, and injustices.

Adolescents are subject to many stresses placed on them by their families, schools, peer groups, and society at large. Adolescents are vulnerable to stress, since they have not yet developed a strong identity with sufficient coping mechanisms to deal with negative stress. Problems such as teen pregnancy, drug abuse, conflict with parents, dropping out of school, or delinquency may result. As our society grows in complexity, there is an increase in potential stress factors to which adolescents are subject. An individual teenager's response to stress may result in growth in personal identity and self-confidence, or in vulnerability to less healthy coping patterns.

Psychosocial Development

According to Erikson, the task of adolescence is the development of ego identity versus the danger of role diffusion. Adolescents become increasingly sensitive to how they think others perceive them as compared with how they perceive themselves. Finding one's own identity is stressful and difficult work. In many ways, it is a lifelong task. If the adolescent can emerge with a reasonably strong sense of his or her own identity, he or she has successfully experienced this stage. If an adolescent does not develop a personal sense of identity, she or he feels an ongoing personal sense of confusion, anxiety, alienation, and incompleteness. The person may then look to a group outside the family for a sense of identity. The peer group becomes an important place for experimentation with various roles outside the family, and the adolescent often feels intense pressure to join one.

Adolescents may also follow or identify with popular entertainers and wear personal apparel or use speech patterns that mark them as part of a group. Because of the vulnerability of young teenagers, the pressures of peer group conformity may be harmful. Individual judgment may often be forfeited to the desires of the group as a whole, creating great stress and anxiety in some adolescents. It is the rare adolescent who has developed enough ego strength to stand alone against the crowd. Teenagers, however, perceive their behavior as highly individualistic or original because it is different from that of adults, even though it may conform to group codes.

During preadolescence, close friendships are important to identity development. During the later teen years, relationships with the opposite sex usually develop. They may take the form of group activities or couple dating. Adolescents begin to experience the possibilities for trust and intimacy with others. Some individuals become aware that they may have a homosexual orientation.

Another important characteristic is the relationship between the parent of an adolescent and his or her peer group of friends. Frequently, values and beliefs of parents are dramatically different from those of the adolescent's friends. This can result in friction between these two influential factions and can be a source of stress, especially if the teenager feels that he or she must make a choice between loved family members and friends.

The emotional life of an adolescent ranges from exhilarating peaks to depressing lows. Much energy goes into this effort to understand the meaning of this shifting complex of feelings. Outwardly these emotional expressions may be a source of tension and conflict. Gradually the emotions even out to some extent, and a sense of balance develops.

■ YOUNG ADULTHOOD: 20 TO 30-35

Leaving adolescence and entering young adulthood means separation from the family and its financial support as well as greater freedom to choose experiences and friends. It is also a time of taking greater responsi-

figure**4.9** Young adulthood.

bility for one's own life. During the first several years of early adulthood, some of the major tasks are to achieve relative independence from parental figures, to establish an independent lifestyle, and to develop a sense of emotional, social, and economic responsibility for one's own life. The young adult faces many complex issues that affect personal and professional growth. Coping mechanisms that were developing during childhood and adolescence are challenged and expanded during the young adult years when choices and responsibilities increase. The young adult must balance the desire to explore options with the need for some stability.

During the middle years of young adulthood, there is often a period of questioning and reflection. Questions the individual reflects on may include: "Why am I doing this, and not something else?" "Where am I going with my life, my career?" or "What other alternatives should I consider?" This is probably the first period of conscious self-examination. Sometimes this search reaffirms the direction a person's life is taking; sometimes change seems desirable. Depending on the set of circumstances, the person may decide to get married, change jobs, get divorced, have children, develop a career as a parent, or return to work.

This period of questioning and transition is often followed by a period of settling in with the choices that have been made. The individual can use energy to develop the chosen lifestyle and find a special place or role in a family and in society. People at this stage invest in home, career, and family.

During the later years of young adulthood the individual may establish a career commitment, form significant relationships, and even take on parenthood.

Developmental Tasks

The major developmental tasks of early adulthood include:
1. Becoming independent from parents
2. Establishing a household
3. Choosing and beginning to establish a career or vocation
4. Developing a personal style of living, including shared living or single living
5. Establishing an intimate relationship
6. Establishing friendships and a social network
7. Choosing activities in social and community organizations
8. Developing parenting behaviors for biological offspring or in the broader framework of social parenting
9. Implementing personal values in home, employment, and community settings

Physical Development

Physical growth reaches its peak during early adulthood. The body is operating efficiently, with good muscle tone, strength, and coordination, and a high energy level. The young adult has the physical strength and stamina for many activities that influence life patterns.

Sexual development is a part of this period of peak physical development. Exploration with sexuality and various sexual roles occurs at this time. During young adulthood the individual establishes a sense of identity with his or her sexual role. This is also the time for decisions on childbearing.

Nutritional needs are no longer for growth, but for maintenance and repair. Weight control becomes a problem for many adults, especially for those who continue to consume food as they did during adolescence, but whose energy expenditure is less than it was during those years.

Cognitive Development

The young adult years are a time of optimal cognitive functioning. The individual is engaged in the mastery of new skills and new knowledge, and the intellect is stimulated by these exciting and challenging events. Cognitive functioning at the level of formal operations, the capacity for abstract thinking, emerged during adolescence. The young adult expands on this base by becoming less egocentric and more realistic and objective. The young adult has an excellent ability to acquire and use knowledge, and to engage in problem-solving and creative endeavors.

For many, education continues during the early years

of young adulthood. College, graduate school, on-the-job training, and/or continuing education classes prepare the young adult to enter some field of work. Depending on the career path chosen, educational preparation may continue well into the 20s.

Psychosocial Development

Erikson's sixth stage, intimacy versus isolation, focuses on one of the tasks of young adulthood: forming an intimate relationship. After establishing self-identity, the individual can enter a relationship with another without losing self-identity. Because neither the development of self-identity nor readiness for an intimate relationship is clearly defined, young adults often experience some fear that they will undergo a loss of personal identity when entering a relationship. Intimacy involves more than physical contact: it is the ability to share personal identity with another without losing one's own unique identity. The desired outcome is mutual satisfaction and support.

Although Erikson focused on the heterosexual marriage relationship, intimate bonds are also formed within a homosexual relationship. Erikson suggested that affiliation or intimacy was expressed as mutuality with a loved partner with whom one is willing and able to share the cycles of work, family life, and recreation. This bond involves the capacity to enter a committed relationship and to stand by it through difficult times.

The danger of this stage is isolation or an avoidance of those persons and settings that promote and provide intimacy. A young adult whose identity work is not well underway may settle for sets of stereotyped interpersonal relationships that lead to a deep sense of isolation. This false "intimacy" is not a love relationship; it bypasses the accomplishment of improved understanding of one's own inner resources and those of others. The person feels isolated, lonely, and withdrawn.

Another of Erikson's stages of ego development, which is important during young adulthood, as well as during middle and late adulthood, is the stage of generativity versus stagnation. Generativity refers to a productive life: productivity within personal relationships (family and friends), a chosen career, and in the community.

Establishing independence

Young adults may move out of the parental home or establish a more equal role with their parents if they stay in it. During difficult economic times, when jobs for high school and college graduates are hard to find, many young adults continue to live in their parents' home until they are able to establish themselves financially. Whether the young adult remains temporarily in the parents' home or moves out to establish an independent living situation, the young adult should work toward emotional, social, and economic independence.

Marriage or singlehood

Marriage is increasingly viewed today in our society as a loving, sharing relationship between two people, rather than as a social institution for creating and rearing a family. While many young adults still choose marriage, singlehood is another viable option. Remaining single may meet the needs of those not ready for the complex interdependent relationship of marriage, or those who by temperament are not suited to the roles of spouse and parent. Single persons may experience pressure from the family. Even people who remain single by choice may have difficulty with feelings of aloneness and lack of companionship. Singlehood, however, may increase the opportunities for career advancement, creative expression, and community service.

Divorce

The expectations for marriage as a close, loving and sharing relationship where both individuals benefit from the union are often unmet. Divorce is a common result in our society. Divorce may be a freeing experience, but initially, it may be quite traumatic as each person deals with feelings of anger, disappointment, grief, and disillusionment. Each person must move on to develop new roles. Financial strain is a frequent problem, most commonly for the woman.

The development of adult maturity includes the quest for independence, willingness to assume responsibility, the ability to deal constructively with frustration and to maintain self-control, sensitivity to others, and the ability to communicate effectively.

Parenting

Parenting tasks may be initiated by bearing children, adopting, becoming a foster parent, or reaching out in other ways, such as coaching children's teams or participating in child development organizations. The decision to raise children involves a major change in a couple's relationship. The arrival of a child is usually a happy event in the life of a couple, yet it can also bring great stress to the marriage. The role of parent is very demanding and requires changes in roles, relationships, and time commitments within and outside the home.

Many individuals raise children as single parents. This may be a deliberate choice to remain single or may occur as a result of desertion, divorce, or the death of a spouse. When divorce and remarriage occur in families with children, the difficult roles of stepparent and stepchild must be worked through and established.

Career, work, and occupation

The young adult also chooses a career or a vocation and may begin to consider how beliefs about self and society affect that choice. During these years work is closely tied with identity. A young adult who feels satis-

fied with her or his work feels challenged, fulfilled, and rewarded. Frustration with work can lead to boredom and apathy. Work satisfaction is important for maturation and mental health. It can provide prestige and social recognition, a sense of self-worth, opportunities for service, creative self-expression, varied interactions, and a means of self-support. The individual is in a position to stand on his or her own, take risks, and accept consequences for personal actions. This can produce both excitement and fear and holds great potential for personal growth.

Organizational participation

During young adulthood, many individuals begin to establish connections with various organizations in the community. These affiliations may be related to commitment to a cause or belief system, development of friendship networks, physical exercise, or social purposes. Group membership serves the important purpose of providing an outlet for self-expression. However, groups may be problematic if they become a substitute for development of the individual. Maintaining a healthy balance within various group memberships and time for self-orientation is important for young adults. Self-direction, or the knowledge of one's own goals, and recognition of what membership with certain adult groups means to those goals are necessary if an individual is to achieve appropriate group affiliation.

■ MIDDLE ADULTHOOD: 30-35 TO 65-70

Middle adulthood is a stage of life when growth is strongest in the areas of personal, social, and emotional development. By this time, individuals have generally chosen a lifestyle, a family or single pattern of living, and an occupation. The span of time considered to cover the middle adulthood years is variable; some consider ages 40 to 65, and others use ages 30 to 70. Stevenson (1977) uses the term *middlescence* to describe this age span of 30 to 70 years. She further subdivides it into two categories: middlescence I from 30 to 50 and middlescence II from 50 to 70. The boundaries of this stage of life must be considered tentative and flexible. Regardless of the parameters used, this is likely to be the longest stage of a person's life.

Developmental Tasks

The categories of early middle age and late middle age are used here to describe major developmental tasks.

The major developmental tasks for people in early middle age, between ages 30 to 35 and 50 to 55, include:

1. Adjusting to the physical changes of aging
2. Continuing to learn in the areas of personal and career interests

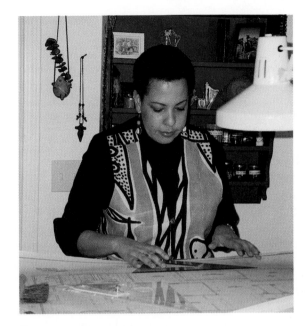

figure**4.10** Middle adulthood.

3. Reviewing, evaluating, and refining career goals (orientation) in light of a personal value system
4. Reaching the desired level of achievement in one's career
5. Working on a maturing relationship with one's spouse or significant other
6. Choosing organizational and civic activities in which to participate
7. Helping younger persons develop as they search for their own identity
8. Coping with the "empty nest" as children leave home
9. Assisting aging parents, or planning for the time when that will be necessary
10. Developing hobby and leisure activities for current enjoyment and for long-range retirement planning
11. Planning for the financial, personal, and social aspects of retirement

The major developmental tasks for people in late middle age, between ages 50 to 55 and 65 to 70, include:

1. Developing supportive, interdependent relationships with grown children, their families, and other members of the younger generation
2. Enhancing the relationship with one's spouse or most significant other person
3. Adjusting to the loss of a spouse or significant other person, if necessary
4. Maintaining an affiliation with some civic, political, professional, religious, and/or social organization(s)
5. Maintaining an interest in current scientific, political, and cultural changes

6. Helping aged parents or other relatives cope with changes in their lives
7. Developing satisfying leisure time activities
8. Preparing for or adapting to retirement, which may include another career, a move, a change in financial status, and numerous other changes
9. Adapting to changes accompanying the aging processes

Physical Changes

During the years of early middle age, physical changes are generally gradual. During the years of late middle age, they become more marked. In our society, aging changes are often the focus of humor, denial, and depression. However, many adults accept the physical changes of aging with grace. Aging changes may begin over a wide span of time. For some people they begin in the early 30s; for others changes do not occur until well into the 40s. The skin loses some of its elasticity: wrinkles gradually begin to form around the eyes and mouth and on the forehead. The skin sags a bit under the eyes and around the chin and jaw. The hair begins to lose pigment and turns gray or white. It may thin somewhat, and in men the hairline often recedes. Because of decreased muscular tone, the abdominal muscles are no longer as firm. Frequently weight gain occurs, especially when the activity level decreases but caloric intake does not. Sensory function remains generally intact except for decreased accommodation for near vision (presbyopia). Internal organ function remains fairly constant in the healthy adult, although some decrease may occur in respiratory and cardiac function. If the individual actively pursues physical fitness, these changes may not occur until later.

During the late 40s or early 50s, women experience menopause. The menstrual cycle becomes irregular in frequency and flow pattern. Periods of heavy bleeding alternate with amenorrhea for 1 to 2 years and finally cease altogether. The decrease in the hormones estrogen and progesterone produces symptoms that may include vasomotor changes (hot flashes and sweating) and mood changes.

Men do not experience such an abrupt halt to their reproductive ability. During the late 50s or during the 60s, testosterone production decreases somewhat, leading to decreased sperm production, longer erection time, and less intense orgasms.

During middle adulthood many individuals experience for the first time the diagnosis of a chronic health problem such as hypertension, diabetes, or arthritis. A history of smoking may lead to cardiovascular or respiratory problems, which are evident for the first time during middle age.

As the individual moves through late middle adulthood and toward late adulthood in the late 60s and into the 70s, many develop more chronic health status changes. While none of them may be life-threatening, together they do take a toll on the energy level and sense of well-being. (See also Chapter 26: Aging Clients.)

Cognitive Development

Cognitive processes in adulthood include learning, problem solving, memory, and creativity.

Learning continues in adulthood. Much of it comes from life experiences that are integrated by thought and reflection. Adult learning is enhanced by interest, motivation, self-confidence, a sense of humor, and flexibility. The middle-aged adult is interested in how knowledge is applied to living and improving life. The growth in continuing education and outreach programs makes ongoing, lifelong learning available to interested adults. These programs enable persons to update their knowledge for their profession or occupation and to develop new personal interest areas. Some adults use middle age as the opportunity to enroll in college for the first time, and others return to earn an advanced degree. Reaction time or speed of intellectual performance is individual and generally stays the same or diminishes during late middle age. Most adults experience no decrease in the ability to learn, though they may need a longer learning period.

Problem-solving abilities remain fairly constant throughout adulthood. The levels of education and intelligence, and the accumulation of life experiences influence the ability to solve problems at this age, as they do at any age. People of various ages will perceive problems and situations differently. Early formative experiences differ somewhat with each generation and affect how people view problems and how they seek resolution. The older the person is, the greater the store of past experiences used to evaluate current situations. Moving through the middle adult years, individuals have the opportunity to broaden their perspectives and deepen their insights.

Memory generally remains intact during the middle adulthood years. Some decrease in recent memory may occur during the late middle years. Memory is aided by the presentation of well-organized material.

Creativity continues and may increase during middle adulthood. The insight needed for many creative thoughts, acts, and productions depends on the range of life experiences accumulated over the years.

Psychosocial Development
Generativity versus stagnation

Erikson believed that the important task for personality development at this stage of life is resolution of generativity versus stagnation. Adults need to contribute to the next generation either by raising children or producing something that can be passed on. The latter may involve creative, socially useful work. The motivation is

to create and/or nurture those who will follow and to leave a mark on the world. Generativity means sharing, giving, and contributing to the growth of others, as well as passing something on to the next generation. For some this means parenthood; for others this means generativity through creative acts of expression in the arts or through community involvement. Stagnation means experiencing boredom and a sense of emptiness in life, which leads to being inactive, self-absorbed, and self-indulgent.

Between the ages of 30 and 50, major life goals and activities concentrate on the areas of self-development, career development, assistance to both the younger and older generations, and organizational endeavors. Individuals feel a need to come to terms with both their own values and society's values. Personal values undergo a major change or numerous minor changes during these years when patterns are beginning to seem set but may not feel comfortable. Individuals move into various roles in a number of settings: in the family, at work, in religious organizations, and in community and civic affairs. In Western society, much of the implementation of the goals of major institutions, such as business, industry, government, education, religion, and charitable agencies, is done by the middle-aged population.

Work/career

Work is a major activity and motivating force during middle age. For some the work itself is rewarding and gratifying; for others the only rewards are a paycheck and fringe benefits. Success in a line of work enhances the self-image; lack of success can damage that image. As the person advances through middle age, she or he becomes more aware of the years remaining before retirement. The person reflects on whether he or she is on schedule with career goals, and whether this is the desired career path for the remaining years of employment. Middle-aged individuals may realize that they have expended time and energy in doing what their family and society felt they "should" do. They may begin to feel too restricted by the career and personal choices made earlier. They may find that other aspects of themselves are struggling to surface and find expression. This reflection may involve an uprooting of the life that seemed well grounded and striking out after a new vision. During the 40s and early 50s individuals may be enjoying success and promotions at work or may harbor a concern that this is the last chance to "make it." Some experience tension from a fear of being passed by and are sensitive to any indications that peers or superiors are losing confidence. While much energy is going into the work setting, the home setting may suffer.

For the working woman, involvement in a career may be a source of strength, if the work brings its own rewards and sense of personal accomplishment. A mother benefits from having an identity outside her family role.

However, it may also be a source of stress, since demands from both work and family may be high. Women in the work world who may already have experienced some discrimination can find promotions increasingly rare and even when they occur, they may be resented by a husband who has not been similarly recognized.

Family roles and relationships

New roles emerge as the middle-aged adult deals with growing children and aging parents. The adult may feel sandwiched between the concurrent needs of the older and younger generations. As the children grow through their own life stages, the parents must switch from a role of great involvement during young childhood, to lesser involvement with continued support as the offspring move through their adolescent years. When the children reach young adulthood, it is healthy for the relationship if the roles of children and parents become more equal. With aging parents, a role change for the middle-aged adult depends to a great extent on the health and dependency needs of the parents. If the parents become weak and frail, requiring more health care and a change in housing arrangements, middle-aged adults often feel as if their roles with their parents have switched; they are now increasingly in charge. When a parent dies, the middle-aged adult may feel lonely, vulnerable, and aware of the limited time to live one's life.

Caring for children

A major family task facing the middle-aged adult with children is to help children live up to their potential and to assist them in their search for personal identity. The parent must adjust to the increasing desire of a child to be independent. As adolescence evolves, the child becomes less involved in family activities and desires increased responsibility and freedom. Some parents nurture the independence and delight in the developing individual. Others tend to be overprotective and controlling. Parents may believe they are protecting their children from the same mistakes they made as youths, but children usually resent overly protective efforts. When the last child moves out of the family home, the middle-aged adult again needs to reconsider her or his role in the family and in the community. For some parents this event leaves a void; for others it presents a new opportunity for growth. A woman who has devoted years to home and family may be eager to get involved in the outside world of school, career, or community activities.

If two parents remain in the home, they need to face one another as a couple again. This opportunity can bring the positive experience of increased closeness and more time and freedom for shared activities. Or the couple may realize that their relationship was based on the children, and that apart from the children, they have

little in common. A reconsideration of the marriage may occur. Changes also occur for the parent in a single-parent household. The single parent may experience loneliness, but this time may also be an opportunity for new relationships or career goals. During late middle adulthood the role of grandparent may be realized.

Midlife transition

The phrase "midlife crisis" has become popular in recent decades, but because the term *crisis* often has a negative connotation, the term *transition* is used here. Many middle-aged individuals are aware of the changes and challenges they must confront but see this more as a period of reassessment and reevaluation than as a period of crisis. This phase may begin in the early 40s, although it may be some years earlier or later. People look at the realities of life and at the goals and dreams they have been carrying. Some of these have or can be met; others must be set aside. It is a time of taking stock, readjusting, and emerging with a new understanding. Questions frequently asked include: "What have I done with my life?" "Is this what I want out of life?" or "Have I set aside my own deepest dreams and desires for practicalities that are not satisfying?" Individuals may move their lives onto a different track, or they may accept the one they are on, adjusting to it with greater understanding.

There may be gender differences in midlife perception of the midlife transition. Men still tend to be more involved in career assessment because their traditional role has been focused on becoming established in the career world. Many women, including those who are employed, still tend to see the family as the central issue. This difference does not mean that family is not important to men, or that career issues are not important to women. Many women have experienced the situation of children growing in independence and leaving home. This affects the women's identity. They feel that they are no longer needed in the same way. Some women see this as liberating, because they can now focus on their own goals with greater energy.

At about age 35, a women may see her youngest child enter school. She may then reenter the workforce, and she may also realize that the biological boundary of childbearing is now in sight. (It must be noted, however, that with the recent developments in fertility technology, it is increasingly possible for women to become pregnant at a later age.) Aging and biology force women to review options that were set aside and that will be closed off in the now foreseeable future. Women with or without children face this review.

Whatever the central issue, all those in midlife transition explore the meaning of their career, their family, and their personal identity. An individual who has spent some years searching for power and responsibility now may crave more inner growth and meaning. Childless couples reconsider having children, whereas those who have spent a number of years raising young children may move toward involvement outside the home. Single people may reconsider the choice of career over marriage. The midlife transition may mean less acceptance of stereotyped roles and acknowledgment that few answers are absolute. The years 35 to 45 are a time of reevaluating choices, purposes, and the expenditure of resources. It is a time of uncertainty and opportunity, a chance to restructure a narrower, earlier identity.

The midlife transition is variable; some may never sense a transition at all, whereas others experience profound searches and changes.

Development of interests outside of work

At some point in middle age, the attitude toward work may change from one of total involvement to one of lesser involvement, with a growing interest in focusing on home and family and/or developing skill in a sport or hobby. Work may become more acceptable and be viewed more in terms of its responsibilities than in terms of power. The meaningfulness of activities is a frequent theme as individuals rethink daily routines at work and home and reevaluate beliefs in religion, politics, and relationships. This situation offers the potential for psychological growth and a reintegration and stabilization of identity. During these years, aspects of the personality and talents that have been latent may begin to emerge.

Coping with physical changes

Part of self-knowledge and self-acceptance is an acknowledgment of the physical, emotional, and intellectual changes that accompany the aging process. Physical changes may be difficult to accept in a culture where the signs of youthfulness are highly acclaimed. Middle-aged adults ideally find some balance between accepting the inevitable changes in appearance while striving to maintain a high level of health with positive approaches toward exercise, diet, and their socioemotional environment. They may also appreciate the changes of added years in terms of the emotional and intellectual benefits that accumulate.

Weight may become an eminent concern; a battle against weight gain may also be a battle against aging and the loss of physical attractiveness, and all that this implies in our culture. Difficulties in this area may well depend on the amount of self-esteem that a person previously derived from physical attractiveness. Gray hair is yet another manifestation of a physical change accompanying aging. The adult may perceive it as a source of distress or as a sign of hard-won wisdom.

Menopause

Menopause, which normally occurs during the 40s or early 50s, involves both physiological and psychological

changes. The hormonal changes may result in episodes of rapid mood shifts, nervousness, irritability, insomnia, hot flashes, diaphoresis, and fatigue. These changes cause some women to experience confusion or depression. Other women experience relatively minor physical and psychological distress. In some cultures menopause is recognized as a time of greater wisdom, creativity, and participation in the life of the community. Menopause may be followed by increased enjoyment of sex, since concerns about pregnancy are now absent.

Loss of peers

Many middle-aged adults are suddenly made aware of the relatively brief and fragile nature of life because of the death of peers. Most deaths that occur during the middle years of adulthood are due to cardiovascular disease and cancer. These events are also cause for reflection and taking stock of the meaning and direction of one's own life.

Personal inner growth

Individuals reexamine many issues during these years of middle adulthood—issues of personal qualities, relationships, commitments, career choices, and organizational affiliations. All of the choices and reflections concerning those choices provide an opportunity for personal growth.

Maintaining interest in current affairs

People in this age group, as in any age group, are confronted with rapid changes in technology and in the social environment. However, they often prefer to advise some caution and restraint in the type and rate of change. Life experiences have brought some sense of wisdom and judgment to the middle-aged; although some younger people may view them as overly cautious and nonprogressive, the balance between the two views is important. At the same time, openness and flexibility continue to be important characteristics to health and well-being. Those who stay current with ideas and trends have a more positive approach to life and less need to maintain a defensive posture. They will probably also be able to communicate more effectively with younger individuals.

Retirement

Preparation for retirement is an important task, both for people who have been employed outside the home and for those who have maintained the household. For a married couple, both must readjust to more shared time. Single individuals need to adjust to more time alone. Preparation through adult education or development of new skills can pave the way for a refocusing of talents and interests. Preparation for retirement is actually lifelong. People bring to retirement all that they have become during their lifetime. During the entire span of middle age, the activities an individual chooses to participate in are worthy of thoughtful consideration. A person should not delay specific planning for retirement until retirement is imminent but should integrate it throughout the adult years.

Special characteristics of late middle age

While many of the issues and characteristics described above continue to affect the years of late middle adulthood, some changes and special characteristics may become more prominent during the 50s and 60s. These individuals have an opportunity to define and integrate the emotional and intellectual growth of the earlier adulthood years. It may be a time of changes outside the family, thus giving the individual time and energy to develop new areas of interest. In the work world, although advancement is still possible, many have attained much or most of what they can. In certain areas, such as in law, business, government, religion, and community service, this period may include the prime years of activity. People in the late middle years occupy many of the highest positions in these areas. Within the family setting, spouses may be back to the couple stage, or fast approaching it, and must readjust to the contracted nuclear family or to life alone if a spouse should die. Grandparenting is a new role that is often acquired during this stage. Parents must reassess their relationships with their children and move from adult-child interactions to adult-adult interactions. Men may become more aware, less fearful, and more accepting of their tendencies to provide care and nurturance, whereas women may accept and develop more fully their assertiveness through an interest in business, politics, or other organizations and activities outside the home. The aging parents of 50- to 70-year-olds often require a great deal of emotional, physical, and/or financial assistance.

■ LATE ADULTHOOD: 65-70 TO 95+

As is the case with other stages of adulthood, the parameters of late adulthood and old age are not easy to determine. Some people seem old at 40, whereas others seem young at 65. Some gerontologists have attempted to deal with this situation by setting apart the years from 60 to 75 as early old age and the years after age 75 as late old age.

Later adulthood has become a subject of increasing interest because of longer life spans and declining death rates in Western society. The elderly are now the fastest-growing portion of the population. The larger numbers of the elderly and the changes that come with aging have created numerous challenges for individuals and for society as a whole. Institutional forms of care have been developed but have often proved unsatisfactory; major pieces of legislation have been passed on behalf of

figure**4.11** Late adulthood.

the elderly, but often this has not eased the passage of time and the financial, social, and emotional problems that develop. The emphasis in our society on youth and their culture, behavior, and attitudes is accompanied by a negative attitude toward those on the other end of the age continuum. This prejudice is known as "ageism," a negative attitude toward aging and discrimination based on age. This attitude characterizes the elderly as burdensome, sick, and senile. It is an indication of much anxiety about aging. This attitude is changing somewhat because the ever-increasing numbers of elderly are commanding more attention to the process of aging. It is often said that in this culture, everyone wants to live long but no one wishes to grow old. This is in marked contrast to other cultures, where old age is respected and even revered. Older adults are not a homogeneous group. Most people become more individualized as their years increase. Each individual's story, responses, and needs are unique.

Developmental Tasks

Late adulthood is similar to all other developmental stages in that individuals must be able to make certain adaptations and achieve certain developmental tasks. These tasks are different from earlier ones in that these are the final ones in life. Among the most significant developmental tasks in late adulthood are:

1. Maintaining and developing activities that enhance self-image, contribute to a sense of worth in society, and help to retain functional capacity
2. Developing new family roles as in-laws and grandparents

3. Accepting retirement and adjusting to reduced income
4. Adapting to changes in physical status and health
5. Adjusting to satisfactory living arrangements
6. Adapting to losses of spouse, other family members, and friends
7. Working on a life review
8. Preparing for one's own death

Physical Changes

Individuals age at different rates. How people age depends on a number of factors, including:

Personal attitude toward aging and life
Level of physical activity
Nutrition
Personal habits
Presence or absence of illness

Even in the absence of illness, some decline in physical function comes with advancing years. Usually this occurs gradually. Reaction times slow, and eyesight and hearing may diminish. In addition, older adults experience an increased incidence of chronic disease, less resistance to acute illnesses, and a slower recovery period. These physical changes produce an increase in use of the health care system.

Some older persons adjust to these changes with an attitude of acceptance and humor. Others become preoccupied with their discomforts and ailments.

Cognitive Changes

There are few predictable changes in intellectual function that accompany aging. No decrease in general knowledge occurs, and an increase in wisdom may come with advancing years. Speed in mental performance and in complex decision making may slow. Maintenance of mental function is affected by many factors, including:

Personal motivation
Interest in the subject
Sensory function, especially vision and hearing
Educational accomplishments
Recency of learning
Personal value on intellectual activity

Psychosocial Development

During the early part of late adulthood, the major life commitments to job and family are nearing completion. Ideally, planning for the next phase of life has been going on for many years. Most older adults have time and energy during the retirement years to further develop interests in many areas. The older adult has an opportunity to develop a new balance with others and society. It can be a time for creative endeavors.

Retirement

As both demands from work and family and living arrangements change somewhat with the onset of retire-

ment, time becomes more available for doing other things. As mentioned previously, advance planning for postretirement activities that enhance self-respect is crucial. Failure to plan can make the change come as a shock, and the hours may seem empty, heavy, or endless. If adults prepare, they can use the time to advantage for developing new careers, hobbies, sporting skills, or community activities. This productive use should enhance self-worth, a sense of usefulness, and functional capacity. Educational opportunities for adults of all ages are increasing. For the older adult, continuing education can provide an opportunity to learn again simply for the pleasure of learning or to develop another set of skills. Both physical and mental well-being depend on continuing involvement in, and contribution to, society.

If one or both elderly spouses have been employed, the marriage relationship is affected by retirement. The couple must adjust to having more shared time and to weaving their lives together effectively. A spouse may have, at least initially, a sense of the other person being more "underfoot" and of losing privacy. Couples can develop a more equal relationship with regard to household and leisure activities.

How a person reacts to retirement is related to the meaning and satisfaction the job held. Feelings of relief and release may be present if the job lacked personal meaning and satisfaction. If the job held much meaning and gave a person satisfaction and authority, the loss is more deeply felt and may lead to depression. In addition to the loss of a job, the retiree also feels the loss of work associates, and the social network and friendships they may have provided.

Retirement usually involves a financial change, typically a decrease in income. This change is difficult because it affects the person's lifestyle in the areas of daily living, home ownership and maintenance, socializing, entertainment, and travel.

New roles

New roles emerge for older adults as their children marry and have children of their own. Acceptance of their children's spouses into the family network is instrumental in the ongoing interaction of the family. Interaction with grandchildren can be a pleasant aspect of aging if it does not become too time-consuming or burdensome. Grandparents can provide a sense of family and history. Another role that may begin in an earlier phase of late adulthood is the caring for elderly parents who may be ill or dependent. One needs to reevaluate personal identity in light of these new roles.

Living arrangements

The older adult may need to change living arrangements for many reasons, including physical status and finances. This may mean giving up a home of many years, with all the comfort and memories that it holds. Some individuals are able to find more suitable arrangements in single homes; others may move in with adult children or to a retirement or nursing home. In our society, the extended family is no longer expected to take care of the elders in their own homes, so a move to a facility may be seen as necessary but not desirable. Such a move usually involves giving up some or many personal belongings and some loss of privacy. These moves can, however, also involve the positive aspects of more efficient accommodations and an increase in socialization with peers.

Losses

Many of the numerous changes that occur in late adulthood are felt as losses. These include employment status, income, deaths of significant people, and changes in physical strength and sensory acuity.

The loss of a job after many years of employment may be one of the greatest developmental and situational crises in an individual's life. As retirement incomes become relatively smaller in an inflationary era, lowered income becomes more of a loss. Homes, entertainment styles, and lifelong travel plans may have to be given up or diminished in scope to meet the costs of food, housing, and health care.

Other losses may include the deaths of friends, a spouse, or other family members. These losses are among the most difficult aspects of later adulthood. Coping with bereavement for the person with whom one has shared life experiences, memories, and plans leaves a great personal void. Ideally, the older adult experiences the profound emotions that accompany the loss and then goes on living and fostering the development of new relationships. This process requires time and patience. Serious illnesses and deaths of people who have been close during life are also a reminder that there is an unknown but limited amount of time left to live.

Older adults may also feel physical changes as losses. Physical strength, energy, and sensory acuity of the eyes and ears typically decline gradually over the years. By age 60, most people are aware of some physical decline, and most have at least one illness or limiting condition. The occurrence of one or more chronic health conditions may affect strength, energy, and self-image. The older adult faces challenges in accepting physical changes and limitations and in using energy most effectively.

Life review

The process of performing a life review is an important developmental task of later adulthood. The goal is to achieve a sense of integrity, acceptance, and wholeness in looking back on the life one has lived. Most older persons do spend some time reflecting on their accomplishments and failures, satisfactions, and disappointments in an effort to integrate and evaluate the di-

verse elements of their life so that they can reach a reasonably positive view of their life's worth. Failure to accomplish this task may lead to serious psychological problems. The life review process is far more than useless reminiscence. It allows for some gratification and also for revision in understanding and clarification of experiences that a person may have poorly understood or accepted when they occurred. It is an inventory that helps put past successes and failures into some perspective. If considered with others, particularly with the younger generation, this review can be mutually beneficial; it gives the older person a sense of usefulness and some credit for age and wisdom and can provide the younger person with a sense of family and history. Today's older Americans have lived through more changes than any other single group in human history.

This developmental task is well described by Erikson as the last ego stage: ego integrity versus despair. Successful consideration leads to the acceptance of one's life as the way it had to be, given the person, the choices, and the circumstances. The inability to come to terms with the life one lived can lead to negative feelings, such as despair, anger, resentment, and hopelessness. Life for most people is complex, so the life review is unlikely to be entirely "good" or "bad." For most, it involves some satisfactions and some disappointments. Some hopes and dreams are realized; some remain unfulfilled. The task is to accept what happened and to accept oneself.

Preparation for death

Preparation for one's own death, views on death, and the possibility of an afterlife are likely to evolve from the life review process. For many, considering the issue of their own death is important, and they want to prepare for it in terms of finishing their business or setting their affairs in order. This preparation takes many forms, including finalizing a will, achieving some goal, resolving some or many interpersonal relationships, and saying farewell to significant family members and friends. If the dying process is prolonged because of some chronic illness, the individual goes through several phases of dealing with eventual death. To die in a way as close as possible to what the individual desires may be thought of as life's final developmental task.

---

sample documentation & diagnoses   CRITICAL THINKING

■ FOCUSED HEALTH HISTORY (SUBJECTIVE DATA)

Ms. W., age 65, has come to the clinic for a periodic blood pressure check. States she is feeling fairly well physically but is experiencing bouts of sadness and loneliness due to her recent retirement from a career in international nursing for over 40 years. States she misses the demands of her job, the many colleagues she now sees less frequently, the travel opportunities, and, in general, the sense of meaning and purpose she had in life. States she was always so busy that she did not plan adequately for retirement and now regrets this. Still feels capable of doing many of the things she has done before, but recognizes that certain tasks do take a bit longer. Asks if she might be referred to a "retirement specialist." Is a single woman, never married, and has 2 siblings and numerous nieces and nephews, all of whom she enjoys, but she does not want to begin interfering in their lives. No recent significant weight loss or gain.

■ FOCUSED PHYSICAL EXAMINATION (OBJECTIVE DATA)

Vital signs: BP 134/82; pulse 66, regular.
Height 5 ft 5 in, weight 140 lb.
General appearance: Asian-American female who appears younger than stated age, in good health, and well nourished; neat appearance. Handshake is warm and strong; speech is clear and articulate. Affect is somewhat sad, although she is responsive, cooperative, and eager to discuss her life situation.

diagnoses

NURSING DIAGNOSES

Altered role performance related to retirement
Defining Characteristic
- Change in usual patterns of responsibilities

Social isolation
Defining Characteristics
- Verbalization of isolation from others
- Lack of contact with significant others
- Perceived inadequacy of significant purpose in life
- Less contact with peers

chapter

5

Nutritional Assessment

Nutrition is a key component in the maintenance of health and in the prevention or treatment of disease. Adequate nutrition provides the fuel and nutrients necessary to keep the body functioning in the optimum state, making it better able to fight off illness or recover from disease.

Less than optimum nutrition is of two main types: overnutrition and undernutrition. Overnutrition is the most common nutritional concern in the United States. Obesity and overweight are indicators of a state of overnutrition, which increases the risk of developing chronic diseases, including heart disease, cancer, hypertension, diabetes, and joint disease. Overnourished clients are also at higher risk for surgical complications, poor wound healing, and venous thrombosis (Detsky, Smalley, and Chang, 1994). Protein calorie malnutrition is a form of undernutrition characterized by too little lean body mass as a result of insufficient energy and/or protein being supplied to the body. Undernourished people, including those with protein calorie malnutrition, are at a higher risk for developing complications when undergoing treatment for illness or disease. Common complications in undernourished persons include poor wound healing, sepsis, abscess formation, and other infections such as pneumonia.

Identifying and addressing nutritional risk is important in all health care settings because of the potential to reduce the severity of a disease or shorten recovery time, leading to better patient outcomes and reduced health care costs. Nutritional screening is the process of identifying characteristics known to be associated with nutritional problems in order to pinpoint individuals who have a poor nutritional status or who are at nutritional risk. Nutritional screening includes the collection of relevant data on risk factors through the use of questionnaires or brief interviews. It can be completed in any setting (the hospital, a clinic waiting room, or a shopping mall or other public site), it facilitates early intervention, and it is cost-effective. For clients identified as having poor nutritional status, nutrition screening reveals the need for nutritional assessment, which is a more in-depth process that may require medical diagnosis and treatment, as well as nutrition counseling, as part of a health care plan (Foltz, Schiller, and Ryan, 1993).

Nutrition screening and assessment are part of a comprehensive approach to defining nutritional status that uses health, nutrition, and medication histories; physical examination; anthropometric measurements; and laboratory data. The clinician conducts a nutritional assessment to identify the presence, nature, and ex-

tent of impaired nutritional status of any type and to obtain the information needed to develop a nutrition care plan. The ideal approach to nutrition screening and assessment involves a health care team that includes a registered dietitian.

■ ELEMENTS OF NUTRITION SCREENING AND ASSESSMENT

The types of information that may be included in the nutrition screening and assessment include health and diet histories, laboratory measurements, and anthropometric measurements. Depending on the situation, part or all of this information may be collected and evaluated. For example, the albumin level, total lymphocyte count, and percentage of weight loss have been identified as the best combination of parameters to determine the risk of protein calorie malnutrition, so these elements would be recommended when undernutrition is suspected (Elmore et al., 1994). However, if the client being assessed is overweight and diabetes is suspected, the blood glucose level, body weight, and meal patterns from the diet history would be more important.

Histories

Histories help establish the context within which the nutritional assessment is taking place and might include a health history, medication history, and/or diet history.

Health history

Nutritional assessment requires a knowledge of the client's health history, since illnesses, symptoms, surgeries, and treatments can affect nutritional status and appropriate food choices. Include any weight gain or loss and any history of nausea, diarrhea, or change in appetite in the health history (Kushner et al., 1994). A menstrual history can be important for clients who are at risk for eating disorders, since irregular menses or amenorrhea may indicate that the client has been restricting food intake or participating in excessive exercise, and that further screening is needed.

Obtain the client's family history, since many diseases that have a nutritional component also have a genetic basis. A strong family history of heart disease would indicate that a careful look at the client's heart disease risk factors is warranted. Gather information on lifestyle habits, such as smoking, exercise, and eating out, since these factors can have a bearing on the client's nutritional status.

Medication history

Drugs can influence nutrient absorption, metabolism, or excretion; likewise, nutrients or foods may interact with drugs in the gastrointestinal tract or affect drug metabolism, action, or excretion. Drugs can also affect the appetite, which will affect the adequacy of the diet.

Assess the use of vitamin, mineral, and other nutrient supplements. Supplements may be required to correct nutrient deficiencies, to prevent deficiencies in situations where food intake is limited, or to reduce the risk of disease. Excessive vitamin supplementation is especially common in the elderly and can interfere with the action of medications. Generally, supplements equal to or less than the Recommended Dietary Allowances (RDAs) are not harmful. Supplements containing several times the RDAs for vitamins or minerals are called megadoses and are often promoted commercially, even though scientific evidence of merit is lacking. Inform clients that megadoses of the fat-soluble vitamins A and D are harmful because they accumulate in the body. Most water-soluble vitamins (the B vitamins and vitamin C) do not accumulate in the body, but there have been reports of toxicity from the use of megadoses of vitamin B_6, and vitamin C in very large doses can increase the risk of kidney stones. Advise clients to approach the use of any megadoses of vitamins and minerals with caution.

Diet history

A diet history includes data about the client's usual food and fluid intake, eating patterns and habits, food preferences and restrictions, problems with eating, and food buying and preparation habits. Information on food choices should include the type and amount of foods eaten. Usual eating patterns and habits include the number and timing of meals and snacks typically eaten, the setting of meals eaten at home (e.g., eaten alone or with other family members), and the frequency and location of meals eaten out. Ask clients about food preferences in order to make reasonable and practical recommendations to the client. Food restrictions may include religious or cultural dietary restrictions, as well as food allergies or intolerances. Problems with eating may involve chewing or swallowing, as well as difficulty cutting or mashing foods because of arthritis or other problems. Ask the client who is responsible for food purchases and find out about financial limitations affecting food selection. Pertinent information regarding food preparation includes the person responsible, the availability of refrigeration and cooking facilities, typical methods used, and the receptivity of the preparer to suggestions for change.

Food intake can be assessed by several methods. The best method depends on the purpose of the assessment, the situation in which the assessment is being conducted, the person conducting the assessment, and the target population for the assessment. Diet histories may be conducted to screen for deficiencies or excesses in the diet, or they may be used to establish a baseline for behavior change counseling with the client. Because food

is a very personal issue and one that can easily elicit feelings of guilt or defensiveness, avoid judgment or criticism in the interview and all subsequent interactions with the client.

Diet recall. The most common type of diet history conducted is the 24-hour recall, or 24-hour diet history. When using this method, ask the client to recall or list everything he or she had to eat and drink on the previous day or to list what the client eats and drinks on a typical day. Begin by asking, "What was the first thing you had to eat or drink yesterday?" or "What is the first thing you usually have to eat or drink?" After the initial response from the client, guide the diet history by asking, "What was the next thing that you had to eat or drink yesterday?" When the recall process is complete, review the day's intake with the client, requesting more detail on serving size, preparation method, and time and location of each meal and snack, as needed.

The advantages of the 24-hour recall method of dietary assessment include the ease of administration, the accuracy from one interviewer to the next, the minimum time requirement, and the ease of client participation. The major disadvantage of this method is that it is not truly representative, because it assesses only 1 day's intake and does not reflect differences from weekend to weekday or from season to season. The recall method relies on memory, so it may not be accurate in groups of people with memory limitations, such as the elderly. Research has shown that clients tend to exhibit some selective memory, so liquids, high-calorie snacks, alcohol, and added fats tend to be underreported. It has also been documented that obese persons substantially underreport their calorie intake (Heitmann and Lissner, 1995).

Food records. Food records are another method of collecting a diet history. When using this approach, ask the client to record his or her intake for a number of days—usually 3 days. Give the client blank forms on which to keep the records, and advise the client to record amounts of food and beverages, preparation methods, and times when meals and snacks are eaten. Clarify the recorded information, as necessary, when the client has completed the food records and returned them to you.

The advantages of food records include a small time investment by the interviewer and a more representative view of the client's diet because more days are included. In addition, the process of keeping food records increases clients' awareness of their food choices and helps them review their dietary habits. The disadvantages of food records include the requirement that clients be literate, a larger time investment by clients, the tendency of clients to optimize their diet during the period of recording, and the delay in collecting the dietary information.

Food frequency. A third method of obtaining a diet history is the food frequency assessment. This assessment usually takes the form of a questionnaire that asks the client to indicate how often, or with what frequency, certain foods have been eaten in the last 6 months. For example, the questionnaire might list ½ cup ice cream and ask the client to indicate whether it is eaten three or more times a week, one or two times a week, less than once a week, or never eaten.

The advantages of the food frequency method include the facts that an interviewer is not required, it is quick to complete, and it provides a view of dietary habits over a longer period of time. In addition, it is possible to design the food frequency assessment so that a score can be calculated as an indication of dietary quality. Disadvantages of the food frequency method include the inability to assess patterns of food intake (number and timing of meals), the need to design a questionnaire that includes questions pertinent to the client population being surveyed, and the difficulty that some clients have completing the form.

A targeted food frequency assessment can be designed and effectively used in specific populations of clients. For example, if clients with heart disease are being interviewed, the food frequency assessment should include significant detail about the type of milk, cheese, meat, and added fats included in the diet, with less emphasis on the type of vegetables or grain products. However, if the population is elderly women at risk of osteoporosis, the food frequency assessment should contain more detail on calcium and vitamin D sources in the diet (milk products, green leafy vegetables, fortified foods).

An approach to dietary assessment that is useful in clinical practice is a combination food record and food frequency assessment. Clients are asked to keep food records for 2 or 3 days and to complete an abbreviated food frequency questionnaire. The detail of the food record is maintained, and the food frequency questionnaire provides information on long-term eating patterns.

Portion-estimate tools are helpful in clarifying serving sizes or recommended amounts with a client. Plastic food models are one type of portion-estimate tool available in many patient education catalogs. Each model represents a specified amount of a particular food and can be shown to a client while the interviewer asks, "How did your serving compare with this?" If food models are not available, a set of measuring cups and spoons and several different sizes of bowls and plates can be beneficial in estimating quantities.

Assessing the diet history. Once the diet history has been collected, it needs to be assessed for adequacy. The Food Guide Pyramid, designed by the U.S. Department of Agriculture, provides a simplified approach

What Counts as One Serving?*

BREADS, CEREALS, RICE, AND PASTA
1 slice of bread
½ cup of cooked rice or pasta
½ cup of cooked cereal
1 oz of ready-to-eat cereal

VEGETABLES
½ cup of chopped raw or cooked vegetables
1 cup of leafy raw vegetables

FRUITS
1 piece of fruit or melon wedge
¾ cup of juice
½ cup of canned fruit
¼ cup of dried fruit

MILK, YOGURT, AND CHEESE
1 cup of milk or yogurt
1½ to 2 oz of cheese

MEAT, POULTRY, FISH, DRY BEANS, EGGS, AND NUTS
2½ to 3 oz of cooked lean meat, poultry, or fish
Count ½ cup of cooked beans, or 1 egg, or 2 tbsp of peanut butter as 1 oz of lean meat (about ⅓ serving)

FATS, OILS, AND SWEETS
Limit calories from these, especially if you need to lose weight

Modified from the *Food Guide Pyramid*, Home and Garden Bulletin No 252, US Department of Agriculture, Human Nutrition Information Service.
*The amount you eat may be more than one serving. For example, a dinner portion of spaghetti would count as two or three servings of pasta.

---

table 5.1   How Many Servings Do You Need Each Day?

	Women, some older adults	Children, teenage girls, active women, most men	Teenage boys, active men
Calorie level*	About 1600	About 2200	About 2800
Bread group	6	9	11
Vegetable group	3	4	5
Fruit group	2	3	4
Milk group	2-3[†]	2-3[†]	2-3[†]
Meat group	2, for a total of 5 oz	2, for a total of 6 oz	3 for a total of 7 oz

Modified from the *Food Guide Pyramid*, Home and Garden Bulletin No 252, US Department of Agriculture, Human Nutrition Information Service.
*These are the calorie levels if you choose low-fat, lean foods from the five major food groups and use foods from the fats, oils, and sweets group sparingly.
[†]Women who are pregnant or breast-feeding, teenagers, and young adults to age 24 need 3 servings.

---

to assessing dietary adequacy (Figure 5.1). The Food Guide Pyramid divides foods into six basic categories:

1. Bread, cereal, rice, and pasta group
2. Fruit group
3. Vegetable group
4. Meat, poultry, fish, dry beans, eggs, and nuts group
5. Milk, yogurt, and cheese group
6. Fats, oils, and sweets

A range of recommended servings is listed for each of the five food groups to represent nutritionally adequate diets for adults and children at three different calorie levels (Table 5.1). The Food Group Pyramid includes a section that describes the size of servings in each of the groups (see box above).

To analyze a diet recall or food record using the Food Guide Pyramid, count the number of servings from each group on the recall or record and compare them with the recommendations on the Food Guide Pyramid. If the number of servings from each group on the diet history meets or exceeds the minimum number of servings recommended from each of the five food groups on the pyramid, the client's diet can be considered nutritionally adequate. A form listing the food groups and recommended number of servings with spaces to fill in the client's servings from each group can be a valuable teaching tool to use with this method of assessment (see box on p. 107). In summarizing the nutritional adequacy of the diet, emphasize to the client that the diet recall addresses only 1 day of the client's intake and does not provide a representative view of the whole diet.

A diet history can also be evaluated using the RDAs, comparing the nutrient content of the client's diet with the recommendations established by the National Research Council of the National Academy of Sciences (Table 5.2). Because the RDAs are designed to meet or exceed the nutritional needs of 95% of the population, a diet is not considered deficient in a nutrient unless the intake of that nutrient consistently falls below two thirds of the RDA values.

The nutrient content of the food record can be analyzed using nutrient composition handbooks (Pennington, 1989), but it is tedious to analyze any more than

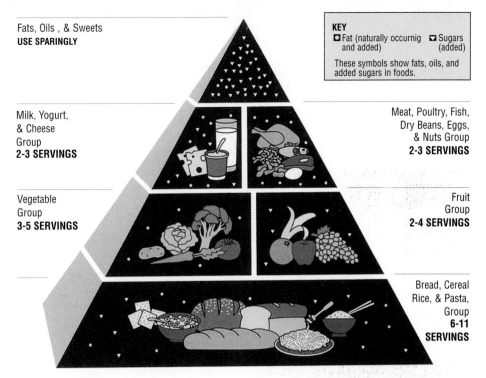

Fats, Oils , & Sweets
USE SPARINGLY

KEY
☐ Fat (naturally occurnig and added)   ☐ Sugars (added)
These symbols show fats, oils, and added sugars in foods.

Milk, Yogurt,
& Cheese
Group
2-3 SERVINGS

Meat, Poultry, Fish,
Dry Beans, Eggs,
& Nuts Group
2-3 SERVINGS

Vegetable
Group
3-5 SERVINGS

Fruit
Group
2-4 SERVINGS

Bread, Cereal
Rice, & Pasta,
Group
**6-11
SERVINGS**

figure **5.1**   Food Guide Pyramid. *(From U.S. Department of Agriculture and U.S. Department of Health and Human Services.)*

Nutrition Prescription

Client's name _____ Date _____

	Bread-cereal	Vegetable	Fruit	Dairy	Meat
Recommended daily servings	6-11	3-5	2-4	2-3	2-3
Your daily servings	_____	_____	_____	_____	_____
Suggested change (+ or −)	_____	_____	_____	_____	_____

PRESCRIPTION FOR DIETARY CHANGES

_____ Eat more foods from the bread, cereal, rice, and pasta group.

_____ Eat more vegetables.

_____ Eat more fruit.

_____ Consume more dairy foods.

_____ Eat more foods from the meat, poultry, fish, dry beans, eggs, and nuts group.

_____ Use low-fat or fat-free dairy products.

_____ Use lean meats, remove poultry skin, and broil or bake meats.

_____ Eat smaller quantities of meat and poultry.

_____ Eat fewer egg yolks (maximum 4 yolks per week).

_____ Use less of added fats (margarine, butter, salad dressing, mayonnaise) or use light varieties of these foods.

_____ Have smaller amounts of desserts or have them less often.

_____ Use fruits, vegetables, or low-fat crackers as snacks.

_____ Reduce intake of sweetened beverages (soda, fruit juices).

_____ Consume less alcohol.

_____ Use less salt and eat smaller amounts of salty foods.

_____ Consume more fluids.

Comments:

Clinician's signature _____

| table 5.2 | *Recommended Dietary Allowances*[a] |

Designed for the maintenance of good nutrition of practically all healthy people in the United States

Category	Age (years) or condition	Weight[b] (kg)	Weight[b] (lb)	Height[b] (cm)	Height[b] (in)	Protein (g)	Fat-soluble vitamins Vitamin A (µg RE)[c]	Vitamin D (µg)[d]	Vitamin E (mg α-TE)[e]	Vitamin K (µg)
Infants	0.0–0.5	6	13	60	24	13	375	7.5	3	5
	0.5–1.0	9	20	71	28	14	375	10	4	10
Children	1–3	13	29	90	35	16	400	10	6	15
	4–6	20	44	112	44	24	500	10	7	20
	7–10	28	62	132	52	28	700	10	7	30
Males	11–14	45	99	157	62	45	1000	10	10	45
	15–18	66	145	176	69	59	1000	10	10	65
	19–24	72	160	177	70	58	1000	10	10	70
	25–50	79	174	176	70	63	1000	5	10	80
	51+	77	170	173	68	63	1000	5	10	80
Females	11–14	46	101	157	62	46	800	10	8	45
	15–18	55	120	163	64	44	800	10	8	55
	19–24	58	128	164	65	46	800	10	8	60
	25–50	63	138	163	64	50	800	5	8	65
	51+	65	143	160	63	50	800	5	8	65
Pregnant						60	800	10	10	65
Lactating	1st 6 months					65	1300	10	12	65
	2nd 6 months					62	1200	10	11	65

From *Recommended Dietary Allowances,* Revised 1989, Food and Nutrition Board, National Academy of Sciences—National Research Council, Washington, DC.

[a]The allowances, expressed as average daily intakes over time, are intended to provide for individual variations among most normal persons as they live in the United States under usual environmental stresses. Diets should be based on a variety of common foods in order to provide other nutrients for which human requirements have been less well defined.

[b]Weights and heights of Reference Adults are actual medians for the U.S. population of the designated age, as reported by NHANES II. The use of these figures does not imply that the height-to-weight ratios are ideal.

one or two nutrients manually. Computer programs provide the opportunity to analyze the nutrient content of a diet record quickly and completely. Many types of programs are available, with varying abilities and costs. Programs may analyze as few as 10 or as many as 50 nutrients, and they present the analysis in a variety of ways. The analysis is usually a list of the nutrient content of the day's food, often combined with the RDA percentage for each nutrient. Some programs may present this information in a bar graph or may rank or sort foods based on their nutrient content. Some programs, such as Nutritionist IV Diet Analysis and Nutrition Evaluation (1993), translate a diet record into number of servings from the Food Guide Pyramid, comparing the client's intake with the recommendations graphically.

Computerized dietary analysis is a time-saver when compared with manual analysis, but computer programs have some disadvantages. First, programs are expensive and are not always necessary. In many situations an

analysis of a diet record using the Food Guide Pyramid is adequate and effective. Second, the information obtained from a nutritional analysis program may be given too much weight because it comes from a computer. Clients may become overly concerned because a 1–day analysis of their diet shows nutrient deficiencies, or they may become too confident because the analysis shows an acceptable, but lower than usual, intake of fat or sodium. The computer analysis is only as good as the data on which it is based, and it will not be representative if it is based on only 1 day. Finally, the accuracy of the analysis is dependent on the accuracy of the database, and some analysis programs have a limited nutrient database (Underbakke, 1989).

Another method of analyzing a dietary assessment is the scoring of the food frequency assessment. Many validated food frequency assessments offer the option of scoring the completed food frequency assessment. The score indicates how close to a set of established dietary

Water-soluble vitamins							Minerals						
Vitamin C (mg)	Thiamin (mg)	Riboflavin (mg)	Niacin (mg NE)[f]	Vitamin B_6 (mg)	Folate (µg)	Vitamin B_{12} (µg)	Calcium (mg)	Phosphorus (mg)	Magnesium (mg)	Iron (mg)	Zinc (mg)	Iodine (µg)	Selenium (µg)
30	0.3	0.4	5	0.3	25	0.3	400	300	40	6	5	40	10
35	0.4	0.5	6	0.6	35	0.5	600	500	60	10	5	50	15
40	0.7	0.8	9	1.0	50	0.7	800	800	80	10	10	70	20
45	0.9	1.1	12	1.1	75	1.0	800	800	120	10	10	90	20
45	1.0	1.2	13	1.4	100	1.4	800	800	170	10	10	120	30
50	1.3	1.5	17	1.7	150	2.0	1200	1200	270	12	15	150	40
60	1.5	1.8	20	2.0	200	2.0	1200	1200	400	12	15	150	50
60	1.5	1.7	19	2.0	200	2.0	1200	1200	350	10	15	150	70
60	1.5	1.7	19	2.0	200	2.0	800	800	350	10	15	150	70
60	1.2	1.4	15	2.0	200	2.0	800	800	350	10	15	180	70
50	1.1	1.3	15	1.4	150	2.0	1200	1200	280	15	12	150	45
60	1.1	1.3	15	1.5	180	2.0	1200	1200	300	15	12	150	50
60	1.1	1.3	15	1.6	180	2.0	1200	1200	280	15	12	150	55
60	1.1	1.3	15	1.6	180	2.0	800	800	280	15	12	150	55
60	1.0	1.2	13	1.6	180	2.0	800	800	280	10	12	150	55
70	1.5	1.6	17	2.2	400	2.2	1200	1200	300	30	15	175	65
95	1.6	1.8	20	2.1	280	2.6	1200	1200	355	15	19	200	75
90	1.6	1.7	20	2.1	260	2.6	1200	1200	340	15	16	200	75

[c]Retinol equivalents. 1 retinol equivalent = 1 µg retinol or 6 µg β-carotene.
[d]As cholecalciferol. 10 µg cholecalciferol = 400 IU of vitamin D.
[e]α-Tocopherol equivalents. 1 mg d-α tocopherol = 1 α-TE.
[f]1 NE (niacin equivalent) is equal to 1 mg of niacin or 60 mg of dietary tryptophan.

recommendations the results of the food frequency assessment are.

Anthropometric Measurement

Anthropometric measurement is the measurement of the size, weight, and proportions of the human body. The purpose of anthropometric measurement is to assess growth and body composition by comparing current measurements with previous measurements obtained for an individual or by comparing current measurements with standardized measurements for clients of similar age and status.

The most common measurements taken are height and weight. Additional measurements that may be taken include skinfold thickness and circumference of various body parts, including the head, chest, arm, waist, and hip. Standardization of equipment and methods is essential to provide accurate results that can be interpreted meaningfully.

Height

Height is recorded in inches or centimeters. In adults and older children, measure height by having the client stand erect, without shoes, against a flat, vertical measuring surface. Measure height on the line where the crown of the head intersects the height scale. For clients who are unable to stand for a height measurement because of mobility impairment or handicap, equations have been developed to predict height from knee height measurement (Chumlea, Guo, and Steinbaugh, 1994).

Weight

Weight is recorded in pounds or kilograms. When serial weights are taken, weigh the client at approximately the same time of day, with similar clothing, to allow an accurate comparison. In clinical settings the preferred instrument for measuring weight is the balance beam scale. For ambulatory clients, weight is determined as they stand on the scale, with minimal clothing and no

| table 5.3 | *1983 Metropolitan Life Table** | | | | | | | | |

	Men					Women			
Height		Small frame	Medium frame	Large frame	Height		Small frame	Medium frame	Large frame
Feet	Inches				Feet	Inches			
5	2	128-134	131-141	138-150	4	10	102-111	109-121	118-131
5	3	130-136	133-143	140-153	4	11	103-113	111-123	120-134
5	4	132-138	135-145	142-156	5	0	104-115	113-126	122-137
5	5	134-140	137-148	144-160	5	1	106-118	115-129	125-140
5	6	136-142	139-151	146-164	5	2	108-121	118-132	128-143
5	7	138-145	142-154	149-168	5	3	111-124	121-135	131-147
5	8	140-148	145-157	152-172	5	4	114-127	124-138	134-151
5	9	142-151	148-160	155-176	5	5	117-130	127-141	137-155
5	10	144-154	151-163	158-180	5	6	120-133	130-144	140-159
5	11	146-157	154-166	161-184	5	7	123-136	133-147	143-163
6	0	149-160	157-170	164-188	5	8	126-139	133-150	146-167
6	1	152-164	160-174	168-192	5	9	129-142	139-153	149-170
6	2	155-168	164-178	172-197	5	10	132-145	142-156	152-173
6	3	158-172	167-182	176-202	5	11	135-148	145-159	155-176
6	4	162-176	171-187	181-207	6	0	138-151	148-162	158-179

From Society of Actuaries, Build Study, 1979, Chicago, 1980, Society of Actuaries and Association of Life Insurance Medical Directors of America, Metropolitan Life Insurance Co., New York, 1983. Courtesy *Statistical Bulletin,* Metropolitan Life Insurance, New York.
*Weight in pounds at ages 29 to 59 years according to build. In shoes and 3 pounds of indoor clothing for women and 5 pounds for men.

shoes. Special platform scales that accommodate wheel chairs are available. The client should transfer out of the wheel chair so that the chair can be weighed separately. Then the client returns to the chair, and both are weighed. The client's weight is the total weight minus the weight of the chair.

Standards for weight are available in the Metropolitan Height and Weight Tables, published first in 1959 and revised in 1983 (Table 5.3). Because the 1983 tables describe higher weight ranges for all heights than do the 1959 tables, it has been suggested that use of the 1983 tables endorses the U.S. population trends toward higher rates of obesity. In general, the tables are simply a reference point and should be only one factor used in determining a "healthy" or "goal" weight for a client. Past weight history, other risk factors for disease, and distribution of body weight should also be considered.

A simple formula can also be used to provide an estimate of appropriate weight for height. For adult women, count 100 pounds for the first 5 feet of height and add 5 pounds for each inch of height above five feet. For adult men, count 106 pounds for the first 5 feet of height and add 6 pounds for each inch of height above five feet. For both men and women, allow a range of 10% over and 10% under the calculated weight value.

The measurement of height and weight and the as-

sessment of growth for infants and very young children are discussed in Chapter 25.

Body mass index

The body mass index (BMI) is an assessment of body weight and height that can be helpful in determining the degree to which obesity or overweight is contributing to the risk of disease. The BMI shows a direct and continuous relationship to morbidity and mortality in studies of large populations. The formula for the BMI is weight in kilograms divided by height in meters squared. A nomogram that can be used to quickly estimate the BMI is presented in Figure 5.2. Classifications of obesity based on the BMI are presented in Table 5.4.

Body weight usually varies less than ¼ pound per day in healthy adults. A loss of weight of more than 1 pound per day indicates either negative energy or water balance or a combination of the two (Heymsfield, Tighe, and Wang, 1994). The percentage of weight change is a helpful indicator of the degree of change and is calculated as follows:

$$\frac{\text{Usual weight} - \text{Actual weight}}{\text{Usual weight}} \times 100$$

A weight change of 5% in the past 6 months is considered small for generally healthy clients. A weight loss

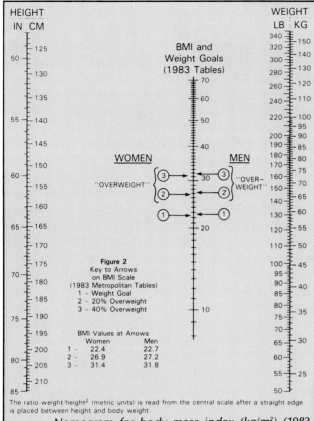

HEIGHT IN CM

WEIGHT LB | KG

BMI and
Weight Goals
(1983 Tables)

WOMEN   MEN

"OVERWEIGHT"   "OVER-WEIGHT"

Figure 2
Key to Arrows
on BMI Scale
(1983 Metropolitan Tables)
1 - Weight Goal
2 - 20% Overweight
3 - 40% Overweight

BMI Values at Arrows

	Women	Men
1 -	22.4	22.7
2 -	26.9	27.2
3 -	31.4	31.8

The ratio weight/height² (metric units) is read from the central scale after a straight edge is placed between height and body weight.

Nomogram for body mass index (kg/m²) (1983 Metropolitan Life Insurance Co. tables   Weights and heights are without clothing. With clothes, add 5 lb (2.3 kg) for men or 3 lb for women, and 1 in. (2.5 cm) in height for shoes.

figure **5.2**   Nomogram for body mass index (kg/m²) 1983 Metropolitan Life Insurance Company tables. Weights and heights are without clothing. With clothes add 5 pounds (2.3 kg) for men or 3 pounds (1.4 kg) for women and 1 inch (2.5 cm) in height for shoes. *(From Burton BT, Foster WR: Health implications of obesity: an NIH consensus development conference,* J Am Diet Assoc 85(9):1117-1121, 1985.)

between 5% and 10% is considered potentially significant for undernutrition, whereas any change of weight greater than 10% over 6 months is significant and warrants further investigation. Note the pattern, as well as the magnitude, of weight loss. Patients may be well nourished despite significant weight loss if there has been a recent stabilization in weight. Ask about weights 1 year ago, 6 months ago, 1 month ago, and at the present time to provide a good picture of the weight pattern.

Weight-change patterns are especially important in clients who may be at risk of eating disorders. Ask about the lowest and highest weights in the past year to provide a helpful picture of the variation that the client has experienced.

table **5.4**   *Classification of Obesity in Adults*

Degree of obesity	% Higher than ideal body weight	Body mass index*	Degree of medical risk
None	<20	20-24	None
Mild	20-40	25-29	Low
Moderate	40-100	30-39	Moderate to high
Severe or morbid	>100 (or >45 kg higher than ideal body weight)	>40	Very high

From Yanovski SV: A practical approach to treatment of the obese patient, *Arch Fam Med* 2:309–316, 1993.
*To calculate body mass index, divide weight in kilograms by height in meters squared.

Body composition

Body weight does not allow assessment of variations in body composition (i.e., the proportion of fat versus muscle mass). Skinfold thickness is one way of assessing body composition, although these measurements are inaccurate in very obese people. For accurate measurement of skinfold thickness, a properly calibrated skinfold calipers and careful technique are required. Reproducibility of skinfold measurements is poor when measurers are untrained or conduct the measurements infrequently. If skinfold measures are required in a clinical setting, have one trained individual conduct the measurements for best results.

The triceps skinfold measurement is most commonly used for screening and assessment for malnutrition (Figure 5.3). Using the nondominant arm, have the client let the arm hang loosely at the side, and determine the point that is halfway between the shoulder and the elbow. Holding the calipers in the right hand, grasp a fold of skin at the midpoint, parallel to the long axis, and pull it away from the underlying muscle. Gently measure the fold with the calipers, and then release and repeat the entire process twice. Take the average of the three measurements for assessment purposes. Tables 5.5 and 5.6 provide norms for triceps skinfold measurements.

Total body composition is most accurately assessed using underwater weighing, but this technique is not available or practical in many clinical settings. Bioelectrical impedance is another technique to estimate body composition that requires special equipment. This method involves the use of electrodes attached to the

figure**5.3** **A,** Measuring triceps skinfold with calipers. **B,** Cross section of arm.

table**5.5** Triceps Skinfold (mm), Males			
	Percentile		
Age (yr)	50th	15th	5th
18-19	8.5	6.0	4.5
20-24	10.0	6.0	4.0
25-34	12.0	6.0	4.5
35-44	12.0	7.0	5.0
45-54	11.0	7.0	5.0
55-64	11.0	6.5	5.0
65-74	11.0	6.5	4.5

Basic data on anthropometric measurements and angular measurements of the hip and knee joints for selected age groups 1-74 years of age, United States, 1971-1975. *National Health Survey,* Vital and Health Statistics Series No 219, US Dept of Health and Human Services, Public Health Service, 1981, pp 20, 26. Reprinted with permission of Ross Laboratories, Columbus, OH 43216, from Nutritional Assessment Summary Sheet G636, © 1987, Ross Laboratories.

table**5.6** Triceps Skinfold (mm), Females			
	Percentile		
Age (yr)	50th	15th	5th
18-19	17.5	12.0	9.0
20-24	18.0	12.0	10.0
25-34	21.0	13.5	10.5
35-44	23.0	16.0	12.0
45-54	25.0	17.0	13.0
55-64	25.0	16.0	11.0
65-74	23.0	16.0	11.5

Basic data on anthropometric measurements and angular measurements of the hip and knee joints for selected age groups 1-74 years of age, United States, 1971-1975. *National Health Survey,* Vital and Health Statistics Series No 219, US Dept of Health and Human Services, Public Health Service, 1981, pp 20, 26. Reprinted with permission of Ross Laboratories, Columbus, OH 43216, from Nutritional Assessment Summary Sheet G636, © 1987, Ross Laboratories.

wrist and the ankle so that a weak current is transmitted and the resistance, or impedance, can be measured. A formula is used to translate the measurement into an estimate of body fat composition.

Skinfold measurements at several locations on the body can be used to estimate total body fat using established formulas to yield a percentage of body fat. These measurements need to be conducted by a well-trained and experienced person in order to be accurate.

Body proportion

The accumulation of fat in different locations on the body presents different degrees of risk. Accumulation of abdominal fat is associated with a much greater risk of chronic disease than accumulation of fat on the hips or legs. In lay terms, the "apple" shape is a greater risk than the "pear" shape. In addition, visceral abdominal fat, the fat accumulating inside the abdominal cavity, carries a much higher risk of chronic disease than does subcutaneous abdominal fat.

The waist/hip ratio is associated with risk in many chronic diseases and is a practical approach to assessment of body proportion. This assessment requires measurement of the waist and hip circumferences and calculation of the waist/hip ratio. A description of the technique to make these measurements is found in the box below. A waist/hip ratio of 1 or lower for men and 0.8 or lower for women is reasonable. A higher value indicates increased health risk.

Circumference measurements are sometimes used as part of the nutritional assessment process. Head and chest circumferences are often used to assess growth and development of infants. Mid-arm and mid-arm muscle circumferences are usually used in the assessment of malnutrition. Circumferences of the chest, waist, hips, and thighs are sometimes used in assessing weight-loss progress and are especially helpful when clients are participating in an exercise program that can increase muscle mass and decrease body fat, without weight loss registering on the scale. Measurement of mid-arm muscle circumference is illustrated in Figure 5.4.

Laboratory Measurements

Laboratory measurements are used to assess nutritional status in conjunction with anthropometric measurements and the health and diet histories. Biochemical measurements commonly used to identify cases of undernutrition include serum albumin, total lymphocyte count (TLC), hemoglobin, and hematocrit values. Fasting blood glucose, serum cholesterol, serum triglyceride, serum low-density lipoprotein, and serum high-density lipoprotein values can be helpful in identifying overnutrition (Council on Practice Quality Management Committee, 1994).

Low serum albumin levels are an indication of protein calorie malnutrition and are associated with higher morbidity and mortality. Hospitalized clients with lower albumin levels tend to stay in the hospital longer and are

---

Accurate Measurement of Waist/Hip Ratio

1. Locate the waist. The waist is defined as the smallest circumference of the torso and is not necessarily at the umbilicus. In obese clients a narrowing at the waist may not be present, and the "waist" should then be defined as the smallest horizontal circumference between the 12th rib and the iliac crest. In obese clients it is often easier to have the client locate the 12th rib.
2. Measure the waist.
   - The client should have no clothing at the waist.
   - The client should be standing with the abdomen relaxed, arms at sides, and feet together.
   - Place a flexible, nonstretchable tape measure horizontally at the waist; do not compress the skin.
   - Measure.
3. Locate the hip (buttocks). The hip is defined as the level of the maximum extension of the buttocks posteriorly. In obese clients the anterior ab-

dominal wall may sag and, by default, have to be included in the measurement.

4. Measure the hip.
   - The client should be wearing only underwear.
   - The client should stand tall but relaxed, with arms at sides.
   - The practitioner should kneel or squat so as to be at eye level laterally with the buttocks.
   - Place a flexible, nonstretchable tape measure horizontally around the buttocks at the point of maximum circumference; do not compress the skin.
   - Measure.
5. Calculate the waist/hip ratio. Divide the waist circumference by the hip circumference. A waist/hip ratio of 1 or lower in men or 0.8 or lower in women is acceptable. Higher ratios indicate increased health risk.

figure**5.4** Measurement of mid–upper arm circumference. *(From Seidel HM et al: Mosby's guide to physical examination, ed 3, St Louis, 1995, Mosby.)*

so it has to be ordered separately. A normal value for the TLC is 1500 to 3000/mm³.

Hemoglobin and hematocrit values are indicators of anemia, and in cases of severe protein malnutrition, the hemoglobin value can be an indicator of protein status. The hematocrit value, also called packed-cell volume, measures the percentage of a blood sample occupied by red blood cells. A low hematocrit value may indicate deficient intakes of iron, vitamin B_{12}, vitamin B_6 (pyridoxine), or folate; chronic blood loss; or overhydration. Increased hematocrit values occur in dehydration, chronic anoxia, and polycythemia.

The fasting blood glucose level is used when screening for the presence of diabetes or glucose intolerance. Glucose levels in the blood are elevated when insulin secreted by the pancreas is insufficient or when an insulin resistance is present in the peripheral tissues. Because glucose levels are altered by a calorie-containing food or beverage, glucose levels must be tested when the patient is fasting (nothing but calorie-free beverages for 8 to 12 hours before the test). A normal value for the fasting blood glucose level is 80 to 120 mg/dl.

Serum lipid levels, including total cholesterol (TCHOL), triglyceride (TG), low-density lipoprotein (LDL), and high-density lipoprotein (HDL) levels, are important determinants of risk factors for coronary heart disease. Elevations of TCHOL, TG, and LDL levels increase the risk of developing atherosclerosis, whereas elevated HDL levels reduce that risk. All adults, as well as children from families at high risk for heart disease, should have a TCHOL test. If the test results fall within normal limits (Table 5.7) and the client has no other risk factors for heart disease (hypertension, smoking, diabetes, family history, or obesity), the TCHOL test does not need to be repeated for 5 years. If the TCHOL level is not normal, or if there are other risk factors present, a lipoprotein panel including TCHOL, TG, HDL, and calculated LDL is recommended. Because serum lipid levels are affected by acute viral illnesses, pregnancy, cancer, and surgery or other trauma (including myocardial infarctions), tests taken during these times may not provide valid results.

more likely to have complications and be readmitted. Low serum albumin levels are associated with inadequate intakes of protein, poor wound healing, and impaired function of the immune system. Serum albumin is available on most laboratory screening panels, which makes it a practical assessment tool. Normal serum albumin levels are 4.0 to 5.5 g/dl. A level under 3.4 g/dl warrants further investigation, and a level below 2.5 g/dl indicates severe protein depletion.

The TLC is used to assess the immune function of the body. Certain nutrient deficiencies and other forms of malnutrition can depress the immune system, leading to a lower lymphocyte count. Conditions other than malnutrition that can reduce the lymphocyte count include viral infections (including acquired immunodeficiency syndrome) and certain medications. The TLC can be increased above normal levels in bacterial infection, sepsis, tuberculosis, and chronic leukemia. The TLC is not usually part of laboratory screening panels,

table 5.7 **Optimum Lipoprotein Levels**		
	Primary prevention— adults without atherosclerosis	Secondary prevention— adults with atherosclerosis	Children and adolescents
LDL cholesterol	<130 mg/dl	<100 mg/dl	<110 mg/dl
Total cholesterol	<200 mg/dl	<160 mg/dl	<170 mg/dl
Triglycerides	<200 mg/dl	<200 mg/dl	<150 mg/dl
HDL	>35 mg/dl	>35 mg/dl	>35 mg/dl

From Taylor R: *Family medicine: principles and practice,* ed 5, New York, 1997, Springer-Verlag.

■ NUTRITION SCREENING AND ASSESSMENT FOR SPECIFIC CLIENT POPULATIONS

This chapter has outlined the data collection that may be a part of nutrition screening and assessment, but the specific elements used in a client interaction will vary depending on several factors. If a client has a diagnosed disease, the nutritional assessment should target issues specific to that disease state and should evaluate whether the client is adhering to appropriate therapy. The following section summarizes important elements to consider in specific client populations at various life stages or with certain chronic diseases.

Healthy Adults and Children

While it may seem that healthy adults and children do not need nutrition screening and assessment, all persons can benefit from a brief review of their eating habits using a general guide such as the Food Guide Pyramid. A healthy person may be eating well enough to prevent obvious signs of nutrient deficiency but may still have a less than optimum dietary intake, which puts the person at risk for developing chronic diseases in the future. Good nutrition plays an important role in the prevention of disease and other health problems, as well as in the treatment of a disease once it has developed. Nutrition screening elements appropriate for a healthy person include height and weight, a blood panel for cholesterol and blood glucose levels, and a diet recall.

The Dietary Guidelines published by the federal government are summarized in the box at right. According to these guidelines, Americans tend to eat too many calories, too much fat, and too little fiber. The average American intake of fat has decreased from 40% of calories in the late 1970s to 34% of calories today. Still, two thirds of Americans continue to eat more fat calories than the 30% recommended. In men excess fat is often provided by meat, cheese, and fried food, whereas women tend to consume extra fat in fried food, salad dressing, and snacks or desserts.

The average fiber intake of Americans is about one half of the recommended 20 to 25 g per day, primarily because of inadequate intakes of fruits and vegetables and whole grains. Less than one third of Americans consume the recommended five servings of fruits or vegetables each day. Nearly half of the population reports eating no fruit in a typical day. Most Americans obtain enough vitamin C and vitamin A from their diet to prevent deficiency symptoms, but the quantities of fruits and vegetables are not large enough to provide what are thought to be adequate amounts of "phytonutrients," including antioxidants, which appear to protect against the development of chronic disease.

Another area of concern in American eating habits is

Dietary Guidelines for Americans

1. *Eat a variety of foods.* Since no food can provide all of the more than 40 nutrients that the body requires, variety is crucial.
2. *Balance the food you eat with physical activity. Maintain or improve your weight.* Being overweight and gaining weight as an adult are linked to high blood pressure, heart disease, stroke, diabetes, certain types of cancer, arthritis, breathing problems, and other illness. If your weight is not in the healthiest range, try to reduce risks through better eating and exercise habits.
3. *Choose a diet with plenty of grain products, vegetables, and fruits.* These foods provide vitamins, minerals, starch, and dietary fiber and are low in fat. Most of the calories in your diet should come from grain products, vegetables, and fruits.
4. *Choose a diet low in fat, saturated fat, and cholesterol.* Some fat is needed for good health, but many Americans eat too much fat, which increases the risk of heart disease and certain cancers. Choose a diet that contains no more than 30% of the calories as fat.
5. *Choose a diet moderate in sugars.* Sugars are carbohydrates, but they contain very few nutrients and can contribute to dental caries. Sugars should be used in moderation by most people and sparingly by people with low caloric needs.
6. *Choose a diet moderate in salt and sodium.* Sodium plays an essential role in regulating fluids and blood pressure in the body, but most Americans consume more sodium than is needed. People with, or at risk of developing, high blood pressure should limit their intake of sodium.
7. *If you drink alcoholic beverages, do so in moderation.* Alcoholic beverages supply calories but no nutrients. The alcohol in these beverages has physiologic drug effects and is harmful when consumed in excess.

Modified from *Nutrition and your health: dietary guidelines for Americans,* ed 4, USDA HG-232, Washington, DC, 1995, Departments of Agriculture and Health and Human Services.

an inadequate consumption of calcium by children and adolescents, at least in part because of increased intakes of soft drinks and fruit-flavored juice drinks. From 1990 to the present, milk consumption has decreased by 16% in children under 5 years of age. The average calcium intake for teenage girls is about 600 mg, well below the 1200 mg RDA for that age group (Wright et al., 1991). Because of the growth and strengthening of bone that occurs at these ages, inadequate calcium intake during childhood, adolescence, and young adulthood can increase the risk of osteoporosis in later life.

Vegetarians

Vegetarian diets are adopted for a variety of reasons, ranging from ethical, to health related, to economic. Vegetarianism can take several forms, but the most common types are total vegetarians, or vegans, who eat no animal products of any type, and lacto-ovo vegetarians, who consume plant foods plus dairy products and eggs. When working with a vegetarian client, it is important to initially define the type of vegetarianism that they adhere to, so you can accurately identify potential nutritional concerns.

Populations that consume vegetarian diets have a lower risk of obesity, lung cancer, hypertension, heart disease, non–insulin-dependent diabetes, and gallstones than meat-eating populations (Dwyer, 1988). To be nutritionally adequate, however, a vegetarian diet must replace the excluded animal foods with vegetable foods that provide similar types and amounts of nutrients (i.e., the iron found in meat must be obtained instead from leafy green vegetables or beans). As more food groups are eliminated from a vegetarian diet, there is a greater chance that some nutrients may not be adequate. For example, the vegan diet, which eliminates dairy products, is more likely to be deficient in calcium than the lacto-ovo vegetarian diet, which includes dairy products.

A daily food guide for both the lacto-ovo and vegan diet is found in Table 5.8. Lacto-ovo vegetarians consume dried beans, such as black beans, navy beans, kidney beans, split peas, and lentils, to take the place of meat, poultry, or fish servings. The number of servings of vegetables, especially the dark green leafy type, should be increased in a vegetarian diet to replace the calcium usually provided by dairy products and the other minerals provided by meats.

A vitamin B_{12} supplement of 2 µg per day is recommended for all vegans because vitamin B_{12} is found only in animal products. Some vegetarians regard fermented foods as an alternative source of Vitamin B_{12}, but these foods are not reliable sources. Other nutrients most likely to be deficient in the vegetarian diet are calcium, iron, and vitamin D.

Because of the increased fiber and bulk in the vegetarian diet, children and pregnant women who follow a

table 5.8 *Vegetarian Food Guides*		
	Servings per day*	
	Vegan diet	Lacto-ovo diet
Breads and cereals	10	9
Legumes (dried peas and beans)	2	2
Vegetables	3	4
Dark green leafy vegetables	2	No amount specified
Fruits	4	3
Nuts and seeds	1	1
Milk and yogurt	0	2
Eggs	0	3-4 per week
Fortified soy drinks and tofu	2	No amount specified

Data from Dwyer JT: Health aspects of vegetarian diets, *Am J Clin Nutr* 48(suppl 3): 712-738, 1988.
*Based on a 2200-calorie diet for an active adult.

vegan diet may have difficulty consuming an adequate number of calories, which could interfere with adequate growth in children and adequate weight gain in pregnant women. Caloric intake is not usually a concern with a lacto-ovo vegetarian diet.

Athletes and Active Children and Adults

There are special recommendations for diets for athletes to help maximize performance and to protect overall health. The general recommendation is that athletes consume a diet consistent with the Dietary Guidelines: 60% to 70% carbohydrate, 20% to 30% fat, and 15% to 20% protein, with adequate calories to maintain a desirable weight. Complex carbohydrate is emphasized because it is recognized as the primary source of muscle glycogen, which is the major source of energy for muscles.

Some athletes, especially those involved with body building, may overemphasize the role of protein in the diet, assuming that very high intakes of protein are necessary to build muscle tissue. Current recommendations are that strength or speed athletes consume 1.2 to 1.7 g of protein per kilogram of body weight per day, whereas endurance athletes consume 1.2 to 1.4 g per kilogram of body weight (Tarnopolsky, 1993). The RDA for protein for adults is 0.8 g per kilogram of body weight, and most Americans consume more protein than this, especially if they are eating enough food to meet the increased caloric needs of the athlete. According to research, athletes can obtain all the nutrition they need from food and do not need, and will not benefit

table 5.9	*Recommended Total Weight Gain Ranges for Pregnant Women Based on Prepregnancy Body Mass Index (BMI)*				

			Recommended total gain[†]	
Prepregnancy weight classification	BMI*	% Ideal body weight	kg	lb
Underweight	<19.8	<85	12.5-18	28-40
Normal weight	19.8-26	100	11.5-16	25-35
Overweight	26-29	120	7.0-11.5	15-25
Obese	>29	>135	At least 7	At least 15

From National Academy of Sciences: *Nutrition during pregnancy,* Washington, DC, 1990, National Academy Press.
*BMI is calculated using metric units. BMI = [prepregnancy weight (lb)/height (in)^2] × 100.
[†]Young adolescents and black women should strive for gains at the upper end of the recommended range. Short women (<157 cm or 62 in) should strive for gains at the lower end of the range.

from, supplements of amino acids or protein powders.

Anemia is not uncommon in athletes, especially women athletes, and is thought to be due to the breakdown of red blood cells in the active muscle tissue and/or losses through the gastrointestinal tract. Athletes may need to increase their intake of iron-rich foods or take supplemental iron to correct the anemia.

Pregnant and Breast-Feeding Women

Pregnancy places increased nutritional demands on a woman's body, since her diet is providing nutrition for herself and for the developing fetus. Caloric needs increase by approximately 300 calories per day for the last two trimesters of pregnancy. This increased caloric intake should facilitate the appropriate weight gain for pregnancy, which varies with prepregnancy body weight, as described in Table 5.9. A healthy pattern of weight gain includes a small gain (2 to 4 pounds) in the first trimester and a gain of approximately ¾ pound per week in the second and third trimesters for the normal-weight woman. Weight gain should be monitored carefully, since it is closely associated with infant birth weight, which is associated with infant morbidity and mortality.

The recommendations for most nutrients increase during pregnancy. Protein requirements increase from 50 to 60 g per day, and calcium recommendations increase by 400 mg per day. Both of these increased requirements can be met by consuming an additional 2 cups of milk each day. The need for folic acid during pregnancy is doubled because of its role in normal cell division. Since rapid cell division begins in the first trimester of pregnancy, adequate folic acid is especially important during this time to prevent neural tube defects (Daly et al., 1995). Because most women do not know they are pregnant until midway through the first trimester, any woman of childbearing age should make an effort to consume adequate amounts of folic acid. Recent government action to require fortification of grain products with folic acid will help the general population achieve adequate intakes of folic acid. Folic acid can be obtained from fortified cereals, liver, nuts and seeds, legumes, green leafy vegetables, and fruits, but supplements are often recommended during pregnancy.

Other vitamin and mineral requirements are increased in pregnancy as well, but these requirements can usually be met without much change in the diet, although a multivitamin mineral supplement may be recommended. Iron is often supplemented in the second and third trimesters because of expanding blood volume and the need for additional red blood cells.

Pregnant women may experience "morning sickness" during pregnancy, usually during the first trimester, but occasionally throughout the pregnancy. The nausea and vomiting associated with morning sickness is not a nutritional problem unless it is constant and interferes with the ability to eat or keep food in the stomach, which could interfere with weight gain and adequate nutrient consumption. If weight gain is inadequate, the priority is to increase caloric intake, which means eating any food that is tolerated, regardless of where it falls in the Food Guide Pyramid, until the nausea subsides.

Breast-feeding also places increased nutritional demands on a woman. To provide the energy needed to manufacture breast milk, caloric requirements increase by approximately 500 calories per day, whereas protein requirements increase by 15 g per day. Adequate fluid intake is important. Women who gained excess weight during pregnancy can safely lose weight during breast-feeding without compromising milk production, as long as the caloric restriction is mild and fluid intake is adequate.

Elderly Men and Women

Risk factors for poor nutritional status in the elderly include inappropriate food intake, poverty, social isolation, dependency and/or disability, acute or chronic diseases or conditions, chronic medication use, and age greater than 80 (Nutrition Screening Initiative, 1991). The more of these factors that are present, the greater the risk of poor nutritional status. The most common nutrition-related problems of the elderly are chronic conditions, such as obesity, cardiovascular disease, diabetes, hypertension, osteoporosis, certain cancers, and gastrointestinal disorders (American Dietetic Association, 1993).

Physiological changes associated with aging affect the nutritional status of the elderly person. Reductions in lean body mass; changes in glucose tolerance, lipid metabolism, and protein synthesis; and alterations in hydration status and blood pressure regulation may change nutrient requirements. Poor dentition, dryness of the mouth, and decreased sense of taste and smell may diminish appetite and reduce food intake, whereas impaired thirst sensitivity may result in dehydration. Lower gastrointestinal motility and reduced production of digestive enzymes can lead to impaired nutrient digestion, absorption, transport, and utilization.

The social environment can also have important ef-

Determine Your Nutritional Health

The warning signs of poor nutritional health are often overlooked. Use this checklist to find out if you or someone you know is at nutritional risk.

Read the statements below. Circle the number in the yes column for those that apply to you or someone you know. For each yes answer, score the number in the box. Total your nutritional score.

	Yes
I have an illness or condition that made me change the kind and/or amount of food I eat.	2
I eat fewer than 2 meals per day.	3
I eat few fruits or vegetables, or milk products.	2
I have 3 or more drinks of beer, liquor or wine almost every day.	2
I have tooth or mouth problems that make it hard for me to eat.	2
I don't always have enough money to buy the food I need.	4
I eat alone most of the time.	1
I take 3 or more different prescribed or over-the-counter drugs a day.	1
Without wanting to, I have lost or gained 10 pounds in the last 6 months.	2
I am not always physically able to shop, cook, and/or feed myself.	2
TOTAL	

TOTAL YOUR NUTRITIONAL SCORE. IF IT'S—

0-2 Good! Recheck your nutritional score in 6 months.

3-5 You are at moderate nutritional risk. See what can be done to improve your eating habits and lifestyle. Your office on aging, senior nutrition program, senior citizens center, or health department can help. Recheck your nutritional score in 3 months.

6 or more You are at high nutritional risk. Bring this checklist the next time you see your doctor, dietitian, or other qualified health or social service professional. Talk with them about any problems you may have. Ask for help to improve your nutritional health.

Courtesy Nutrition Screening Initiative, a project of the American Academy of Family Physicians, the American Dietetic Association, and the National Council on the Aging, Inc., and funded in part by a grant from Ross Products Division, Abbott Laboratories.

fects on the eating habits of the elderly person. Many persons do not enjoy eating alone and do not prepare full meals for themselves, which often leads to the omission of vegetables and meats. There may also be difficulty obtaining food supplies and preparing food. Meal delivery programs such as Meals on Wheels or participation in community meal sites can help the elderly client overcome many of these barriers.

The Nutrition Screening Initiative (NSI) was formed in 1990 as a joint project of the American Academy of Family Physicians, the American Dietetic Association, and the National Council on Aging, Inc., to promote nutrition screening and better nutritional care through the involvement of health professionals along the continuum of care (Nutrition Screening Initiative, 1991). NSI has designed a nutrition screening tool to be used with elderly clients to address risk factors for poor nutritional status (see box on p. 118). If risk factors are noted on this screening tool, a more in-depth assessment should be completed for the client.

Obese Clients

Based on 1990 population estimates, approximately 58 million people—about one third of the U.S. population—are overweight. National surveys indicate that substantial numbers of Americans are trying to lose weight; 40% of women and 24% of men report that they are currently dieting, and approximately 20% of these are using a "fad" diet (Lissner et al., 1992). Nutrition screening and assessment should address the nutritional adequacy of weight loss diets. The major criticism of most fad diets is that they do not change unhealthy eating habits, so although short-term weight loss may occur, it will not be maintained. Any diet that promises quick results with little effort and diverts food choices away from Food Guide Pyramid recommendations should be regarded with caution. The only diets that will produce a true loss of fat tissue are those that create an energy imbalance, with more calories being expended than are being consumed.

Safe dietary changes involve the reduction of caloric intake by approximately 500 calories per day from the client's maintenance caloric level. Maintenance caloric needs can be estimated from a record of the client's typical intake or from an energy expenditure formula (see box at right). A 500-calorie-per-day reduction in intake should produce a weekly weight loss of approximately 1 pound. Experts recommend a weight loss of ½ to 1 pound per week as the safest and most effective rate. Restricting intake to less than 1200 calories per day is not recommended, because it is difficult to eat enough food to meet the Food Guide Pyramid recommendations at this level of caloric intake, and because these very restrictive diets can have a slowing effect on the metabolic rate.

The distribution of macronutrients in a weight-loss diet should follow healthy diet guidelines, with approximately 60% to 70% of calories coming from carbohydrate, 20% to 30% coming from fat, and 15% to 20% coming from protein. A more strict limitation of fat intake, sometimes as low as 10% of calories, has been popular for weight loss in recent years. This approach can be nutritionally adequate and calorically appropriate if fruits, vegetables, low-fat proteins, and whole grains are emphasized. The availability of many desserts and snacks that are low in fat or fat free but moderate to high in caloric content makes it possible to control fat intake to 10% while still consuming too many calories to allow weight loss. In addition, many of the processed foods that are fat free provide few nutrients and little fiber, so a diet of this type could be nutritionally inadequate.

Childhood obesity is a growing concern in this country, with at least 25% of children in this country being obese (Ernst, Obarzanek, 1994). Obese children are more likely to become obese adults, are more likely to experience high blood pressure and high blood choles-

---

Estimating Daily Caloric Needs

First, calculate resting energy expenditure (REE) using the Harris-Benedict equation:

Females: 655 + (9.6 × weight in kilograms) + (1.7 × height in centimeters) − (4.7 × age)

Males: 66 + (13.7 × weight in kilograms) + (5 × height in centimeters) − (6.8 × age)

Second, determine how active the client is and multiply the REE that you calculated for the client by the appropriate activity factor:

Sedentary	1.15
Sedentary work, with three or four 20-minute exercise sessions per week	1.20
Active job on feet, but no exercise program	1.20
Active job plus three or four 20-minute exercise sessions per week	1.25

Sample calculation: Male, 35 years old, weight 84.1 kg (185 lb), height 178 cm (70 in). Has sedentary job; gets no regular exercise.

66 + (13.7 × 84.1) + (5 × 178) − (6.8 × 35) = 1870 calories

Activity factor is 1.15%
1870 × 1.15 = 2150 calories per day to maintain current weight

terol levels earlier in life, and may establish eating habits that will persist throughout their life. Because treatment approaches for childhood obesity must provide an adequate number of calories and adequate nutrients for optimum growth and development, most programs emphasize slowing the rate of gain rather than achieving significant weight loss. Exercise, control of fat intake to approximately 25% to 30% of calories, and increased intakes of fruits, vegetables, and whole grains in line with the Food Guide Pyramid are usually recommended.

Clients with Eating Disorders

Types of disordered eating range from poor eating habits to the defined eating disorders: anorexia nervosa and bulimia nervosa. It is estimated that 8 million American teenagers and adults show some sign of one of these eating disorders. Anorexia nervosa is the chronic, intentional pursuit toward thinness, resulting in weight at least 15% below ideal weight. Bulimia nervosa is a cycle characterized by eating great quantities of food (binges commonly contain 1000 to 15,000 calories) and then purging through the use of vomiting, laxatives, diuretics, enemas, and/or exercise. Compulsive overeating and binge eating disorder are two additional types of eating disorders. The compulsive overeater or binge eater does not purge to maintain normal weight and very often is obese.

Two simple and nonthreatening questions used to screen for eating disorders are (1) "What were your highest and lowest weights in the last year?" and (2) "What do you think your ideal weight is?" Large discrepancies between these numbers and the client's current weight may indicate unhealthy weight control attitudes or practices. Ask women clients about their menstrual history, since irregular menses may indicate a caloric deficiency. An exercise history including frequency, duration, and type of activity may reveal excessive exercise patterns that could raise suspicion.

If an eating disorder is suspected, a more detailed history should be obtained. This history should include questions about the frequency and extent of binge eating; use of diet pills, laxatives, diuretics, and self-induced vomiting; use of medications; use of alcohol, tobacco, and/or other drugs; any family history of eating disorders, obesity, substance abuse, or depression; self-esteem and control issues; symptoms of depression; frequent sore throats or abdominal pain (from frequent vomiting); and diarrhea and constipation (from laxative use) (Joy, Donnell, and Husu, 1995).

Clients with Heart Disease

Approximately 490,000 people died of coronary heart disease in 1993, and it is estimated that about 1.5 million people in the United States had a heart attack in 1995. The risk of heart disease increases with advancing age and the presence of risk factors, including smoking, hypertension, diabetes, abnormal lipid levels, and family history. Nutrition plays a role in reducing the risk of heart disease by helping to control several of these risk factors.

Serum lipid disorders can include elevations of total cholesterol, LDL, and triglyceride levels, or deficiencies of HDL levels. As noted in Table 5.7, lower LDL goal levels are recommended for people with diagnosed heart disease because of the demonstration of reduced mortality in recent studies (Scandanavian Simvastatin Survival Study Group, 1994). Dietary treatment recommendations for lipid abnormalities have been established and are described in Table 5.10 (Expert Panel, 1993).

Low-fat diets are usually described as a percentage of calories, so before a client can implement the diet by reading labels and food composition charts, an estimation of the client's caloric intake and a conversion to fat grams need to be made. The fat gram allowances for several caloric intake and fat percentage levels are listed in Table 5.11. To calculate fat grams from a percentage

table5.10 *Nutritional Plans for Treatment of Lipid Abnormalities*

	Step one diet*	Step two diet*	Very low fat diet
Total fat	Less than 30% of total calories	Less than 30% of total calories	10%
Saturated fat	Less than 10%	Less than 7%	—
Monounsaturated fat	10% to 15%	10% to 15%	—
Polyunsaturated fat	Up to 10%	Up to 10%	—
Carbohydrate	50% to 60%	50% to 60%	70% to 75%
Protein	10% to 20%	10% to 20%	15% to 20%
Cholesterol	Less than 300 mg	Less than 200 mg	5 mg

From Taylor R: *Family medicine: principles and practice,* ed 5, New York, 1997, Springer-Verlag.
*Recommended by the American Heart Association.

table 5.11	*Percentage of Calories as Fat Translated to Daily Fat Gram Allowance*		
Caloric Intake	30% of calories (g)	20% of calories (g)	10% of calories (g)
1500	50	33	17
1800	60	40	20
2000	67	44	22
2400	80	53	27

Modified from Taylor R: *Family medicine: principles and practice*, ed 5, New York, 1997, Springer-Verlag.

of calories as fat for other calorie levels, multiply the usual caloric intake by the fat percentage and divide the resulting number of calories by 9. For example:

$$1800 \text{ calories} \times 30\% = 540 \text{ calories}$$

$$\frac{540 \text{ calories}}{9 \text{ Calories/Fat grams}} = 60 \text{ g of fat}$$

This client could eat up to 60 g of fat per day if the goal was to limit fat intake to 30% of the calories.

A very low fat diet (10% of calories) can be nutritionally adequate and has been recommended by some experts for the treatment of heart disease, but it requires major changes from the typical American diet. This diet includes vegetable proteins in place of most or all of the animal products and limits or eliminates added fats. Most clients would benefit from a visit to a registered dietitian to help them make these major changes in their eating habits.

Clients with Hypertension

Hypertension affects an estimated 43 million Americans and is more common in African-Americans and older adults. Factors that increase the risk of hypertension are obesity, excessive salt intake, excessive alcohol consumption, and lack of exercise. The most effective dietary treatment for hypertension is weight loss. Blood pressures usually improve significantly with the loss of as little as 10 to 15 pounds. A reduction in dietary sodium may be of clinical benefit to persons who either have sodium-dependent hypertension or are likely to develop it (U.S. Preventive Services Task Force, 1996). It is estimated that approximately one half of hypertensive clients are sodium sensitive. Sodium sensitivity can be determined by restricting sodium intake and monitoring improvement in blood pressure.

A sodium restriction to approximately 2000 mg per day is recommended for the hypertensive client. This restriction requires the use of no added salt at the table, little or no salt in cooking, and avoidance of foods processed with large amounts of salt. The restriction of alcohol intake to no more than two drinks per day for men or one drink per day for women can help control blood pressure and may make weight loss more likely because of a reduction in caloric intake. Increased intakes of calcium, potassium, and magnesium have been shown to help reduce blood pressure, but the effects of these dietary components are small and are not clinically significant.

Clients with Diabetes

Approximately 14 million persons in the United States have diabetes mellitus. Non–insulin-dependent, or type II, diabetes accounts for 90% to 95% of all cases of diabetes, whereas insulin-dependent, or type I diabetes, accounts for the remaining 5% to 10% of cases. It is estimated that half of the patients with type II diabetes are currently unaware of their condition (U.S. Preventive Services Task Force, 1996). Individuals at higher risk of diabetes include obese men and women over age 40, those with a strong family history of diabetes, women who have had gestational diabetes, and members of certain ethnic groups (Native Americans, Hispanics, and African-Americans).

For type I diabetes, a meal plan based on the individual's usual diet and nutritional adequacy is determined and used as a basis for integration of insulin therapy. Once this plan is established, consistency from day to day is recommended in order to synchronize food intake and insulin administration. The food exchange system is usually used to establish the eating plan, but guidelines can be generalized if the client has difficulty understanding the concept of exchanges.

For type II diabetes, the emphasis is on achievement of blood glucose, serum lipid, and blood pressure goals. Weight loss is important for diabetic control, but because of the ineffectiveness of traditional approaches emphasizing weight loss, current recommendations do not make weight loss the focus of dietary efforts (Nutrition recommendations, 1994). The initial starting point

should be improvement of food choices, using the Food Guide Pyramid and the Dietary Guidelines. The resulting food choices will be lower in fat, saturated fat, and cholesterol and higher in fiber. Spacing meals and snacks throughout the day rather than eating one or two large meals is also helpful for blood glucose control.

The potential of many carbohydrate foods to raise blood glucose levels has been evaluated and summarized in the form of a glycemic index (Jenkins et al., 1981). This research shows that increases in blood glucose levels are similar whether the carbohydrates consumed are complex (starches) or simple (sugars). For this reason, current guidelines for diabetic diets emphasize total carbohydrates consumption and do not call for elimination of sugar from the diet. Some control of sugar intake is recommended for diabetics, as it is for all Americans, because of excess calories and the lack of nutrients that sugar provides and because of its potential to cause dental caries.

Clients with diabetes are at high risk of developing heart disease, so their diet should limit total fat to no more than 30% of calories and saturated fat to no more than 10% of calories (7% if the LDL level is elevated). A further restriction of fat intake to 20% of calories may be beneficial if weight loss is a goal. Clients who have high triglyceride levels, which is common in persons with diabetes, may actually see an elevation in triglyceride levels if they increase their intake of carbohydrate as they restrict their fat intake. These people will probably have the best response by maintaining a fat intake of 30% fat, emphasizing monounsaturated fats rather than polyunsaturated or saturated fats.

Carbohydrate counting is a dietary approach that may be used in intensive management of diabetes. Carbohydrate is emphasized because it has the greatest impact on blood glucose levels. Clients are taught to count grams of carbohydrate in the meal or snack that they plan to eat and to adjust their insulin dose accordingly (Gregory and Davis, 1994).

Clients with Cancer

Because of both the cancer and the therapeutic regimens, protein-energy malnutrition is more common among cancer patients than in any other patient group. This malnutrition is characterized by anorexia (lack of appetite), early satiety, weight loss, anemia, and skeletal muscle atrophy, as well as impaired wound healing and diminished immune response.

Cancer seems to change taste sensations, making some flavors seem stronger and some less well detected, which can affect food preferences and tolerances. Altered brain neurotransmitters may also be a cause of poor appetite. The effects of chemotherapy on nutrition depend on the specific medication, dose, duration of treatment, and individual tolerance. Radiation therapy may affect the client's ability to consume, digest, and absorb adequate nutrient intake. Radiation to the head and neck present special nutritional problems because of frequent distortion of taste (dysgeusia), difficulty in swallowing (dysphagia), dry mouth, and possible esophagitis or esophageal stricture (Charuhas, 1990).

It is important to perform nutritional assessment as soon after the cancer is diagnosed as possible. The dietary assessment should include special attention to unorthodox nutrition treatment and megavitamin therapy, since cancer patients are vulnerable to unproven dietary regimens and supplements. A careful weight history is important to assess nutritional risk before treatment begins. A weight loss of greater than 5% of usual weight defines a patient as being at nutritional risk. The validity of usual biochemical parameters, such as albumin, hematocrit, hemoglobin, and total lymphocyte count, may be affected by cancer therapy. The creatinine-height index has been demonstrated to be the most sensitive tool for assessing protein-calorie malnutrition and survival in cancer patients (Kouba, 1988).

Caloric requirements for the cancer patient who is losing or has lost weight are usually 1.5 to 2.0 times the REE (see box on p. 119) to account for stress and increased metabolic demands. Maintenance caloric requirements for cancer patients are usually 1.3 to 1.4 times the REE. Protein requirements are increased in the client with cancer and are usually in the range of 1.5 to 2.0 g per kilogram of ideal body weight. Alterations in usual food choices may be necessary in order to address changes in taste, appetite, and food tolerance. The oral route is the preferred one for feeding, but the degree of loss of appetite or other problems may make tube feedings or parenteral nutrition a necessity (Kouba, 1988).

▪ REFERRAL FOR IN-DEPTH NUTRITIONAL ASSESSMENT OR FOLLOW-UP

After an initial assessment it will become apparent that some clients need to be referred to a registered dietitian and/or physician for in-depth evaluation or follow-up. Clients with moderate to severe cases of undernutrition will probably need additional laboratory tests and detailed advice on a plan to reestablish adequate nutrition. Clients affected by overnutrition may need further evaluation of serum lipid levels, blood glucose control, and potential metabolic causes of obesity. A therapeutic approach to overnutrition may include an eating plan designed by the client and a registered dietitian, an exercise plan with input from a physician or exercise

counselor, and behavioral change advice provided by a counselor.

The client will benefit from a comprehensive approach to address nutritional concerns as long as the efforts of health care professionals are well coordinated. Clear and adequate communication between health care providers can help ensure that patients are receiving the care they need in an efficient and effective manner. When clients are referred to another health care professional, information gathered during the initial assessment should be summarized and shared to prevent duplication of effort. Expectations of the referral should be made clear to the referral health care professional, and a summary of the referral visit should be returned to the client's primary care provider to ensure continuity of care.

■ SUMMARY

Adequate nutrition is necessary for good health. Most clients are aware that they should make healthy food choices, but they are more likely to do so with consistent direction and reinforcement from their health care providers. Nutrition screening and assessment is the first step in the process of evaluating the client's nutritional status and emphasizing the importance of good nutrition. Nutrition screening and assessment may include health and diet histories, anthropometric measurements, and biochemical measurements. The use of each of these elements depends on the type of client, the time available, and the expertise of the health care provider. The information gathered during nutrition screening and assessment forms the basis for the development and implementation of an overall nutrition care plan.

---

sample documentation & diagnoses CRITICAL THINKING

■ FOCUSED HEALTH HISTORY (SUBJECTIVE DATA)

Mr. F., a 42-year-old black bus driver, has come to the clinic because of concern over his weight. Client works the day shift in a large metropolitan area and describes his job as "very stressful." Sits 8 hours per day on the job and does not exercise regularly. Does not smoke. A 24-hour diet recall reveals three meals per day that are usually "fast food" with high-fat content and little fruit or vegetable intake. Client relaxes by watching TV. Has not been to a health care provider for 12 years.

■ FOCUSED PHYSICAL EXAMINATION (OBJECTIVE DATA)

Vital signs: BP 138/90, pulse 88, respirations 18, temperature 37°C (98.6° F) (oral).
Weight 250 lb, height 5 ft 11 in, BMI 36, triceps skinfold 18 mm.
Laboratory values: Serum cholesterol 250 mg/dl, HDL 35 mg/dl, LDL 150 mg/dl.
General appearance: Well-groomed moderately obese male who appears somewhat anxious.

diagnoses

HEALTH PROBLEM
Obesity; elevated LDL

NURSING DIAGNOSES

Altered nutrition: more than body requirements related to food intake energy/expenditure imbalance

Defining Characteristics
- Weight 20% over ideal for height and frame
- Sedentary activity level

Altered health maintenance related to failure to seek help to maintain health

Defining Characteristics
- History of lack of health-seeking behaviors
- Expression of interest in improving behaviors

chapter 6

Sleep Assessment

■ PURPOSE OF EXAMINATION

Sleep is a basic human need. It has a restorative function, both physically and psychologically. Adequate sleep is essential to a sense of well-being. Circadian rhythms are those physiological functions that occur within a period of approximately 24 hours. The sleep-wakefulness pattern is a part of this rhythm. People who are sleep-deprived usually have less ability to cope with psychological stressors and physical activities. During illness, the sleep state can be difficult to attain and can be a frustrating accompaniment to the illness.

The purpose of assessing the client's sleep-rest pattern is to incorporate that aspect of the client's daily pattern into your holistic assessment of her or his life, health, and abilities to function and cope. A client's sense of adequate sleep and rest can affect that individual's sense of physical and psychological well-being.

■ CATEGORIES, STAGES, AND CYCLES OF SLEEP

Categories of Sleep

Sleep is divided into two major categories:
1. Nonrapid eye movement (nonREM) sleep, consisting of four stages during which no dreaming occurs
2. Rapid eye movement (REM) sleep during which dreaming occurs

The brain is active and produces electrical patterns during wakefulness and sleep. These electrical patterns can be traced by electroencephalogram (EEG) recordings. Other monitoring devices that are used to differentiate stages of sleep and wakefulness include the electro-oculogram (EOG), which records eye movements, and the electromyelogram (EMG), which monitors muscle tone and activity.

Stages of Sleep

Stage 1 nonREM sleep

Stage 1 occurs as a person falls asleep. It is the transition between wakefulness and sleep and may last only 5 minutes. There is a sensation of drowsiness, drifting, or relaxation. A person may be easily awakened from stage 1 sleep by noise or other stimuli and may state that he or she has not yet fallen asleep. This stage is characterized by:

1. Absence of rapid eye movements (the eyes roll slowly from side to side)
2. Decreasing heart and respiratory rates, relatively high muscle tone, and jerks or sudden twitching in the face or extremities

Stage 2 nonREM sleep

Stage 2 lasts from 10 to 15 minutes and is a deeper sleep state. Awakening a person from this stage is more difficult. There is little eye movement, and body temperature and metabolic rates decrease somewhat.

Stage 3 nonREM sleep

Stage 3 is deeper and more restful sleep. It is dominated by parasympathetic nervous system activity with decreased blood pressure and lowered heart and respiratory rates. Awakening the person is difficult.

Stage 4 nonREM sleep

Stage 4 sleep is the deepest sleep, and awakening the person during this stage is difficult. The sleeper enters it anywhere from 15 to 30 minutes after falling asleep. The eyes remain still. Muscle tone is relaxed, and respiratory rate, heart rate, and blood pressure are lowered. Restorative physiological processes occur during stage 4, including increased protein synthesis and secretion of growth hormone. Sleep quality is often judged by the amount of time spent in stage 4 sleep. People who report that they have not slept well, although the actual time spent sleeping may have been adequate, may not have obtained sufficient stage 4 sleep.

REM sleep

REM sleep differs from nonREM sleep in that it is a relatively active sleep state. It shows bursts of increased sympathetic nervous system activity. This activity is exhibited by muscle twitches and variability in pulse, blood pressure, and respiratory rates. Gastric secretion may increase, and steroid hormones are released. Penile erections may occur in males of all ages during this stage. Paradoxically, during this stage the muscles are relaxed, and deep tendon reflexes are reduced. Thus, during REM sleep, some characteristics associated with wakefulness and others associated with deep sleep are present. Episodic bursts of rapid eye movements associated with dreaming are present. These movements are visible even though the person's eyes are closed. REM sleep varies in duration. People who do not have adequate REM sleep also feel they have had too little sleep.

Sleep Cycles

The sleep stages occur in a cyclical fashion. During an average 8-hour sleep period, an individual may experience four to six sleep cycles. An average cycle is 90 minutes long, and each cycle has varying amounts of REM and nonREM sleep. For example, during early sleep, nonREM sleep is longer, lasting from 70 to 100 minutes, and REM sleep is shorter. During a later part of the sleep period, REM sleep lengthens. The normal sequence varies with age, environment, and the effect of daily activities.

The first sleep cycle generally follows the most orderly progression through each of the sleep stages. The stages proceed from 1 through 4 and then on to REM sleep. During a subsequent cycle, stage 1 may be absent, and the stages may proceed in a different order, such as from stage 4 to stage 2 to REM sleep. At all ages stage 2 accounts for 50% or more of total sleep time, and REM sleep usually arises from stage 2. The number of REM periods varies between four and six per night, accounting for about 20% to 25% of the total sleep time. During a sleep cycle, the length of each stage can be influenced by physical and mental states and by medication. As an individual ages, there is a gradual decrease in stages 3 and 4 of sleep. The elderly have little or no stage 4 sleep. During REM sleep, there is general relaxation of skeletal muscles, including pharyngeal muscles. This may play a role in the development of upper airway obstruction during sleep.

As people age, the sleep cycle changes (Figure 6.1). In general, total sleep time is greatest during infancy, decreases in childhood, may increase again during parts of adolescence, remains relatively stable during the adult years, and declines during the late years of adulthood. The newborn spends 50% of sleep time in REM sleep, and the sleep cycles are 45 to 60 minutes long. Total sleep time for the newborn is 14 to 18 hours a day. By age 1, REM sleep is only 20% to 30%. Stage 4 sleep is greater in duration during childhood, As the child matures, the sleep cycle increases in length and the total sleep time decreases. Sleep patterns of 8 to 10 hours develop during childhood. Many adolescents go through stages of needing increased amounts of sleep. Most healthy adults spend 7 to 9 hours sleeping each day, although many require less than 6 hours of sleep and others require more than 9 hours. Of this time, about 25% of sleep is in REM sleep, 50% is in stage 2 sleep, and 5% to 10% is in stage 1 sleep. The remaining 15% to 20% is a combination of stages 3 and 4. Older adults have a decrease in total sleep time and in stage 4 sleep. The elderly may experience more frequent awakenings during

figure**6.1** Sleep cycles of normal subjects. The sleep of children and young adults shows early preponderance of stages 3 and 4, progressive lengthening of the first three REM periods, and infrequent awakenings. In elderly adults there is little or no stage 4 sleep, REM periods are fairly uniform in length, and awakenings are frequent and often lengthy. *(From Kales A et al: Sleep and dreams: recent research on clinical aspects* Ann Intern Med *68:1078–1104, 1968.)*

the night; some need to compensate for this with rest periods during the day. Some elderly clients view their pattern of diminished sleep with frustration, whereas others accept it as an opportunity to have more time for other activities.

■ EXAMINATION

Health History

Most people take sleep for granted until they have a problem with it. Use open-ended questions to elicit a description of any sleep problem in the client's own words. In this situation it is often appropriate to obtain information about a sleep problem from the client's bed partner or, in the case of a child, from a parent. These observers usually have important information that the client cannot report.

Present health problem

1. Typical daily schedule, including waking and sleep-rest patterns

a. Daytime activities
   b. Difficulty falling asleep, staying asleep, or awakening too early
   c. Time it takes to fall asleep
   d. Time(s) client awakens
2. Onset and duration of symptoms, and pattern since onset (e.g., changes in intensity, changes with season)
3. Stress-related factors at time of onset and at present (home, job, medical), and relationship of these factors to intensity of the symptoms
   a. Current life situation, including situations for which sleep is providing escape or relief for the client
   b. Relationships
   c. Role of work
   d. Sense of meaning, purpose in life
   e. Coping skills in dealing with stress, anxiety, unresolved feelings
   f. Depression
4. Factors that make symptoms better or worse; change in symptoms at time of vacation
5. Impact of sleep problem on client's life
   a. Fatigue
   b. Irritability
   c. Inability to think and/or speak clearly
   d. Daytime sleepiness or napping
   e. Decreased attention span
   f. Memory changes
6. Treatments attempted to date, including prescription and nonprescription medications, and effectiveness of each
   a. Medications
   b. Bedtime rituals, such as reading, music, or beverage
7. Other medications
8. Sleep environment
   a. Sleeping arrangements
   b. Comfort level
   c. Noise, light, and temperature
9. Associated symptoms:
   a. Pain
   b. Nocturia
   c. Shortness of breath
10. Personal beliefs about the value of sleep, rest, and dreams

Information from bed partner or parent

1. Snoring
2. Apneic periods
3. Movements or activities during sleep

Family sleep patterns

1. Family sleep practices and habits
2. Family history of sleep problems

Technique for Examination and Normal Findings

Use the technique of observation to help assess the sleep/rest status of the client. Physical findings are normal in most clients.

1. Client's mental alertness status, thought patterns, speech patterns, facial appearance, gross motor movements, and posture
2. Measure:
   a. Blood pressure
   b. Body weight
3. Inspect:
   a. Nose: Nasal septum may be deviated.
   b. Neck: Clients with sleep apnea syndrome may have a short, thick neck.
   c. Throat: Look for narrow pharyngeal space; bulky, elevated base of the tongue; and a long or edematous uvula. Tonsils and adenoids may be enlarged.

Screening Tests and Procedures

When a sleep disorder is suspected, polysomnography, an overnight sleep study, is conducted for one or two nights. This study includes:

Electroencephalogram (EEG)
Electro-oculogram (EOG)
Electromyelogram (EMG)
Electrocardiogram (ECG)
Measures of oxygen saturation and carbon dioxide values and nasal and oral airflow
Thoracic and abdominal respiratory movements and leg muscle activity

■ VARIATIONS FROM HEALTH

Sleep Apnea Syndrome

Apnea is the temporary cessation of airflow at the level of the nostrils and mouth for at least 10 seconds. Persons with sleep apnea syndrome (SAS) may experience several to hundreds of apneic periods each night, with each period lasting from 10 seconds to 2 minutes. Sleep disruption and sleep deprivation result. Men over age 50 are most frequently affected.

Apnea occurring during sleep may be categorized as:
1. Obstructive sleep apnea (OSA)
2. Central sleep apnea (CSA)
3. Mixed sleep apnea

Obstructive sleep apnea

OSA is the most common form of sleep apnea, accounting for about 95% of sleep apneas. OSA is caused by a physical blockage to the flow of air. It results when the flow of air is obstructed as the soft palate and the tongue move backward against the posterior pharyngeal wall and partially or completely obstruct the pharynx.

Obesity is a risk factor, especially if the neck is short and thick. However, persons of normal weight with normal neck features can also have OSA. Enlarged tonsils, a large tongue, or a narrowed pharyngeal passageway can be causative factors.

In OSA, the neural stimulus is present, so a persistent effort to breathe continues even during the occlusive phase of the cycle. Thus an observer can see thoracic and abdominal movements.

The individual with obstructive sleep apnea exhibits a cyclical breathing pattern in which periods of apnea alternate with arousal and breathing. Sometime after the individual falls asleep, a loss of upper airway muscle tone occurs, creating an airway occlusion. The apneic period ranges from 20 to 120 seconds and results in hypoxemia, which stimulates the respiratory drive. The person arouses to a lighter stage of sleep or may awaken, and the upper airway muscles are activated, resulting in the return of airflow. The individual returns to sleep, and the cycle starts again. The duration of the apneic periods and the degree of hypoxemia increase gradually as the disease progresses, resulting in a higher degree of hypoxemia necessary to stimulate arousal. The increasing stimulus necessary to create arousal may also be a result of the fragmented sleep caused by the disease process.

Central sleep apnea

CSA is the least common form of SAS. It is characterized by cessation of airflow caused by decreased respiratory center output. The neural signal to breathe is interrupted, so that both respiratory effort and airflow are absent. The absence of rib cage and abdominal movement is characteristic. Individuals with central sleep apnea syndrome are usually of normal weight or are underweight. Their reported difficulty tends to be disrupted sleep rather than excessive daytime sleepiness. Clients with CSA generally fall asleep easily and rapidly but subsequently wake up several times during the night with a choking sensation.

Mixed sleep apnea

Mixed sleep apnea occurs when a person experiences both disorders. It starts as central apnea and is followed by upper airway obstruction. Mixed apneas are less common than obstructive apnea but more frequent than central apnea.

Characteristics of sleep apnea syndrome

The primary symptoms of sleep apnea are nighttime snoring and daytime sleepiness and inattentiveness. Other symptoms include abnormal physical movements during sleep, morning headache, nausea, hallucinations, personality changes, deterioration of intellectual capacity, including impaired memory and difficulty acquiring

new information, sexual problems, and altered cardiac function.

Nighttime snoring. The family or sleeping partner may be a better source of information than the client, since the client may not be aware of alterations that occur during the sleep period. The family or partner may report the following about the individual's snoring and other sleep period symptoms:

1. Snores loudly and sometimes irregularly
2. Has multiple apneic periods while sleeping, each lasting more than 10 seconds
3. May or may not make respiratory efforts during the apneic period
4. Awakens or partially awakens coughing and/or choking on secretions in the throat
5. Makes grunting or gurgling noises during sleep
6. Flails about in bed

The incidence of these events increases if the individual consumes alcohol, takes a depressant drug, or has a change in his or her sleeping pattern.

Daytime sleepiness. This is often the symptom that makes an individual seek help, because it interferes with his or her lifestyle. The person experiences excessive drowsiness and a strong urge to sleep at various and often inappropriate times during the day. The client may be resisting the urge to sleep or may be taking short naps, although they are often not restful and may be accompanied by headaches and a sense of fogginess or confusion. These changes may lead to difficulty with work and relationships. These difficulties may lead to depression or other emotional changes. Excessive daytime sleepiness can lead to serious accidents if the individual is operating a car or other machinery. The life of the client and of others in the environment may be endangered.

Abnormal physical movements. Abnormal movements during sleep are usually reported by the sleeping partner or show up on polysomnographic tests. Agitation is evidenced by movement of the extremities or of the whole body. These movements, in addition to the snoring, may be so disruptive to the bed partner that she or he will sleep in a different bed or different room. Other abnormal sleep behaviors may include sleeptalking and sleepwalking. The person may suddenly sit upright in bed, gasping for breath. These movements may or may not awaken the client.

Morning headache. Recurrent morning headache is a complaint of many clients with sleep apnea syndrome. The headache is usually frontal but is occasionally diffuse. It usually diminishes several hours after the patient awakens but may recur if there are episodes of sleep during the day. The headache may be accompanied by some confusion.

Hallucinations. Hallucinatory images may appear during the waking state when the urge to sleep arises.

Although the images usually persist for only a short time, the individual may react to the image before recognizing its hallucinatory nature. For example, if the client visualizes a tree while driving, he or she may swerve or brake to avoid hitting it. Obviously, hallucinatory images pose a threat to the safety of the client and others.

Personality changes. Irritability is an early personality change reported by persons with SAS. Other changes can develop, such as paranoia, confusion, depression, aggressiveness, jealousy, suspicion, and hostility. Emotional and/or psychological assessment is appropriate.

Deterioration of intellectual capacity. Diminished intellectual function, decreased memory retention, poor judgment, and difficulty concentrating may seriously affect job performance and personal life activities.

Sexual problems. Many clients with sleep apnea report a progressive decrease in sexual drive and, for men, difficulty in obtaining erection and ejaculation.

Altered cardiac function. During the apneic period, the client experiences hypoxemia (decreased PaO_2), hypercapnia (increased $PaCO_2$), and acidosis. The hypoxemia may lead to serious cardiac dysrhythmias. Clients with sleep apnea, as a rule, have normal sinus rhythm while awake, but during sleep the ECG shows progressive sinus bradycardia during apnea and sinus acceleration when breathing resumes. ECG abnormalities may include left anterior hemiblock, ST-T wave abnormalities, marked sinus arrhythmias, sinus bradycardia, asystole, second-degree atrioventricular (AV) block, atrial tachycardia, atrial fibrillation, premature ventricular contractions, and ventricular tachycardia. The asphyxia experienced by the individual may result in pulmonary and systemic vasoconstriction. The vasoconstriction may lead to pulmonary hypertension, right-sided heart failure, and systemic hypertension.

Insomnia

Insomnia is the inability to fall asleep or to stay asleep for an adequate period of time. Insomnia may be chronic or may last for only a brief period in an individual's life. It can result from a variety of causes. Insomnia may be due to the sleep interruptions involving the needs of a newborn child. Stressful situations caused by loss, grief, or unresolved emotional pain, and environmental factors, such as uncomfortable temperatures or a change in work schedule, may contribute to insomnia. The noise level in a hospital and the need to awaken patients for treatments or medications may cause insomnia. Drugs such as amphetamines or caffeine, which remain active in the bloodstream for up to 12 hours, may also cause insomnia. Some people who believe they have insomnia may actually be sleeping but do not feel rested or refreshed by their sleep. Insomnia may be a symptom of depression.

Insomnia may occur during any part of the sleep cycle: early, midway, or late. Most people fall asleep within 5 to 15 minutes of the time they lie down to go to sleep. People with initial insomnia need 30 or more minutes to fall asleep. This is the most common sleep disorder in young adults. Autonomic nervous system activity is higher in these clients; stress and anxiety also play a role.

Intermittent insomnia is the most common form of insomnia in all age groups. It occurs when sleep is interrupted midcycle. The person may or may not be aware of a sleep pattern disturbance if she or he falls asleep easily again. Factors causing intermittent insomnia may be environmental, such as a baby crying; they may be physiological, such as pain or the need to void; or they may be an aspect of the sleep state itself, such as nightmares. Some people return to sleep if they stay in bed; others find that getting up for a while to engage in some activity helps them return to sleep more easily.

Insomnia that occurs toward the end of the sleep cycle becomes more common as people age. This type of insomnia is characterized by early awakenings with an inability to return to sleep. The person may report final awakening as early as 3 or 4 AM. End-cycle insomnia may be associated with daytime napping or an early bedtime. It may also be an important sign of depression or other change in emotional state.

The finding of insomnia indicates a need to carefully assess the overall sleep pattern, current life stresses, coping abilities, and self-concept. Individuals experiencing insomnia may interpret it very differently: some find it upsetting, whereas others see it as extra time to accomplish their goals.

Prolonged sleep deprivation for whatever reason typically causes changes in mood and performance. These changes may include fatigue, irritability, anxiety, depression, feelings of persecution, poor concentration, feelings of depersonalization, and increased aggression.

Narcolepsy

Narcolepsy is a disorder of excessive daytime sleepiness. It is characterized by the following:

1. Sudden, irresistible attacks of daytime sleepiness occur and last anywhere from 10 to 30 minutes.
2. Cataplexy, a sudden loss of muscle tone, occurs in response to sudden emotional stimuli. Although the episodes are typically brief, the person is at risk for falls or other accidents because he or she cannot move or speak.
3. Sleep paralysis usually occurs once or twice a week at the time of sleep onset. There is a period of mental alertness, but the person is paralyzed except for respiratory and eye musculature.
4. Hypnagogic (brief, vivid, dreamlike) hallucinations typically occur at sleep onset.

Involuntary daytime sleep attacks may begin in adolescence or young adulthood. People with this problem may have symptoms for years before the disorder is diagnosed. Not all persons with the disorder experience all four symptoms.

Parasomnias

Parasomnias consist of sleep disorders that are not abnormalities of the sleep process but are undesirable phenomena that occur during sleep.

Sleepwalking

Sleepwalking (somnambulism) occurs most often in children; boys are affected more often than girls. It occurs most often in the first third of the sleep period during stage 3 or 4 nonREM sleep. The episode lasts from a few seconds to several minutes. The person usually cannot remember the sleepwalking episode after awakening. It is more likely to occur if the individual is fatigued or under stress or has taken a sedative or hypnotic medication at bedtime. Other predisposing factors include seizure disorders, central nervous system infections, and trauma.

Sleep terror disorder

Sleep terror disorder, or night terrors, most often affect children and are more common in boys than in girls. After a few hours of sleep, the child bolts up in bed, may or may not awaken, shakes, screams, and appears terrified. There is intense anxiety, confusion, agitation, disorientation, and unresponsiveness. Children usually do not remember these episodes. Night terrors occur predominantly in stages 3 and 4 of nonREM sleep. The episodes are extremely variable in frequency. They are more likely to occur if the individual is fatigued, is under stress, or has been given a tricyclic antidepressant at bedtime.

Nocturnal enuresis

Nocturnal enuresis (bed-wetting) is primarily a childhood disorder, occurring more frequently in boys. It may be either primary or secondary. Primary enuresis may persist from birth to age 6 or older. In secondary enuresis, bed-wetting occurs because of psychological factors. Urination usually occurs just before entering REM sleep. The child may wake up as a result of the wet clothing and bed linens. When assessing enuresis, interview both the parent(s) and the child.

Bruxism

Bruxism (teeth grinding) during sleep may be a symptom of tension and may cause the teeth to become chipped. The individual with bruxism may not be aware of it, but it can be quite irritating to the bed partner. It usually occurs during stage 2 nonREM sleep.

■ FOCUSED HEALTH HISTORY *(SUBJECTIVE DATA)*

Mr. N., a 56-year-old male, reports an increasingly disrupted sleep pattern off and on over the past 4 to 5 years. Notices that he is waking up more often with a cough. Is able to fall asleep fairly easily at the time he retires for the night, but wakes up repeatedly, often because of phone calls related to his occupation; but sometimes awakes for no apparent reason. Once awake, may or may not fall asleep again right away. Occasionally wakes up at 4 or 5 AM and is not able to fall asleep again. Has noticed increased daytime sleepiness, with occasional strong urges to "just get away and take a nap." Does not think this has interfered with his work up to this point, but is concerned that ongoing sleepiness may affect his ability to function effectively. No nocturia, pain, or shortness of breath. Adequate rest has always been important to client, though being on call most nights has often made it difficult. Typical sleeping conditions in his home are quiet after about 10:30 PM, and the room is dark; temperature is comfortable. Usually reads for 30 to 60 minutes before sleeping, does not eat or drink heavily 2 hours before retiring, and takes no sleeping or other medications. Reports no irritability or memory changes. No change in his current life situation, including personal relationships or job; no new or unusual stresses. Finds work meaningful, though demanding.

His wife has noted an increase in episodes of apnea during sleep over the past 5 to 6 months. She reports that he stops breathing for 10 to 30 seconds several times during the night, and after several such periods will wake up choking and coughing. He snores occasionally. This situation is causing her to lose sleep.

■ FOCUSED PHYSICAL EXAMINATION *(OBJECTIVE DATA)*

Vital signs: BP 130/82 sitting; pulse 70, strong and regular; respirations 16.

Height 6 ft, weight 175 lb.

General appearance: Healthy male; alert, appears younger that stated age of 56. No gross abnormalities present; in no acute distress. Well-groomed; clear patterns of thought and speech; responsive, cooperative.

Head and neck: Face symmetrical at rest and with movement. Head in normal position; no swelling or unusual movements. Neck not short or thick; full range of motion; strong symmetrically; thyroid not palpable; trachea in midline; no head or neck nodes palpable.

Ears, nose, and throat: Small amount of cerumen in ear canals; drum intact; hearing normal in both ears (finger rub at 3 ft); Weber and Rinne equal in both ears. Nostrils patent; nasal septum slightly deviated to the right; turbinates and membranes—pink, moist, no discharge. Mouth and throat membranes—pink, moist, no lesions; gums—no inflammation; teeth in good repair; palate—intact, moves symmetrically, gag reflex present; tonsils not enlarged; tongue—normal size and strength, moves symmetrically; uvula—somewhat elongated, not edematous.

Heart and neck vessels: Point of maximum impulse in fifth left intercostal space (5LICS), no abnormal pulsations or lifts. Apical pulse 80 and regular; S1 single sound; S2 split with inspiration; no murmurs or extra sounds. Carotid pulses—equal, strong, no bruits. Jugular veins not distended.

Lungs: Thorax oval; anteroposterior (AP) diameter and lateral diameter symmetrical at rest and with movement; excursion equal bilaterally; tactile fremitus equal bilaterally; no masses or tenderness; percussion tones resonant; lungs clear to auscultation.

Central nervous system: Alert, oriented, mood appropriate; cranial nerves II through XII intact; all movements coordinated; deep tendon reflexes (DTRs) +2 (scale of 0 to +4).

diagnoses

HEALTH PROBLEM
Sleep apnea

NURSING DIAGNOSES

Sleep pattern disturbance related to sleep apnea
Defining Characteristics
- Interrupted sleep
- Fatigue during day

Related Factor
- Family stress (wife losing sleep)

Fatigue
Defining Characteristics
- Perceived need for additional periods of rest
- Fatigue during day

chapter **7**

Cultural Considerations in Health Assessment

■ NURSING AND CULTURE

Cultural beliefs and personal characteristics determine health behavior in individuals and families. More than half of all health problems are the result of behavior and lifestyle. If nursing's goal is to promote health while respecting individual value systems and lifestyles, culture-based health behavior must be understood.

Nurses as a group reflect society's cultural mix. In North America the majority of nurses hold values, beliefs, and attitudes that are typical of the dominant middle class. In addition, nurses belong to a separate culture as members of the health care team. When two people of differing cultural backgrounds interact, significant communication barriers may arise unless at least one of the persons is willing and able to recognize and adapt to the other's values. To care for others, nurses must be able to accept a wide diversity of beliefs, practices, and ideas about health and illness, including many that differ from their own.

Acceptance of alternate beliefs about health and illness can be more difficult for nurses than might be initially assumed. As health care professionals educated in and exposed to the established health care system, nurses share certain values, attitudes, and beliefs about health and illness that they may not consciously think about. These ways of thinking have been shaped by more than 2000 years of Western thought broadly known as Hippocratic medicine. Modern health care is based on rational, scientific, biomedical principles directed toward solving human health problems. As part of the dominant culture, the health care culture is interwoven with established social, religious, political, and economic systems. Certain aspects of the health care culture, such as nurse-physician relationships and provider-patient relationships, are governed by a broadly shared set of customs and protocols.

The cultural beliefs of some clients may conflict with the cultural beliefs many nurses share. Nurses cannot hope to plan meaningful health care for their clients without at least understanding their health beliefs. That is why performing a sensitive cultural assessment is necessary (see box on p. 132 on ways to develop cultural sensitivity). A thorough assessment of the cultural as-

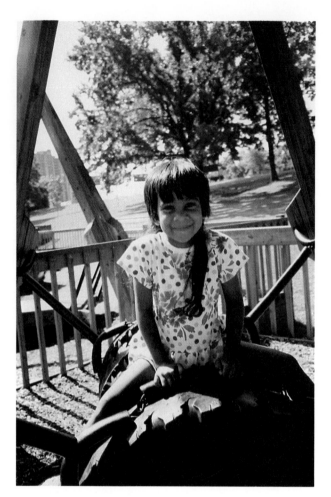

figure **7.1** Cultural beliefs play an important role in molding a child's personality.

From Stulc DM: The family as a bearer of culture. In Cookfair JN: *Nursing process and practice in the community*, St Louis, 1991, Mosby.

Ways to Develop Cultural Sensitivity

1. Recognize that cultural diversity exists.
2. Demonstrate respect for people as unique individuals, with culture as one factor that contributes to their uniqueness.
3. Respect the unfamiliar.
4. Identify and examine your own cultural beliefs.
5. Recognize that some cultural groups have definitions of health and illness, as well as practices that attempt to promote health and cure illness, which may differ from the nurse's own.
6. Be willing to modify health care delivery in keeping with the client's cultural background.
7. Do not expect all members of one cultural group to behave in exactly the same way.
8. Appreciate that each person's cultural values are ingrained and therefore very difficult to change.

pects of a client's lifestyle, health beliefs, and health practices enhances decision making and clinical judgment during care.

■ TERMINOLOGY ASSOCIATED WITH CULTURAL CONSIDERATIONS

Culture is defined as a complex, integrated system that includes knowledge, beliefs, skills, art, morals, law, customs, and any other *acquired* habits and capabilities of a group of people. Culture is characterized by being learned, shared with others, and adapted to the environment. It is stable but subject to, and capable of, change. As a learned set of traits, culture is transmitted from one generation to the next by both formal education and imitation.

Subculture refers to a group of persons within a culture with one or more shared traits. These include age,

socioeconomic status, race, ethnic origin, education, and occupation. Literally thousands of subcultures exist within a culture, and everyone is a member of several. Although subcultures have an identity uniquely their own, they are also related to the overall culture in certain ways. Major subcultural groups in the United States include African-Americans (12.1%), Hispanics (9%), Asian-Americans (2.9%), and Native Americans (0.8%). In Canada, major subcultures include French Canadians (27%) and Natives (2%).

Race refers to the classification of human beings on the basis of physical characteristics, such as skin pigmentation, head form, or stature, that are transmitted through generations. The recognized races are Caucasian, Negroid, and Mongoloid.

Ethnic groups share traits such as a common national or regional origin and linguistic, ancestral, and physical characteristics. Within the major North American subcultures, distinct ethnic groups include African, Haitian, or Dominican (Black); Mexican, Cuban, or Puerto Rican (Hispanic); Japanese, Chinese, Filipino, Korean, Vietnamese, Guamian, or Samoan (Asian); many European ethnic subcultures (German, Italian, Polish, Slavic, Scandinavian, Swiss, French, Dutch, Russian, English, Irish, Scottish); and Native American and Alaska Native subcultures.

Minority group is a frequently misunderstood term. More normative than descriptive, it refers to any group

that receives different and unequal treatment from others in the larger group or society and whose members see themselves as victims of discrimination. This concept is important for caregivers to understand, since many people in our society are discriminated against, and discrimination takes place in the health care system. However, an individual's membership in a minority group is not necessarily related to the individual's cultural affiliations, and this distinction has an important bearing on cultural assessment.

Customs refer to the learned behaviors shared by, and associated with, a particular cultural group. They include dietary practices, communication patterns, family and kinship relations, religious practices, and health behaviors.

Rituals are highly structured patterns of behavior characteristic of cultural groups. They are prescribed ways to define basic human activities within a cultural context. Rituals may govern a group's approach to communication, traditions, taboos, religion, healing and care for the sick, trade, means of travel, sexual activities, or recreation.

Values and norms are judgments that cultural groups apply to behavior. Values are universal to all cultures and define the desirable or undesirable state of affairs within a culture. Norms provide direction for applying values and are the rules that govern human behavior. Cultural norms set limits. Members of a culture are rewarded or punished as they conform or deviate from them. Norms

figure**7.2** Cultural beliefs affect how mothers raise their children.

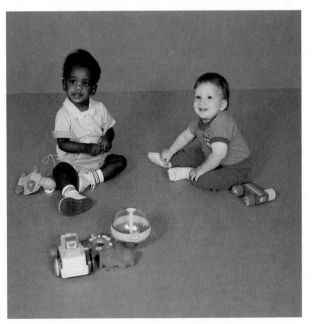

figure**7.3** The nurse will encounter a variety of cultural backgrounds in practice.

perform a number of important functions. They influence a person's perception of others. They direct a person's responses to situations and to others. They provide a basis for self-evaluation. They provide a foundation for forming opinions. They motivate behavior, and they give meaning to life and self-esteem. Values and norms exert a powerful influence over an individual's beliefs, attitudes, and practices. You must explore the client's value system to gain an appreciation for health-related behavior.

Cultural paradigms encompass abstract explanations used by groups to account for major life events. The term is synonymous with the idea of world view. The three dominant cultural paradigms are magico-religious, holistic, and scientific. This concept is crucial to health care professionals because all beliefs and values regarding health are derived from a person's basic world view. Aspects of all three world views are identifiable in most cultures, but one view usually predominates. The magico-religious paradigm offers a mystical cause-and-effect relationship between health and illness. The holistic paradigm provides the basis for a sense of balance and harmony between humans and the larger environment. The scientific view defines health as the absence of disease symptoms.

Enculturation is the process of acquiring one's cultural identity as it is transmitted by the previous generation. The *degree* of enculturation is important to assess before planning care, especially if you anticipate that the client will obtain health benefits by modifying some culturally based aspect of health beliefs, attitudes, or practices. You can also act as an advocate or "culture broker" for the client by educating teachers, other health care workers, or representatives of social agencies about specific cultural beliefs and practices that may influence the client's and his or her family's behaviors or response to recommendations (DeSantis and Thomas, 1992).

Acculturation refers to the process of adapting to a culture different from the one in which a person was enculturated. Because North America is a continent of immigrants, you will frequently encounter clients undergoing acculturation. Culture is a learned group of traits, so it is possible for an individual to acquire a new cultural identity. Again, you must assess the *degree* of acculturation to predict the client's inclination to comply with a desirable modification in health care beliefs, attitudes, or practices. The degree of acculturation has been shown to be related to a variety of health concerns, such as mental health (Rogler, Cortes, and Malgady, 1991), psychosocial distress (Krause and Goldenhar, 1992), and childrearing attitudes (Raugh, Wasserman, and Brunelli, 1990). When a client is undergoing acculturation, you can play a significant role in teaching the sort of acquired health behavior the client is already attempting to learn.

Cultural determinism is simply a term for conveying the notion that a person's behavior is *determined* by cultural beliefs. The concept is central to cultural assessment because one must understand it to formulate client goals. A goal is something the client, not the nurse, wants to achieve. A goal therefore must take into account the client's culturally determined behavior; otherwise, you cannot expect client compliance.

Ethnocentrism is the tendency to view people unconsciously by using one's group and one's own customs as the standard for all judgments. A nurse with this tendency will gather data only selectively in accordance with personal standards, values, and judgments and will not be able to see what the patient has to offer or the different ways in which the patient views the world. This bias will limit the data a nurse gathers and will distort interpretation.

Cultural relativity refers to the attempt to view or interpret behavior of culturally different individuals within the context of those individuals' culture. This perspective acknowledges that behavior that is appropriate in one culture may not be so defined in another culture. Providing nursing care from a perspective of cultural relativity involves viewing behaviors within the context of the client's culture. This approach may provide meaning to behaviors that caregivers might otherwise consider negative or confusing.

Cultural competence refers to a combination of skills in provision of care to clients. Starn (1996) describes five components of culturally competent care: (1) basic knowledge about a family's culture, (2) awareness and acceptance of cultural differences, (3) understanding of the dynamics of cultural differences, (4) awareness of one's own personal and professional cultures, and (5) adaptation of services to respond to a family's culture. Cultural competence is a complex combination of attitude, knowledge, and skills that when integrated promote sensitive and, ideally, more effective interventions (Lipson, Dibble, and Minarik, 1996). Development of cultural competence occurs over time through experiences with clients from other cultures; through knowledge acquisition; through development of specific skills, such as cross-cultural communication and cultural assessment; and through the nurse's own appreciation of, and receptiveness to, the client's values, beliefs and customs. Cultural competence is needed to prevent mistakes such as inadvertently teaching behaviors that are inconsistent with a family's culture (e.g., encouraging a child's open expression of feelings or questioning of elders when such behavior is seen as inappropriate or disrespectful in that family's culture [Starn, 1996]).

Ethnoscience refers to a systematic study of the way of life of a designated cultural group to obtain an accurate account of the people's behavior and how they perceive and interpret their universe. An ethnoscience approach

includes the various ethnic groups' views on health and illness. This chapter takes an ethnoscience approach to cultural assessment because it presents the beliefs of cultural groups as they relate to health and illness. Research by Morse, Young, and Swartz (1991) examines the differences between Cree Indian methods of treating a chronic skin disease (psoriasis) and the Western health care system approach. Using an ethnographic approach, they were able to identify conflicts between the two types of health care and reasons for client dissatisfaction with the Western approach.

Disease, illness, and sickness are similar terms that are frequently used and misused. The distinctions among them are important to cultural assessment. *Disease* is a medical term, arising from the dominant, scientifically based health care subculture. It refers to a pathological process within human structure and function. *Illness* is a subjective term clients may use to describe the symptoms of discomfort. *Sickness,* on the other hand, is a personal state of illness with distinct social dimensions. Depending on the norms within any given culture, role behaviors are modified when a person becomes sick. These modified role behaviors are an important aspect of cultural assessment.

■ MAJOR VARIABLES IN CULTURAL ASSESSMENT

Tripp-Reimer (1992) describes an anthropological model of cultural strata that is useful for examining the variables in cultural assessment (Figure 7.4). As is shown in the model, customs (or behaviors) are based on beliefs, and beliefs are rooted in values. A nurse may observe and describe customs; therefore they are the easiest to assess. People, however, frequently learn values through an unconscious process of socialization; values are the most difficult to assess.

Values

Values provide the foundation for beliefs, attitudes, and behaviors. Often people are unaware of their values,

Comparison of Value Orientations

TIME ORIENTATIONS
Present oriented: Accepts each day as it comes; little regard for the past; future unpredictable
Past oriented: Maintains traditions that were meaningful in the past; worships ancestors
Future oriented: Anticipates "bigger and better" future; high value on change

ACTIVITY ORIENTATIONS
"Doing" orientation: Emphasizes accomplishments that are measurable by external standards
"Being" orientation: Spontaneous expression of self
"Being-in-becoming": Emphasizes self-development of all aspects of self as an integrated whole

HUMAN NATURE ORIENTATIONS
Human being basically evil but with perfectable nature; constant self-control and discipline necessary
Human being as neutral, neither good nor evil

HUMAN-NATURE ORIENTATIONS
Human being subject to environment with very little control over own destiny
Human being in harmony with nature
Human being master over nature

RELATIONAL ORIENTATIONS
Individualistic: Encourages individualism: impersonal relationships occur more with outsiders and less with family
Lineal: Group goals dominant over individual goals; ordered positional succession (father to son)
Collateral: Group goals dominant over individual goals: more emphasis on relationship with others on one's own level

Modified from Kluckhohn F: Dominant and variant value orientation. In Brink P, editor: *Transcultural nursing: a book of readings,* Stamford, Conn, 1976, Appleton & Lange.

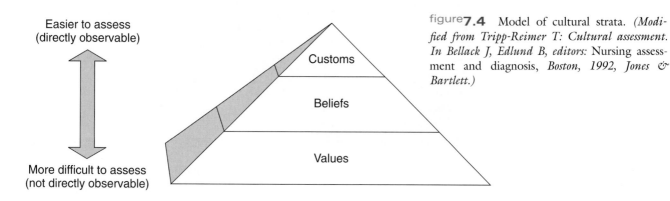

figure**7.4** Model of cultural strata. (*Modified from Tripp-Reimer T: Cultural assessment. In Bellack J, Edlund B, editors:* Nursing assessment and diagnosis, *Boston, 1992, Jones & Bartlett.*)

Easier to assess (directly observable)

More difficult to assess (not directly observable)

Customs

Beliefs

Values

even though they are able to describe their beliefs and customs. They acquire values through socialization early in childhood, and these values guide the individual's goals, aspirations, and behaviors. Kluckhohn (1976) describes values common to all population groups in the box on p. 135. Kluckhohn proposes that variation in value orientation is one of the most important differences among people.

Recognizing the underlying value orientation of the culture of the health care system and the impact it may have on interactions with clients is particularly helpful for nurses. The health care culture tends to have the following value orientations:

1. *Time orientation:* Has a future orientation, which means an expectation for promptness and keeping scheduled appointments.
2. *Activity orientation:* Values individuals for their accomplishments (a "doing" orientation), which may include getting healthy or taking medications as prescribed.
3. *Human-nature orientation:* Views humans as having mastery over nature and values the omnipotence of technology.
4. *Relational orientation:* Is individualistic in its focus, emphasizing autonomy and putting the needs of the individual over the needs of the family.

Be aware of your own values in these areas so that when conflicts with clients arise, you can have an understanding that your expectations (based on the preceding values) may be contributing to the difficulty.

Beliefs

Beliefs include opinions, knowledge, and faith regarding various aspects of the world. Beliefs of particular concern to nurses are those related to illness causation, preferred method of treatment, expected outcomes, and fears about the illness. How the individual defines illness is based on his or her belief system and is largely determined by his or her culture. Tripp-Reimer (1992) notes that an individual with an obvious pathological condition may not consult the "scientific" health care professional because the condition may be ignored, undetected, or attributed to a nonscientific cause.

Many chronic illnesses, such as hypertension and renal problems, may go undetected because they do not exhibit symptoms obvious to a layperson. Illnesses attributed to nonscientific causes are called "folk illnesses." A client usually seeks treatment for folk illnesses from a folk practitioner. Health professionals, such as physicians and nurses, are usually not seen as knowledgeable in these areas, and the client may not mention folk remedies or treatments unless specifically asked. Tripp-Reimer (1992) divides folk illnesses into two categories: naturalistic illness and personalistic illness.

Naturalistic illnesses are caused by impersonal factors that have no regard for the individual. These illnesses usually involve the concept of equilibrium. Problems develop when the balance is disturbed. One of the most common imbalances is between "hot" and "cold." These beliefs exist in Hispanic, Chinese, Filipino, and Arab cultures. In traditional Chinese health beliefs, the forces are called yin (cold) and yang (hot). Treatments

figure**7.5** Values are acquired through socialization early in childhood, guiding the child's goals, aspirations, and behaviors.

usually involve restoring balance by applying opposing forces, (e.g., application of the appropriate "hot" remedy to treat a "cold" illness and vice versa). Hot-cold classifications for treatments and illnesses are culturally determined and have nothing to do with actual temperature. The box below gives examples of hot-cold classifications. Understanding this belief system may help explain a client's desire for, or rejection of, a specific medical treatment. For example, the client may insist on penicillin (a "hot" medicine) or an x-ray (a "hot" treatment) for a viral respiratory infection (a "cold" condition) and may not be satisfied with his care without receiving what he believes to be an appropriate treatment.

Personalistic illnesses result from aggression directed at, or punishment of, the individual. The "evil eye" and witchcraft are two examples of personalistic folk beliefs. The "evil eye" is a concept known throughout Mediterranean (e.g., Greek and Italian cultures) and Spanish-speaking cultures. It is usually caused unintentionally and is related to envy and admiration. Complimenting another person's child may be considered a way to "cast the evil eye," and the symptoms may be interpreted as being related to this. Usually, some general methods can

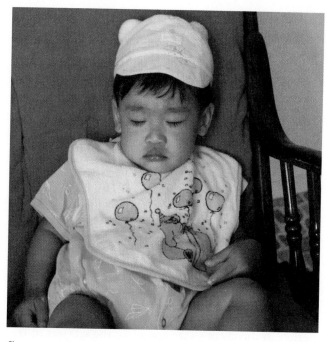

figure**7.6** How an individual perceives a sick child can be based on cultural beliefs.

Hot and Cold Conditions and Their Corresponding Treatment

HOT CONDITIONS	COLD FOODS	COLD MEDICINES AND HERBS
Fever	Fresh vegetables	Orange flower water
Infection	Tropical fruits	Linden
Diarrhea	Dairy products	Sage
Kidney problem	Meats such as goat, fish, chicken	Milk of magnesia
Rash	Honey	Bicarbonate of soda
Skin ailment	Cod	
Sore throat	Raisins	
Liver problem	Bottled milk	
Ulcer	Barley water	
Constipation		
COLD CONDITIONS	**HOT FOODS**	**HOT MEDICINES AND HERBS**
Cancer	Chocolate	Penicillin
Pneumonia	Cheese	Tobacco
Malaria	Temperate-zone fruits	Ginger root
Joint pain	Eggs	Garlic
Menstrual period	Peas	Cinnamon
Teething	Onions	Anise
Earache	Aromatic beverages	Vitamins
Rheumatism	Hard liquor	Iron preparations
Tuberculosis	Oils	Cod-liver oil
Cold	Meats such as beef, waterfowl, mutton	Castor oil
Headache	Goat's milk	Aspirin
Paralysis	Cereal grains	
Stomach cramps	Chili peppers	

From Seidel HM et al: *Mosby's guide to physical examination*, ed 3, St Louis, 1995, Mosby.

protect against the evil eye. Children may wear protective amulets, beads, or gold crosses, for example. Respect these cultural beliefs and help the client determine ways to resolve the situation along with appropriate medical interventions, if they are required.

Belief in witchcraft as a cause of illness is prevalent in many cultures. Snow (1981) noted evidence of this belief in Puerto Ricans, Haitians, and black Americans. He estimated that one third of black clients treated in psychiatric centers in the southern United States believed that they were victims of witchcraft. The common theme Snow noted was that someone had done something to cause another person's injury, illness, or death.

Clients usually seek out a folk healer for treatment of these conditions. For many clients, the practitioner can be most helpful by working in a collaborative and cooperative manner with the folk healer to provide holistic care to the client. An example of this approach is the effort of the Indian Health Service to involve traditional healers in the client's care and make the services of traditional healers accessible to clients even when they are hospitalized (Giger and Davidhizar, 1995). Table 7.1 describes different folk healing practices. Table 7.2 describes different types of folk healers, their preparation, and practice.

While health care practitioners may assess health beliefs in a variety of ways, an assessment model proposed by Kleinman, Eisenberg, and Good (1978) is very useful. These authors suggest the following set of questions to elicit the client's explanatory model:

What do you think caused your problem?

Why do you think it started when it did?

What does your sickness do to you? How does it work?

How severe is your sickness? Will it have a long or a short duration?

What kind of treatment do you think you should receive?

What are the most important results you hope to receive from this treatment?

What are the chief problems your sickness has caused you?

What do you fear most about your sickness?

Customs

Customs are learned behaviors that you can easily assess through observation and direct questioning. However, problems and misunderstandings can arise if you do not assess customs or if you do not validate the meaning of observed behaviors. Customs include dietary practices, communication patterns, family and kinship relations, religious practices, and health behaviors. Tables 7.3 and 7.4 describe examples of behaviors relevant to the health care of different cultural groups, and the implications for health care.

table 7.1   *Folk Healing Practices*

Practice name	Ethnicity	Practice procedure	Purpose
Acupuncture	Asian (Chinese)	Needles in meridians (energy lines), herbs	Pain, sinus problems, injuries, stress, stroke, deafness, epilepsy, and so on
Cao Gio	Vietnamese, Cambodian	Coining produces ecchymosis, petechiae	Coughing, congestion, fever
Curanderismo	Hispanic	Bleeding, herbs, emetics, diuretics, prayers, penance, miracles	Physiologic or psychologic problems, social maladjustment
Folk practitioners	Haitian	Poltices, voodoo	Evil eye lifted
Hilot	Filipino	Faith healing through prayer, herbal medicine, massage, manipulation of bones and tissues	Most illness
Medicine men	Native American	Meditation, sweat lodges, herbal medicine, ritual	Any disease caused by an imbalance with nature
Moxa	Chinese	Burning of a plant on the skin	Mumps, convulsions, epistaxis
Root doctor	African-American	Herbs, laying on of hands	Any illness
Spiritual healer	White	Laying on of hands	Physiologic, psychologic, or social problems

From: Starn J: Family culture and chronic conditions. In Jackson PL, Vessey JA: *Primary care of the child with a chronic condition,* ed 2, St Louis, 1996, Mosby.

table 7.2 *Healers and Their Scope of Practice*

Culture/folk practitioner	Preparation	Scope of practice
HISPANIC		
Family member	Possesses knowledge of folk medicine	Common illnesses of a mild nature that may or may not be recognized by modern medicine.
Curandero	May receive training in an apprenticeship. May receive a "gift from God" that enables her/him to cure. Knowledgeable in use of herbs, diet, massage, and rituals.	Treats almost all of the traditional illnesses. Some may not treat illness caused by witchcraft for fear of being accused of possessing evil powers. Usually admired by members of the community.
Espiritualista or spiritualist	Born with the special gifts of being able to analyze dreams and foretell future events. May serve apprenticeship with an older practitioner.	Emphasis on prevention of illness or bewitchment through use of medals, prayers, amulets. May also be sought for cure of existing illness.
Yerbero	No formal training. Knowledgeable in growing and prescribing herbs.	Consulted for preventive and curative use of herbs for both traditional and Western illnesses.
Sabador (may refer to a chiropractor by this title)	Knowledgeable in massage and manipulation of bones and muscles.*	Treats many traditional illnesses, particularly those affecting the musculoskeletal system. May also treat nontraditional illnesses.
BLACK		
"Old lady"	Usually an older woman who has successfully raised her own family. Knowledgeable in child care and folk remedies.	Consulted about common ailments and for advice on child care. Found in rural and urban communities.
Spiritualist	Called by God to help others. No formal training. Usually associated with a fundamentalist Christian church.	Assists with problems that are financial, personal, spiritual, or physical. Predominantly found in urban communities.
Voodoo priest(ess) or hougan	May be trained by other priests(esses). In the U.S. the eldest son of a priest becomes a priest. A daughter of a priest(ess) becomes a priestess if she is born with a veil (amniotic sac) over her face.	Knowledgeable about properties of herbs; interpretation of signs and omens. Able to cure illness caused by voodoo. Uses communication techniques to establish a therapeutic milieu like a psychiatrist. Treats blacks, Mexican-Americans, and Native Americans.
CHINESE		
Herbalist	Knowledgeable in diagnosis of illness and herbal remedies.	Both diagnostic and therapeutic. Diagnostic techniques include interviewing, inspection, auscultation, and assessment of pulses.

From Hautman MA: Folk health and illness beliefs, *Nurse Pract* 4(4):31, 1979.
*Preparation is for *sabador*, not chiropractor.

table 7.3 *Cultural Behaviors Relevant to Health Assessment*

Cultural group	Cultural variations (Common belief/practice)	Nursing implications
African-Americans	Dialect and slang terms require careful communication to prevent error (i.e., "bad" may mean "good").	Question the client's meaning or intent.
Mexican-Americans	Eye behavior is important. An individual who looks at and admires a child without touching the child has given the child the "evil eye."	Always touch the child you are examining or admiring.
Native Americans	Eye contact is considered a sign of disrespect and is thus avoided.	Recognize that the client may be attentive and interested even though eye contact is avoided.
Appalachians	Eye contact is considered impolite or a sign of hostility. Verbal patter may be confusing.	Avoid excessive eye contact. Clarify statements.
American Eskimos	Body language is very important. The individual seldom disagrees publicly with others. Client may nod yes to be polite, even if not in agreement.	Monitor own body language closely as well as client's to detect meaning.
Jewish-Americans	Orthodox Jews consider excess touching, particularly from members of the opposite sex, offensive.	Establish whether client is an Orthodox Jew and avoid excessive touch.
Chinese-Americans	Individual may nod head to indicate yes or shake head to indicate no. Excessive eye contact indicates rudeness. Excessive touch is offensive.	Ask questions carefully and clarify responses. Avoid excessive eye contact and touch.
Filipino-Americans	Offending people is to be avoided at all cost. Nonverbal behavior is very important.	Monitor nonverbal behaviors of self and client, being sensitive to physical and emotional discomfort or concerns of the client.
Haitian-Americans	Touch is used in conversation. Direct eye contact is used to gain attention and respect during communication.	Use direct eye contact when communicating.
East Indian Hindu–Americans	Women avoid eye contact as a sign of respect.	Be aware that men may view eye contact by women as offensive. Avoid eye contact.
Vietnamese-Americans	Avoidance of eye contact is a sign of respect. The head is considered sacred; it is not polite to pat the head. An upturned palm is offensive in communication.	Limit eye contact. Touch the head only when mandated and explain clearly before proceeding to do so. Avoid hand gesturing.

Modified from Giger JN, Davidhizar RE: *Transcultural nursing: assessment and intervention,* ed 2, St Louis, 1995, Mosby.

Diet and nutrition

Anthropologists have shown that cultural groups differ in their dietary beliefs and practices, but this is obvious to anyone who associates particular foods with specific ethnic groups. The development of national cuisines is a complex process related to the availability of certain kinds of food, the price, the efficiency of its distribution, the subjective preferences of taste and spices, and patterns of trade and commerce. Hotter, spicier food is preferred by groups living relatively closer to the equator, where the climate is warmer, whereas groups living in higher latitudes in more temperate climates prefer relatively less spicy food. The variety of foods available in industrialized countries is greater than that in Third World countries. Moreover, apart from its nutritional value, food carries a range of symbolic meanings. Food that is popular in one society may be rigorously forbidden in another. Food and the social aspects of eating it play a central role in daily life. Consequently, the practitioner should appreciate that dietary beliefs and practices are notoriously difficult to change, even if they interfere with adequate nutrition.

Try to understand the ways in which various cultures view their food, and the ways food is classified, before attempting to change nutrition practices. Food is usually classified into (1) definitions of what is edible and what is not, (2) what is sacred and what is profane, (3) the ways food is grouped, (4) food as medicine, and (5) social food. Rancid butter is not normally considered edible in North American culture, yet it is a standard condiment in tea in many central Asian regions. By the same token, food commonly eaten in North America, such as pork rinds, would be considered repulsive in some other cultures. Snails and eel, for instance, are considered delicacies by some people but inedible by others.

In the United States and Canada, industrialized countries with many immigrants, few foods are generally considered profane. But among specific religious groups, some examples of sacred and profane foods are familiar. Many Jews will not eat pork, and strict Catholics will not eat meat on Fridays (although this has become a less common practice). Apart from religious-based sanctions, many people are vegetarians and other groups eschew highly processed foods.

In American culture, food is classified according to the Food Guide Pyramid, which consists of bread/cereals; fruits, vegetables; dairy; meat/protein; and fats and sweets (see Chapter 5: Nutritional Assessment). Many people regard food in terms of its use by the body—protein, fat, and starch and carbohydrates. We live in a culture strongly influenced by science, and the biochemistry of food is part of our general fund of knowledge. The staples in the diets of a great many North Americans are meat and potatoes, something sweet for

figure**7.7** Cultural groups may differ in their dietary beliefs and practices.

dessert, salads, soups, and fruit juices, all reflecting the conception of a healthy diet as one containing a balance of the food groups widely recognized and accepted as healthy. In other cultures standard dishes might include pastas or rice, sausage, or bread.

Medicinal qualities are ascribed to various foods, rightly or wrongly, across the world. North Americans have their own widely shared beliefs associating food with medicine. Apples keep doctors away. Honey and lemon help reduce congestion. Fish is brain food. Citrus fruits provide protection from colds. Oats unclog arteries.

Finally, all cultures tend to associate foods with social occasions unique to their cultures. Some occasions seem to demand wine, and others seem to demand hot chocolate. Certain foods are consumed at baseball games, whereas other foods are eaten as family traditions on various holidays.

Other cultures are no different from the dominant culture in these broad aspects of food. Only the foods that carry strong cultural preferences or taboos vary from one culture to another.

Communication patterns

Communication patterns are closely intertwined with culture and may be the source of misunderstandings between you and your client. Communication patterns include both verbal and nonverbal behaviors. Verbal behaviors include language, vocabulary, grammatical structure, voice qualities, intonation, speed, pronunciation,

| table 7.4 | *Cross-Cultural Examples of Cultural Phenomena Impacting on Nursing Care* | | |

Nations of origin	Communication	Space	Time orientation
Asian China Hawaii Philippines Korea Japan Southeast Asia (Laos, Cambodia, Vietnam)	National language preference Dialects, written characters Use of silence Nonverbal and contextual cuing	Noncontact people	Present
African West Coast (as slaves) Many African countries West Indian Islands Dominican Republic Haiti Jamaica	National languages Dialect: Pidgin, Creole, Spanish, and French	Close personal space	Present over future
Europe Germany England Italy Ireland Other European countries	National languages Many learn English immediately	Noncontact people Aloof Distant Southern countries: closer contact and touch	Future over present
Native American 170 Native American tribes Aleuts Eskimos	Tribal languages Use of silence and body lan- guage	Space very important and has no bound- aries	Present
Hispanic countries Spain Cuba Mexico Central and South America	Spanish or Portuguese primary language	Tactile relationships Touch Handshakes Embracing Value physical presence	Present

From Giger JN, Davidhizar RE: *Transcultural nursing: assessment and intervention*, ed 2, St Louis, 1995, Mosby; compiled by Rachel Specter, RN, PhD.

and silence. Nonverbal behaviors include touch, facial expression, eye movement, posture, personal space, and distance.

Determining what language is spoken at home is an important part of a cultural assessment. Find out how well the client understands written and spoken English, since this is important for both verbal interactions and for giving the client written information, such as health education pamphlets. Even when the client speaks English, colloquialisms may be confusing. For example, "bad" may have a negative connotation for one group and a more positive connotation for another group. Certain groups may use lay terms such as "high blood" for hypertension and "low blood" for anemia. These may vary among different ethnic groups, so confirm your understanding of the term with the client.

Social organization	Environmental control	Biological variations
Family: hierarchial structure, loyalty Devotion to tradition Many religions, including Taoism, Buddhism, Islam, and Christianity Community social organizations	Traditional health and illness beliefs Use of traditional medicines Traditional practitioners: Chinese doctors and herbalists	Liver cancer Stomach cancer Coccidioidomycosis Hypertension Lactose intolerance
Family: many female, single parent Large, extended family networks Strong church affiliation within community Community social organizations	Traditional health and illness beliefs Folk medicine tradition Traditional healer: root-worker	Sickle cell anemia Hypertension Cancer of the esophagus Stomach cancer Coccidioidomycosis Lactose intolerance
Nuclear families Extended families Judeo-Christian religions Community social organizations	Primary reliance on modern health care system Traditional health and illness beliefs Some remaining folk medicine traditions	Breast cancer Heart disease Diabetes mellitus Thalassemia
Extremely family oriented Biological and extended families Children taught to respect traditions Community social organizations	Traditional health and illness beliefs Folk medicine tradition Traditional healer: medicine man	Accidents Heart disease Cirrhosis of the liver
Nuclear family Extended families Compadrazzo: godparents Community social organizations	Traditional health and illness beliefs Folk medicine tradition Traditional healers: curandero, espiritista, partera, senora	Diabetes mellitus Parasites Coccidioidomycosis Lactose intolerance

Also be aware of cultural norms related to the way you address clients (e.g., whether you address them by their first name or use a more formal title). Proper forms of address may vary according to ethnic or regional groups.

Nonverbal communication may also have different meanings in different cultures. In North American middle-class culture, looking directly at the person with whom you are speaking is important. However, in many cultures (Asian, Native American, Indochinese, Arab, Appalachian), looking directly at another person may be a sign of disrespect or aggression. Touch also has many different interpretations by different cultural groups. Some groups, such as those of Mediterranean descent, use touch to communicate feelings, whereas other groups see touch as an invasion of privacy. Many Asian

groups believe that the head is the most sacred part of the body; therefore obtain permission before touching the client's head. The feet are the lowest part of the body, so showing the bottom of your shoe or pointing your toe at the client is disrespectful.

Family relationships

Attitudes toward family structure and family roles and relationships have been traditionally mediated by cultural considerations. However, over the past 20 years cultural differences related to families, once a defining characteristic of different cultural groups, have been rapidly changing. Our society has become highly mobile and more integrated, tearing down barriers that previously kept family norms intact within subcultures. The media have focused our attention on alternate family arrangements and practices, making them more familiar and thus acceptable.

As of 25 years ago, the concept of the nuclear family was predominant. Typically, young men and women married someone who was raised within 25 miles of them. People married people with whom they shared cultural or group affiliations. Couples tended to share the same race, religion, and socioeconomic status. They had children, and the mother provided child care while the father earned the income. They tended to stay married for life, and they tried to transmit these values to their children. Because of mass communication, easy ac-

cess to cheap and fast transportation, and economic changes promoting urbanization, today's young people often move far away from their parents. More young people attend college and use this opportunity to migrate elsewhere. Far from the daily influences of their families, new group affiliations develop based on common interests, education, and jobs. There has been an increased incidence and acceptance of divorce, dual-income families, single-parent families, teenage parents, and involvement of fathers in child care. The nuclear family is not nearly as prevalent now, and neither are culturally mediated family practices that used to distinguish one cultural group from another.

This is not to say that cultural differences in attitudes toward family structure and role no longer exist. Rather, they cannot be taken for granted. Therefore, avoid making any assumptions about the relationship between family and culture, and take a value-free approach to assessing family dimensions, which can be so important to health and well-being.

A neutral starting point in assessing the client's family is to determine the family structure. Use a simple family tree or family diagram, sometimes called a genogram, to establish who the members of the family are and how the client fits in. Particularly with individuals who live far from their natural families, extend the genogram concept to a broader tool known as an ecomap. This tool maps the network of the client's significant others, including friends, neighbors, peers, and associates who may be more important to the client's health and well-being than are actual family members.

Once the structure is clear, explore roles and relationships to determine whom the client is attached to and how the dynamics of various relationships work. Re-

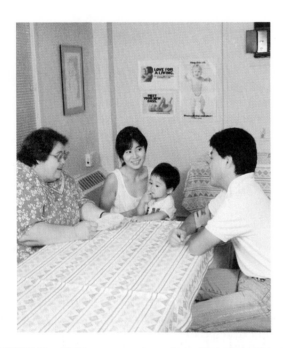

figure**7.8**   Making assumptions about the relationship between family and culture should be avoided, since cultural differences related to families are rapidly changing in today's society.

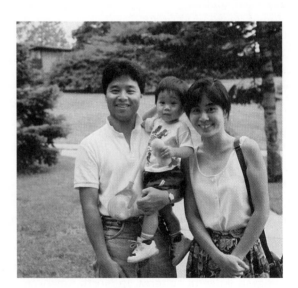

figure**7.9**   A "traditional" nuclear family.

lationships, both within families and in broader associations, can be close or distant, dependent or hostile. In each relationship, the sharing of power and decision making, as well as approaches to problem solving, can vary widely. Assess communication patterns and willingness to express feelings and offer support. Individuality may be submerged or fostered. Many tools exist to provide for an orderly assessment of these roles and functions. A familiar one that assesses the person's satisfaction with relationships in the immediate family (and is both reliable and valid and clinically useful) is the Family APGAR (see box below).

Keep in mind that despite the rapid change in family structure and function associated with distinct cultural groups, cultural considerations remain very important for many individuals.

Religious practices

Religion has an influence on the lifestyles of most cultures and may affect health care practices. Most religions have rituals or ceremonies that mark life cycle stages such as birth, entrance into adulthood, marriage, and death. Religions may have certain dietary restrictions, such as prohibitions against eating pork (Jewish and Muslim religions) or abstaining from specific foods on certain days (Roman Catholic). Religions may prohibit certain types of health care interventions, such as the administration of blood (Jehovah's Witnesses) or use of medications containing caffeine or made from pork products. Table 3.2 describes a variety of religious beliefs that may affect nursing care. Remember that the strictness of adherence to these rules varies among individuals and subgroups within the religion.

Religious beliefs may influence a client's perception of the cause of an illness, its severity, and the type of healer required. The religion and religiosity of the individual determine the role that religious faith plays in the recovery process. In many instances religiosity also affects the response to a specific treatment and the process of healing. Although cultural heritage and religion may

---

Family APGAR

DEFINITION

Adaptation is the use of intrafamilial and extrafamilial resources for problem solving when family equilibrium is stressed during a crisis.

Partnership is the sharing of decision making and nurturing responsibilities by family members.

Growth is the physical and emotional maturation and self-fulfillment that is achieved by family members through mutual support and guidance.

Affection is the caring or loving relationship that exists among family members.

Resolve is the commitment to devote time to other members of the family for physical and emotional nurturing. It also usually involves a decision to share wealth and space.

FUNCTIONS MEASURED BY THE FAMILY APGAR

How resources are shared, or the degree to which a member is satisfied with the assistance received when family resources are needed.

How decisions are shared, or the member's satisfaction with mutuality in family communication and problem solving.

How nurturing is shared, or the member's satisfaction with the freedom available within the family to change roles and attain physical and emotional growth or maturation.

How emotional experiences are shared, or the member's satisfaction with the intimacy and emotional interaction that exists in the family.

How time (and space and money) is shared, or the member's satisfaction with the time commitment that has been made to the family by its members.

RELEVANT OPEN-ENDED QUESTIONS

How have family members aided each other in time of need?

In what way have family members received help or assistance from friends and community agencies?

How do family members communicate with each other about such matters as vacations, finances, medical care, large purchases, and personal problems?

How have family members changed during the past years?

How has this change been accepted by family members?

In what ways have family members aided each other in growing or developing independent lifestyles?

How have family members reacted to your desires for change?

How have members of your family responded to emotional expressions such as affection, love, sorrow, or anger?

How do members of your family share time, space, and money?

Modified from Smilkstein G: The Family APGAR: a proposal for a family function test and its use by physicians, *J Fam Pract* 6:1231–1239, 1978.

be interrelated, do not assume that membership in a particular ethnic or cultural group is equated with membership in a specific religion. For example, although many Mexican-Americans are Catholic, do not assume that your Mexican-American client is Catholic and in a time of crisis offer to contact a priest for support. This approach, although well intentioned, may add to the client's stress and sense of frustration. Gathering initial information about the client's religious affiliation and the role that religious beliefs and practices play in health and illness helps avoid mistaken assumptions and provides information that is important to the client's care.

Health and illness behaviors

Cultures also influence the client's attitudes toward health, response to illness, and even experience of symptoms such as pain. Individuals learn about health behaviors through socialization in their families. Beliefs about illness and alternative types of health care providers are discussed earlier in the section on beliefs. Specific illness behaviors also are culturally determined. Zola (1966) examined the differences in symptoms that caused clients to seek health care by a physician. In his comparison of diagnostically matched clients from different ethnic groups, he found that the definition of an illness and the pattern of response to symptoms varied according to ethnic group. The experience of pain is another symptom that is strongly influenced by culture.

Pain. Pain is among the most common symptoms in clinical practice, yet it is not purely a neurophysiological response. Pain is influenced by social, psychological, and cultural factors.

Culture influences both pain intensity and pain tolerance. Culture determines a person's attitudes toward pain and beliefs about it. Emotions associated with the context in which pain is experienced can have a powerful effect on how pain is felt. Sometimes soldiers are wounded in battle and do not realize it until afterward. In some cultures meditation or religious trances dissipate the sensation of pain, as in the firewalkers of Sri Lanka, who are apparently oblivious to the expected intensity of the pain they experience. Other cultures value the ability to withstand pain without complaint or physical manifestations, as in the case of certain American Indian and African tribes, who demonstrate their adulthood by withstanding painful stimuli.

It is difficult to separate culturally determined pain from pain that is mediated by neurological mechanisms. Nurses often encounter the so-called "placebo effect," in which an inactive drug relieves suffering. A simple belief in the effectiveness of the placebo can release endorphins in the brain, actually providing physiological pain relief.

Culture also determines when pain is abnormal, requiring medical attention and treatment. The extent to which pain is considered a normal part of life also affects a person's willingness to withstand it. Studies show, for instance, that Polish women are far more able to accept the pain associated with childbirth than their American counterparts, who have greater access to anesthesia during labor.

Each culture has its own language of distress, which includes facial expressions, changes in activity, sounds, and words describing feeling. These norms determine acceptable ways clients express pain to others. For example, Zborowski (1952) in a classic study found that Italian-Americans tended to dramatize their pain as a means of allaying anxiety and dissipating the pain. Irish-Americans, by contrast, were more reticent about their bodily complaints. Villarruel and Ortiz de Montellano (1992) identified themes related to the cultural meanings of pain and pain-related behaviors in Mesoamerican cultures (with particular reference to Mexican-Americans).

Pain is a subjective sensation that has physiological, cultural, and emotional components. The actual cause or intensity of pain is difficult to assess. In treating pain, remember that it is the client's experience of pain, as the client feels it, that determines how you treat it. Carefully assess, however, cultural considerations that affect a client's ability or willingness to report pain as a sign of illness, as well as inclination to seek treatment, because of their implications for ascertaining the person's actual degree of illness.

Other Variables to Consider
Heredity

Information concerning ethnic, cultural, or racial heritage is also important for assessing the client's susceptibility to specific genetic disorders. Because of intermarriage within a relatively narrow range of ethnic, geographic, or religious groups, certain traits are passed on that place members of those groups at risk for genetic disorders. (See Table 3.1 for an overview of disorders and genetic traits for a variety of population or ethnic groups.) Knowledge of these susceptibilities is important for screening clients for problems, providing interventions to avoid complications related to problems, and counseling clients who are considering having children and are concerned about the risks of passing on such traits.

Socioeconomic status

Socioeconomic status (SES) is related to education, income, and occupation. A client's SES may have a stronger influence on health and access to health care than ethnic or racial status (Lipson, Dibble, and Minarik, 1996). Public health research shows that people in lower socioeconomic groups have the highest rates of death and disease resulting from virtually every health problem. Thus, although speaking of "a culture of

poverty" is incorrect, socioeconomic status is an important predictor of health and disease.

People in poverty make less use of the health care system. Their choice of providers, as well as their criterion for seeking health care, is different from the frequency and criterion associated with more affluent citizens. Therefore an awareness of a client's economic status has implications for care.

The changing American demographics: the need for cross-cultural care

The American population is becoming increasingly more diverse with a rapid growth in the numbers of ethnic minorities, as well as new immigrants. Since the 1980s the American population has grown about 10%. While groups with a long history in this country grew at a moderate rate, there was a major increase in the number of immigrants, in particular Hispanics and Asians, and refugees (Buchwald et al., 1994). This represents a profound shift in the demographic makeup of the United States. It is estimated that by the year 2000 nearly one third of school-age children will be from minority populations. In some of the Southwestern states, white children are expected to be in the minority by the year 2000 (Starn, 1996). As our population becomes more diverse, the need for an appreciation and understanding of cultural influences on health care becomes increasingly more important. Awareness of the distribution of

table 7.5 *Population Data for Selected Ethnic Groups*

Group	U.S. #	State #1*	State #2	State #3
Arab	716,391	CA: 123,933	NY: 79,600	MI: 65,906
Black/African-American	29,930,524	NY: 2,860,590	CA: 2,198,766	TX: 2,018,543
Brazilian[†]	375,000	NY, NJ, CT: 200,000	FL: 120,000	CA: 20,000
Cambodian	149,047	CA: 71,178	MA: 13,849	WA: 10,757
Chinese	1,647,486	CA: 713,423	NY: 285,322	HI: 68,769
Columbian	378,726	NY: 107,377	FL: 83,634	NJ: 52,210
Cuban	1,053,197	FL: 675,786	NJ: 87,085	NY: 77,016
Ethiopian[†]	123,000	CA	Wash., DC	NY
Filipino	1,419,711	CA: 733,941	HI: 168,232	IL: 67,383
Guatemalan	268,779	CA: 159,177	NY: 21,995	IL: 16,017
Gypsies[†]	300,000	NYC	LA, SF, Bay Area	Cleveland, Seattle
Haitian[‡]	365,000	FL: 125,000	NY: 125,000	MA: 35,000
Hmong	94,439	CA: 49,343	MN: 17,764	WI: 16,980
E. Indian	786,694	CA: 154,122	NY: 132,801	NJ: 79,367
Iranian[§]	285,000	CA	NY	Wash., DC
Japanese	866,160	CA: 320,730	HI: 252,291	NY: 36,488
Korean	797,304	CA: 259,908	NY: 97,111	IL: 41,436
Mexican	13,393,208	CA: 6,070,637	TX: 3,899,518	AZ: 619,435
American Indian	1,937,391	OK: 252,132	CA: 243,736	AZ: 204,150
Nicaraguan	202,658	FL: 79,056	CA: 74,119	NY: 11,011
Pakistanis[†]	500,000	NY	Chicago	CA
Puerto Rican	2,651,815	NY: 1,046,896	NJ: 304,179	FL: 240,673
Russian	2,114,506	NY: 455,162	CA: 327,675	FL: 183,244
Salvadoran	565,081	CA: 388,769	TX: 58,128	NY: 47,350
Samoan	57,679	CA: 28,320	HI: 15,000	WA: 3589
Vietnamese	593,213	CA: 280,233	TX: 69,634	WA: 20,693
West Indian	21,058,345	NY: 452,338	FL: 226,854	NJ: 60,668

From Lipson JG, Dibble SL, Minarik PA: *Culture and nursing care: a pocket guide,* San Francisco, 1996, USCF Nursing Press.

*This column shows the state in which the group is most populous; states #2 and #3 are the second and third most populous states; based on 1990 U.S. Census data unless otherwise indicated.

[†]U.S. Census data for specific group either unavailable or undercounted. Table estimates are provided based on various sources and on in-depth knowledge of the specific population. West Indians include Haitians, Trinidadians, Barbadians, and Jamaicans.

[‡]Stepick A, Stepick CD: *Demographics of the Diaspora: census results of Haitians in the U.S.,* Immigration and Ethnicity Institute, Florida International University.

[§]Bozorgmehr M: Diaspora in the postrevolutionary period, *Encyclopedia Iranica* 7:380-383, 1995.

table 7.6   Sample Format for a Cross-Cultural Assessment of a Family with a Member with a Chronic Condition

Area of concern	Sample questions
Family demographics	Who lives in your family (i.e., members, ages, sexes)? What kind of work do members of the household do? What is your family's socioeconomic status? What kind of health insurance coverage do you have? Which family members are covered? What chronic conditions or symptoms do you have? How would you describe the problems that have brought you here today? Who is the primary care taker in your family?
Orientation	Where were the members of the family born? What is the ethnic background of the family members? How many years have family members lived in the United States? (NOTE: Only ask if appropriate.) In your family is it important to be on time for an appointment or to get to an appointment when possible based on everyone's schedule for that day? Why do you think you have (the above-named) chronic condition (e.g., punishment for a parent's past behavior, such as conceiving a child out of wedlock; the result of a genetic problem; or a gift given because of the family's patience and love)?
Communication	What language(s) and dialect(s) are spoken at home? Who reads English in the family? If no one reads English, in what language would you prefer printed materials? Do parents and children look when spoken to or do they look down? To whom should questions be addressed? (NOTE: Avoid using a child as a translator, if at all possible, because of the strain this task imposes.)
Family relationships	Besides the immediate household, who else makes up the members of this family? Who makes the decisions in this family (e.g., mother-in-law, father, both partners, other family or friends, group decision)? Who cares for the client and the client's medical needs? What are the housing arrangements (e.g., space, number of rooms, members living in the home)? What is the family's usual daily routine like? To whom do you turn when you need help with, or have questions about, your condition?
Beliefs about health	What is the present health status of family members? What illnesses or conditions are present in the current family members? What illnesses or conditions were present in deceased family members? How often and for what reasons have family members used Western medicine in the past? What complementary therapies are used by your family routinely and specifically for the client (e.g., acupuncture, healers, prayer, massage)? What do you do when you are in pain? Is it important to keep the client at home or to use institutional placement? What do you think will help clear up the problem? Are there things that help you get better that the health care providers should know? What problems has your illness caused your family?

Modified from Starn J: Family culture and chronic conditions. In Jackson PL, Vessey JA: *Primary care of the child with a chronic condition,* ed 2, St Louis, 1996, Mosby.

table 7.6	*Sample Format for a Cross-Cultural Assessment of a Family with a Member with a Chronic Condition—cont'd*	

Area of concern	Sample questions
Education	How much schooling have members of the family completed?
	What ways are the best for you to learn about your condition (e.g., pamphlets, videos, direct patient teaching, home visits, return demonstrations)?
	From whom are you most comfortable learning about your condition (e.g., doctor, nurse, social worker, home health aide, other family members)?
Religion	What religion(s) are practiced in your family?
	What religious things do you do to help yourself or your family (e.g., pray, meditate, attend a support group, practice the laying on of hands)?
	What things does your religion say you should *not* do (e.g., have blood transfusions, allow strangers or dangerous circumstances to affect you or your family)?
Nutrition	When are usual mealtimes for your family?
	With whom do you eat?
	What foods do you usually eat?
	What special foods do you eat when you are sick?
	What foods do you *not* eat and when?

populations in this country may also help providers focus their learning on specific cultural groups in their region. Table 7.5 provides regional population data for selected ethnic groups.

■ CULTURAL ASSESSMENT CONSIDERATIONS

Health care providers often want detailed descriptions of characteristics of different cultural groups to help guide their care. There are several excellent texts that present such information (e.g., Giger and Davidhizar, 1995; and Lipson, Dibble, and Minarik, 1996; as well as others listed in the Bibliography). It is important to keep in mind that these descriptions are generalizations meant to be used as guidelines only.

Cultural traits are not uniform and static. How important cultural influences are to health care concerns varies according to the degree of enculturation and acculturation, the type of problem, and the congruence with the health care culture. Knowledge of cultural factors provides a context for understanding behaviors and designing care to meet the client's (or family's) needs. A cultural assessment does not require exhaustive information on every element of the culture. Make sure to identify major values, beliefs, and behaviors related to particular health concerns. Tailor actual assessments and interventions to the individual client and family. Also avoid making assumptions about cultural beliefs and be-

haviors without receiving validation from the client. This assessment involves a shared negotiation between you and the client in which each person is equal in bringing important and relevant information to the interview.

Cultural affiliation cannot be determined by an individual's appearance or surname. Therefore it is important that every client have a cultural assessment. Lipson, Dibble, and Minarik (1996) recommend that at a minimum the following content be included in the cultural assessment of any client.

1. Where was the client born? If an immigrant, how long has the client lived in this country?
2. What is the client ethnic affiliation, and how strong is the client's ethnic identity?
3. Who are the client's major support people: family members, friends? Does the client live in an ethnic community?
4. What are the primary and secondary languages? What is the client's speaking and reading ability in these languages?
5. How would you characterize the client's nonverbal communication style?
6. What is the client's religion? What is its importance in daily life and current practices?
7. What are the client's food preferences and prohibitions?
8. What is the client's economic situation, and is the income adequate to meet the needs of the client and family?

1. The asset model used is based on recognizing cultural differences in child rearing, family strengths, and culturally based coping methods.

   The primary care provider gathers data based on reviewing previous health care records, reading about the specific culture to learn about basic beliefs and values, and asking family members questions. This model asks what the family's strengths are (e.g., family members present, ways the family cares for their child, types of complementary therapies the family has used, ways family members find support or coping techniques, shared caregiving by all family members). These strengths are then built on by the primary care provider to foster care.

2. Primary care providers seek community participation in all stages of program design, development, implementation, outreach, policy making, problem solving, and evaluation.

   Informal and formal community leaders need to be involved in and approve of assessment and intervention approaches. This means talking to church leaders, various traditional healers, and elders who are respected in each ethnic community to learn what they think is culturally appropriate and sensitive care. Primary care providers may also seek out leaders of support groups for clients with special needs.

3. Community outreach to families is ongoing and culturally appropriate.

   Primary care providers and support staff who either speak the language of the clients or are from the same ethnic group are sought. Interpreters are hired when necessary to provide outreach at schools, churches, or ethnic gathering places. Nurses must explain concepts of confidentiality and privacy to interpreters. Nurses should also look at the client/parent when the interpreter is translating, unless direct eye contact is contraindicated in the culture (e.g., Native American or Filipino cultures).

4. Intake systems are sensitive to family and cultural values.

   Primary care providers should ask the family appropriate questions about the family's culture. However, intake may take several visits if privacy and mistrust of outsiders are issues that must be resolved before effective service can begin. Limit the number of professional care providers present. Encourage the family to have those family members who are important to them and the interpreter present. Conduct the meeting in either an informal or a formal manner based on the family's values.

5. Families are involved directly in the family treatment and service plan.

   Families help prioritize the goals. The family decision makers are consulted in determining the plan. The family's orientation to primary care providers as authority figures or joint decision makers is determined before attempting to develop the service plan. Family caregivers and decision makers are involved in the ways that the family deem acceptable when developing the individualized service plan.

6. Family goals permit intracultural variation on a case-by-case basis.

   Standard care plans are altered based on family needs to include alternative modes of therapy, such as healers, acupuncture, or other practices of importance to the family.

7. Emphasis is placed on maintaining and improving the self-esteem, cultural identification, and goal-setting ability of each family to foster self-sufficiency.

   Family decision makers and the caregivers are acknowledged. Family strengths are praised.

8. The teaching of parent-child interaction patterns must fit ideal family cultural values.

   For example, a Filipino or Native American child is not pushed to look at authority figures or to speak up in a disagreement; deference and avoidance of eye contact are culturally appropriate.

9. Team members have ongoing, culturally appropriate training.

   Team members are either of the same cultural background and speak the same language as the family or they have taken workshops given by ethnic leaders or others with expertise in the cultural group receiving care.

10. Educational materials, media, evaluation, and monitoring instruments are field-tested for cultural appropriateness and congruency in language content and emotional meaning.

11. Typical cultural and familial celebrations and symbolism are incorporated within services. Special holidays may be acknowledged by families sharing native foods and holiday traditions with care providers and other families.

12. Continuous evaluation is mandated to ensure cultural appropriateness and program effectiveness. The client's progress is monitored internally and by external evaluators. Assess the family's perceptions of the intervention. Determine whether the family is meeting goals and prioritizing these goals.

Modified from Starn J: Family culture and chronic conditions. In Jackson PL, Vessey JA: *Primary care of the child with a chronic condition*, ed 2, St Louis, 1996, Mosby.

9. What are the health and illness beliefs and practices?

10. What are the customs and beliefs around such transitions as birth, illness, and death?

Table 7.6 provides an example of a more detailed cultural assessment of a family with a chronically ill member. This could be easily modified for an acutely ill client or one with health promotion needs.

Health care providers also need to consider the ways in which the health care system in which they function can be more responsive to the needs of culturally diverse populations. The box on p. 150 provides an excellent summary of the ways providers can promote culturally sensitive health care services. This will become increasingly important given the demographic changes predicted for the future.

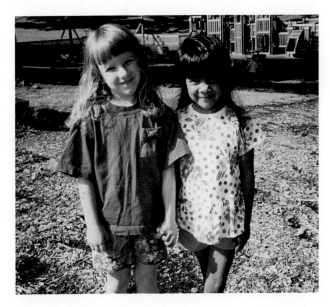

figure **7.10** Knowledge of cultural factors provides a context for understanding behaviors and designing care to meet the client's needs.

Assessment Techniques

▧ PURPOSE OF EXAMINATION

The overall goal of the physical examination is to identify variations from the normal state. This information becomes part of the client's database. The health assessment database consists of both subjective and objective information. Subjective information is the client's verbalized perceptions and interpretations. In the interview, the history and review of systems provide subjective information. This information alerts the nurse to areas to focus on during the examination. The nurse obtains objective information through the physical examination by observation or measurement of data using all of the senses. This information is used to support the subjective information given by the client during the interview.

▧ CONDUCTING THE EXAMINATION

Basic Principles

The examiner's goal is to conduct an efficient and complete examination that involves as little trauma and fatigue to the client as possible. Accomplishing this goal requires a consistent, systematic pattern of performing the examination. Following such a pattern will prevent omitting a step and possibly vital information. The nurse examiner must be thorough and exacting in the examination routine. With experience, he or she will develop an individual examination technique and sequence. However, the following six general principles will help to ensure that the examiner conducts a comprehensive examination in a logical order:

1. Explain the procedures to the client at the begin-

ning of the evaluation and restate them as the examination proceeds. Assist the client in appropriate positioning and warn the client of any uncomfortable maneuvers.

2. Use a head-to-toe approach. The head and face are examined before the genitals or feet because this sequence is generally more acceptable to the adult client.

3. Move from external to internal. Begin with observation, and then use instruments or perform digital examinations. Initial observations are general impressions, such as the client's appearance. Later observations might involve using an instrument such as an otoscope to identify anatomical landmarks of the eardrum, or tympanic membrane.

4. Examine normal or unaffected areas before observing abnormal areas or parts of the body where the client describes symptoms. The regions that are to be examined must be exposed completely to ensure an accurate finding. Be sensitive to the client's anxiety and possible embarrassment when certain areas of the body are exposed.

5. Observe for body symmetry, comparing one side to the other. Although minor asymmetry may be a normal finding, right-to-left differences in leg circumference or joint movement may be the first clue to other problems.

6. Perform the physical examination while standing on the client's right. This consistency of examiner position will help to locate anatomical landmarks while the examination is being performed.

Safety

Health care providers must be aware of the need to protect themselves and their clients from the risk of infection. Whenever a health care provider comes in close physical contact with a client, infection can be transmitted. Hand washing is one of the most effective methods of reducing the transmission of infection and must be done before and after any physical contact with a client during an examination (see box below, left).

Equipment Preparation for Health Assessment

Equipment needed in a comprehensive health assessment is shown in Figure 8.1. The examiner should keep all equipment within easy reach and place it out on a table before beginning the examination. In addition to the equipment shown in the figure, the examiner may use a thermometer and a visual acuity chart during a screening examination. The purpose of each piece of equipment is discussed in detail in the various assessment chapters.

Examination Techniques

The four assessment techniques used in the physical examination are inspection, palpation, percussion, and auscultation. Positioning of the client is sometimes used as a fifth assessment technique. The examiner uses these techniques as an organizing framework for bringing the senses of sight, hearing, touch, and smell into focus. These techniques are explained further in the chapters that deal with their application to specific organs and systems.

Inspection

During inspection the examiner concentrates attention on a thorough and unhurried visualization of the client. Inspection also involves listening to any sounds coming from the client and being aware of any odors that may be present. The inexperienced examiner often moves too quickly to a "hands on" technique and may miss information that can be obtained only through careful observation. Up to 80% of diagnoses are based on data obtained from a history and inspection. Observing for body symmetry is one of the first steps in examining a body system (see Figures 14.8 and 19.14).

Lighting must be adequate for inspection. Either daylight or artificial light is suitable. Tangential lighting is a method of directing light from an adjustable lamp at a right angle to the area being observed. This technique

---

Safety First

The goal of standard precautions is that the health care provider will avoid contact with all of the client's body fluids. This approach involves wearing latex gloves whenever examining an area of the client's body (e.g., mouth, genitals) or obtaining a specimen (e.g., blood, sputum) when there is potential for contact with body fluids. Protective eyewear should be worn when dealing with secretions that can be passed through the air and might come in contact with the examiner's eye (e.g., during suctioning). Protective clothing, such as a fully buttoned lab coat, a disposable gown, or a uniform, should be worn to reduce the risk of transmission of infectious organisms.

Risk of transmission of infection to the practitioner and to housekeeping and maintenance personnel can be reduced by proper disposal of any equipment that has come in contact with the client's body fluids. Needles should not be recapped. Needles and other sharp objects should be disposed of in a "sharps" container to avoid accidental puncture or incision wounds.

figure**8.1** Equipment used during the physical examination. *1,* Nasal speculum; *2,* reflex hammer (two types shown); *3,* dull-end object for sensory examination; *4,* penlight; *5,* flashlight; *6,* ophthalmoscope; *7,* otoscope; *8,* cotton balls; *9,* lubricant; *10,* disposable vaginal speculum; *11,* cervical brush; *12,* cotton-tip applicator; *13,* cervical spatula; *14,* tongue depressor; *15,* disposable gloves; *16,* specimen cup; *17,* stethoscope; *18,* sphygmomanometer; *19,* tuning fork (two types shown); *20,* centimeter rulers (two types shown); *21,* tape measure; *22,* marking pen.

produces shadows that are useful in assessing movements, such as abdominal pulsations or precordial movement.

Palpation

In performing palpation, the skilled examiner uses the most sensitive parts of the hand for each type of palpation (Table 8.1). The examiner's hands should be warm and have well-trimmed nails. Gloves should be worn for any examination of mucous membranes or any area where contact with body fluids or drainage is likely. Touch is used to determine the extent of tenderness and to note any tremor or spasm of muscle tissues. It is also used to elicit crepitus, or crackling, in bones and joints.

> **HELPFUL HINT** *Always palpate areas of tenderness last.*

The examiner may palpate individual structures within body cavities, particularly the abdomen, for position, size, shape, consistency, and mobility. The examining hand can be used to detect masses. Palpation may also serve as a means of evaluating abnormal collections of fluid. Both light and deep palpation are used in the ex-amination. Light palpation involves applying slight pressure to the area being examined to assess skin, tenderness, or pulsations. Deep palpation is done to assess the size or contour of organs, such as the liver or kidney (see Figures 17.24 and 17.25). Light palpation should always be performed first because it is less likely to create discomfort for the client. Touch is used to examine the skin and hair for moisture and texture.

Percussion

Percussion involves tapping on the surface of the skin. This tapping creates a vibration of underlying organs that produces sound. Immediate, or direct, percussion is the striking of a finger or hand directly against the body (see Figure 18.36).

table 8.1	Discriminating Areas of the Hands Used in Palpation
Discriminating sense	**Sensitive regions**
Pulses Fine tactile discrimination	Fingertips
Skin texture	General differences: fingertips
	Fine discrimination: back of the hands and fingers
Position, consistency, and form of a structure or mass	Fingertips using the grasping fingers
Vibration	Palmar aspects of the metacarpophalangeal joints (ball of the hand)
	Alternatively: ulnar side of the hand
Temperature	Dorsa of the hands or fingers (back of the hand)

From Talbot L, Meyers-Marquardt M: *Pocket guide to critical care assessment,* ed 3, St Louis, 1997, Mosby.

A

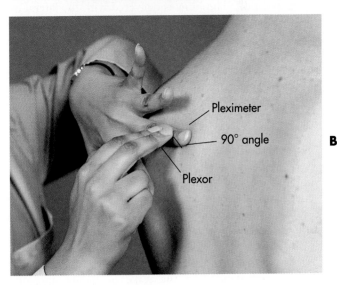

Pleximeter

90° angle

Plexor

B

figure **8.2** Indirect percussion. **A,** Positioning of the hands. **B,** Hand movement. The plexor blow to the pleximeter hand is delivered with a crisp, sharp wrist action.

table **8.2**	*Sounds Produced by Percussion*			
Record of finding	**Intensity**	**Pitch**	**Quality**	**Example of where sounds may be heard**
Tympany	Loud	High	Drumlike	Gastric air bubble
Hyperresonance	Very loud	Very low	Booming	Air-filled lungs (e.g., in emphysema)
Resonance	Loud	Low	Hollow	Normal lung
Dullness	Moderate	Moderate	Thudlike	Liver
Flatness	Soft	High	Flat	Muscle, bone

In mediate, or indirect, percussion the middle finger of the dominant hand (plexor) is used to strike against the middle finger (pleximeter) of the other hand. Only the distal portion of the middle finger of the pleximeter hand is placed firmly against the skin. The middle finger is used to strike at, or immediately distal to, the distal interphalangeal joint. A crisp and sharp blow is delivered with the plexor positioned perpendicular to the pleximeter.

Wrist action controls the speed and force of a blow. The hand is flexed backward on the forearm and brought forward with a quick, snapping motion that follows a fast strike and rapid removal of the plexor to avoiding dampening the vibration (Figure 8.2). The fingernails of the plexor finger must be kept short to avoid cutting the skin of the pleximeter. The vibration produced through percussion involves only the tissue adjacent (3 to 5 cm) to the pleximeter. Other examples of mediate percussion are shown in Figures 15.17, 17.13, and 17.16.

Fist percussion involves striking with the hand in a fisted position. The blow is delivered with the lateral aspect of the hand. The purpose of this type of percussion is to elicit sensation by the vibration of the tissue, which stimulates pain or tenderness of organs (e.g., liver, kidneys). Fist percussion may be direct or indirect. When indirect fist percussion is used, the blow is delivered to the dorsal surface of the opposite hand (see Figure 17.17 and 17.36).

Vibrating structures produce sound. The vibrations generate a series of compression waves in a medium that is capable of sound transmission. For example, solids, liquids, and gases that are sufficiently elastic to convert energy to motion can transmit sound. The examiner evaluates the following characteristics of percussion sounds: intensity, pitch, and quality (Table 8.2).

Intensity. Intensity refers to the loudness of sound. As a sound wave travels, air molecules are compressed and then expanded in the wake of the compression wave. The difference between maximum pressure and minimum pressure is the amplitude of the sound wave.

The greater the displacement of air, the more movement will occur during vibration of the tympanic membrane, and the louder the perception of sound will be. Loudness is a subjective quality. The perception of loudness is affected by the attentiveness of the individual or competing sounds in the environment.

Pitch. Pitch is related to the frequency of sound. It is the number of vibrations of the sound source per second. The waveform of a sound of single frequency is sinusoidal:

with perfectly matched peaks and valleys. The distance from one peak to the next is one cycle. The recording of frequency is done in cycles per second (cps) or hertz (Hz). The human ear can detect sounds in the frequency range of 20 to 20,000 Hz. With advancing age, the human ear becomes progressively less sensitive to the higher sound frequencies. The sounds of speech and music (300 to 3000 Hz) are most frequently lost in elderly persons.

Quality. The term *harmonic* refers to the physical property of sound that causes the effect called quality or timbre. The examiner records the quality in descriptive terms, such as humming, buzzing, or musical.

The more air that the tissue contains (i.e., the less dense the tissue), the deeper and louder the sound will be. The denser the tissue, the higher and fainter the sound will be. The examiner records sounds elicited in percussion in relation to the density of the tissue being vibrated. The least dense tissues produce tympany. Successively denser tissue results in hyperresonance, resonance, dullness, and flatness.

The change from resonance (less density) to dullness (greater density) is more easily perceived than the change from dullness to resonance. Thus percussion should be done from more resonant to less resonant areas.

Auscultation

Auscultation is the process of listening for the sounds that the human body produces. The particularly important sounds are those produced by (1) the thoracic or abdominal viscera and (2) the movement of blood in the cardiovascular system. Direct auscultation involves listening with the unassisted ear (i.e., without any amplifying device). However, auscultation is routinely done with a stethoscope, an instrument developed by René Laënnec in 1816. The purpose of the stethoscope is to exclude environmental sound and to augment internal sound.

The acoustic stethoscope is the type currently used (Figure 8.3). It is a closed cylinder that captures sound waves produced by the sound source. The diaphragm of the stethoscope is most effective in assessing high-frequency sounds such as breath and bowel sounds. The diaphragm is applied firmly to the skin so that it creates a seal between the skin surface and the diaphragm (see Figure 16.25).

The bell-type head of the stethoscope is most effective in detecting low-frequency sounds such as vascular sounds or blood pressure (see Figures 16.24 and 16.28). It is important to avoid pressing the bell too firmly on the skin surface because stretching the skin inhibits vibration by actually converting the tissue to a diaphragm. The bell chestpiece should be wide enough to span an intercostal space in an adult and deep enough that it will not fill with tissue.

Several sizes of earpieces are supplied with better stethoscopes. The examiner should determine which size fits his or her ear most snugly. The earpiece should occlude the external meatus, thus blocking extraneous sound. However, the earpiece should not cause the examiner pain. The binaurals (metal tubing) are angled slightly toward the nose of the wearer to project the sound onto the tympanic membrane. The direction of the angle may be adjusted by the tension spring. The tubing should not be longer than 30 to 35 cm to minimize sound distortion. Longer tubing increases the chance of diminishing the sound.

> **HELPFUL HINT** *Don't wear a stethoscope backwards. Make sure the earpieces, when held in front of you, angle forward.*

Auscultation can also be done using a Doppler monitor. A Doppler monitor is a battery-operated instrument that is placed on the body surface to amplify quiet sounds. A seal is created between the skin and the instrument with a water-soluble gel. A Doppler monitor is commonly used to listen to fetal heart tones.

figure **8.3** Parts of a stethoscope. (From Potter PA, Perry AG: *Basic nursing: theory and practice*, ed 3, St Louis, 1995, Mosby.)

examination step-by-step

Using the techniques of examination in combination for assessment of the lungs would include the following steps:
1. Inspecting the anterior and posterior thorax to observe symmetry of movement.
2. Palpating the posterior and anterior thorax to assess tenderness and vibrations produced by underlying tissues.
3. Using direct percussion over the posterior thorax to assess intensity, pitch, and quality of sound.
4. Auscultating over the anterior and posterior thorax to assess for breath sounds.
5. Positioning the client in a sitting position with the shoulders rounded to expose maximum lung tissue when examining the posterior thorax.

table **8.3** *Positions for Examination*

Position	Areas assessed	Rationale	Limitations
Sitting	Head and neck, back, posterior thorax and lungs, anterior thorax and lungs, breasts, axillae, heart, vital signs, and upper extremities	Sitting upright provides full expansion of lungs and provides better visualization of symmetry of upper body parts.	Physically weakened client may be unable to sit. Examiner should use supine position with head of bed elevated instead.
Supine	Head and neck, anterior thorax and lungs, breasts, axillae, heart, abdomen, extremities, pulses	This is most normally relaxed position. It provides easy access to pulse sites.	If client becomes short of breath easily, examiner may need to raise head of bed.
Dorsal recumbent	Head and neck, anterior thorax and lungs, breasts, axillae, heart, abdomen	Position is used for abdominal assessment because it promotes relaxation of abdominal muscles.	Clients with painful disorders are more comfortable with knees flexed.
Lithotomy*	Female genitalia and genital tract	This position provides maximal exposure of genitalia and facilitates insertion of vaginal speculum.	Lithotomy position is embarrassing and uncomfortable, so examiner minimizes time that client spends in it. Client is kept well draped.
Sims'	Rectum and vagina	Flexion of hip and knee improves exposure of rectal area.	Joint deformities may hinder client's ability to bend hip and knee.
Prone	Musculoskeletal system	This position is used only to assess extension of hip joint.	This position is poorly tolerated in clients with respiratory difficulties.
Lateral recumbent	Heart	This position aids in detecting murmurs.	This position is poorly tolerated in clients with respiratory difficulties.
Knee-chest*	Rectum	This position provides maximal exposure of rectal area.	This position is embarassing and uncomfortable.

From Potter PA, Perry AG: *Basic nursing: theory and practice*, ed 3, St Louis, 1995, Mosby.
*Clients with arthritis or other joint deformities may be unable to assume this position.

Special maneuvers—positioning

Positioning the client can help in using the four modalities described here. For example, positioning the client in a right side-lying position will aid in palpating the spleen. Positioning also makes certain body areas more accessible to the examiner. Table 8.3 summarizes the positions used for assessing different body parts. The inability of a client to assume a position may be an important objective finding. For example, the inability to lie flat may be a sign of a cardiovascular or pulmonary problem.

Special populations

The examiner needs to adapt her or his approach to the physical examination for special populations. For a client with a cognitive deficit, the presence of a familiar person may help to assure cooperation during the examination. For a client who is wheelchair bound, most of the physical examination can be performed with the client sitting. Assistance may be needed for the client to assume a standing or supine position. The length of the examination needs to correlate with the client's mental and physical levels of tolerance. For example, recovery from brain damage is often associated with fatigue.

chapter 9

General Assessment, Including Vital Signs

■ PURPOSE OF EXAMINATION

After obtaining subjective data from the client using methods of interviewing and history taking, the examiner proceeds to the physical examination. Techniques of the physical examination provide the objective measurements of health assessment. The client's and examiner's coordinated efforts lead to the recognition and identification of abnormal phenomena.

The examiner's observations and measurements are essential in verifying the client's description of symptoms and in identifying signs or objective findings. The tools of physical assessment also allow the examiner to explore facets not usually available to the client. Conclusions about an individual's health status are drawn from synthesizing information from the client's description and the physical assessment.

■ GENERAL INSPECTION

General inspection begins with observing the client entering the room, during introductions, and as he or she follows instructions before the interview begins.

General observation is the overall impression given by the client's general state of health and outstanding characteristics.

The survey proceeds from head to toe. The examiner observes thoroughly and discerningly. Inspection is a more detailed observation that includes smell, hearing, and touch, as well as visual inspection. Make observations only in good light, particularly when assessing skin color.

Make every attempt to concentrate on the person being examined. With practice and by carefully guarding against distractions, either from the environment or unrelated thoughts, you will learn to become completely absorbed with the client. Total and focused concentration on the client allows the examiner to process information using all sensory modalities.

The general observations continue throughout the interview. In some cases, the initial impression sets the focus of the interview and the physical examination. For instance, some feature of the client's appearance may point immediately to the problem. Slow speech and a hoarse voice, for example, may indicate the need to look

further for the dry skin and sluggish movements of hypothyroidism.

Although the initial inspection is a scanning procedure, the astute practitioner gathers information that may be used as the basis for planning portions of the examination that deserve special attention.

HELPFUL HINT *Give the client total attention. Do not allow yourself to be interrupted to take phone calls or to be distracted by other responsibilities. Consider the time with the client as precious.*

▪ ASSESSMENT OF BODY MORPHOLOGY AND GAIT

Normal Body Types

Although body morphology, or the size and physical shape of a person, is to some degree genetically determined, the environment plays a significant role in altering body type. Several normal variations in body types are shown in Figure 9.1.

Mesomorphic type

The mesomorphic body type is characterized by average height, well-developed musculature, wide shoulders with a subcostal angle that is approximately a right angle, and a flat abdomen.

Ectomorphic type

The ectomorphic body build is often described as tall and willowy. The musculature and subcutaneous fat are poorly developed. The extremity bones are long and thin. The clavicles, ribs, and spinous processes protrude because of the deficient subcutaneous fat. The chest is long and narrow. Because abdominal muscles are not as well developed, the abdominal wall may sag outward. The stomach is lower in the abdomen and more vertical in position. The neck is long.

Endomorphic type

The endomorphic body build is short, stocky, and the most likely of the body types to be obese. The neck is short and thick. The extremities are large and sturdy. Compared with the mesomorphic and ectomorphic types, the chest is shorter and broader and the costal margin is a wider angle (obtuse). The heart is likely to lie in a transverse position. The abdomen is long and of great capacity. The stomach is higher in the abdomen than it is in the other two body types and more or less in a transverse position.

Symmetry

The arrangement of most structures of the human body is symmetrical; that is, the size and shape of parts correspond. If inspection reveals obvious areas of lack of symmetry, note this and investigate it later.

Posture

Posture is a part of body image. Good body alignment is a sign of good health. Correct posture is the position in which minimum stress will be applied to each joint. Minimum muscular effort is required to maintain an upright posture, which is achieved when the line of the center of gravity bisects the principal weight-bearing joints and is the same distance from each foot. Frequent changes of posture are necessary for comfort. Good posture depends on a normal sense of balance and muscular coordination. Faulty posture is any position that increases stress to joints (Figure 9.2).

🌐 CULTURAL CONSIDERATIONS

EXERCISE INFLUENCES

Some evidence points to appropriate exercise as an aid to maintaining erect posture. Chinese shadowboxing exercises are purported to maintain body awareness and erect posture despite advancing years.

Mesomorphic   Ectomorphic   Endomorphic

Mesomorphic   Ectomorphic   Endomorphic

figure**9.1** Body types.

Aging and posture

Bone and joint changes contribute to the bent posture often seen in the elderly. Joint degeneration and osteoporosis occur with aging. Aging changes, such as widening and flattening of the third cervical vertebrae and drying of the intervertebral disks, may result in a decrease from baseline adult height of as much as 2 to 3 cm.

Although all muscles decline in girth and strength with aging, the muscles of the trunk are particularly affected. Weakness of the abdominal muscles also contributes to the slumped posture of the elderly. (See also Chapter 26: Aging Clients.)

Gait

The phases of normal gait are stance and swing (Figure 9.3). The stance phase occurs when the foot is on the ground and bearing weight. The lower leg supports the body weight, and the body advances over the supporting limb. The five components of stance are (1) initial contact, (2) loading response, (3) midstance, (4) terminal stance, and (5) preswing.

The normal heel strike is quiet and smoothly coordinated with the knee extended. The load response, the movement to full contact of the foot with the floor, should be complete and proceed smoothly. The midstance of the foot is the shift of weight onto the foot. The weight should be supported evenly by all aspects of the foot, and the knee is slightly flexed. In the terminal stance, the metatarsal pushoff is a smoothly coordinated lift off the floor. The swing phase occurs when the foot is non–weight bearing and moving forward. The swing

| Good posture | Relaxed faulty posture | Kyphosis Lordosis | Sway back | Flat back | Round back |

figure**9.2**   Types of faulty posture.

Stance phase   **Swing phase**

| Right initial contact | Loading Response | Midstance | Terminal Stance | Right Preswing | Initial swing (acceleration) | Midswing | Terminal swing |

figure**9.3**   Stance and swing phase of gait. *(Modified from Magee DJ:* Orthopedic physical assessment, *Philadelphia, 1992, WB Saunders.)*

phase allows the toes to clear the floor and the swing leg to advance forward.

Technique for Assessment of Posture and Gait

Develop a protocol for observing the main postures of the body in all its common acts. Watch the client come into the room and sit down, and observe while the client lies on the examining table. It is important to note whether the client sits tensely or slumps in the chair.

The characteristics of the client's walk provide clues to the client's problems. Ask the client to walk a straight line, and observe the client walking a short distance both toward and away from you. Note the speed of the client's step, as well as the smoothness and style of movement.

■ ASSESSMENT OF GENERAL APPEARANCE

Weight

Weight is sometimes considered a vital sign because unexplained weight loss frequently is one of the early signs of illness. With aging, weight tends to increase, and a more sedentary lifestyle may also contribute to weight gain. Body fat distribution changes with age; abdominal and truncal fat increases, and the extremities thin.

Adipose deposition varies by gender. Women have fat deposits over the shoulders, breasts, buttocks or lateral aspect of the thighs, and pubic symphysis. The fat deposits in men are more evenly dispersed throughout the body.

An essential part of the assessment of children or anyone who has not completed the growth cycle is the accurate, serial measurement of height and weight. Growth charts (see Figure 25.20), which are assembled from data gathered from large populations, allow the examiner to compare an individual client's pattern of growth with national standards.

Hair Growth Patterns

Hair growth is influenced by hereditary and racial factors. Excessive hairiness is thought to be a dominant hereditary trait related to the presence of androgens, whereas thinning or absent hair is a recessive trait.

Hair grows at various rates. The most rapid rate of growth is that of the beard, followed by that of the scalp, axillae, thighs, and eyebrows. The rate of hair growth is affected by environmental temperature and by the general state of health. Extremely cold temperatures impede hair growth, whereas hot climates appear to promote increased length.

Axillary and pubic hair growth is initiated by adrenal hormones, ovarian hormones, and testicular hormones. True sexual hair grows on the face, chest, abdomen, back, and extremities. The hair may be classified by the types of hormonal influences the growth receives:

1. Hair dependent on growth hormone (GH) is that which grows on the head, including eyelashes and eyebrows; on the midphalangeal area; on the distal portions of limbs; and, to some extent, on the lumbosacral area.
2. Hair dependent on female hormones is that which grows on the pubic area, axillae, limbs, and hypogastric area. The female pubic hair pattern is triangular, with the base over the mons pubis.
3. Hair dependent on male hormones is that of the beard, mustache, nasal tip, ear, and body hair (particularly on the back). The male pubic hair configuration is that of a diamond, with its superior angle at the umbilicus.

HAIR GROWTH VARIATIONS

Caucasian persons have more abundant and coarser body hair than Asians. Facial hirsutism, or excessive hair growth, occurs in more than 40% of Caucasian women. Asian women, on the other hand, do not develop excessive facial hair growth, and Asian men have sparser beards than Caucasian men. Blacks have kinky hair, whereas Caucasians have straight or wavy to curly hair. Native Americans have straight hair.

A heavier distribution of hair is correlated with darker skin pigmentation; that is, the brunette individual is more likely to have more hair than the blonde person.

Some male hair growth characteristics may be normal for women of certain ethnic or familial groups and could include sideburns; hair growth on the upper lip, abdomen, and lower limbs; and hair growth around the areola of the breasts.

Alopecia (balding) is more frequently noted in individuals with abundant coarse-hair growth on the body. Alopecia is thought to be related to androgen production. Male pattern baldness is recession of the hairline and baldness of the crown. As a rule, women do not bald unless androgens are present in relatively increased amounts or the baldness occurs as a result of disease or chemotherapy.

Technique for Assessment of General Appearance

Weight

Weigh the client and measure his or her height. Compare the client's parameters with actuarial tables of average weights and heights, which are prepared by insurance companies (see Chapter 5: Nutritional Assessment). Record weight in kilograms or pounds and height in centimeters or inches, depending on the requirements of the particular setting.

HELPFUL HINT *Weigh the client with or without clothes; however, note whether or not the client was clothed. The client should not wear shoes when height is measured.*

Hair

Inspect for hair growth on the following body regions: scalp, beard, mustache, ears, hypogastric area, thoracic area, lower limbs, genital area, lumbosacral area, upper back, midphalangeal area, pubis, and axillae. Observe hair for growth characteristics, distribution, density of growth, appearance, and hygiene.

Nails

The nails may indicate the level of concern and care the client has for appearance. Inspect the nails for length, cleanliness, neatness of filing, and the presence of polish. Inspection of the nail is obscured in women who use artificial nails that are glued to the nail bed. Note the texture, thickness, and contour.

Personal hygiene

General cleanliness of the body is an important indication of the individual's self-esteem and access to necessary supplies to maintain good body care. Standards of cleanliness are a sociocultural value. Deodorants are not used in all cultures. Although shaving the legs is normal in some groups of women in the United States, it is not practiced by all women. However, although norms may vary, poor personal hygiene can indicate serious mental or physical illness.

Odors

Note odor of the body and breath. The smell of alcohol on the client's breath should alert one to look for other effects of alcohol, a central nervous system (CNS) depressant. Foul breath points to the possibility of an oral or pulmonary infection or may simply be the result of poor oral hygiene. The odor of ammonia may be detectable in the patient with uremia. Body odor may be related to the activities of the sweat and sebaceous glands and to the general cleanliness of the body.

The odors emanating from the client may provide clues helpful in defining the client's condition. Some diseases are characterized by particular odors emanating from the mouth. The odors known to have diagnostic importance are listed in Table 9.1.

Manner of dress

Note the fit of clothing, as well as its appropriateness to the season or room temperature. General cleanliness and neatness of grooming may provide clues to the client's cultural or socioeconomic status, as well as ego strength and self-image. If a client is unshaven or unwashed, this may be a sign of self-neglect or neglect by relatives or others on whom the client is dependent. Carefully note such signs of neglect.

■ ASSESSMENT OF VITAL SIGNS

The most frequent clinical measurements made by the health practitioner are temperature, pulse, respiratory rate, and blood pressure. These measures provide such valuable data on the client's state of health that they have been termed the vital or cardinal signs. Obtain vital signs at the beginning of any examination.

Variations from the client's baseline values or from the previous measurement are clinically significant. The client's baseline measures are important because there is considerable variability among individuals. The examiner assesses vital signs to establish a database; data obtained on future occasions may then be compared with baseline values.

Bear in mind that your manner of approach to the client may alter the client's vital signs, especially if the client reacts emotionally to your actions. For instance, a curt, impatient, rude interaction or awkward handling of the instruments may upset the client, increasing the pulse rate, respiration rate, blood pressure, and even temperature if the interaction is prolonged.

Temperature

For most individuals the optimum temperature for metabolic function of all cells of the human body is 37° C (98.6° F). The core temperature of the body is maintained within very narrow limits. The normal ranges for temperature are 36.4° to 37.2° C (97.5° to 99.0° F).

table 9.1	Association of Breath Odors to Disease	
Breath odor	**Description**	**Associated condition**
Halitosis, foul	Odor of necrotic tissue	Pyorrhea Poor dental hygiene Tonsilitis Sinusitis Lung abcess Bronchiectasis
Feculent	Odor of feces	Bowel obstruction
Fetor hepaticus	"Fishy" odor	Hepatic failure
Acid	Odor of acid	Peptic disease
Ammonia	Odor of urine	Renal failure
Acetone	Odor of acetone ("fruity")	Diabetic ketoacidosis
Bitter almonds	Odor of almonds	Cyanide poisoning

Factors that influence temperature are described in the box below.

Temperature regulation

Body temperature is an excellent example of both homeostasis and biological rhythms. The hypothalamus serves as the body's thermostat. Two hypothalamic centers trigger heat-dissipating or heat-conserving mechanisms. The delivery of overwarmed blood to thermoreceptors in the anterior hypothalamus results in sweating and redistribution of blood, which dilates surface capillaries and causes flushing. Temperature loss from the skin occurs when blood flow to the skin increases and sweat evaporates. This heat loss is related to the temperature difference between the skin and external environment.

Conduction, convection, radiation, and evaporation are the physical phenomena involved in temperature regulation. Conduction is heat loss from the object of higher temperature to the object of lower temperature.

Convection is the loss of heat to the molecules of air. Conduction and convection occur only when the ambient temperature is lower than the body temperature.

Radiation is the loss of heat by electromagnetic infrared waves. The radiation does not heat the air through which it passes. Evaporation is the conversion of liquid (sweat) to gaseous form. Vaporization of perspiration depends on ambient humidity and does not occur when air is very humid.

Heat-conserving mechanisms are activated when overcooled blood is delivered to thermoreceptors in the posterior hypothalamus. These mechanisms include reducing blood flow to the distal extremities and constricting peripheral capillary beds (blanching). Compensatory heat production is enhanced both at the metabolic level (nonshivering thermogenesis) and through voluntary muscle contraction and shivering. Shivering occurs when vasoconstriction is ineffective in preventing heat loss.

Temperature acclimatization

Clients who have spent a good deal of time in very cold climates show an increased ability to tolerate cold. These individuals show (1) an increased metabolic rate with increased rates of secretion of thyroid hormones, (2) reduction in shivering, and (3) an increased rate of hair growth.

Adaptation to heat changes the secretion of sweat. The amount of sweat produced declines from the profuse, dripping, early response to a quantity that will evaporate on reaching the air.

Temperature recording

Record body temperature in degrees Celsius (°C) or in degrees Fahrenheit (°F) according to the protocol of the practice setting. The metric system is generally the preferred system in health care. Each scale may be readily converted through use of the following formulas:

$$°C = 5/9 \ (°F - 32)$$
$$°F = 9(°C)/5 + 32$$

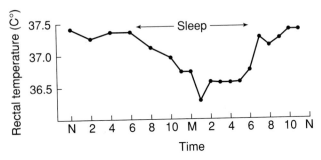

Factors Influencing Temperature

Biological rhythms are reflected in temperature assessment (Figure 9.4). Diurnal variations of up to 1.0° C are observed; the trough occurs in the hours before waking; the peak occurs in the late afternoon or early evening.

Hormones can increase temperature. Increased secretion of thyroid hormone increases body temperature. Progesterone secretion at the time of ovulation correlates with temperature increases of 0.5° C, which continue until the menses.

Environment affects temperature. Body temperature is altered little by seasonal changes in temperature. Hot and cold baths produce temporary changes in temperature.

Exercise increases body temperature because of the physiological changes incurred.

Eating food is associated with a rise in temperature as a result of the specific dynamic action (SDA) of the food.

Age is a factor in temperature assessment. Because heat control mechanisms are not as well established in the child as in the adult, considerable variation in a child's temperature may occur. Normal body temperature declines with age, from 37.2° C (99.0°F) in young children, to 37° C (98.6°F) in adults, to 36° C (96.8° F) in older adults.

---

figure**9.4** Biological rhythms for temperature in a 24-hour cycle. (*From Mountcastle VB:* Medical physiology, *vol 2, ed 14, St Louis, 1980, Mosby.*)

Figure 9.5 equates Fahrenheit and Celsius temperatures in the compatible range for human survival.

Technique for temperature measurement and normal findings

For accurate temperature measurement, insert the glass or electronic thermometer properly and leave in place for the recommended length of time. Explain to the client what is being done. The box below describes the proper placement of a thermometer.

Oral temperature. The oral temperature is the most convenient method for registering body temperature in the alert, adult client. Normal oral temperature in adults is 37° C (98.6° F). Wait 15 minutes before taking a temperature if the client has smoked or ingested hot or iced liquids. Place a glass mercury thermometer in the mouth for 3 to 5 minutes, although the oral thermometer may take as long as 7 minutes to reach maximum registration. An electronic thermometer has the advantage of registering temperature within 30 seconds, in addition to using disposable plastic probe covers.

Rectal temperature. The rectal site for registering temperature is preferable for the client who is confused or comatose, who is unable to close his or her mouth, or who is receiving oxygen. The normal rectal temperature in adults is 37.5° C (99.5° F). The lubricated thermometer placed in the rectum will register within 2 minutes.

Axillary temperature. The axillary method is safe and accurate for infants and small children but is not often used with adult clients unless oral and rectal routes are not accessible. The normal axillary temperature in adults is 36.5° C (97.7° F). It can take up to 10 minutes for the full registration of axillary temperature in adults and about 5 minutes for children.

Tympanic temperature. Tympanic thermography is a noninvasive technique for assessment of body temper-

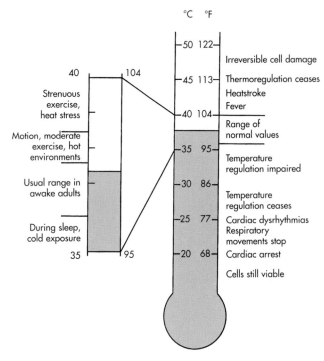

figure**9.5** Body temperature. Diagram, modeled after a thermometer, shows some physiological consequences of an abnormal body temperature. The normal range of body temperature under various conditions is shown in the inset. *(From Thibodeau GA, Patton KT:* Anatomy and physiology, *ed 3, St Louis, 1996, Mosby.)*

ature. It uses an infrared sensor to detect the temperature of blood flowing through the eardrum. The probe tip is shaped like the end of an otoscope, the instrument used to examine the ear. The tympanic thermometer registers an electronic display within 2 seconds (Figure 9.6).

Proper Placement of a Thermometer

ORAL TEMPERATURE
1. Ask the client to open his or her mouth with the tip of the tongue against the upper teeth.
2. Insert the thermometer tip gently under the tongue between the frenulum and the lower gum.
3. Leave in place at least 3 minutes.

RECTAL TEMPERATURE
1. Assist the client to a lateral position with the upper leg flexed.
2. Separate the buttocks to view the anus while instructing the client to breathe deeply.
3. Insert the lubricated thermometer 3 to 4 cm for an adult and 1 to 2 cm for an infant.
4. Leave in place at least 2 minutes.

AXILLARY TEMPERATURE
1. Insert the thermometer into the center of the axilla, and lower the client's arm over the thermometer.
2. Fold the client's arm over his or her chest to keep the thermometer in place.
3. Leave in place at least 5 minutes in children and longer in adults.

figure**9.6** Tympanic temperature measurement.

table **9.2**	**Normal Age Variations in Pulse Rate**
Age	**Pulse rate (beats/min)**
Birth	70-170
Neonate	120-140
1 year	80-140
2 years	80-130
3 years	80-120
4 years	70-115
Adult	60-100
Conditioned athlete	≅ 50

Respiration

Use inspection to assess the rate and effort of respirations. Observe for chest or abdominal movement to assess the rate. Count respirations that occur at regular intervals for 15 seconds. In the normal adult, the resting respiratory rate is 12 to 20 breaths per minute. For irregular respiratory patterns, the rate may need to be assessed over a longer time period of 30 seconds to 1 minute. For clients whose respirations are difficult to observe, lightly place your hand on the client's upper chest to assess the rate. (See also Chapter 15: Respiratory System.)

Pulses

General assessment usually includes assessment of the peripheral (radial) or apical pulse for rate, rhythm, and volume. The nature of the peripheral pulse gives an indication of cardiac function and perfusion of the peripheral tissues.

Pulse rate

The normal heart rate is between 50 and 100 beats per minute. Table 9.2 shows normal variations in pulse rate by age. When obtaining baseline data, count the pulse rate for 1 full minute to accurately evaluate the rate, rhythm, and volume. Normal rhythm is an even tempo. For subsequent measurements, count 15 to 30 seconds if pulses are regular. Auscultate the apical pulse for 1 minute if irregularities are felt. Because of diurnal rhythm, the pulse rate is lowest in the early morning and most rapid in the late afternoon and evening.

Pulse volume

Pulse volume represents the strength of left ventricular contraction, or stroke volume. Estimate pulse volume from the feel of the vessel as blood flows through it with each heartbeat. Bounding is the descriptive term used to describe the full pulse that is difficult to depress with the fingertips. The normal pulse is easily palpable, does not fade in and out, and is not easily obliterated. "Weak," "feeble," and "thready" are descriptive words for the pulse of a vessel with low volume. The artery with low volume is readily compressed.

Technique for Assessment of Vital Signs

The modalities used to assess vital signs include inspection, palpation, auscultation, and the use of instruments to obtain specific measures of physiological functioning.

Inspection

Inspect for changes in color, such as the flush of fever, the pallor in response to cold, or the dusky blueness of cyanosis.

Palpation

Palpation to assess body temperature. Palpate to determine temperature using the dorsal aspect of your hand or fingers, which are more sensitive to temperature variation. Palpation may reveal moisture and texture variations, as well as the vibration of shivering.

Palpation to assess arterial pulses. The pulse is best palpated over arteries that are close to the surface of the body and that lie over a bony surface. Feel bilateral pulses simultaneously to assess symmetry.

Radial pulse. Clinicians most frequently use the radial pulse to initially assess the rate and rhythm of pulsation, the pattern of pulsation, and the shape (consistency) of the arterial wall. The examiner has easy access

figure**9.8**   **A,** Palpation of the radial pulse. The site for palpation of the ulnar artery is also marked. **B,** Palpation of the brachial pulse.

Brachial artery
(palpate pulse here)

Radial artery
(palpate pulse here)

Ulnar artery
(palpate pulse here)

figure**9.7**   Arteries of the upper extremity. *(Modified from Francis CC, Martin AH:* Introduction to human anatomy, *ed 7, St Louis, 1975, Mosby.)*

to this pulse, and its evaluation causes little inconvenience to the client. Other pulses in the upper extremity that are easy to evaluate are the ulnar and brachial pulses (Figure 9.7).

Evaluate the radial pulse by placing the pads of your first and second fingers on the palmar surface of the client's relaxed and slightly flexed wrist medial to the ra-

dius bone (Figure 9.8). (Occasionally the arteries run in a deeper and more lateral course.) Exert sufficient pressure to occlude the artery during diastole yet allow the vessel to return to normal contour during systole.

Brachial pulse. The brachial pulse is palpated and auscultated as part of the blood pressure evaluation. Palpate the pulse over the antecubital fossa (anterior surface of the elbow joint). The brachial artery is medial to the biceps tendon.

The major pulses of the lower extremities are palpated over the femoral, popliteal, dorsalis pedis, and posterior tibial arteries (Figure 9.9). Palpate the femoral pulse midway between the anterosuperior iliac crest and the symphysis pubis, below and medial to the inguinal liga-

figure**9.9** Location of pulses for palpation. *(From Francis CC, Martin AH:* Introduction to human anatomy, *ed 7, St Louis, 1975, Mosby.)*

figure**9.10**   Palpation of various pulses. **A,** Femoral pulse. **B,** Popliteal pulse. **C,** Dorsal pedal pulse. **D,** Posterior tibial pulse.

ment. Palpate the popliteal pulse by pressing deeply into the dorsal aspect of the knee while the knee is slightly bent. Palpate the dorsalis pedis pulse by applying light touch about midway between the ankle and toes on the dorsum of the foot. Palpate the posterior tibial pulse slightly below and posterior to the medial malleolus of the ankle (Figure 9.10).

Blood Pressure
Anatomy and physiology

Blood pressure is the result of the interaction of cardiac output and peripheral resistance and is dependent on the velocity of the arterial blood, the intravascular volume, and the elasticity of the arterial walls. Arterial pressure is the force exerted by the blood against the wall of the artery as the heart contracts and relaxes. Systolic (systole) arterial blood pressure is the force exerted against the wall of the artery when the ventricles are contracted, and diastolic (diastole) arterial blood pressure is the force when the heart is in the filling or relaxed phase. Pulse pressure is the difference between the systolic and diastolic blood pressures. The usual pulse pressure is between 30 and 40 mm Hg (see box at right for normal variations).

Normal Variations in Blood Pressure

The blood pressure in a normal individual varies continually with respiration, autonomic state, emotional levels, and biological rhythms. Furthermore, successive readings of indirect measures of blood pressure by the same or different observers may differ by as much as 10 mm Hg.

In the normal individual, the change from a supine to an erect position causes a slight decrease in systolic blood pressure (less than 15 mm Hg) and a slight rise in diastolic pressure (less than 5 mm Hg).

The blood pressure also shows a circadian pattern; it is higher in the afternoon and evening hours and lower in the late hours of sleep.

Because blood pressure is readily altered by stressful events, an effort should be made to relax the client as much as possible before taking the blood pressure.

The blood pressure in the arm increases when the arm is lower than the level of the heart; conversely, raising the arm above the level of the heart lowers the blood pressure. If you are measuring a standing blood pressure, rest the elbow of the client's arm in your hand, with the weight of his or her forearm on your arm.

The examiner may assess the systemic arterial blood pressure by direct or indirect methods. The direct method requires cannulation of the artery and is not done routinely. Indirect blood pressure measurement can be made without opening the artery. Direct blood pressure standards are used to calibrate indirect pressure instruments.

Indirect measurement of blood pressure

Indirect methods of blood pressure measurement take into account the following three physiological facts: (1) the arterial wall may be occluded by direct pressure, resulting in obliteration of the pulse distal to the compression; (2) oscillations that vary directly with the amount of applied pressure may be measured from the compressed artery; and (3) the normal extremity blanches (pales) when its arterial blood supply is occluded by pressure, and there is flushing or return of color when the pressure is removed.

The most commonly used method of indirect assessment of blood pressure is the auscultatory technique. The proper application of the auscultatory method yields values that are within 4 to 5 mm Hg of the results of the direct method of measurement.

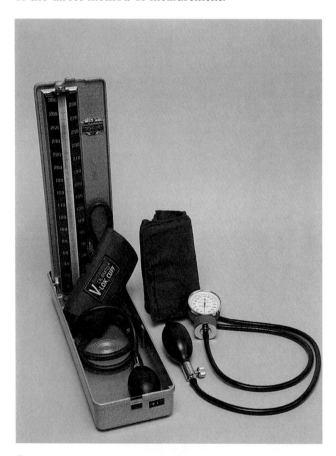

figure**9.11** Mercury column and aneroid sphygmomanometers. (*From Potter PA, Perry AG:* Basic nursing: theory and practice, *ed 3, St Louis, 1995, Mosby.*)

The two types of sphygmomanometers that clinicians commonly use to assess arterial blood pressure are the mercury column (Figure 9.11) and the aneroid instruments (see box below). The preferred instrument is the mercury column sphygmomanometer. Each instrument includes a pressure manometer, an inflatable rubber bladder used to occlude an artery encased in a cloth cuff, and a rubber hand bulb with a pressure control valve. The mercury column sphygmomanometer is considered to be the most accurate and reliable measure when properly used.

Cuff size. If the cuff is too narrow, the blood pressure reading will be erroneously high. Using a cuff that is too small is a common pitfall in blood pressure measurement. A wide cuff increases the risk of an erroneously low reading (Figure 9.12). Cuffs may be obtained in several sizes as shown in Figure 9.13.

Blood Pressure Equipment

A stethoscope is used to listen to sounds produced by each type of the blood pressure measurement devices described below.

The mercury column manometer is a straight glass tube connected to a reservoir of mercury. The reservoir in turn is connected to the pressure bulb so that pressure created on the bulb causes the mercury to rise in the tube. Because the weight of mercury depends on gravity, a given amount of pressure will always support a column of mercury of the same height if the tube is straight and of uniform diameter. The mercury manometer does not need further calibration after the initial setting.

The aneroid sphygmomanometer is made up of a metal bellows connected to the compression cuff. The movement of the bellows rotates a gear that moves a pointer across the calibrated dial. The aneroid sphygmomanometer is calibrated against a mercury manometer because the more complex mechanisms have been shown to need routine and frequent adjustment. This is simply done by using a connecting Y tube between the manometers.

Electronic devices are available for blood pressure measurement and are used for continuous blood pressure monitoring, as well as for self-monitoring of the client's blood pressure at home. The electronic units determine blood pressure by analyzing the sounds of blood flow or measuring oscillations. A cuff is automatically inflated to occlude the artery. Battery-operated units produce a digital readout of the systolic and diastolic measures after the cuff is manually inflated.

A

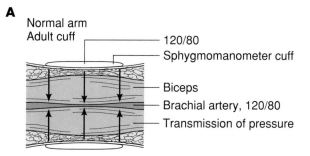

Normal arm
Adult cuff
— 120/80
— Sphygmomanometer cuff
— Biceps
— Brachial artery, 120/80
— Transmission of pressure

B

**Correct
sphygmomanometer cuff**

Thin arm
Child cuff
— 120/80

C

**Incorrect
sphygmomanometer cuff**

Thin arm
Adult cuff
— 110/70
— 120/80

D

Correct
Obese arm
Large cuff
— 120/80

Incorrect
Obese arm
Adult cuff
— 150/100
— 120/80

E

figure**9.12** Longitudinal sections of arms of different diameters to which sphygmomanometer cuffs have been applied. **A,** Normal arm. **B,** Thin arm, correct application. **C,** Thin arm, incorrect application. **D,** Obese arm, correct application using large arm cuff. **E,** Obese arm, incorrect application using adult cuff.

The size of the cuff must always be checked in relation to the size of the arm on which it will be used. The width of the bladder should reach halfway around the arm. The length of the bladder should reach 80% around the arm. To determine the correct cuff size, many manufacturers premark the cuffs with three lines: the index line, and range lines 1 and 2 (Figure 9.14). The index line and range line 1 mark the ends of the rubber bladder. A proper-sized cuff edge should fall between range lines 1 and 2 when the cuff is applied.

Technique for blood pressure measurement and normal findings

Auscultatory method of arterial blood pressure assessment. When the cuff is properly placed on the client's limb, the arterial blood can flow past the cuff only when arterial pressure exceeds that in the cuff. Partial obstruction of arterial blood flow disturbs the lami-

figure**9.13** Blood pressure cuff sizes. **A,** Thigh. **B,** Large adult. **C,** Adult. **D,** Neonate.

Range line 1 · Range line 2 · Edge of bladder · Index line · Inside of cuff

figure**9.14**   Selection of proper cuff size. The index line should reach halfway around the arm diameter. The range lines define the minimum and maximum size arm on which that cuff can be used. The end of the cuff must fall between range lines 1 and 2 when the cuff is applied. *(From American Heart Association of Wisconsin:* Blood pressure measurement education program, *Milwaukee, 1996, The Association.)*

Taking a Blood Pressure Step-by-Step

1. Situate the client in a comfortable sitting position, with the arm resting on a flat surface at heart level and the palm turned upward. Expose the upper arm fully. Have the person rest 5 minutes before taking the blood pressure. Wait 30 minutes if the client has smoked or ingested caffeine.
2. Palpate the brachial artery. Center the bladder of the cuff over the brachial artery with the bottom edge of the cuff 2.5 cm (1 inch) above the antecubital space. Do not rely on cuff markings; find the center by folding the bladder in half.
3. If you do not know the client's usual blood pressure, estimate the systolic pressure first by applying the cuff, palpating the radial pulse, and inflating the cuff until the pulse disappears. The point when the pulse disappears is the estimated systolic pressure. Deflate the cuff completely and wait 30 seconds before measuring the blood pressure.
4. Be sure the cuff is fully deflated. Wrap the cuff evenly and snugly around the upper arm. Place the manometer at eye level.
5. Place the stethoscope over the brachial artery. Apply light pressure to ensure good skin contact. Heavy pressure may distort sounds.
6. Close the valve of the pressure bulb clockwise until tight.
7. Rapidly and steadily inflate the cuff to 30 mm Hg above the client's normal or estimated systolic level.
8. Slowly release the valve, allowing the mercury to fall at a rate of 2 to 3 mm Hg per second.
9. Note the point on the manometer at which the first clear sound is heard (phase I). This is the systolic pressure. Continue to deflate the cuff, noting the point at which sound is muffled (phase IV) and when sound disappears (phase V). In children, record phase IV and phase V for the diastolic pressure. In adults, record phase V.
10. Listen 10 to 20 mm Hg below the last sound, then deflate the cuff rapidly and remove it from the client's arm. If repeating the procedure, wait 1 to 2 minutes.

When initially evaluating a client, take blood pressure measures in both sitting and lying positions on each arm. In the normal client there may be a slight decrease in blood pressure, less than 10 mm Hg, from supine to sitting.

nar flow pattern, creating turbulence. This turbulence produces sounds called Korotkoff sounds, which can be heard over arteries distal to the cuff through a stethoscope (Figure 9.15).

Record the systolic blood pressure at the point when you initially hear Korotkoff sounds. This is also the be-

ginning of *phase I,* which starts with faint, clear, and rhythmic tapping noises that gradually increase in intensity. At this point the intraluminal pressure is the same as the cuff pressure, but it is not great enough to produce a radial pulse.

Phase II is characterized by a murmur, or swishing

figure**9.15** Phases of Korotkoff sounds that would be recorded as a blood pressure of 120/80/50 mm Hg.

Normal diastolic pressure is below 85 mm Hg. Therefore, a client with a systolic blood pressure less than 55 mm Hg, for example, may be considered hypotensive, although there is no numerical guideline to label blood pressure hypotensive. Hypotension in the absence of other signs and symptoms is generally innocent, although the blood pressure must be high enough to perfuse blood to the kidneys, brain, and other tissues.

Blood pressure gradually increases until late adolescence, when adult blood pressure levels are reached. To get the best estimate of a person's usual blood pressure, take two or three readings and average them. A single blood pressure reading can be a very unreliable measure.

Measurement of blood pressure in the leg. Measure blood pressure in the leg with the client lying prone, if possible. Apply a large cuff (thigh) to the lower third of the thigh. Center the bladder of the cuff over the popliteal artery. Auscultate in the popliteal fossa. The systolic blood pressure is normally 20 to 30 mm Hg higher in the leg than in the arm.

Auscultatory gap. Occasionally, as the cuff is deflating, the Korotkoff sounds disappear and then are heard 10 to 15 mm Hg later. This is called an auscultatory gap. When this happens, the examiner may seriously underestimate the systolic pressure or overestimate the diastolic pressure. An auscultatory gap occurs in about 5% of adults and is prevalent in individuals with hypertension. The auscultatory gap will not be a cause for error if the examiner palpates the pulse for disappearance while the cuff is inflated to 30 mm Hg above the point at which the artery is occluded.

sound that is heard as the vessel distends with blood. *Phase III* is the period when the sounds are crisper and more intense. In phase III the vessel remains open in systole but obliterated in diastole.

The muffling of the Korotkoff sounds is the beginning of *phase IV,* and the pressure at this point is the closest to the diastolic arterial pressure measured by a direct method. Phase IV is frequently called the first diastolic pressure.

Cessation of sound is *phase V,* or the second diastolic pressure. During the entire phase V, the vessel remains open.

In children the muffling of sound (phase IV) is regarded as the true diastolic pressure, whereas in adults true diastolic pressure is the disappearance of sound (phase V). An example of a blood pressure recorded for a child might be 96/54/46.

Normal systolic and diastolic pressure. In adults a normal systolic blood pressure is below 130 mm Hg.

> **HELPFUL HINT** *Place the bell lightly over the skin. The bell of the stethoscope transmits low-frequency sounds better than the diaphragm.*

> **HELPFUL HINT** *If you have not inflated the cuff 30 mm Hg above the systolic pressure (obliteration of the pulse) and begin to listen during Phase II, the sounds may be too soft to hear.*

Absent phase V. In some individuals the Korotkoff sounds do not disappear but are heard until the manometer falls to 0 mm Hg. This is especially common in children. In this situation phase IV, or the change in Korotkoff sounds, is a more reliable estimate of the diastolic pressure than phase V. The blood pressure would be recorded as 140/80/0.

■ VARIATIONS FROM HEALTH

General Inspection

Be aware of signs of distress in the client. If you detect distress, you may need to deal with the underlying problem immediately and postpone the full interview and physical examination to a later time. Some of the signs that may indicate a need for immediate intervention are (1) anxiety, indicated by a clenched jaw, fidgety movements, and an apparent inability to process questions normally; (2) pain, indicated by moaning, writhing, facial grimacing, or guarding of the painful part; (3) cardiopulmonary distress, signaled by labored breathing, coughing, cyanosis, and/or pallor; (4) alteration in consciousness; or (5) observable hemorrhage or injury.

Facial expression

Individuals with Parkinson's disease tend to have motionless faces because of limited movement of the musculature. In addition, their blinking rate is slowed so that the client appears to stare.

The facial changes that occur with acromegaly, caused by excessive growth hormone production, include a prominent supraorbital ridge, jutting jaw, and enlarged nose and lips (Figure 9.16).

In myxedema (hypothyroidism) the features are flattened because they are swollen from fluid retention that is caused by the accumulation of mucopolysaccharides. The face appears heavy and coarse.

Posture

Faulty posture is most likely to result from postural or structural problems. Postural problems result from poor posture habits, muscle imbalance, or pain. Examples are the deviation of the spine toward the affected side in sciatica (irritation to the sciatic nerve) and the maintenance of a position that elevates the clavicles, such as leaning forward on extended arms, by the client with chronic obstructive lung disease. Children may have poor postural habits because they do not want to appear taller than their peers.

Occupations that require positions that deviate from normal alignment may result in chronic pain or deformity. Examples include bent shoulders in mine workers and painful shoulders in sewing machine operators.

Structural factors, especially spinal deformities, can also cause faulty posture. Disordered body alignment may lead to changes of the surrounding soft tissue. An example of this is the change in lung volume and ventilation, as well as in circulation, that occurs with scoliosis or lateral curvature of the spine (Figure 9.17).

Weight

Anorexia nervosa is a psychological disorder in which the person has a distorted body image and perceives that he or she needs to lose weight. To lose weight, the person with anorexia nervosa severely restricts his or her food intake. Bulimia nervosa includes cycles of bingeing and purging by vomiting or using laxatives. Anorexia nervosa and bulimia occur mostly in adolescent females and is associated with amenorrhea. Anorexia nervosa is present if the client is at or below 85% of his or her expected weight (Figure 9.18). Although over 40% of

figure**9.16** Acromegaly. Note the prominent jaw and forehead, the large zygomatic arches and supraorbital ridges, enlarged nose, and coarse and oily skin. *(From Mazzaferri EL: Endocrinology case studies, ed 2, Flushing NY, 1975, Medical Examination Publishing.)*

🌐 CULTURAL CONSIDERATIONS

OBESITY VARIATIONS

Race	Gender	% Obesity
White	M	32.0
	F	33.5
Native American	M	33.8
	F	30.3
African-American	M	31.5
	F	49.6
Hispanic	M	39.5
	F	47.9

Modified from 1988–91 (NHanes III) and HHanes 1982–84. In American Heart Association: *Heart and stroke facts 1996,* supplement, Dallas, 1996, The Association.

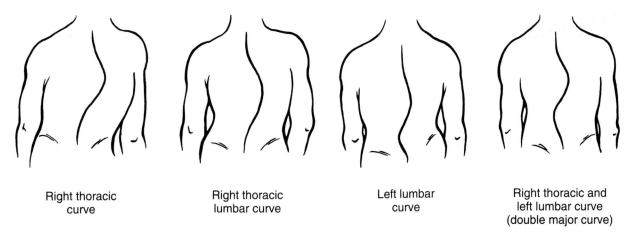

| Right thoracic curve | Right thoracic lumbar curve | Left lumbar curve | Right thoracic and left lumbar curve (double major curve) |

figure**9.17**   Examples of scoliosis curve patterns.

clients recover from anorexia nervosa, it is associated with a fivefold increase in mortality when compared with the general population of the same age and sex.

Obesity is a body weight that is 20% greater than the ideal weight for height. (For ideal body weight values, see Chapter 5: Nutritional Assessment.)

Endocrine disorders

When hypothyroidism begins in infancy it is called cretinism and is characterized by retarded bone maturation and multiple abnormal areas of epiphyseal ossification. Juvenile myxedema is also a cause of retarded growth. In adults hypothyroidism is identified by the presence of generalized signs and symptoms, such as fa-

figure**9.18**   Young female with anorexia nervosa. *(From Ezrin D, Godden JO, Volpe R: Systematic endocrinology, ed 2, New York, 1979, Harper & Row.)*

tigue, modest weight gain, dry skin, cold intolerance, constipation, slowed pulse, and periorbital swelling.

Gigantism is caused by excess growth hormone (GH) before puberty and before the ossification of the epiphyseal plates. The excess results in the overgrowth of the long bones.

Pituitary dwarfism is the result of hyposecretion of GH. Mental development is usually normal. Men are affected twice as often as women.

Acromegaly is a disease caused by hypersecretion of GH secondary to pituitary tumor; it is usually detected in the fourth or fifth decade of life. In most instances growth of the acral (small) parts proceeds so slowly that it is not noticed until the changes are well advanced. Bony changes in the skull are most apparent. The mandible is increased in length and width. There is little increase in height because the epiphyseal plates have closed. The features are exaggerated as a result of the expansion of the facial, molar, and frontal bones. The skull itself, as well as the sinuses, may be markedly enlarged. Arthralgia and arthritis are commonly present in acromegaly.

Cushing's syndrome is a disease caused by an excess of endogenous cortisol or exogenous glucocorticoids. The fat distribution that is characteristic of Cushing's syndrome (hyperadrenalism) or administration of the glucocorticoid hormone is in the facial, nuchal (neck), truncal, and girdle areas. Cushing's syndrome (Figure 9.19) is characterized by thin skin, purplish striae, plethora (red cheeks), muscle weakness, evidence of osteoporosis, redistribution of fat deposits, truncal obesity, "buffalo hump" (cervicodorsal fat), "moon facies" (fat cheeks), and thin extremities.

Hair

In starvation, general protein production is inhibited, which leads to reduced hair growth, dullness in appear-

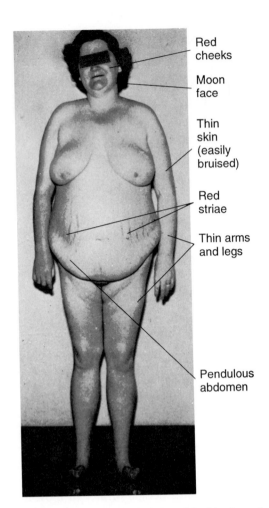

Red cheeks

Moon face

Thin skin (easily bruised)

Red striae

Thin arms and legs

Pendulous abdomen

figure**9.19** Physical characteristics of Cushing's syndrome. Prominent features include moon facies, red cheeks, thin skin, bruisability, red striae, and poor wound healing. Fat distribution is in the trunk with thin arms and legs. *(Modified from Prior JA, Silberstein JS, Stang JM: Physical diagnosis: the history and examination of the patient, ed 6, St Louis, 1981, Mosby.)*

ance, and loss of color. In some ethnic groups, especially those with black or dark brown hair, this loss of hair pigment results in a reddish brown hair color.

Chemotherapeutic drugs inhibit cell division and thereby inhibit hair growth.

Increased hair growth in normal sites has been associated with adrenal tumors.

Hirsutism, the appearance of excessive hair in normal and abnormal sites caused by increased androgens, has been observed in the following pathophysiological conditions: bilateral polycystic ovary, Cushing's syndrome, and ovarian tumor. Hirsutism can be most disturbing to the female client. The degree of overgrowth need not be marked to pose a threat to the client's feelings of femininity. When the examiner notes hirsutism in a fe-

male client, he or she should also be alerted to the presence of other virilizing signs, which include a deepening of the voice, clitoral enlargement, and changes in fat distribution. Because of the identity confusion that may exist in the presence of hirsutism, approach the problem with sensitivity. Fungal infections (tinea capitis) may cause hair loss. The fungal contamination is frequently acquired from pets and contaminated cosmetics.

Chemical and thermal treatment of the hair can cause damage to the surface characterized by breaking and splitting.

Symmetry

Defects of the thoracic cage might change the nature of respiration. Some defects are pectus carinatum, in which the sternum is markedly protuberant (as in a bird); funnel chest, or pectus excavatum, in which the sternum is retracted; and barrel chest (Figure 9.20).

Fever

Fever, or pyrexia, is the elevation of body temperature above normal limits compared with a given individual's basal data. For example, a temperature of 37° C (98.6° F) in a client whose normal temperature is 36.1° C (97° F) would be considered a fever. Fever is described in three stages: cold, hot, and defervescence (decline).

Cold stage

The cold stage is the period of a developing increase in core temperature and is characterized by heat conservation reactions. Cutaneous circulation is decreased, and the skin looks blanched and feels cold. Heat production produces shivering and piloerection ("goose pimples"). Chills and rigor are the extremes of shivering and produce rapid increases in temperature.

Hot stage

The hot stage is the period after the fever has peaked (regulated at the new set point). During this stage blood flow to the periphery is increased. The body radiates excess heat, feels hot, and is flushed.

Defervescence

The stage of defervescence is the period of fever abatement and is characterized by heat-loss mechanisms, particularly vasodilation and sweating. Diaphoresis is diffuse perspiration, which may accompany fever abatement.

Irregularities in Pulse
Tachycardia

Rates that are persistently over 100 beats per minute (tachycardia) suggest some abnormality. Heart rates are

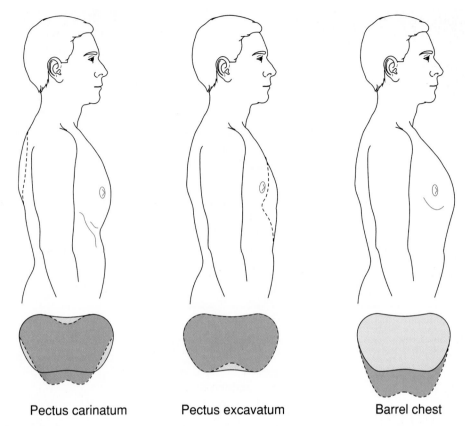

Pectus carinatum   Pectus excavatum   Barrel chest

figure**9.20**   Chest deformities. Lower vertical views show change in chest wall contours with deformity. *(Modified from Magee DJ:* Orthopedic physical assessment, *Philadelphia, 1992, WB Saunders.)*

increased during fever, anemia, hypoxia, and low-volume states (shock). However, tachycardia can also be a result of exercise, anger, anxiety, or fear.

Bradycardia

Bradycardia is a slow heart rate of less than 50 beats per minute. A slow rate may indicate stimulation of the parasympathetic system or failure in the electrical conduction system of the heart. Bradycardia may be caused by overdoses of digitalis. Bradycardia occurs normally in the well-trained athlete. This is due to heart muscle increasing in strength with development of skeletal muscle. This increased strength results in greater stroke volume, which in turn requires fewer beats per minute to maintain cardiac output.

Palpitations

When the client describes feeling his or her heartbeat, this feeling is referred to as a palpitation. Common terms used by clients to describe this phenomenon are "pounding," "thudding," "fluttering," "flopping," and "skipping." Palpitations are more common just before falling asleep or during sleep.

Palpitations may be experienced by the normal individual following strenuous exercise or when that person is aroused emotionally or sexually. In this case the cardiac contraction is of a greater rate and amplitude. A common feature of the anxiety state (arousal) is palpitations caused by the increased adrenergic activity. The relationship between anxiety and palpitations creates some problem for the examiner; because the presence of palpitations frequently creates anxiety, ask questions carefully so as not to cause further anxiety.

Palpitations are also associated with anemia, fever, hypoglycemia, and thyrotoxicosis. Irregularities in cardiac rhythm have also been associated with palpitations, particularly extra systoles and ectopic tachycardia (Table 9.3).

Variations in Blood Pressure
Differences in blood pressure indicating disease

On initial examination, measure blood pressures in both arms. Differences in blood pressure between the two arms may be caused by congenital aortic obstruc-

table 9.3 *Arterial Pulse Abnormalities*

Type	Description	Possible Causes
Diminished, weak, thready	Pulse is difficult to feel, easily obliterated by the fingers, and may fade out Pulse is slow to rise, has a sustained summit, and falls slowly	Hypovolemia Aortic stenosis Decreased cardiac output
Full, strong, bounding	Pulse is readily palpable, not easily obliterated by fingers Pulse is felt as a brisk impact; can occur with or without increased pulse pressure	Anemia Exercise Fever Hyperthyroidism
Water-hammer, collapsing	Pulse has greater than normal amplitude Pulse is marked by rapid rise, followed by a sudden descent	Chronic aortic regurgitation Patent ductus arteriosus
Pulsus bisferiens (double peaked)	Best felt by palpating carotid artery Two systolic peaks can occur in disorders that cause rapid left ventricular ejection of large stroke volume with wide pulse pressure	Aortic regurgitation Patent ductus arteriosus
Pulsus alternans	Pulses have large-amplitude beats followed by pulses of small amplitude Rhythm remains normal	Left-sided congestive heart failure
Bigeminal pulse	Normal pulses are followed by premature contractions Amplitude of premature contraction is less than that of normal pulse Rhythm is irregular	Premature ventricular or atrial contraction

Modified from Canobbio MM: *Cardiovascular disorders,* St Louis, 1990, Mosby.

table 9.3 *Arterial Pulse Abnormalities—cont'd*

Type	Description	Possible Causes
Pulsus paradoxus	Pattern is exaggerated (>10 mm Hg) during inspiration, and amplitude is increased during expiration Heart rate and rhythm are unchanged	Cardiac tamponade Constrictive pericarditis Pulmonary emphysema (noncardiac)

Inspiration   Expiration   Inspiration

tion (coarctation), acquired conditions such as aortic dissection, or obstruction of the arteries of the upper arm.

Marked drops in pressure (greater than 30 mm Hg) incurred when the client stands may indicate a vasopressor defect or hypovolemia.

Sudden changes in blood pressure may produce changes in body function, and sudden drops in normal blood pressure may result in fainting. Fainting is observed in orthostatic hypotension, defined as a systolic blood pressure decrease of 30 mm Hg and an increase in pulse of 10 to 20 beats per minute when moving from a lying to a standing position. In orthostatic hypotension, the blood pressure may be normal when an individual is reclining but drops when he or she rises to a sitting or standing position, particularly when the position change is rapid. Faintness and dizziness from orthostatic hypotension is common in individuals taking antihypertensive medications, or in individuals who are elderly, volume depleted, or confined to bed.

table 9.4 *Classification of Blood Pressure for Adults Age 18 Years and Older**

Category	Systolic (mm Hg)	Diastolic (mm Hg)
Normal[†]	<130	<85
High normal	130–139	85–89
Hypertension[‡]		
Stage 1 (mild)	140–159	90–99
Stage 2 (moderate)	160–179	100–109
Stage 3 (severe)	180–209	110–119
Stage 4 (very severe)	≥210	≥120

*Not taking antihypertensive drugs and not acutely ill. When systolic and diastolic pressures fall into different categories, the higher category should be selected to classify the individual's blood pressure status. For instance, 160/92 mm Hg should be classified as stage 2, and 180/120 mm Hg should be classified as stage 4. Isolated systolic hypertension (ISH) is defined as systolic blood pressure (SBP) ≥140 mm Hg and diastolic blood pressure (DBP) <90 mm Hg and staged appropriately (e.g., 170/85 mm Hg is defined as stage 2 ISH).

[†]Optimal blood pressure with respect to cardiovascular risk is SBP <120 mm Hg and DBP <80 mm Hg. However, unusually low readings should be evaluated for clinical significance.

[‡]Based on the average of two or more readings taken at each of two or more visits following an initial screening.

NOTE: In addition to classifying stages of hypertension based on average blood pressure levels, the clinician should specify presence or absence of target-organ disease and additional risk factors. For example, a patient with diabetes and a blood pressure of 142/94 mm Hg plus left ventricular hypertrophy should be classified as "stage 1 hypertension with target-organ disease (left ventricular hypertrophy) and with another major risk factor (diabetes)." This specificity is important for risk classification and management.

From Joint National Committee on Detection, Evaluation, and Treatment of High Blood Pressure: The fifth report of the Joint National Committee on Detection, Evaluation, and Treatment of High Blood Pressure, *Arch Intern Med* 153:154, 1993.

Hypertension

The screening examination is especially important for recognizing the client who has hypertension (persistently elevated blood pressure). Because hypertension may be present without symptoms, it is known as the silent disease. A client who does not feel ill does not usually come to a clinic or hospital for health care. Thus the screening examination may be instrumental in prompting the hypertensive client to begin early treatment to prevent some of the complications of untreated hypertension.

In their 1993 report, the Joint National Committee on Detection, Evaluation, and Treatment of High Blood Pressure Guidelines defines hypertension as being at least two blood pressure readings that average greater than 140/90 mm Hg (Table 9.4) or as requiring antihypertensive medication to maintain a blood pressure below 140/90. Hypertension should be diagnosed not on the basis of a single blood pressure reading but on the basis of several readings. The timing of subsequent readings should be based on the initial blood pressure level. Table 9.5 presents follow-up criteria for ranges of systolic and diastolic readings.

One in four American adults has high blood pressure. Ninety percent of adults who have high blood pressure have essential or idiopathic hypertension. In essential hypertension, no physiological cause is identified for the elevated blood pressure level. Hypertension is present in about 60% of non-Hispanic whites, 71% of non-Hispanic blacks, and 61% of Mexican-Americans who are age 60 or older.

Obtain a blood pressure measurement with well-child visits beginning at age 3. Blood pressure measurement in children should be obtained on the right arm for two reasons. Initial studies to determine "normal" blood pressure in children were done using the right arm. Also, if a child has a narrowing of the aorta or subclavian artery, the effect on the left-arm blood pressure reading will be greater.

The screening examination may yield an incidence of hypertension in less than 3% of children 4 to 15 years of age. However, early detection of hypertensive children may mean that diagnosis and treatment may be initiated in time to prevent the sequelae of the underlying disease process. (See also Chapter 25: Pediatric Clients.)

---

table 9.5 *Recommendations for Follow-Up Based on Initial Set of Blood Pressure Measurements for Adults Age 18 and Older*

Initial screening blood pressure (mm Hg)*		Follow-up recommended[†]
Systolic	Diastolic	
<130	<85	Recheck in 2 years
130–139	85–89	Recheck in 1 year[‡]
140–159	90–99	Confirm within 2 months
160–179	100–109	Evaluate or refer to source of care within 1 month
180–209	110–119	Evaluate or refer to source of care within 1 week
≥210	≥120	Evaluate or refer to source of care immediately

From Joint National Committee on Detection, Evaluation, and Treatment of High Blood Pressure: The fifth report of the Joint National Committee on Detection, Evaluation, and Treatment of High Blood Pressure, *Arch Intern Med* 153:154, 1993.
*If the systolic and diastolic categories are different, follow recommendation for the shorter-time follow-up (e.g., 160/85 mm Hg should be evaluated or referred to source of care within 1 month).
[†]The scheduling of follow-up should be modified by reliable information about past blood pressure measurements, other cardiovascular risk factors, or target-organ disease.
[‡]Consider providing advice about lifestyle modifications.

■ TEACHING SELF-ASSESSMENT

Maintaining a normal weight reduces the risk of hypertension. Weight loss often results in a substantial decrease in blood pressure even when ideal weight is not achieved. Restriction of daily dietary sodium to 2 g is also recommended. Alcohol consumption should not exceed 1 ounce per day (i.e., 8 ounces of wine or 24 ounces of beer). Other risk-reducing behaviors include avoiding tobacco use, following a regular program of exercise, and using behavior modification therapies such as relaxation and biofeedback.

A client can identify his or her maximal heart rate to measure the amount of exertion in physical exercise. To do this, he or she subtracts his or her age from 220. To exercise aerobically, the pulse must reach 80% of an individual's maximal heart rate. The client should obtain a radial or carotid baseline pulse before exercising by feeling the pulse, counting for 10 seconds, and then multiplying that count by 6. The count should be repeated immediately after exercise to obtain the maximal heart rate and 2 minutes later to assess recovery to baseline. If after 2 minutes the pulse has not returned to near baseline, the exercise involved too much exertion.

---

sample documentation & diagnoses — CRITICAL THINKING

■ FOCUSED HEALTH HISTORY *(SUBJECTIVE DATA)*

Mrs. H. was brought to the emergency room by her daughter, who found her confused and slumped in a chair in an extremely hot apartment. The daughter had tried to call Mrs. H. all evening but no one had answered. When her daughter arrived 12 hours later, Mrs. H. was confused and complained of black spots in front of her eyes, a severe headache, and nausea.

■ FOCUSED PHYSICAL EXAMINATION *(OBJECTIVE DATA)*

Vital signs: BP 100/50 right arm, lying down; pulse 120, weak, regular; respirations 32, labored and shallow; temperature 40° C (104° F) (rectal).

General appearance: Elderly woman who appears weak, unable to stand or sit. Skin is flushed; client is shivering. Daughter is present during examination at request of client.

Physical examination: Skin generally flushed, cool to touch on extremities, warm and dry to touch on trunk. Oral mucosa dry. Peripheral pulses barely palpable.

diagnoses

HEALTH PROBLEM
Hyperthermia

NURSING DIAGNOSES

Hyperthermia related to exposure to hot environment
Defining Characteristics
- Fever
- Flushed skin, warm to touch
- Increased respiratory rate
- Tachycardia

Activity intolerance related to generalized weakness
Defining Characteristics
- Weakness
- Shallow, labored breathing
- Confusion

Altered tissue perfusion related to hyperthermia
Defining Characteristics
- Decreased peripheral pulses
- Cool peripheral skin

chapter

10

Skin, Hair, and Nails

■ PURPOSE OF EXAMINATION

The skin, or integumentary system, is an organ system readily accessible to examination. It provides a membrane barrier between the individual and the external environment. The skin responds to changes in the external environment. It also reflects changes in the internal environment. A careful examination of the skin may yield valuable information about the client's general health. It can provide specific information needed to identify a systemic disease or a skin problem. A description of the skin of the healthy client, as well as a description of the client with a skin problem, is important. The examiner should pay special attention to any deviation from normal.

Examination of the skin requires some understanding of the structure and function of the system and familiarity with the appearance of the skin, hair, nails, and mucous membranes in health and disease. This chapter includes a brief discussion of the anatomy and function of

the skin, hair, and nails; methods for conducting a health history; and the systematic examination of the skin, hair, and nails. (The examination of the sclera and conjunctiva is discussed in Chapter 12, and the examination of the oral mucosa is discussed in Chapter 13.)

■ ANATOMY AND PHYSIOLOGY

The skin, combined with its appendages (the hair, nails, sebaceous glands, and eccrine and apocrine sweat glands), is the largest organ of the body. It has many important functions: it (1) provides a barrier to loss of water and electrolytes; (2) provides protection from external agents injurious to the internal structures; (3) regulates body temperature and blood pressure; (4) acts as a sense organ for touch, pressure, temperature, and pain; (5) maintains body surface integrity by ongoing cell replacement and increased regeneration for wound repair; (6) maintains a buffered protective skin film by

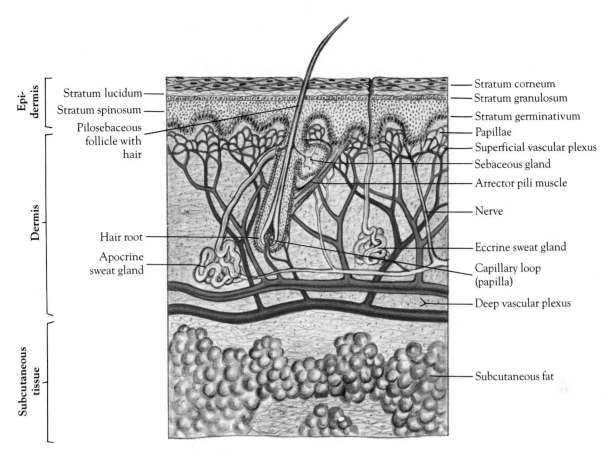

Epidermis
- Stratum lucidum
- Stratum spinosum
- Pilosebaceous follicle with hair

Dermis
- Hair root
- Apocrine sweat gland

Subcutaneous tissue

- Stratum corneum
- Stratum granulosum
- Stratum germinativum
- Papillae
- Superficial vascular plexus
- Sebaceous gland
- Arrector pili muscle
- Nerve
- Eccrine sweat gland
- Capillary loop (papilla)
- Deep vascular plexus
- Subcutaneous fat

figure **10.1**   Structures of the skin. *(From Thompson JM et al:* Mosby's clinical nursing, *ed 4, St Louis, 1997, Mosby.)*

eccrine and sebaceous glands to protect against microbial and fungal agents; (7) participates in production of vitamin D; (8) delays hypersensitivity reactions to foreign substances; and (9) indicates emotion through color change.

Skin

The skin is composed of three distinct layers: the epidermis, the dermis, and the subcutaneous tissue (Figure 10.1).

Epidermis

The epidermis is the outermost layer of the skin and varies from about 0.3 to 1.5 mm thick. It is an avascular, cornified cellular structure that depends on the underlying dermis for its nutrition. The epidermis is continuous with the mucous membranes and the lining of the ear canals. It is stratified into several layers and is composed chiefly of keratinocytes, cells that produce keratin. Keratin makes up much of the horny material in the outermost epidermal layer, the stratum corneum, and is the principal constituent of the harder, kera-

tinized structures of nails and hair. The innermost layer of the epidermis contains melanocytes, the source of melanin, which is the pigment that gives color to the skin and hair. The outermost, or horny, layer is made up of stratified layers of dead keratinized cells. This outer layer is constantly shed in an inconspicuous way and replenished by mitosis of the underlying cells, so that there is almost a complete turnover every 3 to 4 weeks.

Epidermal appendages include the hair, nails, eccrine sweat glands, apocrine sweat glands, and sebaceous glands. These appendages are formed by invagination of the epidermis into the underlying dermis. The eccrine, sebaceous, and apocrine appendages are glandular.

Dermis

The dermis underlying the epidermis constitutes the bulk of the skin. It is often referred to as the "true skin." It is a tough connective tissue that contains lymphatics and nerves and is highly vascular. The dermis consists of predominantly collagen fibers. It supports and nourishes the epidermis.

Subcutaneous tissue

The subcutaneous layer immediately under the dermis is composed of adipose tissue. It stores fat for energy and is important in temperature insulation.

Sebaceous glands

The sebaceous glands usually arise from the hair follicles and produce sebum, which has a lubricating effect on the horny outer layer of the epidermis. Sebaceous glands are on all parts of the body except the palms and soles. They are most abundant on the forehead, face, chin, and scalp. Excessive production of sebum is called seborrhea.

Sweat glands

The eccrine sweat glands open onto the surface of the skin and produce a dilute saline solution, or sweat. They are distributed widely and in great density on the palms and other parts of the hands. They have an important function in the dissipation of body heat as sweat is produced and evaporates. The apocrine sweat glands are found in the axillary and genital areas. They usually open into the hair follicles and produce a milky, viscid fluid or sweat. The sweat produced by the apocrine glands decomposes when it is contaminated by bacteria, resulting in its characteristic body odor. The apocrine glands do not function until a person reached puberty.

Hair

Hair is formed by invagination of epidermal cells into the dermal layers. Hair consists of a root, shaft, and hair follicle. Hair follicles are formed in utero and continue functioning through old age. No new follicles are formed after birth. Hair follicles produce the keratin of mature hair. Adults have two types of hairs: vellus hairs, which are short, fine, nonpigmented hairs; and terminal hairs, which are thick, coarse, and pigmented. Terminal hairs are found most extensively on the scalp, brows, and extremities.

Each hair goes through cyclic growth phases: a growing (anagen) phase, a transition (catogen) phase lasting only a few days, and a resting (telogen) phase. Ninety percent of normal scalp hairs are in the growing (anagen) phase, and 10% are in the resting stage. Hairs in the resting stage are subsequently expelled by the regenerating new hair. Hair growth is different depending on its location. Axillary, pubic, beard, and body hair is influenced by hormones. Hair on the scalp, eyelashes, and extremities does not require hormonal stimulus. Hair loss may be related to factors such as destruction of the hair matrix, slowing of hair growth due to medications or metabolic disorders, and genetic characteristics.

Nails

The nails are keratinized appendages of the epidermis. The nails consist of (1) the nail matrix (root),

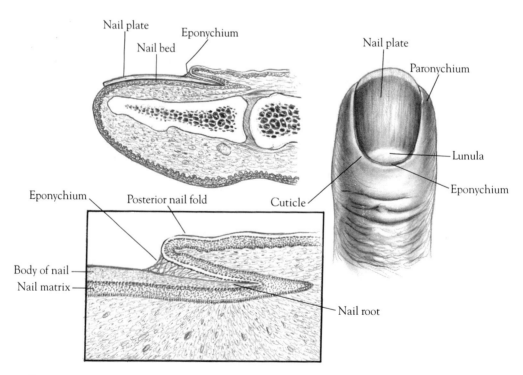

figure**10.2**   Structures of the nail. (*From Thompson JM et al: Mosby's clinical nursing, ed 4, St Louis, 1997, Mosby.*)

wherein the nail plate is developed; (2) the nail plate; (3) the nail bed, which is attached to the nail plate; and (4) the periungual tissue, including the eponychium and the perionychium (Figure 10.2).

The nail matrix is not visible. The lunula, located at the base of the visible nail, has the shape of a half-moon. It marks the end of the nail matrix, the site of nail growth. A bluish hue is visible in the nails of more darkly pigmented individuals. The size of the lunula is variable; it may not be visible in older individuals. The nail plate is a horny, semitransparent structure with a dorsal convexity. The nail bed lies distal to the lunula and is not known to participate in nail formation. The visible nail has a roughly rectangular shape. Normal thickness of the nail is 0.3 to 0.65 mm. It is somewhat thicker in men. The free edge of the nail fold is continuous with the cuticle, which is an extension of the stratum corneum of the dorsum of the finger. The eponychium lies below this and is the anterior extension of the roof of the nail fold on the nail plate. The hyponychium is the portion of the fingertip underlying the free portion of the nail. The perionychium is the epidermis bordering the nail.

The nail plate is formed continuously and uniformly at all points in the matrix. Reports of the fingernail growth rate in the normal adult vary from 0.1 to 1 mm per day. The rate varies with nutrition, age, and activity level. Nail growth also has a circadian and seasonal rhythm. It is greater in the morning, lessening progressively in the afternoon and the night. Nail growth is greater in warm seasons than in cold, and accelerated growth has been observed in warm climates. The growth rate slows with aging. The total time required for reaching the free margin of the nail from the lunula is called the migration time and is normally 130 days. The time required for complete renewal of the fingernail (regeneration time) is 170 days, whereas that of the toenail is 1 to 1½ years.

■ EXAMINATION
Health History
Present health status

1. Chief complaint
2. Allergies: Medications, foods, pollens, seasonal allergens
3. Exposures: Travel; environmental or occupational hazards or irritants; frequent sun exposure; use of tanning salons; frequent hand washing or immersion in water; family members or close contacts with skin problems
4. Medications: Prescribed or over-the-counter; topical or systemic; new or previously taken
5. Skin care habits: Cleansing patterns; skin care prod-

ucts used (soaps, oils, astringents, alcohol, facials, etc.); use of sunscreens; recent changes in skin care habits or products
6. Nail care habits: Difficulty cutting or clipping toenails and/or fingernails; types of instruments used; nail biting; use of adhesives for false fingernails
7. Hair care habits: Cleansing routines; recent changes in routine or products used; use of dyes, hair straighteners, permanents, or other chemical treatments; hair styles that put tension on the hair
8. Diet: Any recent dietary changes; liquid protein diet; new foods
9. Recent life changes, losses, or psychological or physiological stress

Specific Problems

1. Skin
   a. Changes in usual state of health; rashes, sores, lumps; pruritus; pigmentation changes; texture; dryness; odor; changes in or new presentation of wart or mole; lesion that is repeatedly irritated or that is slow to heal
   b. Onset: Sudden or gradual; date of onset
   c. Duration: How long has problem persisted?
   d. Frequency: Previous occurrence or progressive problem
   e. Location: Extensor or flexor surfaces; skinfolds; generalized or localized; any progression of rash or pattern
   f. Precipitating factors: Change in skin care products; use of different perfumes, detergents, or other products that come in contact with the skin; diet changes; exposures (travel; other family members or close contacts with a similar problem; new pet); stress-related reactions
   g. Alleviating factors: Medications, relaxation, not using certain products or avoiding contact with allergens, etc.
   h. Associated symptoms: Recent viral illness, high fever, systemic diseases, relationship to leisure activities or stress
   i. Efforts to treat: Medications or home remedies; response to treatment
2. Hair
   a. Changes in usual state of health; thinning or hair loss; excess hair; distribution of hair; color
   b. Onset: Sudden or gradual; asymmetrical or symmetrical pattern
   c. Duration: How long has problem persisted?
   d. Frequency: Recurrence or progressive problem
   e. Precipitating factors: Dietary changes, dieting (particularly liquid protein diet), malnutrition, hair care products/chemicals
   f. Alleviating factors: Not using particular products; diet; specific actions

g. Associated symptoms: Any other health problems; skin disorders; hormonal changes (medications or menarche, pregnancy, menopause); thyroid disease

h. Efforts to treat: Medications or other preparations used; response to treatment

3. Nails

a. Changes in usual state of health; splitting, breaking, biting, thickening, discoloration; separation from nail bed; inflammation

b. Onset: Sudden or gradual; related to illness or trauma

c. Duration: How long has problem persisted?

d. Frequency: Recurrent or intermittent; how often?

e. Precipitating factors: Exposure to drugs, chemicals; immersion in water; nail care products

f. Alleviating factors: Diet; stopping specific behaviors

g. Associated symptoms: Any other health problems, such as cardiac or respiratory disease, psoriasis, hypothyroidism

h. Efforts to treat: Medications or other remedies used; response to treatment

Past health history

1. Previous occurrences of the problem and its resolution

2. Previous skin problems; history of allergies, eczema, lesions, and their response to treatment

3. Previous hair problems: Loss; unusual growth or distribution; thinning, breakage; response to treatment

4. Previous nail problems: Injury, infections (fungal, bacterial, viral), allergic reactions (to nail care products); response to treatment

5. Systemic health problems: Severe cardiac, endocrine, respiratory, liver, hematologic, or other systemic diseases

6. Tolerance to sunlight; history of sunburns

Family health history

1. History of allergic diseases such as asthma, hay fever, or other sensitivities

2. Dermatologic disorders: Skin cancer; melanoma; psoriasis; eczema; infestations (lice, scabies); fungal, bacterial, or viral infections

---

RISK FACTORS ■ **SKIN CANCER**

Over age 50

Male

Family history of skin cancer, especially melanomas

Fair skin and light-colored hair or eyes

Precancerous skin lesions (dysplastic nevi, certain congenital nevi)

Extended periods of exposure to sunlight (occupational or recreational)

Tendency to burn easily

Geographical location—high altitudes or near equator

Exposure to radium, isotopes, x-rays, ultraviolet (UV) light

Exposure to coal, tar, arsenic, creosote, and/or petroleum products

Repeated skin trauma or irritation

History of childhood sunburns and sunlight exposure

RISK FACTORS **MALIGNANT MELANOMA**

Malignant melanoma is the most rapidly increasing form of cancer in the United States. Surgical treatment of early stages is usually curative, whereas treatment of later stages results in a poor prognosis. Those at high risk for melanoma have one or more of the following:

1. Large number of typical moles

2. Presence of atypical moles

3. Family history of melanoma

4. Prior melanoma

5. History of repeated severe sunburns, ease of burning, freckling, or inability to tan

The NIH Consensus Development Panel on Melanoma (1992) recommends that individuals be taught self-examination of the skin, know the warning signs of melanoma, and contact their health care provider if such signs appear. Warning signs include these ABCDs of melanoma (Figure 10.3):

Asymmetry: Early melanoma is asymmetrical. Most typical or common moles are symmetrical.

Border: Melanomas may have notching, scalloping, or poorly defined borders. Most common moles have very clear-cut borders.

Color: Melanomas are usually variegated. They may have shades of brown, tan, red, white, blue/black, or combinations thereof. Common moles tend to be uniform in color.

Diameter: Melanomas are frequently larger than 6 mm in diameter, although they may be diagnosed at a smaller size. Most common moles are less than 6 mm in diameter (about the size of a pencil eraser).

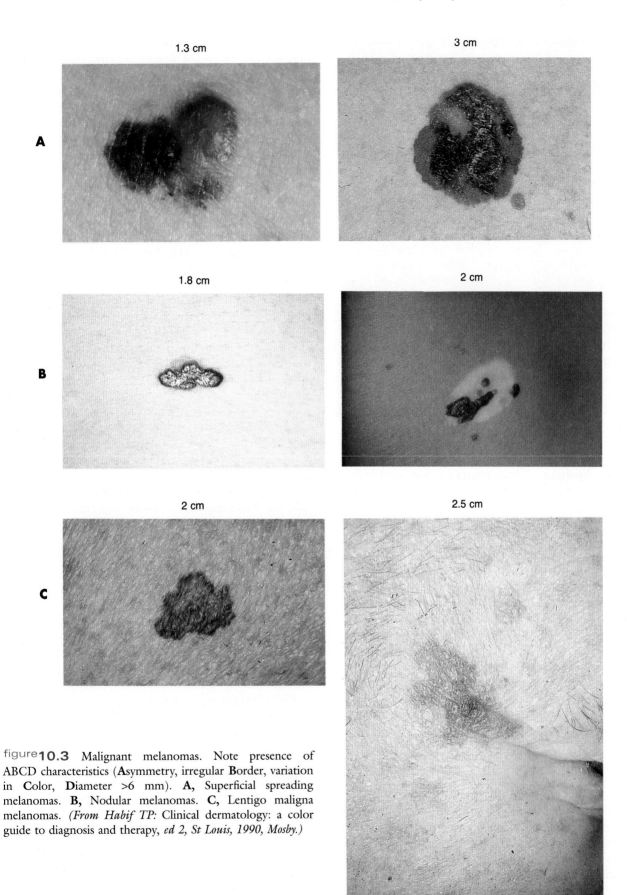

1.3 cm

3 cm

A

1.8 cm

2 cm

B

2 cm

2.5 cm

C

figure**10.3** Malignant melanomas. Note presence of ABCD characteristics (**A**symmetry, irregular **B**order, variation in **C**olor, **D**iameter >6 mm). **A,** Superficial spreading melanomas. **B,** Nodular melanomas. **C,** Lentigo maligna melanomas. *(From Habif TP: Clinical dermatology: a color guide to diagnosis and therapy, ed 2, St Louis, 1990, Mosby.)*

PREPARATION FOR EXAMINATION

EQUIPMENT

Item	Purpose
Metric ruler	To measure lesions
Flashlight	To illuminate lesions
Magnifying glass (optional)	To aid in evaluation of lesions
Disposable latex gloves	To protect examiner when examining lesions
For special procedures:	
Wood's lamp (filtered ultraviolet light)	To assess for tinea capitis
Glass slides and 20% KOH solution	To assess for fungal infection

CLIENT AND ENVIRONMENT

1. Provide a warm room with adequate lighting.
2. Protect the client's modesty while exposing areas to be examined as fully as possible.
3. Explain examination before beginning.
4. Use short, clear instructions.

3. Familial patterns of hair loss, coloration, or distribution

Preparation for Examination: Client and Environment

The examination of the skin is important in the assessment of the client's overall health and as a screening for skin cancer. A complete examination of the skin needs to be a part of every complete physical examination. This requires that you take a brief but careful view of the entire body and then examine specific areas in more detail. Provide a warm examining room with sufficient privacy. Have the client remove clothing so that you can fully view each section of the body. Protect client modesty by draping areas you are not examining.

Technique for Examination and Normal Findings

The examination of the skin and appendages needs to include a general inspection of the entire body, followed by a detailed regional examination. A good source of illumination is necessary; indirect natural daylight is preferred. Consider using a small magnifying glass to aid in examining individual lesions of the skin. Use a clear, flexible measure to assess the size of the lesions. Always wear gloves when examining lesions.

When doing a complete physical examination, you may want to begin the skin examination with areas the client is more used to having exposed (hair, face, hands, and arms). This technique may be less threatening to the client. Then inspect and palpate the skin, mucous membranes, and epidermal appendages of each body part as you examine it. Examine the entire body (with the client disrobed) at the end of the examination when the client is standing. For example, assess the skin on the back, buttocks, and legs before or after the examination of the spine.

Research indicates that detailed full-body examinations reveal several times as many melanomas as less detailed examinations. This is particularly important for clients at risk for melanoma (see Risk Factors box on p. 188).

If the client's main reason for being examined is to evaluate a skin problem, do a full-body inspection first to get an idea of the distribution pattern and extent of any lesions. Follow this with a detailed examination of the specific areas affected. To protect client modesty, drape the client's front as you are examining the back and vice versa.

Compare symmetrical anatomical areas throughout the examination. Also compare sun-exposed areas with non–sun-exposed areas. Examine intertriginous areas (those with skinfolds), which are dark, warm, and moist, such as large breasts, the groin, or an obese abdomen, for signs of irritation and/or infection. Make sure to have the client remove the socks, and examine the feet, between the toes, and toenails.

Skin

Inspection. Inspect the skin for color and vascularity and for evidence of perspiration, edema, injuries, or skin lesions. During the examination, think about the underlying structures and the particular kind of exposure of a body part. Note those changes in the skin that indicate past injuries and habits, such as calluses, stains, scars, needle marks, or insect bites. Also note the grooming of hair and nails.

Color. Skin color varies from person to person and from one part of the body to another. Normally, it is a

> **HELPFUL HINT** *In evaluating skin color, if you notice a color change in the client's skin, consider:*
> - *The lighting in the examination room*
> - *The position of the client or the client's extremity*
> - *The room temperature*
> - *The client's emotional condition*
> - *The cleanliness of the skin*
> - *The presence of edema*

HELPFUL HINT *In assessing dark skin:*

- *Skin color should be observed in the sclera, conjunctiva, buccal mucosa, tongue, lips, nail beds, palms, and soles.*
- *Inspection should be accompanied by palpation, especially if inflammation or edema is suspected.*
- *Findings should always be correlated with the patient's history to arrive at a nursing diagnosis.*
- *Pallor in brown-skinned patients may present as a yellowish brown tinge to the skin. In a black-skinned patient the skin will appear "ashen gray." It can be difficult to determine. Pallor in dark-skinned individuals is characterized by absence of the underlying red tones in the skin.*
- *Jaundice may be observed in the sclera but should not be confused with the normal yellow pigmentation of the dark-skinned black patient. The best place to inspect is in that portion of the sclera that is observable when the eye is open. If jaundice is suspected, the posterior portion of the hard palate should also be observed for a yellowish cast. This is most effective when done in bright daylight.*
- *The oral mucosa of dark-skinned individuals may have a normal freckling of pigmentation that may also be evident in the gums, the borders of the tongue, and the lining of the cheeks.*
- *The gingiva normally may have a dark blue color that may appear blotchy or be evenly distributed.*
- *Petechiae are best observed over areas of lighter pigmentation—the abdomen, gluteal areas, and volar aspect of the forearm. They may also be seen in the palpebral conjunctiva and buccal mucosa.*
- *To differentiate petechiae and ecchymosis from erythema, remember that pressure over the area will cause erythema to blanch but will not affect either petechiae or ecchymosis.*
- *Erythema usually is associated with increased skin temperature, so palpation should also be used if an inflammatory condition is suspected.*
- *Edema may reduce the intensity of the color of an area of skin because of the increased distance between the external epithelium and the pigmented layers. Therefore, darker skin would appear lighter. On palpation the skin may feel "tight."*
- *Cyanosis can often be difficult to determine in dark-skinned individuals. Familiarity with the precyanotic color is often helpful. However, if this is not possible, close inspection of the nail beds, lips, palpebral conjunctiva, palms, and soles should show evidence of cyanosis.*
- *Skin rashes may be assessed by palpating for changes in skin texture.*

From Roach B: Color changes in dark skin, *Nursing 77,* Jan 1977.

whitish pink or a brown shade, depending on race. The exposed areas of the body, including the face, ears, back of the neck, and backs of the hands and arms, are noticeably different from the unexposed areas and may be more damaged after long exposure to the sun and weather. The vascular flush areas are the cheeks, the bridge of the nose, the neck, the upper chest, the flexor surfaces of the extremities, and the genital area. These areas may be involved in a vascular disturbance or may demonstrate increased color caused by blushing or temperature elevation. Compare them with areas of less vascularity.

The pigment-labile areas are the face, the backs of the hands, the flexors of the wrists, the axillae, the mammary areoleae, the midline of the abdomen, and the genital area. These areas may demonstrate normal systemic pigmentary changes, such as during pregnancy.

Other changes in skin color may provide evidence of systemic disease. These changes include the following:

1. Cyanosis, a dusky blue color, may be visible in the nail beds and in the lips and the oral mucosa. It results from decreased oxyhemoglobin binding, or decreased oxygenation of the blood, and can be caused by pulmonary or heart disease, by abnormalities of hemoglobin, or by cold.
2. Jaundice, a yellow or green hue, occurs when tissue bilirubin is increased and may be visible first in the sclerae and then in the mucous membranes and the skin.
3. Pallor, or decreased color in the skin, results from decreased blood flow to the superficial vessels or from decreased amounts of hemoglobin in the blood. Pallor is most evident in the face, the palpebral conjunctiva, the mouth, and the nail beds.
4. Erythema, or an intense redness of the skin, may be generalized or localized. Generalized redness of the skin may be caused by fever, whereas defined areas of redness may be the result of a localized infection or sunburn.
5. Pigmentation changes or alterations in the normal pattern of pigmentation result from changes in

table 10.1 *Conditions Causing Variation in Pigmentation*

Condition	Characteristic color	Location
DIFFUSE HYPERPIGMENTATION		
Addison's disease, ACTH-producing tumors*	Tan to brown, "bronzing"	Generalized, more marked on exposed areas, flexures, mucous membrane of mouth
Arsenic toxicity	Dusky, diffuse, paler spots	Trunk, extremities
Chloasma (mask of pregnancy), phenytoin ingestion	Tan to brown	Forehead—adjacent to hairline, malar prominence, upper lip, chin
Hemochromatosis	Bronze to grayish brown, deposits of hemosiderin	Generalized
Ichthyosis	Tan, fine to coarse scales	Generalized
Malabsorption syndrome (sprue)	Tan to brown patches	Any area of body
Scleroderma	Yellow to tan (may also have depigmentation)	Generalized
Uremia (chronic renal failure)	Yellow-brown, retention of urinary chromogens	Generalized
LACK OF PIGMENTATION		
Vitiligo	Circumscribed lack of pigmentation	
Albinism—hereditary	Complete or partial lack of melanin	Generalized (universal albinism), skin, hair, eyes

*ACTH, Adrenocorticotropic hormone.

the distribution of melanin or in the function of the melanocytes in the epidermis. Either hyperpigmentation or depigmentation can occur. A nevus, or birthmark, is an example of a defined area of hyperpigmentation that may be an innocent manifestation, such as the mongolian spots found on infants, or it may be a more serious finding, such as the numerous cafe au lait spots of neurofibromatosis. Depigmentation of the skin, which occurs in vitiligo, may involve only one or a few areas or may be more generalized. Common sites of vitiligo are the face, neck, axillae, groin, anogenital area, eyelids, hands, and wrists. Table 10.1 lists other conditions causing variations in pigmentation.

It is important to be aware that expression of the above skin color changes will vary depending on the client's racial group. Table 10.2 summarizes the differences in assessment of color changes in light-skinned and dark-skinned individuals.

Other localized changes in color may indicate a problem such as edema, which tends to blanch skin color.

Palpation. Palpate the skin to augment your findings on inspection. In general, perform palpation simultaneously as you examine each body part. Note changes in temperature, moisture, texture, and turgor.

Temperature. Skin temperature increases when blood flow through the dermis increases. Localized elevations in skin temperature occur with a burn or a localized infection. A generalized increase in skin temperature may occur with a fever, which may be due to a localized infection or systemic disease. The temperature of the skin is reduced when blood flow through the dermis decreases. Generalized skin coolness occurs when the client is in shock. Localized hypothermia occurs in conditions such as arteriosclerosis. Always check for bilateral symmetry. Inequality in temperature may indicate circulatory problems or infection.

Moisture. Moisture on the skin varies from one body area to another. The soles of the feet, the palms of the hands, and the intertriginous areas (where two surfaces are close together) contain more moisture than other parts. The amount of moisture found over the entire integument also varies with changes in the environmental temperature, muscular activity, and body temperature. The skin regulates body temperature by producing perspiration that evaporates, thus cooling the body when the temperature increases. The skin is normally drier

table 10.2 *Differences in Color Changes in Light and Dark Skin*

Etiology	Light skin	Dark skin
PALLOR		
Anemia—decreased hematocrit	Generalized pallor, loss of rosy glow in skin, especially in face; skin with natural yellow tones appears more yellow, may be mistaken for mild jaundice	Brown skin appears yellow-brown, dull; black skin loses its red undertones and appears ashen gray; skin loses its healthy glow—check areas with pigmentation, such as conjunctivae, mucous membranes
Shock—decreased perfusion, vaso-constriction		
Local arterial insufficiency	Marked localized pallor (e.g., lower extremities), especially when elevated	Ashen gray, dull; cool to palpation
Albinism—total absence of pigment melanin throughout integument	Whitish pink skin; white or pale blond hair; pink irises	Tan, cream, or white skin; white or pale blond hair; pink irises
Vitiligo—patchy depigmentation from destruction of melanocytes	Patchy milky white spots, often symmetrical, bilaterally, especially around mouth	Patchy milky white spots, often symmetrical bilaterally
CYANOSIS		
Increased amount of unoxygenated hemoglobin	Skin, lips, and mucous membranes look blue tinged; nail beds, and conjunctivae are blue	Skin dark but dull, lifeless; natural skin tone will influence color of cyanotic skin*; cyanosis may be undetectable except for ashen gray lips, tongue, oral mucous membranes, nail beds; conjunctivae may appear pale or blue tinged
Central—chronic heart and lung disease cause arterial desaturation		
Peripheral—exposure to cold, anxiety	Nail beds dusky	Nail beds dusky
ERYTHEMA		
Hyperemia—increased blood flow through engorged arterioles, such as in inflammation, fever, alcohol intake, blushing	Red, bright pink; easily seen anywhere on body; inflammation accompanied by higher temperature at site	Redness may be difficult to detect; localized inflamed areas may appear purple; rely on palpation for increased temperature, hardness, swelling, or edema
Polycythemia—increased red blood cells, capillary stasis	Ruddy blue in face, oral mucosa, conjunctiva, hands and feet	Difficult to detect; check lips for redness
Carbon monoxide poisoning	Bright cherry red in face and upper torso	Cherry red color in nail beds, lips, and oral mucosa
Venous stasis—decreased blood flow from area, engorged venules	Dusky rubor of dependent extremities; a prelude to necrosis with pressure sore	Easily masked; use palpation for warmth or edema

*Gaskin (1986) describes the following changes:

Natural		Cyanotic
black	→	gray
brown	→	dark blue
red	→	purple
tan	→	blue
yellow	→	green
white	→	blue

continued

table 10.2   *Differences in Color Changes in Light and Dark Skin—cont'd*

Etiology	Light skin	Dark skin
PURPURAS		

Ecchymosis (bruise)
Large patch of capillary bleeding into tissue secondary to trauma
	Color goes from:
	  1. Red-blue or purple within 24 hours of trauma
	  2. Blue to purple (1–5 days)
	  3. Green (5–7 days)
	  4. Yellow (7–10 days)
	  5. Brown to disappearing (10–14 days)
		Deeper dark purple, bluish, or black tone; difficult to see unless it occurs in an area of light pigmentation

Petechiae Due to bleeding from superficial capillaries; infection	Lesions appear as small, reddish purple pinpoints; may be seen in mouth, buccal mucosa, and conjunctiva; on skin especially noticeable on abdomen, buttocks, and inner surfaces of arms or legs	In dark skin difficult to see; may be evident in buccal mucosa, sclera, and conjunctiva; also look in areas of lighter melanization, such as abdomen, buttocks, and inner surface of forearm
JAUNDICE		
Increased serum bilirubin, over 2 to 3 mg/dl, due to liver inflammation or hemolytic disease, such as after severe burns and some infections	Generalized; also see yellow in sclera, hard palate, oral mucosa, fingernails, palms of hands and soles of feet	Check sclera for yellow near limbus; do not mistake normal yellowish fatty deposits in periphery under eyelids for jaundice—jaundice best noted in junction of hands and soft palate and also on palms of hands and soles of feet
Carotenemia—increased serum carotene from ingestion of large amounts of carotene-rich foods	Yellow-orange in forehead, palms and soles, and nasolabial folds, but no yellowing in sclera or mucous membranes	Yellow-orange tinge on palms of hands and soles of feet; no yellowing of sclera or mucous membranes
Uremia—renal failure causes retained urochrome pigments in blood	Generalized pallor and yellow or orange-green or gray overlying pallor of anemia; may also have ecchymoses and purpura; does not affect conjunctiva or mucous membranes	Difficult to discern and easily masked; rely on laboratory and clinical findings; does not effect conjunctiva or mucous membranes
BROWN-TAN		
Addison's disease—cortisol deficiency stimulates increased melanin production	Bronzed appearance, an "eternal tan"; most apparent around nipples, perineum, genitalia, and pressure points (inner thighs, buttocks, elbow, axillae)	General deepening of skin tone, but is easily masked; rely on laboratory and clinical findings
RASH		
Various causes	May be visualized, as well as felt with light palpation	Not easily visualized but may be felt with light palpation
SCAR		
Multiple causes	Generally heals, showing narrow scar line	Frequently has keloid development, resulting in a thickened, raised scar

figure **10.4** Testing skin turgor.

during the winter months, when environmental temperatures and humidity are lower, and as the individual ages. Abnormal dryness of the skin occurs with dehydration. In this instance, the skin feels dry even when the temperature increases. Dryness of the skin also occurs in conditions such as myxedema and chronic nephritis.

Texture. Texture refers to the fineness or coarseness of the skin. Changes in skin texture may indicate local irritation or trauma to defined skin areas or may be associated with problems of other systems. The skin becomes soft and smooth in hyperthyroidism and rough and dry in hypothyroidism.

Turgor. Turgor refers to the elasticity of the skin. You can most easily determine turgor by picking up a fold of skin over the abdomen and observing how quickly it returns to its normal shape (Figure 10.4). A loss of turgor is associated with dehydration. The skin demonstrates a laxness and a loss of normal mobility, returning to place slowly. Loss of turgor is also associated with aging; the skin becomes wrinkled and lax from loss of elasticity. Increased turgor is associated with an increase in tension, which causes the skin to return to place quickly when pinched. Increased turgor occurs in progressive systemic sclerosis (PSS), a connective tissue disorder.

Lesions. Perform the initial examination of any skin lesion at a distance of 3 feet or more to determine the general characteristics of the eruption. This first observation provides the opportunity to determine the location, distribution, and configuration of the lesions. Next, carry out a closer examination to determine the color, size, shape, texture, firmness, and morphological characteristics of the individual lesions.

DISTRIBUTION. Describe the distribution of skin lesions according to the location or body region affected and the symmetry or asymmetry of findings in comparable body parts. Keep in mind the characteristic patterns that provide the major clue in the diagnosis of a specific skin problem. Figure 10.5 illustrates a few distribution patterns observed in specific problems.

CONFIGURATION. Note the configuration of skin lesions, which is equally important in defining the problem. Configuration refers to the arrangement or position of several lesions in relation to each other. For example, the skin lesions of tinea corporis, which is ringworm of the body, have an annular configuration that is circular. Use the following terms to describe the configuration of skin lesions, as appropriate:

Grouped	Lesions clustered together
Herpetiform or zosteriform	Multiple groups of vesicles erupting unilaterally following the course of cutaneous nerves
Linear	Lesions arranged in a line
Annular	Lesions arranged in a circle, ring shaped
Polycyclic	Multiple annular arrangements of lesions
Arciform	Lesions arranged in an arc, bow shaped
Reticular	Lesions meshed in the form of a network
Confluent	Lesions merged together, not discrete

Figure 10.6 illustrates some configurations.

TYPE OF LESION. The morphological classification of skin lesions organizes lesions in terms of their structure. It is based on the size, shape, elevation, or depression of the lesions. Determining the morphological structure of the individual lesion (macule, papule, vesicle, etc.) helps identify the specific problem. Table 10.3 provides detailed parameters for classification of skin lesions. Figures 10.7, 10.8, and 10.9 illustrate descriptions and characteristics of lesions.

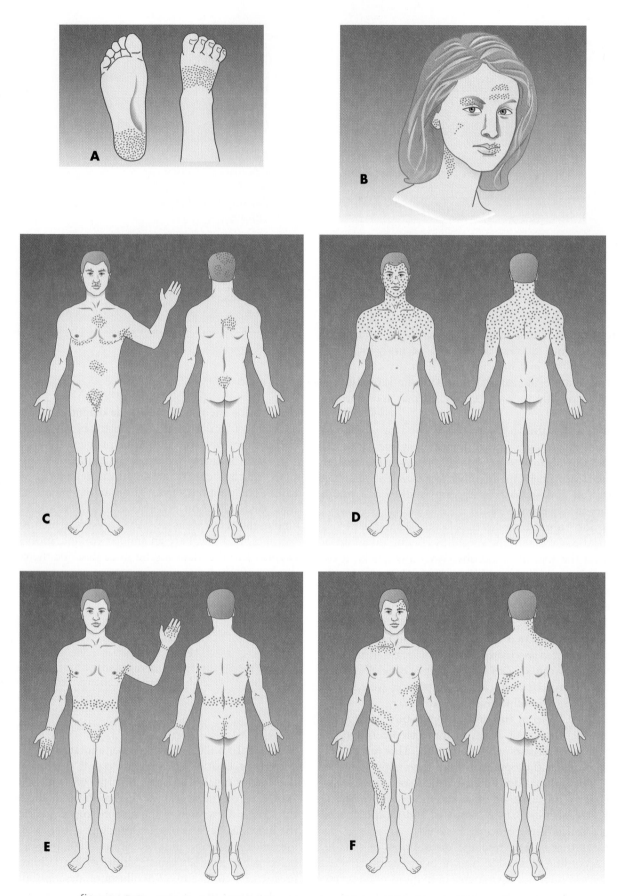

figure **10.5**   Distribution of lesions in selected problems of the skin. **A,** Contact dermatitis (shoes). **B,** Contact dermatitis (cosmetics, perfumes, earrings). **C,** Seborrheic dermatitis. **D,** Acne. **E,** Scabies. **F,** Herpes zoster.

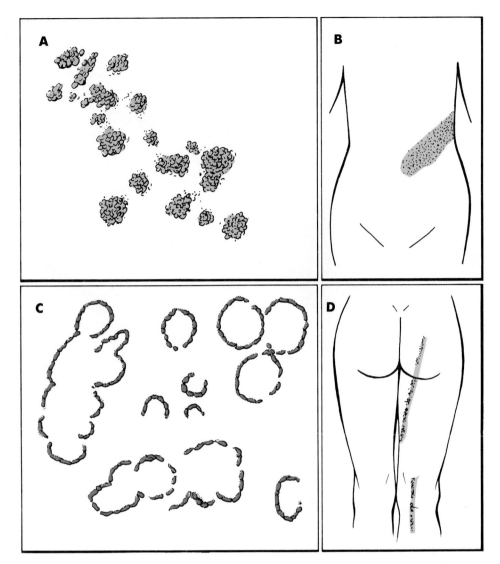

figure **10.6** Examples of different configurations of skin lesions. **A,** Grouped. **B,** Zosteriform. **C,** Annular *(circular)* and arciform *(arc).* **D,** Linear.

Classify lesions as primary, secondary, or vascular. Primary lesions are those that appear initially in response to some change in the external or internal environment of the skin. Secondary lesions do not appear initially but result from modifications such as trauma, chronicity, or infection in the primary lesion. For instance, the primary lesion may be a vesicle, which is a small, circumscribed, elevated lesion containing clear fluid. The vesicle will rupture, leaving a small moist area, which is classified as a secondary lesion called an erosion. Figures 10.7 and 10.8 illustrate some of the primary and secondary lesions. Table 10.4 describes types of skin lesions that characterize stages of dermatitis. Primary and secondary lesions may occur at the same time.

Vascular lesions usually appear as red pigmented lesions. They may be indicative of problems such as bleeding (petechiae and ecchymoses) or liver disease (spider angioma), or they may be due to benign conditions such as telangiectasia. Determining whether or not the lesion blanches will help identify the type of lesion. Place a glass slide over the lesion and apply pressure. If the lesion loses color or fades, it blanches, thus indicating a vascular lesion. Vascular lesions are described in Figure 10.9.

Measure the lesion with a small, clear, and flexible ruler. Report sizes in centimeters (inches may also be used but are less desirable). Measure all the dimensions possible (length, width, height/depth). If possible, draw a diagram with location and dimensions included. This will help you monitor the progression or resolution of

Text continued on p. 203

Macule—flat, circumscribed area that is a change in the color of the skin; less than 1 cm in diameter
Examples: Freckle; flat mole (nevus), petechia; measles, scarlet fever

Plaque—elevated, firm, and rough lesion with a flat-top surface greater than 1 cm in diameter
Examples: Psoriasis, seborrheic and actinic keratoses

Wheal—elevated, irregular-shaped area of cutaneous edema; solid, transient; variable diameter
Examples: Urticaria, insect bite, allergic reaction

Patch—flat, non-palpable, irregular-shaped macule more than 1 cm in diameter
Examples: Vitiligo, port-wine stain, mongolian spot, café au lait spot

Nodule—elevated, firm, circumscribed lesion; deeper in dermis than a papule; 1 to 2 cm in diameter
Examples: Erythema nodosum, lipoma

Papule—elevated, firm, circumscribed area less than 1 cm in diameter (verruca)
Examples: Wart, elevated mole, lichen planus

figure**10.7** Descriptions and characteristics of primary skin lesions. (*Modified from Thompson JM et al:* Mosby's clinical nursing, *ed 4, St Louis, 1997, Mosby.*)

Tumor—elevated and solid lesion; may or may not be clearly demarcated; deeper in dermis; greater than 2 cm in diameter
Examples: Neoplasm, benign tumor, lipoma, hemangioma

Pustule—elevated, superficial lesion; similar to a vesicle but filled with purulent fluid
Examples: Impetigo, acne

Vesicle—elevated, circumscribed, superficial (not into dermis); filled with serous fluid; less than 1 cm in diameter
Examples: Varicella (chicken-pox), herpes zoster (shingles)

Cyst—elevated, circumscribed, encapsulated lesion; in dermis or subcutaneous layer; filled with liquid or semisolid material
Examples: Sebaceous cyst, cystic acne

Bulla—vesicle greater than 1 cm in diameter
Examples: Blister, pemphigus vulgaris

Scar—thin to thick fibrous tissue that replaces normal skin following injury or laceration to the dermis
Example: Healed wound or surgical incision

Scale—heaped-up keratinized cells; flaky skin; irregular; thick or thin; dry or oily; variation in size
Examples: Flaking of skin with seborrheic dermatitis following scarlet fever, or flaking of skin following a drug reaction; dry skin

Keloid—irregular-shaped, elevated, progressively enlarging scar; grows beyond the boundaries of the wound; caused by excessive collagen formation during healing
Example: Keloid formation following surgery

Crust—dried serum, blood, or purulent exudate; slightly elevated; size varies; brown, red, black, tan, or straw in color
Examples: Scab on abrasion; eczema

Excoriation—loss of the epidermis; linear, hollowed-out crusted area
Examples: Abrasion or scratch, scabie

Lichenification—rough, thickened epidermis secondary to persistent rubbing, itching, or skin irritation; often involves flexor surface of extremity
Example: Chronic dermatitis

figure **10.8**   Descriptions and characteristics of secondary skin lesions. (*Modified from Thompson JM et al:* Mosby's clinical nursing, *ed 4, St Louis, 1997, Mosby.*)

Fissure—linear crack or break from the epidermis to the dermis; may be moist or dry
Examples: Athlete's foot; crack at the corner of the mouth

Erosion—loss of part of the epidermis; depressed, moist, glistening; follows rupture of a vesicle or bulla
Examples: Varicella; variola after rupture

Ulcer—loss of epidermis and dermis; concave; varies in size
Examples: Decubitis; stasis ulcer

Atrophy—thinning of the skin surface and loss of skin markings; skin appears translucent and paperlike
Examples: Striae, aged skin

Purpura—red-purple nonblanchable discoloration greater than 0.5 cm in diameter
Cause: Intravascular defects, infection

Petechiae—red-purple nonblanchable discoloration less than 0.5 cm in diameter
Cause: Intravascular defects, infection

Ecchymoses—red-purple nonblanchable discoloration of variable size
Cause: Vascular wall destruction, trauma, vasculitis

Spider angioma—red central body with radiating spiderlike legs that blanch with pressure to the central body
Cause: Liver disease, vitamin B deficiency, idiopathic

Venous star—bluish spider, linear or irregularly shaped; does not blanch with pressure
Cause: Increased pressure in superficial veins

Telangiectasia—fine, irregular red line
Cause: Dilation of capillaries

Capillary hemangioma (nevus flammeus)—red irregular macular patches
Cause: Dilation of dermal capillaries

figure**10.9** Characteristics and causes of vascular lesions. *(Modified from Seidel HM et al:* Mosby's guide to physical examination, *ed 3, St Louis, 1995, Mosby.)*

table 10.3 *Identification of Skin Lesions*

	Name of lesion	Description	<1 cm	>1 cm
Type of lesion:				
Primary	Macule—patch	Flat, circumscribed discoloration	Macule	Patch
	Papule—plaque	Solid, elevated lesion	Papule	Plaque
	Nodule—tumor	Solid, elevated lesion; also has depth	Nodule	Tumor
	Vesicle—bulla	Fluid filled, superficial, elevated	Vesicle	Bulla
Primary of varying size	Pustule	Vesicle or bulla containing pus		
	Wheal	Lesion caused by cutaneous edema; irregular in shape; elevated; transient		
	Telangiectasia	Dilated capillary; fine red line(s)		
Secondary	Scale	Accumulation of loose surface epithelium		
	Crust	Dried surface fluids: serum or pus		
	Excoriation	Scratch mark		
	Erosion	Superficial denuded lesion		
	Scar	First red, then pale, smooth hyaline wound repair; may be flat, depressed, elevated, or hypertrophic (keloid)		
	Ulcer	Loss of tissue from a surface caused by destruction of a superficial lesion		
	Atrophy	Thinning of skin; loss of hair and sweat glands		
	Fissure	Linear crack in skin that extends to dermis		
	Lichenification	Thickening of skin caused by chronic scratching		

Number of lesions: ☐ Single ☐ Numerous ☐ Actual count
Size of lesion: (Measure)
Shape of lesion: ☐ Round ☐ Oval ☐ Umbilicated ☐ Irregular
Color of lesion: ☐ Red ☐ Brown ☐ Black ☐ Gray-blue ☐ White ☐ Purple ☐ Orange
☐ Yellow ☐ Circumscribed? ☐ Diffuse? ☐ Change with diascopy*?
Configuration: ☐ Single ☐ Grouped: ☐ Herpetiform ☐ Linear ☐ Annular ☐ Arciform
☐ Reticular ☐ Scattered
Distribution: ☐ Localized ☐ Generalized ☐ Symmetrical
Site of predilection _____

*Diascopy consists of the application of firm pressure against a microscope slide or clear plastic placed over a skin lesion, allowing identification of capillary dilation and thus differentiating telangiectasia from purpura. The technique also makes lymphoma, sarcoidosis, and tuberculosis of the skin appear yellow-brown.

table 10.4 *Stages of Dermatitis*

Stage	Lesions
Acute	Erythema, edema, vesicles, exudate, crusting
Subacute	Erythema, residual crusting, scaling
Chronic	Scaling, hyperpigmentation, lichenification, fissuring

the lesion. The term used to describe a lesion will vary with its size. For example, a vesicle is a fluid-filled lesion and is less than 1 cm in diameter. If it is greater than 1 cm, it is called a bulla.

Gently palpate lesions to determine the texture and firmness of the individual lesion and in some instances to determine the actual shape of the lesion. Always wear gloves when palpating a skin lesion.

COLOR. Describe the color of the individual lesion. There may be no discoloration, or you may see many colors. For example, with ecchymosis the initial dark red and dark blue colors fade and a yellow color appears. Lesions may be well defined with the color changes limited to the borders of the lesion. These lesions are re-

ferred to as "circumscribed." Lesions may have "diffuse" borders that are undefined, with the color changes spread over a large area. You can use diascopy to observe for color changes of a lesion when pressure is applied. Place a transparent slide against the skin to express blood from the capillaries and superficial venules. Telangiectases will blanch, whereas petechial or purpuric lesions will not.

Hair

Inspection and palpation. Examine the hair over the entire body to determine the distribution, quantity, and quality.

Distribution. Hair may be present on the scalp, lower face, nares, ears, neck, axillae, anterior chest, back and shoulders, arms, legs, buttocks and pubic area, and around the nipples. Coarse terminal hair occurs on the scalp, on the pubic and axillary areas, and in the male's beard. The body is covered with fine vellus hair. A normal male or female hair pattern evolves after puberty. The pattern of hair distribution in the male genital area is diamond shaped, whereas the pattern of hair distribution in the female genital area is an inverted triangle. A deviation may indicate an endocrine problem.

Quantity. Changes in the quantity of the hair are also important. Hirsutism, increased hair growth, occurs in conditions such as Cushing's syndrome, polycystic ovary disease, and acromegaly. Decreased hair growth or loss of hair may be associated with hypopituitarism or a pyogenic infection. Patterns of hair loss may also be hormonally regulated as with male-pattern baldness (Figure 10.10). Table 10.5 lists types of alopecia, or hair loss.

Texture. Hair in the pubic and axillary areas is coarse. Scalp hair may be thick or thin, coarse or fine, straight, curly, or kinky. It should be shiny, smooth, and resilient. This characteristic may be affected by the use of beauty products such as rinses, hair straighteners, dyes, or per-

manents. Texture may also change with systemic illnesses. For example, changes in the texture of hair associated with hypothyroidism include dryness and coarseness, and changes associated with hyperthyroidism include increased silkiness and fineness. Texture and color determine the quality of the hair. Palpate the hair for texture and the scalp for dryness.

Color. Hair color may vary from light blond to black. Changes in color such as graying occur normally with aging. Premature graying may be indicative of underlying disease such as pernicious anemia. Patchy gray hair may develop following nerve injuries. Hair color may also change as a result of malnutrition. Use of dyes, rinses, or permanents will also influence hair color.

Nails

Inspection and palpation. The assessment of the nails is important to determine not only their condition, but also possible evidence of systemic diseases. Examine the nails for shape, normal dorsal curvature, adhesion to the nail bed, regularity of the nail surface, color, cleanliness, and thickness. Examine the skinfolds around the nails for any color changes, swelling, increased temperature, or tenderness (see Figure 10.2). Complete absence of the nail, or anonychia, is usually congenital.

Curvature. The nail surface is usually flat or slightly curved. The nail edges should be rounded and smooth. The normal angle of the nail base is 160 degrees. Clubbing, which is associated with respiratory and cardiovas-

figure**10.10** Male-pattern baldness.

table **10.5**	*Alopecia—Hair Loss*
Type of alopecia	**Description**
Androgen (in female)	Thinning of scalp hair, male pattern; hirsutism on body
Areata	Circumscribed bald areas; sudden onset, usually reversible
Chemical	Hair brittle, breaks off
Cicatricial	Permanent localized loss of hair associated with scarring
Drug or radiation	Generalized loss of hair caused by antineoplastic agents, such as gold, thallium, and arsenic, or by radiation
Male pattern	Receding of anterior hairline, temples, and vertex; hereditary
Mucinosis	Erythmatous papules or plaques without hair
Syphilitic	Generalized thinning of hair or baldness; mucous patches without hair

cular problems, cirrhosis, colitis, and thyroid disease, occurs when the angle of the nail base exceeds 180 degrees (Figure 10.11). With clubbing, the nail becomes thickened, hard, shiny, and curved at the free end. In advanced cases the entire nail is pushed away from the base at an angle greater than 180 degrees and feels "spongy."

Nail adhesion. The nail should be firmly adherent to the nail bed, and the nail base should be firm to palpation. To test for adherence, gently squeeze the nail between your thumb and the pad of your finger (Figure

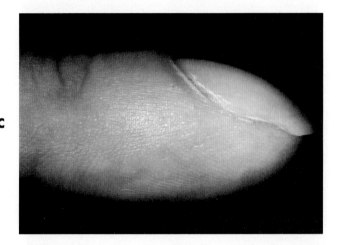

figure**10.11** Finger clubbing. **A,** Normal angle of the nail. **B,** Abnormal angle of the nail seen in late clubbing. **C,** The distal phalanges are enlarged to a rounded bulbous shape. The nail enlarges and becomes curved, hard, and thickened. *(C From Habif TP: Clinical dermatology: a color guide to diagnosis and therapy, ed 3, St Louis, 1996, Mosby.)*

figure**10.12** Palpate the nail to test for adherence.

figure**10.13** Paronychia. **A,** Acute paronychia. Erythema and purulent material occur at the proximal nail fold. **B,** Chronic paronychia. Erythema and swelling of the nail folds. The cuticle is absent. Chronic inflammation has caused horizontal ridging of the nails. *(From Habif TP: Clinical dermatology: a color guide to diagnosis and therapy, ed 3, St Louis, 1996, Mosby.)*

figure**10.14** Longitudinal ridging. Parallel elevated nail ridges are a common aging change and do not indicate any deficiency. *(From Habif TP: Clinical dermatology: a color guide to diagnosis and therapy, ed 3, St Louis, 1996, Mosby.)*

figure**10.15** Lichen planus. Inflammation of the matrix results in adherence of the proximal nail fold to the scarred matrix. *(From Habif TP: Clinical dermatology: a color guide to diagnosis and therapy, ed 2, St Louis, 1990, Mosby.)*

figure**10.16** Pigmented bands occur as a normal finding in over 90% of black individuals. *(From Habif TP: Clinical dermatology: a color guide to diagnosis and therapy, ed 3, St Louis, 1996, Mosby.)*

10.12). Examine the nail folds for swelling, redness, pus, warts, or tumors. Paronychia is an inflammation of the folds of tissue surrounding the nails, leading to erythema, with inflammation, swelling, and induration of the nail fold accompanied by pain and tenderness (Figure 10.13). It is the most common complaint related to the nails.

Nail surface. The nail surface should be smooth and flat. Inspect for grooves, depressions, pitting, and ridging. Longitudinal ridging may be a normal variant (Figure 10.14) or may occur with lichen planus (Figure 10.15). The client may have transverse grooves related to repeated injury to the nail, such as picking.

Nail color. Nail color should be pink, although pigment bands may normally be present in the nail beds of dark-skinned individuals (Figure 10.16). Sudden appearance of a pigment band in white individuals may indicate melanoma.

Nail thickness. Thickening or hypertrophy of the nail is generally caused by trauma. The nail of the small toe is often the only one affected; it takes on a clawlike shape. Thickening of the nails has been associated with psoriasis, fungal infection, a defective vascular supply, and trauma. Thinning of the nail has been linked to defective peripheral circulation and nutritional anemias. Brittleness of the nails is a common sign. Systemic diseases associated with brittle nails are nutritional anemias and impaired peripheral circulation. Prolonged exposure to water and alkaline substances also has been associated with brittle nails.

Sebaceous glands. The sebaceous glands, which are more numerous over the face and scalp areas, normally become more active during adolescence, resulting in increased oiliness of the skin. A sudden increase in the oil of the skin at other ages would not be normal and may suggest an endocrine problem.

Screening Tests and Procedures
Fungal examination

To confirm the presence of a fungal infection, take fungal scrapings from scaling and vesicular lesions. Using a scalpel, collect scales from the edge of a lesion. Place them on a glass slide. Cover the scrapings with 10% to 20% KOH (potassium hydroxide) solution and a coverslip. Gently heat the slide for 20 to 30 seconds and then cool it for 10 minutes. Examine the slide with a microscope using both high and low power. If a fungal infection exists, hyphae and spores will be visible as refractile tubules and oval bodies.

To assess for tinea capitis (ringworm of the scalp), use a Wood's lamp. Darken the room and then shine the light on the suspected area. Tinea capitis will fluoresce a characteristic bright blue-green. Tinea versicolor fluoresces a golden yellow.

examination *step-by-step*

Skin
1. Perform an overall inspection of the entire body.
2. Inspect each area of the body for:
   a. Color
   b. Symmetry
   c. Uniformity
   d. Thickness
   e. Pigmentation
   f. Lesions
3. Palpate the skin in each area of the body for:
   a. Moisture (dry, sweaty, oily, scaly)
   b. Temperature
   c. Thickness
   d. Mobility/turgor
4. Inspect and palpate lesions for:
   a. Size
   b. Color
   c. Surface texture (flat, raised, indurated)
   d. Pattern
   e. Location and distribution
   f. Exudates

Hair
1. Inspect the hair for the following:
   a. Quantity
   b. Distribution
   c. Pattern of loss
   d. Color
2. Palpate the hair for texture.

Nails
1. Inspect the nails for:
   a. Angle
   b. Contour
   c. Color
   d. Ridges
   e. Symmetry
   f. Cleanliness
2. Palpate the nail plate for:
   a. Texture
   b. Consistency
   c. Thickness
   d. Adherence to the nail bed

■ VARIATIONS FROM HEALTH

The particular manifestations of the many skin problems that you may find in practice are too numerous to discuss here. This section presents a few examples of skin problems commonly seen in practice. For more specific details, consult a textbook on dermatology.

Tables 10.6 and 10.7 provide an overview of common skin lesions. Figures 10.17 through 10.43 illustrate common skin lesions and common problems of the hair and nails.

Text continued on p. 227

table 10.6 *Common Lesions of the Skin*

Condition	Lesion	Location
Actinic keratosis	Macule; scaling; red	Areas exposed to sunlight; scalp; ears
Atopic dermatitis	Dry, scaling inflammation; pruritus; excoriated lichenification; abnormally sensitive to environmental irritants	Forehead; cheeks; flexure regions; may be generalized
Contact dermatitis	Erythema; pruritus resulting from environmental irritant	Area of contact
Discoid lupus erythematosus	Discrete with hyperkeratotic plugs; scaling; central atrophy; scarring, red	Paranasal area; eyebrows; upper midback
Eczema		
Allergic	Erythema to exudate	Scalp; nose; forehead; eyelids; neck (from shampoo or hair dye); feet (from shoes); ears (from hearing aids or glasses); hands (from rubber gloves)
Chronic hereditary	Laminated silvery scales, tiny bleeding spots if scale pulled off	Points of trauma; genitalia
Nummular	Round lesions; moist surface; crusting; excoriation	Extensor surfaces of arms and legs
Intertrigo	Moist patches or erosions; borders well demarcated; red; associated with friction; macerated	Skinfolds (warm and moist); breasts; axilla; inguinal regions; between toes; marked in obesity
Pityriasis rosea (unknown cause)	Macules; scaling, oval shape; long axis follows lines of cleavage; red	Herald patch; then generalized
Psoriasis	Early lesion discrete; deep red patches; scaling; later discrete or confluent patches; plaques; gray-white thick scale; scale may appear shiny (disorder of keratin synthesis, hereditary)	May arise in one skin area or may appear as generalized skin involvement
Rosacea	Papules; pustules; oiliness; erythema; telangiectasia may be present	Face
Seborrhea	Noninflammatory dryness and scaling "dandruff" or oiliness	Scalp; face
Seborrheic dermatitis	Inflammation; dryness; scaling (loose, flaky); oiliness; pruritus; may be crushed; eczematous	Scalp; ears; face (nasolabial fold, temples, eyelids); shoulders; navel; perianal region
Seborrheic keratosis	Early lesion—tan macule; progresses to papules, plaques; surface brown, rough	Any area; common on trunk
Scleroderma	Indurated; atrophic; shiny; skin appears tight, fastened down; hyperpigmentation or depigmentation	Generalized; tight facies; claw fingers
Systemic lupus erythematosus	Purpuric lesions; erythema; telangiectasia	Malar prominence; over joints

table 10.6 *Common Lesions of the Skin—cont'd*

Condition	Lesion	Location
VASCULAR		
Nevus flammeus (port wine stain)	Plaque; plexus of capillaries may have rough surface; red or purple	Present at birth; 50% on nuchal area
Nevus vasculosus	Capillary hemangioma; single tumor; rough surface; bright or dark red	75% in head region; appear in first or second month; most disappear by age 7
Spider nevus (arteriolar spider or spider angioma)	Small branching arteriole; red; blanches on pressure	Any area; most common on face, neck, arms, and upper trunk
Telangiectasia	Capillary dilatation; red; blanches on pressure	Lips, tongue, nose, palms, and fingers
EXTRAVASATION OF BLOOD		
Senile purpura	Ecchymoses; large areas blue-black, then green-yellow, then yellow; lesions do not blanch	Usually occurs on dorsum of hand of forearm
NEOPLASIA		
Paget's disease	Crusted dermatitis; moist verrucous surface; pruritus	Nipple and areola (manifestation of deeper intraductal malignancy)
Kaposi's sarcoma (associated with AIDS*)	Reddish brown plaques and nodules often associated with lymphedema	Most commonly seen on lower extremities
SCAR		
Striae	Linear; depressed; red-blue first, then silvery white	Abdomen, buttocks, or breasts; less often on thighs, upper arms, and back
BACTERIAL INFECTION		
Erysipelas	Acute; edematous; red; tender	Face; limbs; abdomen
Impetigo	Yellow crusts; erythematous base; rapid spreading	Facial area; may be localized or may spread
Leprosy	Macules—tan to pink; nodules—yellowish; may ulcerate; incubation about 3 years	
Scarlet fever	Confluent, diffuse, blanching dermatitis; erythematous 1–7 days after—sore throat, fever	Generalized
Syphilis (secondary)	Macules; papules; lymphadenopathy; malaise, myalgia; low-grade fever	Mucous membranes; palms; soles
Syphilitic chancre	Small, round, red macule; erodes to indurated ulcer (1–2 cm); regional lymphadenopathy	Breast, vulva; penis
TRICHOMONAL INFECTION		
Trichomoniasis	Granular vaginal mucosa; bright red; petechiae may be present; discharge "foamy"	Vagina, labia
***CANDIDA* INFECTION**		
Candida	Patch borders well demarcated; flaccid pustules; patches creamy white; erythematous base; curdlike white discharge, pruritus patches; erythema	Inguinal region, vagina; glans penis

*AIDS, Acquired immunodeficiency syndrome.

continued

table **10.6** *Common Lesions of the Skin—cont'd*

Condition	Lesion	Location
VIRAL INFECTION		
Rubella, rubeola, roseola	Macules; discrete; erythematous; fever; lymphadenopathy (rubella); Koplik's spots (rubeola); 2- to 3-week incubation (rubella); then malaise, fever	Appear on trunk first; spread peripherally
Varicella (chickenpox)	Papule; vesicle; erythematous base; first clear fluid, then turbid; crusting on fourth day; 2-week incubation; 24-hour fever; malaise	First on chest and back; then face, arms, and legs
Variola (smallpox)	Macules; erythematous; progress to umbilicated lesions; then pustules, firm, round; then crusting; 2- to 3-week incubation; 5-day prodromal; toxic myalgia; fever	More lesions on face, extremities
HIV[†] INFECTION	Variety of dermatoses (macules, papules, nodules, plaques): bacterial, fungal, parasitic, viral; worsening of psoriasis, seborrheic dermatitis; herpes simplex, herpes zoster, oral candidiasis	Anywhere on body, including all mucosal surfaces
FUNGAL INFECTION		
Tinea corporis (ringworm)	Scaling; red with pale center; vesicular border; pruritic	Face; neck; extremities
Tinea cruris	Scaling; crescentic; red-brown	Axilla; inguinal region
Tinea pedis (fungal infection of foot)	Scaling; circular; vesicular border; red; chronic hyperkeratotic	Feet
INFESTATIONS		
Pediculosis capitis	Pruritus; white concretions on hair—nits	Hair of scalp
VARIATION IN PIGMENTATION		
Café au lait spots	Patches; light tan (six or more larger than 1.5 cm indicative of neurofibromatosis)	Anywhere on skin
Freckle (ephelis)	Discrete; macule; tan to brown	Pigmenting increased in areas exposed to sun
Lentigo		
Juvenile	Discrete macule; brown	Not affected by sun exposure
Senile	Single macule; scaling; yellow-brown; may be dark brown	Exposed surfaces, forehead, cheeks, extensor surfaces of limbs
Malignant	Mottled; irregular macule; enlarging; tan-brown, black-white; may ulcerate—then red	Face; also eyelids, conjunctiva, lips, penis, axilla
Mongolian spots	Patch; irregular; dark blue or purple (chromophobe-like cell in skin)	Sacrum; present at birth; more common with darker-pigmented individuals; disappear spontaneously by age 4
Nevus	Macule; pigmented or nonpigmented; may be present at birth or arise later	
Peutz-Jeghers syndrome	Brown spots; abdominal pain	Lips; fingers; toes
DEPIGMENTATION		
Vitiligo	Circumscribed patch(es) of depigmentation	Face, neck, axillae, groins, anogenital area, eyelids, hands, and wrist
Addison's disease		
Pernicious anemia		
Thyrotoxicosis		

[†]*HIV,* Human immunodeficiency virus.

table 10.7 *Common Raised Lesions*

Condition	Lesion	Location
Acne vulgaris	Comedones; papules; pustules; cysts; scars	Face; back; shoulders; upper arms
Dermatitis herpetiformis (chronic)	Macules; papules; vesicles; excoriated vesicles; pruritus (intense); residual hyperpigmentation; hereditary	Scalp; interscapular; sacral
Leukoplakia	Plaque; thick; indurated; white	Mucous membrane; mouth; labia; vagina
Lichen planus (unknown cause)	Maculopapular lesion; deep red to purple; pruritus; hyperkeratotic	Flexor surfaces of wrists; palms; soles; ankles; abdomen; sacrum
Lichen simplex (chronic)	Plaque; dry; lichenification; hyperpigmentation	Scalp; labia
Seborrheic keratosis	Single plaque; soft lesion with rough surface; brown	Back, chest, scalp, face, backs of hands, and external surfaces of forearms
LIPID DISORDER		
Xanthelasma	Papules or plaques; yellow; lipid deposits	Eyelids
CYSTS		
Epidermoid and sebaceous cysts	Fluctuant, globular lesions	Scalp, face, back, or scrotum
Milia	Pinhead (1–2 mm) white, sebaceous cyst	Infraorbital skin; nose; chin; common in newborn
NEOPLASIA		
Acrochordon (skin tag)	Pedunculated skin tag; skin color	Neck; axilla; groin
Basal cell carcinoma	Nodular—rolled edge; tendency to ulcerate in center	Face, scalp, ears, or neck
Basal cell epithelioma	May follow actinic keratosis; papule or nodule—rolled edge; ulcer—nonhealing	Face, scalp, upper back
Squamous cell carcinoma	Nodule; indurated; ulcer—nonhealing; history of overexposure to sun, x-ray films; often opaque	Often on head (75%); hands (15%)
Dermatofibroma	Tumor; discrete; dome shaped; brown; less than 1 cm	Usually legs
Lipoma	Fatty tumor; soft	Trunk, nuchal area, arms, and thighs
Malignant melanoma	Arises from pigmented nevus; indurated; may be flat or elevated, eroded, or ulcerated	Any area of skin or mucous membrane
Neurofibroma	Pedunculated; soft; flaccid lesion; skin color black, brown, rose, white	Anywhere on skin, including palms and soles
Pigmented nevus	Single or multiple dome-shaped lesions; may be hairy; brown to black; present at birth	Anywhere on skin
VASCULAR		
Angioma (sometimes called senile angioma)	Papule; vascular; cherry red; pinhead (1–3 mm); most adults after climacteric	Usually on trunk
HYPERKERATOSIS		
Clavus (corn)	Hyperkeratosis; hard; tender; shape—inverted cone	Dorsum of toes; most common on fifth toe

continued

table 10.7 *Common Raised Lesions—cont'd*

Condition	Lesion	Location
Cutaneous horn	Horn projection of hyperkeratotic lesion	Face, arms, scalp, and dorsum of hand
WHEALS		
Dermographism	Wheal in response to scratch or pressure; (histamine easily released)	Anywhere on skin
Erythema multiforme (varied causes)	Wheal-like; round, darker, depressed center (target appearance)	Arms and legs first; then on body
Urticaria	Wheal; pale on erythematous base; pruritus; transient	Usually trunk but may appear anywhere on body
BULLAE		
Pemphigus	Bullae; flaccid, moist, fluid-filled rupture easily bleeds; erythematous base; from lack of mucopolysaccharide protein for intercellular cement	Skin—all parts of mucous membranes
FROM BACTERIAL INFECTION		
Chancroid	Vesicopustule; ulcer; ragged, undermined edges; shallow; may be multiple; red; lymphadenopathy	Genitalia—male and female
Folliculitis	Discrete perifollicular papules and pustules; erythematous	Any hairy area
Furuncle	Swelling becomes pustular; red; tender; painful	Any hairy site but most common on neck, buttocks, wrists, and ankles
FROM VIRAL INFECTION		
Herpes simplex	Vesicles; grouped; may be recurrent	Lips; anywhere on face
Herpes zoster	Tenderness, burning; pruritus; vesicles later crusting; erythematous base; hypersensitivity; localized lymphadenopathy	Pathway of a peripheral nerve, may have postherpetic neuralgia
Molluscum contagiosum	Multiple, discrete globules; waxy depression in center	Trunk
Verruca acuminata	Papillary (cauliflower-like); red; soft	Penis; vulva; perianal area
Verruca plantaris (plantar wart)	Circumscribed callus; surrounded by hyperkeratosis; black dots; tender	Plantar surface of foot or toes
Verruca vulgaris (wart)	Single or multiple; tan	Hands
FROM INFESTATION		
Pediculosis corporis (body lice)	Wheal; central hemorrhagic spot; linear excoriations; later dry, scaly pigmentation	Trunk; can be generalized
Pediculosis pubis (pubic lice)	Papules; discrete; excoriated; gray-white dots at base of hair—nits; lice may be seen at base of hairs	Genital region; lower abdomen; chest; axillae; eyebrows; eyelashes
	Gray-blue macules	May be present on abdomen; chest; axillae; eyebrows; eyelashes
Scabies	Vesicles; papules; pruritus	Skinfolds

figure**10.17** Vascular lesions. **A,** Cherry angioma. **B,** Nevus flammeus. **C,** Telangiectasias. **D,** Strawberry hemangioma. **E,** Spider angioma. *(From Habif TP: Clinical dermatology: a color guide to diagnosis and therapy, ed 3, St Louis, 1996, Mosby; courtesy American Academy of Dermatology and Institute for Dermatologic Communication, Schaumburg, Ill.)*

A

B

figure**10.18** Neoplasias. **A,** Squamous cell carcinoma.
B, Basal cell carcinoma. **C,** Kaposi's sarcoma. *(From Habif
TP:* Clinical dermatology: a color guide to diagnosis and ther-
apy, *ed 3, St Louis, 1996, Mosby.)*

C

figure**10.19** Melanocytic growths. **A,** Common typical moles: junction nevus—flat, black, and uniform; compound nevus—center is elevated. **B,** Dysplastic nevi—numerous large nevi are present. *(From Habif TP: Clinical dermatology: a color guide to diagnosis and therapy, ed 3, St Louis, 1996, Mosby.)*

figure**10.20**   Warts. **A,** Verruca vulgaris. **B,** Molluscum contagiosum. *(Courtesy American Academy of Dermatology and Institute for Dermatologic Communication and Education, Schaumburg, Ill.)*

figure**10.21**   Seborrheic keratosis.

figure**10.22**   Actinic keratosis. Early lesions are present on the forehead. A more advanced lesion with yellow scale is on the cheek. *(From Habif TP: Clinical dermatology: a color guide to diagnosis and therapy, ed 3, St Louis, 1996, Mosby.)*

figure**10.23**   Psoriasis. *(Courtesy American Academy of Dermatology and Institute for Dermatologic Communication and Education, Schaumburg, Ill.)*

figure**10.24**   Nummular eczema. *(Courtesy American Academy of Dermatology and Institute for Dermatologic Communication and Education, Schaumburg, Ill.)*

figure**10.25**   Contact dermatitis. **A,** From shampoo. **B,** From shoes. **C,** From application of Lanacaine. *(A and B courtesy American Academy of Dermatology and Institute for Dermatologic Communication and Education, Schaumburg, Ill.; C from Cohen BA:* Atlas of pediatric dermatology, *London, 1993, Mosby-Wolfe.)*

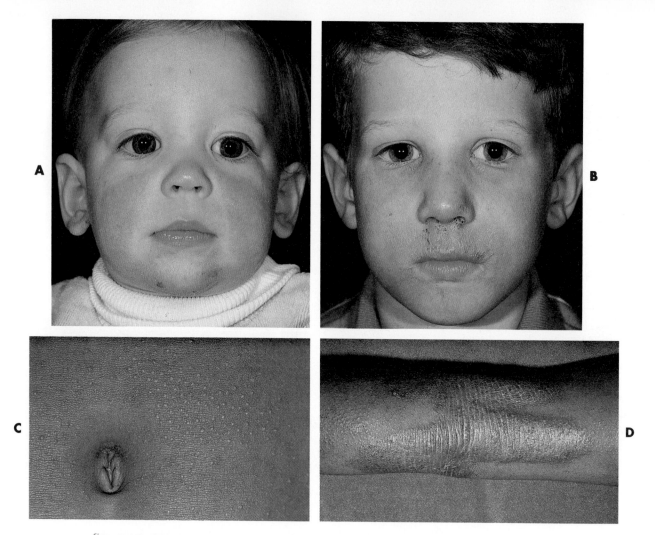

figure**10.26** Atopic dermatitis. **A** and **B,** In light-skinned children. **C,** Follicular hyperkeratosis on the abdomen in a dark-skinned client. **D,** Lichenification of the popliteal fossa from chronic rubbing of the skin in a dark-skinned client. *(A and B from Habif TP:* Clinical dermatology: a color guide to diagnosis and therapy, *ed 3, St Louis, 1996, Mosby; C and D from Weston WL, Lane AT, Morelli JG:* Color textbook of pediatric dermatology, *ed 2, St Louis, 1996, Mosby.)*

figure**10.27** Seborrheic dermatitis. **A** and **B,** In light-skinned clients. **C,** In a dark-skinned client. *(A and B courtesy American Academy of Dermatology and Institute for Dermatologic Communication and Education, Schaumburg, Ill.; C from Cohen BA:* Atlas of pediatric dermatology, *London, 1993, Mosby-Wolfe.)*

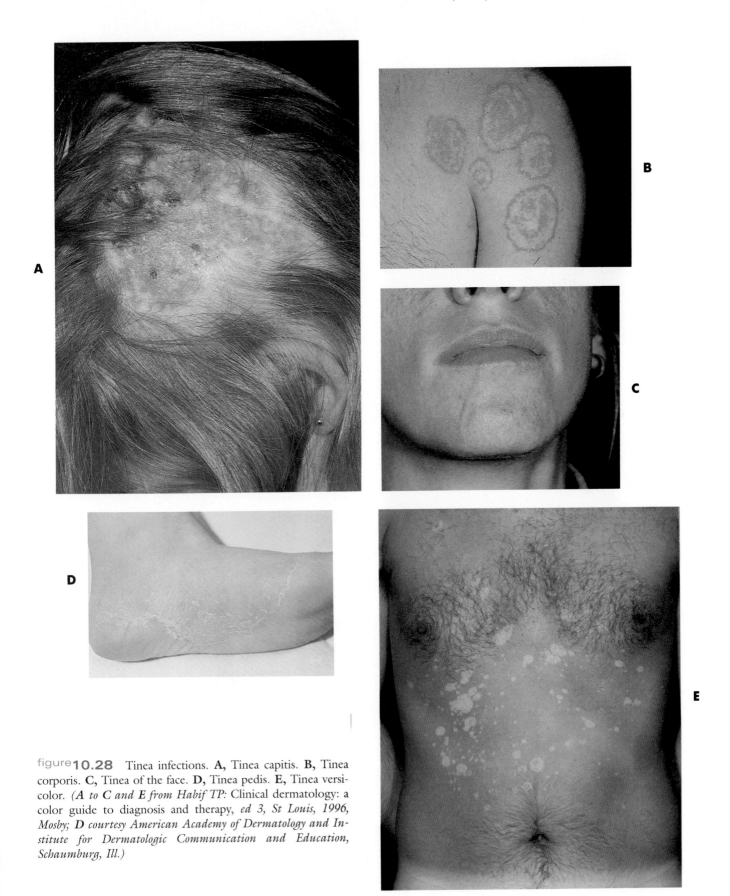

figure**10.28** Tinea infections. **A,** Tinea capitis. **B,** Tinea corporis. **C,** Tinea of the face. **D,** Tinea pedis. **E,** Tinea versicolor. *(A to C and E from Habif TP: Clinical dermatology: a color guide to diagnosis and therapy,* ed 3, St Louis, 1996, *Mosby;* **D** *courtesy American Academy of Dermatology and Institute for Dermatologic Communication and Education, Schaumburg, Ill.)*

figure**10.29** Candidiasis. **A,** *Candida* intertrigo. **B,** Diaper candidiasis. *(From Habif TP: Clinical dermatology: a color guide to diagnosis and therapy, ed 3, St Louis, 1996, Mosby.)*

figure**10.30** Acne. **A,** Acne rosacea. **B,** Acne vulgaris. *(Courtesy American Academy of Dermatology and Institute for Dermatologic Communication and Education, Schaumburg, Ill.)*

figure**10.31** Pityriasis rosea. **A,** Large herald patch on the chest shows central clearing, mimicking tinea corporis. **B,** Oval lesions on the chest. **C,** Back of an African-American client; note the Christmas tree pattern. **D,** Small papular lesions, as well as larger scaly patches, are prominent on the abdomen and thighs. *(From Cohen BA: Atlas of pediatric dermatology, London, 1993, Mosby-Wolfe.)*

figure**10.32**   Lupus. **A,** Discoid lupus erythematosus. **B,** Systemic lupus erythematosus. *(Courtesy American Academy of Dermatology and Institute for Dermatologic Communication and Education, Schaumburg, Ill.)*

figure**10.33**   Vitiligo. *(Courtesy American Academy of Dermatology and Institute for Dermatologic Communication and Education, Schaumburg, Ill.)*

figure**10.34**   Lichen planus. *(Courtesy American Academy of Dermatology and Institute for Dermatologic Communication and Education, Schaumburg, Ill.)*

figure**10.35**   Impetigo. **A,** Impetigo contagiosa. **B** and **C,** Impetigo (bullous). *(Courtesy American Academy of Dermatology and Institute for Dermatologic Communication and Education, Schaumburg, Ill.)*

figure**10.36**   Scars. **A,** Scar on the knee. **B,** Scar from a second-degree burn on the leg.

A

B

A

B

figure **10.40** Infestations. **A,** Lice. **B,** Scabies. *(From Habif TP: Clinical dermatology: a color guide to diagnosis and therapy, ed 3, St Louis, 1996, Mosby.)*

figure **10.41** Hair disorders. **A,** Alopecia areata. **B,** Trichotillomania. **C,** Folliculitis. **D,** Hirsutism. *(A and C courtesy American Academy of Dermatology and Institute for Dermatologic Communication and Education, Schaumburg, Ill.; B and D from Habif TP: Clinical dermatology: a color guide to diagnosis and therapy, ed 3, St Louis, 1996, Mosby.)*

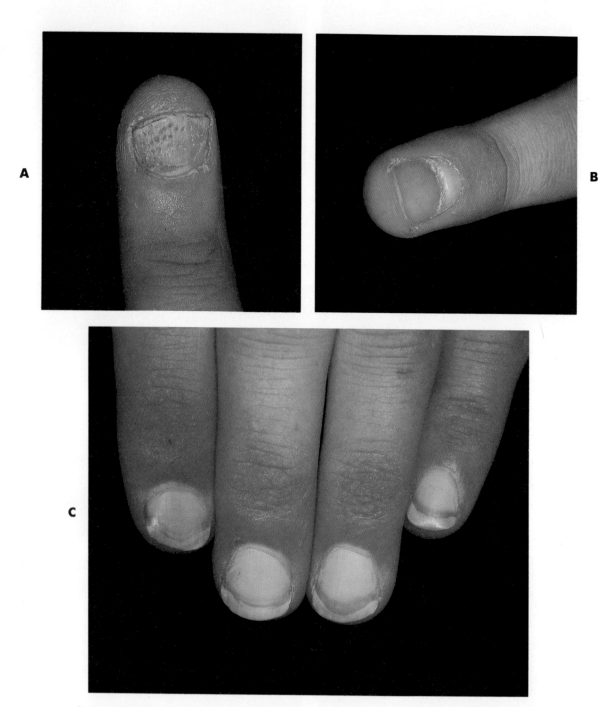

figure**10.42**   Nail changes associated with systemic disease. **A,** Psoriasis. Pitting is the most common change found in psoriasis. **B,** Beau's nails. A transverse depression of the nails occurs several weeks after certain illnesses. **C,** Terry's nails. The nail bed is white with only a narrow area of pink at the distal end. Findings are associated with cirrhosis, congestive heart failure, diabetes mellitus, and aging. *(From Habif TP:* Clinical dermatology: a color guide to diagnosis and therapy, *ed 3, St Louis, 1996, Mosby.)*

■ TEACHING SELF-ASSESSMENT

Several professional organizations recommend teaching the client to do regular, monthly (ideally), self-examination of the skin for abnormal lesions, in addition to annual complete skin examinations by a health care provider. The U.S. Preventive Services Task Force finds no evidence for or against skin self-examination. However, there is agreement that individuals at high risk for melanoma (see Risk Factors box on p. 188) can benefit from close monitoring and self-examination. In addition, organizations such as the American Academy of Dermatology and the U.S. Preventive Services Task Force (1996) recommend that individuals limit their exposure to sunlight, use sunscreen preparations (rated at least 15 SPF), and wear protective clothing when exposed to the sunlight.

Suggestions for individuals for performing self-examination include (from the National Cancer Institute):

1. Use a good light: adjust position to avoid glare.
2. Use a full-length mirror and hand-held mirrors to examine your back and other hard-to-see areas. If possible, ask a relative or close friend to help inspect areas you are unable to see.
3. Begin with your face and scalp and work your way down your body.
4. Concentrate on areas where dysplastic nevi are most common—the shoulders and back, and least common—scalp, breasts, buttocks. Make sure to check between your toes and the soles of your feet.
5. Keep a record, or take pictures, of moles, birthmarks, and other lesions. Note their location, size, and appearance.
6. Compare photographs or your information about your moles to see if there is any change in appearance.
7. Consult your health care provider promptly if you notice:
   a. Any of the ABCDs of Melanomas (see Risk Factors box on p. 188)
   b. Existing moles that have changed in other ways, such as bleeding, or development of an ulcer or nodule
   c. New moles
   d. Sores that do not heal
   e. Persistent swelling or lumps

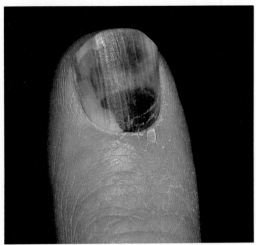

figure**10.43** Nail changes associated with injury or infection. **A,** Ingrown toenail. **B,** Subungual hematoma.

*sample***documentation&diagnoses** C R I T I C A L   T H I N K I N G

■ **FOCUSED HEALTH HISTORY** *(SUBJECTIVE DATA)*

Mr. J., a 50-year-old white male, states that 2 days ago he noticed that a mole at his back waistline had changed color (from brown to blue-black) and bled slightly yesterday. States that his waistband aggravates the mole. Is concerned about skin cancer and has monitored the mole for the past few years. Past measurement of the mole (approximately 2 months ago) was 5 mm in diameter; at that time it was round, flat, and brown. Denies any skin reactions or other lesions, as well as any pain or pruritus, any change in scalp/body hair, or excessive sun exposure. Denies any previous history of atypical moles or skin cancer and any family history of melanoma or skin cancer. States he has been in good health, with no other problems.

■ **FOCUSED PHYSICAL EXAMINATION** *(OBJECTIVE DATA)*

General appearance: Appears quite anxious about change in mole.
Skin: Fair/pink, cool, smooth; elastic turgor. Hyperpigmented macules across shoulders; 5-mm round, raised nevus at waistline—blue-black in color; excoriation with some crusting noted at edges.
Hair: Normal distribution and texture.
Nails: No clubbing, deformities, or change in color. Nail beds pink; brisk capillary refill.

diagnoses

HEALTH PROBLEM

Recent change in mole; rule out skin cancer

NURSING DIAGNOSES

Impaired skin integrity related to mechanical irritation of mole

Defining Characteristics
- Color change in mole
- Bleeding noted from mole
- Waistband rubs against mole, causing irritation

Anxiety related to potential diagnosis of cancer

Defining Characteristic
- Apprehensive with reassurance-seeking behavior

Face, Head, Neck, and Regional Lymphatics

▇ PURPOSE OF EXAMINATION

Facial expression and appearance are likely to be the first observations that a practitioner will make about a client. The initial examination of the client routinely begins with the face, head, and neck. The head and neck provide the protective casing for the special sense organs, brain, and upper spinal column. Many structures and portions of body systems are located in this region, including structures for sensation and expression; skin and hair; and components of the musculoskeletal, vascular, lymphatic, and glandular systems.

This chapter focuses on the elements and factors to be considered in assessment, including the face: appearance, expression, and landmarks; the head: bony structures, position, and scalp; and the neck: muscles, trachea, thyroid gland, and cervical vertebrae. The beginning practitioner will gradually learn to incorporate all of these components into the examination.

For assessment of other structures of the face, head, and neck, see Chapters 10, 12, 13, and 19.

▇ ANATOMY AND PHYSIOLOGY

Face

As an individual grows and develops from infancy throughout mature adulthood, the facial appearance changes. The distribution of underlying fat undergoes modification, nasal cartilage enlarges, and the features become more pronounced.

The external portions of the special sense organs of the face and head are generally symmetrical. These include the eyes, nose, mouth, and ears. The palpebral fissures and the nasolabial folds are also symmetrical. The palpebral fissures are the openings between the margins of the upper and lower eyelids. The nasolabial folds are the creases in the skin extending from the angle of the nose to the corner of the mouth (Figure 11.1).

Two cranial nerves mediate the sensation and motion of the face: the trigeminal nerve and the facial nerve. The trigeminal nerve, cranial nerve (CN) V, carries sensation of the face (Figure 11.2). The trigeminal nerve has three sensory branches: ophthalmic, maxillary, and

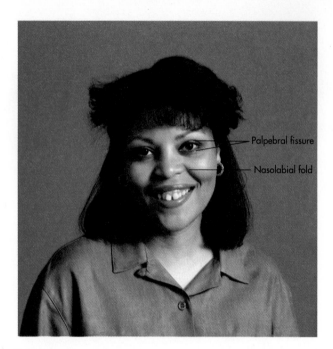

figure**11.1** Palpebral fissures and nasolabial folds.

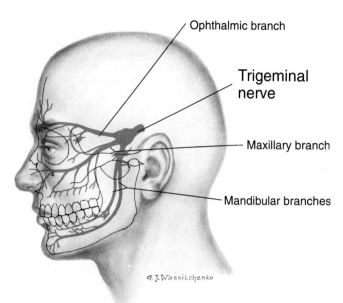

figure**11.2** Trigeminal nerve with innervation to the face by ophthalmic, maxillary, and mandibular branches. *(From Rudy EB: Advanced neurological and neurosurgical nursing, St Louis, 1984, Mosby.)*

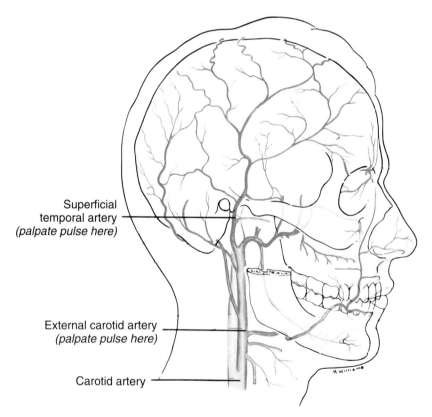

figure**11.3** Temporal artery. *(Modified from Francis CC, Martin AH: Introduction to human anatomy, ed 7, St Louis, 1975, Mosby.)*

mandibular. The facial nerve, CN VII, innervates the muscles of facial expression.

The artery accessible to examination on the face is the temporal artery, which runs anterior to the ear over the temporal bone and onto the forehead (Figure 11.3).

Head

The skull protects the sensitive structures of the brain. In infancy the cranial bones that compose the skull are soft and separated along suture lines, but by adulthood they have become fused along these suture lines (Figure 11.4). These cranial bones are made up of the following:

Frontal
Parietal
Temporal
Occipital

The facial bones give the face its contours, allow jaw mobility, and offer protection for the special sense organs. The fused bones of the face include the following:

Frontal
Nasal
Zygomatic
Lacrimal
Sphenoid
Maxilla

The mandible, or lower jaw bone, is not fused. It is connected to the temporal bone of the skull at the temporomandibular joint.

When you examine the head and face, use the bones as landmarks to identify the regions of the head and their overlying structures.

Neck

The following components are the major structures of the neck:

Sternocleidomastoid and trapezius muscles
Trachea
Thyroid gland
Carotid arteries and jugular veins (see Chapter 16: Cardiovascular System)
Cervical lymph nodes
Cervical vertebrae

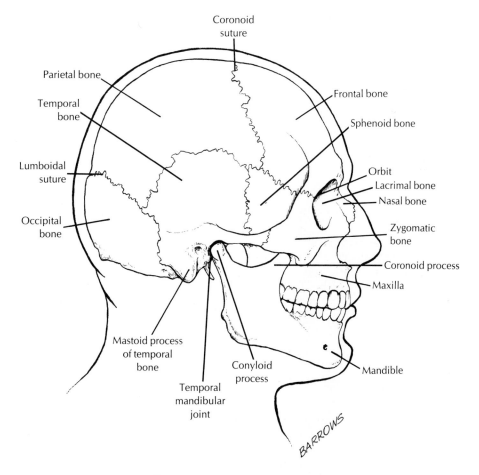

figure**11.4**   Bones of the skull.

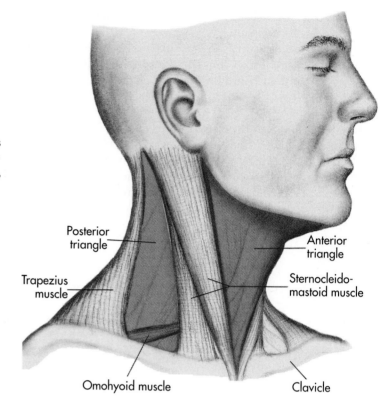

figure**11.5**   Sternocleidomastoid and trapezius muscles. Anterior and posterior triangles. *(From Seidel HM et al:* Mosby's guide to physical examination, *ed 3, St Louis, 1995, Mosby.)*

Posterior triangle

Trapezius muscle

Omohyoid muscle

Anterior triangle

Sternocleido-mastoid muscle

Clavicle

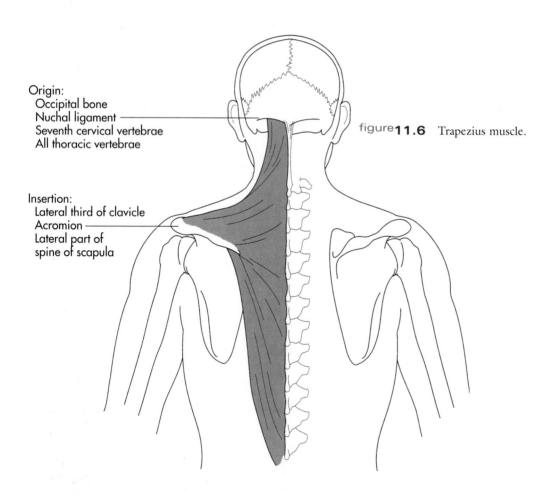

Origin:
  Occipital bone
  Nuchal ligament
  Seventh cervical vertebrae
  All thoracic vertebrae

Insertion:
  Lateral third of clavicle
  Acromion
  Lateral part of spine of scapula

figure**11.6**   Trapezius muscle.

Neck muscles

The two major muscles of the neck are the sternocleidomastoid muscle and the trapezius muscle (Figures 11.5 and 11.6). These symmetrical muscles provide support and allow movement of the neck, enabling it to flex, extend, rotate, and turn laterally. They are innervated by the spinal accessory nerve, CN XI. Both sets of muscles and their position in relation to adjacent bones form triangles that are used to describe anatomical landmarks and physical findings. Each sternocleidomastoid muscle extends from the upper sternum and the proximal portion of the clavical to the mastoid process of the temporal bone behind the ear. This pair of muscles provides for turning and lateral flexion of the head.

The trapezius muscles (Figure 11.6) are large, flat, and triangular. Each one extends from the cervical and thoracic vertebrae and from the spine of the scapula to the occipital bone of the skull. The trapezius muscles are involved in the movements of shrugging the shoulders, pulling the scapulae downward and toward the vertebral column, rotating the head to the side, and extending the head backward.

For the purpose of describing findings, each side of the neck can be divided into two triangles called the anterior and posterior triangles (Figure 11.5). Forming the anterior triangle are the edge of the mandible (superiorly), the sternocleidomastoid muscle (laterally), and the midline of the trachea (medially). Composing the posterior triangle are the sternocleidomastoid muscle (laterally), the trapezius muscle (posteriorly), and the clavicle (inferiorly).

Within the anterior triangle are the anterior cervical lymph nodes, the carotid artery, and the internal jugular vein. Several groups of lymph nodes lie within the posterior triangle.

Midline neck structures

As shown in Figure 11.7, the anterior midline neck structures include the following:
Hyoid bone
Thyroid cartilage
Cricoid cartilage
Tracheal rings
Isthmus of the thyroid gland
The hyoid bone lies just below the mandible at the angle of the floor of the mouth. The thyroid cartilage is shaped like a shield, with a notch at the upper edge that marks the level of bifurcation, or division, of the common carotid artery into the internal and external carotid arteries. The thyroid is the largest of the cartilaginous

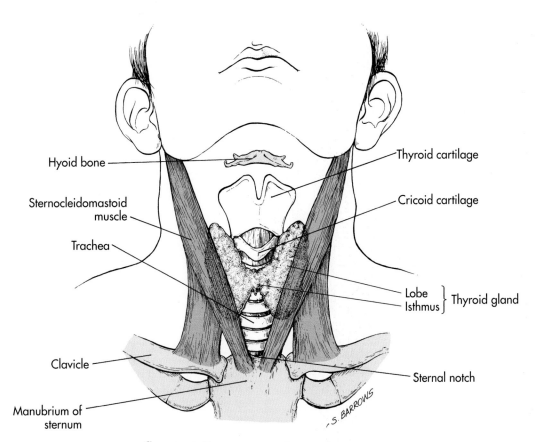

Hyoid bone
Sternocleidomastoid muscle
Trachea
Clavicle
Manubrium of sternum

Thyroid cartilage
Cricoid cartilage
Lobe
Isthmus } Thyroid gland
Sternal notch

S. BARROWS

figure**11.7** Anterior midline neck structures.

structures of the neck. The cricoid cartilage, the uppermost ring of the trachea, lies just below the thyroid cartilage. The isthmus of the thyroid gland is found across the trachea and below the cricoid cartilage. The cartilaginous trachea is located below the cricoid cartilage. It continues to the lungs, where it divides into two bronchi.

Thyroid gland

The thyroid gland (Figures 11.7 and 11.8) is the largest endocrine gland in the body and the only one that is accessible to direct physical examination. It is butterfly shaped with a lobe on each side of the trachea. A connecting isthmus joins the lower part of the lobes just below the cricoid cartilage. The lobes curve posteriorly and are largely covered by the sternocleidomastoid muscles. Each lobe, which is somewhat irregular and cone shaped, is approximately 5 cm long, 3 cm in diameter, and 2 cm thick. The normal consistency of the thyroid can be described as "meaty" or "rubbery." The thyroid arteries supply the highly vascular thyroid tissue.

The thyroid gland produces two hormones: thyroxine (T_4) and triiodothyronine (T_3). The functions of these hormones are essential for normal physical growth and development in infancy and childhood and for the maintenance of metabolic stability throughout life. These hormones influence the concentration and activity of numerous enzymes and the metabolism of substrates, vitamins, and minerals. They also affect the secretion and degradation rates of all other hormones and their target tissue responses. Thus thyroid hormones affect virtually all the tissues and organ systems of the body. It is important to note that changes due to altered thyroid function can occur in other body systems even when there is no change in the thyroid gland that is detectable on physical examination. Thyroid tissue may enlarge retrosternally or in areas that are not accessible to palpation. If a thyroid disorder is suspected, clinical assessment must include other body systems, such as the cardiovascular, gastrointestinal, integumentary, and neurological systems.

Lymph Nodes

In this text, examination of the lymphatic system is described by body region; therefore the system is described in this chapter and also in the chapters on assessment of the ears, nose, and throat (Chapter 13); breasts (Chapter 14); and genitalia (Chapters 20 and 21). Since this text follows a head-to-foot examination format, the first lymph nodes to be examined are those in the head and neck. General material about the lymphatic system is included in this chapter.

The lymphatic system consists of a network through-

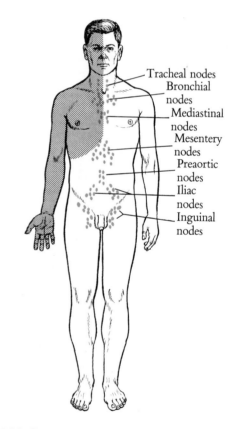

figure **11.9** Lymphatic drainage pathways. Shaded area of the body is drained via the right lymphatic duct, which is formed by the union of three vessels: right jugular trunk, right subclavian trunk, and right bronchomediastinal trunk. Lymph from the remainder of the body enters the venous system by way of the thoracic duct. (*From Seidel HM et al: Mosby's guide to physical examination, ed 3, St Louis, 1995, Mosby; modified from Francis CC, Martin AH: Introduction to human anatomy, ed 7, St Louis, 1975, Mosby.*)

figure **11.8** Thyroid gland. (*From Thompson JM et al: Mosby's clinical nursing, ed 4, St Louis, 1997, Mosby.*)

out the body, including lymph fluid, collecting ducts, lymph nodes, the spleen, the thymus, the tonsils, the adenoids, and small amounts of lymph tissue found in other places in the body, such as the bone marrow, the appendix, and Peyer's patches in the intestinal wall. The lymphatic system is a complete circulatory system distinct from, but closely linked to, the blood circulatory system. The fluid and proteins that compose the lymphatic fluid move from the vascular system into the interstitial spaces. Here they are collected by microscopic lymphatic tubules that return the fluid to the cardiovascular system. Lymphatic vessels originate as microscopic, open-ended tubules that merge to form large collecting ducts. Lymph nodes are small oval clumps of lymphatic tissue occurring in groups along the lymph vessels. Superficial lymph nodes lie in the subcutaneous connective tissues; the deeper nodes are beneath the muscular fascia or in various body cavities. Some nodes have a diameter of 0.5 cm, but most are smaller. The lymphatic ducts merge into two main trunks that drain into the venous system at the subclavian veins. The right lymphatic duct receives the lymphatic fluid from the right side of the head and neck, the right arm, and the right side of the chest wall. It drains into the right subclavian vein. The thoracic duct drains the rest of the body and empties into the left subclavian vein (Figure 11.9)

The lymphatic system has no pumping device of its own. Its movement is much slower than that of the blood circulatory system. Factors affecting the movement of lymph include arterial pulsation; compression of lymphatic vessels by contracting skeletal muscles; and contraction of the smooth muscles in the walls of the lymphatic vessels, lymph nodes, and collecting ducts. Mechanical obstruction slows or stops the movement of lymph, causing the nodes to dilate.

A primary purpose of the lymphatic system is to protect the body from infection by providing immunity against foreign substances. The lymphatic system functions to:

1. Filter and engulf bacteria, certain other cells, foreign particles, or toxins in the lymph nodes, thus providing defensive immunity against microorganisms and abnormal cells
2. Return fluid, proteins, and electrolytes from tissue space to the blood
3. Absorb fat and fat-soluble substances from the intestinal tract
4. Produce lymphocytes in the lymph nodes, tonsils, adenoids, spleen, and bone marrow
5. Produce antibodies

The lymphatic system is also a pathway for the spread of malignancy.

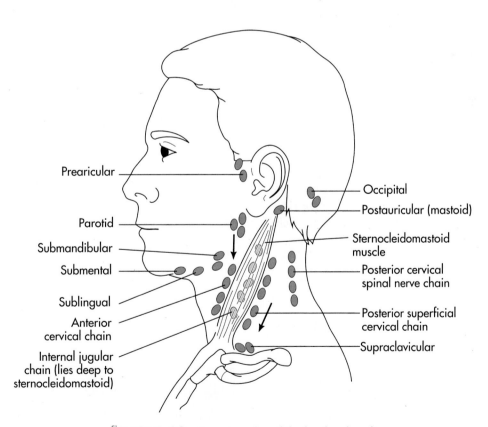

figure**11.10** Lymph nodes of the head and neck.

Lymph nodes of the head and neck

The head and neck are richly supplied with lymph node groups (Figure 11.10). Some of the groups are known by several names. The following is one commonly used system of terms:

Lymph nodes of the head

Occipital—at the base of the skull

Postauricular (mastoid)—behind the ear, slightly anterior to the mastoid process

Preauricular—in front of the ear

Parotid—near the angle of the jaw

Submandibular (submaxillary)—midway between the angle of the jaw and the tip of the mandible

Sublingual—near the midline, beneath the tongue

Submental—in the midline posterior to the tip of the mandible.

Lymph nodes of the neck—lie in the anterior or posterior triangle or under the sternocleidomastoid muscle

Anterior cervical chain—over and anterior to the sternocleidomastoid muscle, in the anterior triangle

Internal jugular chain—behind and largely covered by the sternocleidomastoid muscle

Posterior cervical spinal nerve chain—near the cervical vertebrae (located in the posterior area of the neck)

Posterior superficial cervical chain—along the anterior edge of the trapezius, in the posterior triangle

Supraclavicular—just above the clavicle in the angle formed by the clavicle and sternocleidomastoid muscle.

■ EXAMINATION

Health History
General considerations, lifestyle, and health history

1. Home living environment: Includes potential risks for injury, such as use of handrails, presence of electrical cords, loose rugs
2. Employment: Risk of head injury; use of helmet, protective eye shields; exposure to toxins or chemicals
3. Participation in activities with potential for risk of injury, such as active sports
4. Stress, tension, demands at home, work, or school
5. Nutrition: Eating habits, food intolerances, recent weight gain or loss
6. Use of alcohol or drugs
7. Medications: Analgesics, anticonvulsants, cardiac preparations, thyroid preparations, oral contraceptives

8. History of trauma, injury, surgery, tumor, seizure disorder, radiation to the head, neck, or upper chest

Headache

1. Type or types of headache and extent of time over which they have been occurring
2. Onset: Time of day or night; gradual or abrupt
3. Duration: Minutes, hours, days, weeks
4. Frequency and timing: Occasional, clustering, headache-free periods
5. Location: Entire head, unilateral, one spot, sinus region, behind eyes, "hatband" distribution, neck
6. Character of pain: (a) Throbbing, pounding, boring, shocklike, dull, sharp, nagging, constant, intermittent; (b) effect of motion; (c) change in level of consciousness as pain increases
7. Severity: Same or different with each event. (A graded scale of 1 to 5 or 1 to 10 may be useful in assessing this factor.)
8. Visual prodromal event(s): Scotoma (a defect of vision in a defined area); hemianopia; distortion of size, shape, or location of objects
9. Pattern: Description of headache over course of day, worse or better as day progresses, occurrence during sleep
10. Associated symptoms: Gastrointestinal symptoms, such as nausea, vomiting, diarrhea; visual disturbances, such as photophobia (abnormal sensitivity to light); increased tearing; difficulty falling asleep; nasal discharge; tinnitus; paresthesias; impaired mobility
11. Precipitating factors: Fever, fatigue, stress, food or food additives, fasting, alcohol, seasonal allergies, menstrual cycle, intercourse, oral contraceptives, feelings of anxiety or depression (Inquire about client's activities during 24 hours preceding onset.)
12. Efforts to treat: Medication(s), including analgesics, vasodilators, bronchodilators, oral contraceptives, and stimulants such as caffeine; sleep; meditation; other approaches
13. Family history of headaches
14. Diet: Includes sensitivity to chemicals in food and beverages; alcohol intake
15. Lifestyle: Includes use of tobacco; allergies

A sample headache record, such as the one shown in Table 11.1, is useful in helping the client record the pattern of headaches for a certain amount of time. The record helps to assess the type of headaches that the client is experiencing.

RISK FACTORS	HEADACHE
Exposure to stressful conditions and situations	

table 11.1 *Sample Headache Record*							
Date	Time of onset	Duration	Location	Severity 1 = mild 10 = severe	Efforts to relieve	Results	Possible precipitating factors

Head injury

1. History of traumatic event: State of consciousness, duration of unconsciousness, behaviors after event, other sequelae (It may be useful to have an observer's description of the event in addition to the client's account.)
2. Predisposing factors: Visual changes, light-headedness, fainting, seizure disorder
3. Associated symptoms: Blurred or double vision, change in level of consciousness, change in breathing pattern, discharge from nose or ears, gastrointestinal symptoms, head or neck pain, laceration, local tenderness

Neck pain

1. History of neck injury or strain, head injury, swelling of neck, surgery
2. Duration of symptoms
3. History of bacterial or viral infection or other illnesses

RISK FACTORS   HEAD INJURY

Exposure to potentially traumatic situations in the home, at work, while traveling, or while participating in high-risk sports. If indicated, counsel client on measures to reduce the risk of injury from these sources.

4. Character: Effect of movement on pain; limitation of motion; point of maximum pain; character of pain: burning, cramping, dull, sharp, throbbing; point of origin and radiation patterns to shoulders, arms, and back
5. Neurological symptoms: Clumsiness, numbness, weakness, bowel or bladder dysfunction
6. Emotional stress
7. Efforts to treat and effectiveness of treatment: Heat, cold, medication, movement

Thyroid function

1. History of thyroid dysfunction, radiation, or surgery
2. Change in temperature preference: Altered sensitivity to heat or cold; wearing more or less clothing
3. Swelling in neck; interference with swallowing; redness; pain with touch, swallowing, or hyperextension of neck
4. Change in texture of hair, skin, or nails; increased pigmentation of skin at pressure points
5. Change in emotional stability: Alteration in usual energy level; irritability, nervousness, lethargy, disinterest

RISK FACTORS   THYROID DISEASE

Exposure to upper body radiation

6. Increased prominence of eyes, puffiness in periorbital area, blurred or double vision
7. Cardiorespiratory changes: Dyspnea on exertion, tachycardia, palpitations, cardiac irregularity
8. Change in menstrual pattern
9. Change in appetite, bowel habits, thirst, or frequency of urination; weight loss
10. Family history of thyroid disorders

Lymph nodes

Present health status. First obtain client's own description of her or his health status, including any health problems.

1. Enlarged nodes (client may describe as lumps, bumps, kernels, or swollen glands)
   a. Characteristics: Location, onset, duration, number, consistency, tenderness
   b. Associated symptoms: Pain, fever, redness, warmth, red streaks, itching, ulceration, bleeding (note site and character), fatigue, weakness, weight gain or loss
   c. Predisposing factors: Infection, surgery, trauma
2. Swelling
   a. Location
   b. Unilateral or bilateral, intermittent or constant, pitting or nonpitting, variations during the day, duration
   c. Predisposing factors: Cardiac or renal disorder, surgery, infection, trauma, venous insufficiency
   d. Associated symptoms: Warmth, redness or discoloration, ulceration, fatigue, weakness, weight gain or loss
   e. Treatment efforts and effect: Support stocking, elevation
3. Medications
   Past health history
1. Hodgkin's or other lymphoma
2. Other cancer
3. Chronic illness: Cardiac, renal, tuberculosis, HIV infection

4. Medications, including antibiotics and chemotherapy
5. Surgery: Purpose, time, result, residual effects, including trauma to regional lymph nodes
6. Recurrent infections, including infectious mononucleosis
7. Blood transfusions
8. Environmental exposure to radiation, toxic chemicals, infections
9. Use of intravenous drugs
10. Sexual practices
   Family health history
1. Malignancy
2. Anemia
3. Recent infections
4. Tuberculosis
5. Agammaglobulinemia
6. Hemophilia
   Other considerations
1. Environmental exposure to radiation, toxic chemicals, infection (including HIV)
2. Travel to sites of infectious outbreaks

Preparation for Examination: Client and Environment

The examination room should provide the client with privacy, and the room temperature should be comfortable for the client. The room should be well lighted and quiet.

Technique for Examination and Normal Findings
Face

The techniques of inspection and palpation are used to perform a complete examination of the face.

Inspection. To begin, observe the client's facial expression and appearance. Facial expression is frequently a guide to a person's feelings because it communicates a

---

RISK FACTORS — LYMPHATIC ENLARGEMENT

Inadequate primary defenses, such as broken skin or stasis of body fluids
Inadequate secondary defenses, such as suppressed inflammatory response
Immunosuppression
Chronic disease
Malnutrition
Risk factors for those cancers that involve the lymph nodes, such as lymphomas, breast cancer, lung cancer, and prostatic cancer

---

PREPARATION FOR EXAMINATION

EQUIPMENT

Item	Purpose
Gloves	For palpation of head and hair
Stethoscope	For auscultation of temporal artery and thyroid
Glass of water	For observation and palpation of thyroid
Ruler	To measure enlarged lymph nodes

message. However, it is important to remember that cultures vary in the degree and style of facial expression. Persons from certain cultures use pronounced facial expressions along with hand gestures and words. Those from other cultures are less expressive, particularly with strangers.

Inspect the color and condition of the facial skin and the shape and symmetry of the facial features, including the eyebrows, eyes, palpebral fissures, mouth, and nasolabial folds. The head is normally upright and still. The facial features should be symmetrical at rest and with a change of expression, although a slight degree of asymmetry is common.

Test facial muscular and neurological function by asking the client to elevate and lower eyebrows, frown, close the eyes tightly so that you cannot open them, puff the cheeks, show the teeth, and smile. This test is used to evaluate the function of the facial nerve, CN VII.

Palpation. Palpate the temporal arteries bilaterally just anterior to and slightly above the tragus of the ear (Figure 11.11). Note any thickening, hardness, or tenderness of the vessel. Use the bell of the stethoscope to auscultate the temporal artery for a bruit, which is a soft blowing sound of blood flowing through a stenosed (narrowed) vessel. A bruit is not normally present.

Palpate the temporomandibular joint. To locate this joint, place your fingertips just anterior to the tragus of the ear. Rest your fingertips over this area, and ask the client to open and close the mouth and move the joint from side to side. The temporomandibular joint should

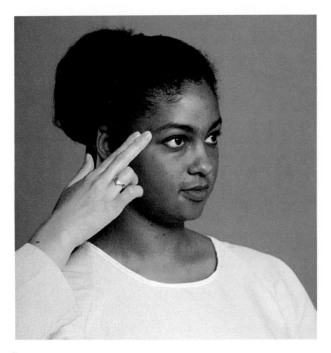

figure**11.11**   Palpation of the temporal artery.

move smoothly up and down and to the right and left. Check for swelling or crepitus.

Head

The techniques of inspection and palpation are used for examination of the head.

Inspection. Observe the head for size, shape, symmetry, position, and any unusual movements. To inspect the scalp, part the hair in several areas. Check behind the ears and along the hairline. Hair condition and styling may be useful indicators of the client's social group identification, emotional status, and personal hygiene.

Palpation. If the client wears a wig or other hairpiece, ask him or her to remove it. Using the pads of the second, third, and fourth fingers, palpate the scalp in several areas with a gentle rotary motion. The scalp should move freely over the skull. Normally, there are no depressions, swelling, or tenderness. Inspect the distribution and texture of the hair, and note the use of coloring or lubricating agents.

Neck

In a case involving traumatic neck injury, do not manipulate or examine the cervical spine. Stabilize the spine until further studies can be performed.

The techniques of inspection, palpation, and auscultation are used for examination of the structures of the neck.

Inspection. Inspect the neck for symmetry of the muscles and trachea, and for stability in normal position. Normally, no masses, muscular asymmetries, scars, discolorations, or lesions are present. The neck muscles should be symmetrical, with no masses or swelling noted. To assess muscular function, ask the client to perform range of motion by flexing the chin to the chest (Figure 11.12, *A*), turning the head in lateral rotation (Figure 11.12, *B*), and *slightly* hyperextending the neck backward (Figure 11.12 *C*). These motions should be smooth and should not cause pain or dizziness. Inspect the midline cartilages, including the thyroid and cricoid cartilages, and the tracheal rings, assessing for symmetry. The trachea should be centered and equidistant from each sternocleidomastoid muscle. Look for fullness at the base of the neck. Inspect the posterior aspect of the neck. The cervical vertebrae should be in alignment. The neck should be symmetrical, and no masses or swelling should be present.

Palpation. Test the sternocleidomastoid muscle by having the client turn the head to one side and then to the other against the resistance of your hand. Test for trapezius muscle strength by asking the client to shrug the shoulders against the resistance of your hands. If the client has pain, palpate the sternocleidomastoid for tenderness, spasm, swelling, and trigger points. When you test the strength of the neck muscles, you are also as-

A　　　　　　　　**B**　　　　　　　　**C**

figure **11.12**　**A,** Flexion of the neck. **B,** Lateral rotation of the neck. **C,** Extension of the neck.

sessing CN XI, the spinal accessory nerve. (The neurological examination of these muscles and their innervation is discussed in Chapter 19.) Gently palpate the midline cartilages. They should be smooth and nontender. Palpate the occipital area, the mastoid process, and the spinous processes of the cervical vertebrae. These should be symmetrical, without tenderness, pain, or swelling.

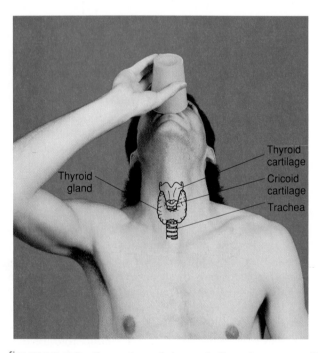

Thyroid gland

Thyroid cartilage

Cricoid cartilage

Trachea

figure **11.13**　Inspection of the neck for enlargement of the thyroid gland.

Thyroid gland. The techniques used to examine the thyroid gland include inspection, palpation, and auscultation. The thyroid is assessed for enlargement, tenderness, nodules, and bruits. The normal thyroid gland is not visible or palpable, or only slightly so. Examining the thyroid is easy if the neck is long and slender. If the neck is short or thick, or if the client has had neck surgery, examination may be difficult. Note that determination of thyroid function includes more than assessment of the neck. Since effects of thyroid activity are widespread, observations of behavior, appearance, skin, eyes, hair, and cardiovascular status are also important.

Inspection. To inspect the thyroid gland, stand in front of the client and observe the lower half of the neck—first in normal position, next in slight extension, and then while the client swallows a sip of water (Figure 11.13). The movements of the cartilages are fairly easy to observe. Note any unusual bulging of thyroid tissue in the midline, at the base of the neck, or of the lobes behind the sternocleidomastoid muscles. Normally, none is seen.

Palpation. Following inspection, palpate the neck for the presence of an enlarged thyroid, for consistency of the gland, and for any nodules. The lobes of the normal thyroid gland are generally not palpable. In a thin neck the isthmus is occasionally palpable. The thyroid is also sometimes palpable during pregnancy. In a short, stocky neck, even an enlarged gland may be difficult to palpate. Palpation may be done with the examiner standing either in front of or behind the client. Although several techniques can be used for palpation of the thyroid, the underlying principles for each technique include the following:

1. Movement of the gland while the client swallows

figure**11.14**   Palpation of the thyroid: posterior approach.

2. Adequate exposure of the gland by tilting the head to one side to relax the muscles
3. Manual displacement of surrounding structures to better expose the gland
4. Comparison of one side with the other

Since the sternocleidomastoid muscles are strong and large, it is important to relax them. The thyroid gland is fixed to the trachea and rises during swallowing. This feature distinguishes the thyroid from other neck structures. Palpate the area where the isthmus and lobes are located to determine the gland's size, consistency, degree of enlargement, presence of nodules, and surface characteristics.

POSTERIOR APPROACH. The posterior approach is easier and less awkward for the practitioner than the anterior approach. Stand behind the client, who is seated on a chair or examining table. Ask the client to lower the chin to relax the sternocleidomastoid muscles. Curve your fingers anteriorly so that your fingertips rest on the lower half of the neck over the trachea below the cricoid cartilage (Figure 11.14). Ask the client to swallow a sip of water while you palpate for any enlargement of the thyroid isthmus. Next, in order to examine each lobe separately, ask the client to lower the chin and turn the head slightly to the right. With the fingers of your left hand, gently displace the thyroid cartilage slightly to the right while you use the fingers of your right hand to palpate the area next to the midline cartilage where the thyroid lobe lies (Figure 11.15). This procedure is then repeated with the client turning the chin to the left while you palpate with the fingers of your left hand. Having the client swallow a sip of water during this procedure may be helpful.

ANTERIOR APPROACH. Stand in front of the seated client. Using the fingertips of your index and middle fingers, palpate below the cricoid cartilage for the thyroid isthmus as the client swallows a sip of water. As in the procedure used for the posterior approach, ask the client to flex the head and turn it slightly to one side and then the other. Palpate the left lobe by displacing the thyroid cartilage slightly toward that lobe with the left hand and examining the thyroid with the right hand. This area can be more deeply palpated by hooking the thumb and fingers around the sternocleidomastoid muscle (Figure 11.16). Measure palpable masses or nodules, and describe their location, tenderness, size, shape, consistency, surface characteristics, and fixation to surrounding tissue.

Auscultation. If enlargement of the gland is detected or suspected, perform auscultation over the lobes of the thyroid by using the bell of the stethoscope (Figure 11.17). Increased blood flow to the thyroid gland produces vibrations that may be heard as a soft rushing sound or bruit.

Lymph nodes

The lymphatic system is not generally accessible to examination in healthy people. When infection or ma-

figure **11.15** Posterior approach to thyroid examination. To examine the right lobe of the thyroid gland, the examiner displaces the trachea slightly to the right with the fingers of the left hand and palpates for the right thyroid lobe with the fingers of the right hand.

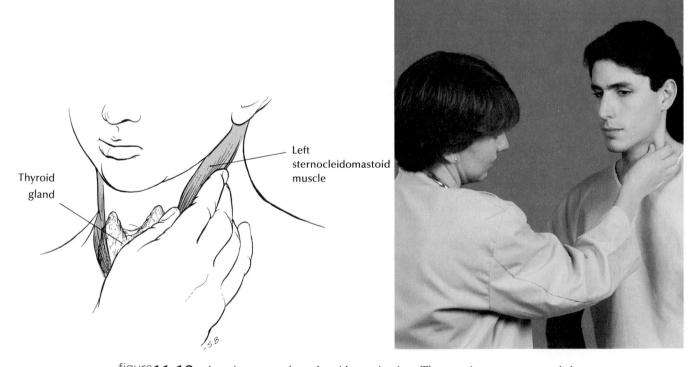

Thyroid gland

Left sternocleidomastoid muscle

figure **11.16** Anterior approach to thyroid examination. The examiner grasps around the left sternocleidomastoid muscle with the right hand to palpate for an enlarged left thyroid lobe.

figure**11.17** Auscultation over the thyroid gland.

figure**11.18** Palpation of preauricular lymph nodes.

lignancy is present, the nodes typically enlarge. Those nodes lying near the surface of the body can be palpated. Some healthy people have a few discrete (separate or distinct), movable, small, nontender nodes present. These are typically less than 1 cm in diameter. They are sometimes referred to as "shotty" nodes.

The techniques of observation and palpation are used to examine the lymph nodes.

Inspection. In the healthy client, lymph nodes are not visible. With infection or neoplasm, the areas where the nodes are located may appear swollen. Inspect the areas where the superficial lymph nodes are located, and observe any swelling, edema, skin lesions, erythema, or red streaks on the skin. Often the enlargement is subtle, so observation is based on a careful history and is carefully integrated with palpation. Observe the areas of the head and neck where lymph nodes are grouped.

Palpation. Palpate those areas of the head and neck using the pads of the second, third, and fourth fingers. Use a gentle, circular motion. Move the skin lightly over the underlying tissues rather than moving the examining fingers over the skin. Press lightly at first, increasing the pressure gradually, if needed. Heavy pressure can push the nodes into the deeper soft tissues so that their presence may be missed. You may palpate the nodes on each side of the head simultaneously. When you palpate the nodes in the neck that lie near the carotid sinus, palpate one side at a time because pressure over the carotid sinus can result in a drop in blood pressure.

To examine the lymph nodes of the head, begin node palpation at the base of the skull (occipital nodes) and move toward the areas posterior and anterior to the ear (postauricular and preauricular nodes, Figure 11.18), along the angle of the jaw (parotid nodes), then along and under the mandible (submandibular, sublingual, and submental nodes).

When examining the neck nodes, ask the client to bend her or his head slightly downward (Figure 11.19). This position reduces muscle tension and enhances accurate palpation. Palpate the node chains superficially and then more deeply in the soft tissues of the anterior triangle (anterior cervical chain, Figure 11.18) and posterior triangle (posterior superficial cervical chain). The internal jugular chain is difficult to examine, particularly if pressed too heavily. Probe gently with your thumb and fingers around the sternocleidomastoid muscle (Figure 11.20).

To examine the supraclavicular nodes, palpate into the soft tissue just above the clavicle (Figure 11.21 *A*). As with the other neck nodes, it is helpful to ask the client to bend his or her head slightly downward (Figure 11.21, *B*).

If any nodes are detected, describe them according to:
1. Location
2. Size
3. Shape
4. Number of nodes
5. Surface characteristics

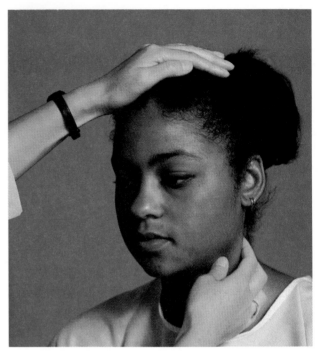

figure**11.19**   Palpation of anterior cervical lymph nodes.

figure**11.20**   Palpation of deep cervical lymph nodes.

A

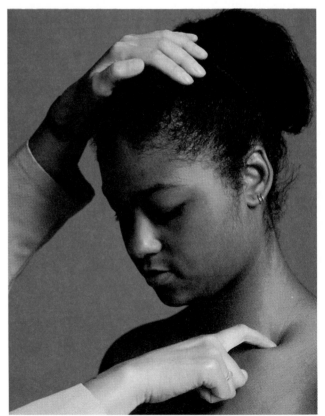

B

figure**11.21**   Palpation of the supraclavicular lymph nodes.

Terms Used to Describe the Characteristics of Enlarged Lymph Nodes

Location: Use imaginary body lines, such as the midclavicular line; bony prominences, such as the mandible; or muscles, such as the sternocleidomastoid, to describe specific location.

Size: Measure in cm.

Shape: Usually oval.

Surface characteristics: Smooth, nodular, irregular, singular or matted (in groups).

Consistency: Soft, firm, hard, rubbery, spongy, cystic.

Mobility/fixation: Describe whether node moves freely or is attached to adjacent structure or underlying tissue.

Tenderness: Describe whether node is painful without palpation and/or tender with palpation.

Signs of inflammation: Erythema, increased warmth.

6. Consistency
7. Tenderness
8. Mobility or fixation to surrounding tissues
9. Discreteness or matting—whether the nodes are palpated as separate from or connected to each other
10. Signs of inflammation

Nodes enlarged because of infection are likely to be tender and matted. Nodes enlarged because of a malignancy are likely to be hard, discrete, asymmetrical, and not tender. When you find enlarged lymph nodes, explore the areas drained by those nodes for signs of infection or malignancy.

HELPFUL HINT *The groups of lymph nodes are not always as distinctive as the drawings indicate. If you are not certain which group you are palpating, describe them by location as precisely as possible. (See box below for terms commonly used to describe some of the characteristics of enlarged nodes.)*

HELPFUL HINT *Whenever a lesion is present, look for involvement of the regional lymph nodes that drain it. Whenever a node is enlarged or tender, look for a source of infection or neoplastic growth in the area that it drains.*

---

table 11.2	Some Tests Used to Determine Altered Thyroid Function	
Test	**Comments**
TSH—thyroid stimulating hormone	Elevated with hypothyroidism
	Lowered with hyperthyroidism
Total serum T$_4$	Elevated with hyperthyroidism
	Lowered with hypothyroidism
Thyroid scan	Evaluates functional status of nodular goiter
Ultrasonography	Evaluates status of single nodules

Screening Tests and Procedures

Listed in Table 11.2 are common laboratory tests used to help evaluate the client who has signs and symptoms of thyroid dysfunction. Since values may differ among laboratories, the normal value range for the specific laboratory that provides the results needs to be determined.

---

examination step-by-step

Make sure that the examination room has good lighting, a comfortable temperature, and privacy for the client. Have the necessary equipment—a stethoscope, glass of water, ruler, and gloves—ready.

Inspection
1. Face: Appearance, expression, symmetry of structure and features, skin color, movements
2. Head: Size, shape, symmetry, condition of skin, hair (distribution, texture, quantity), and scalp (deformities, lesions), unusual movements
3. Neck: Symmetry, mobility, range of motion, neck vessels

Palpation
1. Head: Scalp (tenderness, deformities, lesions), hair (if indicated), temporal artery pulses, temporomandibular joint, lymph nodes
2. Neck: Anterior midline neck structures, thyroid gland, carotid artery pulses, lymph nodes, muscle strength, cervical vertebrae

Auscultation
1. Neck: Carotid arteries and thyroid gland for bruits

■ VARIATIONS FROM HEALTH

Face

Changes in coloration

1. Cyanosis: Occurs with poor circulation to local structures or when the amount of unsaturated hemoglobin in the body tissues is increased, as may occur with cardiac or pulmonary disease. Lips, nose, cheeks, ears, and oral mucosa may become bluish.
2. Pallor: Results from decreased vascular supply, as in shock.
3. Jaundice: Results from decreased liver function or obstruction and increased bilirubin deposits in the skin. Before the yellow color of jaundice is evident in the skin, it may be observed in the sclera of the eyes and mucous membranes of the mouth.
4. Lupus erythematosus: An erythematous discoloration in a butterfly pattern bridges the cheeks and nose.
5. Other: Localized color changes from acne, moles, or scar tissue.

Changes in shape

1. Edema: Excess accumulation of fluid in the tissues may result from cardiovascular or renal disease. Often initially evident in the eyelids, where it is called periorbital edema, this condition can involve the entire face.
2. Protrusion of eyeballs (exophthalmos) and elevation of upper lids: Result of hyperthyroidism; gives face a staring or startled expression.
3. Puffiness with dry skin and coarse features: Result of hypothyroidism; called myxedema facies.
4. Face rounded, cheeks red: Result of increased adrenal hormone production (Cushing's syndrome) or secondary to intake of synthetic adrenal hormones; called moon facies.
5. Face sunken, skin rough and dry: Prolonged illness, dehydration, or starvation may produce this cachectic face. Eyes, cheeks, and temples appear sunken, and nose appears sharp.

Changes in symmetry

1. Asymmetry, abnormal movements, or both, may result from facial nerve lesions or from central nervous system lesion, such as results from a cardiovascular accident.
2. Paralysis of CN VII, or Bell's palsy, causes changes on affected side; eyelid does not close completely, lower eyelid and corner of mouth droop, and nasolabial fold disappears.

Changes in hair distribution

1. For women in some ethnic groups, increased facial hair, often above the upper lip, is a normal finding.
2. Excessive hair growth in moustache, sideburn, and chin areas results from elevated production of adrenal hormones.
3. Thinning of scalp hair and eyebrows is a result of increased thyroid activity.

Pain

1. Trigeminal neuralgia (tic douloureux). This neurological abnormality is caused by degeneration of or pressure on one or all of the three divisions of the trigeminal nerve, CN V (see Figure 11.2 for distribution pattern of this nerve):
   • Ophthalmic (first division)—pain around eyes and over forehead
   • Maxillary (second division)—pain in nose, cheek, and upper lip
   • Mandibular (third division)—pain in lower lip and side of tongue
   The pain is aching, burning, flashing, or stablike, and attacks cause the person to wince with facial contractions. Pain attacks may occur spontaneously or may be evoked by pressure on a trigger zone, cold air, a light touch, biting, swallowing, chewing, laughing, talking, yawning, or sneezing. The pain may last from a few seconds to a few minutes. Cycles of pain and abatement may continue for hours. Trigeminal neuralgia affects persons in middle to late adulthood.
2. Herpes zoster may affect any sensory nerve, but the virus typically tends to invade the posterior root ganglia associated with the thoracic and trigeminal nerves. The pain may be constant or intermittent, superficial or deep.
3. Sinus tenderness results from inflammation of one or more of the paranasal sinuses. The client may experience pressure and pain in the area of the sinuses, headache, fever, and local tenderness to palpation.
4. Temporomandibular joint pain dysfunction syndrome is an abnormal condition marked by painful jaw movement and mandibular dysfunction. The joint may snap, lock, or "pop." The pain may be referred to other points on the face and neck.

Head

Changes in size

1. Abnormally large head in children: Caused by accumulation of fluid in the ventricles of the brain (hydrocephalus).
2. Large head in adults: Results from osteitis deformans (Paget's disease) or acromegaly, which causes an increase in thickness of the skull, lengthening of the mandible, prominence of the nose and forehead, and coarsening of the facial features.

table 11.3 *Characteristics of Primary Headaches*

	Muscle contraction or tension headaches	Migraine headaches	Cluster headaches
Age at onset	Adolescence through adulthood	Childhood, adolescence, or young adulthood	Young to middle adulthood
Sex distribution	Occur more frequent in females	Occur more frequently in females	Occur more frequently in males
Typical onset	Gradual, often following stress	Begins as dull ache, progresses to intense pain, occurs anytime during day, may have aura of warning symptoms	Sudden; reaches peak intensity in several minutes; often occurs during evening or night; may awaken client
Location	"Hatband" distribution; may radiate to occipital area and around eyes	Generally unilateral; may be frontal around eye or cheek, may alternate from side to side with subsequent attacks, or may be bilateral	Unilateral, involving facial area from neck to temple; may be around eye
Character of pain	Dull, bandlike, constricting, persistent, with occasional episodes of severe pain	Intense, pulsating, throbbing, one-sided	Sharp, intense, deep, burning, boring, stabbing, excruciating, steady
Duration	Hours to days or months	Several hours to several days	Several minutes to several hours
Frequency	Varies	Varying intervals from several times per month to several times per year; may have a pattern, as with menstrual cycle	May be daily for several weeks in repetitive clusters several times per year
Associated symptoms	Neck stiffness, shoulder ache, nausea	Photophobia, nausea, vomiting, dizziness, tremors, sensitivity to sound	Tearing of eye and stuffiness of nostril on affected side; facial flushing; modified Horner's syndrome with mild ptosis (drooping of upper eyelid) and miosis (constriction of pupil) on affected side
Precipitating factors	Fatigue, stress, anxiety, depression, or no obvious precipitant	Fatigue, prolonged hunger, menstruation, birth control pills, stress, bright sunlight, foods or drugs containing vasoactive chemicals	Alcohol, vasodilators, cigarette smoke, caffeine
Other factors	Most common type of head pain; may result from depression or anxiety or from organic problems, such as cervical arthritis	Familial	
Prodromal events		Complex of neurological events that may precede the migraine include paresthesias, aura, visual changes such as flashing lights, scotomata (blind spots), hemianopsia (loss of vision on one side), distorted perception of size and shape of objects	

Changes in shape

1. Sebaceous cysts on scalp: Result from occlusion of sebaceous gland ducts; palpable as smooth, rounded nodules attached to the scalp.
2. Trauma or surgical removal of a portion of the skull alters shape.

Changes in hair

1. Coarse, dry, brittle: Results from hypothyroidism.
2. Fine, silky, soft: Results from hyperthyroidism.
3. Thinning or hair loss (alopecia): May be hereditary (especially in men), a side effect of chemotherapy, or a result of prolonged illness or emotional stress.
4. Hair and scalp should be checked for dandruff and parasites.

Pain

Headaches are one of the most common symptoms experienced, resulting more often from tension or emotional distress than from organic disease. They may also be the presenting symptom of an injury or severe illness, such as cerebral hemorrhage, brain tumor, or meningitis. Whatever their cause, headaches are often intense and debilitating. In addition, individuals may suffer from more than one type of headache at a time.

Headaches can be classified in numerous ways. One approach is to divide them into primary headaches with three main groups: (1) muscle contraction or tension headaches, (2) migraine headaches, and (3) cluster headaches (Table 11.3). These headaches are classified as primary because they are not directly related to a specific underlying cause.

Secondary headaches are due to structural or physiological problems. They include traction and inflammatory headaches, which are caused by disease or injury, such as sinus inflammation, cranial hemorrhage, or brain tumor, to some structure of the head or neck (e.g., brain, meninges, arteries, veins, eyes, ears, teeth, nose, paranasal sinuses, jaw, neck joints). Secondary headaches may also be due to a systemic cause, such as allergies, hormones, toxins, infection, or exertion. The nature of the headache depends on the underlying disorder. Secondary headaches occur less frequently than primary headaches. However, it is very important to rule out the underlying, possibly life-threatening, cause(s) of the headache before deciding on a diagnosis of a primary headache.

Sinus headaches are the most common type in this category of headaches. They are caused by inflammation of one or more of the paranasal sinuses. These headaches may be a complication of a respiratory infection, dental infection, allergy, or change in atmospheric pressure (air travel, swimming), or they may result from a structural defect. Swelling of the nasal mucous membranes obstructs the openings from the sinuses to the nose, resulting in an accumulation of secretions. This situation may cause tenderness, pressure, and headache.

Temporal arteritis

Arteritis is an inflammatory condition of one or more layers of an arterial wall. Temporal arteritis usually affects individuals older than 50 years of age and is characterized by flulike symptoms, polymyalgia, ocular symptoms, and headache. The skin over the temporal artery becomes red, swollen, and tender. The temporal pulse may be strong, weak, or absent.

Neck

If traumatic neck injury has occurred, the neck should not be moved.

Neck muscles

Common variations from health of the neck muscles include stiffness and pain caused by tension, cervical arthritis, or meningitis.

Temporomandibular joint disease

Pain in the area of the temporomandibular joint results from dislocation of the condyle, osteoarthritis, rheumatoid arthritis, or a myofacial pain syndrome. Pain is often localized to the neck and ear in the area adjacent to the joint. The client has limited motion of the jaw, muscle tenderness, and, occasionally, joint crepitus.

Polymyalgia rheumatica

This syndrome is characterized by an aching pain, tenderness, and stiffness in the neck and shoulders, which may extend to the upper arms, forearms, hips, and legs. Aching is increased with motion.

Hypothyroidism and hyperthyroidism

In general, with hypothyroidism there is a slowing of body functions; with hyperthyroidism there is an acceleration of body functions. Signs and symptoms of either are initially often subtle. The thyroid gland may have diffuse or local enlargement. Symmetrical enlargement may occur with dietary iodine deficiency. Localized or nodular enlargement consists of one or more nodules and may be found in the lobes or the isthmus. Solitary nodules are suggestive of carcinoma, particularly in young adults. Thyroid dysfunction, either hypothyroidism or hyperthyroidism, cannot be determined by the size of the gland alone. If thyroid dysfunction is suspected, thyroid function studies are necessary. The effects of excessive or inadequate amounts of thyroid hormones on body structures and systems are shown in Table 11.4.

table 11.4   Effects of Hyperthyroidism and Hypothyroidism on Body Systems and Structures

Body system or structure	Hyperthyroidism	Hypothyroidism
General		
Weight	Loss	Gain
Temperature intolerance	Heat	Cold
Energy level	Sense of increased energy and alertness	Fatigue, exercise intolerance
Sleep	Insomnia	Drowsiness, difficulty sleeping, obstructive sleep apnea
Skin	Warm, moist; increased sweating; smooth texture; diffuse pigmentation; erythema; brittle nails	Cool, pale, dry, rough, scaly, itchy, facial edema, decreased sweating
Hair	Fine texture, loss, inability to hold a permanent	Thin, dry, poor growth, loss
Cardiovascular/ pulmonary	Increased cardiac output, increased blood pressure, wide pulse pressure, tachycardia, atrial arrhythmias, systolic murmur, palpitations, angina, dyspnea, edema, increase in rate or depth of respirations, bruit over thyroid	Congestive heart failure, angina, bradycardia, cardiomegaly, pericardial or pulmonary effusions, slow and shallow respirations, upper airway obstruction, dyspnea on exertion
Gastrointestinal	Indigestion, anorexia, polyphagia, diarrhea, increased appetite	Thickened tongue, decreased appetite, constipation, abdominal distention
Renal	Polydipsia, polyuria, urgency	Decreased output
Nervous	Restlessness, irritability, anxiety, memory loss, easy distractability, decreased ability to concentrate, emotional liability, panic attacks, hyperreflexia, tremor	Reduced concentration and memory, irritability, slowed thought processes and speech, inability to concentrate, apathy, depression, slowed motor functions, delayed relaxation of deep tendon reflexes, coma
Muscular	Weakness, tremulousness	Stiffness, aching, pain, weakness, muscle cramps, arthralgias
Eyes	Lid lag and lid retraction (startled look), tearing, conjunctival irritation	Periorbital puffiness
Voice		Deep, hoarse
Hearing		Acuity may diminish
Reproductive		
Women	Hypomenorrhea, amenorrhea	Menorrhagia, amenorrhea, infertility, anovulatory cycles
Men	Decreased libido and potency	Decreased libido and potency

Lymph Nodes
Lymph node enlargement

Enlarged lymph nodes may be due to acute or chronic infections. Examples of acute conditions are infectious mononucleosis, tonsillitis, or streptococcal meningitis. Acute infections may cause lymph nodes to be firm, tender, matted, or discrete. Sharply localized tender nodes suggest infection at a distal focus. More serious illnesses related to the immune system, cancer, and acquired immunodeficiency syndrome (AIDS) may also present clinically in the lymph nodes. For example, the first clinical sign of metastatic disease is the involvement of lymph nodes in the region draining the site of neoplastic growth. The lymph nodes may be hard, fixed to surrounding tissue, and nontender. In a person infected with human immunodeficiency virus (HIV), nodes of any chain may be enlarged, but those of the head and neck are most frequently involved.

Acute infections

Streptococcal pharyngitis. Symptoms of streptococcal pharyngitis usually include a sore throat and runny nose and may include headache, fatigue, myalgias, and abdominal discomfort. Anterior cervical nodes are commonly palpable and tend to be firm, discrete, mobile, and tender.

Epstein-Barr virus mononucleosis. Epstein-Barr virus mononucleosis (infectious mononucleosis) is most common in adolescents and young adults. Lymph node enlargement may be generalized but is most common in the anterior and posterior cervical chains. Nodes vary in firmness, are generally discrete, and may be tender. Early symptoms include pharyngitis, fever, fatigue, and malaise. Splenomegaly, hepatomegaly, and a rash may develop.

Lymphadenitis.
Lymphadenitis is an inflammatory condition of the lymph nodes resulting from bacterial infection, neoplastic disease, or other inflammatory conditions. The nodes may be enlarged, hard, tender, smooth, or irregular. The overlying skin may become edematous, red, and warm. The site of the affected node indicates the site of the origin of the disease.

Metastatic disease.
Malignant lymphomas, including Hodgkin's disease, cause nodes to be large, discrete, nontender, and firm to rubbery in consistency. Such nodes may be localized to any area but are occasionally generalized. Lymphadenopathy, an inflammatory condition of the lymph nodes, may be due to chronic lymphocytic leukemia. Lymph nodes due to metastatic cancer are nontender, have a firm to hard consistency, may be discrete or matted, and tend to be localized initially. The various lymphomas differ in degree of cellular differentiation and content, but the manifestations are similar in all types. Characteristically, the appearance of a painless, enlarged lymph node or nodes in the neck is followed by weakness, fever, weight loss, and anemia.

Hodgkin's disease is a malignant disorder characterized by painless, progressive enlargement of lymphoid tissue, which is usually first evident in cervical lymph nodes. Symptoms include anorexia, weight loss, generalized pruritus, low-grade fever, and night sweats.

Acquired immunodeficiency syndrome.
AIDS is a disease involving a defect in cell-mediated immunity. This syndrome is caused by HIV infection. It is characterized by the loss of T_4 lymphocyte cells, which leads to progressive loss of immune system competency, with the development of opportunistic infections, impairment of the central nervous system, chronic wasting, and often malignancy. Initial symptoms include lymphadenopathy, extreme fatigue, intermittent fever, chills, night sweats, enlarged spleen, anorexia, diarrhea, weight loss, apathy, and depression. As the disease progresses, general malnourishment, decreased energy, and recurrent infections develop. Most people with AIDS are susceptible to malignant neoplasms, especially Kaposi's sarcoma and non-Hodgkin's lymphoma.

■ FOCUSED HEALTH HISTORY *(SUBJECTIVE DATA)*

Ms. O., a 25-year-old graduate student, gives a history of headaches occurring with increasing frequency. Headaches begin in the late morning to early afternoon; they have occurred every 1 to 2 weeks for the past 5 months. Client describes them as "a tight band around my head with throbbing on the sides." Pain and stiffness develop at the base of the head and in the neck and shoulders. Pain is gradual in onset and is typically dull and nagging. Occasionally it becomes so severe that she must stop working for 1 to 2 hours. Associated symptoms include occasional slight nausea. No other GI symptoms and no photophobia, changes in vision, or paresthesias. Client uses aspirin or acetaminophen q 3 to 4 hours with some relief. Is not allergic to any food or drugs, does not smoke, and drinks a glass of wine about twice a month. States she is very concerned about the increasing frequency of the headaches. Is a full-time graduate student and works about 30 hours per week.

■ FOCUSED PHYSICAL EXAMINATION *(OBJECTIVE DATA)*

General appearance: Client appears tired and anxious.

Physical examination: Scalp is clear of lesions; hair is normally distributed. Temporal artery pulse palpable; rhythm regular; no thickening or tenderness.

Eyes: Vision 20/20 in each eye using Snellen; visual fields intact; PERRLA; extraocular movements (EOMs) intact.

Neck: Thyroid not palpable; trapezius muscles stiff and tender; trapezius and sternocleidomastoid strength good bilaterally.

Neurological: Cranial nerves II through XII intact.

diagnoses

HEALTH PROBLEM
Headache

NURSING DIAGNOSIS

Pain

Defining Characteristics
- Facial appearance of pain and fatigue
- Verbal report of pain and stiffness at base of head, neck, and shoulders
- Interference with work schedule

chapter 12

Eyes

■ PURPOSE OF EXAMINATION

Vision is one of our most important mechanisms for experiencing the world. The eyes are complex and delicate structures. They receive visual stimuli and transmit it to the visual cortex in the brain. The optic nerve (cranial nerve [CN] II) directly connects the eye and the brain. Six of the twelve cranial nerves are involved with the eyes. The eyes are balanced and held in place by six sets of extraocular muscles.

A thorough examination of the eyes can reveal a wealth of information about both local and systemic health and about variations from the healthy state.

In conjunction with observation of facial expression and body posture, observation of the eyes frequently provides information about the client's emotional status.

The examination of the eyes includes measurement of visual acuity, evaluation of visual fields, testing of ocular movements, inspection of ocular structures, testing of nerve reflexes, and the ophthalmoscopic examination.

■ ANATOMY AND PHYSIOLOGY

The eyes are located within the bony orbital cavity. The anterior aspect of the eye is exposed, and the remainder is protected within the skull. The structures of the eye described in this chapter include:

Eyelids and eyelashes
Conjunctiva
Sclera
Cornea
Anterior chamber
Lacrimal apparatus
Iris
Pupils
Lens
Vitreous body
Retina
Ocular muscles
Optic nerve
Portions of the retina that are described here include:
Optic disc
Retinal vessels
Macula
Retinal background
The structures of the eyelid and the globe of the eye are illustrated in Figures 12.1 through 12.3.

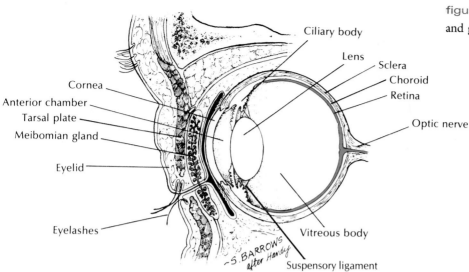

figure**12.1**   Structures of the eyelid and globe of the eye.

Ciliary body

Lens

Sclera

Choroid

Retina

Optic nerve

Cornea

Anterior chamber

Tarsal plate

Meibomian gland

Eyelid

Eyelashes

Vitreous body

Suspensory ligament

~S. BARROWS after Hardy

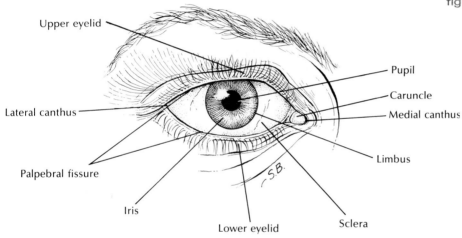

figure**12.2**   Anterior view of the eye.

Upper eyelid

Pupil

Caruncle

Medial canthus

Lateral canthus

Limbus

Palpebral fissure

Iris

Lower eyelid

Sclera

~S.B.

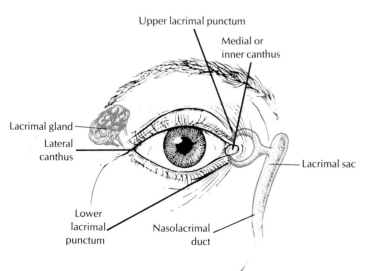

figure**12.3**   Lacrimal system.

Upper lacrimal punctum

Medial or inner canthus

Lacrimal gland

Lateral canthus

Lacrimal sac

Lower lacrimal punctum

Nasolacrimal duct

Ocular Structures

Eyelids and eyelashes

The eyelashes are distributed along the margin of each eyelid and curve outward. The eyelids (palpebrae) serve a protective function, covering the anterior aspect of the eye and distributing tears across the surface of the eye to keep it moist and lubricated. The eyelids also limit the amount of light that enters the eyes and protect the eyes from foreign objects. When the eyes are open, the upper eyelid normally covers a small portion of the iris and the cornea overlying it, located about midway between the limbus and the pupil. The margin of the lower eyelid lies at or just below the limbus. The limbus is the junction line of the cornea and the sclera. The distance between the upper and the lower eyelid margin is called the palpebral fissure. The tarsal plates are thin strips of connective tissue that lie within the eyelid and give it form and consistency.

Conjunctiva

The conjunctiva lines the eyelids and covers the anterior portion of the eyeball. This continuous transparent lining is divided into two portions: palpebral and bulbar. The palpebral portion lines the eyelids; it appears shiny pink or red because it overlies the fleshy vascular structures of the lids. The bulbar portion lies over the sclera. The palpebral conjunctiva recesses into the folds of the eyelids and is continuous with the bulbar conjunctiva, which rests loosely over the sclera to the limbus, where it merges with the corneal epithelium. This portion of the conjunctiva is normally clear; the white color comes from the sclera below. The bulbar portion does, however, contain many small blood vessels. These vessels are normally visible and may become dilated, producing varying degrees of redness. A small fleshy elevation, the caruncle is located in the nasal corner of the conjunctiva. Yellowish triangular deposits, called pinguecula, may occur in the bulbar conjunctiva near the limbus. These essentially normal senile changes are caused by a hyaline degeneration of fibrous tissue. The meibomian glands, which secrete an oily lubricating substance, appear as vertical yellow striations on the palpebral conjunctiva.

Sclera

The globe of the eye is surrounded by three coats: sclera, choroid, and retina. The sclera is the outer fibrous layer. It is visible anteriorly as the white portion of the eye. Several small, distinct conjunctival vessels lie over the sclera, particularly around the periphery. In some dark-skinned persons, small dark-pigmented dots are located on the sclera near the limbus.

Cornea

The cornea is a smooth, moist tissue that covers the area over the pupil and the iris. It is continuous with the conjunctiva. Like the bulbar conjunctiva, the cornea is transparent and permits the passage of light inward toward the retina. The cornea merges with the conjunctiva at the limbus. It separates fluid from the anterior chamber from the external environment. The cornea is sensitive to touch. This sensation is transmitted by the ophthalmic branch of the trigeminal nerve (CN V).

Anterior chamber

The anterior chamber lies posterior to the cornea. It is bounded anteriorly by the cornea, laterally by the sclera and the ciliary body, and posteriorly by the iris and that portion of the lens that is within the pupillary opening. The anterior chamber is filled with aqueous humor, a fluid that is continuously produced by the ciliary body. The relationship between the rate of production of aqueous humor and the resistance to aqueous outflow at the anterior chamber angle determines the intraocular pressure, which is normally 15 mm Hg ± 3 mm Hg.

Lacrimal apparatus

The components of the lacrimal apparatus are the following:
   Lacrimal gland
   Lacrimal puncta
   Lacrimal sac
   Nasolacrimal duct

The lacrimal gland is located above and slightly lateral to the eye (Figure 12.3). It produces tears, which moisten and lubricate the conjunctiva and the cornea. The tears wash across the eye and drain through the upper and lower lacrimal puncta, which are small openings located at the nasal side of both the upper and lower eyelid margins. The tears then pass into the nasolacrimal sac, which is located medial to the eye. From the nasolacrimal sac, the tears pass into the nasolacrimal duct and the nasal meatus. Tearing is also referred to as lacrimation.

Iris

The iris is the circular disc containing pigmented fibrils that give the eye its distinctive color. It is located in front of the lens and behind the anterior chamber. The iris, the ciliary body, and the suspensory ligament form the interior portion of the choroid layer of the eye. Posterior to the layer of fibrils are two groups of muscles, dilator and sphincter muscles. These muscles function in a manner similar to that of the diaphragm of a camera within the image-forming portion of the eye.

Pupil

The pupil is the opening in the iris through which light passes. The size of the pupil is determined by the amount of light entering the eye and the closeness of

the object being visualized. It is regulated by the constriction and dilation of the muscles of the iris. This muscular activity is controlled by the autonomic nervous system. Stimulation of the parasympathetic fibers leads to constriction of the pupils; stimulation of the sympathetic fibers produces dilation of the pupils. The amount of light that is present influences the size of the pupils. Increasing the amount of light causes pupillary constriction. Diminishing the light causes dilation. These changes represent adaptation. The pupils also constrict in response to accommodation, which is the change in focus from a distant to a near object.

The constricting response of the pupils to a bright, direct light is a pupillary reflex. This reflex consists of two aspects: the direct reaction and the consensual reaction, or the consensual light reflex. The direct reaction refers to the constriction of the pupil receiving the increased illumination. The constriction of the pupil that is not receiving increased light is the consensual reaction. The optic nerve (CN II) transmits the stimulus from the eye to the brain. The oculomotor nerve (CN III) transmits the reflex from the brain to both eyes. The presence of both direct and consensual responses indicates the functioning of these two cranial nerves.

Lens

The lens is located directly behind the iris at the pupillary opening. It is the center of the refracting system of the eye. The lens is composed of epithelial cells within an elastic membrane, the lens capsule. The lens is transparent and has no blood vessels, nerves, or connective tissue. The thickness of the lens is controlled by the muscles of the ciliary body. Changes in lens thickness enable the eye to focus on near and distant objects. The coordinated function of the muscles of the iris and the muscles of the ciliary body acting on the lens controls the amount of light permitted to reach the retina and the focusing of objects on the retina.

Vitreous humor

The vitreous humor is a transparent fluid that occupies the area posterior to the lens, which is called the posterior chamber. The vitreous humor is surrounded by the retinal layer of the globe of the eye.

Retina and retinal structures

The retina is the inner coat of the globe of the eye. It contains the neurosensory elements that transform light impulses into the electrical impulses that are carried to the visual cortex by way of the optic nerve and the optic tract. Several important structures are located on the retina, including (1) the optic disc, which is the head of the optic nerve; (2) four sets of retinal vessels, which emerge from the optic disc and travel medially and laterally around the retina; and the macula, where central vision is concentrated (Figure 12.4).

Optic disc and physiologic cup. The optic disc is located on the nasal half of the retina. This round structure is creamy yellow to pink and is lighter than the surrounding retina. The color of both the disc and the retinal background varies from one individual to another; it is somewhat lighter in fair-complected, light-haired people and slightly darker in dark-complected, dark-haired people.

The physiologic cup (physiologic depression) is a small depression within the disc just temporal to the center of the disc. It is yellowish white and slightly lighter in color than the rest of the disc. The physiologic cup does not extend to the disc margins; it occupies one fourth to one third of the area of the disc.

Retinal vessels. Four sets of retinal vessels emerge from the optic disc and extend outward, becoming smaller at the periphery. Each set of vessels, which includes an arteriole and a vein, is named according to the quadrant of the disc in which it is located: superior nasal, inferior nasal, superior temporal, and inferior temporal. The arterioles are brighter red than the veins because they carry oxygenated blood. The veins are darker red because they carry deoxygenated blood. Since the arterioles are approximately 25% smaller than the veins, there is an arteriole/vein ratio (A:V ratio) of about 2:3 or 4:5.

Macula and retinal background. The rods and the cones are neurosensory elements located in the retina. The rods mediate black-and-white vision, and the cones mediate color vision. At a point temporal to the optic disc at the posterior pole of the eye, the retina has a slight depression called the fovea centralis. The cones are most heavily concentrated in this area, making it the point of central vision and most acute color and daylight vision. The retinal area immediately around the fovea centralis is called the macula. The retinal background is reddish orange.

Extraocular muscles and cranial nerves

Six muscles of each eye, working in a coordinated, or yoked, fashion with those of the other eye, control eye movement. The movements of the two eyes normally occur in conjugate, parallel fashion except during convergence. The eyes converge, or come toward each other, when the person focuses on a very close object. The six extraocular muscles are shown in Figure 12.5.

The parallel movement of the eyes makes it possible to have single-image binocular vision. The yoked muscles are the muscles in each eye that work together to move the eyes in parallel motion to any position of gaze (Figure 12.5, *A*). For example, the left lateral rectus and the right medial rectus are yoked muscles that work concurrently to move the gaze to the left.

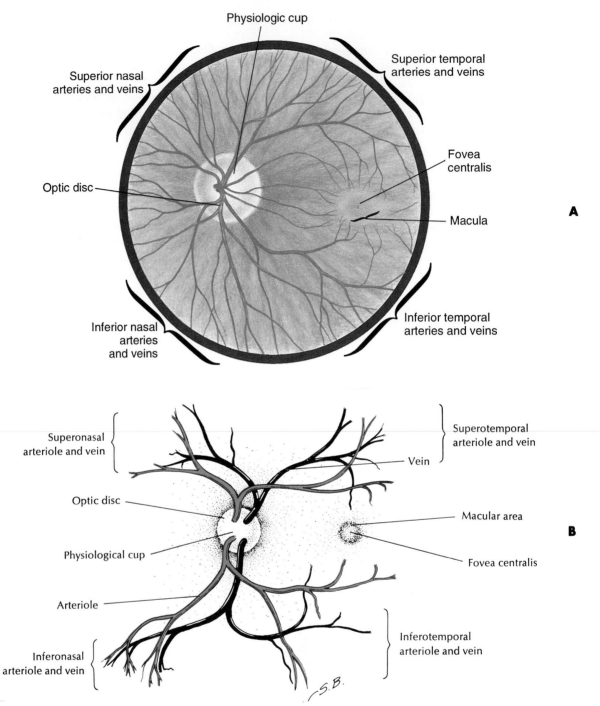

figure **12.4** **A,** Retinal structures of the left eye. **B,** Optic disc, physiological cup, and retinal vessels of the left eye. (*A modified from Seidel HM et al:* Mosby's guide to physical examination, *ed 3, St Louis, 1995, Mosby.*)

The six eye muscles are innervated by three cranial nerves. The oculomotor nerve (CN III) supplies four muscles: the superior, inferior, and medial rectus muscles and the inferior oblique muscle. The trochlear nerve (CN IV) innervates the superior oblique muscle. The abducens nerve (CN VI) supplies the lateral rectus muscle.

Six of the 12 cranial nerves and portions of the cerebral hemispheres are involved in the total neurological innervation of the eye and related structures. Table 12.1 summarizes the relationship of the six cranial nerves to the eye structures and their functions (see also Table 19.1).

figure **12.5**   **A,** Movement of the eyes related to the six sets of extraocular muscles. **B,** Extraocular muscles of the right eye. (**B** *from Thibodeau GA:* Anthony's textbook of anatomy and physiology, *ed 13, St Louis, 1990, Mosby.*)

Physiology of Vision

For someone to perceive a clear visual image, light reflected from an object must pass through several transparent structures: the cornea, anterior chamber, lens, and vitreous fluid. Then the light must focus on the retina, where the neural receptors, the rods and cones, are activated and carry the impulse along the optic nerve and tract to the visual cortex of the brain.

Formation of retinal image

Four processes lead to the formation of a clear image on the retina:

1. Refraction, or bending, of the light rays
2. Accommodation, or change in curvature, of the lens
3. Constriction of the pupil
4. Convergence of the eyes

Refraction is the bending or deflecting of light rays that occurs when the rays pass obliquely from one transparent medium into another of a different density. In the eye these media are the cornea, the aqueous humor, the lens, and the vitreous humor. All of these structures work in conjunction to bring an object into focus on the retina (Figure 12.6).

Accommodation for near vision enables the eye to focus on near objects by increasing the curvature of the lens, constriction of the pupils, and convergence of the eyes. Light rays from close objects are divergent and

table 12.1	*Relationship of Cranial Nerves to Eye Structures and Functions*
Cranial nerve	**Function**
II Optic	Mediates vision
III Oculomotor	Innervates medial, superior, and inferior rectus muscles; inferior oblique muscle; muscles elevating eyelid (levator palpebrae); and muscles of iris and ciliary body
IV Trochlear	Innervates superior oblique muscle
V Trigeminal (ophthalmic division)	Innervates sensory portion of corneal reflex
VI Abducens	Innervates lateral rectus muscle
VII Facial	Innervates lacrimal glands and muscles involved in lid closure (orbicularis oculi)

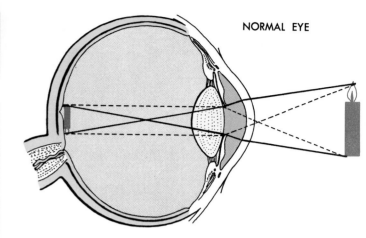

NORMAL EYE

figure**12.6** Formation of a retinal image. In the normal eye, light rays from an object are refracted by the cornea, aqueous humor, lens, and vitreous humor; those rays converge on the fovea of the retina, where an inverted image is clearly formed. *(From Thibodeau GA:* Anthony's textbook of anatomy and physiology, *ed 13, St Louis, 1990, Mosby.)*

must be bent to focus on the retina. The curvature of the lens increases to accomplish this result. Contraction of the ciliary muscle causes the elastic lens to bulge.

The pupils constrict as a result of contraction of the circular fibers of the iris. This constriction prevents divergent light rays from coming into the eye through the peripheral portions of the cornea and the lens. The pupil constricts both for near vision and in the presence of bright light.

Convergence is the movement of the eyes inward to bring together the visual axes on the object being viewed. Single binocular vision requires that light rays from an object fall on corresponding points of the two retinas so that a person sees one object instead of two. The extraocular muscles hold the visual axes of the two eyes parallel.

Visual pathways and visual fields

The images formed on the retina are reversed right to left and are upside down. Thus an object in the upper nasal field of vision is formed on the lower temporal quadrant of the retina. The field of vision is the area that can be visualized when the eye is not moving. Light stimulates neuron impulses that are conducted through the retina, the optic nerve, and the optic tract to the visual cortex of the occipital lobes.

The arrangement of the nerve fibers in the retina is continued in the optic nerve: temporal (lateral) fibers follow the lateral side of the nerve, and nasal (medial) fibers run along the medial portion of the nerve. At the optic chiasm, however, the nasal or medial fibers cross over and join the temporal fibers of the opposite optic tract. Thus the left optic tract contains fibers from only the left half of each retina or only the right half of each field of vision. The right optic tract contains fibers from only the right half of each retina or only the left half of each field of vision. This sequence of pathways and events produces vision. The relationship of visual pathways and fields of vision is illustrated in Figure 12.7.

■ EXAMINATION

Health History
Present health status

1. Adequacy of vision in each eye, use of corrective lenses, date of last eye examination, and results of that examination
2. Difficulty with vision
   a. Near or distant
   b. Central, peripheral, or specific area
   c. Constant or intermittent
   d. Day or night
   e. Presence of floaters, halos around lights
   f. Double vision
   g. Abnormal movements
3. Pain
   a. In or around eye

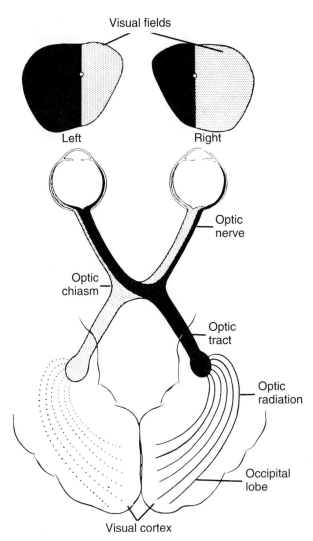

Visual fields

Left   Right

Optic
nerve

Optic
chiasm

Optic
tract

Optic
radiation

Occipital
lobe

Visual cortex

figure **12.7** Representation of the visual field in the optic pathways. *(From Havener WH: Synopsis of ophthalmology, ed 6, St Louis, 1984, Mosby.)*

RISK FACTORS   GLAUCOMA

Glaucoma is the second leading cause of new cases of blindness in the United States. Open-angle glaucoma is the most common form. When symptoms are not present, it may progress until irreversible visual field loss occurs.

Risk factors for glaucoma include diabetes mellitus, myopia, and a family history of glaucoma. African-Americans are at increased risk for glaucoma, which is the leading cause of blindness in this group. Persons over age 75 are also at increased risk for glaucoma.

Clients who are at risk for glaucoma should be referred to an eye specialist for further assessment.

CULTURAL CONSIDERATIONS

EYE DISTINCTIONS

Persons of Asian heritage have a characteristic shape of upward slanting and narrowed palpebral fissures. In non-Asian individuals this finding may indicate Down syndrome. In dark-skinned persons the sclera, iris, and fundus are typically darker than in light-skinned persons.

b. Superficial or deep
c. Onset: Abrupt or gradual
d. Associated symptoms: Itching, burning, photophobia, injection, erythema, other sensations
4. Abnormal secretions
  a. Color
  b. Consistency
  c. Onset and duration
  d. Excessive or decreased tearing
5. Use of eye medications: Type and purpose; frequency and duration of use
6. Trauma or foreign body

Past health history

1. Trauma, injury to eye(s)
  a. History of incident

b. Structures damaged
c. Efforts to correct damage and degree of success
2. Eye surgery
  a. Condition(s) requiring surgery
  b. Date surgery performed
  c. Outcome
3. Variations from health that may affect the eyes
  a. Hypertension
  b. Diabetes
  c. Thyroid disorder
  d. Glaucoma
  e. Cataract
  f. Eye infection

Family health history

1. Nearsightedness (myopia), farsightedness (hyperopia), strabismus
2. Retinoblastoma (cancer of the retina)
3. Color blindness, cataracts, glaucoma, retinitis pigmentosa, macular degeneration, diabetes, hypertension, thyroid disorder
4. Conditions similar to that of client

PREPARATION FOR EXAMINATION

EQUIPMENT

Item	Purpose
Visual acuity charts Snellen or E (for distant vision) Rosenbaum (for near vision)	To assess visual acuity
Opaque card or eye cover	To assess visual acuity, visual fields, and muscle function
Penlight	To assess pupillary light reflex and external structures of eye
Cotton-tipped applicator	To evert upper eyelid
Ophthalmoscope	To assess transparent ocular media and perform retinal examination

CLIENT AND ENVIRONMENT

The examination room must have lighting that can be controlled and comfortable seating for the client. An area for testing visual acuity is needed that allows the client to be 20 feet from the Snellen chart.

General considerations

1. Exposure to irritating chemicals, gases
2. Activities: Participation in sports that could endanger the eyes
3. Use of protective devices when participating in activities that could endanger the eyes

Preparation for Examination: Client and Environment

The examination should be conducted in a room where the lighting can be controlled. A well-lighted room is needed for the visual acuity tests, and it must be possible to darken the room to assess the pupillary reflexes and to perform the ophthalmoscopic examination. A room or hallway where the client can be 20 feet away from the Snellen chart is required for testing visual acuity.

The eye examination involves multiple components, which should be learned in a thorough and efficient arrangement. The order in which the examination is performed should focus on completeness and the comfortable positioning of the client. The client will remain seated during most of the examination. The assessment begins with visual acuity, ocular function, and visual fields. Then the external eye structures are examined. The ophthalmoscopic examination is done last.

Technique for Examination and Normal Findings

In the eye examination, the range of normal findings is broad and variations are numerous. Much time, patience, and practice are needed to learn assessment of the many structures and functions of the eyes. Inspection is the main technique used to examine the eye. Palpation should be done only if a symptom or sign requires further investigation, such as palpating the lacrimal sac if blockage or infection is suspected. A description of the procedures that involve palpation is integrated into the discussion of inspection that follows. NOTE : Abbreviations from Latin are used to refer to the right eye and left eye. *Oculus dexter (OD)* refers to the right eye, *oculus sinister (OS)* refers to the left eye.

Inspection

The components of the examination that involve inspection include the following:

Visual acuity
Visual fields
Extraocular muscle function
External ocular structures
Ophthalmoscopic examination

Visual acuity. The assessment of visual acuity is a simple test of ocular function. Findings in the normal range of visual acuity give an indication of the clarity of the transparent structures (cornea, anterior body, lens, and vitreous humor), the adequacy of macular (central) vision, and the functioning of the nerve fibers from the macula to the occipital cortex.

The Snellen alphabet chart (Figure 12.8, *A*), which has various sizes of letters, is traditionally used to test visual acuity. For clients who are illiterate or those who are unfamiliar with the English alphabet, the E chart is useful. The letter E is shown in different directions, and the client can state or point to which side is open (Figure 12.8, *B*).

The Snellen chart has standardized numbers at the end of each line of letters. These numbers indicate the degree of visual acuity demonstrated when the client reads the chart from a distance of 20 feet. The number above the line or to the left of it is 20, the distance in feet between the chart and the client. This amount is the standard testing distance. The number below the line or to the right of it is the distance from which the normal eye can read the letters on a particular line. The higher the number below the line or to the right, the poorer the visual acuity. For example, 20/20 vision is better than 20/40 vision.

figure**12.8** **A,** Snellen chart for testing distance vision. **B,** E chart for testing distance vision. *(From Seidel HM et al:* Mosby's guide to physical examination, *ed 3, St Louis, 1995, Mosby.)*

Measurement of 20/20 vision in a client indicates normal visual acuity and a functional optic pathway. Measurement of less than 20/20 vision indicates either a refractive error or some other optic disorder.

Be sure that the room is well lighted for the visual acuity test. Have the client stand or sit 20 feet from the Snellen chart. The chart should be located approximately at eye level. To assess visual acuity, initially test only one eye at a time. Cover the other eye with an opaque

card or an eye cover. Do not let the client use his or her fingers to cover the eye. Alternatively, both eyes may be tested together, since binocular vision is the client's functional vision. Test a client who wears corrective lenses both with and without them. This approach allows for an assessment of the adequacy of correction. Since reading glasses blur distant vision, the client should not wear them for this test.

If a client cannot see the largest letter on the chart

ROSENBAUM POCKET VISION SCREENER

			Point	Jaeger	distance equivalent
95					$\frac{20}{800}$
874					$\frac{20}{400}$
2843			26	16	$\frac{20}{200}$
638	ЕШЭ	XOO	14	10	$\frac{20}{100}$
8745	ЭШШ	OXO	10	7	$\frac{20}{70}$
63925	ШЕЭ	XOX	8	5	$\frac{20}{50}$
428365	ШЕШ	oxo	6	3	$\frac{20}{40}$
374258	эшэ	x x o	5	2	$\frac{20}{30}$
937826	шшЕ	x o o	4	1	$\frac{20}{25}$
428739	Ешш	o o x	3	1+	$\frac{20}{20}$

Card is held in good light 14 inches from eye. Record vision for each eye separately with and without glasses. Presbyopic patients should read thru bifocal segment. Check myopes with glasses only.

DESIGN COURTESY J. G. ROSENBAUM, M.D.

PUPIL GAUGE (mm.)

2 3 4 5 6 7 8 9

figure **12.9** Rosenbaum chart for testing near vision. *(From Seidel HM et al: Mosby's guide to physical examination, ed 3, St Louis, 1995, Mosby.)*

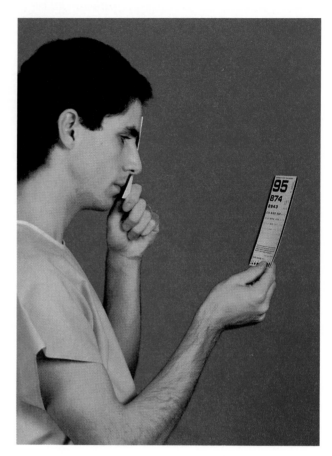

figure **12.10** Assessing a client's near vision with the Rosenbaum chart.

(20/200), check to see if he or she can perceive the movement of your hand at about 12 inches from the eyes or can perceive the light of a penlight directed into the eyes.

Perform a gross assessment of near vision for the client who has difficulty reading. Ask the client to read the letters on a Rosenbaum chart (Figure 12.9) or a newspaper with various sizes of print. Have the client hold the reading material at a distance of approximately 12 to 14 inches (Figure 12.10).

Visual fields confrontation test. The assessment of visual acuity indicates the functioning of the macular area, the area of central vision. It does not test the sensitivity of the other areas of the retina, which perceive the peripheral stimuli. The visual fields confrontation test (Figure 12.11) provides a gross assessment of peripheral vision. In this test you use your own visual fields to make comparisons with the client's visual fields. For this test to be useful, your own visual fields must be normal.

You and the client sit or stand opposite each other about $1\frac{1}{2}$ to 2 feet apart with your eyes at the same horizontal level. The client covers one eye with an opaque card or eye cover, and you cover your own eye that is opposite the client's covered eye. For example, if the client's right eye is covered, then your left eye is covered. This method leaves the same field of vision open for assessment. You and the client stare directly into each other's open eye. Tell the client not to look at the object approaching from the periphery. Hold a small object, such as a penlight or a pen, and gradually move it in from the periphery toward the center from eight

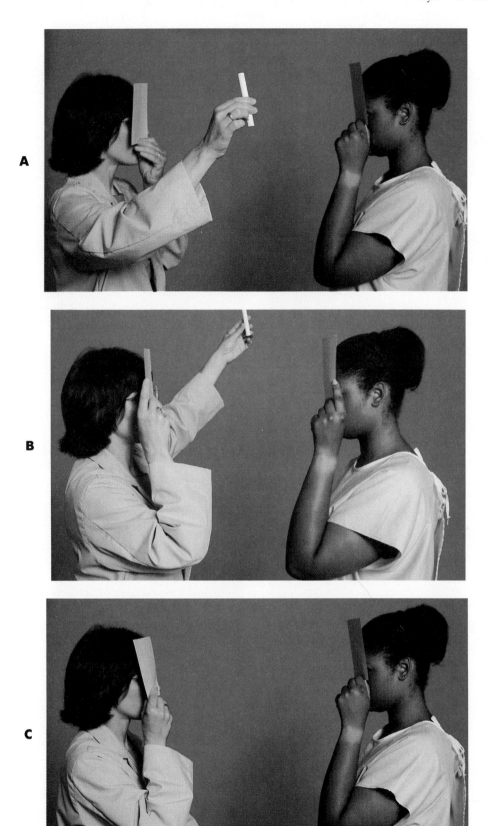

figure 12.11 Visual fields confrontation test. The examiner assesses the client's right field of vision from the nasal direction (**A**), superior direction (**B**), and inferior direction (**C**). (Also tested but not shown: temporal direction.)

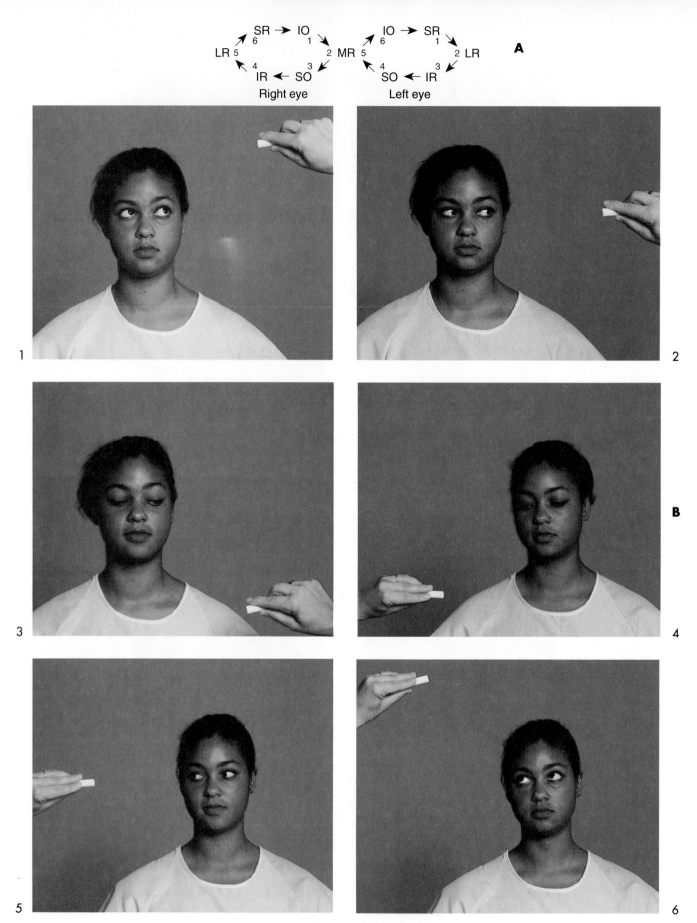

figure**12.12** **A,** The six cardinal positions of gaze. **B,** Examination of the six cardinal positions of gaze.

directions: right and left, above and below, and at the midpoints between each of these directions. At first, the object should be outside the field of vision. Hold the object equidistant between yourself and the client. Bring it in gradually toward the center. You and the client should be able to see the object enter the field of vision at the same time.

> **HELPFUL HINT** *You may find it difficult to move the test object out far enough in the temporal field so that neither you nor the client can see it. If this happens, hold the object slightly closer to the client than to yourself initially, and move it toward a line equidistant between you as you bring the object toward the center.*

This test provides only a crude estimate of visual fields. Although it may demonstrate large field defects, it does not usually detect small changes. Therefore clinical use of this test is limited. If you suspect decreased peripheral vision or loss of vision in certain areas, refer the client to an eye specialist for further testing.

Extraocular muscle function. The assessment of extraocular muscle function has these three components:

Six cardinal positions of gaze

Corneal light reflex

Cover-uncover test

Basic to each of these components is the observation of the parallelism of the eyes and ocular movements.

Six cardinal positions of gaze. To assess the six cardinal positions of gaze (Figure 12.12, *A*), stand in front of the client and ask him or her to watch your finger or a small object as you move it through the six cardinal positions of gaze. Ask the client to hold the head still and to move only the eyes. Move your finger or the object clockwise to each of the six positions shown in Figure 12.12, *B*. Ask the client to hold the gaze briefly at each position. Observe for parallel movements and for slight oscillating movements of the eyes, called nystagmus. A small amount of end-position lateral nystagmus is normal. However, in any other position, nystagmus is abnormal. The eyes should move together in parallel fashion to each position.

After you have examined the extraocular muscles in the six cardinal positions, ask the client to look straight up and then down without moving the head. Observe the relationship of the upper eyelid to the iris as the client's gaze moves. The upper eyelid should overlap the iris slightly throughout this movement. No sclera should show between the iris and the upper eyelid.

Corneal light reflex. You can assess the parallelism of the anterior and posterior axes of the two eyes by ob-

serving the reflection of light from the cornea. Ask the client to stare straight ahead while you shine a penlight toward the bridge of the nose from a distance of 12 to 15 inches. The bright dot of light reflected from the shiny surface of the corneas should be located symmetrically, (e.g., at the 12 o'clock position in both eyes). If the reflected dot of light is not symmetrical, perform the cover-uncover test.

Cover-uncover test. Maintenance of parallelism of the eyes is a result of the fusion reflex that makes binocular vision possible. Normally, both eyes are aligned and centrally fixed and there is no movement of the eyes when they are covered or uncovered. If a muscle imbalance is present and the fusion reflex is blocked when one eye is covered, this weakness can be observed.

Ask the client to look at a specific fixed point, such as the corner of a picture or doorframe. Then cover one of the client's eyes with an opaque card or eye cover; while

A

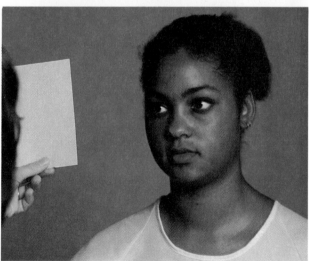

B

figure**12.13** Cover-uncover test.

doing so, observe the uncovered eye to see if it moves to fix on the object (Figure 12.13, *A*). Then remove the cover and observe for any movement of the eye that was just uncovered (Figure 12.13, *B*). When an eye is covered, the appearance of an object on that retina is suppressed. The eye relaxes; if there is a weakness in one of the extraocular muscles, the eye drifts to another resting position. Then, when the eye is uncovered, it pulls back into alignment. Perform this procedure on both eyes.

External eye structures

Eyelids and eyelashes. Inspect the eyelashes to see that they are present and curve outward. The palpebral fissures (distance between the upper and lower lids) should be equal. The margin of the upper eyelid is normally between the upper margin of the pupil and the upper margin of the limbus. Check to see that the client can close the lids completely. Note the position of the globe of the eye: normal, prominent, or sunken. Raised yellow plaques, or xanthelasma, may appear on the lids near the inner canthi. These plaques can be normal variations that grow slowly and may disappear spontaneously.

Conjunctiva. Inspect the bulbar and palpebral portions of the conjunctiva by separating the eyelids widely and having the client look up, down, and to each side. When separating the eyelids, do not exert pressure against the eyeball. Hold the eyelid against the ridge of the bony orbit surrounding the eye (Figure 12.14). Normally, many small blood vessels are visible through the clear conjunctiva. The white sclera is visible through the bulbar conjunctiva.

Although eversion of the upper eyelid is not a necessary part of the physical examination, you should learn a careful technique for performing the procedure. It may be indicated, for example, when you suspect a foreign body in the upper eyelid. Explain the entire procedure to the client before you begin, and provide reassurance as you do it. If you do not show gentleness and care and give reassurance, the client is very likely to become tense when you manipulate the eyelid. When you are everting the eyelid, be aware of those techniques that promote relaxation rather than contraction of the muscles. Perform eversion of the upper eyelid (Figure 12.15) in the following way:

1. Ask the client to look down but keep the eyes slightly open. This maneuver relaxes the levator muscle. Closing the eyes contracts the orbicularis muscle, preventing lid eversion.
2. Gently grasp the upper eyelashes and pull them gently downward. Do not pull the lashes outward or upward, since this action causes muscle contraction.

figure**12.14**   Examination of the conjunctiva.

figure**12.15**   Eversion of the eyelid.

3. Place a cotton-tipped applicator about 1 cm above the eyelid margin and gently push downward with the applicator while still holding the lashes. This maneuver everts the lid.

4. Hold the lashes of the everted eyelid against the upper ridge of the bony orbit, just beneath the eyebrow. Do *not* push against the eyeball.

5. Inspect the eyelid for a foreign object, lesion, swelling, or infection.

6. To return the eyelid to its normal position, move the lashes slightly forward and ask the client to look up and then blink. The lid should return easily to a normal position.

Sclera. Inspect the sclera while you are inspecting the bulbar conjunctiva. The sclera is normally white. However, some pigmented deposits are within the ranges of normal findings.

Cornea. Inspect the cornea by directing the light of a penlight at it obliquely from several positions. The cornea should be transparent, smooth, shiny, and bright. The surface should have no irregularities. The features of the iris should be fully visible through the cornea. In older persons the appearance of arcus senilis may be considered normal. Arcus senilis is a white ring that is located around the periphery of the cornea.

Anterior chamber. Inspect the anterior chamber while you are inspecting the cornea. Use the oblique light from a penlight to assess the anterior chamber (or use the light of the ophthalmoscope). The anterior chamber is a transparent structure. Any visible material is abnormal. Assess the depth of the anterior chamber, which is the distance between the cornea and the iris. Look at the eye from the side, rather than from directly in front, and shine the light across the eye from the opposite side. From a side view, the iris should appear flat and should not be bulging forward (Figure 12.16).

Lacrimal apparatus. Of the several components of the lacrimal apparatus (lacrimal gland, puncta, lacrimal sac, and nasolacrimal duct), you can normally inspect only the puncta. These pinpoint openings are located near the inner canthus on the upper and lower eyelid margins. They should be just barely visible, with no swelling or redness noted. Check for blockage of the nasolacrimal duct by pressing against the lacrimal sac with your index finger or with a cotton-tipped applicator. Press in toward the lower inner orbital rim, not against the side of the nose (Figure 12.17). Then pull the lower lid down gently over the lower margin of the orbital rim to check for regurgitant material. Normally, there is no regurgitation of material through the puncta.

Iris. Inspect the iris for regular round shape. As noted in the discussion of the anterior chamber, the iris should be flat, not bulging into the anterior chamber.

Pupil. Inspection of the pupils includes assessment of the following four components: size, shape, reaction to light, and accommodation. The pupils are normally round and equal in size. Approximately 5% of people do have a slight but noticeable difference in the size of their pupils. Inequality in the size of the pupils is called anisocoria. Although this condition may be normal, regard the finding with some suspicion until you have completely assessed the health status of the client's eyes. The normal pupil is between 2 and 6 mm in diameter. The size of the pupils varies among individuals exposed to the same amount of light. The pupils tend to be smaller in infancy and older age. Nearsighted persons tend to have larger pupils, whereas farsighted persons tend to have smaller pupils. Pupils of less than 2 mm in diameter are called miotic. Those that are more than 6 mm in diameter are called mydriatic.

To assess the pupillary response to light, bring the beam of a penlight in from the side of the client's head and direct it at one eye at a time. First, observe the pupil toward which you are directing the light. Then glance quickly at the pupil of the other eye. Perform this assessment on each eye. The pupils normally constrict in response to light. There are two pupillary responses to light: direct and consensual. The pupil toward which the light is directed should constrict; this reaction is the direct pupillary response to light. The other pupil

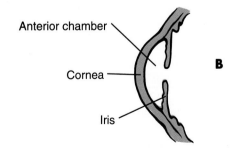

figure **12.16** **A,** Anterior view of the anterior chamber. **B,** Cross section showing a normal anterior chamber. (*A from Seidel HM et al:* Mosby's guide to physical examination, *ed 3, St Louis, 1995, Mosby.*)

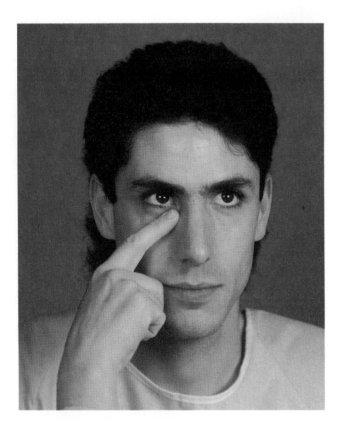

figure**12.17** Examination of the nasolacrimal sac.

should also constrict; this reaction is the consensual response to light. Observe each eye for both direct and consensual response. Normally, both responses are present. The rapidity with which the pupils respond varies among individuals.

> **HELPFUL HINT** *If you are having difficulty seeing the pupillary response, darken the room for a few moments so that the client's pupils will dilate. Shining the light into the client's eye should then show the pupillary constriction more clearly. A bright, sunny room makes it difficult to see the pupils constrict.*

The accommodation response of the pupils consists of convergence of the eyes and constriction of the pupils as the client shifts the glance from a distant to a near object. Ask the client to stare for several moments at an object across the room or at your finger held several feet away from the client. Visualizing a distant object normally causes the pupils to dilate. Then ask the client to switch the gaze to your finger, which you have placed about 6 inches from the client's nose. The normal re-

sponse is pupillary constriction and convergence of the eyes. The rapidity of the pupillary response varies; it is slower in older persons.

Ophthalmoscopic examination. You can inspect the lens, vitreous humor, and retina with the ophthalmoscope (see box on p. 269). Darken the room so that the client's pupils will dilate (this lighting change will make the examination easier to perform). If the client wears corrective lenses, they may be left in place or removed. Try both ways to see which works most effectively for you.

Explain this portion of the examination to the client before you begin. The client's cooperation is essential, since you will be asking him or her to hold the gaze constant and, for part of the examination, to stare into the bright light of the ophthalmoscope.

Ask the client to stare at a fixed point at eye level over your shoulder, such as a light switch or the corner of a picture. Staring at a distant object also helps to dilate the pupils. Tell the client that it is all right to blink, but no more than necessary. If blinking becomes too frequent, you may need to elevate the upper lid and hold it against the upper orbital rim with your free hand. If you elevate the lid, do so for only a few seconds because the cornea can become dry, causing the client discomfort.

Turn on the ophthalmoscope light. Set the lens on 0 diopters. Begin by holding the ophthalmoscope in your right hand with your right index finger on the selector wheel. Hold the aperture of the ophthalmoscope up to your right eye. At a distance of about 12 inches, direct the light toward the client's right eye (Figure 12.20, *A*). When the beam of light falls on the client's pupil, you will see a red reflex, which is a reflection of the color of the retina.

> **HELPFUL HINT** *If you lose sight of the red reflex, you are no longer directing the light through the pupil. Instead, you are directing it on the iris or sclera or away from the eye. If this situation occurs, move your head back from the ophthalmoscope, redirect the beam of light to the pupil, and bring your eye back to the aperture.*

Gradually move in closer to the client's eye until the ophthalmoscope is just a few inches away from the client's eye (Figure 12.20, *B*). Keep the red reflex in your line of vision while turning the selector wheel clockwise toward the positive numbers. This approach enables you to focus on the more anterior structures—the lens and the vitreous body. Both structures should be clear, with no opacities or clouding. Gradually rotate

Ophthalmoscope

The ophthalmoscope (Figures 12.18 and 12.19) is an instrument designed to permit evaluation of certain internal structures of the eye. These structures include the lens, the vitreous humor, and the retinal structures. The ophthalmoscope contains a bright light and lenses of varying magnification that are used to bring the various structures of the eye into focus.

Bring the structures into focus by rotating the lens selector dial until the image becomes clear. You can hold and focus the instrument with one hand (Figure 12.18). Look through the viewing aperture near the top of the ophthalmoscope to focus on the eye structures. Below the viewing aperture is another aperture that shows the number of the lens. The lens numbers go from 0 to +40 when the lens selection dial is rotated clockwise. (These numbers appear in black.) The numbers go to −25 when the lens selection dial is rotated counterclockwise. (These numbers appear in red.) The plus and minus lenses can compensate for nearsightedness or farsightedness in both the examiner and the client. The lens selection dial is located on the side of the ophthalmoscope head. Of the several different apertures, the large full circle of light is used most frequently because it works best for illuminating most of the structures of the eye. (Other apertures that are used less frequently are described in Table 12.2.)

table 12.2 Apertures of the Ophthalmoscope

Aperture	Description
Full aperture	Used most frequently because it provides a wide field of light for retinal examination
Small aperture	Especially useful for examining retina through a small pupil
Red-free filter	A green beam of light is used to examine optic disc for pallor and retina for small hemorrhages
Grid	Used to estimate size of retinal lesions
Slit	Used to examine anterior portion of eye and to determine elevation of retinal lesions

figure**12.18** Holding the ophthalmoscope.

figure**12.19** Ophthalmoscope. *(From Seidel HM et al: Mosby's guide to physical examination, ed 3, St Louis, 1995, Mosby.)*

figure **12.20**   **A,** Ophthalmoscopic examination: finding the red reflex. **B,** Ophthalmoscopic examination: examining the retinal structures.

the selector wheel counterclockwise toward the negative numbers. Look for a structure on the retina, such as the disc or a vessel. When you have found a certain structure, turn the wheel until it is in focus and you can visualize that structure clearly. With a nearsighted person, whose eyeball is more elongated than normal, you will need the more negative lenses in order to focus farther back. With a farsighted client, rotate the wheel toward 0. Focusing has individual variations and depends on the refractive state of both you and the client. If you locate the optic disc first, begin your inspection there. If you find a vessel first, follow that vessel in toward the optic disc. Examine the retinal structures in this order:

1. Optic disc
2. Retinal vessels
3. Retinal background
4. Macular area

Optic disc. Examine the optic disc for size, shape, color, distinctness of its margins, and the physiologic cup. The disc is normally approximately 1.5 mm in diameter and round or slightly oval. It ranges in color from creamy yellow to pink and is lighter than the surrounding retina (see Figure 12.4). The color varies somewhat from one individual to another. The margins of the optic disc are usually sharp and clearly demarcated from the surrounding retina. However, several normal variations occur. Dense pigment deposits may be situated around the disc margins, particularly in dark-complected people. A whitish to grayish crescent of scleral tissue may be located immediately adjacent to the disc, particularly on the temporal side.

The physiologic cup, or physiologic depression, is a small depression just temporal to the center of the optic disc. It normally occupies about one third of the optic disc and is slightly lighter than the remainder of the disc.

The optic disc is a standard measurement device for findings on the retina. For example, a finding can be described as being 2 disc diameters away from the disc itself. Also, the size of the finding can be described in terms of the disc diameter. For example, an abnormality may measure one half of the disc diameter (Figure 12.21).

Retinal vessels. Use the light from the ophthalmoscope to follow each of the four sets of vessels out from the optic disc to the periphery. Inspect the retinal vessels for the following four characteristics:

Color
Arteriolar light reflex
Arteriole-vein (A:V) ratio
Arteriovenous crossing changes

The arterioles are a brighter red and approximately 25% smaller than the veins. The A:V ratio is between 2:3 and 4:5. Usually, the arterioles will have a narrow light reflex from the center line of the vessel. Veins do not show a light reflex. Normally, both arterioles and veins show a gradually and regularly diminishing diameter as they go from the disc to the periphery. They normally cross and intertwine, but where the vessels cross one another, there should be no change in the course or caliber of either vessel. Pulsations are sometimes visible in the veins near the optic disc.

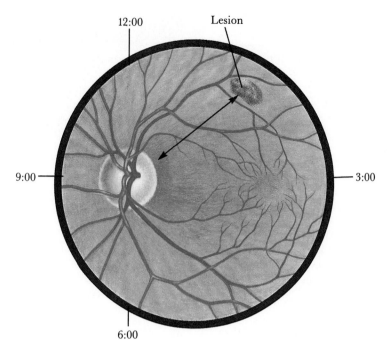

12:00

Lesion

9:00

3:00

6:00

figure**12.21** Method of describing a retinal lesion in terms of the diameter of the optic disc. *(From Seidel HM et al: Mosby's guide to physical examination, ed 3, St Louis, 1995, Mosby.)*

HELPFUL HINT *To follow the course of the retinal vessels out to the periphery and to see more of the retinal background, ask the client to shift the gaze upward, downward, and to each side. This maneuver brings more of the retina into view.*

Retinal background. Inspect the retinal background. It is normally fairly regular in color. Look for any areas that are darker or lighter.

Macular area. Inspection of the macular area should be done at the end of the ophthalmoscopic examination. Ask the client to stare directly at the bright light of the ophthalmoscope. You will then be looking at the macular area. The macula may be so similar in color to the rest of the retinal background that it will be difficult to visualize it as a separate structure, or it may be slightly darker. Learn to do this portion of the retinal examination quickly because the client may feel quite uncomfortable as you direct the bright light at the area of most acute color vision.

The macular area, which is approximately 1 disc diameter in size, is located about 2 disc diameters temporal to the optic disc. At the center of the macula is the fovea centralis. The macula appears as a regularly colored area. A bright spot of light may be reflected from the fovea centralis. The macular area usually has no visible retinal vessels. It is nourished by choroidal vessels and appears slightly darker than the rest of the retinal background.

The retina appears reddish orange because of its deep vascular supply and deeply pigmented layers. The pigment in the posterior layers of the retina also accounts for its slightly stippled appearance. Normally, the color of the retina is uniform, with no patches of light or dark discoloration present.

Screening Tests and Procedures

1. Vision screening to detect amblyopia and strabismus is recommended once for all children before entering school, preferably between ages 3 and 4. Clinicians should be alert for signs of ocular misalignment when examining infants and children.

2. Screening for diminished visual acuity in the elderly with the Snellen visual acuity chart is recommended. There are differences of opinion on the efficacy of vision screening for schoolchildren. In many settings vision screening with the Snellen chart is performed as part of the school physical at required intervals.

3. There is insufficient evidence to recommend routine performance of tonometry by primary care practitioners as an effective screening test for glaucoma. It may be clinically prudent, however, to advise clients at high risk, such as those age 65 or older, to be tested periodically for glaucoma by an eye specialist.

examination step-by-step

Perform examination of the eyes with the client sitting or standing. Equipment needed includes:
Snellen chart
Rosenbaum chart or newspaper
Opaque card or eye cover
Penlight
Cotton-tipped applicator
Ophthalmoscope

A. Measure visual acuity (CN II).
   1. Distant vision using Snellen chart
   2. Near vision using Rosenbaum chart or newspaper
B. Assess visual fields (CN II) using visual fields confrontation test.
C. Assess extraocular muscle function (CN III, IV, VI).
   1. Six cardinal positions of gaze
   2. Corneal light reflex
   3. Cover-uncover test
D. Inspect external eye structures.
   1. Position of globe—normal, protruding, or sunken
   2. Eyelids and eyelashes
      a. Position of eyelids and eyelashes, palpebral fissures
      b. Ability to close lids
      c. Redness, swelling, lumps
   3. Conjunctiva and sclera
      a. Clarity
      b. Eversion of eyelid, if indicated
      c. Redness, discharge
   4. Cornea
      a. Light reflex
      b. Arcus senilis

5. Anterior chamber
   a. Clarity
   b. Depth
6. Lacrimal apparatus
   a. Puncta
   b. Swelling or redness
   c. Regurgitation of material from lacrimal sac
7. Iris
   a. Shape
   b. Fluttering movements
8. Pupil
   a. Size
   b. Shape
   c. Response to light and accommodation
9. Ophthalmoscopic examination
   a. Lens clarity
   b. Red reflex
   c. Optic disc
      (1) Size and shape
      (2) Color
      (3) Margins
      (4) Physiologic cup
   d. Retinal vessels
      (1) Color
      (2) Arteriolar light reflex
      (3) Arteriole/vein ratio
      (4) Arteriovenous crossing characteristics
   e. Retinal background
      (1) Regularity
      (2) Color
      (3) Presence of microaneurysms, hemorrhages, exudates
   f. Macula and fovea centralis
      (1) Regularity
      (2) Color

■ VARIATIONS FROM HEALTH

Variations of Visual Function

Changes in visual function include the following:
1. Diminished visual acuity
2. Decreased vision
3. Blindness
4. Defects in color vision
5. Diplopia (double vision)
6. Faulty adaptation to the dark
7. Visualization of objects within the eye
8. Iridescent vision

Diminished visual acuity

An error of refraction is a common variation from normal vision. It is an inability to focus rays of light on the retina. Common errors of refraction include nearsightedness (myopia), farsightedness (hyperopia), and astigmatism.

Nearsightedness (myopia). In myopia, the eye focuses the image in front of the retina. This situation can occur when the eyeball is too long or the lens is too thick (Figure 12.22, *A*). Nearsighted individuals can see objects that are nearby, but not objects that are far away.

Farsightedness (hyperopia). In hyperopia, the eye focuses the image at a hypothetical distance behind the retina. This situation can occur when the eyeball is too short or the lens is too thin (Figure 12.22, *B*). Farsighted individuals can see objects that are far away but not those that are nearby. As people age, they typically become farsighted as the lens of the eye becomes more rigid, losing its elasticity. The ciliary muscles also be-

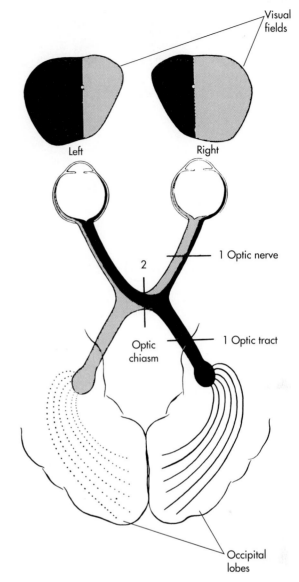

figure**12.22** **A,** The nearsighted, or myopic, eye focuses the image in front of the retina. This condition may occur when the eyeball is too long or the lens is too thick. **B,** The farsighted, or hyperopic, eye can focus the image only at a hypothetical distance behind the retina. This condition may occur when the eyeball is too short or the lens is too thin. *(From Thibodeau GA: Anthony's textbook of anatomy and physiology, ed 13, St Louis, 1990, Mosby.)*

figure**12.23** Visual field defects. *1,* Blind right eye; *2,* bitemporal hemianopia: no temporal vision; *3,* left homonymous hemianopia: no vision in the left field of either eye. *(Modified from Havener WH: Synopsis of ophthalmology, ed 6, St Louis, 1984, Mosby.)*

come weaker, and the lens cannot bulge to accommodate for near vision. This condition is known as presbyopia.

Astigmatism. Astigmatism occurs with uneven curvature of the cornea. Vision is blurred, and use of the eyes may cause discomfort.

Decreased vision

Defects in the field of vision may be caused by lesions of the retina, along the optic nerve, at the optic chiasm (where portions of each nerve cross over to the opposite side), along the optic tract, or in the occipital lobes (Figure 12.23). The resulting defect in vision may be central, peripheral, or specific to portions of the visual fields depending on the nature and location of the lesion. Visual field defects are described according to their location: temporal, nasal, superior, or inferior. The visual field reflects the visual function in the opposite areas of the retina involved. For example, a temporal visual field defect reflects a defect of the nasal retina. A superior field defect reflects an inferior retinal defect. Likewise, an inferior nasal retinal defect would cause a defect in the superior temporal field of vision. The effects of

such lesions on the field of vision are illustrated in Figure 12.24.

Monocular visual defects. If the lesion is located in the retina of one eye or along one optic nerve anterior to the optic chiasm, it affects the vision in that eye.

Bitemporal hemianopsia. Lesions that are found at the optic chiasm, along the optic tract, or in the occipital lobes affect the visual fields of both eyes. This situation occurs because of the crossing and mixing of fibers from both eyes at the chiasm. A lesion at the optic chiasm may be caused by a pituitary tumor. A tumor would produce a loss of vision from the nasal portion of each retina, resulting in a loss of both temporal fields of vision. This condition is called bitemporal hemianopsia.

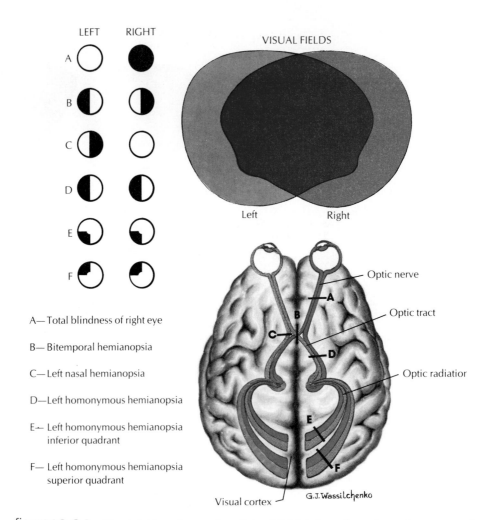

LEFT   RIGHT

VISUAL FIELDS

A

B

C

D

E

F

Left   Right

Optic nerve

Optic tract

Optic radiatior

Visual cortex

G.J.Wassilchenko

A— Total blindness of right eye

B— Bitemporal hemianopsia

C— Left nasal hemianopsia

D— Left homonymous hemianopsia

E— Left homonymous hemianopsia inferior quadrant

F— Left homonymous hemianopsia superior quadrant

figure **12.24** Visual fields and examples of visual field defects along the optic nerve, optic chiasm, optic tracts, and optic radiations in the cortex. *(From Rudy EB: Advanced neurological and neurosurgical nursing, St Louis, 1984, Mosby.)*

Homonymous hemianopsia. Nerve fibers from both eyes mingle behind the chiasm in the optic tracts and in the brain. Lesions along the optic tract or in the temporal, parietal, or occipital lobes will impair the same half of the field of vision in both eyes. For example, a lesion of the right optic tract or the right side of the brain results in visual field defects in the right nasal field and in the left temporal field. Called homonymous hemianopsia, this condition may be caused by occlusion of the middle cerebral artery.

The location of disease on the retina determines the type of resultant visual field defects. Macular defects lead to a central blind area. Localized damage in other areas of the retina causes a loss of vision corresponding to the involved area. A blind spot is called a scotoma. It is an area of blindness surrounded by an area of vision. Advanced diabetic retinopathy may cause macular damage, resulting in a loss of central vision. Increased intraocular pressure, commonly associated with glaucoma, causes decreased peripheral vision. As glaucoma advances, it may also cause a loss of central vision. A retinal detachment causes loss of vision from that portion of the retina where the detachment occurs.

Blindness

A person is considered legally blind when the best visual acuity that can be achieved with corrective lenses in the better eye is 20/200 or less, or when the peripheral visual field is constricted to within 20 degrees. Major causes of blindness in North America are glaucoma, unoperated cataracts, and retinal disorders (mainly diabetic retinopathy and macular degeneration).

Defects in color vision

A variety of conditions may disturb color vision, including diseases of the optic nerve, diseases of the fovea centralis and macular area (where the cones are most concentrated), and nutritional disturbances. In macular

degeneration, the decrease in color vision parallels the loss of visual acuity. The person who is deficient in color vision is unable to see the figures on color plates, which are easily recognizable to the person with normal color vision.

Diplopia

Diplopia, or double vision, occurs whenever the visual axes, the parallel lines of vision, are not directed simultaneously at the same object. It is a cardinal sign of weakness of one or more of the extraocular muscles. Diplopia can be a sign of pressure from a brain tumor or of increased intracranial pressure.

Faulty adaptation to the dark

Night blindness is caused by pigmentary degeneration of the retina, optic nerve disease, glaucoma, or vitamin A deficiency. Deficiency in vitamin A may occur because of inadequate nutrition or cirrhosis of the liver. A client may experience slow recovery of vision during nighttime driving after the headlights of a passing car shine in the eyes.

Visualization of objects within the eye

Translucent specks of various shapes and sizes that float across the visual field and are visible only when the eye is open are called floaters. They are small remnants of the hyaloid vascular system in the vitreous humor. Floaters are visualized as small specks that appear to dart away as the client tries to look at them. Many people experience occasional floaters that have no pathological significance. However, sudden showers of floaters may occur in the periphery of the visual field with vitreous hemorrhage. This occurrence may be the initial symptom of hole formation that precedes retinal separation. The location of the floaters may be helpful in finding the retinal tear. The sudden appearance of a moderately large floater is the main symptom of vitreous detachment. It is important to note that any sudden appearance of floaters is cause for immediate referral to an eye care specialist.

Iridescent vision

Iridescent vision refers to the halos or rainbows that a client sees surrounding bright lights when he or she has corneal edema. This condition may follow a rapid increase in intraocular pressure with acute glaucoma, after prolonged wearing of hard contact lenses, with corneal abrasion, and with cataracts.

Extraocular Neuromuscular Function Variations

Signs of weakness or paralysis of an extraocular muscle or a defect in the nerve supplying it include:

Asymmetrical corneal light reflex

Inability of the eyes to move in a parallel fashion to the six cardinal positions of gaze

Abnormal cover-uncover test

Table 12.3 shows which muscles and cranial nerves are involved when the eye is unable to move to one of the six cardinal positions of gaze.

Examples of the effects of nerve lesions are:

Oculomotor paralysis (CN III): The eye turns down and out, with drooping of the upper lid.

Abducens paralysis (CN VI): The eye turns in toward the nose because of unopposed action of the medial rectus.

Asking the client to look out to the endpoint of the six cardinal positions will exaggerate a defect if one is present. (REMEMBER: The rhythmic twitching motion of nystagmus may be normal at the end of the lateral position, but it is abnormal when the eyes are in any other position.)

Several terms are used to describe weakness of the extraocular muscles:

Phoria: Mild weakness of the extraocular muscles that appears as a deviation of the axes with the cover-uncover test.

Exophoria: Outward (temporal) deviation of the eye.

Esophoria: Inward (nasal) deviation of the eye.

Strabismus: Constant disparity of the eye axes; also termed *tropia.* The two eyes do not focus on an object simultaneously.

Exotropia: Outward (temporal) deviation of the eye.

Esotropia: Inward (nasal) deviation of the eye.

Variations of the Eye and Ocular Structures
Position of the globe of the eye

Exophthalmos. Exophthalmos is a protrusion of the eyeball anteriorly that may be bilateral or unilateral. Bi-

table **12.3** *Muscles and Cranial Nerves Involved When the Eye Is Unable to Move to Cardinal Positions of Gaze*		
Position to which eye will not turn	**Muscle**	**Cranial nerve**
Straight nasal	Medial rectus	III
Up and nasal	Interior oblique	III
Down and nasal	Superior oblique	IV
Straight temporal	Lateral rectus	VI
Up and temporal	Superior rectus	III
Down and temporal	Inferior rectus	III

figure**12.25** Exophthalmos. *(From Stein HA, Slatt BJ, Stein RM: The ophthalmic assistant: a guide for ophthalmic medical personnel, ed 6, St Louis, 1994, Mosby.)*

figure**12.26** Ptosis: drooping upper eyelid. *(From Stein HA, Slatt BJ, Stein RM: The ophthalmic assistant: a guide for ophthalmic medical personnel, ed 6, St Louis, 1994, Mosby.)*

figure**12.27**

figure**12.28** Ectropion. *(From Stein HA, Slatt BJ, Stein RM: The ophthalmic assistant: fundamentals and clinical practice, ed 5, St Louis, 1988, Mosby.)*

lateral exophthalmos is most commonly caused by hyperthyroidism (Figure 12.25). Unilateral exophthalmos may be caused by a tumor located behind the eye. People of Mediterranean or African descent may normally have greater protrusion of the eyes than do Caucasians.

Enophthalmos. Enophthalmos is the backward displacement of the eye in the bony socket, which gives the eyes a sunken appearance. This condition is caused by trauma, starvation, or chronic wasting illness.

Eyelids and eyelashes

Ptosis. With ptosis the eyelid margin is at or below the pupil, and the eyelid appears to be drooping (Figure 12.26). This variation may indicate an oculomotor nerve (CN III) lesion, neuromuscular weakness, or a congenital condition.

Lid lag. When lid lag is present, the eyelid margin is above the limbus, and some sclera is visible (Figure 12.27). This condition may indicate thyroid disease.

Ectropion. In ectropion, the eyelids are loose and roll outward, and the conjunctiva is exposed (Figure 12.28). Tears do not drain through the puncta, and epiphora (tearing) results.

Entropion. In entropion, the eyelids roll inward because of spasm or scar tissue. The lashes may produce corneal irritation. The lower eyelid is usually involved.

Periorbital edema. With periorbital edema, tissue within the eyelid is loosely connected and readily collects excess fluid. The eyelids appear swollen and puffy. This condition may be caused by crying, allergies, heart failure, nephrosis, or thyroid deficiency.

Blepharitis. Blepharitis is a chronic inflammation of the eyelid margins that may begin in childhood and continue intermittently throughout life. It is caused by staphylococcal infection and seborrheic dermatitis. The blood vessels in the eyelid margins become dilated, and the eyelashes become thin, broken, small, and white. Blepharitis is often associated with sties, chalazia, and conjunctivitis.

Hordeolum (sty). A hordeolum (sty) is an infection of the gland of the eyelid. It is located in the hair follicle at the eyelid margin (Figure 12.29). The sty appears painful, red, and swollen.

Chalazion. Chalazion is an infection or retention cyst of the meibomian glands that lies within the posterior portion of the eyelid (Figure 12.30). It is swollen, nontender, firm, and discrete. The skin over the chalazion moves freely.

Xanthelasma. Xanthelasma are raised yellow plaques on the eyelids. They may be a normal variation or may be associated with hypercholesterolemia.

Conjunctiva

Conjunctivitis. Conjunctivitis is an infection or inflammation of the conjunctiva that typically produces

figure**12.29** **A,** Hordeolum, or sty. **B,** Acute sty. (*B from Newell FW: Ophthalmology: principles and concepts, ed 8, St Louis, 1996, Mosby.*)

figure**12.30** **A,** Chalazion. **B,** Chalazion of the right upper eyelid. (*B from Newell FW: Ophthalmology: principles and concepts, ed 7, St Louis, 1992, Mosby.*)

engorgement of the conjunctival vessels and/or a discharge. Clients often experience a foreign body sensation or sensitivity to bright lights. A change in visual acuity is unusual; if present, it is probably due to ocular discharge. Redness of the eye is typically peripheral, not around the limbus. Conjunctivitis may be due to bacterial or viral infections or to allergies. Bacterial conjunctivitis produces a thick, purulent discharge. Viral conjunctivitis typically produces a clear, watery discharge, a burning sensation, photophobia, and sometimes swelling of the lids. Allergic conjunctivitis produces a clear or stringy, mucoid discharge and swollen eyelids.

> **HELPFUL HINT** *If an eyelid infection is present or suspected, you may gently palpate the eyelid surface. Never exert pressure on the eyeball. Use only the bony orbital rims as points over which to slide the eyelids.*

Subconjunctival hemorrhage. This type of hemorrhaging may occur spontaneously or may result from trauma, sneezing, coughing, or lifting. The hemorrhage has sharp borders and appears bright red against the white sclera (Figure 12.31).

Pterygium. Pterygium is an abnormal growth of bulbar conjunctival tissue that usually occurs from the nasal side toward the center of the cornea (Figure 12.32). It may interfere with vision if it covers the pupil.

Pinguecula. Pinguecula, a benign degenerative tumor of the bulbar conjunctiva, appears as a yellowish white, slightly elevated, oval-shaped tissue mass of the cornea. Such tumors, which are usually bilateral and are located on the nasal side, are common with advancing age.

Lacrimal apparatus

Dacryocystitis. Dacryocystitis is an inflammation of the lacrimal sac. Infection and blockage of the lacrimal sac and duct leads to swelling, redness, warmth, and pain below the inner canthus. Pressure on the sac produces purulent discharge through the puncta. To examine for infection in the lacrimal sac, use the examining finger to press against the inner orbital rim, not the nose. Then gently pull the lower eyelid over the lower

figure **12.31** Subconjunctival hemorrhage. *(From Newell FW: Ophthalmology: principles and concepts, ed 8, St Louis, 1996, Mosby.)*

figure **12.32** Pterygium. *(B from Newell FW: Ophthalmology: principles and concepts, ed 8, St Louis, 1996, Mosby.)*

orbital rim to observe for regurgitation of fluid through the puncta. Dacryocystitis is usually unilateral.

Dacryoadenitis. Dacryoadenitis is an inflammation of the lacrimal gland characterized by pain, redness, and swelling developing in the outer third of the upper eyelid. This condition may be associated with mumps, measles, and infectious mononucleosis.

Epiphora. Ectropion, the outward turning of the eyelid, may cause epiphora, or tearing, because of inadequate drainage. Persistent tearing of an infant's eye suggests a blocked tear duct or congenital glaucoma.

Sclera

Changes in the color of the sclera indicate systemic disease.

Scleral icterus. Jaundice manifests its presence in the eyes as a yellow discoloration of the sclera. Excessive bilirubinemia may be evident as scleral icterus before jaundice of the skin becomes apparent.

Bluish sclera. This change is associated with osteogenesis imperfecta, a genetic disorder that involves defective development of the connective tissue and is characterized by abnormally brittle and fragile bones.

Cornea

The cornea is an extremely sensitive structure. Pain and photophobia (sensitivity to light) are common manifestations of corneal disease. Any dullness, irregularities, or opacities of the cornea are abnormal.

Corneal abrasion. This loss of the outer layer of cells of the cornea usually causes severe pain and photophobia. An abrasion may cause the surface to look irregular, but it is usually invisible. The abrasion results from a scratch to the cornea or from improper (usually prolonged) wearing of contact lenses. Since the cornea is

richly supplied with nerve endings, the client with an abrasion feels intense pain and the sensation of a foreign body present. Associated signs include lacrimation, redness, and photophobia. If corneal abrasion is suspected, the client should be referred to an eye care specialist.

Arcus senilis. This extracellular lipid infiltration occurs at the corneal periphery (Figure 12.33). It appears as a grayish white ring around the edge of the cornea separated from the white sclera by a clear interval of 1 mm. Arcus senilis is normal in older people, but in younger clients it may be associated with abnormal lipid metabolism.

Anterior chamber

Abnormalities of the anterior chamber include a decrease in the depth of the chamber and any foreign material that interrupts the normal transparency of the chamber.

Shallow anterior chamber. This characteristic may be a sign of glaucoma, or it may predispose the eye to glaucoma. As increased intraocular pressure causes the iris to become displaced anteriorly, there is less distance between the cornea and the iris. Because of the anterior displacement, light directed obliquely from the tempo-

figure**12.33** Arcus senilis. *(From Newell FW: Ophthalmology: principles and concepts, ed 8, St Louis, 1996, Mosby.)*

figure**12.34** **A,** Anterior view of a normal *(top)* and shallow *(bottom)* anterior chamber. **B,** Cross section of a normal *(top)* and shallow *(bottom)* anterior chamber. *(A from Seidel HM et al: Mosby's guide to physical examination, ed 3, St Louis, 1995, Mosby.)*

ral side illuminates only the temporal side, and the nasal side appears darker or shadowed (Figure 12.34).

Hyphema. Hyphema is an accumulation of blood in the aqueous fluid. It may be caused by trauma or may result from spontaneous hemorrhage. If the hyphema is mild, the red blood cells settle out inferiorly by gravity to a height of a few millimeters. In severe hyphema, the entire anterior chamber may be filled with blood. The blood is bright red in appearance.

Hypopyon. An accumulation of purulent material in the anterior chamber is called hypopyon.

Iris

Iritis. Iritis is an inflammation of the iris. Associated findings include circumcorneal injection (a deep pink to red flush around the cornea), a bulging iris, inequality in the size of the pupils, throbbing pain, photophobia, visual blurring, and a constricted or irregularly shaped pupil. The affected client should be referred to an eye care specialist immediately.

> **HELPFUL HINT** *With iritis, a red flush is present around the iris and cornea. With conjunctivitis, a red flush extends from the periphery toward the iris and cornea.*

Fluttering motion of iris. Removal of the lens takes away the normal support of the iris, leaving it with a tremulous or fluttering motion.

Pupils

Abnormalities of the pupils include alterations in size, shape, and reflexes.

Variations in size and shape

Anisocoria. A difference in the size of the pupils is called anisocoria. Approximately 5% of the population

has a slight but noticeable difference in pupil size. Although this finding may be normal, until the cause is known, it should be regarded with some suspicion because it can be an indication of central nervous system disease.

Dyscoria. Dyscoria is a congenital abnormality affecting the shape of the pupils.

Mydriasis. Mydriasis is an enlargement of the pupils that may result from emotional influences, recent or old trauma, acute glaucoma, a systemic reaction to parasympatholytic or sympathomimetic drugs, or the local use of dilating drops. A unilateral fixed and enlarged pupil may be caused by local trauma to the eye or the head. Oculomotor nerve (CN III) damage results in a pupil that is dilated and fixed; the eye deviates downward and laterally, and the eyelid droops. Fixed dilation of both pupils occurs with deep anesthesia, central nervous system injury, and circulatory arrest.

Miosis. Miosis is constriction of the pupils that is associated with iritis, the use of narcotics, and the use of pilocarpine drops for the treatment of glaucoma.

Variations in reflexes

Argyll Robertson pupil. This condition is a failure of the pupils to react to light with preservation of the accommodation response. It is associated with chronic alcoholism, meningitis, and brain tumor.

Adie's pupil. With this condition, the pupil is dilated and constricts little to light and accommodation. It is often associated with absent deep tendon reflexes in the extremities. The cause of this condition is unknown.

Horner's syndrome. This condition involves sympathetic paralysis of the eye, which includes constriction of the pupil, drooping of the eyelid, and lack of tearing. The paralysis is caused by interruption of the cervical sympathetic chain.

Monocular blindness. In monocular blindness, when light is directed at the blind eye, there is no response to light in either eye. However, when the seeing eye receives illumination, both pupils constrict; this situation occurs because the efferent pupil constriction stimulus via the oculomotor nerve is distributed to both eyes.

Lens

Cataract. A cataract is a gray-white opacity within the lens (Figure 12.35). On ophthalmoscopic examination, the cataract is seen as a dark shadow or black spots within the red reflex or as an absent red reflex because the opacity prevents light from being reflected back to the examiner's eye. Cataracts vary in appearance. They may look like pieces of coral or crystals, or they may have a starlike (stellate) appearance (Figure 12.35, *A*). Cataract formation may accompany aging, or it may be associated with systemic disorders or congenital syndromes.

Senile cataracts occur as a result of various degenerative processes within the lens. These cataracts are the most common type and occur most often after 50 years of age (Figure 12.35, *B*). The tendency to develop cataracts is inherited.

In cataracts associated with diabetes mellitus, the metabolic disturbance results in formation of abnormal lens fiber. These cataracts occur more frequently in young people, are bilateral, progress rapidly, and have a classic snowflake appearance.

Congenital cataracts are usually hereditary. However, they may be caused by viral infection during the first trimester of gestation.

Typical symptoms of cataracts include blurred or cloudy vision, sensitivity to bright light, and, later, distorted or double vision. Untreated cataracts lead to loss of vision.

Retinal structures

Optic disc

Papilledema. Papilledema is a condition characterized by swelling of the optic nerve head that causes the margins of the disc to become blurred and indistinct (Figure 12.36). It is a sign of increased intracranial pressure. This pressure causes decreased venous drainage from the eye and accumulation or leakage of fluid. Papilledema is associated with malignant hypertension, eclampsia of pregnancy, brain tumor, and hematoma.

The nerve head appears to be out of focus with the surrounding retina. The degree of elevation of the optic disc can be assessed by focusing first on the disc and then on the surrounding retina and noting the difference in diopters on the ophthalmoscope.

Cupping of the optic disc. The increased intraocular pressure of glaucoma gradually exerts pressure posteriorly against the optic disc. This pressure causes cupping, an increased posterior curvature of the disc. It may also produce an increase in the cup/disc ratio. The cup may

A   **B**

figure**12.35** Cataract. **A,** Starlike cataract. **B,** Senile cataract. (*A From Donaldson DD:* Atlas of diseases of the eye, *vol 5,* The crystalline lens, *St Louis, 1976, Mosby; **B** from Seidel HM et al:* Mosby's guide to physical examination, *ed 3, St Louis, 1995, Mosby.*)

figure**12.36** Papilledema. (*Modified from Newell FW:* Ophthalmology: principles and concepts, *ed 8, St Louis, 1996, Mosby.*)

enlarge to more than one half the disc diameter. The pressure of glaucoma may also cause pallor of the disc, a sign of optic atrophy.

On ophthalmoscopic examination, cupping may be observed by following carefully the course of the vessels as they emerge over the margin of the optic disc. The increased intraocular pressure causes a vessel to seem to disappear from sight at the disc rim and then to reappear at a slightly different site just past the rim (Figure 12.37).

Cupping of the optic disc and optic atrophy are both late findings of glaucoma. If there is any suspicion of the disease, the client should be referred to an eye care specialist for further testing.

Optic atrophy. Death of the optic nerve fibers leads to the disappearance of the tiny disc vessels that give the disc its normal pinkish color. The affected disc is seen as pale and white, either in a portion of or throughout the disc.

> **HELPFUL HINT** *The scleral crescent, a normal finding, is a pale crescent-shaped area around the rim of the disc only. Do not mistake it for disc atrophy.*

Retinal vessels

Variation in caliber. Variation in the caliber of retinal vessels may occur with hypertension. Since caliber changes may not be evenly distributed along the course of the vessel, it is necessary to follow the vessels out from the disc to the periphery. Arterioles are normally about two thirds to three fourths of the diameter of the corresponding veins. With hypertension, the arterioles may decrease in diameter so that they are only about one half the size of the corresponding vein.

Variation in color. Normally, the color of the vessel is determined by the color of the blood within it. With hypertension, the arterioles may develop sclerotic or sheathing changes, causing them to become opaque and lighter. With arteriosclerosis the width of the light reflex from the arteriolar wall also increases to one third or more of the width of the vessel. In advanced stages the vessels may appear as fine, silvery lines.

Vessel crossing variations. Changes at arteriovenous crossings include an apparent narrowing or blocking of the vein, called nicking, at the point where an arteriole crosses over it (Figure 12.38). This appearance, which is the result of some degree of concealment of the underlying veins by an abnormally opaque arteriole wall, occurs with long-standing hypertension. It is initially apparent as a narrowing or tapering of the vessel at the crossing. Later it appears as a more complete interruption of the vessel.

An embolus in a retinal vessel abruptly impedes the flow of blood and results in the sudden narrowing of an arteriole or dilation of a vein.

Retinal background variations

MICROANEURYSMS. Microaneurysms are outpouchings in the walls of the capillaries that appear as tiny bright red dots on the retina (Figure 12.39). They are frequently associated with diabetes mellitus.

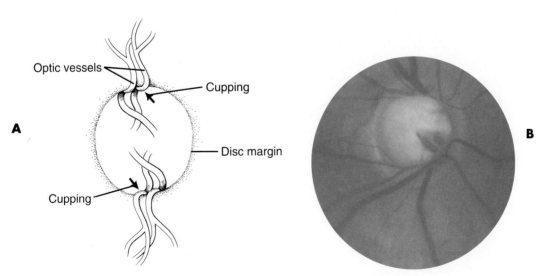

figure **12.37** **A,** Glaucomatous cupping. **B,** Advanced glaucomatous optic atrophy with cupping of the disc and nasal displacement of the retinal vessels. (*B from Newell FW: Ophthalmology: principles and concepts, ed 8, St Louis, 1996, Mosby.*)

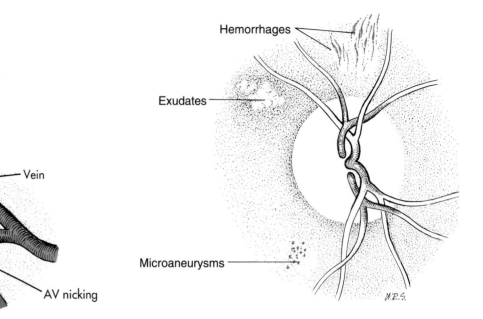

figure**12.38**   Arteriovenous nicking.

figure**12.39**   Microaneurysms.

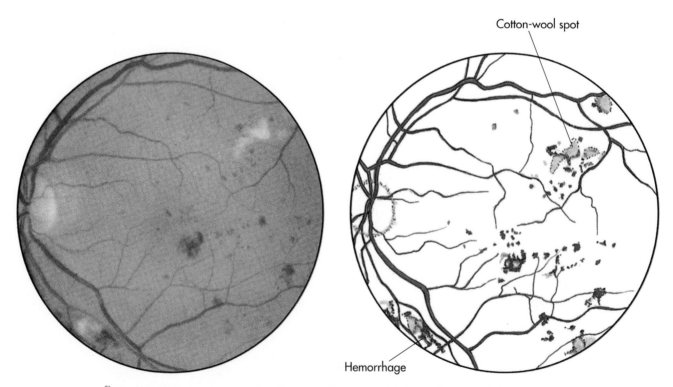

figure**12.40**   Nonproliferative diabetic retinopathy with flame-shaped and dot-blot hemorrhages, cotton-wool spots, and microaneurysms. *(From Yannuzzi LA, Guyer DR, Green WR: The retina atlas, St Louis, 1995, Mosby; courtesy Drs. George Blankenship and Everett Ai and the Diabetes 2000 Program.)*

figure**12.41**   Cotton-wool patches, or exudates, and narrowed arterioles in severe vascular hypertension. *(Modified from Newell FW: Ophthalmology: principles and concepts, ed 7, St Louis, 1992, Mosby.)*

figure**12.42**   Proliferative diabetic retinopathy. *(From Seidel HM et al: Mosby's guide to physical examination, ed 3, St Louis, 1995, Mosby; courtesy John W. Payne, MD, The Wilmer Ophthalmological Institute, The Johns Hopkins University and Hospital, Baltimore, Md.)*

RETINAL EXUDATES. Retinal exudates are whitish yellow infiltrates on the retina (Figures 12.39, 12.40, and 12.41). Both "soft" and "hard" exudates exist. The soft exudates, which look somewhat like a cumulus cloud, are also called "cotton-wool" patches or exudates. Hard exudates have more distinct edges. Retinal exudates are associated with systemic diseases, including diabetes mellitus and hypertension. In addition, they may be associated with inflammatory or degenerative diseases of the retina. Cotton-wool exudates are a common retinal finding in clients with acquired immunodeficiency syndrome (AIDS). Some exudates are resorbed over time.

HEMORRHAGES OF THE RETINA. Retinal hemorrhages are bright to dark red. They may be small and round, as commonly occur with diabetes, or linear and flame shaped, as noted with hypertension (see Figures 12.39 and 12.40).

PROLIFERATIVE DIABETIC RETINOPATHY (Figure 12.42). Numerous new vessels (neovascularization) may proliferate on the retina of a diabetic client. Bleeding from these vessels can lead to blindness.

Retinal changes may affect any part of the retinal background, including the macular area. Changes in central or peripheral vision depend on the location of the lesion.

Variations in Comfort

Numerous relatively minor ocular variations are accompanied by itching, burning, or discomfort of the eyes. These symptoms may result from fatigue, allergy, conjunctivitis, or inadequately corrected refractive error.

Superficial eye pain may be caused by any of the following factors:

Lesion in the eyelid

Foreign body on the cornea or conjunctiva

Loss of corneal or conjunctival epithelium

Deep, severe pain within the eye may result from either of these two conditions:

Inflammation of the iris or ciliary body

Rapid increase in intraocular pressure

Findings accompanying deep eye pain include redness and decreased vision. Immediate referral to an ophthalmologist is required.

Variation in Intraocular Pressure: Glaucoma

Acute glaucoma occurs with a sudden increase in intraocular pressure caused by blocked drainage of aqueous fluid from the anterior chamber.

Findings associated with acute glaucoma include the following:

Intense pain

Photophobia

Blurred vision or halos around lights

Unilateral headache

Diffuse conjunctival injection with a limbal flush

Decreased visual acuity

Dilated pupil that is poorly reactive to light

Cloudy cornea

Shallow anterior chamber

The affected client should be referred to an eye care specialist immediately.

Glaucoma may also be a chronic condition. In this situation symptoms are absent, except for the gradual loss of peripheral vision over a long period of time.

sample**documentation&diagnoses** CRITICAL THINKING

■ FOCUSED HEALTH HISTORY *(SUBJECTIVE DATA)*

Mrs. S., a retired counselor, age 75, states she has noticed that her vision, particularly distant vision, has become increasingly blurred in her right eye over the past 18 to 24 months. Vision in the left eye is unchanged. Reports no pain, itching, inflammation, drainage, or redness in either eye. Wears bifocals—vision is corrected for myopia and presbyopia. Sees an optometrist regularly for eye examinations. Her last eye examination, including a lens prescription, was 2 years ago; new lenses did not correct vision in the right eye as much as previously. Glaucoma testing at that time was normal. Is concerned that her diminished visual acuity is beginning to affect her driving and thus her ability to get together with family and friends, and her ability to read and perform other activities she has enjoyed for many years. Lives alone and is able to care for her own home. History of mild hypertension for 15 years, controlled by diet and medication.

■ FOCUSED PHYSICAL EXAMINATION *(OBJECTIVE DATA)*

Visual acuity: Distant vision (with correction)—OD: 20/100; OS: 20/30. Near vision (with correction)—OD: 20/200 at 14 inches on Rosenbaum; OS: 20/25.
Visual fields: Intact with confrontation test.
Extraocular muscles: Extraocular movements (EOMs) intact; no nystagmus. Corneal light reflex—symmetrical. Cover-uncover test-eyes aligned; no deviation.
External eye: Palpebral fissures equal; lids and lashes normal.
    Conjunctiva: Clear, except for several small blood vessels at cornices.
    Sclera: White.
    Cornea: Clear, bright; arcus senilis present bilaterally.
    Lacrimal apparatus: No excessive tearing; no tenderness.
    Anterior chamber: Iris flat.
    Pupils: Equal, round, react to light and accommodation (PERRLA), though response is somewhat slow.
Ophthalmoscopy
    Red reflex: OS—present; OD—not present (obscured by opacity).
    Lens: OS—clear; OD—cloudy.
    Optic disc: OD—retinal features obscured; OS—optic disc: round, yellowish pink; margins distinct.
    Vessels: OS—arterioles: silver wire appearance; slight nicking of superior temporal vessels, 2 DD from optic disc; A:V ratio: 2:4.
    Retinal background: OS—color regular, no hemorrhages or exudates.

diagnoses

HEALTH PROBLEM
Decreased visual acuity in right eye, possibly due to cataract

NURSING DIAGNOSIS

Sensory/perceptual alteration (visual) related to cataract
Defining Characteristic
  • Presence of uncompensated visual deficits
Related Factors
  • Uncompensated visual loss
  • Early-stage restricted environment

chapter 13

Ears, Nose, Mouth, and Throat

◼ PURPOSE OF EXAMINATION

The examination of the ears, nose, mouth, and throat provides the opportunity to inspect, directly or indirectly, most parts of the upper respiratory system and the first division of the digestive system. Examination of these body orifices provides information about the client's general health and the presence of any local disease. This chapter focuses on three areas: the ears, the nose and paranasal sinuses, and the mouth and oropharynx.

◼ ANATOMY AND PHYSIOLOGY

Ears

The ear is a sensory organ that functions both in hearing and in equilibrium. It is composed of three parts: the external ear, the middle ear, and the inner ear. Figure 13.1 illustrates the structures of the ear.

External ear

The external ear has two divisions: the flap called the auricle, or pinna, and the canal called the external auditory canal, or meatus. Stretching across the proximal portion of the canal is the tympanic membrane (eardrum), which separates the external ear from the middle ear. The auricle is composed of cartilage and skin. The main components of the auricle are the helix, antihelix, crus of the helix, lobule, tragus, antitragus, and concha (Figure 13.2). The mastoid process is not part of the external ear; it is a bony prominence found posterior to the lower part of the auricle.

The external auditory canal, which is approximately 2.2 cm long, has a skeleton of cartilage in its outer third and a skeleton of bone in its inner two thirds. In adults this skeleton curves slightly with the outer one third of the canal and is directed upward and toward the back of the head; the inner two thirds is directed downward and forward. The skin of the outer portion of the auditory

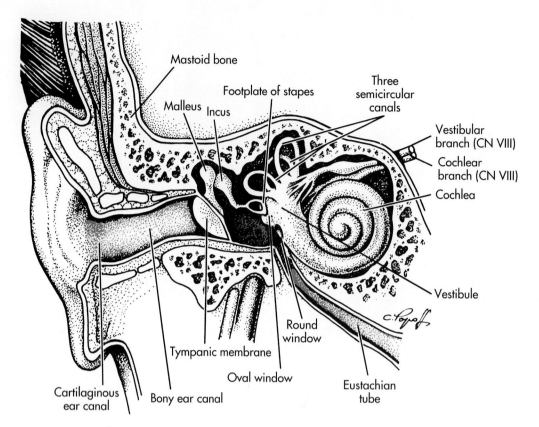

figure **13.1**   External auditory canal, middle ear, and inner ear.

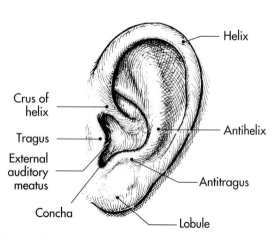

figure **13.2**   Structures of the external ear (pinna).

canal is hairy and contains cerumen (earwax)–producing glands. Ceramen is produced by the sebaceous and apocrine (sweat) glands in the outer third of the lateral auditory canal. The skin of the inner portion of the canal is very thin and sensitive.

Tympanic membrane

The tympanic membrane, which covers the proximal end of the auditory canal, is made up of layers of skin, fibrous tissue, and mucous membrane (Figure 13.3). The mucous membrane is shiny, translucent, and pearl gray. The position of the eardrum is oblique with respect to the ear canal. The anteroinferior quadrant is most distant from the examiner. This positioning results in a reflex of light when a light is directed into the ear. This cone of light is located at the 5 o'clock position in the right ear and at the 7 o'clock position in the left ear.

The tympanic membrane, which is slightly concave, is pulled inward at its center by one of the ossicles of the middle ear, called the malleus. The short process of the malleus protrudes into the eardrum superiorly, and the handle of the malleus extends downward from the short process to the umbo, the point of maximum concavity. Most of the tympanic membrane is taut and is known as the pars tensa. A small part located superiorly is less taut

figure **13.3**   **A,** Usual landmarks of the right tympanic membrane with a "clock" superimposed. **B,** External ear canal partially occluded with cerumen. *(Courtesy Dr. Richard A. Buckingham, Clinical Professor, Otolaryngology, Abraham Lincoln School of Medicine, University of Illinois, Chicago, Ill.)*

and is called the pars flaccida. The dense fibrous ring surrounding the tympanic membrane, except for the anterior and posterior malleolar folds superiorly, is the annulus.

Middle ear

The middle ear is an air-filled cavity located in the temporal bone. It contains three small bones—the malleus, incus, and stapes—which make up the auditory ossicles. The middle ear cavity contains several openings. One, which is from the external auditory meatus, is covered by the tympanic membrane. The two openings into the inner ear are the oval window, into which the stapes fits, and the round window, which is covered by a membrane. Another opening connects the middle ear with the eustachian tube.

The middle ear performs the following three functions:

1. Transmits sound vibrations across the ossicle chain to the inner ear's oval window.
2. Protects the auditory apparatus from intense vibrations.
3. Equalizes the air pressure on both sides of the tympanic membrane to prevent the membrane from being ruptured.

Inner ear

The two components of the inner ear are the bony labyrinth and, inside this structure, a membranous labyrinth. The bony labyrinth consists of three parts: the vestibule, semicircular canals, and cochlea. The vestibule and the semicircular canals are the organs of equilibrium. The cochlea is the organ of hearing. A coiled structure that contains the organ of Corti, the cochlea transmits stimuli to the cochlear branch of the auditory nerve (cranial nerve [CN] VIII).

Pathways of hearing

Hearing occurs when sound waves enter the external auditory canal and strike the tympanic membrane, causing it to vibrate. The auricle does not direct or amplify sound. Its major function is to help perceive the direction of the source of sound (i.e., from behind or ahead). The vibrations are transmitted through the auditory ossicles of the middle ear to the oval window. From the oval window the vibrations travel through the fluid of the cochlea, eventually reaching the round window, where they are dissipated. The vibrations of the membrane cause the delicate hair cells of the organ of Corti to beat against the membrane of Corti, acting as stimuli for impulses carried by the sensory endings of the cochlear branch of the auditory nerve (CN VIII) to the brain.

Nose and Paranasal Sinuses

The nose is the sensory organ for smell. It also warms, moistens, and filters the inspired air. The paranasal sinuses are air-filled cavities that make the skull lighter than it would otherwise be and perform the

same functions as the nose—warming, moistening, and filtering air. These sinuses also aid in voice resonance.

The nose is composed of two parts: external and internal (nasal cavity) (Figure 13.4). The upper third of the nose is bone, and the remainder is cartilage. The nasal cavity is divided into two narrow cavities by the septum (Figure 13.5). The cavities have two openings. The anterior opening, which is the vestibule where the naris is located, is thickly lined with small hairs. The posterior opening, or choana, leads to the throat. The nasal septum forms the medial walls. The lateral walls are divided into the inferior, middle, and superior turbinate bones, which protrude into the nasal cavity. A highly vascular mucous membrane covers the turbinates. Below each turbinate is a meatus named according to the turbinate above it. The nasolacrimal duct drains into the inferior meatus, and most of the paranasal sinuses drain into the middle meatus. A plexus of blood vessels is located in the mucosa of the anterior nasal septum, which is a common site for epistaxis (nosebleeding).

The receptors for smell are located in the olfactory area, which is in the roof of the nasal cavity and the

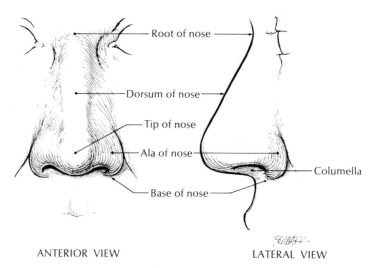

ANTERIOR VIEW   LATERAL VIEW

figure**13.4**   External structure of the nose.

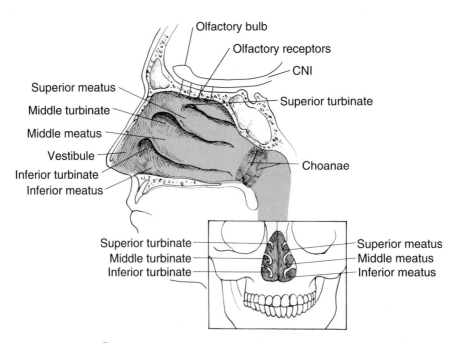

figure**13.5**   Lateral view of the left nasal cavity.

upper third of the septum. The receptor filament cells pass through openings of the cribriform plate, becoming the olfactory nerve (CN I), which transmits neural impulses for smell to the temporal lobe of the brain.

The paranasal sinuses are paired extensions of the nasal cavities within the bones of the skull. They are the frontal, maxillary, ethmoidal, and sphenoidal sinuses (Figure 13.6). Their openings into the nasal cavity are narrow and easily obstructed. The frontal sinuses are located in the anterior part of the frontal bone. The maxillary sinuses, the largest of the paranasal sinuses, are located in the body of the maxilla. The ethmoidal sinuses are small and occupy the ethmoidal labyrinth between the orbit of the eye and the upper part of the nasal cavity. The sphenoidal sinuses are found in the body of the sphenoid.

Mouth and Oropharynx
Mouth

The oropharynx conducts air to and from the larynx and food from the mouth to the esophagus. The structures of the mouth and the oropharynx are illustrated in Figure 13.7. The boundaries of the mouth are the lips (anteriorly) and the soft palate and uvula (posteriorly). The mandibular bone, which is covered by loose, mobile tissue, forms the floor of the mouth. The hard and soft palates comprise the roof of the oral cavity. The soft palate is pink, and the hard palate is lighter. The uvula is a muscular organ that hangs down from the posterior margin of the soft palate. The muscles of mastication (chewing) are innervated by two main nerves: the trigeminal nerve (CN V) and the facial nerve (CN VII). The mouth contains the tongue, gums, teeth, and salivary glands.

Tongue

The tongue is composed of a mass of striated muscles interspersed with fat and many glands. The dorsal surface is rough because of the presence of papillae. The ventral surface toward the floor of the mouth is smooth and shows large veins. The fold of mucous membrane that joins the tongue to the floor of the mouth is called the frenulum. The tongue is innervated by the hypoglossal nerve (CN XII). The sensory receptors for taste are the glossopharyngeal nerve (CN IX) for the posterior third of the tongue and the facial nerve (CN VII) for the anterior two thirds of the tongue.

Gums and teeth

The gums, fibrous tissue covered with a smooth mucous membrane, are attached to the alveolar margins of the jaws and to the necks of the teeth. An adult normally has 32 teeth, 16 in each arch (Figure 13.8).

Salivary glands

Three pairs of salivary glands—parotid, submandibular, and sublingual—secrete into the oral cavity. The largest is the parotid gland, which lies in front of and below the external ear. The parotid (Stensen's) duct opens into the buccal membrane opposite the second molar. The submandibular gland lies below and in

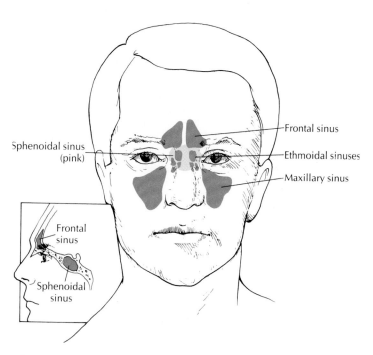

figure **13.6** Anterior view of the frontal and maxillary sinuses.

figure**13.7** **A** and **B,** Structures of the mouth.
C, The mouth and oropharynx.

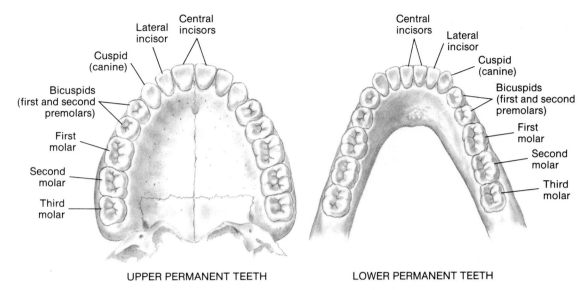

figure 13.8 Upper and lower permanent teeth. *(From Seidel HM et al: Mosby's guide to physical examination, ed 3, St Louis, 1995, Mosby.)*

front of the parotid gland. The submandibular (Wharton's) duct opens at the side of the frenulum on the floor of the mouth. The sublingual gland, the smallest salivary gland, lies in the floor of the mouth and covers its superior surface to form the sublingual fold. The sublingual gland has numerous small openings, which open onto the sublingual fold (see Figure 13.7, *A* and *B*).

Oropharynx

The oropharynx is posterior to the oral cavity and most accessible to examination (see Figure 13.7, *C*). The nasopharynx lies behind the nasal cavities and is superior to the oropharynx. The laryngopharynx is inferior to the oropharynx. Along both lateral walls of the oropharynx are two palatine arches, and between these arches lie the tonsils. The tonsils are usually the same color as the surrounding tissue and do not normally extend beyond the pillars. Tonsillar tissue in children enlarges until puberty, when it shrinks back into the folds of the arches. Consequently, a child's tonsils may normally be larger than an adult's. The posterior pharyngeal wall that is visible during the clinical examination may show many small blood vessels and small areas of pink or red lymphoid tissue.

■ EXAMINATION

Health History

Throughout the health history interview, record the following data about a symptom or problem: (1) onset (specific date, sudden or gradual), (2) duration, (3) frequency, (4) precipitating factors, (5) aggravating or alleviating factors, (6) treatment received or self-care given, and (7) outcome.

Present health status

1. Hearing loss
2. Pain or discomfort in ears, nose, mouth, or throat; pain or pressure around eyes, cheeks, or forehead
3. Drainage from ears or nose
4. Seasonal allergies or allergies to medications or food
5. Condition of teeth and gums—presence of dentures or braces, bleeding gums, ability to chew
6. Reduced ability to smell or presence of unusual odors
7. Unusual tastes or reduced ability to taste
8. Difficulty swallowing
9. Dental hygiene practices; frequency of dental checkups
10. Earwax buildup

Past health history

1. Injury to nose, ears, mouth, or teeth
2. Previous surgery of ears, nose, mouth, or teeth, including tonsillectomy
3. Ringing in ears or dizziness
4. History of frequent nosebleeds
5. History of ear infections

Family health history

1. Family history of hearing loss

PREPARATION FOR EXAMINATION

EQUIPMENT

Item	*Purpose*
Otoscope with various-size speculums	For inspection of tympanic membrane and external auditory canal
Tongue blade	To help visualize oropharynx
4 × 4-inch gauze sponges	To grasp tongue for inspection
Disposable gloves	For palpation of mouth
Tuning fork (512 cycles/sec [cps])	To assess hearing
Penlight	To visualize mouth, nasal turbinates, and oropharynx

OPTIONAL EQUIPMENT

Item	*Purpose*
Dental mirror	To visualize teeth
Nasal speculum	To visualize nasal turbinates

CLIENT AND ENVIRONMENT

The client should be seated near a good light source.

Other considerations

1. Exposure to loud noise
2. Exposure to fumes or dust
3. Use of protective gear for work or hobbies—ear-wear, safety goggles, face mask

Preparation for Examination: Client and Environment

The methods of examination for the ears, nose, mouth, and throat are primarily inspection and palpation.

The client should be seated for this examination. The examiner's head should be at approximately the same level as that of the client. A good light source, such as a gooseneck lamp with a 100- to 150-watt bulb, is helpful.

Tuning fork tests are useful in determining whether the client has a conductive or a perceptive (sensorineural) hearing loss. A fork with frequencies of 512 to 1024 hertz (Hz) is used because it provides an estimate of hearing loss in the speech frequencies of roughly 300 to 3000 Hz. The tuning fork should be held by the base without the fingers touching either of the two prongs. The sound vibrations are softened or stopped entirely when the prongs of the fork are touched or held. The fork is activated by stroking it between the thumb and index finger (Figure 13.9, *A*) or by tapping the tines on the knuckles of the opposite hand (Figure 13.9, *B*). The fork should be made to ring softly.

A   **B**

figure**13.9**   Activating the tuning fork. **A,** Stroking the fork. **B,** Tapping the fork on the knuckle.

Technique for Examination and Normal Findings

Ears

External ear. Begin the examination of the external ear with an inspection of both auricles to determine their horizontal and vertical position, size, and symmetry. The helix should be at or slightly above a line extending from the eye to the occipital area. Next inspect the lateral and medial surfaces of each auricle and the surrounding tissues for skin color and the presence of deformities, lesions, or nodules. Palpate the auricles and mastoid areas for evidence of swelling, tenderness, or nodules.

Manipulation of the auricle can be helpful in detecting tenderness. If pressure on the tragus or gently pulling on the auricle causes pain, the client may have external otitis. Although fairly simple, this part of the examination is frequently neglected (Figure 13.10, *A*).

External auditory canal. Examination of the external auditory canal and tympanic membrane requires an oto-scope for additional lighting (see box on page 294). Before inserting the speculum in the client's ear, carefully inspect the meatus and the auditory canal for cerumen, erythema (redness), swelling, narrowing of the canal, a foreign body, or discharge. Describe the appearance and odor of any discharge.

> **HELPFUL HINT** *For the otoscope to be effective, the batteries should be changed or recharged frequently to ensure good light.*

Inspect the auditory canal for cerumen, erythema, foreign bodies, or swelling. The appearance of the normal canal varies in diameter, shape, and growth of hairs (Figure 13.10, *B*). A small amount of cerumen will not interfere with the examination. You can look past it and visualize the tympanic membrane. However, if cerumen is excessive, removing it may be necessary.

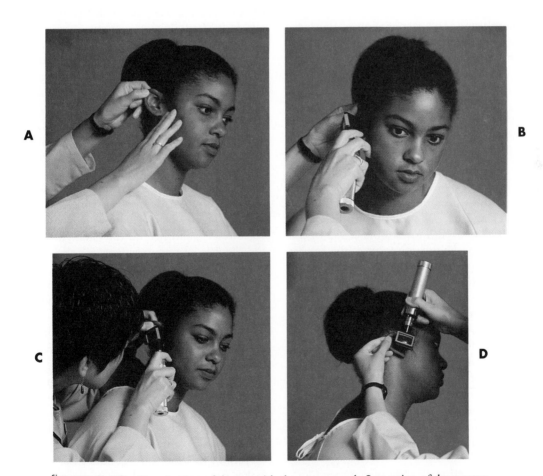

figure **13.10**   Examination of the ear with the otoscope. **A,** Inspection of the meatus. **B,** The client's head is tipped toward the opposite shoulder. **C** and **D,** Two ways of holding the otoscope.

Steps in Using an Otoscope

1. Use the largest speculum that can be inserted in the ear without causing pain.
2. Tip the client's head away from you for easy examination of the canal and the tympanic membrane.
3. In adults, straighten the ear canal by pulling the auricle upward and backward. In young children and infants, straighten the canal by pulling the auricle downward (see Figure 25.41).

4. The inner two thirds of the external meatus is very sensitive to pressure. Insert the speculum gently to minimize discomfort.
5. Vary the angle at which you insert the speculum into the meatus to obtain the best view of the tympanic membrane.

> **HELPFUL HINT** *Racial variations in the color of cerumen occur. Black or brown cerumen will be noted in the client with dark skin coloring. The color of fresh cerumen is light yellow or even pink, as compared with older, drier cerumen, which is a darker yellowish brown.*

Tympanic membrane. The examination of the tympanic membrane (see Figure 13.3, *A*) requires a careful assessment of the color of the membrane and the identification of landmarks. The membrane is usually translucent pearl gray, but when disease is present, it may be yellow, white, red, or dull gray. Some membranes have white flecks or dense white plaques, which are the result of healed inflammatory disease.

Identify landmarks, beginning with the light reflex, which is a triangular cone of reflected light seen in the anteroinferior quadrant of the membrane. This landmark is at the 5 o'clock position on the right tympanic membrane and at the 7 o'clock position on the left. At the top point of the light reflex toward the center of the membrane is the umbo, the inferior point of the handle of the malleus. Anterior and superior to the umbo lies the long process of the malleus, which appears as a whitish line extending from the umbo to the malleolar folds, where the short process of the malleus can be seen. The malleolar folds and the pars flaccida, the relaxed portion of the membrane, are superior and lateral to the short process, respectively. Finally, observe the periphery of the pars tensa. Perforations are frequently noted in the areas close to the annulus.

Normal tympanic membranes vary in size, shape, and color. By examining many normal, healthy membranes, an examiner acquires the ability to recognize the abnormal membrane.

Testing auditory function. Testing of auditory function starts early in the physical examination. Because the client's understanding of the spoken word is the principal use of hearing, an impairment of auditory function may become apparent during the interview. Specific testing of auditory function should be delayed until the end of the examination, after any obvious problems related to hearing have been identified. Although the precise measurement of hearing requires the use of the audiometer, a good estimate of hearing during the physical examination can be made by using the tests discussed in the following sections.

Auditory acuity. Simple assessment of auditory acuity requires that only one ear be tested at a time. Therefore it is necessary to mask the hearing in the ear not being tested. Occlude (or have the client occlude) one of the client's ears by gently placing a finger against the opening of the auditory canal.

Voice tests are frequently used to estimate the client's hearing. Begin testing with a very low whisper. Your lips should be 30 to 60 cm (1 or 2 feet) away from the client's unoccluded ear. Softly whisper numbers that the client is to repeat. If necessary, increase the intensity of the whispered voice. To prevent lipreading during the voice tests, stand behind the client. If being in front of the client is more convenient, ask the client to close his or her eyes.

Air conduction is the transmission of sound through the ear canal, tympanic membrane, and ossicles to the cochlea and the auditory nerve. Bone conduction is sound transmitted through the bones of the skull to the cochlea and the auditory nerve. The client with normal auditory function will hear sound twice as long by air conduction, when the tuning fork is held near the external meatus, than by bone conduction, when the base of the tuning fork is placed on the mastoid bone. Explain these tests to the client before the examination so that he or she can fully cooperate.

Tuning fork tests. To conduct the Weber test, which makes use of bone conduction, place the base of the vibrating tuning fork on the vertex of the skull or on the

table 13.1 *Hearing Tests Using a Tuning Fork*

Hearing	Weber (bone conduction)	Rinne (air and bone conduction)

Normal

Sound is heard equally well in both ears; no lateralization

Air conduction (AC) is heard twice as long as bone conduction (BC); AC:BC 2:1

Conduction loss (problem of external or middle ear, e.g., cerumen buildup or oritis media)

Sound lateralizes to defective ear because it is transmitted through bone rather than air.

Bone conduction is heard longer than air conduction; BC > AC

Sensorineural loss (perceptive problem of inner ear or nerve)

Sound lateralizes to better ear

Air conduction is heard longer than bone conduction (AC > BC) but duration is less than 2:1

figure**13.11** Weber test.

forehead (Figure 13.11). Ask the client if the sound is clearer in one ear or in the other. In a normal Weber test, the client reports hearing sound equally in both ears. In lateralization, sound is detected differently in each ear. In conductive deafness, the sound is lateralized (heard louder) to the deafer ear (Table 13.1). This situation occurs because extraneous sounds in the environment will not disturb the cochlea on the weaker side. Sound is not transmitted because of a problem or defect in the ear canal or middle ear. In sensorineural hearing loss, the sound lateralizes to the better ear because the cochlea or auditory nerve is functioning.

The Rinne test makes use of air conduction and bone conduction. The tuning fork is used to compare the conduction of sound through the mastoid bone and the auditory meatus (Table 13.1). The client who has no conductive hearing loss will hear the sound twice as long (2:1) by air conduction (AC) as by bone conduction (BC). This normal pattern is called a positive Rinne test, recorded as AC > BC or AC : BC = 2:1.

To perform the Rinne test, place the activated tuning fork against the mastoid bone until the client can no longer hear the sound. Then move the fork close to the auditory meatus. The client with no conductive hearing loss will continue to hear the sound by air conduction. A negative Rinne test, a finding in conductive hearing loss, occurs when the client hears sound through bone

A

B

figure**13.12** Rinne test. **A,** Bone conduction. **B,** Air conduction.

conduction as long as or longer than air conduction (AC = BC or AC < BC) (Figure 13.12).

Data from both tests need to be considered together to determine conductive or sensorineural loss. Tuning fork test results are difficult to interpret when hearing loss is mixed.

Nose and paranasal sinuses

Inspect the external portion of the nose for any deviations in shape, size, or color. Check the nares for flaring or discharge. Palpate the ridge and soft tissues of the nose for displacement of the bone and cartilage and for tenderness or masses (Figure 13.13).

Examination of the nasal function includes determination of the ability to smell and the patency of the nasal cavities. To determine patency, ask the client to breathe in through the nose while you occlude one naris with a finger. Repeat the procedure to determine the patency of the opposite naris. To determine the ability to smell, ask the client to close the eyes. Occlude one naris again. Place an aromatic substance, such as coffee or alcohol, close to the client's nose and ask the client to identify the odor. Test each side separately. Olfaction is not routinely tested in a screening examination unless a client describes a change or loss in the ability to smell.

To examine the nasal cavities, use an otoscope with the short, broad nasal speculum. Alternatively, use a penlight to shine a light while using your nondominant thumb to push the tip of the nose upward. The second method is easier to perform and more comfortable for the client (Figure 13.14).

Examination of the nasal cavity through the anterior naris is limited to the vestibule, the anterior portion of the septum, and the inferior and middle turbinates. When the client's head is tipped back, the inferior and middle turbinates can be seen (Figure 13.15). Inspect the septum for deviation, exudate, and perforation. Asymmetry of the nasal septum is normal. Examine the lateral walls of the nasal cavities and the inferior and middle turbinates for polyps, swelling, exudate, and color. The nasal mucosa is normally redder than the oral mucosa. Increased redness indicates infection. Pale turbinates are typical of allergy, whereas redness with edema may indicate localized irritation.

Describe any drainage from the middle meatus, which drains several of the paranasal sinuses. Carefully inspect the floor of the vestibule for evidence of a foreign body. Note the character of nasal secretions. The normal nasal secretion is mucoid. Watery secretions may indicate an acute upper respiratory tract infection or an allergic rhinitis. Purulent, crusty, or bloody secretions are abnormal.

Examination of the paranasal sinuses is performed indirectly. Inspection, percussion, and palpation of the

figure **13.13** Palpation of the external nose.

figure **13.14** Examination of the anterior nasal cavity. Examiner thumb pressure on the tip of the nose enhances visualization.

figure**13.15** Examination of the anterior nasal cavity—view of the inferior and middle turbinates.

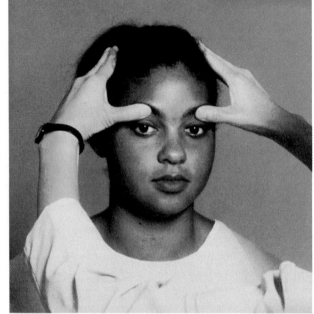

A

overlying tissues and transillumination are used. Only the frontal and maxillary sinuses are accessible for examination. Palpate or percuss the maxillary sinuses over the maxillary areas of the cheeks to elicit any tenderness. By palpating both cheeks simultaneously, it is possible to determine differences in tenderness. Palpate the frontal sinuses by applying finger pressure below the eyebrows (Figure 13.16). Then percuss both the maxillary and the frontal sinuses for tenderness by lightly tapping the area with the index finger.

B

figure**13.16** Palpation of the frontal (**A**) and maxillary (**B**) sinuses.

figure**13.17** Palpation of the temporomandibular joint.

Mouth and oropharynx

Inspect the lips for symmetry, color, edema, or surface abnormalities. Ask the client to open and close the mouth to demonstrate the mobility of the mandible and the occlusion of the teeth. While the client's mouth is opened wide and then closed, palpate the temporomandibular joint for tenderness, crepitus, or deviation (Figure 13.17). Pressure applied to the joint during closing of the mouth may result in referred pain to the ear, often caused by malocclusion. Palpate the lips for induration.

The oral mucosal surfaces are normally light pink and moistened by saliva. Examine the surfaces systematically to ensure that you inspect all areas (Figure 13.18). Use a tongue depressor or your fingers as retractors. With the client's mouth partially open, inspect the mucosa in

figure**13.18** Examination of the lips and oral mucosa. **A,** Palpation of the lips. **B** and **C,** Inspection of the mucosa of the upper and lower anterior area. **D,** Inspection of the mucosa of each cheek with identification of Stensen's duct opening.

the anteroinferior area between the lower lip and gum. With the client's mouth wide open, examine the buccal mucosa and Stensen's duct (the opening to the parotid gland, opposite the upper second molar) of each cheek for patency or inflammation. Next examine the maxillary mucobuccal fold between the upper lip and gum.

HELPFUL HINT *A good source of additional light is essential for examination of the mouth and throat. If the client wears dentures, ask him or her to remove them for the remainder of the examination.*

Inspect the tongue for swelling, variation in size or color, coating, or ulceration. To test the function of the hypoglossal nerve (CN XII), ask the client to extend the tongue and observe for deviation, tremor, or limitation of movement. To inspect the posterior and lateral areas of the tongue, hold the extended tongue with a gloved hand (Figure 13.19). A 4 × 4–inch piece of gauze wrapped around the tip will make this step easier. Move the tongue to each side to inspect the lateral borders. Release the tongue and ask the client to touch the tip of the tongue to the palate. Observe the ventral surface for swelling or varicosities. Inspect the floor of the mouth for abnormalities or swelling. Identify Wharton's ducts (the openings of the submandibular glands), the frenulum, and the sublingual ridge. Because some abnormalities cause little change in the surface and can be detected only by palpation, use a gloved hand to palpate the entire tongue and floor of the mouth carefully.

The examination of the teeth and gums is not a substitute for a dental examination, but it should reveal gross problems that need attention. Use a dental mirror to reflect the surfaces of the teeth and gums that are not readily visible. Systematically inspect the teeth for decay (caries), missing teeth, and malocclusions. Any soft discolorations on the crown of a tooth should be suspected as carious. Inspect the gums for signs of inflammation and hemorrhage (gingivitis). With the client's head tipped back, inspect the palate and the uvula. Depressing the base of the tongue with a tongue blade may be necessary to visualize these structures better. Note the difference in color of the hard and the soft palate and any abnormality of architecture. Ask the client to say "ah," and note the rise of the soft palate and uvula. Any lack of, or asymmetry of, movement indicates impairment of the vagus nerve (CN X) or the glossopharyngeal nerve (CN IX).

These cranial nerves are also tested by touching the posterior wall of the pharynx on each side. The normal response to the second method is a gag reflex.

HELPFUL HINT *When examining the throat, ask the client to open wide and say "ah" with the tongue extended. Most people will be able to lower the tongue and open sufficiently to allow visualization of the pharynx. Use a tongue blade only if necessary, because many clients will involuntarily gag when an object is placed in the mouth. Ask a child to take a deep breath with the mouth open to flatten the tongue.*

Inspect the oropharynx and anterior and posterior arches for inflammation or swelling. Describe the size of the tonsils and note any exudate or postnasal discharge. Note the color of the posterior wall of the oropharynx.

Throughout the examination of the mouth and throat, note any mouth odors, which may result from systemic or oral disease.

Special maneuvers
Cerumen removal

Irrigation is the preferred method for removing cerumen (earwax) buildup. Curettage is indicated if the cerumen is soft or if the tympanic membrane might be perforated. However, this maneuver should be done only by a skilled clinician using an instrument called a curette or a cerumen spoon. The closeness of blood vessels and nerves to the surface of the auditory canal makes it easy to cause bleeding and pain. The risk also

figure**13.19** Examination of the tongue.

examination *step-by-step*

Ears

Inspection

1. Observe the position and shape of the auricle.
2. Whisper in each ear separately at a distance of 30 to 60 cm and have the client repeat what you whispered.
3. Apply a vibrating tuning fork to the middle of the forehead, asking the client to identify in which ear the sound or vibration is heard louder (Weber test) or if it is heard equally in both ears.
4. Apply the vibrating tuning fork to the mastoid process and instruct the client to tell you when the sound stops. Then move the tuning fork close to the auditory meatus. Time the duration in seconds or by the ratio of sound perceived by bone and air conduction (Rinne test). For example, if the bone conduction was heard for 30 seconds and air conduction was heard for 60 seconds, record "AC:BC 2:1 or AC > BC."

Palpation

1. Palpate the pinna, tragus, and mastoid processes for tenderness, lesions, or masses.

Otoscopic Examination

1. Observe the condition of the auditory canal.
2. Note the color of the tympanic membrane.
3. Locate landmarks on the tympanic membrane (e.g., cone of light reflex, umbo, long and short processes of malleus, pars tensa, pars flaccida, and annulus).

Nose and Paranasal Sinuses

Inspection

1. Observe the face for symmetry or swelling from a front and profile view.

Percussion

1. Directly percuss over the maxillary areas of both cheeks and over the middle of each eyebrow to assess tenderness.

Palpation

1. Apply pressure over the maxillary areas of both cheeks and below the eyebrows to assess tenderness.

Mouth and Throat

Inspection

1. Using a tongue blade, penlight, and gloves, inspect the lips, gums, teeth, buccal mucosa, sublingual areas, tongue, parotid duct openings, hard palate, pharnyx, and tonsils for color, condition, and presence of lesions.
2. Observe movement of the soft palate and uvula when the client says "ah."

Palpation

1. With gloved hands, palpate with fingers over the lips and sublingual area to assess for tenderness or lumps.

---

exists of perforating the tympanic membrane if the client moves or if the curette is used too vigorously. Use irrigation when the cerumen is dry and hard, but do not irrigate if the tympanic membrane might be perforated. Use lukewarm water for the irrigation, which is done by repeatedly injecting the water from a syringe toward the posterosuperior canal wall. This procedure may make the client feel dizzy.

Nasal speculum

To use a nasal speculum for inspection of the nasal mucosa and the turbinates, hold the instrument in the nondominant hand and place the index finger on the side of the client's nose to stabilize the position of the speculum. Use the dominant hand to position the client's head and hold the light. Be careful not to apply pressure on the nasal septum because of its great sensi-

tivity. However, open the blades of the nasal speculum as far as possible (see Figure 13.15). Ask the client to tilt the head back. This change in position increases visualization of the middle turbinate.

■ VARIATIONS FROM HEALTH

External Ear

Otitis externa, or "swimmer's ear," is an infection of the external auditory canal. It is most often caused by trauma to the ear canal from cleaning ears with sharp objects or from a moist environment, such as swimming, which favors bacterial or fungal growth. The meatus of the external ear canal is often swollen shut, and foul-smelling discharge may be present. Manipulation of the pinna of the affected ear causes pain.

Tympanic Membrane

Fluid in the middle ear may sometimes be identified by air bubbles or a fluid level seen through the tympanic membrane (Figure 13.20, *A*).

Bulging of the tympanic membrane may occur when fluid forms in the middle ear. The pressure increases, and the membrane may bulge outward, obliterating some or all of the landmarks. The light reflex may be lost or displaced, and the membrane appears amber or a dull blue-gray.

Increased pressure in the middle ear or trauma can cause a perforation of the membrane (Figure 13.20, *C* and *D*).

Retraction of the tympanic membrane occurs when pressure is reduced from obstruction of the eustachian tube, usually associated with an upper respiratory system infection or allergies. The retraction of the membrane accentuates the landmarks. The light reflex may appear less prominent.

Acute otitis media (AOM) (Fig. 13.20, *B*) is the most common cause of ear pain in children, with most cases of AOM occurring in children under 6 years of age. AOM with effusion refers to inflammation of the tympanic membrane with a collection of fluid in the middle ear that results in a visible fluid line or bulging of the tympanic membrane. AOM often occurs after an upper respiratory tract infection. Symptoms include severe earache of sudden onset. Pain may be suddenly relieved if the pressure creates a rupture of the tympanic membrane with drainage of the fluid from the middle ear.

Inner Ear Disorders

Meniere's disease affects the vestibular labyrinth, leading to sensorineural hearing loss. Symptoms are episodic and include a sensation of fullness in one ear with some hearing loss, tinnitus, and severe vertigo. Hearing improves after an attack but deteriorates over time.

Labyrinthitis is an inflammation of the labyrinthine canal of the inner ear and occurs as a complication of an upper respiratory tract infection. Symptoms include vertigo that is more severe with head movement.

Nose

Allergic rhinitis is a recurrent pattern of symptoms of rhinorrhea, sneezing, and pruritis caused by exposure to

figure**13.20** **A,** Air fluid levels in the upper middle ear. **B,** Acute otitis media—red, bulging membrane with loss of bony landmarks and light reflex. **C,** Centrally perforated tympanic membrane. **D,** Perforated membrane that has healed. (*Courtesy Dr. Richard A. Buckingham, Clinical Professor, Otolaryngology, Abraham Lincoln School of Medicine, University of Illinois, Chicago, Ill.*)

an allergen. Nasal turbinates are pale and swollen (Figure 13.21).

Mouth

Pyorrhea is a serious periodontal disease involving the bones and ligaments that anchor the tooth in its socket (Figure 13.22). Note stains, tartar (calculus), or loose teeth as signs of periodontal disease.

Malocclusion is present when two teeth occupy the space for one, teeth overlap, and/or missing teeth create wide spaces. As a result, the lower front teeth are positioned outside the upper front teeth (underbite), or the upper front teeth protrude and hang over the lower front teeth (overbite). Normal occlusion or malocclusion can be demonstrated at oral examination while palpating the temporomandibular joint during opening and closing of the mouth (Figure 13.23).

An exostosis (torus palatinus) is frequently found in the midline of the posterior two thirds of the hard palate (Figure 13.24). This smooth, symmetrical bony structure results from the down-growth of the palatine processes. This type of growth is benign.

The uvula may be bifid and part of a submucosal cleft palate.

Additional variations from health noted in the mouth are shown in Figures 13.25 through 13.27.

Pharynx

Pharyngitis is an inflammation of the mucous membranes of the pharynx, usually of viral or bacterial origin. The posterior pharnyx is erythematous and sometimes has a white coating (exudate). Tonsils, if present, are enlarged (Figures 13.28 and 13.29).

Paranasal Sinuses

Sinusitis is an infection or inflammation of one or more of the paranasal sinuses. Examination reveals tenderness to palpation or percussion over one or more of the sinuses. The nasal mucosa is swollen, pale, or dull red.

figure **13.22** Advanced pyorrhea. (*From DeWeese DD et al:* Otolaryngology—head and neck surgery, *ed 7, St Louis, 1988, Mosby.*)

figure **13.23** Malocclusion. (*From Seidel HM et al:* Mosby's guide to physical examination, *ed 3, St Louis, 1995, Mosby; courtesy Drs. Abelson and Cameron, Lutherville, Md.*)

figure **13.24** Exostosis. (*From Prior JA, Silberstein JS, Stang JM:* Physical diagnosis: the history and examination of the patient, *ed 6, St Louis, 1981, Mosby.*)

figure **13.21** Allergic rhinitis.

figure**13.25** Epidermal carcinoma—lip. *(Courtesy Dr. Edward L. Applebaum, Head, Department of Otolaryngology, University of Illinois Medical Center, Chicago, Ill.)*

figure**13.26** Drug reaction—tongue. *(Courtesy Dr. Edward L. Applebaum, Head, Department of Otolaryngology, University of Illinois Medical Center, Chicago, Ill.)*

figure**13.27** Smooth tongue resulting from vitamin deficiency. *(From Seidel HM et al: Mosby's guide to physical examination, ed 3, St Louis, 1995, Mosby.)*

figure**13.28** Acute viral pharyngitis. *(Courtesy Dr. Edward L. Applebaum, Head, Department of Otolaryngology, University of Illinois Medical Center, Chicago, Ill.)*

figure**13.29** Tonsillitis, pharyngitis. *(Courtesy Dr. Edward L. Applebaum, Head, Department of Otolaryngology, University of Illinois Medical Center, Chicago, Ill.)*

sample documentation&diagnoses   CRITICAL THINKING

■ FOCUSED HEALTH HISTORY *(SUBJECTIVE DATA)*

Mr. B., a 19-year-old black male, complains of experiencing a sore throat for the past 2 days. The discomfort is described as a dull ache that increases in intensity with swallowing. Client has also noticed clear mucus draining from his nose since yesterday. Has taken acetaminophen 650 mg prn for symptoms but without relief. Discomfort is slightly relieved with throat lozenges. Denies earaches, otorrhea, lethargy, or cough. Reports that his girlfriend has had similar symptoms for the past week.

■ FOCUSED PHYSICAL EXAMINATION *(OBJECTIVE DATA)*

Ears: Auricles properly positioned without lesions or tenderness on palpation. Able to hear whispered voice bilaterally at 15 feet. Weber and Rinne tests not done. Otoscopic examination reveals small amount of yellow in each ear; tympanic membranes pearly gray with slight injection. Cone of light in proper position.

Nose: Nasal septum slightly deviated to left. Nostrils patent bilaterally. Mucosa of inferior and middle turbinates pale pink with clear liquid mucus present. Frontal and maxillary sinuses nontender to percussion and palpation.

Mouth and throat: Lips dry and cracked. Gums pink and firm. Teeth in good repair and alignment. Tongue midline with thin white coating, no lesions. Buccal mucosa pink without lesions. Parotid and submaxillary gland orifices without swelling. Tonsils absent. Soft palate rises symmetrically on phonation. Uvula midline. Oropharynx reveals erythematous mucosa with lymphedema of posterior pharynx. No exudate visible.

diagnoses

HEALTH PROBLEM

Pharyngitis

NURSING DIAGNOSES

Impaired swallowing related to irritated oropharyngeal cavity
Defining Characteristics
- Observed evidence of difficulty in swallowing
- Complaints of pain when swallowing
- Edema of oropharyngeal cavity

Pain related to biological injuring agent of oropharyngeal cavity (pharyngitis)
Defining Characteristic
- Communication of pain when swallowing

Breasts and Regional Lymphatics

■ PURPOSE OF EXAMINATION

Breast examination is part of the assessment of sexual development and reproductive function. Because cancer of the breast is a major cause of morbidity and mortality in women, and because early detection and treatment of breast cancer improves survival rates, the breast examination is an important component of screening for cancer and an opportunity to teach breast self-examination.

Breast examination and the teaching of breast self-examination are essential components of health assessment for all women after puberty. Breast examination offers an excellent opportunity for breast and reproductive health education and for the identification of minor problems that would be amenable to early intervention, as well as the identification of breast cancer, which can occur in women of all ages.

Screening for breast cancer is the focus of one of the national health promotion and disease prevention objectives proposed in *Healthy People 2000* (U.S. Department of Health and Human Services, 1991). The objective is to increase (1) to at least 80% the proportion of women age 40 and older who have ever received a clinical breast examination and a mammogram, and (2) to at least 60% those age 50 and older who have received these screening tests within the preceding 1 to 2 years. (Baseline: 36% of women age 40 and older "ever" in 1987; 25% of women age 50 and older "within the preceding 2 years" in 1987.)

■ ANATOMY AND PHYSIOLOGY

The breast is a modified sebaceous gland that is paired. It is located on the anterior chest wall between the second and third ribs (superiorly), the sixth and seventh costal cartilages (inferiorly), the anterior axillary line (laterally), and the sternal border (medially). The breast is composed of three types of tissue: (1) glandular tissue; (2) fibrous tissue, including suspensory ligaments; and (3) adipose tissue. Subcutaneous and retromammary fat compose much of the bulk of the breast. The breast, which is fairly mobile, is supported by a layer of subcutaneous connective tissue and by Cooper's ligaments (Figure 14.1, *B*). The latter are multiple fibrous bands that begin at the breast's subcutaneous

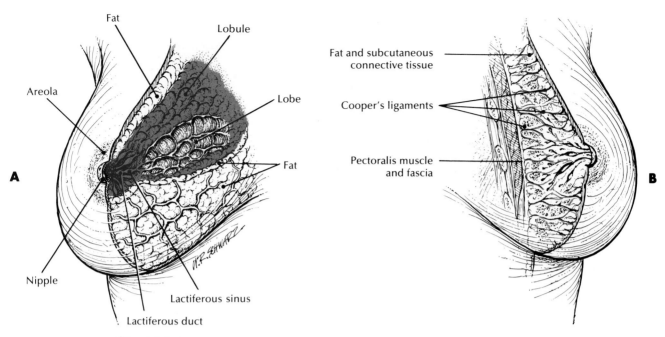

figure**14.1** Female breasts. **A,** Internal structures. **B,** Supportive tissue structures.

connective tissue layer, run through the breast, and are attached to muscle fascia.

The functional components of the female breast are the acini (milk-producing glands), a ductal system, and a nipple (Figure 14.1, *A*). The glandular tissue units, called lobes, are situated in a circular, spokelike fashion around the nipple and are embedded in adipose tissue. Each breast has 15 to 25 lobes. A lobe is composed of 20 to 40 lobules, each containing 10 to 100 acini. Lactiferous ducts drain milk or other fluid from the lobes to the surface of the nipples. The nipples, composed of epithelium intertwined with circular and longitudinal smooth muscle fibers, are located centrally on the breasts. These muscle fibers contract in response to tactile, sensory, and autonomic stimuli, producing erection of the nipple and emptying of any material in the lactiferous ducts. The nipples are round, hairless, pigmented, protuberant structures. Their size, color, and shape vary among women and in an individual woman, depending on the state of contraction. Usually nipples are directed, "pointing" slightly upward and laterally. This position of the nipples places them in an ideal angle for breast-feeding an infant.

Inversion of the nipple is an invagination or depression of its central portion. Inversion can occur congenitally or as a response to an invasive process. The areolae are pigmented areas surrounding the nipples. Their color varies from pink to brown, and their size differs greatly among individuals. Several to many sebaceous glands, termed Montgomery's glands (also called tuber-

cles or follicles), appearing as small bumps, may be present on the areolar surface.

The largest portion of glandular breast tissue is found in the upper lateral quadrant of each breast. From this quadrant there is a cone-shaped anatomical projection of breast tissue into the axilla. This projection is termed the axillary tail of Spence (Figure 14.2). The majority of breast tumors are located in the upper lateral breast quadrant and in the tail of Spence.

On general appearance, the normal breasts are reasonably symmetrical in size and shape, although they are not usually absolutely identical. This symmetry remains constant at rest and with movement. The skin of the breast is the same as that of the abdomen or back. In adults a small number of hair follicles may be scattered around the areola. In light-complected persons a horizontal or vertical vascular pattern may be observed. This pattern, when normally present, is symmetrical.

During early embryonic development, longitudinal ridges appear, extending from the axilla to the groin. Called "milk lines" (Figure 14.3), these ridges usually atrophy, except at the level of the pectoral muscles, where a breast will eventually develop. In some women, the ridges do not entirely disappear, and portions of the milk lines persist. This occurrence is manifested by the presence of a nipple, a nipple and a breast, or glandular breast tissue only. This congenital anomaly is called a supernumerary breast or nipple.

Knowledge of the lymphatic drainage of the breast is important because of the common metastasis of breast

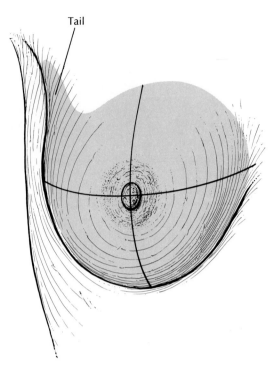

figure**14.2** Four breast quadrants and the axillary tail of Spence.

figure**14.3** Milk lines.

cancer throughout this system. Lymph drainage from the breast is directed toward numerous groups of nodes, with most of the drainage routed to the ipsilateral axillary nodes. However, depending on the site of the lesion, drainage might also be directed into the infraclavicular and supraclavicular nodes, the chest, the abdomen, or the opposite breast.

Two sets of lymph nodes are examined in conjunction with the breast examination: axillary lymph nodes and supraclavicular lymph nodes. Five groups of lymph nodes are located in the axillary fossa (Figure 14.4). All drain upward and medially toward the main lymph-collecting channels. The central axillary nodes are the most frequently palpable. Nomenclature commonly used describes either the area of the axilla in which the nodes are located or their location in relation to one of the adjacent bones or blood vessels.

1. *Anterior axillary* (pectoral) nodes lie in the anterior aspect of the axilla and include a superior group of several nodes found in the region of the third rib and the second and third intercostal spaces, and an inferior group located over the fourth to sixth ribs. The ducts entering these nodes are from the breast and front and side of the costal wall, and from the skin and muscles of the abdominal wall above the umbilicus. They lie along the lateral edge of the pectoralis major muscle, just inside the anterior axillary fold.

2. *Lateral axillary* (brachial) nodes lie along the humerus, inside the upper arm. They receive lymph from the upper extremity, deltoid region, and anterior wall of the chest, including part of the breast.

3. *Posterior axillary* (subscapular) nodes lie in the posterior aspect of the axilla along the lateral edge of the scapula. They drain the posterior wall of the chest and the lower posterior aspect of the neck.

4. *Central axillary* (intermediate) nodes lie high in the middle of the axilla over the ribs. They receive ducts from the anterior axillary (pectoral), lateral axillary (brachial), and posterior (subscapular) lymph nodes draining the chest wall, breast, and arm. Lymph drains from them into the infraclavicular and supraclavicular nodes.

5. *Apical axillary* (infraclavicular or subclavian) nodes lie below the clavicle and receive ducts from the arm, breast, and chest wall.

Drainage flows from the central axillary nodes into the apical axillary (infraclavicular) and supraclavicular

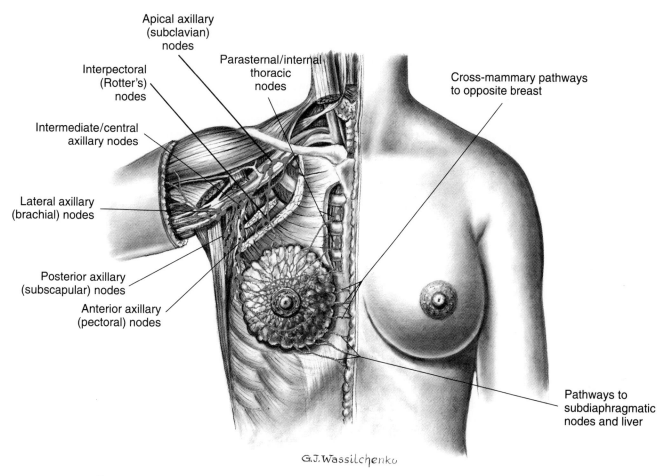

Apical axillary
(subclavian)
nodes

Parasternal/internal
thoracic
nodes

Interpectoral
(Rotter's)
nodes

Cross-mammary pathways
to opposite breast

Intermediate/central
axillary nodes

Lateral axillary
(brachial) nodes

Posterior axillary
(subscapular) nodes

Anterior axillary
(pectoral) nodes

Pathways to
subdiaphragmatic
nodes and liver

G.J.Wassilchenko

figure**14.4**   Lymphatic drainage of the breast. (*From Bobak IM, Jensen MD, Zalar MK: Maternity and gynecologic care: the nurse and the family,* ed 4, St Louis, 1989, Mosby.)

nodes. (See also Chapter 11 on examination of the neck for additional information about infraclavicular and supraclavicular lymph nodes.) A small amount of lymphatic drainage goes directly to the apical axillary (infraclavicular) nodes, deep into the chest or abdomen, or directly across to the opposite breast. Depending on the location of a lesion in the breast tissue, drainage may go to the axillary nodes, to the infraclavicular nodes, into deep channels in the chest or abdomen, or even to the opposite breast. Some nodes are deep and not accessible to examination. The following are accessible to examination. Note that the first five groups are axillary lymph nodes, and the sixth is in another area.

1. Anterior axillary (pectoral) nodes
2. Lateral (brachial) nodes
3. Posterior axillary (subscapular) nodes
4. Central axillary (intermediate) nodes
5. Apical axillary (infraclavicular) nodes
6. Supraclavicular nodes

Other groups that receive lymphatic drainage (but are not palpable) from the breast include:

1. Interpectoral (Rotter's or mammary) nodes lie within the pectoral muscle about the breast.
2. Parasternal (internal thoracic) nodes lie next to the sternum.

The gross appearance and size of the normal female breast vary both among individuals and for an individual at various phases of development. The following paragraphs describe breast development throughout a woman's life span (Figure 14.5).

1. *Appearance before age 10.* Gross appearance of male and female breasts differs little. The nipples are small and slightly elevated. No palpable glandular tissue or areolar pigmentation exists.

2. *Appearance between ages 10 and 14.* The mammary tissues adjacent to and beneath the areola grow, resulting in an increased diameter of the areola and the formation of a "mammary bud." The nipple and breast protrude as a single mound. Breast development may begin bilaterally or may occur unilaterally. Next, the general mammary growth and increases in diameter and pigmentation of the areola continue, resulting in

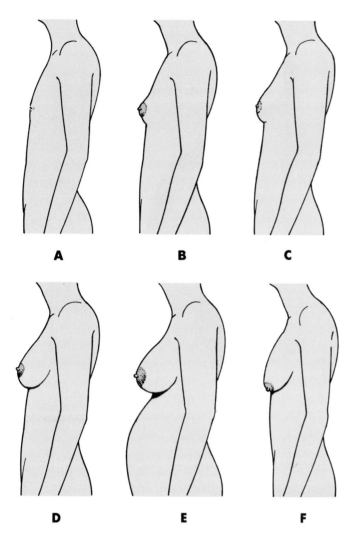

figure **14.5** Appearance of the female breast in various life periods. **A,** Appearance before age 10. **B** and **C,** Appearance between ages 10 through 14. **D,** Appearance of the nulliparous, adult breast. **E,** Appearance of the breast during pregnancy. **F,** Appearance of the breast after menopause.

further elevation of the breasts. The nipple begins to separate from the areola. Growth continues in the mammary tissues. The nipple and areola form a mound that is distinct from the globular shape of the rest of the breast.

3. *Appearance after age 14.* The shape of the adult female breast gradually forms. The areola recedes into the general contour of the breast, and only the nipple protrudes. Heredity, individual sensitivity to hormones, and nutrition influence the size of the adult female breast.

4. *Appearance during reproductive years.* In response to hormonal changes during the menstrual cycle,

a cyclic pattern of breast size change, nodularity, and tenderness occurs. These changes are maximal just before menses. The breast is smallest in days 4 through 7 of the menstrual cycle. Three to 4 days before the onset of menses, many women experience mammary tenseness, fullness, heaviness, tenderness, and pain because of hormonal changes and fluid retention. Total breast volume is significantly increased at this time.

5. *Changes in pregnancy.* Changes in the breast are noted as early as the second month of pregnancy. The breast increases in size, sometimes reaching two to three times the usual size. The areolae and nipples become more prominent and more deeply pigmented. The veins become engorged, Montgomery's glands become more apparent, and striae often develop. During palpation the breasts feel more nodular, and after the fourth month, colostrum can be expressed from the nipples.

6. *Menopausal changes.* After menopause the breast's glandular tissue gradually involutes, and fat is deposited in the breasts. The flattening of structures and decreased elasticity make structures more palpable. The lactiferous ducts especially are more distinctly palpable, feeling firm and stringy. The breast formation becomes flabby and flattened.

The male breast contains a nipple and an areola. Beneath the nipple is a small amount of breast tissue, which usually cannot be clinically differentiated from the other subcutaneous tissues.

■ EXAMINATION

Health History

The foci of the health history are self-examination practices and identification of problems that require assessment. Throughout the health history, the following data about a symptom or problem are recorded: (1) onset (specific date, sudden or gradual), (2) duration, (3) frequency, (4) precipitating factors, (5) aggravating or alleviating factors, (6) treatment received or self-care given, and (7) outcome.

Present health status

1. Breast self-examination
   a. Frequency
   b. Timing with menstrual cycle
2. Changes in breast characteristics and their relationship to menstrual cycle—pain, tenderness, heaviness, swelling, lumps, discharge, and changes in appearance, size, or shape
3. Mammography
   a. Age at first mammography
   b. Date of last mammography and findings
4. Risk factors for breast cancer.

RISK FACTORS — BREAST CANCER

HIGH RISK*
FAMILY HISTORY
Premenopausal breast cancer in mother and sister
PERSONAL HISTORY
Atypical hyperplasia in breast biopsy or aspirated
   sample

MODERATE RISK†
FAMILY HISTORY
Premenopausal breast cancer in mother or sister
PERSONAL HISTORY
Hyperplasia without atypia in breast biopsy or
   aspirated sample
History of previous breast cancer
Older women of the white race

LOW RISK‡
FAMILY HISTORY
Postmenopausal breast cancer in first-degree
   relative
PERSONAL HISTORY
Previous cancer of the ovary or uterine endo-
   metrium
Predominant nodular densities in mammogram
Obesity (in women over age 50)
Excess ionizing radiation to chest wall or breasts
High alcohol consumption
High socioeconomic status
Never pregnant (women under age 40)
Delayed first childbirth
Short duration of breast-feeding of children
Onset of menstruation before age 12
Onset of menopause after age 49
Prolonged use of oral contraceptives (women
   under age 45)
Prolonged estrogen replacement therapy

Modified from Stoll BA, editor: *Reducing breast cancer risk in women,*
Boston, 1995, Kluwer Academic.
*Risk increased more than 4 times.
†Risk increased 2 to 4 times.
‡Increase in risk up to 2 times or findings inconsistent among studies.

*Present illness**

1. Breast discomfort or pain
   a. Pattern
   b. Onset
   c. Duration
   d. Severity

*Common symptoms are listed.

   e. Character
   f. Associated symptoms
   g. Contributory and alleviating factors
2. Swelling and lumps
   a. Location
   b. Size
   c. Changes in surface characteristics of breast
   d. Mobility
   e. Time when first noted
   f. Changes over time
   g. Changes related to menses
   h. Associated symptoms
3. Discharge
   a. Color
   b. Consistency
   c. Amount
   d. Odor
   e. Factors associated with onset, recent injuries
   f. Reproductive status
4. Current medications

Past health history

1. Previous diagnoses of breast disease and injuries
2. Previous breast surgeries
3. Lactation history
4. Mastitis
5. Cancers in other sites

Associated systems

1. Reproductive and menstrual history
2. Medication history, especially hormones
3. Nutrition history, especially caffeine intake
4. Problems noted in axilla

Family health history

1. Breast cancer
2. Benign breast disease

Preparation for Examination: Client and Environment

   Some girls and women are embarrassed while under-
going a breast examination. Their reasons for embarrass-
ment may include a sense of modesty or dissatisfaction
with their breast development. Take care to ensure priva-
cy during the examination and avoid unnecessary expo-
sure of the breasts. With young adolescents, teaching
about the normal sequence of breast development may be
reassuring. Avoid making comments about the client's
breast development that could be misinterpreted. Explain
the components of the examination to relieve the client's
discomfort and provide important health education.
   During the health history preceding the physical ex-

PREPARATION FOR EXAMINATION

EQUIPMENT

Item	Purpose
Small pillow or folded towel	For placement under back of side being examined to spread breast tissue more evenly on chest
Centimeter ruler	To measure position and size of any masses located
Glass slide and cytological fixative	To prepare specimen of any abnormal drainage for microscopic examination (Drainage; which is often thin and accellular, is most effectively collected on a frosted or albumin-coated slide to prevent runoff.)
Teaching aids	For instruction regarding breast self-examination

CLIENT AND ENVIRONMENT

Setting
Well lit
Private
Warm
Client
Stripped to waist
Seated for first portion of examination; lying down for second portion
Examiner
Standing at front of client for first portion; at right side of client for second portion

figure**14.6** Observation of the breasts. These breasts have several characteristics that are deviations within normal limits: (1) the left breast is slightly larger than the right; (2) the nipples are directed in slightly different directions; (3) the left breast has a superficial skin lesion appearing as a dark area medial to the areola; and (4) both breasts have striae.

amination, assess the woman's level of knowledge and practice regarding breast self-examination. The examination provides an excellent opportunity for reviewing the client's technique or for teaching breast self-examination.

Some adolescent or adult male clients may not have had a breast examination previously and may be concerned that the examiner will notice a problem. Explaining to male clients that breast lesions are possible in men and that the breast examination is a routine component of a complete health assessment will help to alleviate any worry and embarrassment. Some male clients have perspiration in the axilla and may be embarrassed

when an examiner palpates this dampened area; it is helpful to offer the male client a tissue for drying the area before the examination is begun.

Technique for Examination and Normal Findings
Inspection

Inspection and palpation are the techniques used to examine the breast. For initial inspection, the client is seated on the side of the examination table and is uncovered to the waist. If the client reports that she has noticed a lump or a change in one of the breasts, ask her to point out the area and demonstrate the technique she used to feel the lump or change. Take special note of that area during the examination.

Observe the breasts, including the nipples and areolae, for symmetry of shape and size, surface characteristics, and abnormal amount or distribution of hair. As with inspection of all paired organs, use the client as her own control and compare both breasts to determine what is "normal" for that individual and to detect any unusual findings for a given individual. Lack of symmetry always indicates a need for additional assessment.

Symmetry of shape and size. Normal female breasts are bilaterally similar in shape and size. However, frequently one breast is somewhat smaller than the other (Figure 14.6). In males the breasts are normally even with the chest wall, except for obese men, whose

breasts assume a bilaterally convex shape similar to that of female breasts.

Surface characteristics. The surface characteristics of breasts may include hyperpigmentation, moles and nevi, edema, retraction, dimpling, focal vascularity, and lesions. The skin of the breasts should appear smooth, and the surface contour should be even and uninterrupted. Normally, only the areola and the nipple are hyperpigmented. Other portions of the breast are normally a color that is uniform with the individual's skin in other covered parts of the body. Focal hyperpigmentation is an abnormal finding. Moles and nevi are common. The client should be questioned about changes or problems, with any skin lesion noted.

Edema of the breast, usually caused by blocked lymph drainage, produces exaggeration of the skin pores, creating an orange-peel appearance called peau d'orange (Figure 14.7, *B*).

Retraction, or dimpling, appears as a depression or pucker on the skin (Figure 14.7, *A*). It usually is caused by the fibrotic shortening and immobilization of Cooper's ligament by an invasive process.

Vascular patterns should be diffuse and symmetrical. Hypervascular patterns may be noted in pregnant, obese, and very fair-skinned individuals. Focal or unilateral patterns are abnormal and may be produced by dilated superficial veins from increased blood flow to a malignancy (Figure 14.7, *A*).

The elastic fibers of the dermis may be damaged whenever the skin of the breasts is stretched rapidly, and observable striae, or stretch marks, are produced. Newly created striae are reddish, but they become white with age.

Areolar area and nipple characteristics. The areolar area can range from light pink to dark brown, depending on the client's genetic skin color and hormonal influences. In pregnancy, the areolae enlarge and darken. The areolar area is normally round or oval and bilaterally similar. Irregular placement of Montgomery's tubercles is common and normal.

After puberty, women may normally have a scattering of coarse, curly hair on the breasts, mostly near the areola. After puberty, males often have a dense mass of chest hair around the areola. Male hair patterns in female clients are abnormal. The areolar areas should be inspected for size, shape, symmetry, color, surface characteristics, bulging, and lesions. Size, shape, and color can normally vary greatly in symmetrical patterns. Any asymmetry, mass, or lesion should be considered abnormal.

If the breasts are symmetrical, both nipples should be pointing laterally in the same way. The nipples should be inspected for size, shape, ability to become erect, color, discharge, and lesions. The nipples should be round, equal in size, and homogeneous in color, and they should have convoluted surfaces, which produce a

---

CULTURAL CONSIDERATIONS

BREAST VARIATIONS

Breast size, color, and configuration vary widely among women. Asian women tend to have smaller breasts than other groups. Women of African heritage have a higher prevalence of supernumerary nipples than others.

---

wrinkled appearance. They should appear soft and smooth and have no crusting, cracks, or discharge.

Inversion of one or both nipples, if present from puberty, is normal. However, this condition may interfere with breast-feeding. Recent inversion of the nipple is probably retraction (Figure 14.7, *A*) and should be investigated.

Supernumerary nipples and areolae may appear along the milk lines in about 1% of the population (see Figure 14.3). These lesions can vary in size. They are the color of the individual's actual areolae and are often mistaken for moles. Occasionally, glandular tissue may accompany these lesions.

Paget's disease, a malignant condition requiring prompt therapy, appears as a red glandular erosion of the nipple or as a nipple that is dry, scaly, or friable. The areola may also be affected.

Breast secretions are normal in pregnancy or lactation. Other causes of discharge are mechanical nipple stimulation, drug influence, hypothalamic and pituitary disorders, and malignant and benign breast lesions. The discharge can be milky, watery, purulent, serous, or bloody. The method for determining the origin of discharge production is discussed in the section on palpation.

Sitting positions for breast inspection. There are four basic sitting positions used for breast inspection. Every adult female client should be examined in each position:

1. *Client is seated with arms at sides* (see Figure 14.6). Observe the breasts at rest and without movement to establish a baseline for comparison. Observe men in this position only, unless they have unusually large breasts, in which case the other inspection positions are also used.
2. *Client is seated with arms abducted over head* (Figure 14.8, *A*). This maneuver creates tension on the suspensory ligaments and may accentuate asymmetry, retraction, and fixation.
3. *Client is seated and pushes hands into hips* (or pushes palms together) (Figure 14.8, *B* to *C*). This action contracts the pectoral muscles and can reveal dimpling and deviations in symmetry.

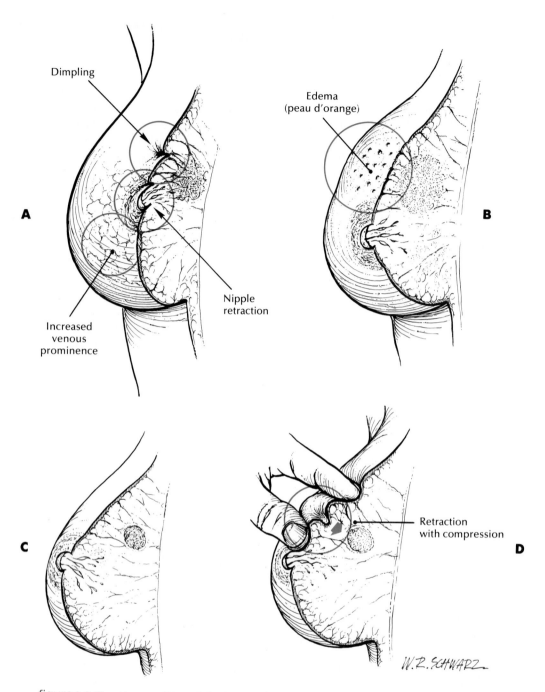

figure **14.7** Abnormalities of the breast. **A,** Breast with dimpling, nipple retraction, and increased venous prominence. **B,** Breast with edema (peau d'orange or pigskin appearance). **C,** Breast with tumor; no retraction is apparent. **D,** Breast with tumor; retraction is apparent with compression.

4. *Client is seated and leans over* (Figure 14.8, *D*). The examiner assists in supporting and balancing the client during this maneuver. The breasts should hang evenly and symmetrically. This approach is especially useful in examining the movement and contour of large breasts.

While the client is performing these maneuvers, carefully observe the breasts for symmetry, bulging, retraction, and fixation. An abnormality may not be apparent in the breasts at rest (Figure 14.9, *A*), but a mass may cause a breast, through invasion of suspensory ligaments, to fix, preventing it from upward or forward

figure **14.8** Observation of the breasts in several positions. **A,** Observation with the client's arms overhead. **B,** Observation with the client contracting her pectoral muscles by pressing her hands into her waist. **C,** Alternate method of observing the client with pectoral muscle contraction—the client's hands are pressed together in front. **D,** Observation with the client leaning forward.

movements (Figure 14.9, *B*). Tension in the breasts through contraction of the pectoral muscles assists in eliciting dimpling if a mass has infiltrated and shortened suspensory ligaments.

Finally, observe the breasts while the client is lying down, before performing palpation.

Palpation

This portion of the breast examination begins with palpation for axillary, subclavicular, and supraclavicular lymph nodes. This step is most effectively performed with the client in a sitting position. The location and

palpation of the subclavicular and supraclavicular nodes are described in Chapter 11. To emphasize the importance of an adequate axillary area examination being done with each breast examination, this procedure is reviewed here.

To examine the axilla, the tissues can be best appreciated if the area muscles are relaxed. Contracted muscles may obscure slightly enlarged nodes. To achieve this relaxation while abducting the arm, support the ipsilateral arm (Figure 14.10). Visualize the axilla as a four-sided pyramid and thoroughly palpate the following areas:

1. *Anterior axillary nodes* (pectoral) lying in the an-

figure**14.9** **A,** The breasts appear symmetrical at rest. **B,** The breasts do not move symmetrically with arm elevation. The right breast is immobilized.

terior aspect of the axilla and including several nodes found in the region of the third rib and the second and third intercostal spaces and over the fourth and sixth ribs

2. *Lateral axillary nodes* (brachial) along the inside of the humerus (upper arm)
3. *Posterior axillary nodes* (subscapular) lying in the posterior aspect of the axilla along the lateral edge of the scapula
4. *Central axillary nodes* (intermediate) lying high in the middle of the axilla over the ribs
5. *Apical axillary nodes* (infraclavicular or subclavian) located below the clavicle

Develop a routine system for axillary node examination. Palpate the apical nodes last, since their deep location will require extra pressure in examination. Normally, nodes should not be palpable.

The primary purpose of the palpation of the breasts is to discover masses. If a mass is discovered, assess it according to the characteristics noted in the box on p. 317 and shown in Figures 14.11 and 14.12.

The range of normal breast consistency is wide. The normal breast feels somewhat granular and "lumpy." This granularity is generalized and becomes more prominent with age. Breast lumpiness results from the configuration of the breast lobes, the fat and connective tissue between and supporting the lobes and other structures, and the irregular density of lobules. Thus the consistency of breasts is not uniform. However, this variation in consistency should be noted uniformly throughout the breasts of an individual client.

The breasts feel relatively homogeneous in the young adolescent. After menarche the presence of proges-

figure**14.10** Palpation of the axillary lymph nodes. (Note that the client's arm is supported on the examiner's arm.)

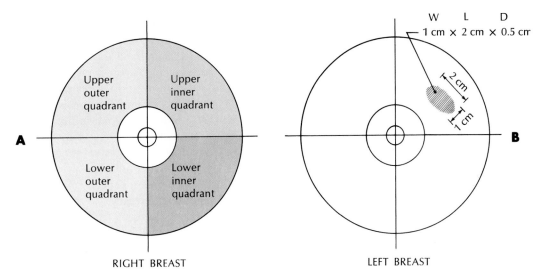

figure **14.11**   **A,** The four quadrants of the breast. **B,** Diagram of a mass within a breast.

Assessment of Breast Masses

1. *Location:* Masses are designated according to the quadrant in which they lie: upper outer, lower outer, upper inner, or lower inner (see Figure 14.11, *A*). To describe the mass in the client's record, it may be helpful to draw the mass within a diagram of the breast (see Figure 14.11, *B*). Another method of describing location is to visualize the breast as the face of a clock with the nipple at the center. A mass can be designated, for example, as being "5 cm from the nipple in the 8 o'clock position."

2. *Size:* The size should be approximated in centimeters in all its planes. For example, a mass may be ovoid, 3 cm wide, 2 cm long, and 1 cm thick.

3. *Shape:* The shape may be round, ovoid, irregular, or matted. Matting occurs in the presence of multiple lesions.

4. *Consistency:* The palpable consistency of a breast lesion may be soft, hard, solid, or cystic. One way to evaluate the consistency of a breast lesion is to palpate over the lesion with the pads of the index and middle fingers of the palpating hand (see Figure 14.12, *A*).

5. *Discreteness:* The borders of a mass are assessed to determine if they are sharp and well defined or irregular. To assess discreteness, an attempt is made to palpate all the borders of the mass with the thumb and index finger of the palpating hand (see Figure 14.12, *B*).

6. *Mobility:* The movability of the mass within the breast is assessed as freely movable or fixed. To assess mobility, the thumb and index finger of the examining hand are used to "hold" the mass, and then the mass is moved in all directions possible (see Figure 14.12, *C*).

7. *Tenderness:* The client is questioned regarding any discomfort with palpation.

8. *Erythema:* The area of skin overlying the mass is inspected for erythema.

9. *Dimpling over the mass:* The tissue over the mass is compressed to determine if this maneuver produces dimpling (see Figure 14.7, *D*).

10. *Depth of mass:* The location of the mass is determined in reference to the surface of the breast. Is the mass close to the surface at midlevel or deep against the chest wall?

figure **14.12** **A,** Palpating for consistency of breast lesion. **B,** Palpating for delineation of borders of breast mass. **C,** Palpating for mobility of breast mass.

terone in pregnancy and premenstrually causes the breasts to feel generally nodular. Hormonally induced nodularity is bilateral and diffuse.

The breasts are palpated most effectively with the client in a supine position. Because of time constraints on most physical examinations, it is not advised that all clients also undergo palpation in a sitting position. However, certain groups of clients should also have breast palpation done in the sitting position: women with present or past complaints of breast masses, women at high risk of breast cancer, and women with large and/or pendulous breasts.

If the breasts are to be examined with the client in a sitting position, small breasts can be examined by using one hand to support the breast and the other hand to palpate the tissue against the chest wall. For palpation of pendulous breasts, use a bimanual technique (Figure 14.13). Support the inferior portion of the breast in one hand while using the other hand to palpate breast tissue against the supporting hand.

With the client lying down, palpate the breasts while they are flattened against the rib cage. If the breasts are large, several methods can be used to enhance flattening. A small pillow or a rolled towel can be placed under the ipsilateral upper back, or the client can abduct the ipsilateral arm and place her hand under her neck (Figure 14.14). Both maneuvers shift the breast medially. For all clients, the humerus should be at least slightly abducted to allow for thorough palpation of the tail of Spence.

Thoroughly palpate the breasts and the tail of Spence areas with the palmar surfaces of the three middle fingers held together (Figure 14.15, *A*). The movements should be smooth and should be done in a back-and-forth or circular motion. Press firmly enough to fully appreciate the underlying tissue, but not so firmly that the tissue is compressed against the rib cage.

Develop a system of breast examination and habitually start and end at a fixed point on the breasts. The important principle is development of a system that ensures a thorough examination of all breast tissues. Several examination patterns have been recommended:

1. The breast is visualized as a round wheel with multiple spokes. Palpation is done along each spoke until the breast has been thoroughly surveyed (Figure 14.16, *A*).
2. The breast is viewed as a group of concentric circles with the nipple as the center. Palpation is performed along the circumferences of the circles, starting at the outermost circle, until the total breast area has been adequately surveyed (Figure 14.16, *B*).
3. Palpation of the breast is done in vertical or horizontal sections, starting immediately below the clavicle at the sternal border and proceeding

A

B

figure**14.13** Bimanual palpation of the breasts.

figure**14.14** Use of a towel to shift breast tissue evenly over the chest for effective palpation.

downward and upward, parallel to the sternal border, or side-to-side until the entire breast has been surveyed.

Whatever system and sequence of examination is used, a thorough examination of all breast tissue and the tail of Spence is critical. Special attention should be fo-cused on the upper outer quadrant area and the tail of Spence because approximately half of all breast cancers develop there (Figure 14.17).

Carefully palpate the areolar areas to determine the presence of underlying masses (see Figure 14.15, *B*). Gently compress each nipple to assess for the presence of masses and discharge (see Figure 14.15, *C*). If discharge is noted, milk the breast along its radii to identify the lobe from which the discharge is originating. Compression of the discharge-producing lobe will cause discharge to exude from the nipple. If the nipple discharge is not associated with normal changes in pregnancy or the postpartum period, collect a specimen of the discharge on a slide. Nipple discharge, which is often thin and cellular, is most effectively collected on a frosted or albumin-coated slide to prevent runoff. When discharge is present on the nipple, bring the slide in contact with the nipple and rub it across the nipple, allowing the discharge to collect across the slide. Fix the slide immediately with cytology fixative.

If a client reports a breast mass, examine the "normal" breast first so that the baseline consistency of that breast will serve as a control for palpation of the reportedly abnormal one.

Mammary folds, or crescent-shaped ridges of breast tissue found at the inferior portions of very large or pendulous breasts, may be confused with breast masses, but they are nonpathological.

The complete sequence of the breast examination is illustrated in Figure 14.18.

figure**14.15** Palpation of the breasts. **A,** Glandular areas. **B,** Areolar area. **C,** Compression of the nipple.

figure**14.16** Two methods of systematic breast palpation. **A,** Palpation in wedge sections from breast periphery to center. **B,** Palpation along concentric circles from periphery to center.

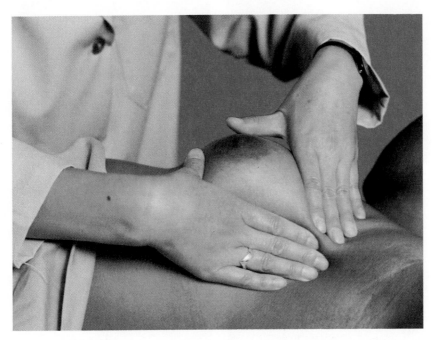

figure**14.17**   Palpation of the axillary tail of Spence.

Special breast examinations

The male breast. The routine male breast examination consists of the following steps:

1. Inspection of the breasts while the client is in a sitting position
2. Palpation of the axillary nodes
3. Palpation of the breasts while the client is lying down

Observe the breast with the client sitting with arms at rest. The other sitting positions used with the woman are unnecessary unless the man has large breasts. Perform the axillary examination using the same technique as described for women. Palpate the breasts, nipples, and areolae while the client is supine, as with the female client.

Occurring most frequently in the areolar area, male breast cancer accounts for approximately 1% of all breast cancers. Every male client should be given a thorough breast examination with an adaptation of the technique used for female clients.

Gynecomastia, or enlargement of the male breast, is a frequently occurring, multicausal condition. Causes include pubertal changes, hormonal administration, cirrhosis, leukemia, thyrotoxicosis, and drugs.

Client who has had a mastectomy. The client who has had a mastectomy has special examination needs. This client may be embarrassed about the condition of the surgical site and apprehensive about the examination of the remaining breast. Perform the inspection and palpation portions of the examination on the unaffected side as described for the routine examination. Inspect the mastectomy scar, surrounding areas, and axilla for swelling, lumps, redness, color changes, and skin lesions. Note the extent of muscle mass and edema and the general appearance and condition of the scar. Palpate the scar with the palmar surface of two fingers of the examining hand with a back-and-forth or circular motion to detect any swelling, lumps, and tenderness. Then systematically and thoroughly palpate the axillary and chest lymph node areas and surrounding tissue. Emphasize the importance of breast self-examination with these clients.

Client who has had breast reconstruction, augmentation, or a lumpectomy. Examine the breasts in the usual manner, giving special attention to scars. Emphasize the need for breast self-examination with these clients.

Screening Tests and Procedures

Further evaluation of breast masses is accomplished through the use of the following techniques:

1. Mammography is a technique of breast examination that involves low-energy radiography.
2. Xeromammography is mammography done with a xerographic plate instead of film. The advantages of this technique are that radiation doses are smaller than with conventional mammography and the images produced are more distinct.

figure**14.18** Sequence of the breast examination. **A,** Observation of the breasts at rest. **B,** Observation with client's arms overhead. **C,** Observation with client contracting pectoral muscles by pressing hands into waist. **D,** Observation with client leaning forward. **E,** Palpation of axillary nodes. **F,** Palpation of the glandular area. **G,** Palpation of the areolar area. **H,** Palpation of the nipple.

Mammography is the major method of detecting nonpalpable breast lesions. Since nonpalpable lesions are generally small, and local when found early, survival rates are increased through early detection. The performance and interpretation of mammograms require specialized skill.

During the past 10 years, mammographic techniques have been improved tremendously in terms of safety and effectiveness. Often mammography is offered through a community-based screening program.

Since the initiation of mammographic screening services, recommended schedules for mammography have changed as research has produced new knowledge related to the detection of breast cancer.

New knowledge about the development of breast cancer and safe mechanisms for early detection and treatment may affect future guidelines for mammography screening schedules. The practitioner working with adult women clients should be alert to possible changes in screening guidelines.

■ VARIATIONS FROM HEALTH

The most common variations in breast health are noted in the form of breast lumps. The various causes of breast lumps are listed in Table 14.1, and the most common causes are discussed in this section.

Breast Cancer

Although certain breast lesions have characteristic findings on inspection and palpation, diagnosis is not made by clinical examination but by surgical procedures and laboratory examinations. Therefore the practitioner is encouraged to learn the distinguishing characteristics of breast lesions but not to rely on them for diagnosis.

The lesions of breast cancer are often solitary, unilateral, solid, hard, irregular, poorly delineated, nonmobile, painless, nontender, and located in the upper outer quad-

---

examination *step-by-step*

Client: Seated and uncovered to waist
Examiner: Standing in front of client

Inspection
1. Skin of anterior thorax
2. Breast and areolar size, configuration, symmetry, and surface characteristics
3. Nipple configuration and plane
4. Symmetry of movement when arms are raised over head
5. Retraction of breast tissue when pectoral muscles are contracted by pushing arms into hips or pushing hands together
6. Symmetry of movement and retraction when client leans forward
7. Skin of axilla

Palpation
1. Axillary nodes: Begin along inner aspect of arm and proceed to chest wall, anterior axilla, posterior axilla, and apex of axilla. (Supraclavicular and infraclavicular nodes can be palpated in conjunction with axillary nodes or with the head and neck examination.)
2. Palpate breasts (1) if unusual symptoms or inspection findings are noted, (2) if client is at risk for breast disease, or (3) if breasts are unusually large.

Client: Lying on back
Examiner: To right of client

Inspection
1. Skin of thorax
2. Surface characteristics of breasts

Palpation
1. Palpate breasts to determine consistency of tissue and presence of masses.
2. Palpate areolar areas for masses.
3. Palpate nipples to determine presence of discharge.

Teaching
1. Review client's technique of breast self-examination or teach breast self-examination.

table 14.1	**Causes of Breast Lumps**	
Origin	**Lesion type**	**Frequency**
Normal structures	Nodularity	Common
	Prominent fat lobule	Less common
	Prominent rib	Less common
	Intramammary lymph node	Rare
	Edge of biopsy wound	Less common
	Accessory breast	Rare
Aberrations of normal development and involution	Fibroadenoma	Common
	Cyclical nodularity	Common
	Cyst	Common
	Galactocele	Rare
	Sclerosing adenosis	Less common
	Stromal fibrosis	Rare
Inflammatory processes	Chronic infected abscess	Rare
	Fat necrosis	Rare
	Foreign body granuloma	Rare
	Mondor's disease	Rare
Benign tumor	Duct papilloma	Less common
	Giant fibroadenoma	Rare
	Lipoma	Rare
	Granular cell myoblastoma	Rare
Intermediate tumor	Phyllodes tumor	Rare
	Carcinoma in situ	Less common
Malignant tumor	Primary tumor	Common
	Secondary tumor	Rare
Lesions of nipple and areola	Squamous papilloma	Less common
	Leiomyoma	Rare
	Retention cyst	Rare
	Papillary adenoma	Rare
Skin lesions	Sebaceous cyst	Less common
	Hidradenitis	Rare
	Benign and malignant skin tumors	Rare

Modified from Hughes LE, Mansel RE, Webster DJT: *Benign disorders and diseases of the breast,* London, 1989, Baillière Tindall.

rants. Breast cancer is a leading cause of death in women in the United States and also a leading cause of cancer morbidity. On average, 1 of every 8 to 10 women will develop breast cancer. Knowledge of the factors indicating that a woman is at a higher than usual risk of cancer can assist in decision making about screening programs and the frequency of general physical examinations.

A summary of risk factors for breast cancer in women is presented in Table 14.1. For women at increased risk, monthly self-examination should be emphasized. Such women should receive a thorough breast screening examination at least once a year.

Benign Lesions

The most commonly seen benign breast lesions are those associated with fibrocystic disease and fibroadenomas.

Fibrocystic disease, noted as an exaggeration of the normal changes in the breasts during the menstrual cycle, is eventually characterized by the formation of single or multiple cysts in the breasts. Fibrocystic disease develops in three stages:

1. The first stage, called mazoplasia, occurs in the late teens and early 20s. It is characterized by painful, tender, premenstrual breast swelling

(chiefly in the axillary tails) that subsides after menses.

2. The second stage occurs in the late 20s and early 30s. The breasts exhibit multinodular changes, and sometimes a dominant mass occurs, which is usually described as a thickness rather than a lump.

3. The third stage involves the development of cysts. The onset of cyst formation is often preceded by a sudden dull pain, a full feeling, or a burning sensation in the breast.

The lesions of fibrocystic disease are commonly bilateral, multiple, painful, tender, well delineated, and slightly mobile. The associated tenderness and the size of the lesions increase premenstrually.

Fibroadenomas are benign lesions that contain both fibrous and glandular tissues. They are usually solitary and unilateral. In general, they are palpated as mobile, solid, firm, rubbery, regular, well-delineated, nontender, painless lumps. Fibroadenomas are usually found in women between the ages of 15 and 35 and do not change with the menstrual cycle.

■ BREAST SELF-EXAMINATION

Despite improved mammographic techniques and their availability, a substantial portion of malignant breast lesions are found by women themselves. Women who perform regular breast self-examinations become very familiar with the inspection and palpatory findings within their own breasts and can note any changes immediately.

Therefore the health-oriented examiner should assess each client's level of knowledge and practice related to monthly breast self-examination. During examination of the breasts, the examiner describes the steps of the examination and the rationale for each step. Use of visual aids, models, pamphlets, and other materials can be valuable additions to demonstrations. A return demonstration by the client on her own breasts reinforces the client's learning and memory of the procedure.

The U.S. Preventive Services Task Force (1996) recommends the following schedule for routine breast cancer screening:

Women ages 50 to 69: Routine screening for breast cancer every 1 to 2 years with mammography alone or mammography and annual clinical breast examination (CBE).

Women ages 40 to 49 or age 70 and older: Insufficient evidence exists to recommend for or against the use of CBE alone or the teaching of breast self-examination. Women with increased risk may require more frequent or additional screening. The American Cancer Society is moving toward recommending yearly mammograms for women starting at age 40. At present, the following screening schedule is commonly recommended in clinical practice:

Mammogram	From ages 40 to 50, once every 1 to 2 years
	From age 50, every year
Clinical breast examination	Done in conjunction with the mammogram
Self-examination	Monthly

Teaching Breast Self-Examination

The following points should be emphasized in the teaching of breast self-examination:

1. The majority of breast lumps are not cancerous.
2. The majority of cancerous breast lesions are curable.
3. Breasts should be examined each month between the fourth through the fourteenth day of the menstrual cycle, when the breasts are least congested. If, for any reason, menses are not present, a specific date of each month should be chosen for the monthly breast examination (e.g., the date of the client's birthday).
4. Visual inspection and palpation should be done.
5. Visual inspection should be done in four arm positions with the woman stripped to the waist and looking at herself in a mirror. The four arm positions are arms at rest; hands on hips and pressed into hips, contracting chest muscles; hands over head; and arms forward with the torso leaning forward.
6. Many women prefer to do palpation in the shower because the soap and water help the hands to glide easily over the skin. However, the examination of large breasts and the axilla are better done in a supine than in a standing position; therefore an examination done in the supine position is recommended in addition to the examination done in the bath or shower.
7. Each entire breast should be palpated in a systematic way.
8. Specific palpation of the nipple (through compression for discharge) and the areola (through palpation) should not be forgotten.
9. Any change should be reported to a health care provider as soon as possible.

■ **FOCUSED HEALTH HISTORY** *(SUBJECTIVE DATA)*

Mrs. R., a 40-year-old white female, noted a small lump, about the "size of a dime," in the areolar area of the right breast 2 weeks ago in breast self-examination, routinely done on day 7 of the menstrual cycle. No change in the lump since discovery. Denies pain, swelling, change in appearance of the breast, or discharge. No history of breast lesions. No hormonal medications taken. Last clinical breast examination was 9 months ago. Has never had a mammogram. Menses are regular; onset was at age 13. Had two pregnancies, delivered at full term 7 (age 33) and 5 (age 35) years ago, and successfully breast-fed for 6 months. One maternal aunt had breast cancer at age 50 and died within 1 year of diagnosis. Is very concerned about breast cancer.

■ **FOCUSED PHYSICAL EXAMINATION** *(OBJECTIVE DATA)*

Inspection: Right breast slightly larger than left breast. Bilaterally similar in surface characteristics, plane of nipple, and mobility. Skin smooth with no unusual vascular patterns. No lesions, erythema, dimpling, or retraction.

Palpation: Right breast—regular, round, movable mass, approximately 0.25 × 0.25 × 0.5 cm, palpated in left lower quadrant at 5 o'clock position approximately 1 cm from center of nipple. Borders are well defined; mass is soft and cystic. Appears to be very close to skin surface. Not tender on palpation or movement. Left breast—Soft, slightly nodular throughout. No masses or tenderness.

Lymph nodes: No axillary, infraclavicular, or supraclavicular nodes palpated. No tenderness in lymph node areas.

diagnoses

HEALTH PROBLEM

Mass in right breast

NURSING DIAGNOSIS

Anxiety related to concern about breast cancer

Defining Characteristics

- Fear of diagnosis of cancer
- Concern about family history of breast cancer

Respiratory System

■ PURPOSE OF EXAMINATION

The purpose of the respiratory examination is to assess the organs and structures of the respiratory system and the functioning of the system as a whole. Because the respiratory system functions in close relationship with the cardiovascular system, these systems are often examined together. The examination is accomplished through various methods, including inspection, percussion, palpation, and auscultation.

■ ANATOMY AND PHYSIOLOGY

The major functions of the respiratory system are to supply the body with oxygen and to eliminate carbon dioxide. These tasks are accomplished through the complex cooperation of many body systems that, in wellness, act in harmony. The actual transfer of oxygen and carbon dioxide between environmental gas and body liquid occurs in the alveoli, which are not accessible to clinical examination. However, assessment of respiratory efficiency is accomplished by direct and indirect appraisal of structures that support alveolar function.

Thoracic Cage

The Thoracic Cage is a semirigid structure consisting of a skeleton of 12 thoracic vertebrae, 12 pairs of ribs, the sternum, the diaphragm, and the intercostal muscles (Figure 15.1). The skeletal components of the thoracic cage are the ribs, the sternum, and the vertebrae. The ribs are paired. Anteriorly, the costal cartilages of the first seven ribs articulate with the body of the sternum. The costal cartilages of the eighth to the tenth ribs are attached to the costal cartilages immediately superior to the ribs. The eleventh and twelfth ribs, the "floating ribs," are unattached anteriorly. The tips of the eleventh ribs are located in the lateral thorax; the tips of the twelfth ribs are found in the posterior thorax. Posteriorly, all ribs articulate with the thoracic vertebrae.

In the adult, the sternum is approximately 17 cm long and consists of three parts: the manubrium, the body, and the xiphoid process. The manubrium of the sternum articulates with and supports the clavicle. The manubrium and the body of the sternum articulate with the first seven ribs. None of the ribs articulates with the xiphoid. An important anatomical landmark, the angle

327

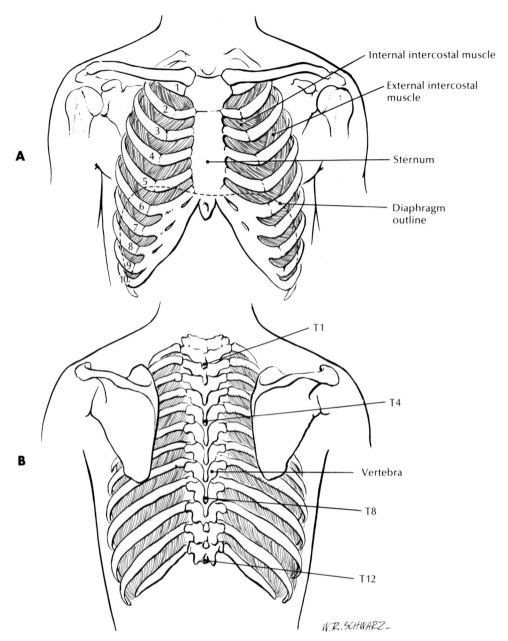

figure **15.1** Thoracic cage. **A,** Anterior thorax. **B,** Posterior thorax.

of Louis is the junction of the manubrium and the body of the sternum (manubriosternal junction). The second rib attaches to the sternum at the angle of Louis.

The spaces between the ribs are termed intercostal spaces. Each space is named according to the rib immediately superior to it; for example, the space between the second and third ribs is designated as the second intercostal space.

Thoracic Cavity and Contents

The thoracic cavity and contents are divided into two distinct (right and left) pleural cavities, which are sepa-

rated by the mediastinum, which contains the heart and the other structures that connect the head with the abdomen. The pleural cavities are lined by serous membranes—the parietal and visceral pleurae. The parietal pleura lines the chest wall and the diaphragm; the visceral pleura covers the outside of the lung. The potential space between the pleurae contains a small amount of lubricating fluid.

The lungs are paired, asymmetrical, conical organs that conform to the shape of the thoracic cavity. The right lung contains three lobes, and the left lung has two lobes.

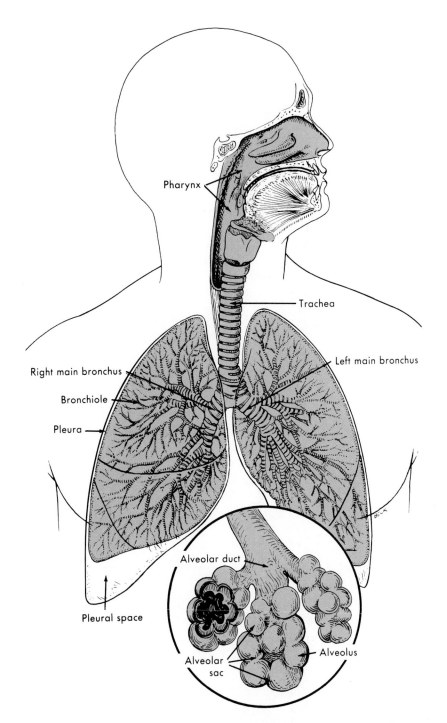

figure**15.2**   Pharynx, trachea, and lungs. Alveolar sacs in inset. *(From Thibodeau GA:* Anthony's textbook of anatomy and physiology, *ed 13, St Louis, 1990, Mosby.)*

Air reaches the lungs through a system of flexible tubes. It enters through the mouth or the nose, passes through the respiratory portion of the larynx, and reaches the trachea. The trachea, approximately 10 to 11 cm long in the adult, begins at the lower border of the cricoid cartilage in the neck and divides into a left and right bronchus, usually at the level of T4 or T5 pos-

teriorly and slightly below the manubriosternal junction anteriorly.

The right bronchus is shorter, wider, and more vertical than the left bronchus. The bronchial structures are subdivided into increasingly smaller bronchi and bronchioles. Each bronchiole opens into an alveolar duct from which multiple alveoli radiate (Figure 15.2).

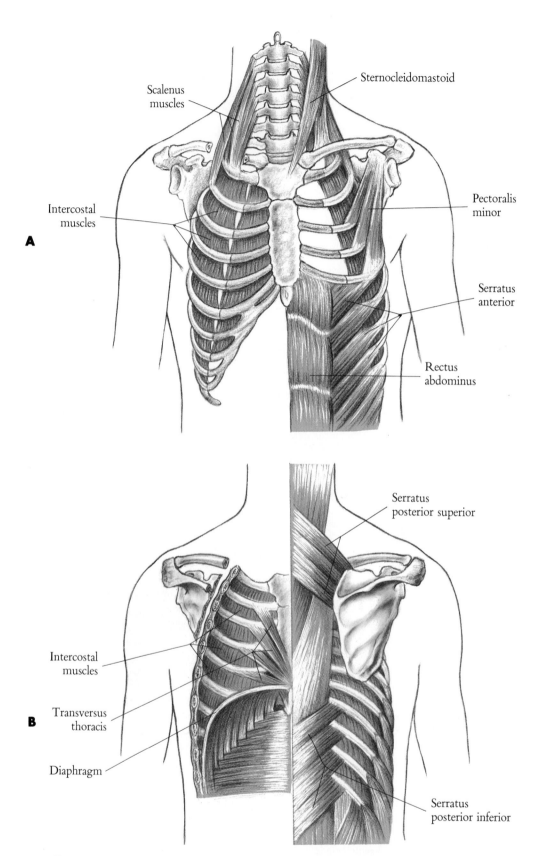

figure**15.3**   Muscles of ventilation. **A,** Anterior view. **B,** Posterior view. *(From Seidel HM et al: Mosby's guide to physical examination, ed 3, St Louis, 1995, Mosby.)*

In the adult, the lungs contain approximately 300 million alveoli.

The bronchi have both transport and protective purposes. They form the pathway through which air is transported into and out of the lungs. In addition, they protect the respiratory system by filtering the air. The bronchial cavities contain mucus, which entraps foreign particles. This mucus is continuously swept into the throat by ciliary movement and then is eliminated.

Two types of muscles are used in respiration: primary and accessory (Figure 15.3). The diaphragm and the external intercostal muscles are the primary muscles of respiration. The accessory muscles of respiration can be used to facilitate or increase inspiration (i.e., assist in raising the ribs and the sternum) or to force expiration in both health and disease. The accessory muscles of respiration are the scalene muscles and the parasternal intercostal muscles.

The thoracic cage is perpetually moving throughout the inspiratory and expiratory phases of respiration (Figure 15.4). During inspiration, the diaphragm descends and flattens, and the intercostal muscles contract. Both the diameter and the length of the thorax are increased. These maneuvers produce differences in pressure among the areas of the mouth, the alveoli, and the pleural cavities, and air moves into the lungs. The intrathoracic pressure is decreased, the lungs are expanded, and the ribs flare, increasing the diameter of the thorax. The second to the sixth ribs move around two axes in a motion commonly termed the "pump handle" movement. The lower ribs move in a "bucket handle" motion. Because of the length and positioning of the lower ribs and because the lower interspaces are wider, the amplitude of movement is greater in the lower thorax.

Expiration is a relatively passive phenomenon. At the completion of inspiration, the diaphragm relaxes and the elastic recoil properties of the lungs expel air and pull the diaphragm to its resting position.

Topographical Anatomy

The topographical, or surface, landmarks of the thorax are helpful in identifying the location of the internal underlying structures and in describing the exact location of physical findings (Figure 15.5).

Manubriosternal junction (angle of Louis)

The manubriosternal junction is the articulation between the manubrium and the body of the sternum. Also called the angle of Louis, this junction is a visible and palpable angulation of the sternum. It is an extremely useful aid in the location of underlying structures. Just under the angle of Louis, the trachea bifurcates into the right and left main bronchi.

The superior border of the second rib articulates with the sternum at the manubriosternal junction. Palpation can be started at this junction, with distal ribs and rib interspaces counted from this point. As noted earlier, the number given to an intercostal space corresponds to the number of the rib immediately superior to that space. In palpation done for rib identification, the sec-

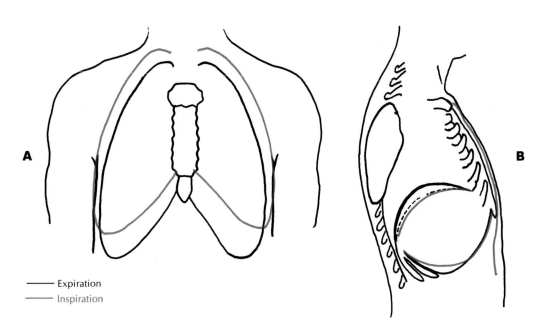

———— Expiration
———— Inspiration

figure **15.4**   Movement of the thorax during respiration. **A,** Anterior thorax. **B,** Lateral thorax.

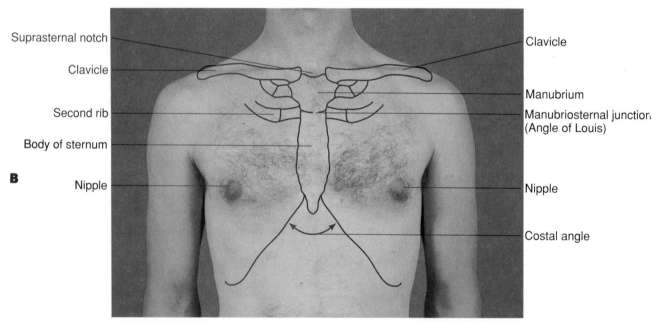

figure **15.5**   Topographical landmarks. **A** and **B,** Anterior thorax.

ond intercostal space should first be identified at the sternum. Then palpation should be done along the midclavicular line, rather than at the sternal border, for the remaining ribs and interspaces. The rib cartilages are very close at the sternum and consequently are difficult to differentiate; the cartilages of only the first seven ribs attach directly to the sternum.

Suprasternal notch

The suprasternal notch is the depression above the manubrium at the top of the sternum.

Costal angle

The costal angle, which is formed by the intersection of the costal margins, normally measures 90 degrees or less.

figure**15.5, cont'd** **C,** Posterior thorax. **D,** Lateral thorax.

Midsternal line

The midsternal line is an imaginary line drawn through the middle of the sternum.

Midclavicular lines

The midclavicular lines are left and right imaginary lines drawn through the midpoints of the clavicles and parallel to the midsternal line.

Anterior axillary lines

The anterior axillary lines are left and right imaginary lines drawn vertically from the anterior axillary folds, along the anterolateral chest, and parallel to the midsternal line.

Vertebra prominens (seventh cervical vertebra)

When the client flexes the neck anteriorly and the posterior thorax is noted, a prominent spinous process can be observed and palpated. This structure is the seventh cervical vertebra. If two spinous processes are observed and palpated, the superior one is C7 and the in-ferior one is T1. The counting of ribs is more difficult on the posterior thorax than on the anterior thorax. The spinous processes of the vertebrae can be counted relatively easily from C7 to T4. From T4 the spinous processes project obliquely, causing the spinous process of the vertebra to lie over the rib below it rather than over its correspondingly numbered rib. For example, the spinous process of T5 lies over the body of T6 and is adjacent to the sixth rib.

Midspinal line

The midspinal line is an imaginary line that runs vertically along the posterior spinous processes of the vertebrae.

Scapular lines

The scapular lines are left and right imaginary lines that lie vertically and are parallel to the midspinal line. They pass through the inferior angles of the scapulae when the client stands erect with the arms at the sides.

Posterior axillary lines

The posterior axillary lines are imaginary left and right lines drawn vertically from the posterior axillary folds along the posterolateral wall of the thorax when the lateral arm is abducted directly from the lateral chest wall.

Midaxillary lines

The midaxillary lines are imaginary left and right lines drawn vertically from the apices of the axillae. They lie approximately midway between the anterior and the posterior axillary lines and run parallel to them.

Underlying Thoracic Structures

When examining the respiratory system, it is important to maintain a mental image of the placement of the organs and organ parts of the respiratory system and the other systems located in the thoracic area (Figures 15.6 through 15.9).

Lung borders

In the anterior thorax the apices of the lungs extend approximately 2 to 4 cm above the clavicles. The inferior borders of the lungs cross the sixth rib at the midclavicular line. In the posterior thorax the apices extend to T1. The lower borders vary with respiration and usually extend from the spinous process of T10 on expira-

tion to the spinous process of T12 on deep inspiration. In the lateral thorax the lung extends from the apex of the axilla to the eighth rib of the midaxillary line.

Lung fissures

The right oblique (diagonal) fissure extends from the area of the spinous process of the third thoracic vertebra laterally and downward until it crosses the fifth rib at the right midaxillary line. It then continues anteriorly and medially to end at the sixth rib at the right midclavicular line. The right horizontal fissure extends from the fifth rib slightly posterior to the right midaxillary line and runs horizontally to the area of the fourth rib at the right sternal border. The left oblique (diagonal) fissure extends from the spinous process of the third thoracic vertebra laterally and downward to the left midaxillary line at the fifth rib. It continues anteriorly and medially until it terminates at the sixth rib in the left midclavicular line.

Borders of the diaphragm

Anteriorly, on expiration, the right dome of the diaphragm is located at the level of the fifth rib at the midclavicular line, and the left dome is situated at the level of the sixth rib. Posteriorly, on expiration, the diaphragm is at the level of the spinous process of T10; laterally it is at the eighth rib at the midaxillary line. On nonlabored inspiration, the diaphragm moves approximately 1.5 cm downward, with the right side being slightly higher than the left side because of the placement of the liver. With forced inspiration and expiration, the diaphragmatic excursion can be increased to 3 to 5 cm.

Trachea

The bifurcation of the trachea occurs approximately just below the manubriosternal junction anteriorly and at the spinous process of T4 posteriorly.

■ EXAMINATION

Health History

If a possible respiratory system problem is being investigated, the history of the respiratory system and the cardiovascular system should be taken together because of the symbiotic nature of the two systems, their sharing of the thoracic region of the body, and the potential effect that intervention directed at one system may have on the other system. However, the health history presented here focuses on the respiratory system.

Throughout the health history interview, record the following data about a symptom or problem: (1) onset (specific date, sudden or gradual), (2) duration, (3) frequency, (4) precipitating factors, (5) aggravating or alle-

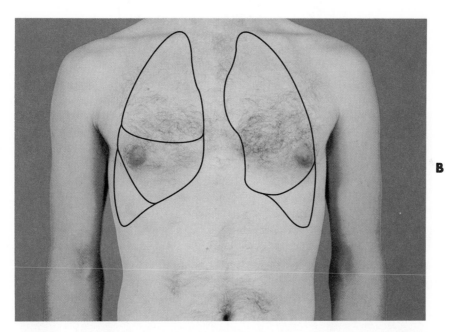

figure **15.6**   Anterior thorax. **A,** Internal organs and structures. **B,** Lung borders.

viating factors, (6) treatment received or self-care given, and (7) outcome.

Present health status

1. Allergies
2. Tobacco use
   a. Type of tobacco(s) smoked, age at which smoking was started, amount of smoking (packs per day), duration of habit (number of years) (A smoking index can be determined by multiplying the num-
   ber of years of smoking by the number of packs smoked per day.)
   b. Exposure to smoke of others
   c. History of attempts to quit and cessation methods tried.
3. Medications: Types and patterns of use
4. Use of aerosols or inhalants for any purpose
5. Recent screening or diagnostic assessments: Allergy test, skin test, chest x-ray examination
6. Nutritional data

figure **15.7** Posterior thorax. **A,** Internal organs and structures. **B,** Lung borders.

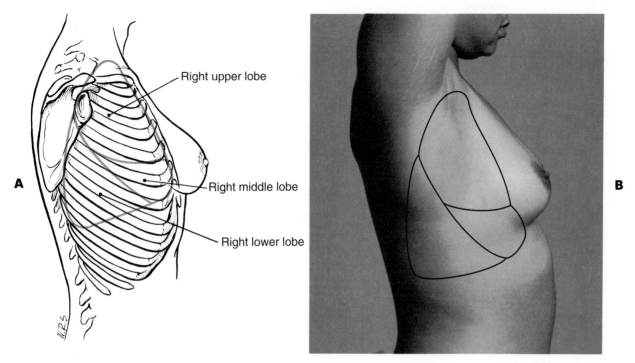

figure**15.8** Right lateral thorax. **A,** Internal organs and chest structures. (Note the relationship of the breast to chest organs and structures.) **B,** Lung borders.

figure**15.9** Left lateral thorax. **A,** Internal organs and chest structures. **B,** Lung borders.

Tools for Assessing Dyspnea

BORG CATEGORY–RATIO SCALE FOR RATING PERCEIVED BREATHLESSNESS

Score	Code
0	Nothing at all
0.5	Very, very slight
1	Very slight
2	Slight
3	Moderate
4	Somewhat severe
5	Severe
6	
7	Very severe
8	
9	
10	Very, very severe

To use: Enlarge the scale on an 8.5 by 11 inch sheet. Ask the client to identify the number which most closely describes the intensity of dyspnea. This scale may be rated differently by various clients, so is not useful as a clinical measure across clients. However, the scale may be useful for measuring changes in individual clients as a result of disease or in response to treatment.

ATS-DLD SCALE FOR RATING BREATHLESSNESS

Score

1. Are you troubled by shortness of breath when hurrying on the level or walking up a slight hill?
2. (If yes) Do you have to walk slower than people of your age on the level because of breathlessness?
3. (If yes) Do you ever have to stop for breath after walking at your own pace on the level?
4. (If yes) Do you ever have to stop for breath after walking about 100 yards (or after a few minutes) on the level?
5. (If yes) Are you too breathless to leave the house or breathless on dressing or undressing?

To use: Score by the highest level of breathlessness experienced.

From Hoeman SP: *Rehabilitation nursing: process and application,* ed 2, St Louis, 1996, Mosby. Scales modified from Borg G, Holmgren A, Linblad I: Quantitative evaluation of chest pain, *Acta Med Scand* 644: 43–45, 1981; and Ferris BG: Recommended respiratory disease questionnaires for use with adults and children, *Am Rev Respir Dis* 118:7–53, 1978.

a. Sudden weight loss
b. Obesity
7. Exercise patterns
8. Use of alcohol and other mind-altering drugs

Present illness*

1. Cough
   a. Type: Dry, moist, wet, productive, nonproductive, bubbling, hoarse, hacking, barking, whooping
   b. Onset: Sudden or gradual
   c. Duration
   d. Pattern: Regular or occasional; relationship to activities, time of day, weather, talking
   e. Severity: Effect on activities of daily living
   f. Associated symptoms: Shortness of breath, chest pain, fever, gagging, choking, changes in respiratory system, sputum production
   g. Efforts to treat: Medications and other interventions; pattern of use and effectiveness
2. Sputum production
   a. Amount
   b. Color
   c. Presence of blood
   d. Odor
   e. Consistency
   f. Pattern of production
3. Shortness of breath (dyspnea; see box at left)
   a. Onset: Sudden or gradual
   b. Frequency: Persistent or intermittent
   c. Pattern: Position when condition occurs; position most comfortable; relationship to exercise, other activity, time of day, eating
   d. Tolerance of activity: How many flights of stairs can be climbed before dyspnea occurs?
   e. Differences between inhalation and exhalation
   f. Severity: Effect on activity during which shortness of breath occurs and on activities of daily living
   g. Associated symptoms: Anxiety, pain, discomfort, cough, fever
   h. Response to treatment
   i. Special situations: (1) Dyspnea that begins or increases when client lies down (orthopnea)—determine number of pillows that client uses; (2) sudden onset of dyspnea after a period of lying down that is relieved by sitting upright (paroxysmal nocturnal dyspnea); (3) dyspnea that increases when client is upright (platypnea)
4. Chest pain
   a. Onset
   b. Pattern
   c. Severity
   d. Duration

*Investigation of common symptoms is outlined.

e. Associated symptoms: Trauma, coughing, infection, fever, anxiety, pain

f. Efforts to treat: Medications, heat, splinting

Past health history

1. Respiratory infections and diseases: Type, frequency, pattern, and treatment (Specific inquiry should include past history of tuberculosis, chronic obstructive pulmonary diseases, e.g., asthma, emphysema, chronic bronchitis.)
2. Trauma to respiratory system or area
3. Surgery to respiratory system or area
4. Chronic conditions of other systems: Cardiac diseases, malignancies, renal diseases

Family health history

1. Tuberculosis
2. Emphysema
3. Lung cancer
4. Allergies, asthma

Other considerations

1. Employment and employment history: Place and nature of work; exposure to chemicals, vapors, dust, allergens, animals, and other possible pulmonary irritants; presence of such possible irritants in the home environment (e.g., types of heating, cooling, and ventilation)
2. Current and past residence and travel to places where exposure to uncommon respiratory disease may have occurred
3. Hobbies that might involve exposure to respiratory irritants

RISK FACTORS　RESPIRATORY DISEASE

Smoking: A major risk factor, contributing to a large portion of lung cancer cases

Sedentary lifestyle or recent immobilization

Age: Respiratory problems increase with aging

Environmental exposures: Especially occupational exposure to certain carcinogens

Extreme obesity

Weakened chest muscles for any reason

History of frequent respiratory infections for any reason

Family history of familial respiratory disease

Preparation for Examination: Client and Environment

Adequate respiratory examination requires a warm, well-lighted, quiet room. In addition to adequate room lighting, a mechanism for supplementary lighting is essential to aid in close inspection of specific areas.

Privacy is important because of the need to examine the entire chest area. Female clients may wish to have a gown or towel to cover their breasts while the posterior thorax is being examined. If the breasts are large, tell clients that you will be asking them to move their breasts to the side so that you will be better able to palpate, percuss, and auscultate the anterior thorax.

Before starting the examination, teach the client how to sit and how to breathe during the auscultation of the posterior thorax. For examination of the posterior thorax, instruct the client to hunch forward slightly and cross the arms over the chest (see Figure 15.16) so that the greatest amount of lung surface is available for examination. Also, instruct the client to breathe deeply and quietly, slowly inhaling and exhaling through the open mouth.

The male client can be seated throughout the examination and stripped to the waist. Female clients can use a towel or gown to cover their breasts when the posterior and lateral portions of the chest are being examined.

The examination of the respiratory system generally is done in the traditional sequence—inspection, palpation, percussion, and auscultation.

PREPARATION FOR EXAMINATION

EQUIPMENT

Item	Purpose
Stethoscope with diaphragm	Auscultation of thorax
Marking pencil	Measurement of diaphragmatic excursion
Metric ruler	Measurement of diaphragmatic excursion

CLIENT AND ENVIRONMENT

Client

Stripped to waist

Gown and sheet covering remainder of body

Covering available for female client to cover chest when not being examined

Instructed regarding breathing and position for examination of posterior thorax

Setting

Warm

Private

Technique for Examination and Normal Findings

Inspection

Inspection is performed to (1) measure and assess the pattern of respirations and (2) assess the skin and the overall configuration, symmetry, and integrity of the thorax.

The approach to the physical examination is regional and integrated. The examination of systems is combined in body regions when appropriate. Because the client is uncovered to the waist during the examination, a large portion of skin and tissue is accessible to inspection. The observation of the skin and underlying tissue provides information about the client's general nutritional state. Common thoracic skin findings are the spider nevi associated with cirrhosis and seborrheic dermatitis (see Chapter 10: Skin, Hair, and Nails).

Lips and nails. Inspection of the respiratory system includes observation of lips and nail beds for color and observation of the nails for clubbing (see Chapter 10 and Chapter 16: Cardiovascular System).

Thoracic configuration. The first point of observation is the general shape of the thorax and its symmetry. Although no individual is absolutely symmetrical in both body hemispheres, most individuals are reasonably similar from side to side. Using the client as his or her own control whenever paired parts are examined is an excellent habit and often yields important findings. The normal thoracic configuration in adults is oval. The anteroposterior diameter of the thorax in the normal adult is less than the transverse diameter at an approximate ratio of 1:2 to 5:7 (Figure 15.10). In the normal infant, in some adults with pulmonary disease, and in elderly adults, the thorax is essentially round. This condition is called barrel chest. The barrel chest is characterized by horizontal ribs, slight kyphosis of the thoracic spine, and a prominent sternal angle. The chest appears as though it is in the continuous inspiratory position.

Other observed abnormalities of thoracic shape include the following:

1. *Retraction of thorax:* The retraction is unilateral, involving only one side.
2. *Pigeon or chicken chest (pectus carinatum):* Sternal protrusion anteriorly. The anteroposterior diameter of the chest is increased, and the resultant configuration resembles the thorax of a fowl.
3. *Funnel chest (pectus excavatum):* Depression of part or all of the sternum. If the depression is deep, it may interfere with both respiratory and cardiac function.
4. *Spinal deformities (scoliosis, kyphosis, lordosis):* The respiratory examination offers an excellent opportunity to initiate inspection of the spine (see Chapter 18: Musculoskeletal System).

Ribs and interspaces. Retraction of interspaces on inspiration may indicate some obstruction of free air inflow. Bulging of interspaces on expiration occurs when air outflow is obstructed, or it may be a result of tumor, aneurysm, or cardiac enlargement.

Normally, the costal angle is less than 90 degrees, and the ribs are inserted into the spine at approximately a 45-degree angle (see Figure 15.1). In clients with obstructive lung disease, these angles are widened.

Pattern of respiration. Normally, men and children breathe diaphragmatically, and women breathe thoracically or costally. A change in this pattern might be significant. If the client appears to have labored respiration, it is important to observe for the use of the accessory muscles of respiration in the neck (sternocleidomastoid, scalenus, and trapezius muscles) and for supraclavicular retraction. Impedance to air inflow is often accompanied by retraction of the intercostal spaces during inspiration. An excessively long expiratory phase of respiration is characteristic of outflow impedance and may be accompanied by the use of abdominal muscles to aid in expiration.

In the normal adult, the resting respiratory rate is 12 to 20 breaths per minute and is regular and unlabored. The ratio of respiratory rate to pulse rate normally is

A   **B**

Angle of rib slope

figure **15.10**   **A,** Normal thoracic configuration. **B,** Increased anteroposterior diameter. Note contrast in the angle of the slope of the ribs.

1:4. Tachypnea is an adult resting respiratory rate of more than 20 breaths per minute. Bradypnea is an adult respiratory rate of less than 10 breaths per minute. Dyspnea is a subjective phenomenon of inadequate or distressful respiration. Many more abnormal patterns of respiration exist. Some of the commonly noted respiratory patterns are listed in Table 15.1.

Palpation

Palpation is performed to (1) further assess abnormalities suggested by the health history or by observation, such as tenderness, pulsations, masses, or skin lesions; (2) assess the skin and subcutaneous structures; (3) assess thoracic expansion; (4) assess tactile fremitus; and (5) assess tracheal position.

In examination of the thorax, four parts of the thorax need consideration: the posterior chest, anterior chest, right and left lateral chest, and apices. During the examination, move from the area of one hemisphere to the corresponding area on the other side (right to left, left to right) until all four major parts have been surveyed. During palpation for assessment of fremitus and all subsequent procedures for examination of the respiratory system, examine all areas meticulously and systematically. It is common for the practitioner to examine the apices, posterior chest, and lateral areas while standing behind the client. However, some examiners prefer to examine apices and lateral chest areas from the front. Either approach is effective. The important point is that no portion of the thorax should be overlooked.

A very helpful landmark for location of points on the thorax, especially the counting of ribs and interspaces, is the angle of Louis, the junction of the manubrium and the body of the sternum. It is also important to remem-

table 15.1	*Characteristics of Commonly Observed Respiratory Patterns*		
Type of respiration	**Diagram**		**Discussion**
Normal			12-20 respirations/min in adults; regular in rhythm; ratio of respiratory rate to pulse rate is 1:4
Hyperventilation or Kussmaul respiration			Increase in both rate and depth; hyperpnea is an increase in depth only
Periodic respiration			Alternating hyperpnea, shallow respiration, and apnea; sometimes called Cheyne-Stokes respiration; frequently occurs in the severely ill
Sighing respiration			Deep and audible; audible portion sounds like a sigh
Air trapping			Present in obstructive pulmonary diseases; air is trapped in the lungs; respiratory level rises, and breathing becomes shallow
Biot's breathing			Shallow breathing interrupted by apnea; seen in some central nervous system disorders and in healthy persons

ber that the second rib connects with this palpable bony prominence and that the second interspace lies immediately below it.

General palpation. First, assess the temperature and turgor of the skin. Then palpate the thoracic muscle mass and the thoracic skeleton. If the client has no complaints in relation to the respiratory system, a rapid, general survey of anterior, lateral, and posterior thoracic areas is sufficient. If the client has respiratory complaints, meticulously palpate all chest areas for tenderness, bulges, or abnormal movements. Palpate areas of abnormality or tenderness last. Inform the client that these areas will be palpated last. To avoid muscle guarding throughout the entire procedure, inform the client again immediately before these sensitive areas are palpated.

Crepitations. In subcutaneous emphysema, the subcutaneous tissue contains fine beads of air. As this tissue is palpated, audible crackling sounds are heard and popping sensations are noted under the skin. These sounds, elicited by palpation, are termed crepitations. Crepitations may be localized or noted diffusely throughout the thorax.

Assessment of thoracic expansion. The degree of thoracic expansion can be assessed from the anterior or posterior chest (Figure 15.11). Anteriorly, place your hands over the client's anterolateral chest with the thumbs extended along the costal margin, pointing to the xiphoid process. Posteriorly, place the thumbs at the level of the tenth rib and place the palms on the posterolateral chest. In either position, the thumbs will be approximately 3 to 5 cm apart before inspiration, depending on the client's size. The amount and symmetry of the thoracic expansion can be felt during quiet and deep respiration. First, feel thoracic expansion during normal, quiet respiration. Next, ask the client to take a deep breath in slowly and then exhale. The symmetry of

A

B

C

D

figure **15.11**   Palpation of the thoracic expansion.

figure **15.12**   Palpation for assessment of tactile fremitus. **A,** Use of the palmar surface of the fingertips. **B,** Simultaneous application of the fingertips of both hands. **C,** Use of the ulnar aspect of the hand. **D,** Use of the ulnar aspect of the closed fist.

respiration should be felt between the left and the right hemithoraces as the thumbs are separated an additional 3 to 5 cm during the deep inspiration.

Assessment of tactile fremitus. Fremitus is vibration that is perceptible on palpation. Tactile (sometimes also called "vocal") fremitus is palpable vibration of the thoracic wall produced by phonation.

Ask the client to repeat "one, two, three" or "ninety-nine" while you systematically palpate the thorax. Use the palmar bases of the fingers, the ulnar aspect of the hand, or the ulnar aspect of the closed fist (Figure 15.12). You can use two hands to assess both sides of the chest simultaneously or one hand moving alternately to compare one side of the chest with the other. See Figure 15.13 for areas of assessment of tactile fremitus. If one hand is used, move it from one side of the chest to the corresponding area on the other side. If two hands are used, place them simultaneously on the corresponding areas of each thoracic side.

Table 15.2 presents information about interpreting tactile fremitus. Fremitus is decreased or absent when the distance between the palpating hand is increased or when there is interference with sound transmission. Distance is increased and sound transmission is decreased in the following conditions: pneumothorax with lung collapse, fluid in the pleural space (pleural effusion), pleural thickening, tumors or masses in the pleural space, em-

physema, bronchial obstruction, and a thick, muscular chest wall. Fremitus is increased in conditions that decrease the distance between the lungs and the palpating fingers and that favor the sound transmission in the chest (e.g., in pneumonia with consolidation, atelectasis [with open bronchus], lung tumors, pulmonary infarction, and pulmonary fibrosis.) Before palpating, visually inspect the trachea for a visual shift.

Assessment of tracheal deviation. The trachea is assessed by palpation for lateral deviation. Place the index finger of your dominant hand on the trachea in the suprasternal notch, then move the finger laterally left and right in the spaces bordered by the upper edge of the clavicle, the inner aspect of the sternocleidomastoid muscle, and the trachea. These spaces should be equal on both sides. In diseases such as atelectasis and pulmonary fibrosis, the trachea may be deviated toward the abnormal side. The trachea may be deviated toward the normal side in conditions such as neck tumors, thyroid enlargement, enlarged lymph nodes, pleural effusion, unilateral emphysema, and tension pneumothorax.

An alternate method of examining for tracheal deviation is as follows: Stand in front of the seated client and place both hands around the client's neck with the thumbs in the spaces lateral to the trachea. Normally, both thumbs should palpate the straight borders of the trachea and assess equality of spaces bilaterally.

A   B

figure **15.13**   Areas of assessment for palpation of tactile fremitus and auscultation of vocal resonance. **A,** Anterior thorax. **B,** Posterior thorax.

table 15.2 *Characteristics of Normal and Abnormal Tactile Fremitus*

Fremitus	Description
Normal (moderate) fremitus	Varies greatly from person to person and depends on intensity and pitch of voice, position and distance of bronchi in relation to chest wall, and thickness of chest wall; is most intense in second intercostal spaces at sternal border near area of bronchial bifurcation
Increased tactile fremitus Area of consolidation	Is observed with conditions that increase density of lung tissue; a dense mass (e.g., consolidation of pneumonia) conducts vibrations with greater intensity than a porous medium (e.g., normal lung); for increased fremitus to occur, there must be a patent bronchus and consolidation must be close to thoracic wall; may be observed in pneumonia, compressed lung, lung tumor, or pulmonary fibrosis
Decreased or absent tactile fremitus Collapsed lung — Air	Is observed when anything obstructs transmission of vibrations, results in a decreased production of sounds, or creates a barrier between lung and thoracic wall; may be observed in pleural effusion, pleural thickening, pneumothorax, bronchial obstruction, or emphysema
Pleural friction rub	Vibration produced by inflamed pleural surfaces rubbing together; is produced when inflammation of pleura creates a decrease in fluid normally lubricating surfaces; is felt as a grating, is synchronous with respiratory movements, and is more commonly felt on inspiration
Rhonchal fremitus	Coarse vibrations produced by passage of air through thick exudates in large air passages; often can be decreased or altered by coughing

Percussion

Percussion is the tapping of an object to set underlying structures in motion and thus produce a sound called a percussion note and a palpable vibration. Percussion penetrates to a depth of approximately 5 to 7 cm into the chest. This technique is used in the thoracic examination to determine the relative amounts of air, liquid, or solid material in the underlying lung and to determine the positions and boundaries of organs. The techniques of percussion, along with other assessment techniques, are discussed thoroughly in Chapter 8.

Mediate (indirect) percussion is used in assessment of the respiratory system. It involves the striking of an object held against the area to be examined. For position in performing mediate percussion on the thorax, see Figure 15.14.

With your forearm and shoulder stationary and all movement done at the wrist, strike the pleximeter sharply with the plexor. Aim the blow at the portion of the pleximeter that is exerting maximum pressure on the thoracic surface, which is usually the base of the terminal phalanx, the distal interphalangeal joint, or the middle phalanx. Execute the blow rapidly, and immediately withdraw the plexor. The plexor strikes with the tip of the finger at right angles to the pleximeter. Strike

one or two rapid blows in each area assessed. Avoid bony areas. Use interspaces for percussion. Compare one side of the thorax with the other.

With experience and study, one learns to differentiate among the five percussion tones commonly elicited from the human body. In the study of tones, the determination of four characteristics will assist in assessment and labeling:

1. *Intensity (amplitude):* Loudness or softness of the tone.
2. *Pitch (frequency):* Relates to the number of vibrations per second. Rapid vibrations produce high-pitched tones; slow vibrations produce low-pitched tones. The greater the density of an object, the higher the frequency.
3. *Duration:* Amount of time a note is sustained.
4. *Quality:* Subjective phenomena relating to the innate characteristics of the object being percussed.

Table 15.3 lists and explains the commonly used descriptive terms for tones elicited by percussion over the thorax and the normal location of such sounds in the thoracic region. Hyperresonance is an abnormal percussion tone in adults. Table 15.6 describes clinical assessment findings in several common respiratory system problems and provides examples of abnormal occurrence of the various percussion tones.

General percussion survey. Figure 15.15 is a percussion map for the normal chest. The procedure for thoracic percussion is as follows:

1. Percuss the apices to determine if the normal 5-cm area of resonance is present between the neck and the shoulder muscles (Figure 15.15), an area approximately 3 to 4 cm above the inner third of the clavicles.
2. Position the client with the head bent and the

A B

figure**15.14**   Indirect percussion. **A,** Positioning of the hands. **B,** Hand movement.

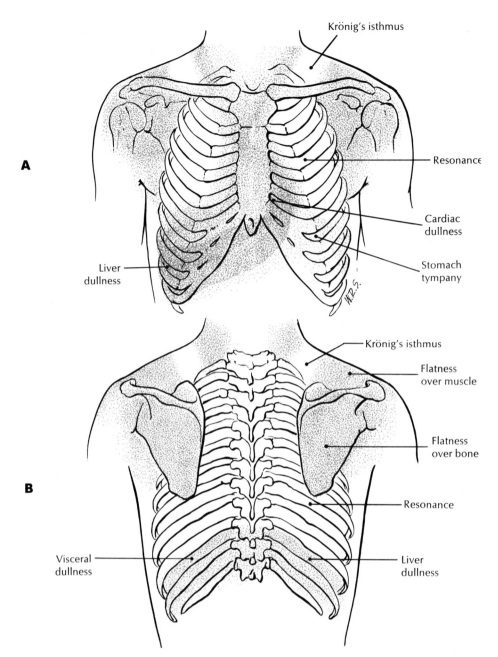

figure **15.15** Percussion areas. **A,** Normal anterior chest. **B,** Normal posterior chest.

table **15.3** *Description of Percussion Tones*

Tone	Intensity	Pitch	Duration	Quality	Normal location
Hyperresonance	Very loud	Very low	Long	Booming	Child's lung
Resonance	Loud	Low	Long	Hollow	Peripheral lung
Tympany	Loud	High	Medium	Drumlike	Stomach
Dullness	Medium	High	Medium	Thudlike	Liver
Flatness	Soft	High	Short	Extreme dullness	Muscle

arms folded over the chest (Figure 15.16). With this maneuver, the scapulae move laterally and more lung area is accessible to examination. On the posterior chest, percuss systematically at about 5-cm intervals from the upper to lower chest, moving left to right, right to left, and avoiding scapular and other bony areas.

3. Percuss the lateral chest with the client's arm positioned over the head (Figure 15.17).

4. On the anterior chest, percuss systematically, as done for the posterior chest.

Diaphragmatic excursion. If the client's breathing is shallow or painful, the measurement of diaphragmatic excursion is indicated. Various pulmonary and abdominal lesions, ascites, or trauma may limit the movement of the diaphragm. The following is the procedure for assessing diaphragmatic excursion:

1. Instruct the client to inhale deeply and hold the breath in.

2. Percuss down the scapular line on one side, starting at T7 or at the end of the scapula, until the lower edge of the lung is identified. Sound will change from resonance to dullness.

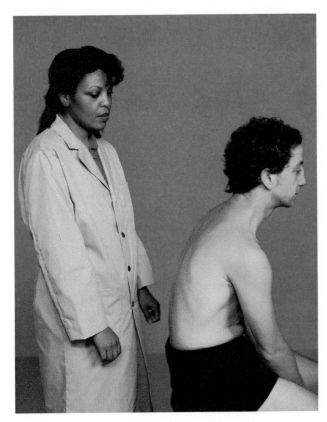

figure**15.16**   Position of the client for examination of the posterior thorax.

figure**15.17**   Position of the client for percussion of the lateral thorax.

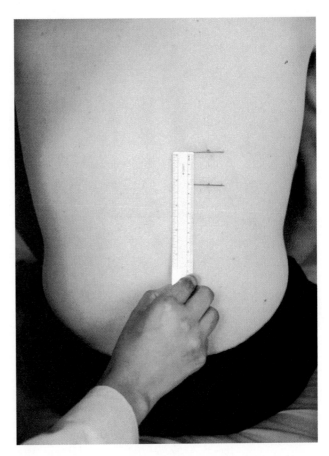

figure**15.18**   Assessment of diaphragmatic excursion.

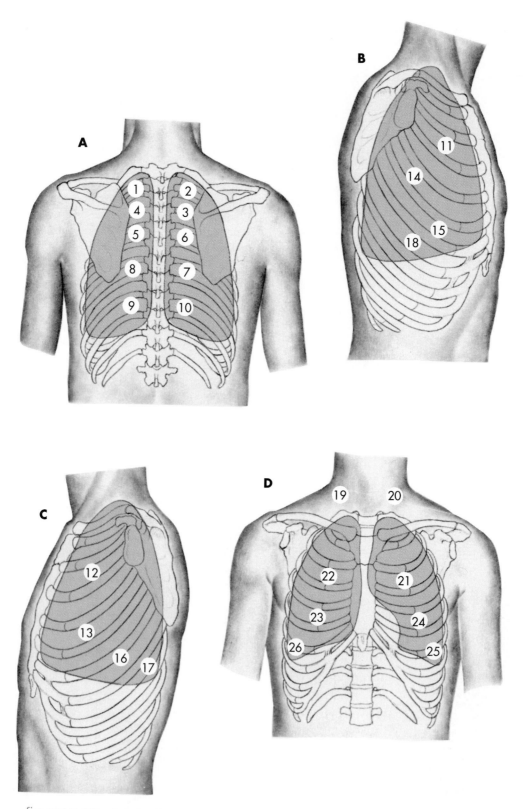

figure**15.19** Routine for systematic percussion and auscultation of the thorax. Numbers indicate a recommended sequence for percussion and auscultation during a routine screening examination. **A,** Posterior thorax. **B,** Right lateral thorax. **C,** Left lateral thorax. **D,** Anterior thorax. *(Modified from Seidel HM et al: Mosby's guide to physical examination, ed 3, St Louis, 1995, Mosby.)*

3. With a skin-marking pencil, mark the point of change at the scapular line. This point is the edge of the diaphragm at full inhalation.

4. Instruct the client to take a few normal breaths.

5. Instruct the client to take a deep breath, exhale completely, and hold the breath at the end of the expiration.

6. Proceed to percuss upward from the previously marked point at the midscapular line. Mark the point where dullness of the diaphragm changes to the resonance of the lung. This point is the level of the diaphragm at full expiration.

7. Repeat the procedure on the opposite side.

8. Measure and record the diaphragmatic excursion, the distance between the upper and lower marks in centimeters for each side of the thorax.

An alternate method of determining the level of the diaphragm at full exhalation is to percuss down along the scapular line and note where the resonance of the lung changes to the dullness of the diaphragm.

The diaphragm is usually slightly higher on the right side because of the location of the liver on that side. Diaphragmatic excursion, which is normally 3 to 5 cm bilaterally, is usually measured only on the posterior chest (Figure 15.18).

In the actual examination, the apices and the posterior and lateral chest would be examined before percussion of the anterior chest is done. A recommended sequence for examination of the posterior, lateral, and anterior thoracic areas is illustrated in Figure 15.19.

Auscultation

Through auscultation, information can be obtained about the functioning of the respiratory system and about the presence of any obstruction in the passages. For auscultation of the lungs, a stethoscope is used. The diaphragm of the stethoscope is commonly used for the thoracic examination because it covers a larger surface than does the bell. Also, the diaphragm is designed to transmit the usually higher pitch of abnormal breath sounds.

Place the stethoscope firmly, but not tightly, on the skin. Avoid client or stethoscope movement because movements of muscle under the skin or movements of the stethoscope over hair produce confusing extrinsic sounds.

The auscultatory assessment includes (1) analysis of breath sounds, (2) detection of any abnormal sounds, and (3) examination of the sounds produced by the spoken voice, or vocal resonance. As with percussion, use a zigzag approach, comparing the finding at each point with the corresponding point on the opposite hemithorax.

Analysis of breath sounds. Before beginning auscultation, instruct the client to breathe through the mouth and more deeply and more slowly than in usual respiration. Then, systematically auscultate the apices and the posterior, lateral, and anterior chest (see Figure 15.19). At each application of the stethoscope, listen to at least one complete respiration. Observe the client for signs of hyperventilation and alter the procedure if the client becomes light-headed or faint.

Normal breath sounds. Breath sounds are produced by the movement of air through the tracheobronchoalveolar system. These sounds are analyzed according to pitch, intensity, quality, and relative duration of inspiratory and expiratory phases. Table 15.4 outlines the types of sounds heard in the thorax.

The sounds heard over normal lung parenchyma are called vesicular breath sounds. The inspiratory phase of the vesicular breath sounds is heard better than the expiratory phase and is about 2.5 times longer. These sounds have a low pitch and soft intensity.

Bronchovesicular breath sounds are normally heard in the areas of the major bronchi, especially in the apex of the right lung and at the sternal borders anteriorly and posteriorly between the scapula. Bronchovesicular breath sounds are characterized by inspiratory and expiratory phases of equal duration, moderate pitch, and moderate intensity. When bronchovesicular breath sounds are heard over the peripheral lung of an adult, an underlying pathological condition is likely to be present.

Bronchial breath sounds are normally heard over the trachea and indicate a pathological condition if heard over lung tissue. They are high-pitched, loud sounds associated with shortened inspiratory and lengthened expiratory phases. A gap of silence audibly separates the inspiratory and expiratory phases.

Figure 15.20 shows the various areas for assessing breath sounds of the anterior and posterior thorax. Absent or decreased breath sounds can occur in (1) any condition that causes the deposition of foreign matter in the pleural space, (2) bronchial obstruction, (3) emphysema, or (4) shallow breathing.

Increased breath sounds, as from vesicular to bronchovesicular or bronchial, can occur in any condition that causes a consolidation of lung tissue.

Adventitious breath sounds. Adventitious sounds are not alterations in breath sounds but abnormal sounds superimposed on breath sounds. Classification of these sounds varies among authorities; consequently, the

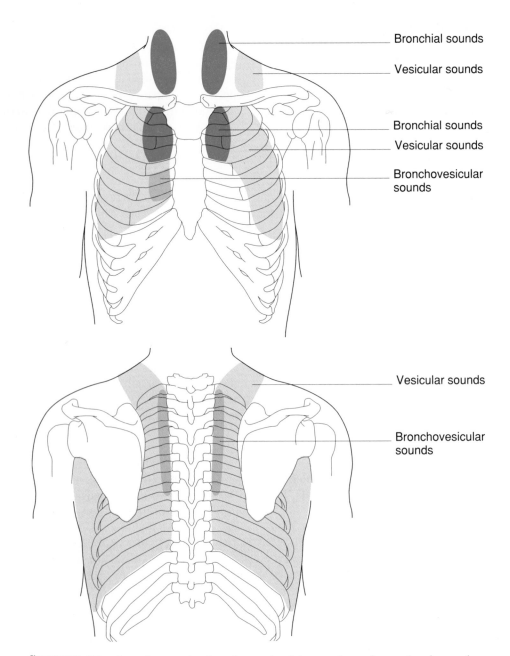

Bronchial sounds

Vesicular sounds

Bronchial sounds
Vesicular sounds
Bronchovesicular
sounds

Vesicular sounds

Bronchovesicular
sounds

figure 15.20   Areas for assessing breath sounds of the anterior and posterior thorax. Areas more darkly colored indicate normal point for auscultation of bronchial and bronchovesicular breath sounds.

nomenclatures are somewhat inconsistent. The commonly used terms for adventitious sounds are described in Table 15.5.

A crackle (or "rale," a term used in older texts) is a short, discrete, interrupted, crackling or bubbling sound that is most commonly heard during inspiration. The sound of crackles is similar to that produced by hairs being rolled between the fingers while close to the ear. The exact mechanism by which crackles are produced is not fully understood. Crackles are thought to be pro-

duced by air passing through moisture in the bronchi, bronchioles, and alveoli or by air rushing through passages and alveoli that were closed during expiration and abruptly opened during inspiration. The pitch and location in the inspiratory phase of the crackles are thought to indicate their site of production. Low-pitched, coarse crackles occurring early in inspiration are thought to originate in the bronchi, as in bronchitis. Medium-pitched crackles in midinspiration occur in diseases of the small bronchi, as in bronchiectasis. High-pitched,

table 15.4 Characteristics of Breath Sounds

Sound	Duration of inspiration and expiration	Diagram of sound	Pitch	Intensity	Normal location	Abnormal location
Vesicular	Inspiration > expiration 2.5:1		Low	Soft	Peripheral lung	Not applicable
Bronchovesicular	Inspiration = expiration 1:1		Medium	Medium	First and second intercostal spaces at sternal border anteriorly; posteriorly at T4 medial to scapulae	Peripheral lung
Bronchial (tubular)	Inspiration < expiration 1:2		High	Loud	Over trachea	Lung area

table 15.5 Origin and Characteristics of Adventitious Sounds

Sound	Diagram of sound	Origin	Characteristics
Crackles*— fine to medium		Air passing through moisture in small air passages and alveoli	Discrete, discontinuous; inspiratory; have a dry or wet crackling quality; not cleared by coughing; sound is simulated by rolling a lock of hair near ear
Crackles*— medium to coarse		Air passing through moisture in bronchioles, bronchi, and trachea	As above; louder than fine crackles
Rhonchi (sonorous wheezes)		Air passing through air passages narrowed by secretions, swelling, tumors, and so on	Continuous sounds; originate in large air passages; may be inspiratory and expiratory but usually predominate in expiration; loud, low-pitched, moaning or snoring quality; coughing may alter sounds
Wheezes— sibilant		Same as rhonchi	Continuous sounds; originate in the small air passages; may be inspiratory and expiratory but usually predominate in expiration; high-pitched, wheezing sounds
Friction rubs		Rubbing together of inflamed and roughened pleural surfaces	Creaking or grating quality; superficial sounding; inspiratory and expiratory; heard most often in the lower anterolateral chest (area of greatest thoracic expansion); coughing has no effect

*Crackles are also called rales or crepitations.

Voice Sound Assessment Techniques

Client vocalization	Normal auscultatory finding	Abnormal auscultatory finding
"Ninety-nine" spoken	Muffled, nondistinct sound	"Ninety-nine": bronchophony
"Ninety-nine" whispered	Barely audible, nondistinct sound	"Ninety-nine": whispered pectoriloquy
"e- e- e" spoken	Muffled, nondistinct sound	"a- a- a": egophony

fine crackles are found in diseases affecting the bronchioles and alveoli and occur late in inspiration.

Rhonchi are continuous sounds produced by the movement of air through narrowed passages in the tracheobronchial tree. They predominate in expiration because bronchi are shortened and narrowed during this respiratory phase. However, they can occur in both the inspiratory and the expiratory phase of respiration, suggesting that lumina have been narrowed during both respiratory phases. As with crackles, the pitch and location of sonorous wheezes in the expiratory phase are thought to indicate their origins. Rhonchi heard in early expiration probably originate in the larger bronchi.

Wheezes are produced by mechanisms similar to those producing rhonchi. Wheezes, however, are high pitched and musical. They can occur throughout the respiratory cycle but are usually more prominent on expiration.

A pleural friction rub is a loud, dry, creaking or grating sound indicative of pleural irritation. It is produced by the rubbing together of inflamed and roughened pleural surfaces during respiration (e.g., in pleurisy). Therefore it is heard best during the latter part of inspiration and the beginning of expiration. Because thoracic expansion is greatest in the lower anterolateral thorax, pleural friction rubs are most often heard there.

If the client has crackles, listen for several respirations in the areas in which the crackles are heard to determine the effects of deep breathing. Also, ask the client to cough and note the changes in adventitious sounds after coughing. Crackles do not usually change with coughing, but ronchi will often do so.

If the client has complained of respiratory difficulty and no adventitious sounds are heard, ask him or her to cough; often, adventitious sounds are noted after coughing.

Vocal resonance. The same mechanism that produces tactile fremitus produces vocal resonance. Resonance is the transmission of voice sounds as heard through the stethoscope placed on the chest wall. Normal vocal resonance is heard as muffled, nondistinct sounds. It is loudest medially and is less intense at the periphery of the lung.

Auscultation Summary

General survey for breath sounds, adventitious sounds
Assessment of vocal resonance

Vocal resonance should be assessed if any respiratory system abnormality has been detected on observation, palpation, percussion, or auscultation. The routine is the same systematic one previously used in assessing tactile fremitus (see Figure 15.13). The client says "one, two, three" or "ninety-nine" while the examiner does an auscultatory survey of the thorax.

Bronchophony is an increase in loudness and clarity of vocal resonance. Special vocal resonance techniques are used when resonance is increased. These include tests for whispered pectoriloquy and egophony.

Whispered pectoriloquy is exaggerated bronchophony. The client is instructed to whisper a series of words. The words as heard through the stethoscope on the chest wall are distinct and understandable.

In egophony, the intensity of the spoken voice, as heard through the stethoscope applied to the chest wall, is increased and the voice has a nasal or bleating quality. If the client says "e- e- e," the transmitted sound will be "a- a- a."

Decreased vocal resonance occurs in the same clinical situations in which tactile fremitus is decreased and breath sounds are absent. Vocal resonance is increased and whispered pectoriloquy and egophony may be present in any condition that causes a consolidation of lung tissue.

Screening Tests and Procedures

A variety of radiological, functional, and chemical diagnostic tests are used in assessing respiratory health. It is beyond the capabilities of this text to describe these various tests fully. However, some of the major ones are mentioned here.

Chest x-ray examination

The chest x-ray examination is a common means of determining the health of lung parenchyma.

Pulmonary function tests

Pulmonary function tests are procedures requiring some respiratory effort by the client. The effort includes blowing air into a spirometer designed to measure lung volumes and flow rates. This assessment is generally done by specialized technicians in a designated laboratory. Spirometry readings are commonly expressed in volumes and capacities. Volumes are single compartments in the lung. The addition of two or more volumes together results in a capacity. Volumes and capacities are expressed as a percentage of normal. Generally, the normal range is plus or minus 20% of the predicted value of all volumes and capacities (Figure 15.21).

The following are common spirometric assessments:

1. *Tidal volume:* Volume of air exhaled or inhaled during quiet breathing.
2. *Minute volume:* Volume of gas expired over 1 minute.
3. *Total lung capacity:* Sum of the vital capacity and the residual volume.
4. *Vital capacity:* Maximum amount of air a person can exhale. It is usually measured after forceful exhalation and termed *forced vital capacity.*
5. *Residual volume:* Amount of gas left in the lung after exhaling all that is physically possible. This

measurement is expressed as a ratio of total lung capacity to vital capacity.

6. *Expiratory reserve volume:* Volume that can be maximally exhaled following a passive exhalation.
7. *Functional residual capacity:* Sum of the residual volume and the expiratory reserve volume.
8. *Forced expiratory volume in 1 second (FEV₁):* Measurement of the maximum volume of air exhaled during the first second of expiration.
9. *FEV₁/FVC:* Ratio of forced expiratory volume in 1 second to forced vital capacity.
10. *Peak flow:* Measurement of the maximum flow rate achieved during the forced vital capacity maneuver.
11. *Diffusing capacity:* Ability of gas to diffuse across the alveolar-capillary membrane.

Arterial blood gases

The measurement of arterial blood gases provides valuable information about the physiological functioning of the respiratory system. Some of the commonly used tests are listed here.

Oxygenation status is measured by the following values:

1. PaO_2: Partial pressure of oxygen in arterial blood.
2. SaO_2: Percent of saturation of oxygen on hemoglobin in arterial blood.
3. CaO_2: Content of oxygen in arterial blood expressed in ml/100 ml of blood.

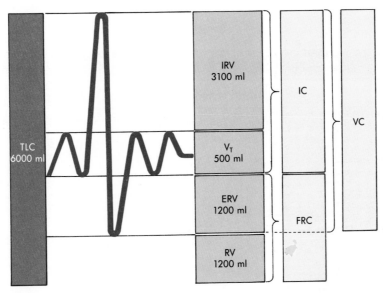

TLC = Total lung capacity

IRV = Inspiratory reserve volume
V_T = Tidal volume
ERV = Expiratory reserve volume
RV = Residual volume

IC = Inspiratory capacity
FRC = Functional residual capacity
VC = Vital capacity

figure **15.21** Components of lung capacity. (*From Wilson SF, Thompson JM: Respiratory disorders, St Louis, 1990, Mosby.*)

examination step-by-step

The examination described here is for a client who is able to sit during the procedure. The approach would need to be adapted for a client who was unable to sit during the examination. In general, the examiner moves around the client, completing one aspect of assessment before initiating the next. Traditional organization of inspection, palpation, percussion, and auscultation is followed.

The client is stripped to the waist and seated so that all areas of the thorax are visible.

A. Inspect all areas of the thorax, noting especially:
1. Breathing rate, pattern, inspiratory-expiratory ratio, audible adventitious sounds
2. Use of accessory muscles of respiration
3. Condition of skin and underlying structures
4. Presence of bulging
5. Skin color and superficial venous patterns
6. Size, shape, and symmetry of thorax

B. Examine the posterior, lateral, and apical thorax.
1. Palpate the thorax.
a. General assessment of skin tone, temperature, tenderness, unusual sensations
b. Thoracic expansion
c. Tactile fremitus
2. Percuss the thorax.
a. Percussion survey of thorax, including assessment of appropriateness of various tones for their location
b. Diaphragmatic excursion
3. Auscultate with the diaphragm of the stethoscope from apex to base, from side to side.
a. Appropriateness of type of breath sound for location
b. Adventitious sounds
c. Vocal resonance

C. Examine the anterior thorax.
1. Palpate the thorax.
a. General assessment of skin tone, temperature, tenderness, unusual sensations
b. Position of trachea
c. Thoracic expansion
d. Tactile fremitus
2. Percuss the thorax. The percussion survey of the thorax includes assessment of the appropriateness of various tones for their location.
3. Auscultate with the diaphragm of the stethoscope from apex to base, from side to side.
a. Appropriateness of type of breath sound for location
b. Adventitious sounds
c. Vocal resonance

---

table 15.6   *Assessment Findings Frequently Associated with Common Lung Conditions*

Condition*	Breath sounds	Description
Normal lung	Inspiration > expiration Pitch—low Intensity—soft Adventitious sounds—none	Tracheobronchial tree and alveoli are clear; pleurae are thin and close together; chest wall is mobile

*Although some disease conditions are bilateral, one diseased lung and one normal lung are illustrated for each condition to provide contrast. When an abnormality is illustrated, the pathological condition is illustrated on the left side and the normal lung is on the right side of the illustration.

4. PvO$_2$: Partial pressure of oxygen in mixed venous blood.

Acid-base balance is measured by the following values:

1. pH: Hydrogen ion concentration in the blood.
2. PCO$_2$: Partial pressure of carbon dioxide in arterial blood.
3. HCO$_3$: Plasma bicarbonate concentration.
4. Base excess.

Sputum examination

Sputum contains exfoliated cells and organisms that are being expelled from the lungs. Therefore examination of sputum can be a valuable component of the respiratory assessment. Sputum specimens can be examined with Gram stain, cultures, and culture sensitivity tests for the presence of various organisms and by cytological examination for the presence of malignancies.

■ VARIATIONS FROM HEALTH

Despite the heavy reliance on laboratory and x-ray findings in the diagnosis of respiratory problems, reasonably sound diagnostic probabilities can be derived by compiling and analyzing the physical assessment data. Table 15.6 outlines the usual assessment findings in a variety of common lung conditions.

General Screening Tests

SCREENING FOR LUNG CANCER

Routine screening for lung cancer with chest x-ray study or sputum cytology in asymptomatic persons is not recommended. All patients should be counseled against tobacco use.

SCREENING FOR TUBERCULOSIS

Persons at high risk for tuberculosis should be screened for exposure to tuberculosis using the PPD (purified protein derivative). Those at high risk include HIV-positive persons; close contacts of persons with known or suspected tuberculosis; health care workers; persons with medical risk factors associated with tuberculosis; immigrants from countries with high tuberculosis prevalence; medically underserved, low-income populations; alcoholics; injection drug users; and residents of long-term care facilities.

Data from US Preventive Services Task Force: *Guide to clinical preventive services*, ed 2, Alexandria, Va, 1996, International Medical Publishing.

Inspection	Palpation	Percussion	Auscultation
Good, symmetrical rib and diaphragmatic movement Anteroposterior diameter < transverse diameter Respirations 12-20/min and regular	Trachea—midline Expansion—adequate, symmetrical Tactile fremitus— moderate and symmetrical No lesions or tenderness	Resonant Diaphragmatic excursion—3 to 5 cm	Breath sounds—vesicular Vocal resonance— muffled Adventitious sounds— none, except for a few transient crackles at bases

continued

| table 15.6 | Assessment Findings Frequently Associated with Common Lung Conditions—cont'd | |

Condition	Breath sounds	Description
Asthma Bronchospasm	Inspiration = expiration Pitch—moderate Intensity—soft Adventitious sounds—expiratory sibilant wheezes 	Asthma is characterized by intermittent episodes of airway obstruction caused by bronchospasm, excessive bronchial secretion, or edema of bronchial mucosa; resultant airway resistance, especially during expiration, produces symptoms of wheezing, dyspnea, and chest tightness
Atelectasis Collapsed portion of lung	*Over empty area* Inspiration > expiration Pitch—low or absent Intensity—soft or absent Adventitious sounds—fine, high-pitched crackles over terminal portion of inspiration if bronchus patent NOTE: Over consolidated lung—bronchial breath sounds, crackles, and wheezes	Atelectasis is collapse of alveolar lung tissue, and findings reflect presence of a small, airless lung; this condition is caused by complete obstruction of a draining bronchus by a tumor, thick secretions, or an aspirated foreign body, or by compression of lung
Bronchiectasis Dilated bronchi	Inspiration > expiration Pitch—low Intensity—soft Adventitious sounds—crackles (sometimes disappear after coughing) 	Bronchiectasis is abnormal dilation of bronchi or bronchioles or both

Inspection	Palpation	Percussion	Auscultation
Cyanosis Air trapping with audible wheezing Use of accessory muscles of respiration Increased respiratory rate	Tactile fremitus—decreased	Hyperresonant	Breath sounds—distant Vocal resonance—decreased Adventitious sounds—wheezes
Less chest motion on affected side Affected side retracted, with ribs appearing close together Cough Rapid, shallow breathing	Trachea—shifted to affected side Expansion—decreased on affected side Tactile fremitus—decreased or absent	Dull to flat over collapsed lung Hyperresonant over remainder of affected hemithorax	Breath sounds—decreased or absent Vocal resonance—varies in intensity, usually reduced or absent in affected area Adventitious sounds—fine, high-pitched crackles may be heard over terminal portion of inspiration
If mild, respirations are normal If severe, tachypnea Less expansion of affected side Cough with purulent sputum	Trachea—midline or deviated toward affected side Expansion—decreased on affected side Tactile fremitus—increased	Resonant or dull	Breath sounds—usually vesicular Vocal resonance—usually muffled Adventitious sounds—crackles

continued

table 15.6	Assessment Findings Frequently Associated with Common Lung Conditions—cont'd	

Condition	Breath sounds	Description
Bronchitis—acute Bronchial inflammation and constriction	Inspiration > or = expiration Pitch—low Intensity—soft Adventitious sounds— localized crackles, expiratory sibilant wheezes	Acute bronchitis is inflammation of bronchial tree characterized by partial bronchial obstruction and secretions or constrictions; it results in abnormally deflated portions of lung
Emphysema Abnormally distended alveoli	Inspiration = expiration Pitch—low to very low Intensity—soft to very soft Adventitious sounds— occasional rhonchi and/or sibilant wheezes; fine inspiratory crackles	Emphysema is a permanent hyperinflation of lung beyond terminal bronchioles, with destruction of alveolar walls; airway resistance is increased, especially on expiration
Pleural effusion and thickening Pleural effusion and thickening Normal Fluid in the pleural space	Inspiration > expiration Pitch—low to absent Intensity—soft to absent Adventitious sounds— occasional pleural friction rub	Pleural effusion is a collection of fluid in pleural space; if pleural effusion is prolonged, fibrous tissue may also accumulate in pleural space; clinical picture depends on amount of fluid or fibrosis present and rapidity of development; fluid tends to gravitate to most dependent areas of thorax, and adjacent lung is compressed

Inspection	Palpation	Percussion	Auscultation
If severe, tachypnea and cyanosis Rasping cough with mucoid sputum	Tactile fremitus—normal to increased	Resonant	Breath sounds—vesicular Vocal resonance—moderate Adventitious sounds—localized crackles, sibilant wheezes
Dyspnea with exertion Barrel chest Tachypnea Use of accessory muscles of respiration	Expansion—limited Tactile fremitus—decreased	Resonant to hyperresonant Diaphragmatic excursion—decreased	Breath sounds—decreased intensity; often prolonged expiration Vocal resonance—muffled or decreased Adventitious sounds—occasional wheezes; often fine crackles in late inspiration
Tachypnea Decrease in definition of intercostal spaces on affected side Dyspnea	Trachea—deviation toward normal side Expansion—decreased on affected side Tactile fremitus—decreased or absent	Dull to flat No diaphragmatic excursion on affected side	Breath sounds—decreased or absent Vocal resonance—muffled or absent; if fluid compresses lung, sounds may be bronchial over compression, and bronchophony, egophony, and whisper pectoriloquy may be present Adventitious sounds—pleural friction rub sometimes present

continued

table 15.6   **Assessment Findings Frequently Associated with Common Lung Conditions—cont'd**

Condition	Breath sounds	Description

Pneumonia with consolidation
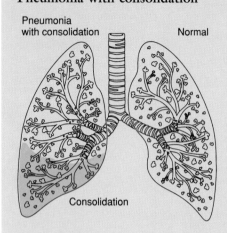
	Inspiration = expiration
	Pitch—high
	Intensity—loud
	Adventitious sounds—
	  inspiratory crackles in
	  terminal third of inspiration
	
		Pneumonia with consolidation occurs when alveolar air is replaced by fluid or tissue; physical findings depend on amount of parenchymal tissue involved

Pneumothorax 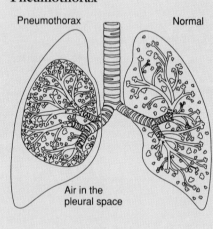	Inspiration > expiration Pitch—low to absent Intensity—soft to absent Adventitious sounds—none 	Pneumothorax implies air in pleural space There are three types of pneumothorax: (1) closed—air in pleural space does not communicate with air in lung; (2) open—air in pleural space freely communicates with air in lung; air in pleural space is atmospheric; and (3) tension—air in pleural space communicates with air in lungs only on inspiration; air pressure in pleural space is greater than atmospheric pressure Physical signs depend on degree of lung collapse and presence or absence of pleural effusion
Pulmonary fibrosis—diffuse 	Inspiration = expiration Pitch—low to absent Intensity—soft to absent Adventitious sounds—crackles 	Pulmonary fibrosis is presence of excessive amount of connective tissue in lungs; consequently, lungs are smaller than normal and less compliant; lower lobes are usually affected most

Inspection	Palpation	Percussion	Auscultation
Tachypnea Guarding and less motion on affected side Tachypnea	Expansion—limited on affected side Tactile fremitus—usually increased, but may be weak if a bronchus leading to affected area is plugged	Dull to flat	Breath sounds—increased in intensity; bronchovesicular or bronchial breath sounds over affected area Vocal resonance—increased bronchophony, egophony, whisper pectoriloquy present Adventitious sounds—inspiratory crackles terminal third of inspiration
Restricted lung expansion on affected side If large, tachypnea Bulging in intercostal spaces on affected side Cyanosis	Trachea—deviated toward normal side Expansion—decreased on affected side Tactile fremitus—absent	Hyperresonant Decreased diaphragmatic excursion	Breath sounds—usually decreased or absent; if open pneumothorax, have an amorphous quality Vocal resonance—decreased or absent Adventitious sounds—none
Dyspnea on exertion Tachypnea Thoracic expansion diminished Cyanosis	Trachea—deviated to most affected side	Resonant to dull	Breath sounds—reduced or absent, bronchovesicular or bronchial Vocal resonance—increased, whisper pectoriloquy may be present Adventitious sounds—crackles on inspiration

sample documentation & diagnoses — CRITICAL THINKING

■ FOCUSED HEALTH HISTORY *(SUBJECTIVE DATA)*

This is a regular, health maintenance clinic visit for Mr. T., a 65-year-old black male with the chief complaint of "low energy." Was diagnosed with emphysema 3 years ago. Is always short of breath, but has been worse for the past 2 days during hot, humid weather. Stays at home with fans, but home is not air-conditioned. Denies chest pain, fever, or change in sputum production. Is unable to climb more than one flight of stairs without resting. Has difficulty walking on flat ground for more than 2 blocks. Uses oxygen at home at 2 L/min after meals, at night, and during physical exertion. Complains of insomnia and restlessness at night—sleeps with 3 pillows. Has moist cough several times daily that produces about 1 to 2 tablespoons of white or yellow sputum. When sputum is yellow, takes ampicillin as directed. Color of sputum has always cleared after medication. Sputum has been white for the past several months. Smoked 2 to 3 packs of cigarettes a day for 50 years, but stopped 3 years ago when emphysema was diagnosed. Diagnosis verified per clinic record. Denies allergies and exposure to lung irritants. Denies TB, cancer, familial lung disease, allergies, heart disease, and renal disease.

■ FOCUSED PHYSICAL EXAMINATION *(OBJECTIVE DATA)*

Inspection: Respirations regular at 22/min. After minimal exercise (walking around examination room ×2) 30/min. Respirations deep—uses accessory muscles of respiration. Chest is barrel shaped. Thorax moves symmetrically; no bulges or retractions.

Palpation: Trachea in midline. Thoracic expansion symmetrical at 3 cm. No areas of bulging or tenderness. Percussion tones resonant and symmetrical. Tactile fremitus decreased throughout lung fields.

Percussion: Diaphragmatic excursion 2 cm bilaterally. Percussion sounds hyperresonant throughout thorax.

Auscultation: Diminished vesicular breath sounds throughout peripheral lung. Expiration sometimes prolonged. Fine crackles and occasional rhonchi noted throughout respiratory cycle in right and left lungs.

diagnoses

HEALTH PROBLEM

Chronic emphysema

NURSING DIAGNOSES

Activity intolerance related to imbalances between oxygen supply and demand

Defining Characteristics

- Complains of shortness of breath when walking >2 blocks or climbing 1 flight of stairs
- Sleep orthopnea

Ineffective breathing pattern related to decreased lung expansion

Defining Characteristics

- Dyspnea on exertion
- Tachypnea with activity
- Tactile fremitus decreased
- Prolonged expiratory phase
- Increased anteroposterior diameter
- Use of accessory muscles

Ineffective airway clearance related to tracheobronchial restriction

Defining Characteristics

- Abnormal breath sounds—crackles throughout all lung fields
- Tachypnea with exercise
- Dyspnea

Anxiety related to change in health status

Defining Characteristics

- Restlessness
- Insomnia
- Expressed concern regarding changes in life events

chapter 16

Cardiovascular System

■ PURPOSE OF EXAMINATION

The cardiovascular system is composed of the heart and an extensive system of blood vessels. The purpose of examination of this system is to assess the function of the heart as a pump and the function of the arteries and veins throughout the body in their role in transporting oxygen and nutrients to the tissues of the body and in transporting waste products and carbon dioxide from those body tissues.

Assessment of the heart, the vessels of the neck, and some aspects of the peripheral vessels is discussed in this chapter. For assessment of the blood pressure and pulse, and their variations from health, see Chapter 9: General Assessment, Including Vital Signs. Assessment of the cardiovascular system is closely related to assessment of the respiratory system, which is discussed in Chapter 15.

■ ANATOMY AND PHYSIOLOGY

Several chest wall landmarks and lines are used to describe the anatomical position of the heart, its movements, and the sounds produced (Figure 16.1). The area of the chest that overlies the heart and the great vessels is called the precordium. The suprasternal notch lies at the top of the sternum. The angle of Louis is the area where the manubrium of the sternum meets the body of the sternum. The ribs and intercostal (between-the-ribs) spaces are numbered from the first rib, with each space taking its number from the rib directly above it.

The imaginary lines used for description (and their abbreviations) include:

The midsternal line (MSL) runs down the center of the sternum.

The midclavicular line (MCL) runs down from the center of the clavicle.

The anterior, middle, and posterior maxillary lines (AAL, MAL, PAL) run down from the axilla.

Other abbreviations commonly used include:

2 LICS—second left intercostal space

2 RICS—second right intercostal space

5 LICS—fifth left intercostal space

LSB—left sternal border

For a more thorough discussion of thoracic landmarks, see Chapter 15: Respiratory System.

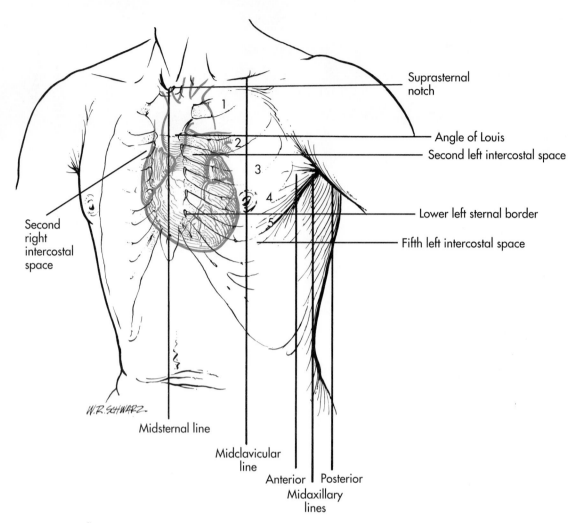

figure**16.1** Location of the heart and chest wall landmarks of the precordium.

Heart and Great Vessels
Location and position of the heart

The heart is located behind the sternum and between the lungs in the mediastinum. It lies mostly to the left of the midsternal line, above the diaphragm. It occupies the space from the second to the fifth intercostal spaces and from the right side of the sternum to the left midclavicular line (Figure 16.2).

The position of the heart can vary somewhat according to the body build, chest configuration, and level of the diaphragm. In persons of average build, the heart lies obliquely: one third of it lies to the right of the midsternal line, and two thirds lies to the left of this line. In short, stocky persons, the heart is usually positioned more horizontally. If the diaphragm is positioned higher, as occurs with pregnancy, the heart also lies more horizontally. In tall, slender individuals, the heart hangs more vertically. With the rare condition of dextrocardia, the position of the heart is reversed, and the heart lies on the right side of the chest.

The heart is shaped like an inverted cone. The upper portion is broader and is called the base of the heart. The lower portion is narrower and is called the apex.

Structure of the heart

Pericardium. The heart is encased in and protected by the pericardium, a double-walled fibrous sac of elastic connective tissue. The pericardium contains several cubic centimeters of fluid that permit the smooth, low-friction movement of the heart.

Heart wall. The heart wall has three main layers: the epicardium, myocardium, and endocardium (Figure 16.3). The epicardium is the thin, outermost serous membrane layer. It covers the surface of the heart and the great vessels. The myocardium is the thick, muscular middle layer that forms the bulk of the heart. This layer is the contractile tissue that pumps the blood. The endocardium is the thin inner layer of epithelial tissue that lines the inner surface of the heart and heart valves.

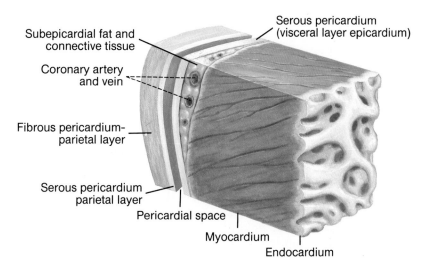

BASE

Aorta

Pulmonary
artery

Superior
vena cava

Left
atrium

Left
ventricle

Right
atrium

Right
ventricle

APEX

figure**16.2**   Position of the heart and great vessels.

Subepicardial fat and
connective tissue

Serous pericardium
(visceral layer epicardium)

Coronary artery
and vein

Fibrous pericardium-
parietal layer

Serous pericardium
parietal layer

Pericardial space

Myocardium

Endocardium

figure**16.3**   Cross section of cardiac muscle. *(From Canobbio MM: Cardiovascular disorders, St Louis, 1990, Mosby.)*

Heart chambers. The heart is composed of four chambers: the right and left atria and the right and left ventricles (Figure 16.4). The two atria lie at the top, or base, of the heart. The two ventricles form the lower portion of the heart. The right atrium and ventricle form the right side of the heart, and the left atrium and ventricle form the left side of the heart. The right and left sides of the heart are separated by a septum; the interatrial septum separates the two atria, and the interventricular septum divides the ventricles. The two atria are thin-walled chambers that receive blood from the body and lungs by way of the major veins. The two ven-

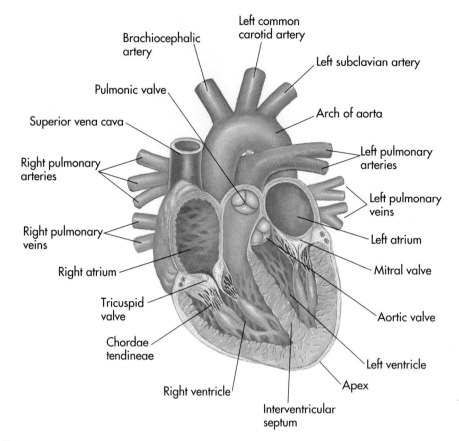

figure **16.4** Frontal section of the heart. *(From Seidel HM et al:* Mosby's guide to physical examination, *ed 3, St Louis, 1995, Mosby.)*

tricles are thick-walled chambers that pump blood out to the body and lungs by way of the major arteries.

Within the mediastinum, the heart is rotated so that the right ventricle composes most of the anterior surface of the heart and the left ventricle forms most of the posterior surface. The right ventricle lies behind the sternum and extends to the left of it. The left ventricle is located posterior to the right ventricle and extends farther to the left, forming the left anterior border of the heart. The right atrium lies slightly above and to the right of the right ventricle, and the left atrium occupies a posterior position on the heart (Figure 16.5).

Abbreviations commonly used for the heart chambers are:

RA—right atrium
RV—right ventricle
LA—left atrium
LV—left ventricle

Heart valves. The heart valves are structures through which blood flows either from the atria to the ventricles or from the ventricles to the great vessels. These valves function to permit the forward flow of blood and to prevent the backward flow of blood during the cardiac cycle. Their closure produces the normal heart sounds. The opening of heart valves is normally silent. The heart chambers and great vessels are separated by two sets of valves: the atrioventricular (AV) valves and the semilunar (SL) valves. The AV valves separate the atria and ventricles; the SL valves separate the ventricles and great vessels (Figure 16.6). The term *competent* is used to describe a properly functioning valve.

Atrioventricular valves. The AV valve on the right side of the heart between the right atrium and right ventricle is called the tricuspid valve. It has three cusps, or leaflets. The AV valve on the left side of the heart between the left atrium and left ventricle is called the mitral valve. It is a bicuspid valve with two cusps. The AV valves open as a result of lower ventricular pressure during ventricular diastole. During ventricular systole, the pressure in the ventricle builds, and the cusps on each of these valves meet and close to form a seal so that no blood flows back into the atria. The valve cusps are anchored by strong, fibrous strands, the chordae tendineae, to the papillary muscles, which are attached

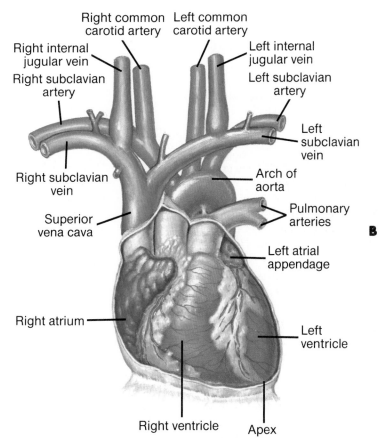

figure**16.5** **A,** Location of the great vessels. **B,** Heart and great vessels. (*B from Canobbio MM:* Cardiovascular disorders, *St Louis, 1990, Mosby.*)

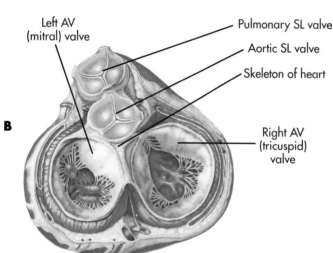

figure**16.6** **A,** Anatomical location of the heart valves and their relationship to the great vessels. **B,** Valves of the heart viewed from above. The atria are removed to show the mitral and tricuspid valves. (*A from Seidel HM et al: Mosby's guide to physical examination, ed 3, St Louis, 1995, Mosby; B from Thibodeau GA, Patton KT: Anthony's textbook of anatomy and physiology, ed 15, St Louis, 1996, Mosby.*)

to the ventricles. The chordae tendineae prevent prolapse of the AV valves into the atria during ventricular contraction (see Figure 16.4).

Semilunar valves. The SL valves are located between the ventricles and the great arteries. Each has three cusps. On the right, the pulmonic valve separates the right ventricle from the pulmonary artery. On the left, the aortic valve separates the left ventricle from the aorta. When the ventricles contract during ventricular systole, these valves open to permit the flow of blood out from the heart into the pulmonary artery and the

aorta. During ventricular diastole, when the ventricles are filling with blood, these valves are closed, preventing the backward flow of blood from the pulmonary artery and the aorta into the ventricles.

There are no valves between the venae cavae and the right atrium or between the pulmonary veins and the left atrium. Therefore, abnormally elevated pressure on the right side of the heart leads to congestion in the neck veins and abdomen, and abnormally elevated pressure on the left side of the heart leads to pulmonary congestion.

Great vessels

The large arteries and veins that lie in a cluster at the base of the heart are called the great vessels. The arteries include the pulmonary artery and the aorta, and the veins include the superior and inferior venae cavae and the pulmonary veins (see Figure 16.5). These vessels circulate blood to and from the body and lungs. The superior and inferior venae cavae return unoxygenated blood from the upper and lower body to the right atrium. The pulmonary artery leaves the right ventricle, bifurcates almost immediately, and carries the unoxygenated blood from the right ventricle to both lungs. The pulmonary veins return the oxygenated blood from the lungs to the left atrium. The aorta receives the blood from the left ventricle and carries it to the body.

The aorta ascends from the left ventricle, arches back at the level of the sternal angle, and descends behind the heart. Several major arteries branch off along the aortic arch. (Blood is supplied to the myocardium by the coronary arteries, which are the first arteries to branch off the aorta.)

Blood circulation

When blood is ejected from the ventricle, it flows through two circulatory systems—the pulmonary and the systemic—simultaneously (Figure 16.7). Unoxygenated blood returning from circulation throughout the body—the systemic circulation—passes through the superior and inferior vena cavae and enters the heart at the right atrium. From there, it crosses the tricuspid

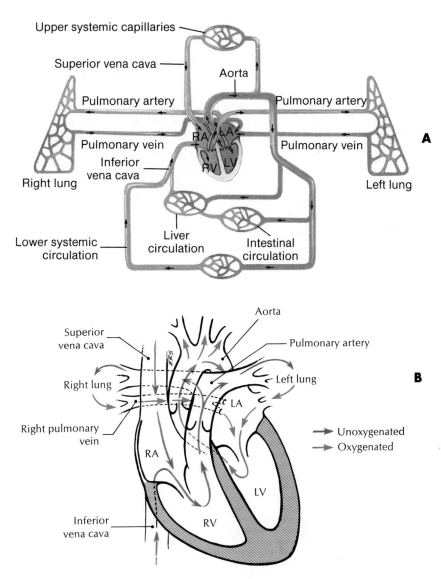

figure **16.7** **A,** Circulatory system. **B,** Route of blood flow through the chambers of the heart and great vessels. (*A from Canobbio MM:* Cardiovascular disorders, *St Louis, 1990, Mosby.*)

valve and enters the right ventricle. When the ventricles contract, the blood flows from the right ventricle over the pulmonic valve and enters the pulmonary artery. The pulmonary circulation carries blood to the lungs, where it releases carbon dioxide and is reoxygenated. The blood returns to the heart through the pulmonary veins and enters the left atrium. From there, it flows across the mitral valve and into the left ventricle. When the ventricles contract, the blood flows from the left ventricle across the aortic valve and enters the aorta. The arterial system carries the blood throughout the body. The blood then returns through the venous vasculature to the superior and inferior venae cavae and into the right atrium. To summarize, a single red blood cell that started its route at the right atrium would follow this pathway: right atrium → tricuspid valve → right ventricle → pulmonary valve → pulmonary artery → lung → pulmonary vein → left atrium → mitral valve → left ventricle → aortic valve → aorta → systemic circulation → vena cava → right atrium.

Cardiac cycle

The heart contracts and relaxes rhythmically, permitting it to fill and then to eject blood, which circulates throughout the body. This occurs at the rate of about 72 times per minute; the normal range is 60 to 100 times per minute. The average time for each cardiac cycle is about 0.8 second. The cardiac cycle describes the events of one complete cycle of the contraction and relaxation of the atria and ventricles. Pressure gradients within the heart and great vessels change with the rhythmic pumping of the heart. Blood flows from areas of higher pressure to areas of lower pressure. There are

two phases to the cardiac cycle: diastole, or relaxation, and systole, or contraction. In general, the terms *diastole* and *systole* refer to the actions of the ventricles, although the atria also have their own phases of relaxation and contraction.

The mechanical events described in this section must be in synchrony with the electrical stimulation of the heart, described in the next section.

Ventricular diastole (Figure 16.8). During ventricular diastole the ventricles relax, and the AV valves open. Pressure in the atria is higher than in the ventricles, so blood flows rapidly across the AV valves into the ventricles. This first, passive filling phase is called early or protodiastolic filling. About 70% of the blood in the atria enters the ventricles during this time. Toward the end of this phase, the atria contract (atrial kick) and eject the remaining 30% of the blood out of the atria and into the ventricles. This is called atrial systole.

> **HELPFUL HINT** *Note that atrial systole occurs at the same time as ventricular diastole. This may be confusing initially, but it is helpful to remember that the upper chambers—the atria—contract while the lower chambers—the ventricles—relax in order to receive the blood. Similarly, ventricular contraction occurs at the same time as atrial relaxation and filling.*

Ventricular systole (Figure 16.9). During systole the ventricles contract, ejecting blood from the right ventricle into the pulmonary artery and from the left ventricle

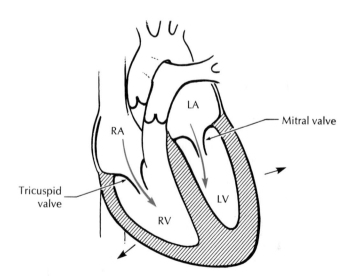

figure**16.8** Ventricular diastole. The ventricles relax, and the mitral and tricuspid valves open, allowing blood to flow from the atria to the ventricles.

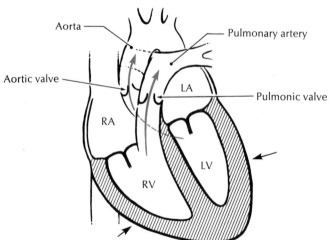

figure**16.9** Ventricular systole. The ventricles contract, forcing the aortic and pulmonic valves to open; blood flows into the aorta and the pulmonary artery.

into the aorta. When the ventricles have filled with blood, ventricular pressure is higher than atrial pressure. The mitral and tricuspid valves snap shut, preventing any backflow of blood into the atria. Briefly, all four heart valves are closed. The ventricle walls then begin to contract, building pressure inside the ventricles. This is the period of isovolumic (same-volume) contraction: the volume of blood within the ventricles does not change. When the pressure in the ventricles exceeds the pressure in the pulmonary artery and the aorta, the pulmonic and aortic valves open and blood is rapidly ejected into the pulmonary artery and the aorta. After the blood is fully ejected from the ventricles, pressure within the ventricles is less than the pressure in the pulmonary artery and the aorta. The pulmonic and aortic valves close. While the ventricles have been contracting, the atria have been filling again with blood from the

lungs and the body. Atrial pressure is again higher than ventricular pressure, the AV valves open, and the cycle begins again.

When the ventricles fill during diastole, they must respond to the force under which filling occurs; this force is called preload. During systole the ventricles eject the blood through the pulmonic and aortic valves against the force in the pulmonary artery and aorta; this force is called afterload.

The relationships of the left ventricular pressure curve, the heart sounds, and the electrocardiogram (ECG) are illustrated in Figure 16.10.

Differences between events on the right and left sides of the heart. Although the same events are occurring simultaneously on both sides of the heart, the pressure relationships are different on each side of the heart. Pressures on the right side are lower than those

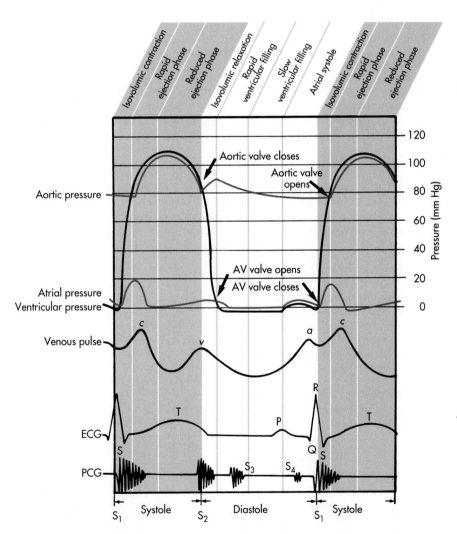

figure **16.10** Events of the cardiac cycle, showing aortic, atrial, and ventricular pressure curves; the venous pulse wave; and the ECG and phonocardiogram tracings during systole and diastole. *(From Seidel HM et al: Mosby's guide to physical examination, ed 3, St Louis, 1995, Mosby.)*

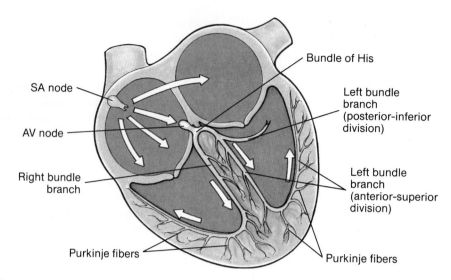

figure **16.11**   Cardiac electrical conduction. *(From Canobbio MM: Cardiovascular disorders, St Louis, 1990, Mosby.)*

on the left side. The right side is pumping blood to the lungs while the left side is pumping blood to the rest of the body. As a result, there are two distinct components to each of the heart sounds; however, the difference is more distinct with the second heart sound. For the first heart sound (S_1), the mitral valve (M_1) closes just before the tricuspid valve (T_1). With the second heart sound (S_2), the aortic valve closure (A_2) occurs slightly before the pulmonic valve closure (P_2).

The four heart valves producing the normal heart sounds of S_1 and S_2 are located close to each other anatomically. However, the sound produced by each valve is best heard at various areas of transmission across the precordium. These auscultation sites are described in this chapter under Technique for Examination and Normal Findings.

Electrical stimulation and conduction in the heart

The heart is distinguished by the feature of automaticity; that is, it is stimulated and contracts by itself. The heart contracts in response to an electrical impulse that spreads through the heart, activating and coordinating the mechanical pumping events of each cardiac cycle. The electrical current depolarizes as it is conveyed along the conduction system. In other words, when in the resting state, the cardiac cell is more positively charged on the outside of the cell and more negatively charged on the inside of the cell. When the electrical current normally initiated in the sinoatrial node flows across the atria and ventricles, depolarization occurs. As a result, the inside of the cardiac cell becomes more pos-

itively charged. Contraction of the atria and then the ventricles follows the electrical stimulation. After contraction, the cardiac cells repolarize: the inside of the cells returns to a more negatively charged state.

The electrical discharge originates at specialized cells in the sinoatrial (SA) node, located near the vena cava in the right atrium (Figure 16.11). This node is also called the pacemaker. The electrical stimulus flows through the heart in an orderly sequence: from the sinoatrial node through the atria to the AV node, located low in the atrial septum. The impulse is normally briefly delayed at the AV node and then proceeds through the bundle of

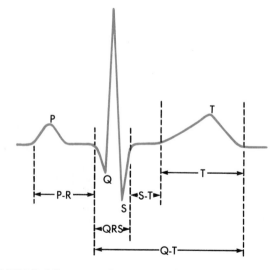

figure **16.12**   Normal ECG waveform. *(From Berne RM, Levy MN: Physiology, ed 3, St Louis, 1993, Mosby.)*

table 16.1 *PQRST Relationship to ECG Phases*	
ECG segment	**Correlating component of the cardiac cycle**
P wave	Spread of impulse through atria—atrial systole (atrial depolarization)
PR interval	From beginning of P wave to beginning of QRS complex; passage of impulse from SA node through atria to AV node; time from initial stimulation of atria to initial stimulation of ventricles
QRS complex	Spread of impulse through ventricles—ventricular systole (ventricular depolarization)
ST segment and T wave	Ventricular muscle returns to resting state (ventricular repolarization)
QT interval	Period from beginning of ventricular depolarization to moment of repolarization: ventricular contraction

His and its branches, reaching the Purkinje fibers in the ventricular myocardium, where it stimulates myocardial contraction. The SA node normally discharges between 60 and 100 electrical impulses per minute.

A small portion of this electrical activity spreads to the skin, where it can be recorded as an ECG (Figure 16.12). The letters *PQRST* stand for the components of the electrical impulse as it spreads through the heart. The relationship of these letters of the ECG to the phases of the cardiac cycle is shown in Table 16.1.

The passage of the electrical impulse as traced by the ECG and its relationship to the pressure curves and heart sounds are illustrated in Figure 16.10.

The electrical stimulation briefly precedes the mechanical response of the myocardium. Because of the pattern in which cardiac depolarization occurs, events on the left side of the heart normally take place slightly before those on the right side of the heart.

Heart sounds

Events in the cardiac cycle produce sounds that can be heard over the chest wall through a stethoscope. The heart sounds include the normal S_1 and S_2, extra sounds, and murmurs. In some persons a third or fourth heart sound, S_3 or S_4, is a normal finding, as are certain kinds of murmurs.

Variations from normal that occur with all of the heart sounds and murmurs, as well as other sounds that are virtually always abnormal, are described in greater detail in this chapter under Variations from Health.

Characteristics. All cardiovascular sounds have the following characteristics:

Frequency: The pitch or tone at which a sound is heard. Frequency is a measure of the number of vibrations in cycles per second (cps). Heart sounds are described as high or low pitched. Since all cardiovascular sounds are actually low pitched, these terms are relative.

Intensity: The loudness of the sound, determined by the amplitude of the vibrations, the source generating the sound, the distance the vibrations must travel, and the medium through which they travel. Some cardiovascular sounds can be heard with the stethoscope barely touching the chest wall; others can be heard only with great concentration. The loudness of the sound is modified by the amount of tissue or space that lies between the sound at its origin and the outer chest wall. The heart sounds are typically very clear in a thin-chested individual but seem diminished or distant in the client who is very muscular or overweight or who has emphysema.

Quality: The overtones of a sound determine its quality, such as whether it is musical, blowing, or harsh.

Duration: Normal cardiovascular sounds are of short duration, the silent phases are longer. Abnormal sounds may be of short duration; such as clicks or snaps, or of longer duration, such as some murmurs.

Timing in the cardiac cycle: During systole (between S_1 and S_2) or during diastole (between S_2 and S_1).

First heart sound: S_1 (Figure 16.13). The first heart sound results from closure of the AV valves. S_1 signals the beginning of ventricular systole. S_1 can be heard over the entire precordium, but it is best heard at the apex, where it is usually louder than the second heart sound. Because pressure is higher and depolarization occurs slightly earlier on the left side of the heart, mitral valve closure occurs slightly before tricuspid valve closure. However, both components of S_1 are usually heard as one sound. Occasionally, both components of S_1 will be audible. This is known as a split first sound.

Second heart sound: S_2 (Figure 16.13). The second heart sound results from the closure of the two semilunar valves: the pulmonic and the aortic. When ventricu-

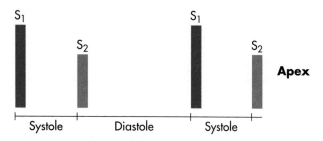

figure**16.13** Relative loudness of S_1 and S_2 as heard over the base and the apex of the heart.

figure**16.14** Normal splitting of S_2 (heard best at the second left intercostal space).

lar systole is completed, pressure in the aorta and pulmonary artery exceeds ventricular pressure, and the semilunar valves are forced closed. S_2 signals the end of ventricular systole and the beginning of ventricular diastole. Diastole is normally the longer interval between the heart sounds. S_2 is audible over the entire precordium, but it is best heard at the base of the heart, where it is louder than S_1. S_2 is slightly higher in pitch and longer in duration than S_1. The two components of S_2 are A_2 (aortic valve closure) and P_2 (pulmonic valve closure). Pressure on the left side of the heart is higher than on the right, making aortic valve closure louder than pulmonic valve closure. Closure of the aortic valve is the loudest component of S_2 across the base of the heart, at both the left and right second intercostal spaces. Normally, the sound produced by the pulmonic valve can be heard only in a small area centering around the second left intercostal space. P_2 can be heard separately from A_2 when splitting of the second heart sound occurs. Remember, in the production of S_1, mitral valve closure (M_1) briefly precedes tricuspid valve closure (T_1). Similarly, in the production of S_2, aortic valve closure (A_2) briefly precedes pulmonic valve closure (P_2).

Effect of respiration on the second heart sound: splitting of S_2 (Figure 16.14). Although the volume of the right and left ventricles is about equal, respiration does affect the volume of blood returned to the right atrium from the vena cava. This increases the stroke volume of the right ventricle and delays the P_2 component of S_2. Also during inspiration, a slightly greater amount of blood remains in the lungs, which decreases the amount of blood returned to the left side of the heart

from the pulmonary veins. This permits the aortic valve to close a bit sooner. With the aortic valve closing a bit earlier and the pulmonic valve closing a bit later, the two distinct components of the second heart sound—a split S_2—can be heard. This is known as normal physiological splitting. A split S_2 is most marked at the peak of the inspiratory phase of normal respiration. In healthy adult clients A_2 and P_2 are separated by 0.04 to 0.05 of a second during inspiration. During expiration the disparity between the blood return to the two ventricles is equalized, and the semilunar valves close nearly synchronously, producing a single S_2. If the client holds his or her breath during inspiration, the ejection times of both ventricles become nearly equal again and the split sound becomes single. If a split S_2 is audible, it may be so in either the supine or sitting position.

Extra heart sounds

Third heart sound: S_3 (Figure 16.15). Diastole is usually a silent phase of the cardiac cycle. Two phases of rapid ventricular filling occur during diastole. The first, which takes place early in diastole, is a passive rapid filling phase. This occurs when the AV valves open after the second heart sound. The blood stored in the atria flows rapidly into the ventricles. This rapid distention of the ventricles causes vibrations of the ventricular walls. These vibrations may produce a third heart sound (S_3). S_3 is low in pitch and loudness and is best heard at the apex of the heart. This sound is common in children and young adults and in such instances is known as a physiological S_3. It is often heard in hyperkinetic states producing increased cardiac output, such as hyperthyroidism, exercise, pregnancy, and anxiety-related tachycardia. When it is heard in middle-aged adults, it is usually abnormal. When the third heart sound originates from the right ventricle, it is diminished during expiration and augmented during inspiration. When it originates from the left ventricle, it is augmented during expiration and diminished during inspiration.

Fourth heart sound: S_4 (Figure 16.16). The second phase of rapid ventricular filling that occurs during ven-

figure**16.15**   S₃, an early diastolic sound.

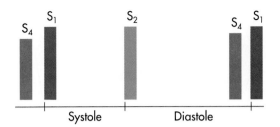

figure**16.16**   S₄, a late diastolic sound.

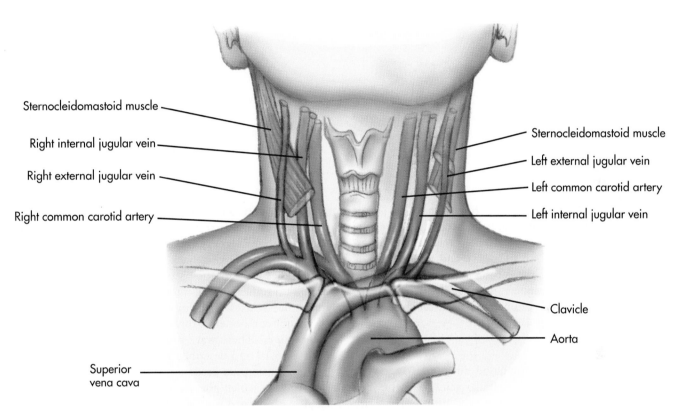

Sternocleidomastoid muscle

Right internal jugular vein

Right external jugular vein

Right common carotid artery

Superior
vena cava

Sternocleidomastoid muscle

Left external jugular vein

Left common carotid artery

Left internal jugular vein

Clavicle

Aorta

figure**16.17**   Neck vessels.

tricular diastole results from the contraction of the atria and is the active rapid filling phase. The atrial contraction, or atrial kick, causes the blood remaining in the atria to rapidly enter the ventricles. This can create vibrations that produce a fourth heart sound (S_4). S_4 occurs just before S_1. Like S_3, it is a soft, low-pitched sound. When the fourth heart sound originates from the right ventricle, it is diminished during expiration and augmented during inspiration. When it originates from the left ventricle, it is augmented during expiration and diminished during inspiration. A physiological S_4 may be heard in middle-aged adults with thin-walled chests, especially after exercise, but it is less likely to be found in a well client than is a physiological S_3.

Neck Vessels
Carotid arteries

The carotid arteries lie in the neck in the groove between the trachea and the sternocleidomastoid muscles. They are lateral to the trachea and medial to and alongside the sternocleidomastoid muscles (Figure 16.17). The pulse wave in the carotid arteries results from ventricular systole. Because of the proximity to the heart, the carotid arteries are easy to palpate, and the pulse wave is commonly visible.

The normal carotid pulse wave consists of a single positive wave followed by a dicrotic notch (Figure 16.18). The curve of the wave is a reflection of left ventricular activity. The upstroke is smooth and rapid, the

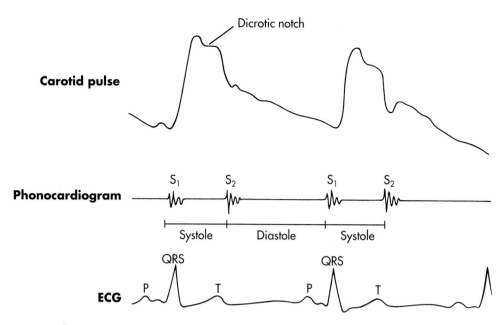

figure **16.18** Carotid pulse wave in relation to S_1 and S_2, and the ECG.

summit is dome shaped, and the downstroke is less steep than the upstroke. The peak occurs just after the first heart sound. Figure 16.18 illustrates the relationship of the carotid pulse to S_1, S_2, and the ECG. The size and amplitude of the carotid pulse are determined by several factors, including the left ventricular stroke volume, ejection rate, peripheral vascular resistance, vessel distensibility, and pulse pressure.

Jugular veins

The jugular veins empty blood directly into the vena cava. No valves separate the jugular veins from the vena cava or the vena cava from the right atrium. Therefore the jugular veins reflect the activity on the right side of the heart, providing an indication of the competency of right-sided heart function. They reflect changes in right atrial volume and filling pressure. There are two sets of jugular veins: the external jugular veins and the internal jugular veins (Figure 16.17). The external jugular veins are smaller, more superficial and discrete, and visible bilaterally above the clavicles, lateral to the insertion of the sternocleidomastoid muscles. The internal jugular veins are larger and lie beneath and medial to the sternocleidomastoid muscles and lateral to the carotid arteries. Because of their superficial location, the external jugular veins are often easier to see and may be particularly prominent in individuals who have chronic elevation of venous pressure. The internal jugular veins are less accessible to inspection, but reflection of their activity may be visible as diffuse pulsations on the skin overlying the lower part of the neck.

Jugular venous pulse. Normal jugular venous pulsations are low-pressure impulses or waves that resemble the pressure changes in the right atrium. The pulsations are waveforms moving back from the right side of the heart. They indicate the pressure and volume changes as the blood returns to the right atrium and the heart contracts and relaxes. The jugular venous pulse wave has five major components: three upward waves and two descent slopes. These wave components are illustrated in Figure 16.19 and described in Table 16.2.

Jugular venous pressure. Jugular venous pressure is the level at which the jugular veins appear full. In a client with normal right-sided heart function, any filling of the jugular veins is not evident until the person is nearly in a supine position. If the jugular veins appear full when the client's head is elevated to a higher position, this indicates less competent function on the right side of the heart.

Venous hum. The venous hum is a continuous, low-pitched humming sound heard over the major veins at the base of the neck in many children and in some adults. It usually has no pathological significance. It is produced by turbulent blood flow in the internal jugular veins. The venous hum is most audible over the supraclavicular spaces, more commonly on the right.

Peripheral Vessels

The arteries and viens of the peripheral vascular system are illustrated in Figure 16.20.

Arteries and veins differ somewhat in their structure, which reflects their functions. Arteries are subject to

figure**16.19** Jugular venous pulse waves in relation to S_1 and S_2, and the ECG.

table16.2 *Jugular Venous Pulse Wave Components*

Jugular pulse component	Reflects	Produced by	Timing
a wave	Atrial contraction	Brief backflow of blood to vena cava during right atrial contraction—normally highest wave in cycle	Peaks just before S_1
c wave	Ventricular contraction	Upward bulging of tricuspid valve early in ventricular systole	Occurs at end of S_1
x descent	Atrial relaxation	Downward pull on right atrium when ventricles contract during systole	Occurs just before S_2
v wave	Atrial filling before tricuspid valve opens	Continuous filling and increased pressure in right atrium	Peaks after S_2
y descent	Passive ventricular filling	Fall in right atrial pressure after tricuspid valve opens; blood flows from right atrium to right ventricle	Follows v wave after S_2

higher pressures; their walls are tougher and less distensible. The venous system involves lower pressures; the vein walls are less tough and more distensible. Lower extremity veins contain valves to prevent the backflow of blood. If blood volume increases, the veins can become distended to hold some of the excess blood; this decreases the workload of the heart. Because of their ability to stretch and accommodate the majority of the total blood volume, veins are also known as capacitance vessels. Veins lie closer to the surface of the skin than do arteries. The variation in structure between veins and arteries is illustrated in Figure 16.21. ■

A

figure**16.20** Systemic circulation. **A,** Arteries. *(From Seidel HM et al: Mosby's guide to physical examination, ed 3, St Louis, 1995, Mosby.)*

B

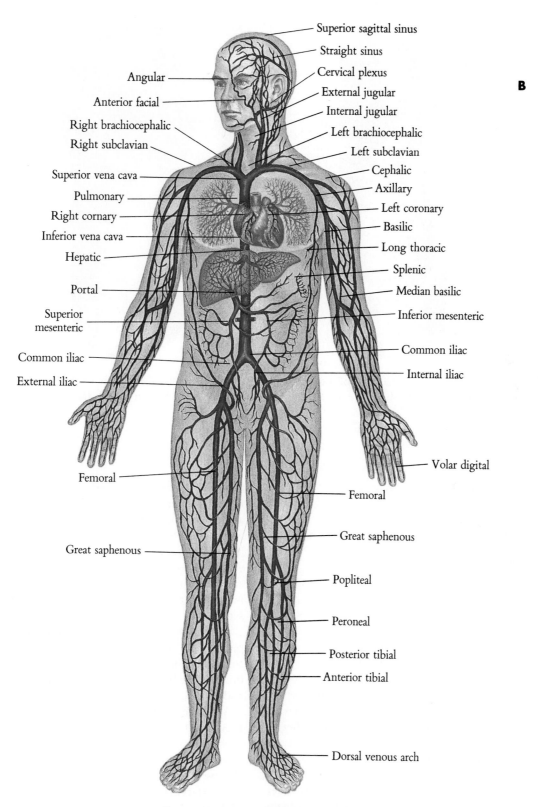

figure**16.20—cont'd** B, Veins.

ARTERY   VEIN

Endothelium
(tunica intima)

Valve

Elastic membrane
(thinner in veins)

Smooth muscle layer
(tunica media)
(thinner in veins)

Connective tissue
(tunica adventitia)
(thickest layer)

figure **16.21** Structure of arteries and veins. Note the relative thickness of the arterial walls. *(From Thompson JM et al:* Mosby's clinical nursing, *ed 3, St Louis, 1993, Mosby.)*

■ EXAMINATION

Health History

For each symptom, describe the following characteristics in the health history:

Onset
Character
Duration
Location
Associated symptoms
Precipitating and aggravating factors
Setting in which the symptoms occur
Effort(s) to relieve and effectiveness

Special features of cardiovascular problems are included in the history outline that follows. Always try to have the client explain or describe the situation in her or his own words before suggesting descriptive terms of your own. Information from family members and/or friends may also be useful in understanding the client's level of health or disability and can provide a broader perspective on the impact of a cardiovascular problem on both the client and the family.

Present health status

Dyspnea. An abnormally uncomfortable awareness of breathing and shortness of breath, dyspnea is one of the principal symptoms of cardiac disease. Dyspnea is normal in healthy persons when it is caused by moderate to strenuous exertion. It is considered abnormal when it occurs at rest or at a level of physical exertion not expected to cause distress. It is associated with a wide variety of diseases of the heart, lungs, chest wall, and respiratory muscles, and with anxiety. Therefore it is important to gather a careful and precise history on this symptom.

Orthopnea is shortness of breath that occurs when a person is lying flat and that is relieved by sitting or standing. Paroxysmal nocturnal dyspnea is shortness of breath that begins several hours after the onset of sleep and that is relieved by sitting or getting up.

When assessing dyspnea; inquire about:

1. Amount of activity or exertion required to cause shortness of breath (number of blocks, number of stairs); compare with 3 and 6 months ago
2. Onset: Sudden or gradual
3. Interference with activities of daily living or with sleep
4. Duration: Constant or intermittent
5. Number of pillows required to sleep
6. Pattern of awakening from sleep
7. Effect of position
8. Alleviating factors

Chest pain, tightness, or discomfort. Chest pain can be due to problems with noncardiac structures (e.g., thoracic structures, tissues of the neck and thoracic wall, and some abdominal organs).

1. Character: Aching, sharp, dull, tingling, burning, stabbing, cramping, crushing, viselike, pressing, squeezing, strangling, constricting, bursting. (Note the client's use of the clenched fist over the sternum to describe the character and location of the pain.)
2. Onset: Sudden or gradual; precipitating factors— eating, physical exertion, rest, stressful situation, emotional experience, coughing, cold temperature, sexual intercourse
3. Duration: Time episode(s) lasted
4. Location: Area of chest wall—may occur on both sides of the chest wall and substernally
5. Radiation: Arms, shoulders, neck, scapula, jaw, teeth, upper abdomen
6. Severity: Degree of interference with activity; need to stop all activity; sleep disruption
7. Associated symptoms: Diaphoresis; nausea/vomiting; dyspnea; palpitations; dizziness; faintness; fatigue; cold, clammy skin; cyanosis of lips, ears, nail beds; pallor; anxiety
8. Efforts to relieve and effectiveness: Rest; position change; medications, including nitroglycerin (number of tablets), other cardiac medications, and analgesics
9. Aggravating factors: Activities that make the pain worse—moving the arms or neck, breathing, lying flat
10. History of intermittent claudication, transient ischemic attack, or stroke

Palpitations. An unpleasant awareness of the forceful or rapid beating of the heart, palpitations may be caused by changes in cardiac rhythm or rate, high cardiac output states. Episodes may be described as "skipped beats" or a "flopping sensation" (most commonly due to extrasystoles), or the client may say that the heart has "stopped beating" (often a result of the compensatory pause after a premature contraction).

1. Onset: Sudden or gradual
2. Duration
3. Precipitating factors: Exertion, excitement, stress
4. Relieving factors: Rest, position change, vomiting
5. Associated symptoms: Throbbing of the neck, syncope, dizziness, tingling in the hands, angina

Cough

1. Characteristics: Dry, hacking, hoarse, productive (color, amount, odor, presence of blood in sputum)
2. Onset and duration
3. Frequency, time of day
4. Relationship to position, activity, talking, exercise
5. Effort to treat and effectiveness: Rest, activity, change in position, medication(s)

Fatigue

1. Onset and duration; unusual or typical; recent change
2. Inability to keep up with family, co-workers
3. Limitation of usual activities
4. Time of day fatigue occurs
5. Bedtime earlier than customary, naps
6. Associated symptoms: Dyspnea, orthopnea, chest pain, palpitations, anorexia, nausea, vomiting, weakness, weight loss, nocturia, visual changes
7. Medications: Prescription and nonprescription

Edema

1. Location: One or both legs, abdomen, face, neck, upper arms, generalized
2. Duration
3. Amount of swelling
4. Changes over 24-hour period
5. Effects of standing, leg elevation, rest
6. Use of support hose
7. Presence of leg pain, sores
8. Weight gain
9. Accompanying symptoms: dyspnea, jaundice, ulceration and pigmentation of the skin of the legs

Leg pain or cramps—intermittent claudication

1. Onset with activity or rest, effect of leg elevation
2. Location
3. Duration
4. Character of pain, radiation
   a. Burning in toes, pain when pointing toes, pain in thighs or buttocks, "charley horses," aching, pain over specific location; effect of activity
   b. Skin changes: Coldness, pallor, hair loss, sores, redness or warmth over vein, visible veins
   c. Fatigue or limping—effect of walking
   d. Waking with pain or cramps

Nocturia

1. Onset and duration
2. Recent changes

Syncope. Syncope (loss of consciousness) results most commonly from reduced perfusion of the brain. It may be due to ventricular fibrillation with AV block, other cardiac arrhythmias, valvular disease, hypotension, stroke, or seizure disorders.

1. Onset: Sudden or gradual
2. Precipitating factors: Exertion, position change, bleeding
3. Preceding sensations: Light-headedness, vertigo, weakness, aphasia, confusion, sudden movements, visual changes, emotional disturbance
4. Associated symptoms: Nausea, chest pain, diaphoresis, palpitation, confusion, numbness, hunger, extra or unusual exertion, sudden turning of neck (carotid sinus effect), change in posture
5. Time taken to regain consciousness

Cyanosis. Cyanosis is a bluish discoloration of the skin and mucous membranes.

1. Onset
2. Location
3. Precipitating factors: Exertion, exposure to cold air or water

Past health history

1. Hypertension
2. Coronary artery disease
3. Elevated lipids (cholesterol, triglycerides)
4. Arrhythmias
5. Previous myocardial infarctions
6. Congenital heart defect
7. Murmurs
8. Cardiac disease
9. Cardiac surgery or hospitalization for cardiac disorder
10. Palpitations
11. Dizziness
12. Dependent leg edema
13. Rheumatic fever, unexplained fever, swollen joints
14. Diabetes mellitus
15. Most recent ECG, stress ECG, or other heart test

Family history

1. Angina
2. Heart disease (heart failure, valvular disease)
3. Myocardial infarction
4. Stroke
5. Diabetes mellitus
6. Hyperlipidemia
7. Hypertension
8. Obesity
9. Sudden death, particularly of young and middle-aged relatives
10. Congenital heart defects
11. Peripheral vascular disease
12. Symptoms such as dyspnea, fatigue, leg pains after exertion, palpitations, syncope

Other considerations

1. Exercise pattern: Type, frequency, duration, intensity, regularity
2. Nutritional status
   a. Usual diet: Proportion of fat, use of salt, intake of caffeine products, food preferences (a dietary log may be useful in gathering this information over time)
   b. Weight: Loss or gain, history of dieting
3. Tobacco use
   a. Type (cigarettes, cigars, pipe, chewing tobacco, snuff), duration, amount, age started, efforts to quit (NOTE: Pack-years of smoking are calculated by multiplying the number of years of smoking by the number of packs smoked each day.)

RISK FACTORS CARDIOVASCULAR DISEASE

CORONARY ARTERY DISEASE
PRINCIPAL MODIFIABLE RISK FACTORS
Elevated serum cholesterol level (greater than 200 mg/dl) and lowered high-density lipoprotein (HDL) level (less than 35 mg/dl)
Smoking
Hypertension
Obesity
Excessive dietary intake of calories and fat, especially saturated fat
Diabetes mellitus
Sedentary lifestyle
Long-term use of oral contraceptives
Personality characteristics such as intensity, compulsivity, hostility
PRINCIPAL NONMODIFIABLE RISK FACTORS
Increasing age
Gender: Men at greater risk; postmenopausal women at greater risk because of loss of protective effect of estrogen
Family history of cardiovascular disease, diabetes, hyperlipidemia, hypertension, or sudden death in young adults.

CEREBROVASCULAR DISEASE
Hypertension
Obesity
Smoking
Coronary artery disease
Atrial fibrillation
Diabetes mellitus
Increased age

PERIPHERAL ARTERY DISEASE
Smoking
Diabetes mellitus
Age over 50

HYPERCHOLESTEROLEMIA
Obesity
Excessive dietary intake of fat, especially saturated fat
Menopause

VARICOSE VEINS
Prolonged standing or sitting
Obesity
Sedentary lifestyle
Gender: Women at greater risk than men, particularly during pregnancy
Increasing age
Race: White Americans at greater risk than African-Americans

b. Exposure to passive smoke
4. Alcohol consumption: Amount per day or week, frequency, duration of current consumption
5. Personality assessment
   a. Perceived level of stress in life
   b. Type and intensity of work
   c. Compulsive behaviors
   d. Hostile attitudes
6. Relaxation habits
   a. Routine activities
   b. Hobbies
   c. Exercise: Type, amount, frequency, intensity
   d. Stress reduction practices
   e. Use of alcohol, drugs
   f. Sexual activity
7. Medications: Antihypertensives, beta-blockers, calcium channel blockers, digoxin, diuretics, oral contraceptives, aspirin, anticoagulants, over-the-counter drugs, street drugs (Ask about dosage, frequency, when began and why, side effects, compliance.)

Preparation for Examination: Client and Environment

A quiet environment is essential for a thorough examination of the cardiovascular system. All heart sounds are quiet and of relatively low pitch. They are very difficult to hear when any extraneous noises are present. A room temperature that is comfortable for the client is also important to prevent chilling and subsequent interference with hearing the heart sounds. For inspection of the subtle motions of the precordium and the neck vessels, good lighting in the room is required, including both standard examination room lighting and a movable light that can be directed at an angle across the precordium and neck vessels. Respect the client's need for privacy. Provide a drape, and uncover only those portions of the body being examined as you proceed.

Other considerations: components, sequence, and integration with other systems

The examination of the cardiovascular system includes the following: (1) peripheral pulse assessment and (2) blood pressure measurement (see Chapter 9); (3) inspection of the neck vessels: the jugular veins and carotid arteries; (4) inspection, palpation, and auscultation of the heart; and (5) inspection of the peripheral veins.

Several changes of position are required of the patient during the cardiovascular examination, so it is very important to organize the various parts of the physical examination in a sequence that is comfortable for the client and that does not involve unnecessary movement. Remember that the cardiovascular examination relates

---

PREPARATION FOR EXAMINATION

EQUIPMENT

Item	Purpose
Examining table large enough for client to change position easily	Client needs to be able to move to left lateral recumbent position for auscultation of the heart
Penlight or lamp with movable arm	Tangential lighting for inspection of precordium and jugular venous pulsations
Sphygmomanometer with appropriate-size cuff	Measurement of blood pressure
Stethoscope with diaphragm and bell	Auscultation of heart and large arteries
Metric ruler	Measurement of jugular venous pressure
Tape measure	Measurement of edematous extremities

CLIENT AND ENVIRONMENT

1. Ensure privacy for the client (provide a drape).
2. Make sure the room, your hands, and the stethoscope are warm during the examination.
3. Ensure a quiet room.
4. Ensure good lighting.

---

to findings in other body systems, such as rales in the lungs, engorgement of the liver, hypertensive changes in the vessels of the retina, a barrel chest, or the bruit of an abdominal aortic aneurysm.

Discussion of the cardiovascular examination in this chapter is divided into three parts: the heart, the neck vessels, and the peripheral vessels.

Technique for Examination and Normal Findings

Begin the cardiovascular examination by assessing the client's general appearance; some of this you have already done while taking the history. Assess the general build, skin color, respiration pattern, position, and movements.

Examination of the heart

For a thorough examination of the heart, you must examine the client in the sitting, supine, and left lateral recumbent positions. Inspection and palpation are performed with the client primarily in the sitting and

supine positions; auscultation must be performed with the client in the sitting, forward-leaning, supine, and left lateral recumbent (also called left lateral decubitus) positions. Examination of the heart in these various positions improves audibility of heart sounds by bringing the heart closer to the chest wall. Always be aware of the client's ability to move and of his or her comfort in the various positions, particularly when examining the client in the supine and left lateral recumbent positions. Clients with a compromised respiratory or cardiovascular system may not be able to tolerate all positions.

The techniques of inspection, palpation, and auscultation are used to examine the heart. Although it is tempting to auscultate the heart first, be sure to inspect and palpate the precordium before placing the stethoscope on the chest wall. You will gain much information that will enhance your auscultation. All the techniques used for examining the heart are affected by the amount and type of tissue lying between the heart and the chest wall. In clients with more developed musculature, more adipose tissue, or a barrel chest, precordial findings may not be visible or palpable, and the sounds will seem more distant.

Inspection. With the client in the supine or sitting position, inspect the chest wall. You will need a tangential light to observe the subtle movements of the chest. Observe the chest first for size and symmetry and for any deformities of the thoracic cage. Note the frequency, depth, and regularity of respirations. Then look for any visible pulsations, retractions, heaves, or lifts.

Apical impulse. The thrust of the contracting left ventricle may produce a visible pulsation in the area of the left midclavicular line at the fifth intercostal space. This is the apical impulse. It occurs nearly synchronously with the carotid pulse and the first heart sound; simultaneous palpation of a carotid artery is helpful in identifying it. When it is visible, the apical impulse helps to identify an area very near the cardiac apex, thus giving some indication of cardiac size. (The apical beat was previously called the point of maximal impulse [PMI]; since other pulsations may be more prominent than the apical beat, this term is no longer used.)

> **HELPFUL HINT** *The apical impulse is visible in only about half of the adult population.*

Retraction. A retraction is a pulling in of some of the tissues on the precordium related to the position and activity of the heart. A slight retraction of the chest wall just medial to the midclavicular line in the fifth intercostal space is a normal finding. It is more evident when the chest wall is thin.

Lifts and heaves. A lift is a more sustained thrust of the ventricle during systole. A heave is an excessive thrust of the heart against the chest wall. A lift or heave may be present with ventricular hypertrophy as a result of an increased workload. A left ventricular lift or heave is seen or palpated in the apical area; a right ventricular lift or heave is seen or palpated at the left sternal border.

Palpation. Use the technique of palpation to build on and expand the findings obtained during inspection. Take time to "tune in" to the movement over the precordium. Most of these movements are subtle and are better perceived after careful inspection. Varying the hand pressure you apply only slightly, use a light and gentle touch, allowing any movements of the chest to come toward your hand. The sensitivity of your hand decreases as the pressure you use increases. Palpate the precordium while the client is sitting, while the client is lying in the lowest position that he or she is able to tolerate, and while the client is in the left lateral decubitus position.

Stand on the right side of the client. Palpate the precordium in three areas, moving either from the apex to the base or from the base to the apex; develop a methodical system. (In this text we will use the apex-to-base approach.) Either way, you will palpate the apical area, along the left sternal border, and at both the left and right second intercostal spaces.

Using the palmar surface of your right hand and fingers, begin at the fifth left intercostal space in the midclavicular line, where the apical impulse is normally located (Figure 16.22, *A*). You will feel this as a slight tap of short duration against your fingers. This pulsation is approximately 1 cm in diameter. On occasion, the apical impulse is located lateral to the midclavicular line (e.g., in association with a high diaphragm, such as occurs with pregnancy). The outward tap of the normal apical impulse is felt only during early systole. Next, place your hand along the left sternal border (Figure 16.21, *B*), then at the base of the heart at the right and then the left sternal borders in the second intercostal spaces (Figure 16.21, *C*). Palpate in these locations for any pulsations, vibrations, heaves, or thrills. None should be palpable against the palm of your hand.

> **HELPFUL HINT** *A thrill is the rushing sensation of blood moving through the heart or a major artery. It is like the sensation transmitted to your fingers when they are placed over the neck of a purring cat. A thrill may be felt over a large murmur.*

The amplitude of the apical impulse may seem to be increased in normal individuals with thin chest walls. In clients with high cardiac output states, such as anemia,

figure **16.22**   Palpation of the precordium. **A,** Apex. **B,** Left sternal border. **C,** Base.

anxiety, fever, or hyperthyroidism, the apical impulse often increases in amplitude and duration. In persons who are obese, have thick chest walls, or have emphysema, you are unlikely to be able to palpate the apical impulse. Left ventricular hypertrophy and/or dilation displaces the apical impulse downward and to the left, and may also increase the size of the impulse.

If significant movements are palpable over the precordium, you should palpate other areas extending beyond the standard areas, including the left anterior axillary area, the epigastrium, and the right sternal border.

Note the timing of any abnormal palpable movements, using the carotid artery pulsation as a guide.

Auscultation. Although heart sounds are described as being "high pitched" or "low pitched," these terms are relative. All heart sounds are low pitched and in a range that is difficult for the human ear to hear. A quiet room and careful use of the stethoscope make it possible to hear the sounds of the heart.

Stethoscope. Review the material on the use of the stethoscope in Chapter 8: Assessment Techniques. Use both the diaphragm and the bell of the stethoscope to auscultate heart sounds. Use the diaphragm to listen to the high-pitched sounds, such as S_1 and S_2. Use the bell to listen to the low-pitched sounds, such as S_3 and S_4. (See Table 16.3 to learn which sounds are best heard with the diaphragm and which ones are best heard with the bell.)

> **HELPFUL HINT** *If you apply too much pressure to the bell of the stethoscope, the underlying skin becomes tight and the skin itself then acts as a diaphragm. Place the bell very lightly on the chest wall, with just enough pressure applied to seal the edge.*

table 16.3	*Use of the Bell and Diaphragm of the Stethoscope for Cardiac Auscultation*
Sounds best heard with the diaphragm	**Sounds best heard with the bell**
High-frequency sounds First heart sound Second heart sound Systolic clicks High-pitched murmurs of valvular regurgitation Ejection clicks Opening snap of mitral valve Pericardial friction rub	Low-frequency sounds Third heart sound Fourth heart sound Diastolic murmurs originating from mitral and tricuspid valves

Auscultatory areas. Although the four heart valves are located close to one another in a small area behind the sternum, the areas on the chest wall where their closure sounds are most audible are not located directly over the valves, but rather in the direction of the flow of blood. The area where the closure of each valve can normally be heard best is summarized in Table 16.4 and illustrated in Figure 16.23.

While these are the main areas for auscultation, do not limit your auscultation to these areas only. Listen in an area around each of the areas described above. Important findings are sometimes present in other loca-

figure**16.23** Anatomical location of the heart valves and transmission of closure sounds from the heart valves.

tions, such as the right parasternal region, axilla, neck, and epigastrium.

Complete auscultation includes listening with the client in the sitting, leaning-forward, supine, and left lateral decubitus positions. Begin auscultation by standing on the right side of the client. The client may be in the sitting or supine position as you begin. A systematic method of auscultation is essential, as with palpation. Begin either at the apex or at the base of the heart. (We will begin at the apex in this description.) Start at the fifth left intercostal space in the midclavicular line (Figure 16.24, *A*). Inch your stethoscope toward the lower left sternal border (Figure 16.24, *B*). Move upward along the left sternal border to the base of the heart. Listen at the base of both the second left intercostal

space at the sternal border (Figure 16.24, *C*) and the second right intercostal space at the sternal border (Figure 16.24, *D*). Repeat this pattern using first the diaphragm and then the bell of the stethoscope. If any sounds radiate beyond the standard area of auscultation, follow them with the stethoscope by inching the stethoscope along in the direction of the sound. For example, sounds may radiate to the area of the anterior axillary line or up to the carotid arteries.

Listen selectively to one sound at a time. As with palpation, the process of auscultation requires a period of "tuning in." Use the following sequence for listening:

1. Note the rate and rhythm of the heartbeat.
2. Identify S_1 and S_2.
3. Focus on S_1; note the intensity, the effect of respiration, and any variations.
4. Focus on S_2; note the intensity, splitting with respiration, and any variations.
5. Focus on systole, then on diastole, noting any extra sounds or murmurs.

table**16.4**	*Areas Where Valve Closures Are Best Heard*
Valve	**Area**
Mitral	Fifth left intercostal space at the midclavicular line
Tricuspid	Left sternal border, fourth left intercostal space
Pulmonic	Left sternal border, second left intercostal space
Aortic	Right sternal border, second right intercostal space

HELPFUL HINT *Listen selectively to each sound and phase of the cardiac cycle—both the sounds and the silences. It is impossible to listen for everything at once.*

Any variations mentioned in this section are more fully described later in this chapter under Variations from Health. They are mentioned here to give you

figure**16.24** Auscultation of the precordium. **A,** Apex. **B,** Left sternal border. **C,** Second left intercostal space. **D,** Second right intercostal space.

some idea of what types of sounds you might anticipate hearing.

If you began auscultation with the client supine, ask her or him to roll to the left side (Figure 16.25). Apply the bell of the stethoscope lightly at the apex and listen for any low-frequency diastolic sounds, such as:

S_3, an early diastolic ventricular filling sound
S_4, a late diastolic ventricular filling sound
A mitral valve murmur

If you began with the client in the sitting position, ask him or her to lean slightly forward. Press the diaphragm of the stethoscope firmly against the client's chest and listen at both the second left and right intercostal spaces near the sternal border to detect any high-pitched diastolic murmurs of aortic or pulmonic valve insufficiency (Figure 16.26). Listen during normal respiration and then ask the client to hold his or her breath in deep expiration.

Rate and rhythm. The normal heart rate ranges from 60 to 100 beats per minute. (Review assessment of the pulse in Chapter 9.) The rhythm is normally regular; however, sinus arrhythmia occurs normally in some children and young adults. With sinus arrhythmia, the rhythm varies with breathing, increasing at the peak of inspiration and slowing with expiration. Note any other irregular rhythm and whether there is a pattern to the irregularity or if it is totally irregular. If you notice any irregularity, check for a pulse deficit by auscultating the apical beat while simultaneously palpating the radial pulse. Each apical beat should be followed by a radial

figure**16.25** Auscultation at the apex of the heart with the client in the left lateral recumbent position.

figure**16.26** Auscultation at the base of the heart with the client leaning forward.

beat. If there are fewer radial pulse beats, count each for 1 minute and subtract the radial rate from the apical rate. The remainder is the pulse deficit.

S_1 and S_2. Distinguish the first and second heart sounds. At heart rates under 100, S_1 is clearly the first of the pair of sounds making up the "lub-dub" of each heartbeat. S_1 is louder at the apex than S_2; S_2 is louder at the base than S_1 (see Figure 16.13). S_1 is very nearly synchronous with the carotid pulse (see Figure 16.18). Note whether each heart sound is normal, accentuated, diminished, or split.

CHARACTERISTICS OF S_1

Caused by closure of the AV valves (mitral and tricuspid)

Beginning of ventricular systole

Can be heard over the entire precordium but is loudest at the apex

Best heard with the diaphragm of the stethoscope

Split S_1 (mitral and tricuspid components heard separately) may be normal, but that is rare; split S_1 is best heard along the lower left sternal border—the tricuspid area.

CHARACTERISTICS OF S_2

Caused by closure of the semilunar valves (pulmonic and aortic)

Beginning of ventricular diastole

Can be heard over the entire precordium but is loudest at the base

Best heard with the diaphragm of the stethoscope

Split S_2 toward the end of inspiration is normal. The split-second sound is heard only in the area where pul-

monic valve closure is loudest (i.e., in the second left intercostal space). Inspiration affects the return of blood to the heart, causing the closure of the pulmonic valve (P_2) to be slightly delayed; thus A_2 occurs slightly before P_2. If the S_2 is split, you will hear a brief double sound near the end of inspiration. During expiration, blood return to the heart equalizes, and the two sounds are heard as one. Asking the client to hold her or his breath during inspiration will equalize the blood return and ejection times, and inspiratory splitting will disappear. To help with your timing, focus on the rise and fall of the client's chest during normal respiration.

Note whether S_1 and S_2 are normal, including the normal splitting of S_2. Note if there is a fixed splitting of S_2 (split remains and is not affected by respiration) or paradoxical splitting (the reverse occurs: S_2 splits on expiration and comes together on inspiration).

Extra heart sounds during systole and diastole. Systole is normally silent. The midsystolic ejection click of mitral valve prolapse is the most common extra sound heard during systole. The third and fourth heart sounds, which occur during diastole, may be normal or abnormal.

Venous hum. A venous hum, caused by turbulent blood flow in the jugular veins, is common in healthy children and is not pathologically significant. Use the

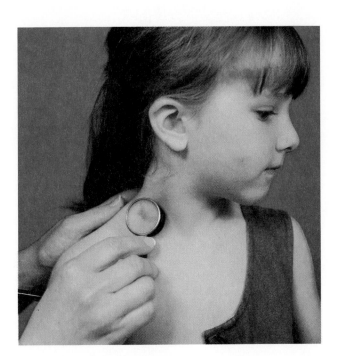

figure**16.27** Venous hum. A continuous, low-pitched hum noted over the neck in many children, it is often best heard over the right supraclavicular space.

bell of the stethoscope to auscultate over the supraclavicular area on the right side. Auscultation can be improved by turning the client's head away and slightly upward from the side being auscultated. The hum is loudest during diastole. Because it is produced by blood flow in the jugular veins, the hum can be stopped by applying gentle pressure over the internal jugular vein in the neck between the trachea and the sternocleidomastoid muscle at approximately the level of the thyroid cartilage Figure 16.27.

Murmurs. A murmur is a blowing, swooshing sound that occurs with turbulent blood flow in the heart or great vessels. Murmurs can be categorized as:

1. Innocent murmurs, which are always systolic and occur without evidence of physiological or structural abnormalities
2. Functional murmurs, which are associated with physiological alterations such as high cardiac output states (e.g., exercise, anemia, hyperthyroidism, or increased blood volume associated with pregnancy)
3. Pathological murmurs, which are always caused by structural abnormalities

Because some murmurs are within the range of normal findings, some basic information on murmurs is presented in this section. Certain murmurs are common in healthy children or adolescents and are termed inno-

cent or functional. The contractile force of the heart is greater in children; this increases blood flow velocity. The increased velocity plus a smaller chest measurement makes a murmur audible. An innocent murmur is generally soft (grade I to II), midsystolic, short, and crescendo-decrescendo, with a vibratory or musical quality. Also, the innocent murmur is heard at the second or third left intercostal space and disappears with sitting. The young person has no associated signs of cardiac dysfunction.

Although it is important to distinguish innocent murmurs from pathological ones, it is best to suspect all murmurs as pathological until they are proved otherwise. Diagnostic tests such as the ECG, phonocardiogram, and echocardiogram are needed to establish an accurate diagnosis.

If you hear a murmur, describe it according to the following characteristics.

TIMING IN THE CARDIAC CYCLE. The timing of a murmur within systole or diastole is the basis for its classification. First, note whether the murmur occurs during systole or diastole, or both. There are three basic categories of murmurs: systolic, diastolic, and continuous. A continuous murmur begins in systole and continues into all or part of diastole. Note during which portion of systole or diastole the murmur occurs:

Early, mid-, or late systole or diastole (Early diastolic murmurs are referred to as protodiastolic, and late diastolic murmurs are called presystolic.)
Throughout systole (pansystolic or holosystolic) or throughout diastole (pandiastolic or holodiastolic)

DURATION. The duration of different murmurs varies from short to long, with gradations in between.

PITCH (FREQUENCY). Describe the pitch as high, medium, or low. The pitch depends on the pressure and the velocity of blood flow producing the murmur. Generally, when the rate of flow is rapid, a high pitch results; when the velocity is slower, the pitch is low.

LOUDNESS (INTENSITY). Describe the intensity in terms of six grades:

Grade I	Faintest that can be detected; audible only in a quiet room and then with special effort
Grade II	Faint but clearly audible
Grade III	Moderately loud; easy to hear
Grade IV	Loud; may be associated with a thrill palpable on the chest wall
Grade V	Very loud; heard with one edge of the stethoscope lifted off the chest wall; thrill may be palpable
Grade VI	Loudest possible; still audible with the entire stethoscope lifted just enough to remove it from contact with the chest wall; thrill may be palpable

When considering the loudness of the murmur, also note whether it muffles or obscures the heart sounds.

PATTERN (SHAPE, CONFIGURATION). The terms *crescendo* and *decrescendo* describe the pattern of loudness reflecting changes in the rate of blood flow. The intensity follows a pattern: growing louder (crescendo), tapering off (decrescendo), or increasing to a peak and then decreasing (crescendo-decrescendo). Some murmurs have a flat or nearly flat configuration (see Figure 16.41).

QUALITY. Several descriptive terms are used to describe the quality, including "musical," "blowing," "harsh," or "rumbling."

LOCATION. Describe the area of maximum intensity of the murmur by using the anatomical landmarks of the area where you hear it best. Some murmurs are localized to small areas; others are heard over large portions of the chest wall.

RADIATION. The murmur may be transmitted downstream in the direction of blood flow and may be heard in another place on the precordium, the neck, the back, or the axilla. Factors affecting radiation include the direction and velocity of the blood flow and the sound transmission through various tissues.

POSITION. Some murmurs disappear or are enhanced by a change in position, such as standing, leaning forward, or lying supine.

EFFECT OF RESPIRATION. Respiration, with its intrathoracic pressure changes, affects filling on the right side of the heart. Venous return to the right side increases with inspiration and decreases with expiration. Murmurs originating in the right side of the heart may be influenced by these factors.

After auscultating in the supine position, have the client roll on the left side. Listen with the bell at the apex for the presence of any diastolic filling sounds of S_3 or S_4. After auscultating in the sitting position, have the client lean forward slightly and exhale. Listen with the diaphragm firmly pressed at the second right and then left intercostal spaces. Listen for the soft, high-pitched murmurs of aortic or pulmonic regurgitation. S_3, S_4, and the semilunar valve regurgitant murmurs may be heard only with these changes in position.

Examination of the neck vessels

The techniques of inspection, palpation, and auscultation are used to examine the carotid arteries. The technique of inspection is used to examine the jugular veins.

figure **16.28** Palpation of the carotid artery pulse.

Carotid arteries

Inspection. Inspect the neck for the amplitude of the carotid pulsation. Note unusually large, bounding pulsations or small, weak pulsations.

Palpation (Figure 16.28). See Chapter 9 for pulse assessment.

Auscultation. Use the bell of the stethoscope to listen for bruits over the carotid arteries (Figure 16.29). A bruit is a blowing sound heard over an artery. It indicates increased flow through the artery or stenosis of the artery.

Jugular veins

Jugular venous pulse. Direct tangential lighting at an angle across the neck where the jugular veins are located (Figure 16.30). The jugular venous pulse (JVP) can be recognized by its location in the neck and by its characteristic pulsation. However, the distinct a, c, and v waves are not always clearly visible. The normal jugular venous pulse may appear as a gentle, undulant wave. In the client with a healthy cardiovascular system, the venous pulse will not be visible until she or he is in, or nearly in, the supine position. To evaluate the JVP, lower the client's head and thorax until the venous pulsations are visible.

The jugular veins lie close to the carotid arteries, and their pulsations need to be distinguished from each other. There are five ways to distinguish venous from arterial pulsations:

1. *Character of the pulse.* The venous pulse is more undulating than the brisk arterial pulse. The carotid pulse has one upstroke, whereas the venous pulse has three. Palpate the carotid pulse on

figure**16.29** Auscultation of the carotid artery.

one side of the neck while observing the jugular pulse on the other side.

2. *Effect of position.* Arterial pulsations do not change when the client's position changes. In the healthy individual, the venous pulsations are visible only in the supine position.

3. *Effect of respiration.* Venous pulsations change with respiration; arterial pulsations do not. With inspiration, intrathoracic pressure decreases, blood flow into the right atrium increases, and the level of the pulsation in the neck veins descends. During expiration, it rises.

4. *Effect of venous compression.* You can easily eliminate the pulsation of the jugular veins by applying gentle pressure over the external jugular vein at the base of the neck above the clavicle. This maneuver blocks the transmission of the venous pulse wave, leaving only the arterial pulsation.

5. *Effect of abdominal pressure (hepatojugular reflux).* The hepatojugular reflux technique may reveal some degree of heart failure when the jugular veins are not obviously distended. With the client in the supine or low Fowler's position, moderate pressure is applied over the upper right quadrant of the abdomen for about 30 seconds. In the client with normal heart function, a slight rise in the venous pulsation may occur but diminishes quickly. In an individual with right-sided heart failure, the jugular venous pressure increases as venous return to the heart increases. Sustained distention suggests right-sided heart failure or chronic lung disease. (The hepatojugular reflux is further described under Variations from Health.)

Jugular venous pressure. Inspection of the jugular veins for the height of the column of blood provides a gross estimate of right-sided heart pressure. When a healthy client is in the sitting position, no neck veins are visible. They become visible only when the client is in the supine position. When the venous pressure is greatly elevated, the jugular veins become evident when the client is sitting.

One method of measuring the height of the venous column is illustrated in Figure 16.31. Before attempting to do this assessment, determine the client's comfort level and ability to have his or her head and chest lowered. Have the client's head and thorax at the level needed to see the upper level of venous pulsations. Use the sternal angle (angle of Louis), the juncture of the manubrium, and the body of the sternum as a reference point. Place a centimeter ruler at the sternal angle and place another ruler perpendicular to the first at the top of the level of jugular venous distention. Note the angle of the client's head and thorax, and the level in centimeters of the pulsation. The lower you place the client's head before the pulsations are visible, the lower the pressure; the higher the client's head when you can identify the upper level of pulsation, the higher is the pressure.

Examination of the peripheral vascular system

The techniques of inspection, palpation, and auscultation are used to examine the peripheral vascular system. The peripheral vasculature is examined over the entire body during the course of the complete physical examination; learn a systematic way of integrating this assessment into the complete examination.

Inspection

1. Skin color changes: Pallor, cyanosis, rubor (redness).

2. Hair distribution: Lack of hair growth may indicate inadequate circulation.

3. Size and symmetry: Atrophy, swelling, edema. If swelling or edema is present, measure both legs at the widest part with a tape measure, noting differences in size and at precisely what distance from a bony landmark (such as the patella or medial malleolus) the measurement is taken. Inspect for pretibial edema. Normally, none is present, although mild edema may be noted in a healthy client who is pregnant or who has been standing all day.

4. Venous patterns: The venous pattern is normally flat and only slightly visible; look for varicosities.

5. Lesions, ulcerations. None are present on healthy skin; if present, they may be due to an inadequate blood supply.

6. Nails: Capillary refill time, clubbing.

   a. Assess capillary refill time by placing the client's hands near the level of the heart; depress and blanch the nail beds, then release and note the

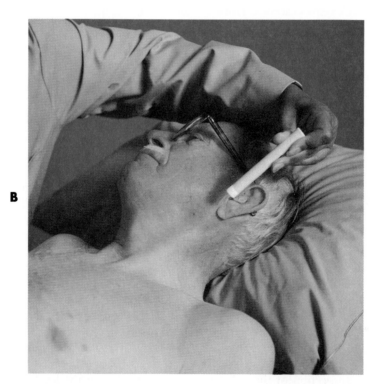

figure**16.30** Inspection of the external jugular vein, directing the light across the neck in order to see the venous pulse wave.

figure **16.31** Measurement of jugular venous pressure. Arrows indicate the height of the jugular venous pressure in centimeters.

figure **16.32** Assessing for pitting edema. *(From Canobbio MM:* Cardiovascular disorders, *St Louis, 1990, Mosby.)*

CULTURAL CONSIDERATIONS

CARDIOVASCULAR DISEASE

Heart disease and stroke are two of the major causes of death among people from various cultural backgrounds, accounting for about 30% of mortality.

Heart disease

Among African-Americans and Native Americans, the incidence of death from heart disease is approximately twice as high as that for all other Americans.

Stroke

African-American males are twice as likely to die of a stroke as are white males, and among all African-American adults, death from coronary artery disease is higher than among other Americans.

Diabetes mellitus

Diabetes mellitus is ranked as the seventh leading cause of death in the United States. It is a major factor in heart disease. The incidence of diabetes mellitus varies greatly among various cultural groups. It is high among some Native American groups, African-Americans, Hispanics, and Chinese-, Japanese-, and Filipino-Americans.

Varicose veins

White Americans are at greater risk for varicose veins than African-Americans because African-Americans have more venous valves in the lower legs than do whites.

time it takes for normal color to return. This should occur in less than 1 to 2 seconds. Remember that a cool room can increase refill time.

b. Check for clubbing of the fingernails by inspecting the fingers from the side. The normal nail bed angle is 160 degrees. Look for roundness and swelling at the tips of the fingers.

Palpation

1. Edema. The degree of edema can be graded on a scale of 1+ to 4+ as follows (Figure 16.32):

   1+ Slight pitting; no visible change in the shape of the extremity; disappears rapidly

   2+ Somewhat deeper pitting; no marked change in the shape of the extremity; disappears in 10 to 15 seconds

   3+ Noticeably deep pitting; full and swollen extremity; may last for more than a minute

   4+ Very deep pitting; very swollen and distorted extremity; lasts as long as 2 to 5 minutes

2. Skin temperature and turgor (see Chapter 10: Skin, Hair, and Nails).
3. Peripheral pulses (see Chapter 9: General Assessment, Including Vital Signs).

Auscultation

1. Blood pressure (see Chapter 9).

Screening Tests and Procedures*
Screening for asymptomatic coronary artery disease

1. Measure blood pressure.
2. Assess modifiable cardiac risk factors, such as cigarette smoking, physical inactivity, and excessive dietary intake of fat and cholesterol.

Screening for high blood cholesterol

Periodic measurement of the total serum cholesterol level is important for men ages 35 to 65 and women ages 45 to 65; over age 65 it may be considered on a case-by-case basis. For adolescents and young adults who have a family history of very high cholesterol levels, premature coronary heart disease (CHD) in a first-degree relative (before age 50 in men or age 60 in women), or major risk factors for CHD, screening may be recommended. Periodic screening is most important when cholesterol levels are increasing (e.g., in middle-aged men, perimenopausal women, and persons who have gained weight). All clients should receive periodic assessment regarding dietary intake of fat, especially saturated fat, and regarding weight control.

*Data from U.S. Preventive Services Task Force: *Guide to clinical preventive services: an assessment of the effectiveness of 169 interventions,* ed 2, Baltimore, 1996, Williams & Wilkins.

Serum cholesterol levels normally undergo substantial physiological fluctuations; therefore a single blood test may not be representative. Levels of serum cholesterol are described as:

High: 240 mg/dl and above
Borderline: 200 to 239 mg/dl

Screening for hypertension

See Chapter 9.

examination step-by-step

1. Before beginning the examination, be sure that the room is quiet and the temperature is comfortable for the client.
2. Have equipment ready: stethoscope, penlight or flashlight for tangential lighting, metric ruler, tape measure, sphygmomanometer.
3. Explain the examination to the client.
4. If possible, position the client in the sitting position to begin the examination. Be sure to examine the client in the sitting, leaning-forward, supine, and left lateral recumbent positions. Proceed from neck to precordium to peripheral vasculature. (The sequence may vary but must include all components.)

Neck Vessels

1. Carotid arteries
   a. *Inspection:* Amplitude of pulsations
   b. *Palpation:* Check pulse in each carotid separately
   c. *Auscultation:* Bruits
2. Jugular veins
   a. *Inspection:* Pulsations and pressure level

Precordium—Heart

1. *Inspection:* Pulsations, heaves, retractions
2. *Palpation:* Fifth left intercostal space, left sternal border, and second left and right intercostal spaces; for apical impulse, lifts, heaves, thrills
3. *Auscultation:* Fifth left intercostal space, left sternal border, second left and right intercostal spaces, and other areas of the precordium as indicated by the history or findings; for normal heart sounds, extra heart sounds, and murmurs (Use both the diaphragm and the bell to auscultate all areas.)

Peripheral Vascular System

1. *Inspection:* Venous vasculature, varicose veins, skin and peripheral tissues for adequacy of vascular delivery of nutrients and clearance of metabolic by-products and fluids
2. *Palpation:* Peripheral pulses

■ VARIATIONS FROM HEALTH

Heart

Variations with inspection

Finding	Possible cause(s)
1. Prominent pulsations in:	Enlargement of:
Apex	Left ventricle
Left parasternal region	Right ventricle
Second left intercostal space	Pulmonary artery
Second right intercostal space	Aorta
2. Thrusting apex exceeding 2 cm in diameter	Left ventricular enlargement
3. Retraction of tissues around apex	Constrictive pericarditis
4. Pulsations visible lateral to and/or inferior to midclavicular line	Cardiac enlargement
5. Shaking of entire precordium with each heartbeat	Severe valvular regurgitation, large left-to-right shunts, complete AV block, hypertrophic obstructive cardiomyopathy, various hyperkinetic states

Variations with palpation

REMINDER: Palpate with the client in both the supine and left lateral decubitus positions.

Finding	Possible cause(s)
1. Prolonged apical thrust during systole; may be accompanied by retraction in left parasternal area	Moderate to severe left ventricular hypertrophy. Aortic regurgitation
2. Systolic impulse displaced laterally and downward into the 6th or 7th intercostal space	Left ventricular enlargement
3. Apical impulse not palpable	Hypovolemia, pericardial effusion, acute myocardial infarction
4. Systolic movement along left sternal border	Right ventricular enlargement, pulmonary hypertension, pulmonic stenosis
5. Exaggerated motion of entire parasternal area	Atrial septal defect, tricuspid regurgitation
6. Prominent systolic impulse in second left intercostal space	Pulmonary hypertension, increased pulmonary blood flow
7. Left parasternal movement	Enlarged left atrium, large posterior left ventricular aneurysm, severe mitral regurgitation with expanding left atrium
8. Right parasternal movement	Aneurysm of aorta, marked enlargement of right atrium

Finding	Possible cause(s)
9. Thrill	Loud, harsh heart murmur of grade IV or greater

The degree of displacement of the apical impulse generally correlates with the extent of cardiac enlargement. Displacement tends to be maximal when both hypertrophy and dilation of the ventricle are present. Conditions associated with volume overload, such as mitral and aortic regurgitation and left-to-right shunts, tend to produce hypertrophy and dilation.

Variations with auscultation

Variations that are audible with auscultation include changes in heart sounds (S_1 and S_2), extra heart sounds, and murmurs.

Normal first and second heart sounds are largely the result of competent heart valves. Valves that fail to prevent the backflow of blood are described as incompetent, insufficient, or regurgitant. Valves that restrict the forward flow of blood are described as stenosed.

The position of the client has an effect on which abnormal sounds can be heard. Most murmurs and gallop rhythms are louder in the recumbent position because of increased venous return to the heart. They can be further increased by raising the client's legs. Mitral murmurs and early and late diastolic gallop rhythms become more audible when the client is in the left lateral recumbent position because this brings the apex closer to the chest wall.

Variations in the carotid artery pulse are discussed in Chapter 9.

Variations in the heart sounds: S_1 and S_2

Variations in S_1. Variations in the first heart sound include splitting (discussed earlier in this chapter under Anatomy and Physiology), and changes in loudness. Changes in S_1 depend on:

1. The status of the pulmonary and systemic circulation
2. Structure of the heart valves
3. Valve leaflet position when ventricular contraction begins
4. The force of the contraction

INCREASED S_1. If systole begins with the mitral valve completely open, the valve closes shut more vigorously, producing a louder S_1. This occurs with:

1. Increased blood velocity found with hyperkinetic states, such as anemia, anxiety, fever, hyperthyroidism, and exercise
2. Stenosis of the mitral valve where greater ventricular pressure is needed to overcome the increase in atrial pressure (Increased closing pressure and more abrupt closure result.)

DIMINISHED S_1. Causes include:

1. A mitral or tricuspid valve that is so fibrosed or calcified that only limited motion is possible, pro-

ducing closure with less force; this may result from rheumatic fever.

2. Systemic or pulmonary hypertension leads to more forceful atrial contraction. If the ventricle is noncompliant, the contraction may be delayed or diminished.

3. An increase in the overlying substance, including fat, fluid, or air, such as occurs with obesity, pericardial fluid, and emphysema, obscures S_1.

VARYING S_1. The loudness of S_1 varies when the valves are in varying positions at the beginning of each beat. Changes in the loudness of S_1 are produced by:

1. Incomplete heart block in which the PR interval is changing, the atria and ventricles beat independently, and the position of valves changes from beat to beat

2. Gross disruption of rhythm, such as occurs during fibrillation

Variations in S_2. Variations in S_2 include changes in loudness, and splitting that is not normal physiological splitting.

INCREASED S_2. Louder closure sounds result from:

1. Higher closing pressure due to systemic hypertension—may result in S_2 having a ringing sound.

2. Exercise and excitement—increase pressure in the aorta, producing an increase in the A_2 component of S_2.

3. Conditions associated with pulmonary hypertension, such as mitral valve stenosis and congestive heart failure—may produce an increase in the P_2 component of S_2.

4. Semilunar valves that are injured but still flexible; the component of S_2 affected depends on which valve is injured.

DIMINISHED S_2. Quieter closure results from:

1. A decrease in systemic blood pressure, such as occurs with shock; A_2 is diminished.

2. Injured valves that are thickened, calcified, and less mobile; the component of S_2 affected depends on which valve is compromised: aortic stenosis affects A_2; pulmonic stenosis affects P_2.

3. Overlying fat, fluid, or air—mutes S_2.

Variations in the splitting of S_2. Variations in the splitting of S_2 include wide splitting, fixed splitting, and paradoxical splitting (Figure 16.33).

WIDE SPLITTING. With wide splitting of S_2, splitting is present with expiration and is even wider with inspiration. Conditions causing delayed electrical stimulation of right ventricular contraction or delayed emptying of the right ventricle result in delayed closure of the pulmonic valve. This occurs with right bundle-branch block, which splits both S_1 and S_2, causing a delay in pulmonic valve closure. Wider splitting also exists with pulmonary hypertension, which delays ventricular emptying.

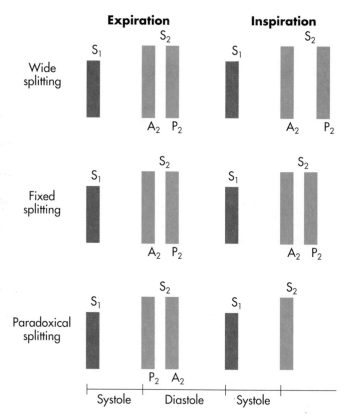

figure **16.33** Variations in splitting of S_2.

FIXED SPLITTING. Splitting of S_2 is described as fixed when it is unaffected by respiration. It is associated with atrial septal defect and right ventricular failure. Pulmonic closure is delayed because with each beat the right ventricle is ejecting a larger volume than is the left ventricle. Right-sided filling cannot be further increased by inspiration, so the split sound remains fixed.

PARADOXICAL SPLITTING. Delayed closure of the aortic valve in left bundle-branch block results in narrowed splitting, or splitting where the normal sequence of sounds is reversed: pulmonic closure precedes aortic valve closure. Paradoxically, inspiration results in the two sounds coming closer together and even fusing into a single sound, and expiration results in more widely separated sounds.

Extra heart sounds

Extra heart sounds during systole	Extra heart sounds during diastole
Ejection click of aortic and tricuspid valve	Opening snap of mitral or pulmonic valve
	S_3
	S_4

Extra sounds in systole. Extra sounds are not normally present during systole. Therefore hearing any sound after the first heart sound should cause you to consider whether a patient has heart disease.

figure**16.34** Ejection click of the aortic valve following S₁.

figure**16.35** Opening snap of the mitral valve following S₂.

AORTIC OR PULMONIC EJECTION SOUNDS (Figure 16.34). Semilunar valve ejection sounds are sharp, high-pitched, and clicking; they are best heard with the diaphragm of the stethoscope. They occur just after the first heart sound, early in systole at the end of isovolumic contraction when the semilunar valves open. Ejection clicks are caused by opening of the stenotic semilunar valves or from the ejection of blood into a dilated aorta or pulmonary artery. They may also be due to systemic or pulmonary hypertension.

Aortic valve ejection clicks are more common than pulmonic valve ejection clicks. The aortic ejection sound is often well heard at the cardiac apex and second right intercostal space. Its intensity does not significantly change with respiration.

The pulmonic ejection sound also is a sharp sound following the first heart sound and is often best heard at the second and third left intercostal spaces along the sternal border. It may decrease in intensity during inspiration and increase during expiration.

Extra sounds in diastole

OPENING SNAPS (Figure 16.35). A mitral or tricuspid valve that is stenotic but mobile produces an opening snap as the valve opens at the beginning of diastole. It may be heard at the apex and second right intercostal space. Opening snaps are high pitched and best heard through the diaphragm. Opening snaps precede third heart sounds and are higher pitched. Their earlier timing and higher frequency can prevent their being misinterpreted as a physiological third heart sound.

THIRD AND FOURTH HEART SOUNDS. Although they may be normal heart sounds, when S₃ and S₄ are abnormal, they are called gallop sounds. Third and fourth heart sounds are low-pitched sounds best heard with the bell of the stethoscope. They are intensified by the recumbent position and by exercise. At heart rates above 100 beats per minute, when both S₃ and S₄ sounds are present, they may fuse, producing a loud sound called a summation gallop.

S₃ (see Figure 16.15) occurs as passive ventricular filling begins. It is best heard with the client in the left lateral recumbent position and during expiration. Left-sided S₃ sounds are best heard at the apex; those originating from the right ventricle are best heard at the left sternal border and are accentuated with inspiration. Auscultate at the apex, placing the bell of the stethoscope lightly against the skin, with just enough pressure to form a seal. Then move to the left sternal border. The pathological S₃ indicates decreased compliance of the ventricles, such as with congestive heart failure, and may also occur with conditions of volume overload, such as with mitral, tricuspid, or aortic regurgitation.

S₄ (see Figure 16.16) occurs late in diastole when the atria contract—the rapid ventricular filling phase. Vigorous atrial contraction is necessary to produce an audible S₄. It is best heard with the client in the left lateral recumbent position and with the bell of the stethoscope gently applied to the chest wall. An S₄ originating from the right ventricle as a result of tricuspid regurgitation or right ventricular failure is heard best along the lower

left sternal border. An abnormal S_4 results from an increased resistance to filling secondary to decreased compliance of the ventricle, such as follows a myocardial infarction, or from systolic overload, including obstruction to outflow from the ventricle, such as occurs with aortic stenosis and systemic hypertension.

When both phases of rapid ventricular filling become audible events as S_3 and S_4, a quadruple rhythm with four audible components results. If the heart rate increases and diastole is shortened, S_3 and S_4 come closer together and may be heard as one sound during diastole: the summation gallop. It may be louder than S_1 and S_2.

Sounds that may occur during both systole and diastole

PERICARDIAL FRICTION RUB. Inflammation of the pericardial sac causes the parietal and visceral surfaces of the roughened pericardium to rub against each other. This action produces an extra cardiac sound having a to-and-fro character and both systolic and diastolic components. This sound is high pitched and can be best heard with the diaphragm. It resembles the sound of squeaky leather and is often described as grating, scratching, or rasping. The sound seems very close to the ear and may seem louder than, or even mask, the other heart sounds. Pericardial friction rubs can usually be heard best be-

table 16.5	*Characteristics of Extra Heart Sounds*			
Sound	**Timing in cardiac cycle**	**Location—bell/diaphragm**	**Qualities**	**Causative factors**
Ejection click of aortic or pulmonic valve	Early systole, after S_1	Apex and second right intercostal space Diaphragm	Sharp, high pitched, clicking	Stenotic aortic or pulmonic valve; or ejection of blood into dilated aorta or pulmonary artery
Opening snap of mitral valve	Early diastole, after S_2, before S_3	Medial to apex and second right intercostal space Diaphragm	High pitched	Stenotic but still mobile mitral valve
S_3	Early to mid-diastole	Apex, left lateral position, during expiration Bell	Low pitched	Heart failure, volume overload, pulmonary or systemic hypertension; also heard in hyperkinetic states
S_4	Late diastole/ presystole	Apex, supine or left lateral position Bell	Low pitched	Increased resistance to ventricular filling due to decreased compliance of ventricle or obstruction to outflow due to valve stenosis, systemic or pulmonary hypertension
Summation gallop	Mid-diastolic	Apex, supine or left lateral recumbent Bell	Intense	S_3 and S_4 with tachycardia
Pericardial friction rub	May occupy all of systole and diastole	Apex to left sternal border Diaphragm	Intense, grating, to-and-fro scratching like shoe leather; may obliterate heart sounds	Inflammation of pericardium

table 16.6 Differentiating a Split S₂ from S₃

Split S₂	S₃
Heard best at base	Heard best at apex or lower left sternal border
High pitched; heard best with diaphragm	Low pitched; heard best with bell
Varies with respiration	Not affected by respiration

table 16.7 Differentiating S₂ from an Opening Snap of the Mitral Valve

S₂	Opening snap of mitral valve
Occurs before opening snap	Occurs after S₂, during diastole
Heard best at base	Heard best at apex to lower left sternal border; may radiate toward base
Lower pitch than opening snap	Higher pitch than S₂
Varies with respiration	Does not vary with respiration

table 16.8 Differentiating S3 from an Opening Snap of the Mitral Valve

Opening snap	S₃
Occurs earlier than S3	Occurs after opening snap
Heard best with diaphragm	Heard best with bell

tween the apex and the sternum, where the pericardium comes in close contact with the chest wall. A pericardial friction rub is common after a myocardial infarction.

Differentiating heart sounds is difficult and challenging. Tables 16.5 through 16.8 present some of the differentiating characteristics of the extra heart sounds, both normal and abnormal, some of which are very close to each other in the cardiac cycle. Table 16.5 summarizes the characteristics of the extra heart sounds. Tables 16.6 through 16.8 highlight the auscultatory differences between a split S₂, S₃, and the opening snap of mitral stenosis.

Murmurs. Heart murmurs are relatively prolonged sounds that occur during systole or diastole. Some murmurs occur in the presence of normal structures when blood flow is increased because of a hyperkinetic condition. Others are caused by defects in the heart valves, major vessels, or blood flow through an abnormal opening. The abnormal sounds are produced by some turbulence of the blood flow as it enters, passes through, or leaves the heart. The sounds heard on auscultation of a murmur depend on numerous cardiovascular compo-

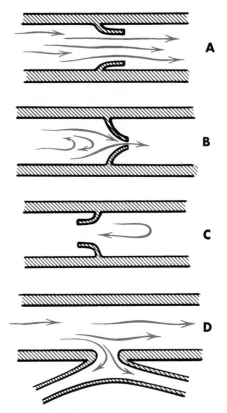

figure 16.36 Mechanisms of murmur production. **A,** Increased flow across a normal valve. **B,** Forward flow through a stenotic valve. **C,** Backflow (regurgitation) through an incompetent valve. **D,** Flow through an abnormal opening, such as a septal defect or an arteriovenous fistula (patent ductus arteriosus).

nents, including the adequacy of valve function, the size of openings between structures, the rate of blood flow, and the health of the myocardium, and on extracardiac factors, such as the thickness and consistency of the overlying tissues through which the sound of the murmur travels. Four mechanisms of murmur production are illustrated in Figure 16.36.

Diseased valves that either do not open or do not close well are a common cause of murmurs. Stenosis is the condition in which the leaflets are thickened and the passage is narrowed, thus restricting the forward flow of blood. Regurgitation is the condition in which the valve leaflets, which are intended to fit together snugly, no longer do so and the incompetent (or insufficient) opening allows the backward flow of blood.

In general, systolic murmurs caused by valvular disease are due to stenotic aortic or pulmonic valves (Figure 16.37) or incompetent mitral or tricuspid valves (Figure 16.38), and in general, diastolic murmurs caused by valvular disease are due to incompetent aortic or pulmonic valves (Figure 16.39) or stenotic mitral or tricuspid valves (Figure 16.40). Stenosis or incompetence can affect any of the four heart valves, but problems with the aortic and mitral valves are the most common.

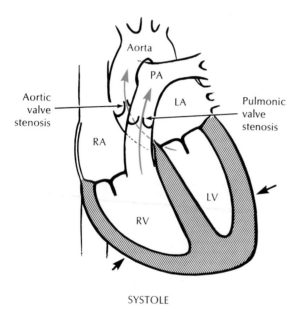

figure**16.37**   Aortic or pulmonic valve stenosis.

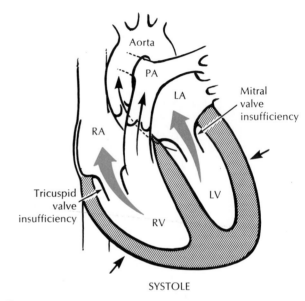

figure**16.38**   Mitral or tricuspid valve insufficiency.

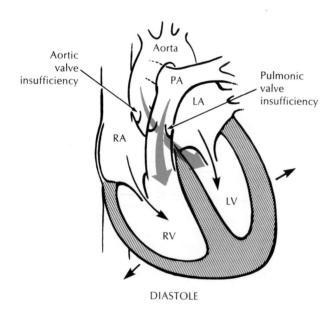

figure**16.39**   Aortic or pulmonic valve insufficiency.

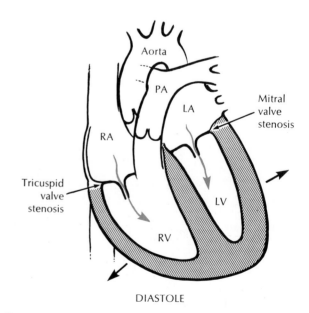

figure**16.40**   Mitral or tricuspid valve stenosis produces a diastolic murmur.

table 16.9 *Systolic Murmurs*

Type	Description of murmur	Other examination findings	Mechanism of production
MIDSYSTOLIC MURMURS*			

Type	Description of murmur	Other examination findings	Mechanism of production
Aortic stenosis	Heard best with diaphragm at second right intercostal space or at third left intercostal space with client sitting up and leaning forward, breath held in expiration; may radiate to carotids or left sternal border; loudness varies; medium pitch; harsh; midsystolic; crescendo-decrescendo; intensifies when client lies flat; if murmur is loud, may be heard over entire thorax; the more severe the stenosis, the later the crescendo of the murmur during systole	May be accompanied by a thrill; S_1 may disappear if stenosis is severe; S_2 diminished; S_4 may be present; early ejection sound at second right intercostal space; slowly rising carotid pulse wave; narrow pulse pressure; with left ventricular hypertrophy, apical impulse is prolonged and shifts downward and to left	Fibrosed or calcified aortic valve cusps make it difficult for blood to flow from left ventricle to aorta; caused by congenitally defective valves, rheumatic heart disease, atherosclerosis
Pulmonic stenosis	Heard best at second or third left intercostal space; may radiate to left side of neck; louder on inspiration; systolic; medium pitch; coarse; crescendo-decrescendo	Thrill may be present; S_1 often followed by ejection click; S_2 widely split and often diminished; P_2 soft or absent; S_4 common in right ventricular hypertrophy	Calcification of pulmonic valve restricts forward flow of blood; usually congenital
Atrial septal defect	Heard best at base, second left intercostal space; systolic; medium pitch (This murmur is not caused by the shunt, but by the increased blood flow through the pulmonic valve.)	Sternal lift; S_2 has fixed split; P_2 often louder than A_2	Abnormal opening in atrial septum resulting in left-to-right shunt, causing large increase in pulmonary blood flow

Illustrations for atrial septal defect and ventricular septal defect are from Wong DL: *Whaley and Wong's nursing care of infants and children,* ed 5, St Louis, 1995, Mosby; all other illustrations are from Thompson JM, Wilson SF: *Health assessment for nursing practice,* St Louis, 1996, Mosby.
*Caused by the forward flow of blood through the semilunar valves.

continued

table 16.9   *Systolic Murmurs—cont'd*

Type	Description of murmur	Other examination findings	Mechanism of production
PANSYSTOLIC MURMURS[*]			

Systole Diastole

S₁ S₂   S₁ S₂   S₁ S₂

Type	Description of murmur	Other examination findings	Mechanism of production
Mitral regurgitation	Heard best around apical area with diaphragm; high pitched; harsh or blowing quality; often loud; radiates from apex to base or to left axilla; does not vary with respiration	Apical impulse displaced down and to left; apical lift; thrill may be palpable at apex; S₁ diminished; S₂ more intense, with P₂ often accentuated; S₃ at apex often present; S₃-S₄ gallop common in late disease	Mitral valve incompetence permits backflow of blood from left ventricle to left atrium; results from rheumatic fever, myocardial infarction, rupture of chordae tendineae, or papillary muscle
Tricuspid regurgitation	Heard best at lower right and left sternal borders; increases with inspiration; pansystolic; soft, blowing	Enlarged jugular veins with large wave, enlarged liver; lift at sternum if right ventricular hypertrophy present; may be thrill at left lower sternal border; S₃ may be present	Incompetent tricuspid valve permits backflow of blood from right ventricle to right atrium; caused by pulmonary hypertension, cardiac trauma, congenital defects, or bacterial endocarditis
Ventricular septal defect	Heard best at lower left sternal border; loud; harsh; pansystolic; large defects also have soft diastolic murmur at apex because of increased blood flow through mitral valve	May be accompanied by a thrill	Abnormal opening in septum between ventricles; size and location vary

[*]Caused by backward flow of blood from area of higher pressure to one of lower pressure across incompetent AV valves.

table 16.10 *Diastolic Murmurs*

Type	Description of murmur	Other examination findings	Mechanism of production

EARLY DIASTOLIC MURMURS

Systole Diastole

S_1 S_2 S_1 S_2 S_1 S_2

Type	Description of murmur	Other examination findings	Mechanism of production
Aortic regurgitation	Heard best with diaphragm at second or third left intercostal space at base, with client sitting up and leaning forward; ask client to hold breath at end of expiration; early diastolic (starts almost simultaneously with S_2); decrescendo; high pitched; soft; blowing; radiates down; duration varies; low-pitched, rumbling murmur at apex is common (Austin-Flint murmur)	Early ejection click sometimes present; S_1 soft; S_2 may have tambourlike quality; S_3-S_4 gallop common; with left ventricular hypertrophy, prominent prolonged apical impulse displaced down and to left; bounding water-hammer pulse in carotid, brachial, and femoral arteries; pulse pressure wide; pulsations in cervical and suprasternal area; aortic stenosis often a concurrent problem	Incompetent aortic valve permits blood to flow back from aorta to left ventricle during diastole; decrescendo pattern of murmur reflects progressive decline in volume and rate of backflow during course of diastole; left ventricle dilates and hypertrophies as a result of increased stroke volume; caused by rheumatic heart disease, hypertension, endocarditis, congenital heart disease, syphilis, or cardiac trauma
Pulmonic regurgitation	Murmur has similar timing and characteristics as that of aortic regurgitation: high pitched, blowing, and decrescendo; heard best at second left intercostal space; may radiate to left lower sternal border; increases with inspiration		Incompetent pulmonic valve permits backflow of blood from pulmonary artery to right ventricle; caused by pulmonary hypertension or bacterial endocarditis

Illustrations are from Thompson JM, Wilson SF: *Health assessment for nursing practice*, St Louis, 1996, Mosby.

continued

table 16.10 *Diastolic Murmurs—cont'd*

Type	Description of murmur	Other examination findings	Mechanism of production

MID- TO LATE DIASTOLIC MURMURS

Systole Diastole

S_1 S_2 S_1 S_2 S_1 S_2

Type	Description of murmur	Other examination findings	Mechanism of production
Mitral stenosis	Heard best with bell held lightly at apex, with client in left lateral position; low-pitched diastolic rumble, more intense in early and late diastole; does not radiate; with increased stenosis, atrial contraction may force more blood across valve at end of ventricular diastole, giving murmur a late diastolic (presystolic) pattern	Systole usually quiet; diastolic thrill commonly palpable at apex in late diastole; apical lift; S_1 increased; S_2 split often with accentuated P_2, heard over wide area of precordium; opening snap follows P_2 closely, followed by murmur; arterial pulse amplitude decreased; pulse often irregular; often occurs with systolic murmur of mitral regurgitation	Calcified mitral valve does not open adequately, thus restricting forward flow of blood from left atrium to left ventricle during diastole; left atrium becomes enlarged; caused by rheumatic fever or calcification
Tricuspid stenosis	Heard best with bell at lower left sternal border with client in left lateral position; low-pitched diastolic rumble; louder with inspiration; does not radiate; similar to murmur of mitral stenosis; may be hard to differentiate	Diminished arterial pulse, prominent jugular venous pulse	Calcified tricuspid valve restricts forward flow of blood from right atrium to right ventricle during diastole; caused by rheumatic heart disease

CONTINUOUS MURMURS

Result of abnormal link between two parts of circulatory system, such as patent ductus arteriosus; with exception of normal venous hum, continuous murmurs are always pathological; typical continuous murmur begins in systole and spills over into diastole, thus sounding like a single murmur; best heard in second left intercostal space lateral to pulmonary area and may radiate down sternal border

S_1 SM S_2
Midsystolic ejection murmur

S_1 SM S_2
Early systolic murmur

S_1 SM S_2
Pansystolic murmur

figure **16.41** Shapes of murmurs.

table 16.11   *Timing of Cardiac Sounds: Sounds Heard During Systole, Diastole, or Both*

Systolic sounds	Diastolic sounds	Both
Aortic and pulmonic ejection clicks	Third heart sound	Pericardial friction rub
Click of mitral valve prolapse	Fourth heart sound	
Functional murmur	Mitral stenosis murmur	
Aortic stenosis murmur	Tricuspid stenosis murmur	
Pulmonic stenosis murmur	Aortic regurgitation murmur	
Mitral regurgitation murmur	Pulmonic regurgitation murmur	
Tricuspid regurgitation murmur	Summation gallop	

The blood flow patterns of the various murmurs produce murmurs of three basic shapes (Figure 16.41):

1. The crescendo-decrescendo, or diamond-shaped, pattern of systolic functional murmurs and murmurs of aortic or pulmonic stenosis
2. The decrescendo pattern of the diastolic murmurs of aortic or pulmonic regurgitation
3. The flat pattern of the pansystolic (holosystolic) murmurs of mitral and tricuspid regurgitation

The greater the blood flow, the greater the intensity of the murmur.

Table 16.9 summarizes the characteristics of six systolic murmurs. Table 16.10 summarizes the characteristics of four diastolic murmurs. Table 16.11 reviews the extra heart sounds and murmurs heard during systole and diastole, and the box on p. 405 reviews the sounds to listen for over each area of the precordium.

Other cardiac disorders

Left ventricular hypertrophy. Increased resistance to the emptying of blood from the left ventricle into the aorta occurs with systemic hypertension, aortic stenosis, and volume overload. The left ventricle hypertrophies as a result of the extra workload. It is sometimes displaced laterally and downward, and the apical impulse may be palpable over a larger area than usual.

Myocardial infarction. Ischemia and necrosis of the myocardium are caused by an abrupt obstruction of circulation to some portion of the heart. The left ventricle is most frequently affected, but damage may extend to either the right ventricle or either atrium. Infarction is characterized by severe pain involving the central area of the chest, commonly with radiation to the left arm, jaw, neck, back, or abdomen. Associated symptoms may include sweating, weakness, nausea, vomiting, dyspnea, light-headedness, restlessness, coolness of the extremi-

Sounds to Listen for over Each Area of the Precordium

APEX
First and second heart sounds
Aortic ejection click
Opening snap of mitral stenosis
Systolic murmur of mitral regurgitation
High-pitched murmur of aortic regurgitation
Diastolic murmur of mitral stenosis (left lateral recumbent position)

LOWER LEFT STERNAL BORDER—FOURTH AND FIFTH INTERCOSTAL SPACES
First and second heart sounds
Aortic ejection click
Opening snap of mitral or tricuspid stenosis
Diastolic murmur of tricuspid stenosis (left lateral recumbent position)
Systolic murmurs of aortic stenosis, tricuspid regurgitation, and ventricular septal defect

LEFT STERNAL BORDER—SECOND AND THIRD INTERCOSTAL SPACES
Both components of second heart sound
Pulmonary ejection click
Systolic murmur of pulmonic stenosis
Diastolic murmurs of aortic and pulmonic valve regurgitation
Systolic murmur of atrial septal defect

RIGHT STERNAL BORDER—SECOND INTERSPACE
First and second heart sounds
Systolic murmur of aortic stenosis

ties, and anxiety. Underlying causes include atherosclerotic coronary disease and embolus to the coronary arteries.

Physical examination findings vary but may include the following:

Pulse: Thready

Blood pressure: Variable

Heart: Dysrhythmias; normal or diminished heart sounds; S_4, sometimes an S_3; soft, systolic, apical murmur of mitral regurgitation; pericardial friction rub

Congestive heart failure. Congestive heart failure (CHF) is a condition in which the heart cannot pump blood forward in the normal pattern, resulting in congestion of the pulmonary or systemic circulation. It may result from some defect in the heart or in the rhythmicity pattern. Heart failure may be predominantly right sided or left sided. Right-sided failure leads to peripheral edema, liver congestion, and jugular venous distention. Left-sided failure leads to pulmonary congestion and dyspnea. Pulmonary hypertension can lead to right-sided hypertrophy and right ventricular failure. This condition is known as cor pulmonale. Heart dysfunction produces changes in other organs, including the lungs, kidneys, and liver. It may develop gradually, such as with hypertension, or suddenly as a result of myocardial infarction.

Symptoms may include dyspnea, orthopnea, paroxysmal nocturnal dyspnea, edema, cough, fatigue at rest, and frequent nocturnal urination.

Physical examination findings may include:

Pulse: Weak, rapid

Blood pressure: Varies

Skin: Cool, moist, pale, or cyanotic

Neck: Jugular venous distention

Heart: Tachycardia, lifts, heaves, displacement of the apical impulse downward and to the left; S_3, S_4

Lungs: Moist rales, crackles, bronchial wheezing

Abdomen: Ascites, liver enlargement

Extremities: Dependent, pitting edema in the legs and sacral area

Jugular Venous Pulse
Variations in the jugular venous pulse waves

Variations in the a wave. The a wave is the highest of the venous waves. It is increased when it is more difficult for the contracting right atrium to empty into the right ventricle. This occurs with tricuspid valve stenosis or decreased compliance of the right ventricle due to right ventricular hypertrophy, pulmonary hypertension, or pulmonic stenosis. Intermittently enlarged a waves, called cannon a waves, result when the atrium contracts against a closed tricuspid valve. This can occur during a

premature ventricular beat or during complete AV block.

Variations in the x descent and in the c and v waves. An incompetent tricuspid valve permits backflow of blood from the right ventricle to the right atrium during atrial filling and ventricular systole. This increased backflow obliterates the x slope, which is replaced by an enlarged combined c-v wave. With severe disease, the wave may become as large as a bounding carotid pulsation.

Variations of the y descent. The tricuspid valve opens shortly after S_2, and the rapid filling phase of ventricular diastole begins. The characteristics of the y descent depend on right-sided pressure and volume and on resistance to flow across the tricuspid valve. Tricuspid stenosis produces a slow y descent because it obstructs right atrial emptying. In clients with severe heart failure in whom the right atrial pressure is extremely high, an exaggerated y wave is produced.

Peripheral Vasculature
Arterial occlusion and insufficiency

Arteries in any location can become occluded or traumatized, making them unable to perform their task of delivering blood and other nutrients to the tissues. Arterial occlusive disease can be an acute condition in which a thrombus or an embolus suddenly occludes an artery, or a chronic condition caused by the buildup of atherosclerotic plaque and resulting in arterial wall thickening, hardening, and loss of elasticity; it can lead to arterial obstruction.

A decrease in arterial circulation results in findings related to the:

1. Site of the problem
2. Degree of occlusion or trauma
3. Ability of collateral channels to compensate
4. Rapidity with which the problem develops

Arterial disease pain can be acute or chronic.

Arterial insufficiency. Pain or a sharp, cramplike sensation distal to the affected artery is the first symptom that results from inadequate blood supply to the muscle. With chronic insufficiency, intermittent claudication is experienced as a dull ache with muscle fatigue and cramping. It typically appears during sustained exercise, such as walking or climbing stairs. A brief rest usually relieves it. Other characteristics of chronic arterial insufficiency may include localized pallor and cyanosis; weak, thready, or absent pulses; ulceration; hair loss; trophic changes of the toenails; diminished sensation; and some degree of atrophy. With more severe insufficiency, pain may occur when the person is supine and may be relieved by lowering the feet, which improves the perfusion pressure and oxygen supply to the distal tissues.

Arterial occlusion. Arterial occlusion is due to either a thrombus or an embolus. The development of a thrombus can follow chronic insufficiency in the area as a result of the atherosclerotic process. An arterial embolism can be due to stagnant blood flow within the heart, such as occurs with a diseased mitral valve, from bacterial endocarditis, or with atrial fibrillation. An acute obstruction results in excruciating pain that is more severe distally and is followed after several hours by numbness and cold. Distal pallor and cyanosis are present when the extremity is raised above the level of the heart, and pulses are weak or absent distal to the occlusion.

Increased capillary refill time. Capillary refill time lasting more than 2 seconds can be due to anemia, peripheral edema, or vasoconstriction or decreased cardiac output due to hypovolemia, shock, or CHF.

Arterial aneurysm. An aneurysm is a localized dilation of an artery resulting from weakness of the arterial wall. The aorta is the most common site for an aneurysm, but an aneurysm may also occur in other peripheral vessels. A bruit, thrill, or visible pulsation may be present over the site of the aneurysm, or it may be palpated as a pulsating mass. Atherosclerosis, which weakens the middle layer of the arterial wall, is a common cause of an aneurysm.

Coarctation of the aorta. Coarctation is a localized narrowing of the aorta. It results in increased pressure proximal to the narrowing and decreased pressure distal to the narrowing. Other symptoms and signs include dizziness, headaches, fainting, epistaxis, reduced or absent femoral pulses, and muscle cramps in the legs. Blood pressure in the arms is higher than in the legs.

Raynaud's syndrome (Figure 16.42). In Raynaud's syndrome, intermittent spasm of the arterioles causes ischemia of the extremities, especially the fingers, toes, ears, and nose. There is a classic tri-colored sequence of events in Raynaud's attack. Exposure to cold, vibrating tools, certain repetitive motions, smoking, or emotional stress causes spasm of the local arteries and arterioles, resulting in severe pallor due to decreased capillary perfusion. The pallor is followed by cyanosis as the small vessels dilate somewhat, allowing a small amount of blood into the capillary bed. Redness follows as an increasing amount of blood enters the area, and the attack terminates with the relaxation of arterial spasm and the return of normal blood flow and perfusion. This condition may be accompanied by numbness, tingling, burning, and pain. The attack may last from minutes to hours. The skin may eventually become smooth, shiny, and tight, and ulcers may appear on the fingertips. When the condition is a benign primary disease, it is called Raynaud's disease. When it is secondary to another disease, such as lupus or scleroderma, it is called Raynaud's phenomenon.

figure **16.42** Raynaud's syndrome.

Venous insufficiency and obstruction

Venous disease results from incompetence of the venous valves or from obstruction.

Venous insufficiency. Incompetent valves lead to overstretched veins and increased venous pressure and stasis. Clients with this condition experience aching, throbbing discomfort during the day, particularly when the legs are in a dependent position. Accumulation of metabolic wastes in the tissues can lead to aching or cramping pain at night. Pain is a frequent symptom and is typically described as diffuse, dull, and aching; it increases as the day progresses. Long periods of standing exacerbate it, whereas leg elevation and the use of support hose may relieve it. Swelling may develop toward the end of the day and be resolved by elevating the legs. Examination findings typically include edema, cyanosis of the affected leg, brown discoloration, and varicosities of the greater and lesser saphenous veins. Pulses are usually normal, although they may be difficult to palpate if edema is present.

Thrombophlebitis. Thrombophlebitis is inflammation of a superficial vein. It is characterized by redness, thickening, and tenderness along the vein. It occurs most commonly as a result of trauma to the vessel wall; hypercoagulability of the blood; infection; chemical irritation; postoperative venous stasis; prolonged sitting, standing, or immobilization; or a long period of intravenous catheterization.

Deep vein thrombosis. Thrombus formation is the main cause of obstructed venous flow. Three causative factors of deep vein thrombosis (DVT) include:

1. Changes in the lining of the vessel
2. Changes in blood flow (stasis)
3. Changes in blood constituents (hypercoagulability)

Signs and symptoms include local tenderness, pain, increased tissue turgor, swelling, and increased skin temperature. Swelling of the legs, or ankle edema, may also be noted. Test for a positive Homan's sign by flexing the client's knee slightly with one hand while dorsiflexing the foot with the other hand. Calf pain is a positive Homan's sign indicating thrombosis. (However, this calf pain can be confused with Achilles tendon pain.)

Edema. Edema is an accumulation of fluid in the tissues that changes the shape of the area affected. Right-sided heart failure leads to increased fluid volume, which in turn leads to edema in dependent parts of the body. Edema caused by CHF is bilateral. Pitting edema is not usually accompanied by thickening or pigmentation of the overlying skin. Edema accompanied by some thickening and ulcerations of the skin is associated with deep venous obstruction or valvular incompetence.

Varicose veins (Figure 16.43). Varicose veins result from incompetent venous valves, weakened vessel walls, or obstruction in a proximal vein. Inside the veins there is a decreased flow rate and an increased intravenous pressure. Superficial varicosities are readily visible on in-

figure**16.43** Varicose veins.

spection, especially when the client is standing. The veins look dilated, swollen, and tortuous.

The Trendelenburg test is used to evaluate venous incompetence when varicose veins are present. With the client in the supine position, lift the affected leg above the level of the heart until the veins empty, then tie a tourniquet around the upper thigh. Ask the client to stand, and observe the venous filling pattern. Normally, the superficial veins should fill from below. With incompetent valves, the veins will fill rapidly from above. Remove the tourniquet and check to see if the veins fill rapidly from above. Normally, they do not: sudden filling indicates incompetent valves.

Clubbing. Clubbing of the distal portions of the fingers is characterized by a flattening of the normal nail bed angle from a 160-degree angle to a 180-degree angle. It occurs in subacute bacterial endocarditis, cor pulmonale, and cyanotic congenital heart disease.

■ FOCUSED HEALTH HISTORY *(SUBJECTIVE DATA)*

Mr. Y., a 58-year-old Native American male, complains of shortness of breath with exertion after walking 2 to 3 blocks or 2 flights of stairs; also has swollen ankles. Symptoms have been increasing gradually over the past 2 months. This is a significant change for him, since he is a carpenter accustomed to heavy work, and until several months ago, jogged during his leisure time. Dyspnea is relieved after about 10 minutes of rest; swelling is relieved by elevating his feet overnight. Gets up 2 or 3 times during the night to urinate. Sleeps well using 1 pillow. States he is very concerned about these symptoms and about feeling slightly more fatigued than usual. No chest pain or discomfort, palpitations, cough, leg cramps, or cyanosis. Usual weight about 175 lb.

History of diabetes—onset at age 49; controlled with daily insulin injection and diet. History of hyperlipidemia—250 three years ago; 210 one year ago—monitors his saturated fat consumption carefully. History of hypertension—takes beta-blocker bid. No history of myocardial infarction (MI), murmurs, other cardiac diseases, or surgery. Family history of heart disease and diabetes mellitus. Father died of MI at age 59; paternal uncle died of MI at age 64.

■ FOCUSED PHYSICAL EXAMINATION *(OBJECTIVE DATA)*

Vital signs: BP 150/96; pulses—radial: 80, strong, rhythm regular; brachial, ulnar, and femoral: normal; posterior tibial and pedal: slightly diminished.

Weight 180 lb, height 5 ft 11 in.

Skin: Normal turgor, no cyanosis.

Heart: Left ventricular heave palpable—apical area. Apical impulse 2 cm left of MCL, 5 LICS. S_1 loudest at apex; S_2 loudest at base, split at 2 LICS. No S_3 or S_4. No extra sounds or murmurs.

Lungs: Clear to percussion and auscultation.

Neck vessels: Carotid pulsations visible, no bruits. Jugular pulse wave visible when client supine; pattern normal; disappears when sitting.

Hepatojugular reflux: No jugular venous distention on compression of liver.

Extremities: 1^+ edema bilaterally over ankles.

diagnoses

HEALTH PROBLEM

Shortness of breath on exertion and peripheral edema, probably caused by congestive heart failure

NURSING DIAGNOSES

Fluid volume excess related to increased preload, decreased contractility, and decreased cardiac output secondary to congestive heart failure

Defining Characteristics

- Edema
- Shortness of breath

Activity intolerance secondary to congestive heart failure

Defining Characteristic

- Verbal report of dyspnea on exertion and fatigue

chapter

17

Abdomen

■ PURPOSE OF EXAMINATION

Because the abdominal cavity contains many of the body's vital organs, the abdominal examination provides information about a variety of systems. It yields direct and indirect information about the functioning of the gastrointestinal system and the genitourinary system. The examination may also reveal specific vascular anomalies, such as an aortic aneurysm, and inflammatory processes affecting various organs.

The screening examination includes a general survey of the organs for signs of tenderness, enlargement, masses, and other indications of dysfunction. Specific maneuvers allow the examiner to determine the source of symptoms such as abdominal pain and to delineate more clearly the characteristics of masses and other abnormal findings. Although directly examining many of the abdominal organs is difficult, some of the examination techniques provide indirect information about organ function. When abnormal findings are present, further diagnostic studies and laboratory tests need to be conducted.

This chapter focuses on the abdominal portion of the gastrointestinal system. Chapter 13 addresses the mouth and throat examination and Chapter 22 describes assessment of the anus and rectum.

■ ANATOMY AND PHYSIOLOGY

The abdomen, the largest body cavity, extends from the diaphragm to the lesser pelvis. It is bounded anteriorly by the abdominal muscles, the costal border, and the superior border of the pelvis and posteriorly by the vertebral column and the lumbar muscles. The abdomen contains many of the body's vital organs—the stomach, small and large intestines, liver, gallbladder, pancreas, spleen, kidneys, bladder, adrenal glands, uterus (in women), and major blood vessels (Figure 17.1). Because many major body organs are contained in this single cavity, susceptibility to organ dysfunction is increased. Methodical and systematic evaluation is vital to distinguish variations from the norm.

Intestines

The small intestine fills a major section of the abdominal cavity and extends from the pyloric sphincter to the ileocecal valve. It consists of three segments: the duodenum, the top portion; the jejunum, the middle portion; and the ileum, the lower portion. At the duodenum, bile and pancreatic secretions are received from the common bile duct for digestion. Absorption then takes place through the walls of the small intestine.

The large intestine extends from the ileocecal valve to the anus. It is composed of three segments: the cecum (with the vermiform appendix), the colon, and the rectum.

The cecum is located in the lower right quadrant of the abdomen. The vermiform appendix is a process extending from the lower part of the cecum. It is subject to infection and inflammation that can cause a rupture, expelling bacteria-laden substances into the abdominal cavity.

The colon frames the abdominal cavity. The ascending colon advances upward on the right side to the hepatic flexure. The transverse colon passes along the top of the abdominal cavity anterior to the liver and the stomach. The colon curves downward at the splenic flexure. The descending colon progresses to the brim of the pelvis, where it unites with the sigmoid colon and proceeds to the rectum and anus.

Liver

The liver lies primarily within the right hypochondrium and epigastrium, with a small portion situated in the left hypochondriac region. It is situated beneath the diaphragm. The rib cage covers a substantial part of the liver, with only the lower margin left exposed. The liver spans the upper quadrant of the abdomen from the fifth intercostal space to slightly below the costal margin.

The liver performs the following functions:
1. Produces and secretes bile
2. Plays a major role in regulating blood glucose levels
3. Maintains an important part in protein, carbohydrate, and lipid metabolism
4. Stores vitamins—A, B_{12} and other B-complex vitamins, and D—and various minerals such as iron and copper
5. Synthesizes most plasma proteins, such as serum albumin, serum globulin, fibrinogen, and blood-clotting factors
6. Is instrumental in the detoxification of many substances, including drugs

Gallbladder

The gallbladder is located on the inferior surface of the liver. A pear-shaped sac, it acts as a reservoir for bile secreted from the liver. The gallbladder concentrates the bile by absorbing excess water through its walls.

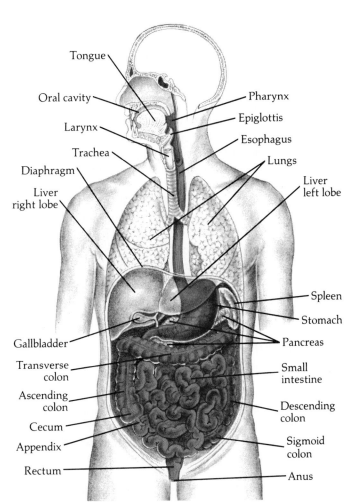

figure **17.1**   Anatomy of the gastrointestinal system. *(From Thompson JM et al: Mosby's clinical nursing, ed 4, St Louis, 1997, Mosby.)*

Labels: Tongue, Oral cavity, Larynx, Trachea, Diaphragm, Liver right lobe, Gallbladder, Transverse colon, Ascending colon, Cecum, Appendix, Rectum, Pharynx, Epiglottis, Esophagus, Lungs, Liver left lobe, Spleen, Stomach, Pancreas, Small intestine, Descending colon, Sigmoid colon, Anus

Stomach

The stomach is located in the left upper quadrant of the abdomen, directly below the diaphragm. It is separated into three areas: (1) the fundus, located above and to the left of the cardiac sphincter; (2) the body, found directly below the fundus; and (3) the pyloric antrum, positioned proximal to the pyloric sphincter.

Two sphincters regulate the flow of substances into and out of the stomach. The cardiac sphincter controls the inflow of food from the esophagus into the stomach. The pyloric sphincter regulates the outflow of chyme to the duodenum.

The primary functions of the stomach are to store food, to mix digestive enzymes and hydrochloric acid, and to liquify food into chyme. Protein breakdown is initiated with the conversion of protein to peptones.

The gallbladder is drained by the cystic duct. The cystic duct unites with the hepatic duct to form the common bile duct, which passes downward into the duodenum.

Pancreas

Immediately below the liver lies the pancreas. The pancreas is situated posterior to the greater curvature of the stomach in front of the first and second lumbar vertebrae.

The pancreas has both an exocrine and an endocrine function. The endocrine secretions from the islets of Langerhans produce insulin, glucagon, and gastrin, which are used in carbohydrate metabolism. The exocrine secretions from the acinar cells produce bicarbonate and pancreatic enzymes necessary for digestion and absorption in the small intestine.

Spleen

Located to the left of the stomach and directly above the kidney in the left upper abdominal quadrant is the spleen. The spleen has numerous functions, but its four primary ones are as follows:

1. Acts as a blood reservoir for 1% to 2% of the red blood cell mass
2. Removes old or agglutinated red blood cells and platelets
3. Is partially responsible for iron metabolism
4. Helps produce erythrocytes outside the bone marrow in the fetus and during bone marrow depression

Kidneys, Ureters, and Bladder

Covered by peritoneum and embedded in fat, the kidneys are located in the dorsal part of the abdomen between the twelfth thoracic and third lumbar vertebrae. The right kidney is slightly lower than the left one. The kidneys measure approximately 11 cm long, 5 to 7.5 cm wide, and 2.5 cm thick.

The nephron is the working unit of the kidney. Its structure consists of the glomerulus and the tubular system. Filtration occurs at the glomerular membrane, whereas reabsorption and secretion of essential materials takes place in the tubular system.

The kidneys are drained by the ureters and empty into the bladder. The ureters pass anteriorly along the psoas major muscles toward the pelvis. These tubes enter the bladder at the posterolateral aspect. Peristaltic action propels the urine downward to the bladder.

Located behind the symphysis pubis in the anterior half of the pelvis is the bladder, which has a maximum storage capacity of 1000 to 1800 ml. Moderate distention is felt when the bladder contains approximately 250 ml of urine, and discomfort is experienced with 400 ml. When distended, the bladder will rise above the level of the pubic bone.

Peritoneum

The peritoneum is a serous membrane that covers and protects the abdominal cavity. It is divided into two layers: the parietal and the visceral peritoneum. The parietal peritoneum lines the abdominal wall, and the visceral peritoneum covers the organs in the abdomen. The mesentery and the omentum are two folds of the peritoneum. The mesentery encircles the jejunum and the ileum and attaches them to the posterior abdominal wall. In addition, it supports blood vessels, lymphatic vessels, lymph nodes, and nerves. The greater omentum is connected to the upper border of the duodenum, to the lower edge of the stomach, and to the transverse colon. Its function is to protect and insulate. The lesser omentum is attached between the liver and the stomach.

Peritonitis is an inflammation of the peritoneum, often associated with rupture of an intraabdominal viscus such as the appendix.

■ EXAMINATION

Health History

The health history related to the abdominal examination focuses on concerns related to the digestive system. The interviewer needs to ask both general questions about the client's health and specific questions that will vary according to the client's symptoms and the organs affected. Determining the client's primary concern is important because it guides the interview and will also influence the client's receptiveness to care. Because a client's nutritional practices, habits, and level of stress influence many gastrointestinal complaints, eliciting information about the client's lifestyle, perceived level of stress, and means of coping with stress is also important.

Chief complaint

The chief complaint is the client's immediate concern—the problem that he or she wants dealt with at this time.

Present health status

1. Nutrition: Appetite, recent change in eating pattern, recent (intentional or unintentional) weight loss or gain, food preferences, food intolerances, cultural influences on eating (foods commonly served or forbidden), lifestyle influences on intake, special diets, 24-hour dietary recall
2. Allergies (food, medications)
3. Alcohol intake: Usual amounts, frequency
4. Medications: Prescription and over-the-counter drugs; laxatives, antiemetics, stool softeners, antidiarrheal agents, or antacids; high doses of aspirin, acetaminophen, or nonsteroidal antiinflammatory agents; corticosteroids, diuretics, or antihypertensives

5. Cigarette smoking (number of packs/day and number of years of habit)
6. Stool characteristics: Frequency, consistency, color, odor
7. Urinary characteristics: Frequency, urgency, color, odor, pain (dysuria, suprapubic, flank), ease of starting stream, force of stream, ability to empty bladder, dribbling, episodes of incontinence
8. Exposure to infectious diseases: Flu, hepatitis, gastroenteritis, family members or companions with similar symptoms, travel history
9. Recent stressful life events: Social, psychological, and physical changes
10. Possibility of pregnancy: Date of last menstrual period, use of contraceptives, unprotected intercourse

Specific problems

Abdominal pain

1. Onset and duration: Specific date, sudden or gradual, persistent or recurrent, specific time of day or unpredictable
2. Character: Burning, knifelike, cramping, aching
3. Location: Radiation, change in location
4. Quality: How bad is pain on a scale of 1 to 10 (with 10 being the worst pain)? Does it interfere with daily activities?
5. Course: Getting better or worse
6. Associated symptoms: Vomiting, diarrhea, constipation, flatulence, belching, jaundice, fever, weight loss
7. Alleviating or precipitating factors: Efforts to treat, medications or other interventions, patterns and effectiveness

Nausea

1. Onset and duration: Related to particular stimuli (odors, time of day); relationship to food intake; date of last menstrual period
2. Associated symptoms: Vomiting, dizziness, headache

Vomiting

1. Onset and duration: Sudden or preceded by nausea; time elapsed since last meal; frequency
2. Character: Nature of emesis (coffee grounds or fresh blood, color, undigested food), quantity, ability to keep fluids or solids in stomach, force (projectile)
3. Associated symptoms: Nausea, fever, headache, previous meal, weight loss, abdominal pain
4. Exposures: Any family members or companions experiencing similar symptoms

Indigestion

1. Onset: Relationship to meals, time of day or night; sudden or gradual
2. Character: Bloated feeling after eating; excessive belching or flatulence; heartburn; loss of appetite; severe pain
3. Location: General or localized; radiation to shoulders or arms
4. Associated symptoms: Vomiting, headache, diarrhea

5. Alleviating or precipitating factors: Association with type or quantity of food; response to antacids, rest, activity, other self-care measures

Diarrhea

1. Onset and duration: Gradual or sudden; frequency of stools; number per day; any change in usual pattern of bowel movements
2. Characteristics: Watery; explosive; color; presence of mucus, blood, undigested food, or fat; odor
3. Course: Improving or getting worse
4. Associated symptoms: Fever, chills, weight loss, abdominal pain, thirst, recent course of antibiotics
5. Alleviating or precipitating factors: Follows a specific pattern related to food intake or stressful encounters; self-care measures attempted and their effectiveness

Constipation

1. Onset and duration: Recent occurrence or long-standing problem; sudden or gradual; last bowel movement
2. Character: Dry, hard stools; number of bowel movements per week; change in size or pattern of stools; black or tarry or associated with bright blood; accompanied by abdominal or rectal pain, alternating with diarrhea
3. Associated symptoms: Abdominal pain, depression
4. Course: Continuous or intermittent problem
5. Alleviating or precipitating factors: Diet (recent change in intake, increase or decrease in fiber, fluid intake); use of enemas, laxatives, or stool softeners; response to self-care measures

Dysuria

1. Onset: Gradual or sudden
2. Character: Pain or burning; at start of stream, at midstream, or throughout stream; force of stream; frequency; urgency; color; presence of blood (internal or external)
3. Course: Improving or increased discomfort
4. Associated symptoms: Abdominal pain, flank pain, fever, chills, labial or scrotal pain

Urinary incontinence

1. Character: Amount, frequency, constant or intermittent, dribbling versus saturation
2. Course: Associated with sneezing, exertion, urgency, continuous versus intermittent
3. Associated symptoms: Fever, chills, dysuria, frequency

Past health history

1. Previous gastrointestinal problems, such as peptic ulcer, ulcerative colitis, polyps, intestinal obstruction, pancreatitis, gallbladder disease, hepatitis, or cirrhosis of the liver
2. Abdominal or urinary tract surgery or injury
3. Past history of urinary tract infections (number, how many in the past year, treatment) or renal calculi (number, treatment)
4. History of major illnesses, such as cancer (type),

arthritis (specify steroid or aspirin use), kidney disease, cardiac disease, respiratory disease (steroid use)
5. Any blood transfusions
6. Hepatitis vaccination status

Family health history

1. Kidney problems
2. Colon cancer

3. Malabsorption syndromes (cystic fibrosis, celiac disease)
4. Gallbladder disease
5. Colitis
6. Familial polyposis

Preparation for Examination: Client and Environment

Helping the client to relax is an important prerequisite to performing a thorough examination of the abdomen. The client should have an empty bladder before the examination begins. He or she needs to be in a comfortable supine position with arms at the sides. To help the client to relax the stomach muscles, place a small pillow under the head and ask the client to flex the knees slightly. A pillow can also be placed behind the knees to support them in a slightly flexed position. The examination room should be warm enough so that the client will not shiver (thereby tensing the abdomen). The abdomen must be fully exposed. For both warmth and modesty, drape the client's chest and groin area.

Have the client breathe quietly and slowly through the mouth. Your hands and the diaphragm of the

---

RISK FACTORS   COLON CANCER

Age older than 50 (Risk increases markedly after age 40, but 90% of cancers occur after age 50.)
First-degree family member (parent or sibling) with colorectal cancer
Personal history of endometrial, breast, or ovarian cancer
Previous diagnosis of inflammatory bowel disease, adenomatous polyps, or colorectal cancer
Family history of hereditary polyposis or hereditary nonpolyposis colorectal cancer

---

RISK FACTORS   HEPATITIS B

The following individuals are at risk for infection and should consider vaccination against hepatitis B virus (HBV):
Persons with occupational risk, such as health care workers and public safety workers who may be exposed to blood or other body fluids
Clients and staff in institutions for the developmentally disabled
Hemodialysis patients
Recipients of blood or blood products
Household contacts and sexual partners of persons with an active or ongoing case of HBV or HBV carriers
Adoptees from countries where HBV is endemic (e.g., China, Southeast Asia)
International travelers, particularly those visiting regions where HBV is endemic
Injecting drug users
Sexually active homosexual and bisexual men
Sexually active heterosexual men and women with a history of (1) more than one partner in 6 months, (2) sexually transmitted diseases, or (3) prostitution
Inmates of long-term correctional facilities
Children and household contacts or populations of high HBV endemicity

---

PREPARATION FOR EXAMINATION

EQUIPMENT

Item	Purpose
Stethoscope (with bell and diaphragm)	To listen to bowel and vascular sounds
Metric ruler	To measure liver span
Marking pen	To mark borders of organs
Small pillows	To position client

CLIENT AND ENVIRONMENT

1. Assemble needed equipment (stethoscope, ruler, marking pen, pillows).
2. Make sure that the room is comfortably warm.
3. Explain the steps of the examination to the client.
4. Position the client in a comfortable supine position with arms at the sides, head supported by a pillow, and knees slightly flexed.
5. Completely expose the abdomen from the costal border to the symphysis pubis, draping the client's chest and pubic area for modesty and warmth.
6. Ask the client to point to any tender areas and reassure the person that you will examine those areas last.
7. Watch the client's facial expressions for signs of discomfort during the examination.

stethoscope should be warm, and your fingernails should be short. Talk to the client in a slow and gentle manner. Avoid any sudden movements. Explain what you will be doing during the examination. Have the client point to any tender areas, and tell the client that you will examine those areas last. Observe the client's facial expression as you conduct the examination. The stoic client may not admit to discomfort, but his or her facial expression may show when that person feels tenderness. You can then confirm this observation with the client and modify your examination accordingly.

Technique for Examination and Normal Findings

The physical assessment of the abdomen includes all four methods of examination (inspection, auscultation, percussion, and palpation). However, in the abdominal examination, auscultation is done before percussion and palpation because stimulation by pressure on the bowel can alter bowel motility and heighten bowel sounds. Palpation is the technique most useful in detecting pathological conditions of the abdomen.

Anatomical mapping

To describe clearly the location of organs and the areas of pain or tenderness, the abdomen can be divided into either four quadrants or nine regions. The most frequently used method is division into four quadrants

(Figure 17.2). An imaginary vertical line is drawn from the sternum down to the pubic bone through the umbilicus, and a second line is drawn perpendicular to the first line through the umbilicus. In general, abdominal structures will be located in one of these quadrants (see box at right of figure). Loops of the small bowel are found in all four quadrants. The bladder and the uterus are located at the lower midline.

The second, less frequently used, method of establishing zones of the abdomen involves nine sections (Figure 17.3). This division is accomplished by drawing two imaginary vertical lines from the midclavicle to the middle of Poupart's (inguinal) ligament, analogous to the lateral borders of the rectus abdominis muscles. At right angles to these lines, two imaginary parallel lines cross the border of the costal margin and the anterosuperior spine of the iliac bones. Essentially, the abdominal structures correlate with the zones shown in Figure 17.3 (see box at right of figure).

Certain anatomical structures are used as landmarks to facilitate the description of abdominal signs and symptoms (Figure 17.4). The following landmarks are useful for this purpose: the ensiform (xiphoid) process of the sternum, the costal margin, the midline (drawn from the tip of the sternum through the umbilicus to the pubic bone), the umbilicus, the anterosuperior iliac spine, Poupart's (inguinal) ligament, and the superior margin of the pubic bone.

Abdominal structures protected by the rib cage that are examined in health assessment are the liver, stomach, and spleen (Figure 17.5). These structures are evaluated by palpation and percussion.

figure **17.2** Four quadrants of the abdomen. *RUQ,* Right upper quadrant; *LUQ,* left upper quadrant; *RLQ,* right lower quadrant; *LLQ,* left lower quadrant.

Anatomical Correlates of the Four Quadrants of the Abdomen

RIGHT UPPER QUADRANT	LEFT UPPER QUADRANT
Liver and gallbladder	Left lobe of liver
Pylorus	Spleen
Duodenum	Stomach
Head of pancreas	Body of pancreas
Right adrenal gland	Left adrenal gland
Portion of right kidney	Portion of left kidney
Hepatic flexure of colon	Splenic flexure of colon
Portions of ascending and transverse colon	Portions of transverse and descending colon

RIGHT LOWER QUADRANT	LEFT LOWER QUADRANT
Lower pole of right kidney	Lower pole of left kidney
Cecum and appendix	Sigmoid colon
Portion of ascending colon	Portion of descending colon
Bladder (if distended)	Bladder (if distended)
Ovary and salpinx	Ovary and salpinx
Uterus (if enlarged)	Uterus (if distended)
Right spermatic cord	Left spermatic cord
Right ureter	Left ureter

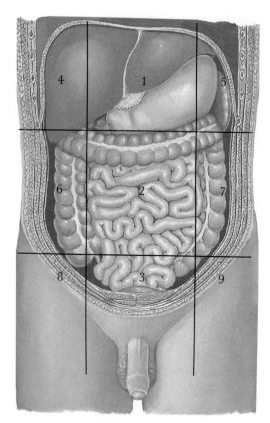

Anatomical Correlates of the Nine Regions of the Abdomen

RIGHT HYPO-CHONDRIAC	EPIGASTRIC	LEFT HYPO-CHONDRIAC
Right lobe of liver	Pyloric end of stomach	Stomach
Gallbladder	Duodenum	Spleen
Portion of duodenum	Pancreas	Tail of pancreas
Hepatic flexure of colon	Portion of liver	Splenic flexure of colon
Portion of right kidney		Upper pole of left kidney
Suprarenal gland		Suprarenal gland
RIGHT LUMBAR	**UMBILICAL**	**LEFT LUMBAR**
Ascending colon	Omentum	Descending colon
Lower half of right kidney	Mesentery	Lower half of right kidney
Portion of duodenum and jejunum	Lower duodenum	Portions of jejunum and ileum
	Jejunum and ileum	
RIGHT INGUINAL	**HYPOGASTRIC**	**LEFT INGUINAL**
Cecum	Ileum	Sigmoid colon
Appendix	Bladder	Left ureter
Ileum (lower end)	Uterus (in pregnancy)	Left spermatic cord
Right ureter		Left ovary
Right spermatic cord		
Right ovary		

figure **17.3**   Nine regions of the abdomen. *1,* Epigastric; *2,* umbilical; *3,* hypogastric (pubic); *4* and *5,* right and left hypochondriac; *6* and *7,* right and left lumbar; *8* and *9,* right and left inguinal. *(From Seidel HM et al:* Mosby's guide to physical examination, *St Louis, 1995, Mosby.)*

figure **17.4**   Landmarks of the abdomen.

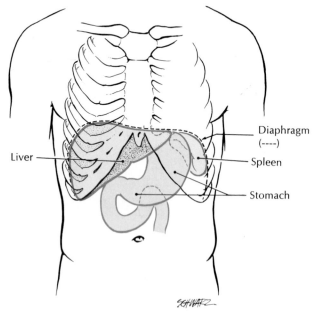

figure **17.5**   Abdominal structures protected by the rib cage. The liver, stomach, and spleen are examined by palpation and percussion.

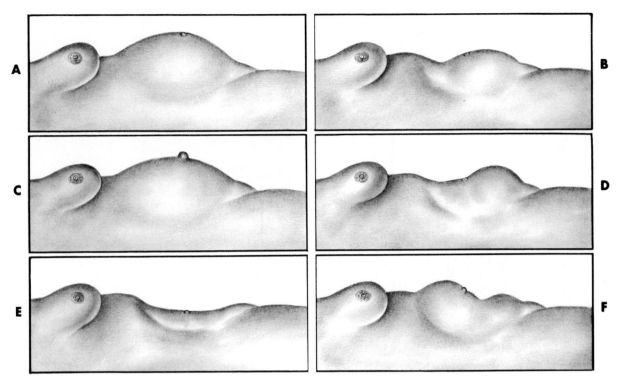

figure **17.6** Abdominal profiles. **A,** Fully rounded or distended, umbilicus inverted. **B,** Distended lower half. **C,** Fully rounded or distended, umbilicus everted. **D,** Distended lower third. **E,** Scaphoid. **F,** Distended upper half. *(From Seidel HM et al: Mosby's guide to physical examination, ed 3, St Louis, 1995, Mosby.)*

Inspection

A good source of light is necessary for inspection of the abdomen. Direct the light at a right angle to the long axis of the client, or focus the light lengthwise over the client, shining it from the foot to the head. Assume a sitting position, *generally at the right side of the client.* To enhance shadows, your head should be only slightly higher than the client's abdomen. Shadows highlight small changes in contour, thus increasing the likelihood of detecting a pathological condition.

Note the position that the client assumes voluntarily. The individual with abdominal pain frequently draws up the knees to reduce tension on the abdominal muscles and to alleviate intraabdominal pressure. The client with generalized peritonitis lies almost motionless with the knees flexed. Marked restlessness has been associated with biliary and intestinal colic, renal colic, and intraperitoneal hemorrhage.

Familiarity with the normal topography of the abdomen is important to avoid identifying normal contours as masses (Figure 17.6). Carefully focus attention on the abdomen to describe accurately the presence or absence of symmetry, distention, masses, visible peristaltic waves, and respiratory movements. If the presence of peristalsis is in question, carefully study the abdomen for several minutes.

To detect masses, such as an enlarged liver or spleen, ask the client to take a deep breath. This action forces the diaphragm downward and decreases the size of the abdominal cavity, which makes masses become more obvious.

The rectus muscles (Figure 17.7) are prominent landmarks of the abdominal wall. Diastasis recti abdominis is a separation of the rectus abdominis muscles. The separation may be palpated and may be observed as a ridge between the muscles when the intraabdominal pressure is increased by raising the head and shoulders. This defect does not pose a threat to the functions of the abdominal structures. Diastasis recti abdominis generally occurs as a result of pregnancy or marked obesity.

Next, inspect the abdomen from a standing position at the foot of the bed or examining table. Asymmetry of the abdominal contour may be more readily detected from this position.

Skin. The abdomen is an especially valuable area for dermatological observation because it encompasses a relatively large expanse of skin. Inspection of the abdominal skin for pigmentation (particularly jaundice),

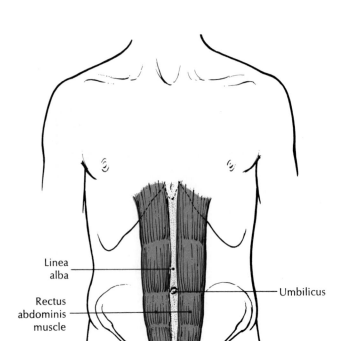

figure **17.7**   Rectus abdominis muscles. Separation of these muscles is called diastasis recti and may be detected by observation or palpation.

figure **17.8**   Striae. *(From Seidel HM et al:* Mosby's guide to physical examination, *ed 3, St Louis, 1995, Mosby.)*

lesions, striae, scars, dehydration, general nutritional status, venous patterns, and the condition of the umbilicus can yield valuable information about the client's general state of health.

Pigmentation. Because clothing frequently protects the skin of the abdomen from the sun, abdominal skin may serve as a baseline for comparison with the pigmentation of the more tanned areas. Jaundice is more readily observed in this less exposed skin. Irregular patches of faint tan pigmentation may be a result of von Recklinghausen's disease.

Lesions. The observation of skin lesions is of particular significance because gastrointestinal alterations are frequently associated with skin changes. Although the presence of small, hard, painless nodules over a wide area of the abdomen may be caused by metastasis of a malignancy, the nodules are generally not the result of carcinoma of the abdominal viscera. Tense and glistening skin is often correlated with ascites or edema of the abdominal wall.

Striae. Lineae albicantes (striae) are atrophic lines or streaks that may be seen in the skin of the abdomen following rapid or prolonged stretching that disrupts the elastic fibers of the reticular layer of the cutis. Striae of recent origin are pink or blue but progress to silvery

white. Striae occurring as a result of Cushing's disease, however, remain pink-purple. The stretching of abdominal skin may occur as a result of pregnancy (striae gravidarum) (Figure 17.8), an abdominal tumor, ascites, or obesity.

Scars. Inspection of the abdomen for scars may yield valuable data concerning previous surgery or trauma. The size and shape of scars are best described through the use of a drawing of the abdomen on which the landmarks or quadrants are shown and the dimensions are noted in centimeters.

If the cause of the scar is not elicited through the history, this information should be sought through inspection. The fact that the client has experienced a previous surgery should alert the examiner to the possibility that adhesions may be present.

Deep, irregular scars may indicate burns. Some individuals produce a dense overgrowth, or hypertrophy, of fibrous tissue in the healing process. This overgrowth, which is called a keloid, consists of large, essentially parallel bands of dense collagenous material separated by bands of cellular fibrous tissue. Keloid formation most frequently occurs following a traumatic injury or burn. Increased prevalence of keloid formation has been noted in African-American individuals and those of Asian extraction.

Veins. A fine venous network is often seen in the abdominal wall. Dilated veins are observed in vena cava

obstruction that is usually related to congested portal circulation.

Umbilicus. The umbilicus should be observed for signs of vena cava obstruction (dilated veins), umbilical hernia, metastatic carcinoma, and dampness or the smell of urine (patent urachus).

Contour. Contralateral areas of the normal abdomen are symmetrical in contour and appearance. The contour is determined by the abdominal profile from the rib margin to the pubic bone as viewed from a right angle to the umbilicus with the client in a recumbent position (see Figure 17.6). The contour of the normal abdomen is described as flat, rounded, or scaphoid.

A flat contour is seen in the muscularly competent and well-nourished individual. A rounded or convex contour is normal in the infant or toddler, but in the adult it is generally caused by poor muscle tone, excessive subcutaneous fat deposits, or both. The rounded abdomen is often called the "spare tire" or "bay window" of middle age (see Figure 17.6, *A*). A scaphoid, or concave, contour may be seen in thin clients of all ages. This type of contour reflects a decrease in fat deposits in the abdominal wall and relaxed or flaccid abdominal musculature (see Figure 17.6, *E*).

Unusual stretching of the abdominal wall is referred to as distention. Abdominal distention may result from fat (obesity), feces or flatus (constipation or intestinal obstruction), a fetus (pregnancy), fluid (ascites), a fibroid tumor, or a fatal tumor. The presence of distention generally implies disease and therefore warrants further investigation. Asymmetrical distention of the abdominal wall may be caused by a hernia, tumor, cysts, or bowel obstruction. A mnemonic device for classifying the six most common causes of distention are fluid, flatulence, fat, feces, fibroid tumor, and fetus—the six Fs.

Generalized, or symmetrical, distention of the abdomen with the umbilicus in its normal inverted position is generally a result of obesity or recent pressure of fluid or gas within the hollow viscera. If the umbilicus is in an everted position (umbilical hernia), ascites or an underlying tumor may be the cause (see Figure 17.6, *C*). An ovarian tumor, distended bladder, or pregnancy may be suspected if the distention is confined to the area between the umbilicus and the symphysis pubis (see Figure 17.6, *B*). Distention of the lower third of the abdomen suggests an ovarian tumor, uterine fibroid tumor, pregnancy, or bladder enlargement (see Figure 17.6, *D*). Possible causes of distention of the upper half of the abdominal wall include a pancreatic cyst or tumor and gastric dilation (see Figure 17.6, *F*).

Movement

Respiratory movement. Observation of respiratory movement has more significance in the male client because men exhibit predominantly abdominal movement with respiration. Women exhibit mainly costal movement. Therefore, limited abdominal respiratory action in the male client may be indicative of peritonitis or other abdominal infection or disease. Abdominal breathing is also common in a child less than 6 or 7 years of age. The presence of abdominal respiratory movements in an older child may indicate respiratory problems. The absence of abdominal respiratory movements in the child who is younger than 6 years suggests peritoneal irritation. Retraction of the abdominal wall on inspiration, called Czerny's sign, is associated with certain central nervous system diseases, such as chorea.

Visible peristalsis. In lean individuals motility of the stomach and intestines may be seen as movement of the abdominal wall even in the absence of disease. However, when strong contractions are visible through an abdominal wall of average thickness, investigate the possibility of bowel obstruction. Sit at the client's side and gaze across the abdomen for several minutes. Percussing the abdomen may augment weak peristalsis. Peristaltic waves of the stomach and small intestine may be seen as elevated oblique bands in the upper left quadrant that move downward to the right. Several of these peristaltic waves occurring in rapid succession may produce a series of parallel bands, or a "ladder effect."

Reverse peristalsis, observed in the upper abdomen in an infant, is seen as an undulation moving from left to right. This observation indicates the presence of pyloric stenosis or, less commonly, duodenal stenosis or malrotation of the bowel.

Pulsation. In thin persons pulsation of the abdominal aorta is visible throughout most of its length. However, in most persons it is visible in the epigastrium.

Auscultation

Auscultation of the abdomen precedes percussion because bowel motility, and thus bowel sounds, may be increased by palpation and percussion. Both the stethoscope and the examiner's hands should be warm. If they are cold, they may initiate a contraction of the abdominal muscles.

Auscultatory findings of diagnostic significance are those sounds originating from the viscera, the arterial system, the venous system, muscular activity, or parietal friction rubs. Gently place the stethoscope on the abdomen to auscultate (Figure 17.9). Light pressure on the stethoscope is sufficient to detect bowel sounds and bruits. Use the diaphragm of the stethoscope, which accentuates the higher-pitched sounds, to listen to the relatively high-pitched abdominal intestinal sounds. Use the bell of the stethoscope to listen for low-pitched arterial bruits and venous hums.

Peristaltic sounds. Normal bowel sounds are high-pitched, gurgling noises that occur approximately every 5 to 15 seconds. Some authorities suggest that the number is as high as 15 to 20 per minute, or roughly

figure**17.9** Auscultation for bowel sounds. The diaphragm of the stethoscope is used to listen to the relatively high-pitched intestinal sounds.

figure**17.10** Auscultation for bruits is performed with the bell of the stethoscope held lightly against the abdomen.

one bowel sound for each breath sound. The duration of a single sound may be less than 1 second or may extend over several seconds. The frequency of sounds is related to the presence of food in the gastrointestinal tract or to the state of digestion. Because the passage of fluids and gases through the intestine causes bowel sounds, uninterrupted bowel sounds may be heard over the ileocecal valve 4 to 7 hours following a meal. A silent abdomen (i.e., the absence of bowel sounds) indicates the arrest of intestinal motility. Flicking the abdominal wall with a finger (direct percussion) will stimulate peristalsis. Because peristaltic sounds may be quite irregular, listening for at least 5 minutes is essential before concluding that no bowel sounds are present. When evaluating for absence of sounds, it is important to auscultate each of the four quadrants for at least 1 minute so that no sounds will be missed and so that specific sounds can be localized.

The two significant alterations in bowel sounds are (1) the absence of any sound or extremely soft and widely separated sounds; and (2) increased sounds with a characteristically high-pitched, loud, rushing sound (borborygmi).

Decreased bowel sounds. Diminished or absent bowel sounds accompany inhibition of bowel motility. Decreased motility occurs with inflammation, gangrene, or paralytic ileus. Decreased peristalsis frequently accompanies peritonitis, electrolyte disturbances, the aftermath of surgical manipulation of the bowel, and late bowel obstruction. In addition, diminished bowel sounds are often correlated with lower lobe pneumonia.

Increased bowel sounds. Loud, gurgling borborygmi accompany increased motility of the bowel, such as with diarrhea. Sounds of loud volume also are heard over areas of a stenotic bowel. Sounds from an early bowel obstruction are high pitched. These may be splashing sounds, similar to the emptying of a bottle into a hollow vessel. Fine, metallic, tinkling sounds are emitted as tiny gas bubbles break through the surface of intestinal juices. Increased motility may be caused by the use of a laxative or by gastroenteritis. Common pathological conditions associated with increased bowel sounds are gastroenteritis and subsiding ileus.

Vascular sounds

Arterial sounds. Bruits are heard when an artery is partially obstructed, causing turbulent flow. A bruit that is heard with the bell of the stethoscope held lightly against the abdomen while the client is in a variety of positions may indicate a dilated, tortuous, or constricted vessel (Figure 17.10). Loud bruits detected over the aorta suggest the presence of an aneurysm. Auscultation of the aorta should be done superior to the umbilicus. The locations of the aorta, renal arteries, and iliac arteries are illustrated in Figure 17.11. Soft, medium- to low-pitched murmurs resulting from renal arterial stenosis may be heard over the upper midline or toward the flank.

For the hypertensive client, listen carefully over the center epigastrium and posterior flank for a bruit in the arterial tree. An epigastric bruit radiating laterally suggests renal artery stenosis.

Venous hums. A normal hum originating from the

Right renal artery

Right Iliac artery

Right femoral artery

Aorta

Left renal artery

Left Iliac artery

Left femoral artery

figure**17.11**   Sites to auscultate for bruits: renal arteries, iliac arteries, aorta, and femoral arteries.

inferior vena cava and its large tributaries is continuously audible with a stethoscope. Its tone is medium pitched and is similar to a muscular fibrillary hum. In the presence of obstructed portal circulation, as from a cirrhotic liver, an abnormal venous hum may be detected in the periumbilical region. Pressure on the bell may obscure the hum. A palpable thrill may accompany the hum. Angiomas may produce hums that can be auscultated over the liver.

Peritoneal friction rub. Peritoneal friction rub creates a rough, grating sound that resembles two pieces of leather being rubbed together. Because the liver and the spleen have large surface areas that are in contact with the peritoneum, these two structures are most often the originating sites of peritoneal friction rubs.

Common causes of friction rubs include splenic infection, abscess, and tumor. These sounds are heard best over the lower rib cage in the anterior axillary line. Deep respiration may emphasize the sound. Metastatic disease of the liver and abscess are the usual causes of peritoneal friction rubs located over the lower right rib cage.

Muscular activity sounds. A fibrillating muscle produces a hum that can be heard with a stethoscope. Both voluntary and involuntary contractions (e.g., muscle guarding of a painful area) produce this sound. Palpation of the tender area often accentuates the hum.

Percussion

Percussion of the abdomen is done to detect fluid, gaseous distention, and masses and to assess the position and size of solid structures within the abdomen. Percussion can be done independently or in conjunction with

palpation. For example, in a client with a tumor, percussion should be done before deep palpation in order to establish a sense of the size and location of the enlarged organ.

Lightly percuss the entire abdomen for a general picture of the areas of tympany and dullness. Tympany predominates because of the presence of gas in the large bowel and the small bowel. Solid masses will percuss as dull, as will organs such as a distended bladder.

Establish a systematic pattern or route to use each time you percuss abdominal structures (Figure 17.12). This will lessen the chance of omitting any portion of the examination.

Assessment of the liver span. To determine the size of the liver, begin percussion in the right midclavicular line at a level below the umbilicus (Figure 17.13, *A*). Start percussion over a region of gas-filled bowel (tympany) and progress upward toward the liver. The first dull percussion note indicates the lower border of the liver. (Be careful not to confuse the costal border with the liver border. Both are dull, but the costal border is easily palpable.) Mark the lower border on the abdomen. To determine the upper border of liver dullness, start percussion in the midclavicular line and examine from an area of lung resonance down to the first dull percussion note (generally the fifth to seventh interspace [Figure 17.13, *B*]). Mark this spot and measure the distance between the two marks in centimeters (Figure 17.13, *C*). Other sites for percussion and measurement when the liver appears enlarged are the anterior axillary line and the midsternal line.

The descent of the liver can also be assessed. Ask the

client to take a deep breath and hold it while you percuss upward from the abdomen to detect the lower liver border. The liver will normally descend 2 to 3 cm with inspiration. This maneuver can help to guide placement of your hands for palpating the liver border.

The suggested ranges of normal values are 6 to 12 cm in the midclavicular line and 4 to 8 cm in the midsternal line (Figure 17.14). A direct correlation exists between body size (lean body mass) and liver span. It is important to remember that men have larger livers than women. The mean midclavicular liver span in men is 10.5 cm, whereas it is 7 cm in women. A midclavicular liver span of 11 cm may indicate hepatomegaly in a 5-foot, 100-pound woman, but it may be within normal limits for a man.

figure**17.12** Systematic route for abdominal percussion.

A

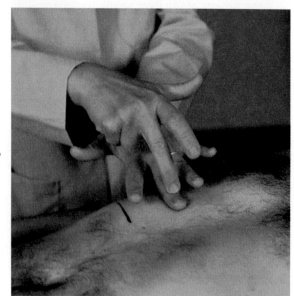

B

figure**17.13** **A,** Liver percussion route. **B,** Percussion method of estimating the size of the liver in the midclavicular line. Lower border percussion is begun over a region of air- or gas-filled bowel and carried upward to the dull percussion note of the liver. The spot is marked. Upper border percussion is performed over the midclavicular line from an area of lung resonance to the first dull percussion note (generally the fifth to seventh interspace). The spot is marked. **C,** The distance between the two marks measured in estimating the liver span in the midclavicular line is normally 6 to 12 cm.

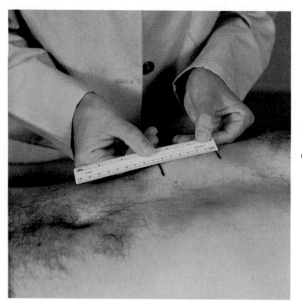

C

Error in estimating the liver span can occur when pleural effusion or lung consolidation obscures the upper liver border or when gas in the colon obscures the lower border. On inspiration, the diaphragm moves downward. This movement shifts the normal span of liver dullness inferiorly 2 to 3 cm. Pulmonary edema may also displace the liver downward. Ascites, massive tumors, or pregnancy may push the liver upward. The liver assumes a more square configuration in cirrhosis of the liver, and the midclavicular and midsternal measurements may approach equality. Percussion of liver dullness is important in detecting atrophy of the liver, such as might occur in acute fulminating hepatitis.

Percussion for tympany and dullness

Spleen. Splenic dullness can be percussed from the level of the seventh to the eleventh rib just posterior to or at the midaxillary line on the left side. Begin percussion at the tenth rib just posterior to the midaxillary line. Percuss in several directions from dullness to resonance or tympany to outline the edges of the spleen (Figure 17.15). The span of normal splenic dullness does not exceed 7 cm. When the spleen has normal dimensions, tympany may be percussed over the lowest left intercostal space between the anterior and midaxillary lines during both inspiration and expiration. However, a finding of tympany on expiration and dullness on inspiration probably denotes splenic hypertrophy. A full stomach, an enlarged kidney, or a colon packed with

feces may elicit dullness and therefore can mimic splenic enlargement. Gastric or colonic air may also obscure normal splenic dullness.

Stomach. The percussion note of the gastric air bubble is lower-pitched tympany than that of the intestine. Percuss in the area of the left lower anterior rib cage and in the left epigastric region to define the area occupied by the bubble (Figure 17.16). The percussion sounds of the stomach vary with the time the last meal was eaten.

Fist percussion. Another percussion method used in the abdominal examination is fist percussion, which causes the tissue to vibrate rather than produce sound (Figure 17.17). Place the palm of the left hand over the region of liver dullness and strike a light blow to the left hand with the fisted right hand. Tenderness elicited by this method is usually associated with hepatitis or cholecystitis. Fist percussion done at the costovertebral angle (CVA) is also used to assess renal tenderness. Common causes of tenderness are pyelonephritis and renal calculi.

Palpation

Palpation is the most important part of the abdominal examination. It is used to substantiate findings noted from careful inspection, auscultation, and percussion and to explore the abdomen further. Palpation allows for evaluation of the major organs of the abdomen in terms of shape, position, mobility, size, consistency, tenderness, and tension. Thorough and systematic screening is performed to detect areas of tenderness, muscular spasm, masses, or fluid.

Make sure that the client is comfortable and that your hands are warm. The client's abdominal muscles

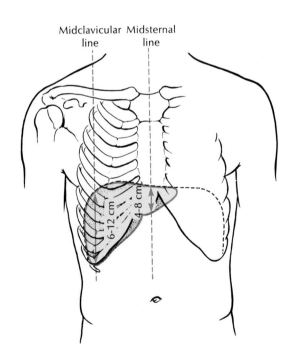

figure**17.14** The range of liver span in the midclavicular and midsternal lines. The size of the liver shows a direct correlation to lean body mass. Thus the mean clavicular liver span is 10.5 cm in men and 7.0 cm in women.

figure**17.15** Spleen percussion route.

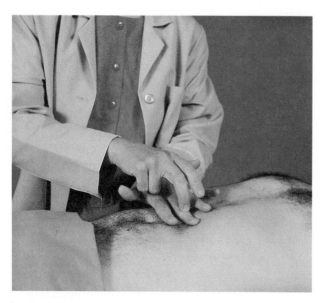

figure**17.16** Percussion of the abdomen for evaluation of fluid, gaseous distention, and masses within the abdominal cavity.

figure**17.18** Light palpation is performed with the hand parallel to the floor and the fingers approximated. The fingers depress the abdominal wall about 1 cm. This method of palpation is recommended for eliciting slight tenderness, large masses, and muscle guarding.

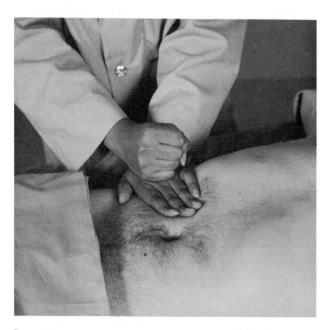

figure**17.17** Fist percussion of the liver. The palm of the hand is placed over the region of liver dullness, and a light blow is struck with the fisted right hand. Tenderness elicited by this method is usually a result of hepatitis or cholecystitis.

should be relaxed. You may need to use relaxation techniques to help the client achieve the appropriate level of relaxation. If the client is unable to relax the abdominal muscles despite these maneuvers, try exerting downward pressure on the lower sternum with the left hand

while palpating with the other hand. The deeper inspiration that results inhibits abdominal muscle contraction. You can also ask the client to put his or her hand on the abdomen so that you can palpate on top of the client's hand.

Light palpation. Light palpation is gentle exploration performed while the client is in the supine position. It is helpful in identifying regions of tenderness, large or superficial masses, and muscle guarding. Frequently, an enlarged or distended structure may be noted through a sense of resistance. Areas of tenderness or guarding, or both, should alert you to proceed with caution in more vigorous manipulation of these structures during deep palpation.

Begin palpation at a site distant from areas described as painful or expected to be tender. Elicitation of pain may result in the client's refusing further examination. Stand at the client's right side. Place the palm of your hand lightly on the client's abdomen with your fingers extended and approximated (Figure 17.18). Press the fingertips gently into the abdominal wall approximately 1 cm. Use a light dipping motion (avoid a digging action). Move systematically from one quadrant to another. The abdomen should feel smooth and soft. Watch the client's face for signs of pain elicited by palpation and confirm this verbally with the client.

Tensing of the abdominal musculature may occur because (1) the examiner's hands are too cold or are pressed too vigorously or deeply into the abdomen, (2) the client is ticklish or guards involuntarily, or (3) a subjacent, generally inflammatory, pathological condition exists. If resistance occurs, try to determine whether it is

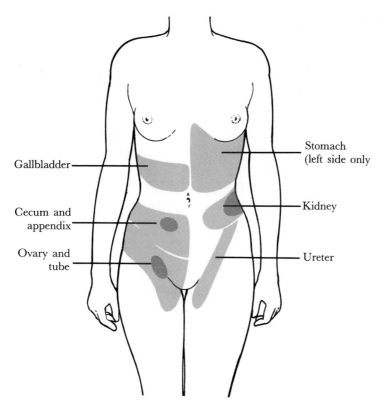

Gallbladder

Cecum and appendix

Ovary and tube

Stomach (left side only

Kidney

Ureter

figure**17.19** Head's zones of cutaneous hypersensitivity. *(From Seidel HM et al:* Mosby's guide to physical examination, *ed 3, St Louis, 1995, Mosby.)*

an involuntary spasm or voluntary tensing by feeling for the rectus muscle, which should normally relax as the client exhales. If the rigidity remains unaltered, it is probably an involuntary response to localized or generalized rigidity. Rigidity is a boardlike hardness of the abdominal wall overlying peritoneal irritation. In generalized peritonitis, rigidity may be constant and hard.

> **HELPFUL HINT** *To examine the ticklish client:*
> - *Ask the client to rest his or her hand on the back of your examining hand and follow it around the abdomen. This method works because tickling yourself is difficult.*
> - *Exert downward pressure on the lower sternum with the left hand while palpating with the right hand. This distraction may decrease the ticklish response.*

Assessment of cutaneous hypersensitivity. When tenderness is noted, testing for cutaneous hypersensitivity can help to delineate the areas of peritoneal irritation. Zones of hypersensitivity of sensory nerve fibers of the skin are thought to reflect specific areas of peritoneal

irritation (Figure 17.19). Although research has not provided proof for all the zones, the clinical consensus is that hypersensitivity in the area of the appendix is associated with appendicitis and hypersensitivity in the middle epigastrium is associated with an active peptic ulcer.

Hypersensitivity can be evaluated in two ways. One method is to stimulate the skin gently with the sharp end of an open safety pin, a wisp of cotton, or the fingernail (Figure 17.20). The second method is to gently lift a fold of skin away from the underlying musculature (Figure 17.21). The alert client will perceive pain or an exaggerated sensation in response to this stimulation. Look for changes in facial expression (grimacing), which may also indicate the increased sensation that the individual is experiencing.

Moderate palpation. Moderate palpation is an intermediate step for gradually approaching deep palpation. After light palpation, apply moderate pressure with the palm of the hand to continue to survey the four quadrants (Figure 17.22). Alternatively, use the side of the hand rather than the fingertips for moderate palpation (Figure 17.23). This technique avoids the tendency to dig into the abdomen with the fingertips. The sensation produced by palpating with the side of the hand is particularly useful in assessing organs that move with respi-

figure **17.20** Assessment of superficial pain sensation of the abdomen.

figure **17.21** Assessment of hypersensitivity by lifting a fold of skin away from the underlying musculature.

ration, such as the liver and the spleen. Feel the organ during normal breathing and then as the client takes a deep breath. On inspiration, the organ will be pushed downward against your hand. Tenderness not elicited by gentle palpation may be perceived by the client when moderate pressure is applied. This stage allows you to gradually prepare the client for deep palpation.

Deep palpation. To assess abdominal organs thoroughly and to detect masses, use deep palpation. Deeply press the palmar surfaces of the fingers into the abdominal wall (Figure 17.24). Systematically palpate all four quadrants. The abdominal wall may slide back and forth while the fingers are moving back and forth over the organ being examined. Deeper structures, such as retroperitoneal organs (the kidneys), or masses may be felt with this type of palpation. This method may uncover tenderness of organs that cannot be elicited by light or moderate palpation. In the absence of disease, the pressure produced by deep palpation may produce tenderness over the cecum, the sigmoid colon, and the aorta.

Bimanual palpation

Superimposition of one hand. Use bimanual palpation when additional pressure is necessary to overcome resistance or to examine a deep abdominal structure. In this method one hand is superimposed on the other so that pressure is exerted by the upper hand while the lower hand remains relaxed and sensitive to the tactile sensation produced by the structure being examined. If you are right-handed, apply pressure with your right (top) hand while concentrating on feeling with your left (bottom) hand (Figure 17.25).

Trapping technique. Use both hands to determine the size of a mass. Trap the mass between your hands for measurement. Clearly describe a mass in terms of location, size, shape, consistency, tenderness, mobility, pulsation, and movement with respiration.

Detection of a pulsatile mass. Place the fingertips of both hands on either side of the mass. Pulsation may be sensed in the fingertips as they feel the motion of a pulsatile flow expanding a structure such as the aorta. Pulsation may also be felt in a mass held between the hands. This palpatory finding indicates that the structure being felt is pulsating rather than transmitting pulsation.

Examination of specific abdominal structures

Palpation is a useful technique for identification and assessment of the specific abdominal structures. Use a systematic approach, always beginning at the same area, so that you do not skip any part of the abdomen. Because you are approaching the client from the right, the liver may be the most convenient structure to palpate first.

Liver. Two types of bimanual palpation are recommended for examination of the liver. In the first method, place your left hand beneath the client at the level of the eleventh and twelfth ribs. Apply upward pressure with your left hand to throw the liver forward, toward your right hand. Place the examining hand below the costal margin and palpate for the liver border with deep inspiration. There are two methods of positioning your right hand. Either place the palmar surface

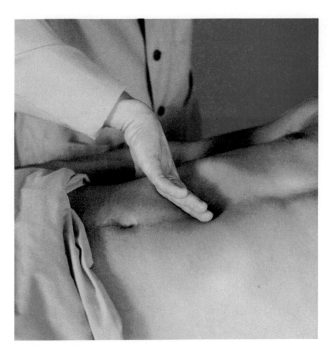

figure**17.22** Moderate palpation. Use moderate pressure with the palm of the hand to continue to survey the four quadrants.

figure**17.23** Moderate palpation performed with the side of the hand. This method of palpation is particularly useful in assessing organs that move with respiration, such as the liver and spleen.

figure**17.24** Deep palpation. Press palmar surfaces of the extended fingers deeply and evenly into the abdominal wall.

figure**17.25** Deep bimanual palpation. Apply pressure with the upper hand while concentrating on feeling structures with the lower hand.

A   **B**   **C**

figure**17.26** **A,** Palpating the liver with the fingers parallel to the costal margin. **B,** Palpating the liver with the fingers extended along the right midclavicular line. **C,** Palpating the liver with the fingers "hooked" over the costal margin.

of your right hand parallel to the right costal margin (Figure 17.26, *A*) or place your right hand on the abdomen, with the fingers pointing toward the head and extended along the right midclavicular line below the level of liver dullness (Figure 17.26, *B*). Ask the client to breathe normally for two or three breaths and then to breathe deeply. The diaphragm is exerted downward on inspiration and will push the liver toward the examining hand (Figure 17.26, *A*).

The liver usually cannot be palpated in the normal adult. However, in extremely thin but otherwise well individuals, it may be felt at the costal margin on inspiration. When the normal liver margin is palpated, it feels smooth, regular in contour, and somewhat sharp. Descriptions of the abnormal liver are provided in Table 17.1.

In the second technique, frequently referred to as the "hooking technique" or "Middleton's technique," place your hands side by side on the client's right costal margin below the border of liver dullness. Stand on the right side facing the client's feet. Press in with your fingers and up toward the costal margin. Ask the client to take a deep breath. As the client inspires, the liver may be felt to descend toward your fingers (Figure 17.26, *C*). Regardless of the technique that is chosen, palpation of the liver should be done slowly, carefully, and gently so that the liver margin is not missed.

To demonstrate tenderness over the liver, place the palm of one hand over the lateral costal margin and deliver a blow to that hand with the ulnar surface of the other hand, which has been curled into a fist (fist percussion) (see Figure 17.17).

Scratch test. The scratch test is useful when the usual techniques for determining the lower liver border

have been unsuccessful. This test makes use of the difference in sound over solid, as opposed to hollow, organs. Actually a percussion technique, the scratch test can be used to assess the size of the liver. Place the stethoscope over the liver while using the opposite hand to scratch lightly over the abdominal surface with short, transverse strokes (Figure 17.27). When the scratch is done over the liver, the sound is magnified. Although this test is of questionable accuracy, it may be of some value in assessing the individual with abdominal distention or spastic abdominal muscles.

Spleen. The spleen is not usually palpable in the normal adult because it is normally soft and is located in the retroperitoneal area. If the spleen is palpable, it is probably enlarged. Turning the client on the right side (to gain gravitational advantage) brings the spleen downward and forward and thus closer to the abdominal wall; therefore this position is often employed in the examination.

While standing at the supine client's right side, extend your left hand and place it beneath the client's left costovertebral angle. Exert an upward pressure with your left hand to displace the spleen anteriorly. Feel for the spleen by pressing your right hand gently under the left anterior costal margin (Figure 17.28). Have the client take a deep breath, and palpate as the client exhales. Repeat the examination with the client lying on the right side with the hips and knees slightly flexed. It is important to remember that the enlarged spleen can rupture with vigorous palpation. If splenic enlargement is suspected, first percuss the splenic area and then palpate very gently and carefully.

Splenic enlargement is described by the number of

table 17.1	Characteristics of Hepato-megaly Related to Common Pathological Conditions

Description of liver	Possible pathological condition
Smooth, nontender	Portal cirrhosis
	Lymphoma
	Passive congestion of liver
	Portal obstruction
	Obstruction of vena cava
	Lymphocytic leukemia
	Rickets
	Amyloidosis
	Schistosomiasis
Smooth, tender	Acute hepatitis
	Amebic hepatitis or abscess
	Early congestive cardiac failure
Nodular	Late portal cirrhosis
	Tertiary syphilis
	Metastatic carcinoma
Hard	Carcinomatosis

figure 17.27 Scratch test in assessment of liver size. Place the stethoscope over the liver while the other hand scratches lightly over the abdominal surface with short, transverse strokes; when the scratch is done over the liver, the sound is magnified.

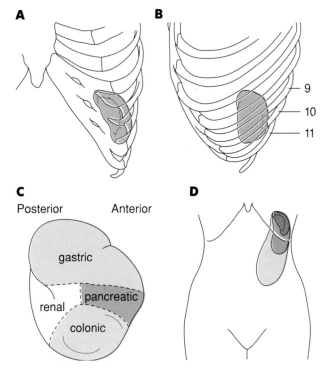

figure 17.29 Normal (A, B, C) and enlarged (D) spleen. A, Anterior view. B, Left lateral view. C, Regions of the spleen (anterior view) that touch other viscera. D, Directions of splenic enlargement.

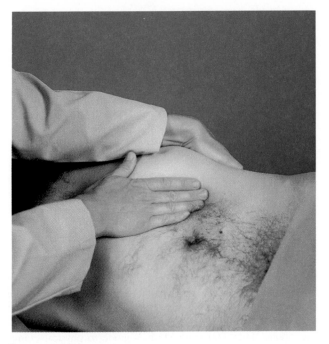

figure 17.28 Palpation of the spleen.

centimeters that the spleen extends below the costal margin: (1) slight—1 to 4 cm below the costal margin; (2) moderate—4 to 8 cm below the costal margin; or (3) great—more than 8 cm below the costal margin. As previously mentioned, the spleen may be percussed to assess enlargement. Normally, splenic dullness may be percussed from the seventh to the eleventh rib in the midaxillary line or posterior to the line.

To best describe splenic enlargement, draw the anterior abdomen, indicating the relative size and shape of the spleen in relation to the costal border and the umbilicus (Figure 17.29).

Gallbladder. The normal gallbladder cannot be felt. However, a distended gallbladder can be palpated below the liver margin at the lateral border of the rectus muscle. The cystic nature of the mass helps to identify the gallbladder. However, the location of the left border varies greatly. It may be found either more medially or more laterally.

An enlarged, tender gallbladder indicates cholecystitis, whereas a large but nontender gallbladder suggests obstruction of the common bile duct. Murphy's sign, elicited through a bimanual technique, is helpful in determining the presence of cholecystitis. While performing deep palpation, ask the client to take a deep breath. As the descending liver brings the gallbladder in contact with the examining hand, the client with cholecystitis will experience pain and will stop the inspiratory movement. Pain may also occur in the client with hepatitis.

Pancreas. The pancreas cannot be palpated in the normal client because of its small size and retroperitoneal position. However, a pancreatic mass may occasionally be felt as a vague sensation of fullness in the epigastrium.

Urinary bladder. The urinary bladder is not palpable in the normal client unless it is distended with urine. A distended bladder is felt as a smooth, round, and rather tense mass. Percussion can be used to define the outline of the distended bladder, which may extend upward as far as the umbilicus.

Umbilicus. Observe the umbilicus for its relationship to the skin surface, hernia, inflammation, or signs of bleeding. The normal umbilicus is recessed below the skin surface.

Umbilical hernia. The umbilical hernia noted in children is seen directly at the umbilical opening, which is centrally located in the linea alba. In the adult, this defect is often apparent above an incomplete umbilical ring and is referred to as paraumbilical. Examine for an umbilical hernia by pressing your index finger into the navel. The fascial opening may feel like a sharp ring with a soft center. The umbilicus may be everted by marked intraabdominal pressure from masses, pregnancy, or large amounts of ascitic fluid.

Abdominal reflexes. To elicit the abdominal reflex, use a key, the base end of an applicator, or your fingernail to stroke the abdominal skin gently over the lateral borders of the rectus abdominis muscles toward the midline (Figure 17.30). Repeat this maneuver in each quadrant. With each stroke, observe contraction of the rectus abdominis muscles, coupled with pulling of the umbilicus to the stimulated side. The abdominal reflex may be weak or absent in the individual who has sustained a good deal of stretching of the abdominal musculature. Thus you may be unable to obtain the abdominal reflex in the multiparous or obese client. In addition, the reflex may be absent in the normal aging client. Its absence may also indicate a pyramidal tract lesion. Absence of the upper abdominal reflex suggests problems at the spinal levels of T7, T8, and T9. Absence of lower abdominal reflexes indicates problems at the spinal levels of T10 and T11.

Aorta. With the client in a supine position, press firmly and deeply in the upper abdomen slightly to the left of midline and palpate for aortic pulsations. In an older individual (over age 50), try to assess the width of the aorta to screen for an aneurysm. Press deeply in the upper abdomen with one hand on either side of the aorta (Figure

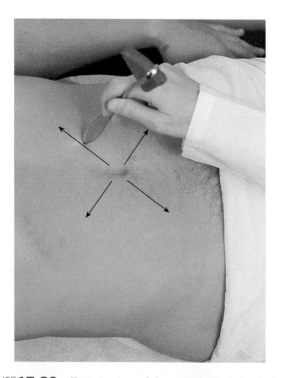

figure **17.30** Examination of the superficial abdominal reflexes. One of several approaches is illustrated. Stroke the upper abdominal area upward, away from the umbilicus, and the lower abdominal area downward, away from the umbilicus. *(From Seidel HM et al: Mosby's guide to physical examination, ed 3, St Louis, 1995, Mosby.)*

17.31). The normal aorta is approximately 1.3 to 3 cm wide, whereas an aneurysm is much broader (>4 to 5 cm).

As noted previously, a bruit is generally heard over an aneurysm. The most common physical finding in clients with an abdominal aneurysm is the presence of an expanding, pulsating mass. More than 95% of such masses are located below the renal arteries but generally at or above the umbilicus. Femoral pulses are usually present but are markedly damped in amplitude. Since more than half of clients with abdominal aneurysms are asymptomatic, the mass may be discovered during a screening physical examination. Although more than 80% of abdominal aneurysms can be palpated, small aneurysms in the markedly obese client may not be felt. If you observe a pulsating abdominal aortic mass and auscultate a bruit, refrain from palpation.

Changes in vascular patterns: venous engorgement. In a healthy person, the veins of the abdominal wall are not prominent. However, in the malnourished individual, the veins are more easily visible because of decreased adipose tissue. The venous return to the heart is cephalad in the veins above the umbilicus and caudal below the navel. The visibility of veins is not useful. However, the direction of flow in visible veins can be helpful to assess obstruction of the vena cava (Figure 17.32). To demonstrate the direction of flow, place the index fingers side by side over a vein, pressing laterally and separating the fingers. A section of the vein may be emptied. Remove one finger and measure the time for filling. "Milk" the blood from a short section of the

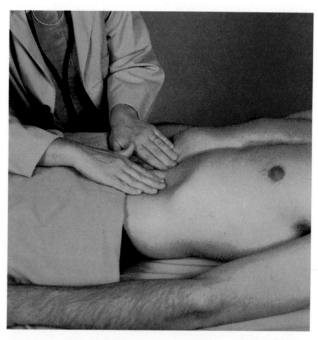

figure**17.31** Palpation of the aorta. Press fingers deeply with one hand on either side of the aorta and feel for pulsation.

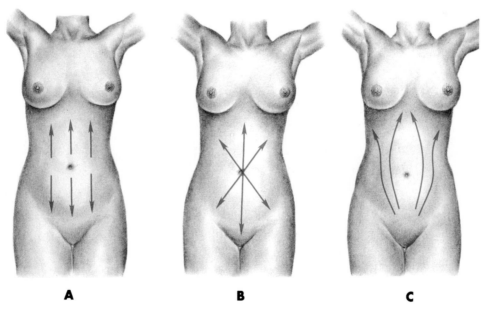

A **B** **C**

figure**17.32** Abdominal venous patterns. **A,** Normal. **B,** Portal hypertension. **C,** Inferior vena cava obstruction. *(From Seidel HM et al: Mosby's guide to physical examination, ed 3, St Louis, 1995, Mosby.)*

vein, remove the other index finger, and measure the time for filling from this side. The flow of venous blood is in the direction of the faster-filling side.

Reversal of flow or an upward venous flow in the veins below the umbilicus accompanies obstruction of the inferior vena cava. Superior vena cava obstruction promotes downward flow in the veins above the navel.

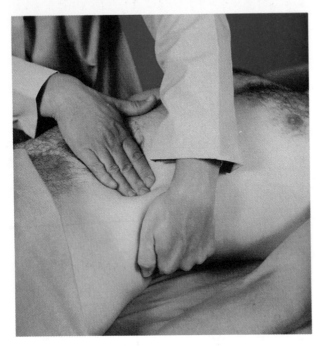

figure**17.33** Palpation of the left kidney.

A pattern of engorged veins around the umbilicus, called caput medusae, is occasionally seen as an accompaniment to emaciation or to obstruction of the superior or inferior vena cava, the superficial vein, or the portal vein.

Kidney. When palpating the kidneys, stand at the client's right side with the client in a supine position. To examine the left kidney, reach across the client with your left arm and place your hand behind the client's left flank (Figure 17.33). Elevate the left flank with your fingers, displacing the kidney anteriorly. Then use the palmar surface of your right hand to palpate the kidney deeply.

To examine the right kidney, remain on the client's right side. Elevate the right flank with the left hand. Use the right hand to palpate the right kidney deeply. The lower pole of the right kidney may be felt as a smooth, rounded mass that descends on inspiration.

The kidneys are usually not palpable in the normal adult. In very thin persons, only the lower pole of the right kidney can be felt. In the elderly, as muscle tone decreases and elastic fibers are lost, the kidneys may be more readily palpated. The left kidney is generally not palpable.

Percussion may be used to differentiate between splenic and left kidney enlargement. The percussion note over the spleen is dull because the bowel is displaced downward. Resonance is heard over the kidney because it is located behind the bowel (Figure 17.34). In addition, the free edge of the spleen is sharp in contour and tends to enlarge caudally and to the right.

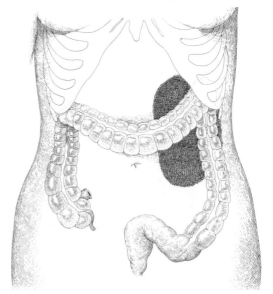

figure**17.34** Differentiation of enlarged spleen **(A)** from enlarged left kidney **(B)**. (*From GI series: physical examination of the abdomen, Richmond, Va, 1981, AH Robins Co.*)

Back. The final step in the abdominal examination includes inspection and fist percussion of the back for renal problems. The client should be in the sitting position for this portion of the examination. In the normal individual, the flanks are symmetrical. Fullness or asymmetry may be a result of renal disorders. Ecchymoses of the flanks (Grey Turner's sign) are associated with retroperitoneal bleeding and may indicate hemorrhagic pancreatitis. Unilateral flank pain or tenderness suggests renal or ureteral disease, such as a stone, tumor, infection, or infarct.

Fist percussion in each costovertebral angle is done to evaluate kidney tenderness. Figure 17.35 demonstrates the relationship of the kidney to the costovertebral junction. For indirect percussion, place the palm of one hand in the costovertebral angle and strike it with the ulnar surface of the fist of your other hand (Figure 17.36, *A*). Direct percussion is demonstrated in Figure 17.36, *B*. In either type of percussion, use enough force for the client to perceive a painless jarring or a thud. Fist percussion should not cause pain in the normal person. Pressure from your fingertips in the costovertebral angle may be enough to reveal tenderness in the client with a kidney infection. Frequently, this maneuver is integrated into the back examination, or it is done at the end of the posterior lung examination for increased efficiency and client comfort.

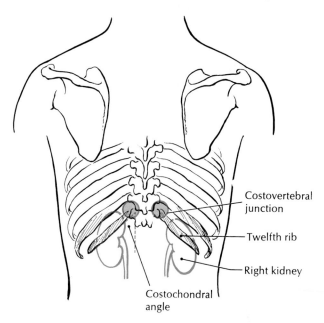

figure**17.35** Relationship of the kidney to the twelfth rib. Note the costovertebral junction.

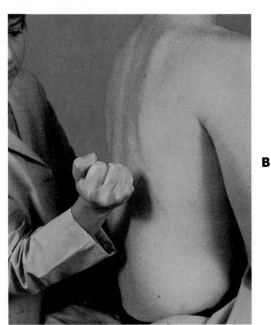

figure**17.36** **A,** Indirect percussion of the costovertebral angle to elicit tenderness related to the kidney. **B,** Direct percussion of the costovertebral angle to elicit tenderness related to the kidney.

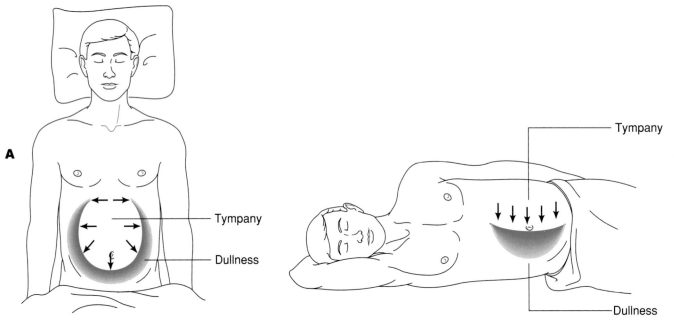

figure**17.37**   Assessment of ascites. **A,** In the supine client, ascites fluid will sink with gravity and give a dull percussion note. Mark borders between tympany and dullness. **B,** To test for shifting dullness, ask the client to turn on one side. Ascites fluid will flow with gravity. Dullness shifts to the dependent side while tympany shifts to the top. Percuss and mark the new line and measure the change.

Special maneuvers

Evaluation of ascites (free fluid). Ascites should be considered in the client with a protuberant abdomen and bulging flanks. This condition is caused by (1) diseases of the liver, such as cirrhosis and hepatitis; (2) diseases of the heart, such as congestive failure and constrictive pericarditis; (3) pancreatitis; (4) cancer, such as peritoneal metastases and ovarian tumors; (5) tuberculous peritonitis; and (6) hypoalbuminemia.

A technique for differentiating ascites from cysts or edema fluid in the abdominal wall is the percussion test for shifting dullness. Palpation of a fluid wave is another method to assess for ascites.

Shifting dullness. Place the client in the supine position. Percuss for areas of dullness and resonance. Ascites will sink with gravity and will produce a dull percussion note in dependent areas (Figure 17.37, *A*). Gas-filled loops of bowel will rise to the upper areas and have a resonant note. Mark the borders between tympany and dullness. Next, test for shifting dullness (Figure 17.37, *B*). After marking the borders, ask the client to turn on one side. The ascites will flow with gravity to shift the line of dullness closer to the umbilicus on the client's dependent side. Percuss and mark a new line, and measure the change in centimeters. In a person without ascites, the borders will remain relatively constant. A vol-

ume of free fluid in the peritoneal cavity greater than 2 L can be detected by methods of shifting dullness.

Fluid wave. The presence of large amounts of fluid within the peritoneal cavity allows the elicitation of a fluid wave (Figure 17.38). To test for the presence of a fluid wave, place the client in a supine position. Ask the client or an assistant to place the edge of one hand and lower arm firmly in the vertical midline of the client's abdomen. This maneuver will help to stop vibrations that might otherwise be transmitted through fat. Place the palmar surface of one of your hands firmly against the lateral abdominal wall and tap the other side with your other hand. An easily felt fluid wave suggests ascites. However, this sign is often negative until ascites becomes obvious. The fluid wave may sometimes be felt in individuals without ascites.

Ballottement. Ballottement (Figure 17.39) is an advanced palpation technique used to assess a floating object. Fluid-filled tissue is pushed toward the examining hand so that the object will float against the examining fingers. This technique is used to determine by abdominal palpation whether the head or the breech of the fetus is in the fundus of the uterus (Leopold's maneuver).

Single-handed ballottement. Single-handed ballottement is performed with the fingers extended in a straight line with the forearm and positioned at a right

angle to the abdomen. Move the fingers quickly toward the mass or organ to be examined and hold them there. As fluid or other structures are displaced, the mass will move upward and be felt at the fingertips. Some examiners prefer this technique for examination of the spleen.

Bimanual ballottement. To perform bimanual ballottement, use one hand to push on the anterior abdominal wall to displace the contents to the flank while the other hand receives the mass or structure pushed against it and feels its dimensions.

Palpation to elicit rebound tenderness. Rebound tenderness is a symptom of peritoneal irritation. To provoke rebound tenderness, hold your hand with the fingers extended at a 90-degree angle. Push your fingers gently but deeply in a region remote from the area of suspected tenderness and then rapidly remove them. The maneuver, when performed over McBurney's point (as illustrated in Figure 17.40), may elicit rebound tenderness related to appendicitis. The rebound of the structures indented by palpation causes a sharp, stabbing sensation of pain on the side of the inflammation. This sensation following the withdrawal of pressure is a sign of peritoneal irritation. The test may be repeated on the side of the suspected disease. It is best performed near the conclusion of the examination because the production of severe pain or muscle spasm may interfere with subsequent examination. Voluntary coughing by the client may produce the same results.

Many examiners consider the elicitation of rebound tenderness by palpation to be a crude and painful tech-

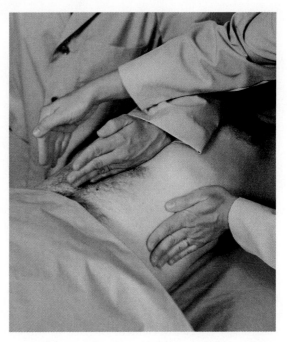

figure**17.38** Testing for a fluid wave. Place the palmar surface of one hand against the abdominal wall and tap the other side with the other hand. An easily felt fluid wave suggests ascites.

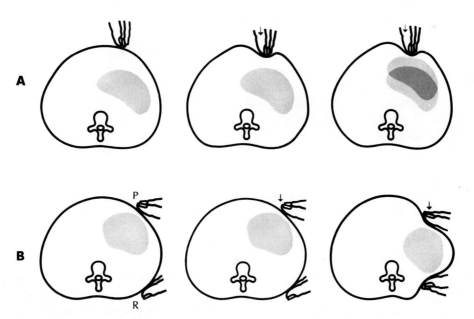

figure**17.39** Ballottement. **A,** Single-handed ballottement. **B,** Bimanual ballottement. *P,* Pushing hand; *R,* receiving hand. *(From* GI series: physical examination of the abdomen, *Richmond, Va, 1981, AH Robins Co.)*

A   **B**

figure**17.40**   Palpation to elicit rebound tenderness. **A,** Deep pressure is applied to the abdominal wall. **B,** On release of pressure, a sensation of pain would indicate peritoneal irritation. This is a test for appendicitis.

nique. The resultant severe pain and muscle spasm not only interfere with subsequent examination but also may adversely affect the element of trust in the client-physician relationship. Light percussion can be used to produce vibration, which causes a mildly uncomfortable response in the presence of peritoneal inflammation. This technique is reputed to be able to localize very small areas of peritoneal inflammation, in some instances an area as small as a quarter.

Palpation for abdominal masses. One of the goals of abdominal palpation is to determine the presence of

table 17.2	*Characteristics of Abdominal Masses Related to Common Pathological Conditions*

Description of mass	Possible pathological condition
Descends on inspiration	Liver, spleen, or kidney mass
Pulsatile mass	Abdominal aneurysm, tortuous aorta
Movable from side to side, not head to foot	Mesenteric or small bowel mass
Complete fixation	Tumor of pancreatic or retroperitoneal origin

abdominal masses. (Palpation techniques are described in detail in the preceding sections.) Once a mass has been found, carefully describe its characteristics. Of particular importance are consistency, regularity of contour movement with respiration, tenderness, and mobility (Table 17.2). A sketch of the anterior abdominal wall with all its bony landmarks and the umbilicus may be the most efficient way to convey location, shape, and size.

To determine whether a palpable mass is located in the anterior abdominal wall or is situated in an intraabdominal position, ask the client to raise the head and shoulders from a supine position or to flex the abdominal muscles. Masses in the subcutaneous tissue will continue to be palpable, whereas those in the peritoneal cavity will be more difficult to feel or will be pushed out of reach altogether.

Normal abdominal structures that are occasionally mistaken for masses are the following (Figure 17.41):

1. Lateral borders of rectus abdominis muscles
2. Uterus
3. Feces-filled ascending colon
4. Feces-filled descending colon and sigmoid colon
5. Aorta
6. Common iliac artery
7. Sacral promontory

Palpable bowel segments. The presence of feces within the bowel frequently contributes to the examiner's ability to palpate the cecum, ascending colon, descending colon, and sigmoid colon. The feces-filled cecum and ascending colon produce a sensation suggestive of a soft, boggy, rounded mass. The client may

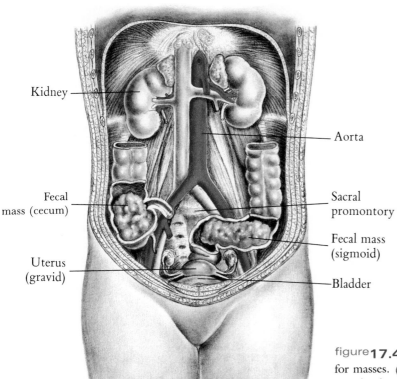

figure**17.41** Abdominal structures frequently mistaken for masses. *(From Seidel HM et al: Mosby's guide to physical examination, ed 3, St Louis, 1995, Mosby.)*

complain of cramps resulting from stimulation of the bowel by the movements of palpation.

Tests for irritation resulting from appendicitis

Iliopsoas muscle test. An inflamed or perforated extrapelvic appendix may cause contact irritation of the lateral iliopsoas muscle. To elicit an indication of involvement, place the client in a supine position. Ask the client to flex the leg at the hip. As the client is flexing, simultaneously exert a moderate downward pressure over the lower thigh (Figure 17.42). With psoas muscle inflammation, the client will describe pain in the lower quadrant. A more sensitive test of psoas muscle irritation is performed with the client lying on the left side. Pain is elicited through all positions of full extension of the right lower limb at the hip.

Obturator muscle test. A perforated intrapelvic appendix or a pelvic abscess adjacent to it can cause irritation of the internal obturator muscle. This pain is demonstrated with the client in the supine position. Ask the client to flex the right extremity at the hip and at the knee to 90 degrees. Grasp the ankle and rotate it internally and externally (Figure 17.43). A complaint of hypogastric pain indicates obturator muscle involvement.

Test for diastasis recti or abdominal hernia. If an umbilical or incisional hernia or diastasis recti abdominis is suspected, instruct the client to raise the head from the pillow, thus increasing the intraabdominal pressure, which may cause the hernia to protrude. Asking the

figure**17.42** Iliopsoas muscle test.

figure**17.43** Obturator muscle test.

examination*step-by-step*

Inspection

1. Observe the surface of the abdomen for the following factors:
   a. Skin color
   b. Scars
   c. Venous network
   d. Umbilicus—placement, contour, surface characteristics
   e. Symmetry (view from the right side at eye level and from behind the client's head)
   f. Contour
   g. Surface characteristics
   h. Surface motility—peristalsis, pulsations

Auscultation

1. Listen to all four quadrants and the epigastrium using the diaphragm of the stethoscope; note the timing and quality of sounds.
2. Listen for arterial vascular sounds (abdominal aorta, renal and femoral arteries). Use the bell of the stethoscope to pick up low-pitched sounds such as a venous hum.
3. Listen for a friction rub, most commonly heard over the liver or the spleen.

Percussion

1. Lightly percuss all four quadrants.
2. Percuss the liver borders at the midclavicular and midsternal lines. Mark the upper and lower borders with a pen and measure the liver span.
3. Percuss the spleen at the left midaxillary line.
4. Percuss the "gastric bubble" at the left lower rib cage.

Palpation

1. Use light palpation with the pads of the fingertips to survey all four quadrants for tenderness, muscle tone, and masses.
2. Use moderate palpation with the palm and the sides of the hands to continue to assess all four quadrants for tenderness, muscle tone, masses, and the general location of major structures.
3. Use deep palpation to survey all four quadrants for tenderness, masses, and the location of deeper structures.
4. Palpate specific organs:
   a. Liver: Deeply palpate by placing the left hand under the eleventh and twelfth ribs and the right hand parallel to the right costal margin. Have the client breathe normally and then take a deep breath. Palpate on inspiration.
   b. Spleen: While standing on the client's right side, extend your left hand and place it beneath the client's left costovertebral angle. Feel for the spleen by pressing your right hand gently under the left anterior costal margin.
   c. Aorta: With the client in the supine position, deeply palpate slightly to the left of midline to feel for the aortic pulsation.
   d. Palpate the umbilicus with the fingertips for bulges, nodules, and the umbilical ring.
   e. Kidneys: With the client supine, palpate each kidney. *Left kidney:* Extend the left hand across the client to elevate the left flank, then deeply palpate the kidney with the right hand (the left kidney is usually not palpable). *Right kidney:* Place the left hand under the right flank and palpate deeply with the right hand.

To assess kidney tenderness, have the client sit up and use fist percussion at the right and left costovertebral angles.

---

client to cough will also cause a hernia to bulge outward. When the client raises the head from the pillow, the rectus muscles contract and will reveal a separation of the muscles. Diastasis recti may be congenital or may be acquired as a result of weakening of the muscles by conditions such as pregnancy and obesity.

Assessment of muscle spasticity. Involuntary muscle contraction or spasticity may indicate peritoneal irritation. Further palpation is done to determine whether the spasticity is unilateral or present on both sides of the abdomen. Generalized and boardlike contraction is thought to be typical of peritonitis. Ask the client to raise the trunk from a horizontal position without arm support. The experience of unilateral pain in response to this maneuver may further pinpoint the areas of spasticity. This mechanism may also help to differentiate mus-

cle contraction from abdominal mass. As the head is raised, the examining hand would be moved away from an abdominal mass. Rigidity and tenderness over McBurney's point, and in some cases over the entire right side, strongly suggest appendicitis. Acute cholecystitis is frequently accompanied by rigidity of the right hypochondrium.

▪ VARIATIONS FROM HEALTH

Tables 17.3 through 17.6 list the history, signs, and symptoms of various conditions associated with the abdomen. The signs and symptoms of intestinal obstruction and of peritoneal irritation are shown in the boxes on p. 441.

Condition	History	Symptoms	Signs
Appendicitis	Children (except infants) and young adults	Anorexia Nausea Pain—early, vague epigastric, periumbilical, or generalized pain after 12-24 hours; RLQ at McBurney's point	Signs may be absent early Vomiting Localized RLQ guarding and tenderness after 12-24 hours Rovsing's sign—pain with pressure in RLQ, iliopsoas sign Obturator sign White blood cell count 10,000 mm^3 or shift to left Low-grade fever Cutaneous hyperesthesia in RLQ Signs are highly variable
Mesenteric adenitis	Young person with history of respiratory infection	Lower abdominal pain May have normal appetite	Tenderness in RLQ Peritoneal irritation signs rare
Perforated duodenal ulcer	Prior history	Abrupt onset of pain in epigastric area or RLQ	Tenderness in epigastric area or RLQ Signs of peritoneal irritation Heme-positive stool Increased white blood cell count
Cecal volvulus	Seen most frequently in the elderly	Abrupt severe abdominal pain	Distention Localized tenderness Tympany
Strangulated hernia	Any age Women—femoral Men—inguinal	Severe localized pain If bowel obstructed, generalized pain	If bowel obstructed, distention

Ectopic pregnancy (1% of all pregnancies)	Woman of childbearing age
	Previous tubal pregnancy or pelvic inflammatory disease
	Missed menstrual period
	Spotting
		Symptoms of pregnancy (i.e., breast changes)
		Lower abdominal pain
		Referred pain to shoulder
		Nausea
			Unruptured:
			  Tenderness—cervical
			  Mass—adnexal or cul-de-sac
			Ruptured:
			  Shock
			  Distention
			  Rigidity
			Mass—cul-de-sac
			Fever

Pelvic inflammatory disease	Woman
	
	Exposure to infection
		Lower abdominal pain
		
		Dyspareunia
			Tenderness—adnexal and cervical (chandelier sign)
			Cervical discharge
			Endocervical smear
			  Gonococcus in one third to one half of cases
			  Chlamydial and anaerobic bacteria cause remainder

Tubal abscess	Woman Exposure to infection Dyspareunia	Lower abdominal pain Mass—adnexal	Fever

RLQ, Right lower quadrant.

table **17.4**   *Conditions Associated with the Right Upper Quadrant of the Abdomen*

Condition	History	Symptoms	Signs
Liver hepatitis	Any age, often young blood product user	Fatigue Malaise Anorexia	Hepatic tenderness Hepatomegaly Bilirubin elevated Jaundice
	Drug addict	Pain in RUQ Low-grade fever May have severe fulminating disease with liver failure	Lymphocytosis in one third of cases Liver enzymes elevated Hepatitis A or B or antibodies to these viruses may be found
Acute hepatic congestion	Usually elderly with congestive heart failure Pericardial disease Pulmonary embolism	Symptoms of congestive heart failure	Hepatomegaly Congestive heart failure
Biliary stones, colic	"Fair, fat, forty" (90%) but can be 30 to 80 years of age	Anorexia Nausea Pain severe in RUQ or epigastric area Episodes last 15 minutes to hours	Tenderness in RUQ Jaundice
Acute cholecystitis	"Fair, fat, forty" (90%) but may be 30 to 80 years of age	Severe RUQ or epigastric pain Episodes prolonged up to 6 hours	Vomiting Tenderness in RUQ Peritoneal irritation signs Increased white blood cell count
Perforated peptic ulcer	Any age	Abrupt RUQ pain	Tenderness in epigastrium and/or right quadrant Peritoneal irritation signs Free air in abdomen

RUQ, Right upper quadrant.

table **17.5**   *Conditions Associated with the Left Lower Quadrant of the Abdomen*

Condition	History	Symptoms	Signs
Ulcerative colitis	Family history Jewish ancestry	Chronic, watery diarrhea with blood, mucus Anorexia Weight loss Fatigue	Fever Cachexia Anemia Leukocytosis
Colonic diverticulitis	Over age 39 Low-residue diet	Pain that recurs in LLQ	Fever Vomiting Chills Diarrhea Tenderness over descending colon

LLQ, Left lower quadrant.

table 17.6	*Conditions Associated with the Left Upper Quadrant of the Abdomen*		
Condition	**History**	**Symptoms**	**Signs**
Splenic trauma	Blunt trauma to LUQ of abdomen	Pain—LUQ pain of abdomen often referred to left shoulder (Kehr's sign)	Hypotension Syncope Increased dyspnea X-ray studies show enlarged spleen
Pancreatitis	Alcohol abuse Pancreatic duct obstruction Infection Cholecystitis	Pain in LUQ or epigastric region radiating to back or chest	Fever Rigidity Rebound tenderness Nausea Vomiting Jaundice Cullen's sign Turner's sign Abdominal distention Diminished bowel sounds
Pyloric obstruction	Duodenal ulcer	Weight loss Gastric upset Vomiting	Increasing dullness in LUQ Visible peristaltic waves in epigastric region

LUQ, Left upper quadrant.

Signs and Symptoms of Intestinal Obstruction

GENERAL SIGNS
Distention
Hyperactive bowel sounds of high-pitched, tinkling character
Minimum rebound tenderness
Pain

SIGNS OF PROXIMAL OBSTRUCTION
Acute onset
Vomiting (marked)
Frequent bouts of pain
Distention (minimal)

SIGNS OF DISTAL OBSTRUCTION
Onset may be more gradual
Less marked vomiting
Less frequent bouts of pain
Distention (marked)

Signs and Symptoms of Peritoneal Irritation

Boardlike, increased rigidity of abdominal wall
Silent bowel sounds
Tenderness and guarding
Severe focal pain
Palpable abdominal rigidity
Positive obturator test
Positive iliopsoas test
Nausea, vomiting
Shock-diaphoresis (requires emergency attention)
Hypotension

table 17.7 *Nature of Abdominal Pain*

Description of pain	Possible pathological condition
Burning	Ulceration (peptic)
Cramping	Biliary colic
Severe cramping (colic)	Appendicitis with fecalith
Aching	Appendiceal inflammation
Knifelike	Pancreatitis
Radiation of pain	See Figure 17.44

table 17.8 *Onset of Abdominal Pain*

Description of pain	Possible pathological condition
Gradual onset	Infection
Acute onset— awakening client from sleep	Duodenal ulcer
Loss of consciousness	Acute pancreatitis
	Perforated ulcer
	Ruptured ectopic pregnancy
	Intestinal obstruction (strangulated)

table 17.9 *Symptoms or Signs Elicited in Other Systems That May Focus the Abdominal Examination*

Symptom or sign	Possible pathological condition	Symptom or sign	Possible pathological condition
Shock	Acute pancreatitis, ruptured tubal pregnancy	Flank tenderness	Renal inflammation, pyelonephritis
Mental status deficit	Hemorrhage—duodenal ulcer		Renal stone
	Abdominal epilepsy		Renal infarct
Hypertension	Aortic dissection		Renal vein thrombosis
	Abdominal aortic aneurysm	Leg edema	Iliac obstruction, pelvic mass
	Renal infarction		Renal disease
	Glomerulonephritis		Renal vein thrombosis
	Vasculitis	Lymphadenopathy	Hepatitis
Orthostatic hypotension	Hypovolemia—blood loss, fluid loss		Lymphoma
			Mononucleosis
Pulse deficit	Aortic dissection	Jaundice	Liver-biliary disease
	Aortic aneurysm or thrombosis		Excessive hemolysis
Bruits	Aortic dissection	Dark yellow to brown urine	Liver-biliary disease
	Aortic aneurysm		Blood resulting from kidney stone, infarct, glomerulonephritis, or pyelonephritis
	Dissection or aneurysm of arteries—splenic, renal, or iliac		
Low-output cardiac symptoms— atrial fibrillation	Ischemia of mesentery	Fever (39.4° C [103° F]) and chills	Peritonitis
			Pelvic infection
			Cholangitis
Valvular disease, congestive heart failure	Embolus		Pyelonephritis
		White blood cell count >10,000 mm^3 or shift to left (more than 80% polymorphonuclear cells) >20,000 mm^3	Appendicitis (95%)
			Acute cholecystitis (90%)
			Localized peritonitis
Pleural effusion	Esophageal rupture		Bowel strangulation
	Pancreatitis		Bowel infarction
	Ovarian tumor		

Abdominal Pain

Tables 17.7 and 17.8 list possible pathological conditions based on descriptions of abdominal pain and its onset.

Referred Pain or Somatic Pain from Intraabdominal Structures

Pain related to abdominal structures may be sensed in remote body surface regions (Table 17.9). The explanation for this phenomenon is that as pain is intensified, increased afferent impulses lower the client's pain threshold and excite secondary sensory neurons in the spinal cord. Thus contact may be established between afferent visceral fibers and somatic nerves of the same embryological dermatome. An example of this phenomenon is pain sensed in the top of the shoulder that is caused by abdominal lesions or peritonitis. The diaphragm, which is irritated in this situation, originates in the region of the fourth cervical nerve and derives its nerve supply from the third, fourth, and fifth cervical nerves. The shoulder is innervated by the fourth cervical nerve. Thus shoulder pain may be a valuable clue in diagnosing a perforated ulcer, hepatic abscess, pancreatitis, cholecystitis, a ruptured spleen, pelvic inflammation, or hemorrhage into the peritoneum. Other examples of referred pain are noted in Figure 17.44.

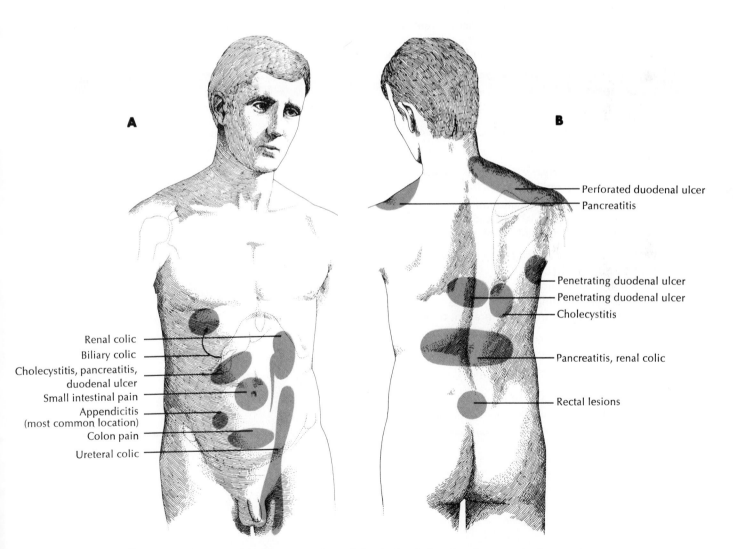

figure **17.44**   **A,** Common areas where abdominal pain is referred or perceived—anterior view. **B,** Common areas where abdominal pain is referred or perceived—posterior view. *(From GI series: physical examination of the abdomen, Richmond, Va, 1981, AH Robins Co.)*

*sample*documentation&diagnoses CRITICAL THINKING

■ **FOCUSED HEALTH HISTORY** *(SUBJECTIVE DATA)*

Mr. M., a 45-year-old white male, complains of severe abdominal cramping, nausea, vomiting, and diarrhea since yesterday. States he ate lunch out yesterday at a local restaurant ("some type of pasta salad and fish dish") and 4 to 5 hours later noted cramping, diarrhea, and vomiting. Has had watery, brownish stools about every hour since yesterday. No longer vomiting. Tried eating bland foods (tea and crackers) without improvement. Denies blood, pus, or mucus in stools. States is usually healthy. No chronic illnesses. Denies history of constipation, indigestion, weight changes, or change in appetite. Has not taken any medications recently (prescription or over-the-counter). No family history of liver, peptic ulcer, or kidney disease. Smokes 1½ packs/day × 15 years; drinks 2 to 3 alcoholic beverages weekly in social setting. Denies increased stress or major life changes; states family situation is "good"—lives with wife and 2 children, ages 6 and 10.

■ **FOCUSED PHYSICAL EXAMINATION** *(OBJECTIVE DATA)*

Vital signs: BP 122/80, pulse 88, respirations 18, temperature 37.7° C (99.9° F).

Skin: Turgor somewhat diminished.

Abdomen:

  Inspection: Flat no visible masses, pulsations, or peristalsis.

  Auscultation: Hyperactive bowel sounds in all four quadrants.

  Percussion: Tympany in all four quadrants.

  Palpation: Tenderness over epigastric area; slight tenderness in all four quadrants; no masses or organomegaly; no costovertebral angle tenderness; negative Murphy's sign, negative McBurney's sign.

Rectal examination: stool negative for occult blood.

diagnoses

HEALTH PROBLEM

Acute gastroenteritis; rule out food poisoning

NURSING DIAGNOSES

Pain related to irritation of gastric mucosa

Defining Characteristics

- Subjective communication of pain
- Grimacing of face when abdomen palpated
- Guarding behavior of upper abdomen

Altered nutrition: less than body requirement related to nausea, vomiting, and pain

Defining Characteristics

- Abdominal pain
- Aversion to eating at present time
- Lack of interest in food at present time

Diarrhea related to irritation of gastric mucosa

Defining Characteristics

- Abdominal pain
- Cramping
- Increased frequency of bowel movements
- Increased frequency of bowel sounds

Musculoskeletal System

■ PURPOSE OF EXAMINATION

The purpose of the musculoskeletal examination is to perform a systematic functional assessment of the musculoskeletal system as it relates to activities of daily living and detection of common dysfunctions.

The musculoskeletal system provides support for the body, protection for the internal organs, mobility to engage in physical activities, production of red blood cells, and storage of minerals. It includes bones, muscles, ligaments, tendons, cartilage, and joints. Because the central nervous system coordinates muscle and bone function, understanding how these two systems interrelate is important. The neurological examination is detailed in Chapter 19.

Musculoskeletal concerns vary at different ages. Injuries, however, are the most common musculoskeletal disorders seen in clinical practice, particularly in children and young adults. Middle-aged and older adults (and, to a lesser degree, children) are also affected by inflammatory, degenerative, and rheumatic conditions. In addition, neurological problems may also affect the mus-

culoskeletal system. A particular symptom, such as difficulty walking, may be caused by a musculoskeletal injury or a cerebellar defect.

■ ANATOMY AND PHYSIOLOGY

Skeleton

The skeleton is made up of 206 bones that are shaped according to their function (Figure 18.1). Bones provide support, allowing the individual to stand erect. They protect the tissues and the internal organs (e.g., skull, rib cage, and pelvis). They assist movement in coordination with muscles and joints. Bones provide storage areas for minerals and serve as sites for the formation of red blood cells (hematopoiesis).

The appendicular skeleton consists of the bones of the shoulders, arms, legs, and pelvis. The axial skeleton is composed of the bones of the face, skull, auditory ossicles, hyoid bone, vertebrae, ribs, and sternum (Figures 18.2 and 18.3).

figure**18.1** Bones that compose the skeleton. *(From Mourad LA:* Orthopedic disorders, *St Louis, 1991, Mosby.)*

figure**18.2** Bones of the upper and lower extremities. *(From Mourad LA:* Orthopedic disorders, *St Louis, 1991, Mosby.)*

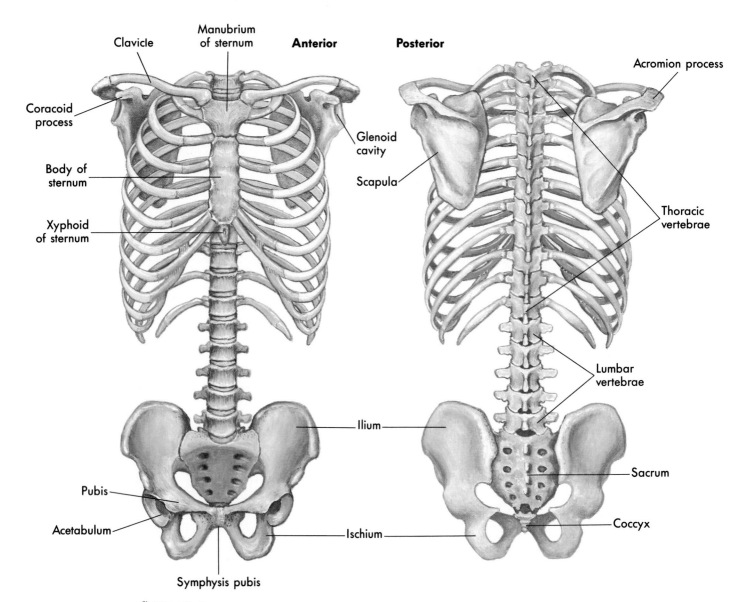

Clavicle

Manubrium
of sternum

Anterior

Posterior

Acromion process

Coracoid
process

Glenoid
cavity

Body of
sternum

Scapula

Xyphoid
of sternum

Thoracic
vertebrae

Lumbar
vertebrae

Ilium

Pubis

Sacrum

Acetabulum

Coccyx

Ischium

Symphysis pubis

figure**18.3** Bones of the trunk and pelvis. *(From Mourad LA:* Orthopedic disorders, *St Louis, 1991, Mosby.)*

Muscles

The musculoskeletal system is composed of more than 600 voluntary, or striated, muscles (Figure 18.4). It constitutes the principal organ of movement and is a repository for metabolites. There are three types of muscles: visceral (smooth, involuntary), cardiac, and skeletal (striated, voluntary). This discussion concerns only skeletal muscle. Skeletal muscle mass accounts for 40% to 45% of body weight. The partial contracture of skeletal muscle makes possible all the characteristic postures of human beings, including the upright position that distinguishes the anthropoid. Muscles are attached at each end to a bone, tendon, ligament, or fascia. The fixed end of the muscle is called the origin. The more movable end is known as the muscle insertion. Muscles are normally full and supple. Aging may bring a loss of muscle fiber and an increase in connective tissue that causes loss of muscle strength. Nutrition, exercise, gender, and genetic constitution account for variations in muscle strength among individuals.

Sternocleidomastoid
Trapezius
Pectoralis major
Deltoid
Serratus anterior
Biceps brachii
Internal oblique
Rectus abdominis
External oblique
Brachioradialis
Transversus abdominis
Flexor carpi radialis
Tensor of fascia lata
Iliopsoas
Sartorius
Pectineus
Adductor magnus
Adductor longus
Iliotibial tract
Gracilis
Vastus lateralis
Rectus femoris
Tendon of rectus femoris
Vastus lateralis
Patella
Patellar ligament
Peroneus longus
Tibialis anterior
Gastrocnemius
Extensor digitorum longus
Soleus

figure**18.4** Muscles of the body. **A,** Anterior view. (*From Thompson JM et al: Mosby's clinical nursing, ed 4, St Louis, 1997, Mosby.*)

continued

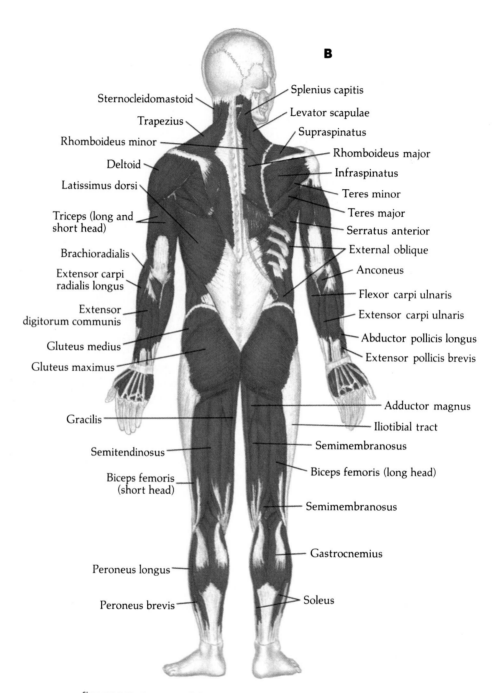

figure**18.4, cont'd** Muscles of the body. **B,** Posterior view.

Ligaments

Ligaments are strong, dense, flexible bands of connective tissue that join bones to one another. They may add strength and stability to a joint by encircling it, as with the hip joint, or they may hold on to the joint obliquely or lie parallel to the ends of bones across the joint, as with the knee joint (Figure 18.5). Ligaments allow movement in some directions and restrict movement in other directions. They may be injured by partial tears (sprains), or they may become detached from the bones (avulsion).

Tendons

Tendons are strong, dense bands of connective tissue at the end of muscles. They attach muscles to the periosteum, the fibrous membrane that covers the bone (Figure 18.5). Tendons enable bones to move when skeletal muscles contract. They are capable of transmitting great force from the contractile muscles to the bone or cartilage without being injured themselves. Most tendons are small (2 to 3 cm in length). The

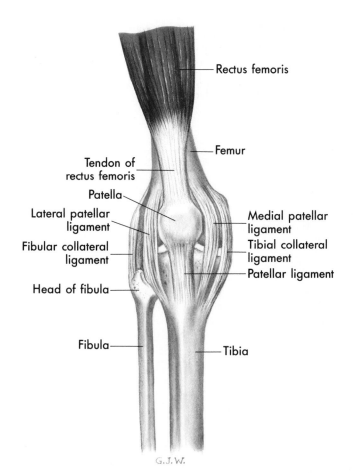

figure **18.5** Ligaments and tendons of the knee joint. *(From Mourad LA:* Orthopedic disorders, *St Louis, 1991, Mosby.)*

Labels on figure:
- Rectus femoris
- Femur
- Tendon of rectus femoris
- Patella
- Lateral patellar ligament
- Medial patellar ligament
- Fibular collateral ligament
- Tibial collateral ligament
- Head of fibula
- Patellar ligament
- Fibula
- Tibia
- G.J.W.

Achilles tendon is the longest and largest in the body (10 to 14 cm long).

Cartilage

Cartilage is a semismooth layer of elastic, gel-like supporting tissue found at the ends of bones. It forms a cap over the ends of bones to protect and support the bone during weight-bearing activities. The outer layer of cartilage is avascular and receives its nourishment from synovial fluids forced into it during movement and weight-bearing activity. Cartilage must have weight-bearing activity and joint movement to remain healthy. It may fray or wear unevenly if joints are abnormally shaped or unstable.

Joints

Joints are locations where two surfaces of bone come together or where two bones are joined to each other. There are three types of joints, classified by their degree of movement and the material that separates them. Synarthrotic joints are immovable. This type of joint separates bones with a thin layer of cartilage. An example is the cranial suture. Amphiarthrotic joints are slightly movable and separate bones with cartilage, such as the symphysis pubis or the manubriosternal joint, or with a fibrocartilaginous disk, such as the joints between the vertebral bodies (Figure 18.6, *A*). Diarthrotic joints are freely movable. They are lined with a synovial membrane that secretes a lubricating synovial fluid. Diarthrotic joints, which are frequently called synovial joints, include the ankle, wrist, knee, hip, or shoulder joints. Most joints are freely movable, or synovial, joints. These joints are supported by a casing that surrounds them, called the joint capsule. Ligaments also add strength by encasing the capsule (Figure 18.6, *B*).

Range of Motion

The degree of movement of a joint is called its range of motion. Diarthrotic, or freely movable, joints are the only joints that have one or more ranges of motion (Figure 18.7). Seven types of joint motion have been defined as follows:

Flexion is the bending forward of the joint to decrease the angle between the bones that it connects.

Extension is the straightening of a limb to increase the joint angle.

Abduction is the movement of a limb away from the midline of the body.

Adduction is the movement of a limb toward the central axis of the body or beyond it.

Internal rotation is the turning of the body part inward toward the central axis of the body.

External rotation is the turning of the body part away from the midline.

A   **B**

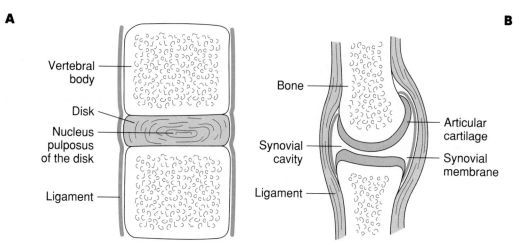

figure **18.6**   Structure of a joint. **A,** Intervertebral joint. **B,** Synovial joint.

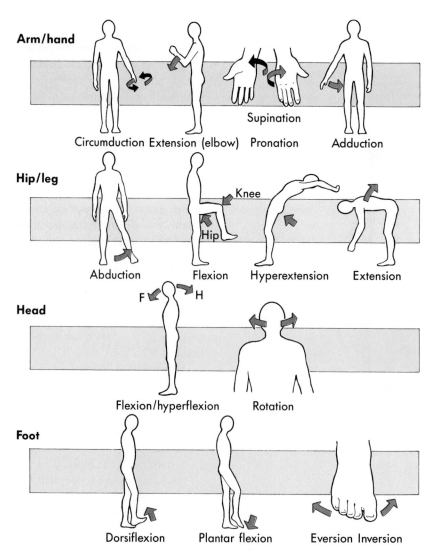

figure **18.7**   Body movements provided by synovial (diathrotic) joints. *(From Mourad LA:* Orthopedic disorders, *St Louis, 1991, Mosby.)*

Circumduction is the movement of a body part in a circular pattern. It is not a singular motion but a combination of motions.

Muscles are categorized according to the type of joint movement produced by their contraction. Therefore they are called flexors, extensors, adductors, abductors, internal rotators, external rotators, or circumflexors. Muscles shorten on contraction and in so doing exert pull on the bones to which they are attached. This action moves them closer together. Most muscles attach to two bones that articulate at an intervening joint. Generally, one bone moves while the other is held stable. This effect is caused by simultaneous shortening of other muscles. The body of the muscle that produces movement of an extremity generally lies proximal to the bone that is moved.

■ EXAMINATION

Health History

The health history for the musculoskeletal system includes information about the client's current concerns, general health, and specific lifestyle factors that may affect his or her physical condition. Lifestyle factors include information about employment, activity level, and any recent or past injuries. Common complaints include pain, loss of mobility, deformity, swelling, inflammation, and weakness. The client's chief complaint may indicate the direction for emphasis in the physical assessment. The individual with a chief complaint of body deformity, paralysis, weakness, or pain associated with movement causes the examiner to focus attention on the bones, joints, and muscles as the possible sites of disorder.

Pain assessment

Pain is the symptom that most frequently causes the client to seek help. In the assessment of musculoskeletal pain, there is particular information from the symptom analysis format that can provide a clearer picture of the cause of the pain (see Chapter 3: The Health History).

Character. Understanding the character of the pain may be helpful in determining its cause and in guiding the physical assessment of the involved joints.

Precipitating events. The client should be encouraged to try to recall those events that occurred before the onset of pain. Most individuals tend to forget minor injuries or unusual physical activity in the weeks before the pain began. The client also is unlikely to correlate symptoms and signs of infection in the preceding months with current joint pain.

Onset. The nature of the onset of pain also needs to be determined. For example, rheumatoid symptoms begin gradually, whereas gout-related attacks are characterized by sudden onset that frequently awakens the client from sleep.

Location. A client frequently has difficulty in localizing the pain associated with joint disease. The client's description may involve large areas of the body (e.g., "my neck" [while moving the hand from the head to the thoracic vertebra], "my back," or "all down my arm"). This difficulty in localizing the pain may be related to whether the pain is deep or superficial and whether a nerve is involved.

The location or distribution of the pain will provide valuable information. Rheumatoid involvement is migratory (i.e., involving first one joint, which improves, then another). On the other hand, most infectious arthritis is confined to one joint. The joint involvement in rheumatoid arthritis tends to be symmetrical, whereas that of gout, psoriatic arthritis, and Reiter's syndrome tends to occur initially in one or two joints but becomes polyarticular in the later stages. Spondylitis is first detected in the spine and then spreads to peripheral joints (centrifugal spread), whereas rheumatoid arthritis starts peripherally in the hands and feet and then involves the large joints of the hips, shoulders, and spine in the later stages of the disease (centripetal spread).

Timing. The time that pain occurs may also be diagnostic. The individual with osteoarthritis generally reports that the pain is worsened by increased use of the affected joint; therefore the affected person frequently has pain later in the day or when tired. The individual with rheumatoid arthritis generally reports that stiffness and pain occur early in the morning and notes some improvement after exercising the part.

Referred pain. Ask the client to describe any referred pain. Individuals frequently feel spinal nerve root involvement in peripheral tissues. For instance, the client may experience lumbosacral nerve root irritation (sciatica) as pain in the thigh or the knee on the involved side. The area of referred pain corresponds with the segmental innervation of the structures. The description of this type of pain may include words associated with paresthesias, such as "prickling," "like an electric shock," "pins and needles," and "numbing." The client may describe pain of muscle origin as "pulled" or "charley horse." Joint pain descriptions may range along a spectrum from dull, aching, or stiff to excruciating and intolerable.

Alleviating factors. Note also those measures that are known to alleviate the pain (e.g., exercise for rheumatoid arthritis and rest for osteoarthritis).

Present health status

1. Chief complaint: Concern(s) client wants to deal with at this time
2. Current and previous employment: Risk of accidental injury, lifting, repetitive motion activities, safety precautions
3. Activities of daily living: Ability to perform personal care (bathing, dressing, grooming, eating, elimina-

tion), household tasks, walking, shopping, communication

4. Exercise: Walking, specific regimen of exercise or sports activity (type, frequency, duration, special equipment, safety measures), overall conditioning
5. Weight: Recent changes, overweight or underweight
6. Nutrition: Calcium and vitamin D intake
7. Cigarette smoking (number of packs/day/number of years)
8. Alcohol intake
9. Medications: Calcium supplements, nonsteroidal anti-inflammatory agents, muscle relaxants, hormone replacement therapy

Specific complaints

1. Joint
   a. Character: Which joint(s) affected, number of joints involved, pain or ache, stiffness or limitation of movement, redness, increased warmth, or swelling
   b. Onset: Specific date of first episode (or age when it occurred), sudden or gradual
   c. Duration: Length of episode
   d. Frequency: Change in pattern, similar episodes in the past
   e. Precipitating factors: Specific movements, prolonged activity, rest, injury, weather, time of day, specific foods, medications (e.g., diuretics), alcohol intake
   f. Alleviating factors: Rest, movement
   g. Associated symptoms: Fever, weight loss, fatigue, malaise, rash, chronic diarrhea
   h. Efforts to treat and their effectiveness: Medications, heat and/or ice, exercise, weight reduction, splints, home remedies
2. Skeletal
   a. Character: Pain associated with particular movement or weight bearing; localized tenderness; swelling crepitus; limping; numbness; tingling or pressure; deformity or change in skeletal contour
   b. Onset: Specific date, sudden or gradual
   c. Duration: Length of episode
   d. Frequency: Change in pattern, similar episodes in the past
   e. Precipitating factors: Injury, sudden movement, repetitive movement, stress
   f. Alleviating factor: Rest
   g. Associated symptoms or conditions: Fever, weight loss, fatigue, malaise, past history of cancer, circulatory problems
   h. Efforts to treat and their effectiveness: Medications, heat and/or ice, exercise, weight reduction, splints, home remedies
3. Muscular
   a. Character: Localized or generalized pain, weak-

ness, limitation of movement, paralysis, spasms, wasting, tremor
   b. Onset: Specific date, sudden or gradual
   c. Duration: Length of episode
   d. Frequency: Change in pattern; similar episodes in the past
   e. Precipitating factors: Injury, muscle contraction, sudden movement, repetitive movement, stress
   f. Alleviating factor: Rest
   g. Associated symptoms or conditions: Fever, malaise
   h. Efforts to treat and their effectiveness: Medications, heat and/or ice, exercise, weight reduction, splints, home remedies
4. Injury
   a. Mechanism of injury: What happened—direct trauma, overuse, overstretching, fall
   b. Character: Location of pain; any noise with injury (popping, click, tearing); numbness; tingling; loss of sensation, strength, or mobility; warmth or coldness; swelling (immediate or gradual)
   c. Onset: Sudden, gradual
   d. Duration: Length of episode
   e. Frequency: Similar episodes in the past

RISK FACTORS   **OSTEOARTHRITIS**

Age over 50
Family history of osteoarthritis
Obesity
Joint abnormality
History of trauma, rheumatoid arthritis, or other degenerative process

---

RISK FACTORS   **OSTEOPOROSIS**

Advanced age
Gender (female)
Family history of osteoporosis
Estrogen deficiency due to menopause, surgical removal of the ovaries, or anorexia accompanied by amenorrhea
Small stature
Race (white)
Northern European descent
Heavy cigarette and/or alcohol use
Poor diet with low calcium intake
Periods of immobilization
Use of steroids
Sedentary lifestyle

f. Precipitating factors: Sudden movement, repetitive movement, stress
g. Alleviating factors: Rest, position of comfort
h. Associated symptoms or conditions: Loss of consciousness, other injuries
i. Efforts to treat and their effectiveness: Medications, heat and/or ice, splints, immobilization, home remedies

Past health history

1. Previous occurrences of the problem and their resolution
2. Past history of trauma to bones, joints, nerves or soft tissue, residual problems, or infections
3. Orthopedic surgery
4. Congenital deformities
5. Chronic illnesses: Arthritis, osteoporosis, cancer, renal or neurological problems

Family history

1. Arthritis: Osteoarthritis, rheumatoid, gout, ankylosing spondylitis
2. Congenital hip or foot disorders
3. Scoliosis or back problems

PREPARATION FOR EXAMINATION

EQUIPMENT

Item	Purpose
Nonstretchable tape measure	To measure length of extremities and limb circumference
Goniometer	To measure joint range of motion

CLIENT AND ENVIRONMENT

1. Provide a warm room with adequate lighting.
2. Protect the client's sense of modesty while exposing as fully as possible the areas to be examined.
3. Explain each procedure before beginning to perform it.
4. Use short, clear instructions.
5. Arrange for extra examination time for older or debilitated clients.
6. Stabilize the joints by having the client sit or lie down.
7. Properly sequence the examination to minimize position changes from sitting to lying.
8. If there is pain, always examine the unaffected side first.

Preparation for Examination: Client and Environment

Thorough assessment of the musculoskeletal system requires appropriate exposure of the client. Have the ambulatory individual wear shorts or underwear, which will allow the extremities and the spine to be available for examination. Allow the female client to wear a bra or some other abbreviated form of chest cover. Make an effort to protect the client's sense of modesty, but recognize that you cannot accurately examine a fully clothed client.

For each examination, position the client in a way that provides the greatest stability for the joints.

Technique for Examination and Normal Findings

The examination of neuromuscular coordination begins when you first meet and observe the client. It continues as the client advances into the room, sits, rises from a sitting position, climbs onto the examining table, lies down, and rolls over. Note the client's speed, coordination, and strength of motion. In particular, note any clumsy, awkward, or involuntary movements and tremor or fasciculation. Assess the client's handshake to gain an estimate of muscle strength.

Explore musculoskeletal structure and function through inspection and palpation of the joints and muscles, assessment of active and passive ranges of motion, and tests for muscle strength.

Use the cephalocaudal (head-to-toe) organization for examination of the bones, joints, and muscles. This organization provides order and helps avoid omissions. Use side-to-side comparison as the basic criterion for assessment. When injury or discomfort is involved, examine the unaffected side first.

Inspection

General inspection of the musculoskeletal system includes a visual scanning for symmetry, contour, size, involuntary movement of the two sides of the body (tremors or fasciculations), gross deformities, areas of swelling or edema, and ecchymoses or other discoloration (Figure 18.8). Inspect the muscles for symmetry of size and contour. Measure asymmetry, noted as hypertrophy or atrophy, for verification.

Examine the posture, or stance, and body alignment from both in front of and behind the client. Note the structural relationships of the feet to the legs and the hips to the pelvis. For the upper extremities, compare the shoulder girdle and the upper trunk.

A deformity is an abnormality in appearance. *Varus* and *valgus* are terms used to describe an angular deviation from the normal structure of an extremity. The reference point is the midline of the body. Genu varum

A   B   C

figure **18.8**   Inspection of overall body posture for symmetry of contour and size, gross deformities, swelling, and alignment of extremities. **A,** Anterior view. **B,** Posterior view. **C,** Lateral view.

(bowleg) is the lateral deviation of the leg from the midline (Figure 18.9). Genu valgum (knock-knee) is deviation of the leg toward the midline (Figure 18.10).

Palpation

Palpate all joints, bones, and associated muscles. Palpate joints for the presence of tenderness, swelling, increased temperature, and crepitation. Gently palpate painful and tender joints and always examine the pain-free side first. Palpate muscles to detect swelling, localized temperature changes, tone, and marked changes in shape. Note the consistency or tone of the muscle on palpation.

Measurement of extremities

The musculoskeletal examination frequently includes measurement of the extremities for length and circumference. Take length measurements to verify the symmetry of two limbs or to determine whether the limbs are in the normal range. Take measurements with the client lying relaxed on a hard surface (examining table)

with the pelvis level and the hips and knees fully extended and with both hips equally adducted. Frequently, apparent discrepancies in limb size are a result of position.

The length of the upper extremity is the distance from the tip of the acromion process to the tip of the middle finger; the shoulder is adducted, and the other joints are at neutral zero (anatomical position: limb in extension). The length of the lower extremity is the distance from the lower edge of the anterosuperior iliac spine to the tibial malleolus (Table 18.1).

Measurement of muscle mass

Examine the muscles for gross hypertrophy or atrophy. Only in the markedly obese client are changes in muscle mass difficult to assess. The difference between the firm, hypertrophic muscle of the athlete and the limp, atrophic muscle of the paralytic is obvious both on inspection and on palpation with the finger. Although muscle size is largely a function of use or disuse of the muscle fibers, changes in the size of muscles may indi-

Normal   Genus varus deformity

figure**18.9**   Varus deformity of the leg: lateral deviation from the midline (bowleg).

Normal   Genus valgus deformity

figure**18.10**   Valgus deformity of the leg: deviation of the leg toward the midline (knock-knee).

cate disease. Malnutrition and lipodystrophy tend to reduce muscle size and markedly weaken the strength of contraction. Lack of neural input resulting from lesions of the spinal cord or the peripheral motor neuron may reduce muscle size by as much as 75% of the normal volume. Such a decrease may occur over as short a time as 3 months. Measuring limbs at their maximal circumference may provide a baseline for comparison when swelling or atrophy is suspected on subsequent routine examination.

Make sure that the limbs are in the same position and the muscles are in the same state of tension each time you take measurements. Several corresponding points may be measured above and below the patella and the olecranon process. To provide uniformity, some clinics routinely measure at 10 cm below and at points 10 and 20 cm above the middle patella. Regardless of the points you select, draw a small diagram showing the points measured (Figure 18.11) in order to ensure consistency in future measures. Differences in symmetry or variations in limb size of less than 1 cm, noted at different times, are not significant (Figure 18.12). The dominant side is usually slightly larger than the nondominant side.

Measurement of range of joint motion

A standardized method for measuring and recording joint motion has been published by the American Academy of Orthopaedic Surgeons (1965). This method describes the range of motion in degrees of deviation from

figure**18.11**   The sites at which a limb is measured are carefully noted to establish accurate location for future comparative measurements.

table 18.1	Anatomical Guideposts for Measuring Extremities	
Area	**From**	**To**
Entire upper extremity	Tip of acromion process	Tip of middle finger
Upper arm	Tip of acromion process	Tip of olecranon process
Forearm	Tip of olecranon process	Styloid process of ulna
Entire lower extremity	Lower edge of anterosuperior iliac spine	Tibial malleolus
Thigh	Lower edge of anterosuperior iliac spine	Medial aspect of knee joint
Lower leg	Medial aspect of knee	Tibial malleolus

figure**18.12**   **A,** Measurement of upper midarm circumference. **B,** Measurement of midgastrocnemius circumference.

a defined neutral zero point for each joint. The position of neutral zero is that of the extended extremity or the anatomical position.

Goniometry and *arthrometry* are terms that describe the measurement of joint motion. It is important to learn to use the goniometer to measure the range of motion and to communicate findings to other health team professionals.

The two arms of the goniometer are a protractor and a pointer that are joined at the zero point of the protractor (Figure 18.13). The hinge should provide sufficient friction so that the instrument remains in position when you pick it up to read it after placing it against the joint. You should be able to read the scale easily from a distance of 18 inches. Some goniometers have full-circle scales, whereas others have half-circle scales. For the sake of portability, the length of the arms is generally about 6 inches.

Describe range of motion as active when the client moves the joint and as passive when you provide the motion.

Active motion. In active range of motion, the joint movement is smooth and painless through its complete range and generally indicates the absence of any advanced lesion. Less muscle tension and joint compression are produced by the voluntary movement of the joints through their range of motion than when the joints are moved against resistance, as in the strength tests. Therefore range of active motion should be assessed before muscle strength because the more marked

contraction may induce pain in the client, which may skew the test results.

If the active range of motion of a given joint is less than the passive range of motion, further investigation should focus on true weakness, joint stability, pain, malingering, or hysterical weakness as possible causes.

Passive motion. Move the relaxed joint through the limits of its movement. When the range of motion is limited, explore further to determine whether (1) excess fluid is within the joint; (2) loose bodies, such as pieces of cartilage, are present in the joint; or (3) joint surface irregularity or contracture of the muscle, ligaments, or capsule exists. Moving the joint through the range of its motion may also reveal hypermobility of the joint. In such a situation, further examination should be directed toward differentiating among (1) a connective tissue disruption, such as the relaxation of the ligaments that occurs in Marfan's syndrome; (2) a ligamentous tear; and (3) an intraarticular fracture. An example of how this information might aid in diagnosis is a joint that can be flexed to a smaller angle with passive movement than with active flexion. Such a finding probably indicates a problem related to the musculature rather than a problem within the joint that causes a block in the flexion.

Recording range of motion. The box on p. 460 summarizes joint movements and the maximal expected angles of movement. Record limited joint movement from the angle of the starting position to the maximal angle reached during movement (i.e., from 20 degrees to 50 degrees).

Screening Examination

Assessment of the full range of motion may not be part of the screening examination unless the history or other parts of the physical examination indicate that muscular or neural dysfunction is a possible problem for the client. Note that movement of the neck and the trunk may be examined by functional groups, rather than by individual joints, to determine joint range of motion and muscle strength.

In the screening examination, carry joints actively through the ranges of motion and describe the results as full range of motion. In joints that do not exhibit full range of motion, measure with the goniometer and record the results. Expect limitations in full range of motion in older individuals.

Examination of bones, joints, and muscles

Bones. Examine bones for deformity and tumors. Also examine bones for integrity by testing resistance to a deforming force. Palpate the bone to assess the presence of pain or tenderness. Tenderness of a bone may indicate tumor, inflammation, or the aftermath of a trauma. Frequently, traumatic injuries are associated

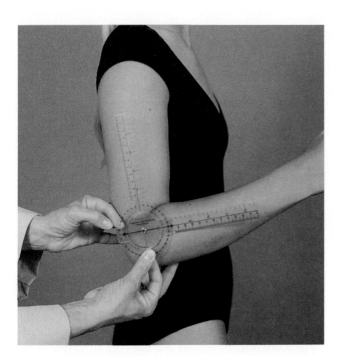

figure**18.13** Use of a goniometer to measure range of motion of a joint.

Recording Range of Motion in Degrees

CERVICAL SPINE			FINGERS		
Flexion		45	Flexion—distal interphalangeal joint		90
Extension		50	Flexion—proximal interphalangeal joint		100
Rotation (right)		70	Flexion—metacarpophalangeal joint		90
Rotation (left)		70	Extension—metacarpophalangeal joint		45
Lateral bending (right)		40	Hyperextension—distal interphalangeal joint		10
Lateral bending (left)		40	Abduction (measure from tips of fingers)		Varies
SPINE			Adduction		Varies
Forward flexion (C7 to S1 = 4 in)		70	**HIP**		
Extension (standing)		30	Flexion (knees bent)		110-120
Extension (lying)		20	Extension		30
Rotation (right)		45	Abduction		45
Rotation (left)		45	Adduction		30
Lateral bending (right)		35	Internal rotation (hip and knee flexed)		40
Lateral bending (left)		35	External rotation (hip and knee flexed)		45
SHOULDER			**KNEE**		
Forward flexion		180	Flexion-extension		135
Backward extension		60	Hyperextension		10
Horizontal flexion		130-135	**ANKLE**		
Horizontal extension		40	Dorsiflexion		20
Abduction		180	Plantar flexion		50
Adduction		50	Inversion hind foot (passive)		5
Internal rotation		90	Eversion hind foot (passive)		5
External rotation		90	Inversion		30
ELBOW			Eversion		20
Flexion-extension		150	Abduction forefoot (passive)		10
Hyperextension		0-15	Adduction forefoot (passive)		20
FOREARM (ELBOW AND WRIST)			**GREAT TOE**		
Pronation		80-90	Flexion—metatarsophalangeal joint		45
Supination		80-90	Extension—metatarsophalangeal joint		70
WRIST			Flexion—interphalangeal joint (passive)		90
Extension		80	**LATERAL FOUR TOES**		
Flexion		70	Flexion—distal interphalangeal joint		60
Radial deviation		20	Extension—distal interphalangeal joint		30
Ulnar deviation		30	Flexion—proximal interphalangeal joint		35
THUMB			Flexion—metatarsophalangeal joint		40
Abduction		50	Extension—metatarsophalangeal joint		40
Flexion—interphalangeal joint		80	Abduction		Varies
Flexion—metacarpophalangeal joint		50	Adduction		Varies
Flexion—carpometacarpal joint		15			
Opposition to tip or base of little finger					

with damage to both bone and nerve. Paralysis of the ulnar and median nerves in the hand is frequently the result of a hand injury and may produce a clawlike posture of the hand.

Joints

Signs and symptoms of disorders. Pain, tenderness, swelling, partial or complete loss of mobility, stiff-ness, weakness, and fatigue are the signs and symptoms most frequently associated with disorders of the joints. Joint disease may be indicated by skin that feels warm, is red, has lesions, or is ulcerated. In psoriatic arthritis, skin lesions and pitting of the nails are involved in approximately 50% of cases. Pitting is the most commonly recognized change. Isolated pitting of a single nail may

occur or the pitting may be uniformly distributed across the nails.

Limitation of range of motion. The client may voluntarily limit the motion of a joint in response to pain. Spasm of the muscles involved in the movement of a joint may limit its motion. Mechanical obstruction to movement may accompany bony overgrowth and scar tissue. Limitation of motion in a joint is accompanied by weakness and atrophy of the muscles that are involved. Decreased range of motion occurs in joints in which there is inflammation of surrounding tissues, arthritis, fibrosis, or bony fixation (ankylosis).

Deformity. Deformities of the joint include absorption of tissues, flexion contracture, and bony overgrowth. Absorption may produce a flail joint, which makes the joint move erratically. Deformities result from scarring phenomena following inflammation and infection.

Swelling. The amount of swelling of the joint may range from difficult to detect to visually evident fluid within the joint (i.e., visible or palpable as a bulging of the joint capsule). Pressure on the sac at one point causes the fluid within it to shift and may lead to bulging at another site. The sac may vary from soft to tense, and the involvement may be symmetrical or unilateral. Frequently, the swelling is fusiform. Redness, warmth, swelling, and pain in a joint are the classic descriptors of an inflammatory process. The inflammation may be within the joint itself or in the soft tissue surrounding it. Swelling may also result from intraarticular effusion, synovial thickening, or bony overgrowth. In addition, swelling may result from the deposition of fat in the region adjacent to the joint. The synovial membrane is not palpable in normal joints. The palpation of a "boggy" or "doughy" consistency generally indicates a thickened or otherwise abnormal synovial membrane.

Tenderness. Injury and inflammatory processes cause joints to be tender. Arthritis, tendonitis, bursitis, and osteomyelitis are associated with tenderness in and around a joint. Therefore it is important to attempt to determine the anatomical structure that is tender.

Increased temperature. Heat noted over a joint indicates inflammation and suggests rheumatoid or septic arthritis. Compare symmetrical joints for temperature when one joint is hot. Use the backs of the fingers when comparing temperature.

Redness. Vasodilation or inflammation occurs in the skin overlying a tender joint that is affected by septic arthritis and gouty arthritis.

Crepitation. Crepitation (crackling or grating sounds) produced by motion of the joint is caused by irregularities of the articulating surfaces. The coarseness of the surface may involve the cartilage or the bony capsule.

Inspection and palpation. Either make a systematic assessment of individual joints during the performance of the head-to-toe physical examination, or examine all the joints at a preselected time during the examination. As with all bilateral structures, compare the paired joints.

The sequence for performing the examination of the joints is inspection, palpation, active range of motion, passive range of motion, and muscle strength testing. Use this sequence in a coordinated examination of each joint.

Begin the assessment with inspection of the joint for swelling, redness, deformity, subcutaneous nodules, or tumors. Let the presence of any observed abnormalities guide you in palpation. Palpate joints for the presence of pain with movement, tenderness, swelling, increased temperature, and crepitation. Palpate painful and tender joints lightly.

Give special consideration to the temporomandibular, sternoclavicular, manubriosternal, shoulder, elbow, wrist, hip, knee, and ankle joints.

Recording joint problems. To conveniently summarize the results of examination of the joints, circle the joint involved on a diagram (Figure 18.14) and briefly note any pathological condition.

Muscles. Examine muscles in symmetrical pairs (i.e., first one and then the other) for equivalence in size, contour, tone, and strength. Position the contralateral, matching muscle pairs uniformly while you examine them. Examine the muscles both at rest and in a state of contraction.

The assessment sequence is inspection, palpation, and testing of muscle strength. You may incorporate the examination of functional muscle groups into the examination of the joints.

Inspection and palpation. Inspect the muscles for symmetry of size and contour. Measure asymmetry, noted as hypertrophy or atrophy, for verification.

Use palpation to detect swelling, localized temperature changes, and marked changes in shape. Note the consistency of the muscle on palpation.

Muscle tone is the tension present in the resting muscle. You will also notice it in the slight resistance you feel when you passively move the relaxed limb. While palpating the muscle, be alert to fasciculations, which are involuntary contractions or twitching of groups of muscle fibers.

Ask the client to tell you of any sensation while you feel the muscles and tendons. Then record the client's descriptions of pain or tenderness on palpation.

Tendon stretch reflexes, included as part of the neurological assessment discussed in Chapter 19, are generally altered in muscle disease, especially if the peripheral nerves are involved. For instance, the tendon reflexes are diminished in muscular dystrophy and polymyositis in proportion to the loss of muscle strength. A length-

ened reflex cycle is characteristic of hypothyroidism, whereas a shortened period indicates the hypermetabolic state.

Recording muscle strength. Examiners frequently use the criteria in Table 18.2 for recording the grading of muscle strength.

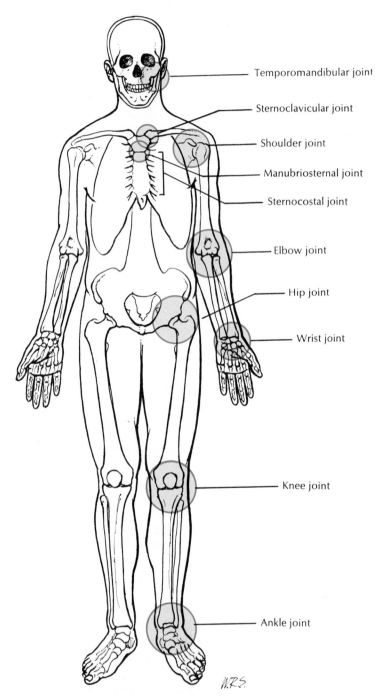

Temporomandibular joint

Sternoclavicular joint

Shoulder joint

Manubriosternal joint

Sternocostal joint

Elbow joint

Hip joint

Wrist joint

Knee joint

Ankle joint

figure**18.14** Results of the examination of joints may be summarized by circling on a diagram the joints involved and briefly noting the pathological condition.

Some examiners prefer to use simple descriptive words such as *paralysis, severe weakness, moderate weakness, minimum weakness,* and *normal.* Disability is considered to exist if (1) the muscle strength is less than grade 3; (2) external support may be required to make the involved part functional; and (3) activity of the part cannot be achieved in a gravity field.

Muscle strength is expected to be greater in the dominant arm and leg. Movements should be coordinated and painless.

The examiner performs only a musculoskeletal screening test unless he or she suspects a musculoskeletal problem.

Screening test for muscle strength. Muscle weakness in adults is generally mild and transitory. However, it may be the outcome of musculoskeletal, neurological, metabolic, or infectious problems. Therefore an evaluation is necessary.

Although you can assess muscle strength throughout the full range of motion for each muscle or group of muscles, there are several simple screening tests that will allow you to find muscle or reflex abnormalities. One brief but effective approach is to observe the client carefully as he or she walks into the examining room and undresses. Watch for cues to neurological and motion deficit. This approach may also help you ascertain whether physical evidence can verify the chief complaint.

table**18.2**	*Criteria for Grading and Recording Muscle Strength*		
Functional level	**Lovett scale**	**Grade**	**Percent of normal**
No evidence of contractility	Zero (0)	0	0
Evidence of slight contractility	Trace (T)	1	10
Complete range of motion with gravity eliminated	Poor (P)	2	25
Complete range of motion with gravity	Fair (F)	3	50
Complete range of motion against gravity with some resistance	Good (G)	4	75
Complete range of motion against gravity with full resistance	Normal (N)	5	100

Table 18.3 gives an example of a formal screening examination.

The usual method of testing is manual and subjective. Place the client in the position that best allows movement through the full range. Apply resistance to the muscles. Grade the muscle contractions according to your judgment of the client's responses. The test allows for a systematic testing of muscle groups from head to toe.

Specific joints and muscles

Temporomandibular joint. The temporomandibular joint is the articulation between the mandible and the temporal bone (Figure 18.15). The joint is divided into two cavities as a fibrocartilaginous disk.

INSPECTION AND PALPATION. Swelling appears as a tumescence over the joint, but it must be considerable to be visible. Palpate the joint by placing the fingertips anterior to the external meatus of the ear. In the normal joint there is a depression over the joint. Swelling may make this indentation difficult to feel. Palpate the jaw while the client moves it through its range of motion.

RANGE OF MOTION. To test range of motion, ask the client to:
1. Open and close the mouth
2. Project the lower jaw (jutting of jaw)
3. Move the jaw from side to side (Figure 18.16)

The normal range of distance between the upper and lower incisors is 3 to 6 cm. Measure lateral motion of

---

table 18.3 *Screening Test for Muscle Strength*

Muscles tested	Client activity	Examiner activity	Muscles tested	Client activity	Examiner activity
Ocular musculature			Biceps	Flex arm	Pull to extend arm
Lids	Close eyes tightly	Attempt to resist closure	Triceps	Extend arm	Push to flex arm
Yoke muscles	Track object in six cardinal positions		Wrist musculature	Extend hand	Push to flex
				Flex hand	Push to extend
Facial musculature	Blow out cheeks	Assess pressure in cheeks with fingertips	Finger muscles	Extend fingers	Push dorsal surface of fingers
	Place tongue in cheek	Assess pressure in cheek with fingertips		Flex fingers	Push ventral surface of fingers
	Stick out tongue, move it to right and left	Observe strength and coordination of thrust and extension		Spread fingers	Hold fingers together
			Hip musculature	In supine position raise extended leg	Push down on leg above knee
Neck muscles	Extend head backward	Push head forward	Hamstring, gluteal, abductor, and adductor muscles of leg	Sit and perform alternate leg crossing	Push in opposite direction of crossing limb
	Flex head forward	Push head backward			
	Rotate head in full circle	Observe mobility, coordination	Quadriceps	Extend leg	Push to flex leg
	Touch shoulders with head	Observe range of motion	Hamstring	Bend knees to flex leg	Push to extend leg
Deltoid	Hold arms upward	Push down on arms	Ankle and foot muscle	Bend foot up (dorsiflexion)	Push to plantar flexion
				Bend foot down (plantar flexion)	Push to dorsiflexion
			Antigravity muscles	Walk on toes	
				Walk on heels	

figure**18.15** Temporomandibular joint. A fibrocartilaginous disk divides the articulation point into two synovial cavities. Note the proximity at this joint to the external acoustic meatus.

figure**18.16** Lateral motion is determined by asking the client to move the lower jaw from side to side. The distance measured is the amount that the midline of the lower lip deviates in each direction. The midline of the stationary upper lip may be used as the baseline.

figure**18.17** The sternoclavicular joint is divided into two synovial cavities. Movement of the shoulder girdle may cause pain when these joints are diseased. Manubriosternal joint examination is done largely by inspection and palpation, since these joints move minimally.

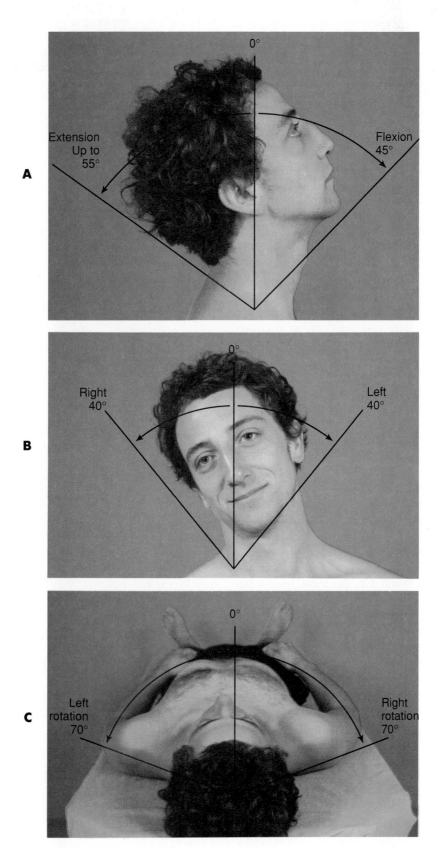

figure**18.18** Range of motion of the cervical spine. **A,** Flexion and hyperextension. **B,** Lateral bending. **C,** Rotation.

the jaw when the client projects the jaw and moves it from side to side. Measure the distance that the midline of the lower lip deviates in each direction. The normal range of motion is 1 to 2 cm. Audible "clicks" on movement may be heard and are considered normal.

MUSCLE STRENGTH. To test muscle strength, ask the client to:

1. Bite down hard while you palpate the masseter muscles.
2. Clench the teeth while you apply downward pressure on the chin.

These maneuvers also test the motor function of cranial nerve (CN) V.

Sternoclavicular joint. The sternoclavicular joint is located at the juncture of the clavicle and the manubrium of the sternum. This joint is divided into two synovial cavities by a disk of cartilage and fibrous material. The joint is reinforced by a fibrous capsule and ligaments (Figure 18.17). The obtuse angle formed by the junction of the manubrium and the body of the sternum, called the angle of Louis, is used as a landmark for counting the ribs.

INSPECTION. Inspection of this joint is easy because little tissue overlies it. Swelling, redness, bony overgrowth, and dislocation are not difficult to see. Swelling of the joint appears as a smooth, round bulge. Although this joint is often overlooked, it is frequently involved in problems following surgery of the neck.

PALPATION. Palpate the joint with your fingertips. Movements of the shoulder depend on the normal function of this joint. Inflammation of the sternoclavicular joint may result in pain on movement of the shoulder girdle.

Cervical spine. The cervical vertebrae are the most mobile of the spinal vertebrae. Flexion and extension occur between the skull and C1. Rotation occurs between C1 and C2.

INSPECTION. Inspect the neck from both an anterior and a posterior position for deformities or abnormal posture. Note the alignment of the head with the shoulders. The cervical spine should be straight with the head erect. The normal spinal curvature should be concave in the cervical area.

PALPATION. Palpate the spinous processes of the cervical spine, including the trapezius, paravertebral, and sternocleidomastoid muscles. There should be symmetry in size, good tone, and no tenderness or muscle spasm.

RANGE OF MOTION. To evaluate range of motion, ask the client to:

1. Touch the chin to the chest.
2. Extend the head backward as far as possible (Figure 18.18, *A*).
3. Bend the head laterally toward each shoulder (touch the ear to the shoulder without raising the shoulder) (Figure 18.18, *B*)

A

B

C

figure **18.19** Examining the strength of the sternocleidomastoid and trapezius muscles. **A,** Rotation against resistance. **B,** Flexion with palpation of the sternocleidomastoid muscle. **C,** Extension against resistance.

4. Rotate the head from side to side (pointing the chin toward each shoulder) (Figure 18.18, *C*)

MUSCLE STRENGTH. To evaluate muscle strength, ask the client to:

1. Push the cheek against your hand (right and left sides). This maneuver also tests the motor function of CN XI (sternocleidomastoid muscle) (Figure 18.19, *A*)
2. Push the forehead against your hand (Figure 18.19, *B*)
3. Push the head back against your hand (Figure 18.19, *C*)

Shoulders. The shoulder joint is a ball-and-socket joint that is the articulation of the humerus and the glenoid fossa of the scapula (Figure 18.20). The joint is protected by the muscles and the ligaments. A fibrous capsule surrounds the joint completely. Overlying these structures is the subacromial bursa. The portion of the bursa that lies beneath the deltoid is called the subdeltoid bursa. The clavicle and the acromion process of the scapula are articulated by the acromioclavicular joint.

INSPECTION. Inspect the shoulders, including the muscles and the acromioclavicular joint, with the client standing with his or her back to you. Look for equality of shoulder height, and contour and shape of the shoulders. Inspect the scapulae and related muscles. Inspection may reveal anterior dislocation of the shoulder as a flattening of its lateral aspect. Swelling of the joint resulting from fluid collection may be visible only when the amount of fluid is moderate to large. Visible swelling generally appears over the anterior aspect of the shoulder.

PALPATION. Palpate the joint and the bursal sites. Sites to palpate include the acromium process, clavicle, scapulae, acromioclavicular joint, greater tubercle of the humerus, sternoclavicular joint, biceps groove, and area muscles. If you suspect neoplasia or infection, palpate the axilla for lymph nodes. Give special attention to the tendons of the teres minor and infraspinatus muscles (rotator cuff). Palpate these tendons for swelling, nodes, tears, and pain.

RANGE OF MOTION. To test for range of motion, ask the client to (Figure 18.21):

1. Extend both arms forward (forward flexion).
2. Extend both arms backward (hyperextension).
3. Put the hands behind the back as if one were going to reach up to touch the shoulder blade (internal rotation).

figure**18.20**   Shoulder joint.

figure**18.21** Range of motion of the shoulder. **A,** Forward flexion and hyperextension. **B,** Abduction and adduction. **C,** Internal rotation. **D,** External rotation.

figure**18.22** Assessment of biceps muscle strength. The client flexes her arm while the examiner attempts to pull the arm into extension.

figure**18.23** Assessment of triceps muscle strength. The client attempts to extend her arm while the examiner tries to push the arm into a flexed position.

figure**18.24** Assessment of trapezius muscle strength. The client shrugs his shoulders while the examiner attempts to push them down.

4. Put the hands behind the head (external rotation).

MUSCLE STRENGTH. To test for muscle strength, ask the client to:

1. Hold the arms upward while you try to push them down (deltoid muscles).
2. Extend the arms and then try to flex them while you try to pull them into extension (biceps muscle) (Figure 18.22).
3. Flex the arms and then extend them while you attempt to push them into a flexed position (triceps muscle) (Figure 18.23).
4. Shrug the shoulders while you try to push down on them (CN XI, trapezius muscle) (Figure 18.24).

figure**18.25** Elbow joint (posterior view).

Humerus

Medial epicondyle

Olecranon

Coronoid process

Ulna

Olecranon bursa

Lateral epicondyle

Annular ligament

Radius

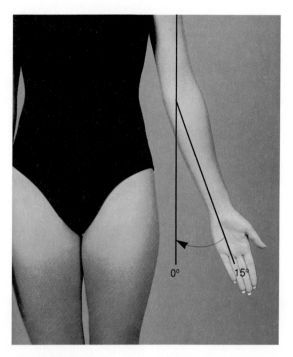

figure**18.26** The expected carrying angle of the arm is between 5 and 15 degrees in the adult.

0° 15°

A

B

figure**18.27** **A,** Examination of the extensor surface of the elbow with the client in the supine position. **B,** Examination of the extensor surface of the elbow joint with the client in the sitting position.

Elbow. The elbow is the articulation of the humerus, the radius, and the ulna (Figure 18.25). The three articulating surfaces are enclosed in a single synovial cavity. The synovial membrane is generally palpable only on the posterior aspect of the joint. Radial and ulnar ligaments provide protection to the joint. The olecranon bursa is the largest bursa of the elbow, although several smaller bursae are present. Swelling and redness are easily visible over the posterior aspect of the elbow.

INSPECTION. Inspect the size and contour of the elbow in flexion and extension. Note deviations in the carrying angle of the arm while the arm is passively extended with the palm facing forward (Figure 18.26). The carrying angle is between 5 and 15 degrees in adults. Variations in the carrying angle are cubitus valgus (forearm farther outward than the arm) and cubitus varus (forearm carried more inwardly). These variations can be caused by acute injury, posttraumatic arthritis, or other forms of arthritis.

PALPATION. With the client's arm flexed to approximately 70 degrees, palpate the elbow with the tips of the fingers while applying pressure on the opposite side of the joint with the thumb of the dominant hand. Support the arm with your other hand. Palpate the lateral and medial condyles, the olecranon process, and the grooves on either side of the olecranon process. Joint swelling is most often palpable in the medial groove (Figure 18.27).

RANGE OF MOTION. To test range of motion (Figure 18.28), ask the client to:

1. Bend and straighten the elbow.
2. Turn the hand face up (supination); face down (pronation).

MUSCLE STRENGTH. To test muscle strength, use the tests for the biceps and triceps muscles described in the section on shoulders.

Wrists, hands, and fingers. The wrist joint contains the points of articulation between the distal radius and the proximal portions of the following carpal bones: scaphoid (navicular), lunate, and triangular (Figure 18.29). An articular disk divides the radius from the ulnar bone and also separates the radius from the wrist joint. The wrist joint is protected by a fibrous capsule and ligaments. The joint is lined by synovial membrane.

INSPECTION. Inspect the wrist and the hands for position, contour, symmetry, smoothness, edema, atrophy or hypertrophy, and deformity. Swelling of the wrist joint most frequently appears on the dorsal surface distal to the ulnar tip. Swelling is easily visible over the dorsal surface of the hand because little tissue covers the joints.

figure**18.28** Range of motion of the elbow. **A,** Flexion and extension. **B,** Pronation and supination.

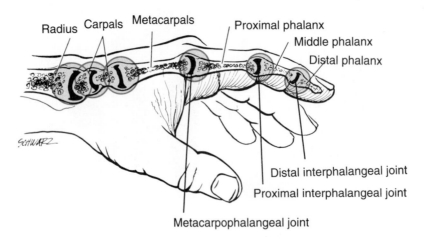

figure**18.29** Joints articulating the bones of the wrist and hand.

PALPATION. Use two hands for palpation of the wrist so that the thumbs and the index fingers are opposed on either side of the wrist. Apply enough pressure to outline bony and soft tissue structures. Palpate the joints between the carpal, metacarpal, and phalangeal bones. Use your thumbs and index fingers to palpate each of these joints (Figure 18.30).

RANGE OF MOTION. To test range of motion of the hands and wrist (Figure 18.31), ask the client to:

1. Spread the fingers apart and bring them back again.
2. Make a fist.
3. Touch the thumb to each fingertip and to the base of the little finger.
4. Bend the fingers up and down at the metacarpophalangeal joint.
5. Bend the hand up and down at the wrist.
6. With the palm facing down, turn the hand to the

A

B

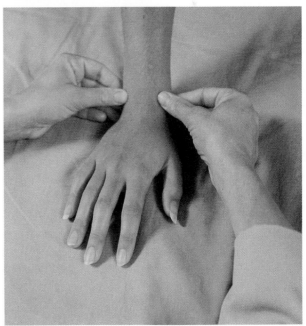

C

figure**18.30** Palpation of joints of the hand and wrist. **A,** Interphalangeal joints. **B,** Metacarpophalangeal joints. **C,** Radiocarpal groove and wrist.

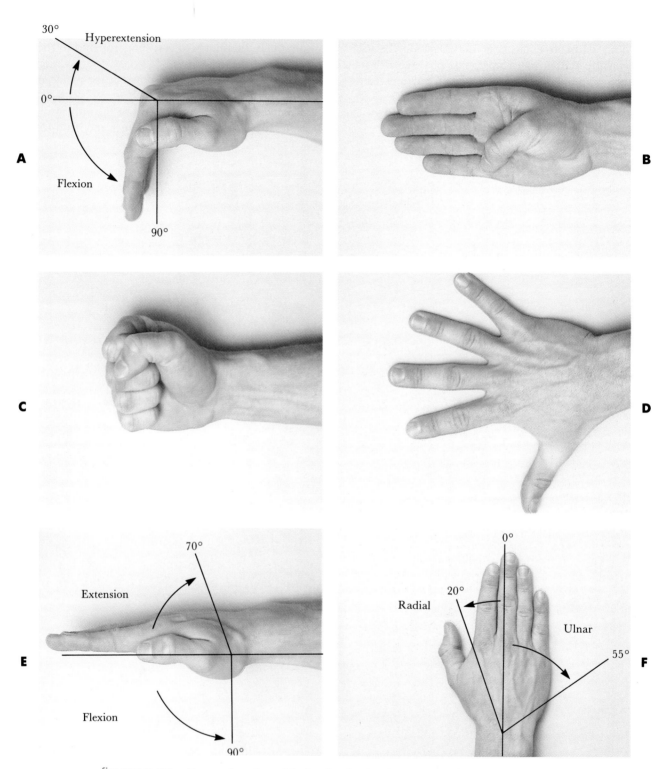

figure **18.31** Range of motion of the hand and wrist. **A,** Metacarpophalangeal flexion and hyperextension. **B,** Finger flexion: the thumb to each fingertip and to the base of the little finger. **C,** Finger flexion: fist formation. **D,** Finger abduction. **E,** Flexion and hyperextension of the wrist. **F,** Radial and ulnar movement of the wrist. *(From Seidel HM et al: Mosby's guide to physical examination, ed 3, St Louis, 1995, Mosby.)*

figure**18.32** To assess wrist strength, the client attempts to extend her wrist while the examiner tries to flex it.

figure**18.33** Assessment of grip strength.

right (radial deviation) and to the left (ulnar deviation).

MUSCLE STRENGTH. To assess wrist strength, ask the client to:

1. Maintain wrist flexion while you try to extend the wrist.
2. Try to extend the wrist as you try to flex it (Figure 18.32).

To assess grip strength, ask the client to squeeze your first two fingers as hard as he or she can (Figure 18.33). If you cross your fingers, you will not feel as much discomfort if the client is exceptionally strong.

To assess finger strength, ask the client to:

1. Extend the fingers while you push down on the dorsal surface.
2. Flex the fingers while you push up on the ventral surface.
3. Spread the fingers as far apart as possible while you try to push them together (Figure 18.34).
4. Push the fingers as close together as possible while you try to pull them apart.

SPECIAL TESTS. Many tendons cross the wrist and hands to their insertions on the fingers. Thickening of the flexor tendon sheath of the median nerve (seen in carpal tunnel syndrome) is a common problem. It may lead to feelings of numbness, burning, and paresthesia along the distribution of the median nerve. The thickness of the sheath may be visible on the palmar surface of the wrist. Two tests may elicit these altered sensory phenomena. In the first of these tests, Phalen's test, the client is asked to maintain palmar flexion for 1 minute (Figure 18.35). The experience of numbness and pares-

figure**18.34** Assessment of finger strength.

thesia over the palmar surface of the hand and the first three fingers and part of the fourth is called Phalen's sign. The symptoms resolve quickly after the hand returns to the resting position. The second test, Tinel's test, consists of tapping over the median nerve (palmar aspect of wrist). The client's sensation of tingling or prickling is known as Tinel's sign (Figure 18.36).

Hips. The hip joint is the articulation of the acetabulum and the femur (Figure 18.37). It is a ball-and-socket joint that is protected by a fibrous capsule and

ligaments. Three bursae reduce friction in the hip: (1) the trochanteric, between the posterolateral greater trochanter and the gluteus maximus; (2) the iliopectineal, between the anterior surface of the joint and the iliopsoas muscle; and (3) the ischiogluteal, situated over the ischial tuberosity.

INSPECTION. Inspect the hips anteriorly and posteriorly while the client stands. Look for symmetry in the iliac crest height, size of the buttocks, and number and level of gluteal folds. Inspection of the hip joint includes an assessment of gait. A smooth and even gait indicates equal leg length and functional hip motion. Antalgic limp is characteristic of disease that produces pain in a hip joint; the body tilts toward the involved diseased hip in such a way that the weight of the body is directly over the hip. This limp decreases the need for abductor muscle movement and thus may alleviate muscle spasm. If

figure**18.35** Phalen's test for carpal tunnel syndrome.

Flexor retinaculum

Carpal canal (sulcus carpi)

Median nerve

figure**18.36** Elicitation of Tinel's sign. *(From Seidel HM et al: Mosby's guide to physical examination, ed 3, St Louis, 1995, Mosby.)*

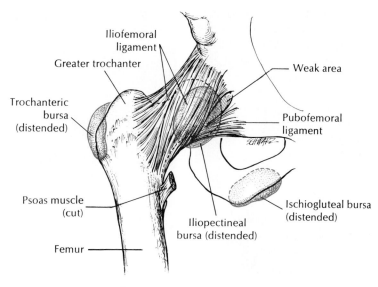

Iliofemoral
ligament

Greater trochanter

Trochanteric
bursa
(distended)

Weak area

Pubofemoral
ligament

Psoas muscle
(cut)

Ischiogluteal bursa
(distended)

Iliopectineal
bursa (distended)

Femur

figure**18.37** Hip joint.

the abductor muscles are weak (i.e., unable to support the pelvis), the unaffected hip may move downward in such a way that the weight is borne on that side. This condition is called Trendelenburg's limp.

PALPATION. With the client supine, palpate the hips and the pelvis for stability, tenderness, or crepitus. The bursae are not palpable unless they are swollen. Swelling and tenderness are the diagnostic findings of pathological conditions of these structures.

RANGE OF MOTION. To test range of motion of the hips (Figure 18.38), ask the client to do the following:

1. While supine:
   a. Raise the leg above the body with the knee extended.
   b. Bring the knee to the chest while keeping the other leg straight.
   c. Swing the leg laterally and medially while keeping the knee straight.
   d. Place the side of the foot on the opposite knee and move the flexed knee down toward the examining table (external rotation).
   e. Flex the knee and rotate the leg so that the flexed knee moves inward toward the opposite leg (internal rotation).
2. While either prone or standing, swing the straightened leg behind the body.

MUSCLE STRENGTH. To test muscle strength in the hips, place the client in a supine position. Then ask the client to:

1. Raise the extended leg while you attempt to hold it down.
2. Push both legs against your hands while your hands are placed on the bed on either side of the client's knees.

3. Bring both legs together while your hands are placed on the bed between the client's knees.

To assess muscle strength in the hamstring, gluteal, abductor, and adductor muscles, ask the client to sit and perform alternate leg crossing (Figure 18.39).

Knee. The knee joint is the articulation of the femur, the tibia, and the patella (Figure 18.40). The lining of the joint is a fibrous membrane. Synovial membrane covers the articular surface of the femur and the tibia with folds to the patella. The medial and lateral menisci are fibrocartilaginous disks whose outside edges (horns) are attached to the tibia and are continuous with the articular capsule. The medial convexity of the femur rotates with the inner portion of the meniscus that is attached to it. A spiral distortion of the menisci occurs on rotation, making these disks susceptible to rupture. The surfaces of the menisci have no synovial membrane. They are thought to aid the spread of synovial fluid, and this function may account for their existence. An anterior pouch in the knee joint that separates the patella and quadriceps tendon and muscle from the femur is called the suprapatellar pouch.

The bursae of the knee are numerous. On the anterior knee the prepatellar bursa lies immediately in front of the patella. The superficial infrapatellar bursa lies anterior to the patellar ligament, and the deep infrapatellar bursa is behind the ligament. The bursae of the posterior knee include the two gastrocnemius bursae. One separates the lateral head of the gastrocnemius muscle from the articular capsule. The other divides the medial head of the gastrocnemius muscle from the articular capsule. In addition, a large bursa separates the medial head of the gastrocnemius muscle from the semimembranous muscle.

figure 18.38   Range of motion of the hip. **A,** Hip flexion, leg extended. **B,** Hip hyperextension, knee extended. **C,** Hip flexion, knee flexed. **D,** Abduction. **E,** Internal rotation. **F,** External rotation.

INSPECTION. Inspect the knee with the client walking (to observe gait), sitting, and supine with knees extended. Be familiar with the normal contour of the knee because loss of contour may occur with swelling. The client may voluntarily maintain the knee at 15 to 20 degrees of flexion because the knee joint is at maximal capacity at this angle and thus pain is reduced. Swelling as a result of synovitis is most apparent at the suprapatellar pouch. Swelling caused by meniscal cysts appears at the lateral or the medial joint surface. Popliteal swelling is more obvious when the knee is extended. Swelling of the knee observed on the anterior aspect of the knee is called prepatellar bursitis or "housemaid's knee."

PALPATION. Palpate the knee with the client in the sitting or supine position, whichever is more comfortable for the client. Apply downward pressure over the suprapatellar pouch to localize the synovial fluid in the lower portion of the articular cavity. Use the examining hand to palpate the lateral and medial joint surfaces with the fingers while using the thumb for stability (Figure 18.41).

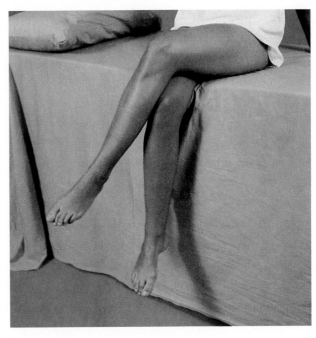

figure **18.39** Alternate leg crossing for assessment of hamstring, gluteal, abductor, and adductor muscle strength.

figure **18.40** Knee joint.

figure**18.41**   **A,** Knee effusion. **B,** Examination of the knee.

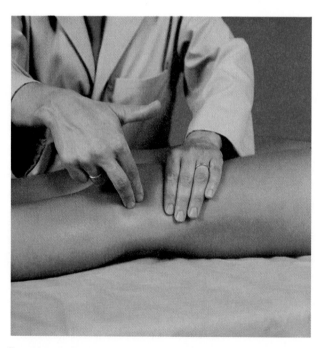

figure**18.42**   Testing for the bulge sign. After milking the medial aspect of the knee, the lateral side of the patella is tapped. The medial side is then observed for the presence of a bulge.

figure**18.43**   Ballottement of the patella. **A,** Sitting. **B,** Supine.

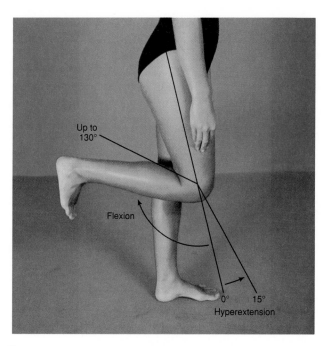

figure**18.44** Range of motion of the knee: flexion and extension.

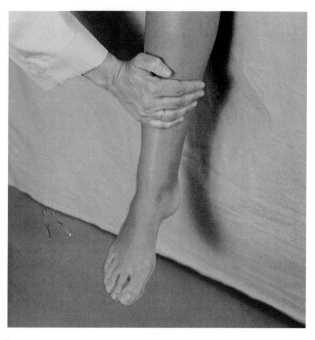

figure**18.45** Assessment of quadriceps muscle strength. The client attempts to straighten the leg while the examiner tries to flex it.

In a second procedure for the examination of the knee, palpate the suprapatellar pouch with the thumb and the fingers of one hand while the other hand pushes the contents of the articular cavity upward. To do this, place your thumb on one side of the patella with the rest of your fingers on the other side to form an arch below the patella. Apply an inward and upward pressure to move any fluid upward into the suprapatellar bursa. Place the examining hand about 10 cm above the patella and move it gradually toward the patella.

SPECIAL TESTS. A test for small effusions in the knee joint is called the bulge sign. Take the ball of your hand and firmly milk the medial aspect of the knee upward two to three times to displace fluid. Then press or tap behind the lateral margin of the knee (Figure 18.42). A positive bulge sign will show a swelling or bulge of fluid in the hollow area medial to the patella. The bulge sign is useful for assessing small effusions, but it may be absent in large effusions.

When considerable fluid is present in the suprapatellar pouch, ballottement of the patella may be possible (Figure 18.43). Ballottement involves applying downward pressure with one hand while pushing the patella backward against the femur with a finger of the opposite hand. Examine the popliteal region with the client in the prone position or while standing. Swelling of the joint in the popliteal region, which is called Baker's cyst, is generally an extension of the articular cavity.

RANGE OF MOTION. To test range of motion of the knee (Figure 18.44), ask the client to:

1. Bend the knee.
2. Straighten and stretch the leg.

MUSCLE STRENGTH. To test muscle strength in the knee, ask the client to:

1. Extend the leg as you try to bend it (quadriceps muscle strength) (Figure 18.45).
2. Bend the knees as you try to straighten them (hamstring muscle strength) (Figure 18.46).

TESTS FOR LIGAMENT INJURY. Sprains or tears of the ligaments are the most common injuries of the knee. Two sets of ligaments play a role in movement of the knee. They are the anterior and posterior cruciate ligaments and the medial and lateral collateral ligaments. The anterior cruciate ligament limits extension and rotation, whereas the posterior cruciate ligament stabilizes the femur against forward dislocation. The collateral ligaments prevent lateral and medial dislocation of the knee. Abnormal movements of the knee may indicate dislocation. You may be able to palpate the tears in the assessment of the knee.

To test the stability of the anterior and posterior cruciate ligaments, use the drawer test (Figure 18.47) or the Lachman test (if you are assessing the anterior ligament). For the drawer sign, have the client lie in a supine position with the knee flexed to 90 degrees and the foot flat on the examining table. Position yourself on the edge of the table so that you can stabilize the foot by sitting on it. Cup your hands around the tibia.

figure**18.46** Assessment of hamstring muscle strength. The client flexes his knees while the examiner tries to straighten them.

To test the stability of the anterior cruciate ligament, pull the tibia toward you. If it slides forward from under the femur, the drawer test is positive and suggests a tear in the anterior ligament. To test the posterior cruciate ligament, push the tibia posteriorly. If it moves backward, the ligament is probably damaged. This test is usually performed in one continuous motion. Test the other knee to compare findings.

The Lachman test is thought to be a better indicator of injury to the anterior cruciate ligament (Magee, 1992). Have the client lie in a supine position with the involved leg beside you. Place the client's knee between 20 and 30 degrees of flexion (close to the functional position of the knee). Stabilize the femur with one hand while you move the proximal aspect of the tibia forward with the other hand. If there is a soft or "mushy" feel and the infrapatellar slope disappears when the tibia is moved forward on the femur, the Lachman test is positive. This sign indicates damage to the anterior cruciate ligament, especially the posterolateral band. Test the other knee to compare findings.

TESTS FOR MENISCUS DAMAGE. Indications of pathological conditions of the meniscus include (1) pain or tenderness on the lateral surfaces of the knee joint; (2) popping, snapping, or grating sounds with movement; and (3) inability to fully extend the knee ("locking"). The medial meniscus is more often injured than is the lateral. The two tests commonly used to aid in the diagnosis of a torn meniscus are the Apley test and the McMurray test.

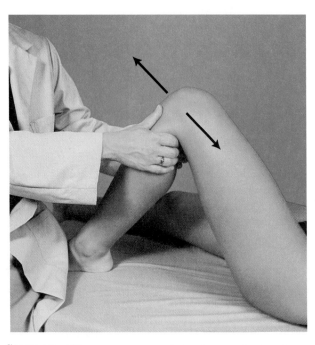

figure**18.47** Examination of the knee with the drawer test for anterior and posterior stability.

figure**18.48** Elicitation of Apley's sign with compression.

Attempt to elicit Apley's sign (Figure 18.48) in the client you suspect of having a loose object in the knee joint or one who has given a history of knee joint locking. Have the client assume the prone position with the suspected knee flexed to 90 degrees. Exert downward pressure on the foot so that the tibia is firmly opposed to the femur. Rotate the leg externally and internally. Locking of the knee, pain with the maneuver, or the sound of clicks is a positive sign and may indicate that a loose body, such as torn cartilage, is trapped in the articulation. Clicks or popping sounds are generated as the object escapes. Repeat the maneuver using distraction rather than downward pressure (compression) on the foot. If the pain is worse when rotation plus compression is used, there is probably a meniscus injury. Pain that is worse when rotation plus distraction is used is probably ligamentous.

When the client states that he or she "feels something in the knee joint" or complains that "sometimes it just won't bend," attempt to elicit McMurray's sign (Figure 18.49). Perform this test with the client in the sitting position with the knee flexed to 90 degrees or in the supine position. Have the client internally rotate the leg while you slowly extend it with one hand. Use the other hand to provide resistance at the medial aspect of

figure**18.49** Elicitation of McMurray's sign to test the lateral meniscus.

the knee. This maneuver tests the medial meniscus. Extension of the knee may not be possible (positive sign) if a loose body impedes its movement. Repeat the procedure by employing external rotation and applying resistance to the lateral aspect of the knee. This maneuver tests the lateral meniscus.

Ankles and feet. The ankle joint is the articulation of the tibia, the fibula, and the talus (Figure 18.50). The capsule is lined with synovia. The ankle joint is protected by ligaments on the medial and lateral surfaces but not on the anterior or posterior surfaces. The joint between the talus and the calcaneus bones is called the talocalcaneal, or subtalar, joint. The forward extension of the joint cavity is the articulation of the talus and the navicular bones. Articular capsules lined with synovial membrane separate the remainder of the tarsal, metatarsal, and phalangeal bones of the foot.

INSPECTION. Inspect the ankle and the foot with the client standing, walking, and sitting (not bearing weight). To best evaluate for swelling, examine the dorsal aspect of the foot because there is less tissue over the bone. Hallux valgus is a lateral deformity of the great toe in which it may lie above or below the second toe. The metatarsophalangeal joint is distorted in such a way that the first metatarsal bone is angled medially. A callus or bursal distention generally occurs at the joint. Hammer toe is a result of hyperextension of the metatarsophalangeal joint and flexion of the proximal phalangeal joint (Figure 18.51).

PALPATION. Palpate the anterior aspect of the ankle joint with your thumbs to assess for bogginess, swelling, or tenderness. Palpate the Achilles tendon for tenderness and nodules (Figure 18.52). Palpate the metatarsal and phalangeal joints with the fingers on the anterior surface and the thumb on the sole of the foot. Note any tenderness.

RANGE OF MOTION. To test range of motion of the ankle and foot (Figure 18.53), ask the client to:
1. Point the foot up toward the ceiling.
2. Point the foot down toward the floor.
3. With the foot bent at the ankle, point the medial side of the foot toward the floor (eversion) and repeat with the lateral side (inversion).
4. Rotate the ankle in order to turn the foot away from and then toward the other foot.

MUSCLE STRENGTH. To test muscle strength in the ankle and foot, ask the client to:
1. Flex the foot upward against your hand.
2. Push the foot down against your hand (Figure 18.54).

Thoracic and lumbar spine

INSPECTION. Inspect the shape of the spine and its structural relationship to the shoulder girdle, thorax, and pelvis. The normal spinal curvatures are concave at the cervical area, convex at the thoracic area, and con-

figure**18.50** Bones and joints of the ankle and foot. *(From Seidel HM et al:* Mosby's guide to physical examination, *ed 3, St Louis, 1995, Mosby.)*

figure**18.51** Hammer great toe. *(From Mann RA, Coughlin MJ:* Surgery of the foot and ankle, *ed 6, St Louis, 1993, Mosby.)*

figure**18.52** Examination of the ankle joint.

A   **B**   **C**

figure **18.53**   Range of motion of the ankle and foot. **A,** Dorsiflexion and plantar flexion. **B,** Inversion and eversion. **C,** Abduction and adduction.

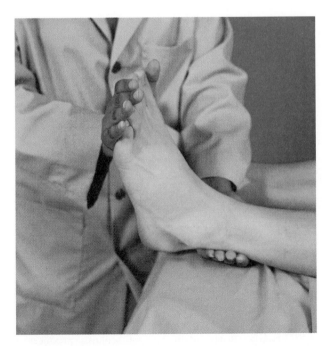

figure **18.54**   Testing muscle strength in the ankle and foot.

cave at the lumbar area. Note any differences in heights of the shoulders and the iliac crests. Unusual heights of the iliac crests suggest uneven leg lengths. Variations in spinal curvature may indicate a structural problem.

Scoliosis is a deformity of the spine that appears as a lateral deviation (Figure 18.55). This angling of the spine produces a downward slant of the thoracic cage on the affected side and an upward tilt of the pelvis on the contralateral side. A rotary deformity of the rib cage also occurs. The ribs protrude posteriorly on the convex side of the spine. A hump or "razorback" may be visible. The protrusion may become more obvious when the client bends over.

SCOLIOSIS ASSESSMENT. To assess for scoliosis, ask the client to stand with the feet approximately 6 inches apart and bend over slowly to touch the toes. Stand behind the client and observe the movement of the spine as the client bends and comes back to an upright position (Figure 18.56). This maneuver provides a "skyline" view of the spine. Structural scoliosis, which is caused by vertebral rotation, tends to become more prominent as the client bends forward. Functional scoliosis, which compensates for structural abnormalities other than those associated with the vertebral column, disappears when the client bends forward. Also note symmetry of the muscles, movement, protrusions, or sharp angulation.

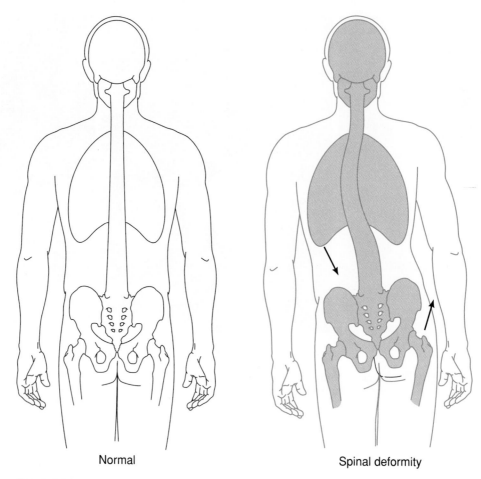

Normal   Spinal deformity

figure**18.55** Deformity of the spine. Scoliosis is a lateral deviation of the spine. Arrows indicate the direction of the thoracic and pelvic tilt.

Kyphosis (humpback) is a flexion deformity (Figure 18.57, *B*). When the angle of the defect is sharp, the apex is called a gibbus.

Lordosis (swayback) is an extension deviation of the spine, commonly in the lumbar area (Figure 18.57, *C*).

PALPATION. Palpate the spinal processes as the client bends over to touch the toes (Figure 18.58). Palpate paravertebral muscles for symmetry, tenderness, and spasm. You may want to percuss for tenderness over the spinous process.

RANGE OF MOTION. To assess range of motion of the spine (Figure 18.59) ask the client to:

1. Bend back as far as possible (hyperextend the spine).
2. Bend to the right and left side as far as possible (lateral bending). You may need to stabilize the client's pelvis.
3. Turn to the right and left in a circular motion (while you stabilize the pelvis).
4. Slowly bend forward at the waist and try to touch the toes (while you watch from behind the client and observe for signs of scoliosis).

figure**18.56** Rotary deformity of scoliosis produces a humpback or "razorback" deformity. This deviation is best demonstrated by asking the client to bend at the waist.

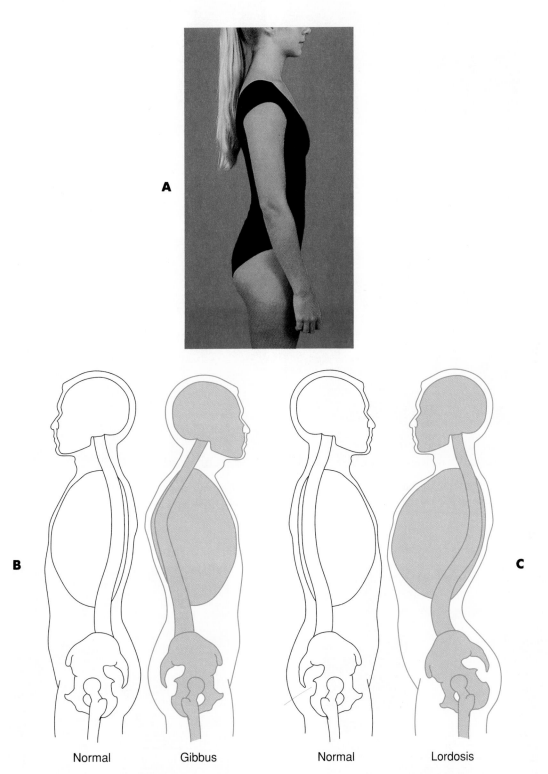

Normal   Gibbus   Normal   Lordosis

figure **18.57** **A,** Normal curvature of the spine. **B,** Kyphosis, a flexion deformity of the spine. **C,** Lordosis and extension deformity of the spine.

figure**18.58**   Range of motion of the thoracic and lumbar spine. **A,** Flexion. **B,** Hyperextension. **C,** Lateral bending. **D,** Rotation of the upper trunk.

figure**18.59**   Palpation of the spinal processes as the client bends over.

figure**18.60**   Assessment of gait.

Assessment of gait. Evaluate gait in both phases—stance and swing—for rhythm and smoothness (Figure 18.60). Stance is considered to consist of three processes: (1) heel strike—the heel contacts the floor or ground; (2) midstance—the body weight is transferred from the heel to the ball of the foot; and (3) push-off—the heel leaves the ground (see Chapter 9: General Assessment, Including Vital Signs).

The swing phase also consists of three processes: (1) acceleration; (2) swing-through—the lifted foot travels ahead of the weight-bearing foot; and (3) deceleration—the foot slows in preparation for the heel strike.

To describe the client's gait, include phase (conformity), cadence (symmetry, regular rhythm), stride length (symmetry, length of swing), trunk posture (related to phases), pelvic posture (related to phases), and arm swing (symmetry, length of swing).

If pain is present, describe it in relation to the phases of gait.

To assess gait, ask the client to walk naturally for a short distance so that you can observe the gait (if you have not already done so). Then ask the client to take a few steps on the toes and a few steps on the heels.

Special maneuvers

Straight leg–raising test. The straight leg–raising test, which is also known as Lasègue's test (Figure 18.61), is useful in determining that a herniated lumbar disk is the cause of sciatic nerve pain. Perform the test for clients who complain of low back pain or pain that radiates down the leg. Have the client lie on the back on a firm surface with the leg and thigh as relaxed as possi-

ble. Slowly raise the foot, keeping the knee straight until the client complains of pain. Then dorsiflex the foot. A positive test includes the following responses: (1) pain is produced before 70 degrees is reached; (2) dorsiflexion aggravates the pain; and (3) pain relief occurs with flexion of the knee. Pain induced in this manner is caused by pressure on the dorsal roots of the lumbosacral nerves and is characteristic of a herniated disk. Repeat this maneuver with the other leg and compare the results. Nerve root irritation is suggested by pain in the lumbar area, hip, or posterior leg or by muscle spasm. If

A

figure**18.61** Straight leg–raising test.

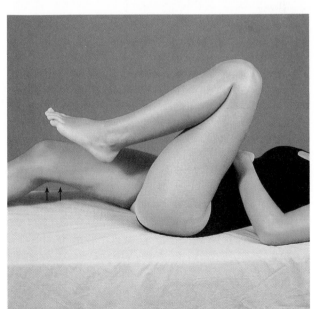

B

figure**18.62** Thomas test. **A,** Negative. **B,** Positive.

examination step-by-step

1. Observe the client for gait, ease of movement, ability to change positions, and signs of discomfort as the client enters the room and interacts during the examination.
2. Observe body alignment and stature with the client standing erect (front, back, and side). Note any deformities, spinal curvatures, atrophied or hypertrophied limbs, or age-related variations in posture and body size.
3. With the client sitting on the examination table, proceed with the examination.

Head

1. Inspect the musculature for facial symmetry of skinfolds, muscles, and wrinkles.
2. Palpate the temporomandibular joint while the client opens and closes the mouth.
3. To test range of motion, ask the client to:
   a. Open and close the mouth.
   b Project the lower jaw.
   c. Move the jaw from side to side.
4. To test muscle strength, ask the client to:
   a. Bite down hard while you palpate the masseter muscles (CN V).
   b. Clench the teeth while you apply downward pressure on the chin.

Cervical Spine

1. Inspect the neck for alignment and symmetry of skinfolds and muscles.
2. Palpate the cervical spine.
3. To evaluate range of motion, ask the client to:
   a. Touch the chin to the chest.
   b. Extend the head backward as far as possible.
   c. Bend the head laterally to each shoulder (touch the ear to the shoulder without raising the shoulder).
   d. Rotate the head from side to side (pointing the chin toward each shoulder).
4. To evaluate muscle strength, ask the client to:
   a. Push the cheek against your hand (right and left sides) (test CN XI).
   b. Push the forehead against your hand.
   c. Push the head back against your hand.

Shoulders

1. Inspect the shoulders, including the muscles and the acromioclavicular joint, for contour and equality.
2. Palpate the shoulders and the bursal sites.
3. To test for range of motion, ask the client to:
   a. Extend both arms forward (forward flexion).
   b. Extend both arms backward (hyperextension).
   c. Put your hands behind your back as if you were going to reach up to touch your shoulder blade (internal rotation).
   d. Put your hands behind your head (external rotation).

4. To test for muscle strength, ask the client to:
   a. Hold the arms upward while you try to push them down (deltoid muscles).
   b. Extend the arms and then try to flex them while you try to pull them into extension (biceps muscle).
   c. Flex the arms and then try to extend them while you attempt to push them into a flexed position (triceps muscle).
   d. Shrug the shoulders while you try to push down on them (trapezius muscle, CN XI).

Elbows

1. Inspect the elbows in both flexed and extended positions for carrying angle and contour.
2. Palpate the extensor surface of the ulna for nodules, the olecranon process and grooves, and the lateral epicondyles of the humerus for tenderness.
3. To test range of motion, ask the client to:
   a. Bend and straighten the elbow.
   b. Turn the hand face up (supination) and face down (pronation).

Hands and Wrists

1. Inspect the dorsal and palmar surfaces of the hands for position, shape, contour, and number and completeness of digits. Inspect the wrists.
2. Palpate the hand and wrist joints.
3. To test range of motion of the hands and wrist, ask the client to:
   a. Spread the fingers apart and bring them back again.
   b. Make a fist.
   c. Touch the thumb to each fingertip and to the base of the little finger.
   d. Bend the fingers up and down at the metacarpophalangeal joint.
   e. Bend the hand up and down at the wrist.
   f. With the palm facing down, turn the hand to the right and to the left.
4. To test strength in the muscles of the hands and wrist, ask the client to:
   a. Maintain wrist flexion while you try to extend the wrist.
   b. Try to extend the wrist as you try to flex it.
   c. Squeeze your first two fingers as hard as he or she can.
   d. Extend the fingers while you push down on the dorsal surface.
   e. Flex the fingers while you push up on the ventral surface.
   f. Spread the fingers apart while you try to push them together.
   g. Push the fingers together while you try to pull them apart.

examination *step-by-step* —cont'd

Hips

1. Inspect the hips for symmetry in iliac crest height and level of gluteal folds.
2. Palpate the hips and the pelvis for stability, tenderness, and crepitus.
3. To test range of motion of the hips, ask the client (while supine) to:
   a. Raise the leg above the body with the knee extended.
   b. Bring the knee to the chest while keeping the other leg straight.
   c. Swing the leg laterally and medially while keeping the knee straight.
   d. Place the side of the foot on the opposite knee and move the flexed knee down toward the examination table (external rotation).
   e. Flex the knee and rotate the leg so that the flexed knee moves inward toward the opposite leg (internal rotation).
4. Ask the client (while either prone or standing) to swing the straightened leg behind the body.
5. To test muscle strength in the hips, ask the client (while supine) to:
   a. Raise the extended leg while you attempt to hold it down.
   b. Push both legs against your hands while your hands are placed on the bed on either side of the client's knees.
   c. Bring both legs together while your hands are placed on the bed between the client's knees.
6. To assess muscle strength in the hamstring, gluteal, abductor, and adductor muscles, ask the client to sit and perform alternate leg crossing.

Knees

1. Inspect the knees for natural concavities and swelling.
2. Palpate the joint space and the popliteal space.
3. To test range of motion of the knee, ask the client to:
   a. Bend the knee.
   b. Straighten and stretch the leg.

4. To test muscle strength in the knee, ask the client to:
   a. Extend the leg as you try to bend it (quadriceps muscle strength).
   b. Bend the knees as you try to straighten them (hamstring muscle strength).

Ankles and Feet

1. Inspect the ankles and the feet during weight bearing and non–weight bearing for position, size, contour, and number of toes.
2. Palpate the ankle joint, Achilles tendon, and metatarsophalangeal joints.
3. To test range of motion of the ankle and foot, ask the client to:
   a. Point the foot up toward the ceiling.
   b. Point the foot down toward the floor.
   c. With the foot bent at the ankle, point the medial side of the foot toward the floor (inversion) and repeat with the lateral side (eversion).
   d. Rotate the ankle in order to turn the foot away from and then toward the other foot.
4. To test muscle strength in the ankle and foot, ask the client to:
   a. Flex the foot upward against your hand.
   b. Push the foot down against your hand.

Thoracic and Lumbar Spine

1. Inspect the spine for alignment.
2. Palpate the spinous processes and the paravertebral muscles for tenderness and spasm.
3. To assess range of motion of the spine, ask the client to:
   a. Bend back as far as possible (hyperextend the spine).
   b. Bend to the right and to the left side as far as possible (lateral bending; you may need to stabilize the client's pelvis).
   c. Turn to the right and to the left in a circular motion (while you stabilize the pelvis).
   d. Slowly bend forward at the waist and try to touch the toes and then return to an upright position (watch from behind the client, take a "skyline view" of the spine, and observe for signs of scoliosis).

one leg is raised and pain is felt in the opposite side, then a large herniated disk is likely.

Thomas test. The Thomas test evaluates flexion contractures of the hip. With the client in the supine position, ask the client to pull one knee up toward the chest as far as possible (Figure 18.62, *A*). In the individual with normal hip function, when the hip is flexed, the opposite leg remains flat on the examination table. For the individual with an immobile hip, the opposite hip and leg flex in response to flexion of the leg. Approxi-

mate the extent of the flexion contracture by noting the degree of flexion of the opposite leg (the angle between the client's leg and the table) (Figure 18.62, *B*).

■ VARIATIONS FROM HEALTH

Osteoarthritis

Osteoarthritis is a degenerative joint disease characterized by a progressive loss of articular cartilage and for-

mation of new bone at the joint surfaces and subchondral area. It occurs primarily in people older than 50 years, and the onset of signs and symptoms is insidious.

Bony overgrowths that feel like hard, nontender nodules frequently occur in the fingers (Figure 18.63).

Bouchard node   Heberden node

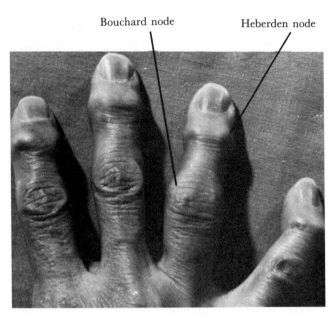

figure **18.63** Nodules of the hand associated with osteoarthritis. *(From Swanson AB: Flexible implant resection arthroplasty in the hand and extremities, St Louis, 1973, Mosby.)*

When located in the distal interphalangeal joints, they are called Heberden's nodes (nodules). When located in the proximal interphalangeal joints, they are called Bouchard's nodes. Bony spurs, particularly in the knees, are also typical of osteoarthritis. Most symptoms are related to weight bearing and are relieved by rest.

Rheumatoid Arthritis

Rheumatoid arthritis is a chronic, systemic, inflammatory disorder that affects individuals of all ages, although its onset is most common in the 30s and 40s. It affects symmetrical joints. Deformities are related to inflammatory destruction of the joint with marginal bone erosion. Systemic complaints include fatigue and malaise in addition to joint pain. Joint inflammation is common, with marked edema, tenderness, pain, and limitation of movement. Stiffness early in the day is common. On palpation, joints will feel "boggy." Common deformities related to rheumatoid arthritis are deviation of the fingers, swan neck, and boutonnière deformities of the fingers (Figure 18.64).

Gout

Gout is a crystal-induced arthritis related to abnormalities in purine metabolism that result in prolonged hyperuricemia and subsequent deposition of uric acid crystals in the joint space. It can be caused by an overproduction of uric acid or an interference in uric acid excretion. It most commonly occurs in men older than 40 years. Joint involvement is usually monarticular. Classically, the proximal phalanx of the great toe is the

figure **18.64** Unilateral ulner deviation of the metacarpophalangeal joints of the **right** hand secondary to rheumatoid arthritis. *(From Prior JA, Silberstein JS, Stang JM: Physical diagnosis: the history and examination of the patient, ed 6, St Louis, 1981, Mosby.)*

figure **18.65** Inflammatory response of acute gout of the great toe. *(From Prior JA, Silberstein JS, Stang JM: Physical diagnosis: the history and examination of the patient, ed 6, St Louis, 1981, Mosby.)*

joint affected (Figure 18.65). However, joints of the foot, ankle, and knee may also be affected. Pain is typically constant and severe (often called "exquisite") during an acute attack and is characterized by marked erythema, swelling, warmth, and tenderness. Tophi or urate crystal deposits may also occur on the ears and in the joints.

Osteoporosis

Osteoporosis is a systemic condition in which a decrease in bone mass occurs because bone resorption exceeds bone deposition. The bones become fragile, and fractures may occur even with minor trauma or during routine activities. The hips, vertebrae, and wrists are the most common fracture sites. Osteoporosis is most common in women (4:1, women/men). A decrease in calcium intake, decrease in estrogen production in women, lack of weight-bearing activities and exercise, and sedentary lifestyle are among the contributing factors (see Risk Factors box on p. 454).

Muscle Weakness

The client who has difficulty in walking up steps or getting up from a sitting position or the client who is able to rise only by pushing off with the hands and arms or by pulling up by grasping some nearby furniture may have a problem involving the shoulder or hip girdle musculature. Further tests are necessary to ascertain the presence of muscular dystrophy, myasthenia gravis, parkinsonism, or polymyositis.

Myasthenia gravis should be strongly suspected if the following are true: (1) the client who has difficulty rising can rise easily after being instructed to sit back and relax for a few minutes; (2) the client is a woman in her 20s or a man in his 50s or 60s; (3) muscle atrophy is not present; and (4) the client has ptosis or extraocular muscle weakness resulting in diplopia.

Polymyositis is a progressive inflammatory disease that occurs in children and adults. It involves progressive symmetrical weakness of the limb girdles, neck, and pharynx. The client who has polymyositis may have pain, muscle atrophy, or a rash, particularly around the eyelids, and low-grade fever.

Parkinsonism may be the underlying cause when the aging client has difficulty rising from a chair. This impression is substantiated if the client says stiffness is a problem. In such a case, it is important to be alert for signs of flexion posture, slow and intermittent movement, frequent tremor, masked facies, or movement of several joint units at one time because these signs are also characteristic of Parkinson's disease.

The client who complains of intermittent bouts of muscle weakness requires methodical and careful investigation for ischemic attacks, disorders of glucose metabolism (diabetes), anemia, and serum electrolyte disturbances, particularly of potassium or calcium ion concentrations.

Transient ischemic attacks may cause a focal episode of motor dysfunction related to vascular disease, such as arteriosclerosis or essential hypertension. Listening for bruits over the neck vessels in the elderly client with muscle weakness is particularly important, since these bruits might strengthen the impression of vascular disease.

Clinical correlation of signs of muscle weakness and disease entities have shown that each neuromuscular disease has a general predilection for a particular group of muscles. A given pattern of weakness, then, suggests the possibility of a certain disease and excludes others. An example lies in the adage that peripheral muscle involvement in the extremities is of muscular origin, whereas distal disease is of neuropathic origin. Further explanation of the correlation of assessment data with underlying disease processes is presented in Table 18.4.

Hypokalemia

Since the ratio of the concentrations of potassium ions of the intracellular environment to the extracellular fluid determines the rate of cell firing, a deficit of this ion is accomplished by disorders of structure and function in muscular and neural tissues. Both skeletal and smooth muscles are affected by hypokalemia. The client complains of varying degrees of weakness and lassitude. Extreme hypokalemia may be accompanied by muscular paralysis. Some other signs that will help confirm hypokalemia as the cause of muscle weakness are abnormalities in motor and secretory activities of the gastrointestinal tract, changes in electrocardiograms, and

table 18.4 *Topographical Patterns of Muscle Palsy*

Muscle weakness or paralysis	Signs	Possible cause
Ocular	Diplopia Ptosis Strabismus	Myasthenia gravis Thyroid disease Ocular dystrophy and botulism
Bifacial	Inability to smile Inability to expose teeth Inability to close eyes	Myasthenia gravis Facioscapulohumeral dystrophy Guillain-Barré syndrome
Bulbar	Dysphonia Dysarthria Dysphagia Hanging-jaw facial weakness (may or may not be present)	Myasthenia gravis Myotonic dystrophy Botulism Diphtheria Poliomyelitis Early polymyositis
Cervical	Inability to lift head from pillow (hanging-head syndrome) Weakness of posterior neck muscles	Polymyositis Dermatomyositis Progressive muscular dystrophy
Bibrachial	Weakness, atrophy, and fasciculations of hands, arms, and shoulders (hanging-arm syndrome)	Amyotrophic lateral sclerosis
Bicrural	Lower leg weakness Floppy feet Inability to walk on heels and toes	Diabetic polyneuropathy
Limb-girdle	Inability to raise arms Inability to rise from sitting position Difficulty in climbing stairs without use of arms Waddling gait	Polymyositis Dermatomyositis Progressive muscular dystrophy
Distal limb	Footdrop with steppage gain Weakness of all leg muscles Wristdrop—weakness of handgrips ("claw hand"; later sign)	Familial polyneuropathy
Generalized or universal	Limb and cranial muscle weakness (acute in onset and periodic) Slow onset and progressive paralysis Atrophy Fasciculations of limb and trunk muscles No sensory loss Paralysis developing over several days Mild degree of generalized weakness	Electrolyte imbalance Hypokalemia Hypocalcemia Hypomagnesemia Motor system disease Guillain-Barré syndrome Glycogen storage diseases Vitamin D deficiency
Single muscles or groups of muscles	Inability to contract affected muscles	Thyrotoxic myopathy (almost always neuropathic)

dilute urine. Some of the conditions known to be correlated with a deficiency of potassium ion are diarrhea, excessive losses in the urine resulting from the use of chlorthiazide, mercurial diuretics, or steroid hormones; Cushing's syndrome; and primary aldosteronism.

Involuntary Contraction of Skeletal Muscles
Fasciculations

Fasciculations are the visible, spontaneous contractions of a number of muscle fibers supplied by a single motor nerve filament. Visible dimpling or twitching may occur, although there is usually insufficient power generated to move the joint.

Fasciculations that occur during muscular contraction (twitching) are associated with conditions of irritability that result in poorly coordinated contraction of small and large motor units. Benign fasciculation occurs in the normal individual and is characterized by normal muscle strength and size. Rarely, myokymia, a rippling appearance of the muscle occasioned by numerous fasciculations, is noted in a normal individual.

Fascicular twitches noted during rest in a client with exaggerated muscular weakness and atrophy are charac-teristic of a peripheral motor neuron disorder. Generalized fascicular twitching that occurs in a progressive, wavelike pattern over an entire muscle and progressing to complete paralysis is characteristic of certain types of poisoning (organic phosphate) and of poliomyelitis.

Cramps and spasm

Muscular spasm, or tremor (Table 18.5), may occur at rest or with movement and may be noted in the normal individual with metabolic and electrolyte alterations. Cramping is a common complaint following excessive sweating and with hyponatremia, hypocalcemia, hypomagnesemia, and hyperuricemia. Diseases that magnify these alterations are correlated with the presence of muscle spasm. A continuous spasm that is heightened by attempts to move the affected muscles occurs in tetanus and following the bite of the black widow spider. Paravertebral muscle spasm is often responsible for low back pain.

Tetany

Hypocalcemia and hypomagnesemia may cause the involuntary spasms of skeletal muscle that resemble cramping. The calcium deficit causes depolarization of the distal segments of the motor nerve. Furthermore, a

table**18.5** *Tremor Classification*		
Cause	**Type and rate of movement**	**Description**
Anxiety	Fine, rapid, 10 to 12/sec	Irregular, variable Increased by attempts to move part; decreased by relaxation of part
Parkinsonism	Fine, regular, or coarse, 2 to 5/sec	Occurs at rest May be inhibited by movement Involves flexion of finger and thumb "pill rolling" Accompanied by rigidity, "cogwheel" phenomena, bradykinesia
Cerebellar tremor	Variable rate	Evident only on movement (most prominent on finger-to-nose test) Dysmetria (seen when client is asked to pat rapidly; pats are of unequal force and do not all arrive at same point)
Essential or senile	Coarse, 3 to 7/sec	Involves the jaw, sometimes the tongue, and sometimes the entire head
Metabolic		Disappears on complete relaxation or in response to alcohol Variable Client is obviously ill; if illness is a result of hepatic failure, client will have other signs, such as palpable liver, spider nevi

change occurs within the muscle fibers themselves, since nerve section or block does not prevent these tetanic contractions. Tetanic cramps can be elicited by percussing the motor nerve leading to a muscle group at frequencies of 15 to 20 per second. Chvostek's sign is the spasm of the facial muscles produced by tapping over the facial nerve near its foramen of exit. The instability of the neuromuscular unit is heightened by hyperventilation (alkalosis) and hypoxia (ischemia). Tetany in its mildest form affects the distal musculature in the form of carpopedal spasm, but it may involve all the muscles of the body except those of the eye.

Muscle cramp

Muscle cramp frequently occurs after a day of vigorous exercise. As the feet cool, a sudden movement may trigger a strong contraction of the foot and leg. The musculature is visible, and the muscle feels hard on palpation. The spasm will cease in response to stretch of the fibers. In the case of the gastrocnemius muscle, the stretch can be achieved by dorsiflexion of the foot. Occasionally, massage is helpful in relaxing the spasm.

Fasciculations frequently appear before and after the cramp. They are further evidence of the hyperexcitability of the neuromuscular unit. Muscle spasms occur more frequently when the client is dehydrated or sweating and in the pregnant client.

The cause of the pain associated with muscle cramp has not been determined, but some believe it is due to increased metabolic needs of the hyperactive muscles and the collection of the metabolic waste products, such as lactic acid, within the muscle.

Myalgia

"I hurt all over" is frequently the chief complaint of the client with diffuse muscle pain that accompanies many types of systemic infection (e.g., influenza, measles, rheumatic fever, brucellosis, dengue fever, or salmonellosis). Soreness and aching are other descriptions given for this type of involvement. Little is known of the cause of myalgia.

Fibromyositis is inflammation of the fibrous tissue in muscle, fascia, and nerves. The client may complain of pain and tenderness in a muscle after exposure to cold, dampness, or minor trauma. Firm, tender zones, occasionally several centimeters in diameter, may be found on palpation. Palpation, active contraction, or passive stretching increases the pain.

Intense pain localized to a smaller group of muscles may be a result of epidemic myalgia, also called pleurodynia, "painful neck," or "devil's grip." Intense pain at the beginning of neurological involvement may occur in poliomyelitis and herpes zoster.

The pain of poliomyelitis is described as marked during the initial involvement of the nerve, whereas the later sensation of the paralyzed muscle is one of aching. The segmental pattern of the intense pain of herpes zoster is caused by the inflammation of spinal nerves and dorsal root ganglia that occurs 3 to 4 days before the skin eruption.

The initial symptoms of rheumatoid arthritis may be diffuse muscular soreness and aching, which may antedate the joint involvement by weeks or months. The muscles are tender, and the client describes the pain as occurring not at the time of activity but hours later. An increased sedimentation rate or a positive latex fixation test may support the conclusion of rheumatoid involvement.

sample documentation & diagnoses CRITICAL THINKING

■ FOCUSED HEALTH HISTORY (SUBJECTIVE DATA)

Ms. L., a 50-year-old executive secretary, complains of swelling and burning in both hands on and off for the past 2 weeks. States, "My hands hurt and the swelling is so bad in the morning, I can hardly type." States joints in hands feel warm, swollen, and tender. Pain and stiffness are worse in the morning, lasting about 1 to 2 hours. Improves over the course of the day. Has noticed increased fatigue, especially in the afternoon. Takes ibuprofen 600 mg for pain as needed. States has been in good health; no recent illnesses or change in weight. Denies any chronic illnesses or family history of arthritis. Is single and lives with her sister, who is in good health.

■ FOCUSED PHYSICAL EXAMINATION (OBJECTIVE DATA)

General appearance: 50-year-old white female who grimaces when hands are touched, tends to pull away, and guards both hands.

Extremities: Normal range of motion (ROM) in shoulders, elbows, hips, and knees; ROM of wrists is diminished—10 degrees radial, 25 degrees ulnar. Hands warm to touch; veins engorged with spindle-shaped swelling of the proximal interphalangeal (PIP) joints, 3rd digits bilaterally. Ulnar deviation of metacarpophalangeal (MCP) joints noted.

Laboratory values: Erythrocyte sedimentation rate (ESR) elevated—25 mm/hr; white blood count mildly elevated with normal differential; red blood cell count slightly decreased (normocytic anemia); rheumatoid factor—positive.

diagnoses

HEALTH PROBLEM

Probable rheumatoid arthritis; needs further evaluation

NURSING DIAGNOSES

Pain related to inflammatory process

Defining Characteristics

- Subjective communication of pain
- Self-focusing
- Guarding behavior
- Grimaces in pain

Activity intolerance related to anemia and disease state

Defining Characteristics

- Verbal reports of fatigue and weakness especially in early afternoon
- Verbal reports of loss of energy

Impaired physical mobility related to joint and systemic involvement

Defining Characteristics

- Limited range of motion of hands
- Decreased muscle strength and control of hands and wrist
- Impaired coordination of hands

chapter **19**

Neurological System, Including Mental Status

■ PURPOSE OF EXAMINATION

The neurological system integrates all the functions of the body. It controls cognitive and voluntary behavioral processes, as well as subconscious and involuntary body functions. The major functions of the neurological system are reception (sensory), integration, and adaptation; that is, the normal nervous system receives stimuli from the environment, adjusts body functions to the environment, and effects changes to ensure homeokinesis, or survival.

The mental status examination is an integral part of the neurological examination. In the context of the total health assessment, this appraisal begins with the initial contact with the client. Most examiners make assessments of mental status while obtaining the client's history and perform special tests of cognitive function immediately afterward.

For the purpose of facilitating learning of this complex system, this chapter is organized with the physical assessment portion of the neurological examination presented first, followed by techniques for examination of mental status. This organization, however, is not the usual order for conducting the assessment; in practice, the mental status examination begins when the practitioner first encounters the client (see Chapter 2: Interviewing Skills and Techniques).

■ ANATOMY AND PHYSIOLOGY

All components of the neurological system are highly interconnected and integrated in function. Maturation of the nervous system continues throughout childhood until early adolescence. For instructional purposes the nervous system is divided into two major parts: (1) the central nervous system, which consists of the brain and spinal cord, and (2) the peripheral nervous system, which is composed of (a) the cranial nerves, (b) 31 pairs of spinal nerves that emerge from the spinal cord, and (c) the autonomic nervous system. The autonomic nervous system is divided into the sympathetic (thoracolumbar) and parasympathetic (craniosacral) nervous systems. It is considered part of the peripheral nervous system because in most parts of the body innervated by these systems, their structures appear together.

Central Nervous System
Brain

The brain is made up of gray and white matter. Gray matter contains cell bodies, and white matter includes myelinated nerve fibers. The brain consists of the cerebrum, the largest part of the brain, which is composed of two hemispheres; the brainstem (midbrain, pons, and medulla); the diencephalon (thalmus, hypothalmus, epithalmus, and subthalmus); and the cerebellum (Figure 19.1). The left side of the brain controls language, whereas the right side is the nonverbal, or perceptual, hemisphere. Ninety percent of the population has a dominant left hemisphere, and these individuals are right-handed. The cerebral functions interact with the

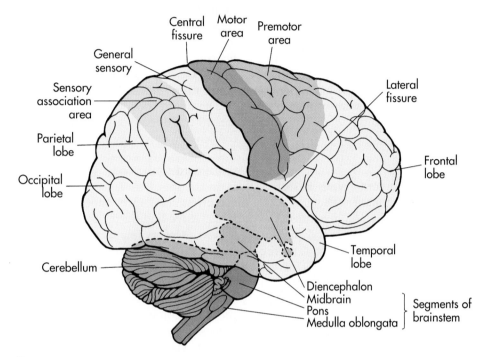

figure**19.1**   Lateral view of the brain. *(Modified from Smith CG:* Serial dissections of the human brain, *Baltimore, 1981, Urban & Schwarzenberg.)*

figure**19.2**   Functional subdivisions of the cerebral cortex.

reticular activating system, located in the upper brainstem and diencephalon, to control conscious movement, thought, and perception. The major cerebellar functions influence mechanisms of equilibrium, muscle tone, and coordinated movement, such as control of gait (Figure 19.2).

Approximately 20% of the oxygen consumed by the body is used to provide energy to the brain. Since the brain depends totally on glucose for metabolism, a lack of oxygen for 2 to 5 minutes can result in irreversible brain damage. The circle of Willis, located at the base of the brain, is an arterial communication between the right and the left cerebral circulation. Its function is to equalize blood flow to various parts of the brain. Superficial and deep veins drain into the system of sinuses of the dura mater, which empties into the internal jugular vein.

Spinal cord

A cross section of the spinal cord reveals H-shaped gray matter surrounded by white matter. The gray matter is made up of cell bodies, axons, and dendrites. The gray matter also contains posterior (dorsal) and anterior (ventral) horns. The actual shape and extent of the white and gray matter vary at different levels of the cord. Figure 19.3 shows a cross section of the spinal cord, with a labeling scheme of laminae (layers) from I to X, as described by Rexed, to show the major longitudinal columns. The columns are identified according to similarity in appearance and function. For example, lamina V receives dorsal root afferent fibers from sensory fibers, such as those that transmit pain, temperature, and light touch (spinothalamic tract).

Motor and sensory pathways

Neurons that transmit impulses can be motor, sensory, or mixed. Motor neurons, or efferent neurons, carry impulses from the central nervous system to effectors, located in muscles, organs, and glands. Sensory neurons, or afferent neurons, carry impulses from receptors to the central nervous system. General sensory afferent fibers involve conscious sensation, such as pain and light touch. General visceral afferent fibers carry sensory impulses from the viscera.

The dorsal roots carry sensory impulses from receptors to the dorsal root ganglia, in which cell bodies of the sensory nerves are located, to the spinal cord. Ventral roots carry efferent (motor) impulses from the spinal cord to the body.

In the spinal cord, descending tracts (pyramidal and extrapyramidal) carry motor impulses away from the brain. Ascending tracts (dorsal columns or spinothalamic) carry sensory impulses to the brain.

Sensory pathways. Sensory impulses travel from the receptors through afferent fibers in the peripheral nerve, through the dorsal root, and to the spinal cord. Various types of receptors are stimulated by pain and temperature, position and movement, or visceral sensations of fullness or cramping. In the spinal cord, sensory impulses travel via two major pathways to higher levels of the

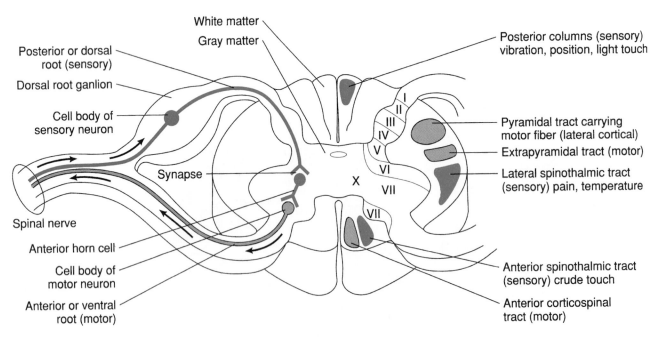

figure**19.3** Cross section of the spinal cord. Spinal nerve roots and their neurons appear on the left side. Spinal nerve tracts appear in the white matter on the right side. All tracts and nerves are bilateral.

nervous system: via the posterior columns or the spinothalamic tract. The lateral spinothalamic tract contains sensory fibers that transmit the sensations of pain, temperature, and light touch. Fibers in the posterior columns transmit stimuli involved with position, vibration, and manipulation with digits, such as stereognosis and graphesthesia (see Figure 19.3).

Motor pathways

Pyramidal system. The pyramidal system (corticospinal tracts) consists of neurons of spinal cord white matter arranged in long columns, or fiber tracts, lateral to the gray matter. The majority of these columns cross to the contralateral side at the level of the medulla. Those that do not cross in the medulla continue as the

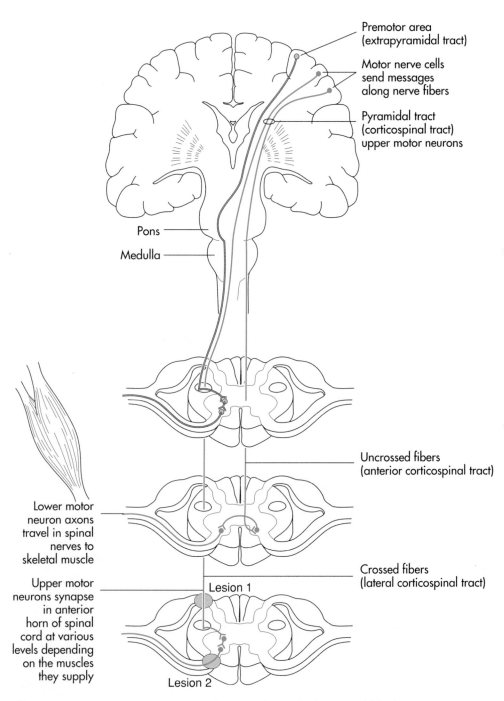

figure **19.4**   Major motor pathways between the cerebral cortex and lower motor neurons in the spinal cord. *Lesion 1*: Upper motor neuron with motor damage on the contralateral side. *Lesion 2*: Lower motor neuron with motor damage on the ipsilateral side.

anterior corticospinal tract and cross over at the cervical or thoracic level of the cord. The pyramidal tract uniquely transmits stimuli concerned with voluntary movements and temporal (time) and spatial (e.g., perceiving change over time) qualities (Figure 19.4).

Upper and lower motor neurons. A model of a two-neuron chain is used here to simplify understanding of the basic structure of the pyramidal tract. The chain begins in the motor area of the cerebral cortex, located anterior to the central sulcus. The size of the cortical area correlates with the degree of skilled function carried out

by a particular body part (Figure 19.5). Note that the face and hands cover the largest areas. This neural chain travels to skeletal muscle and is contained in one of the many ascending and descending pathways in the spinal cord.

The upper motor neuron cell bodies are located in the cerebral cortex, and their axons cross over to the opposite side (contralateral) at the level of the medulla to synapse with the lower motor neuron cell body in the cranial nerve motor nuclei or the anterior horn of the spinal cord (Figure 19.4). The axon of the lower motor

figure**19.5** Representation of specific body parts in the motor strip of the frontal lobe. *(From Seeley RR, Stephens TD, Tate P: Anatomy and physiology, ed 2, New York, 1992, Mc-Graw-Hill.)*

neuron becomes the peripheral nerve. Because upper motor neurons affect motor activity only through the lower motor neurons, the latter are referred to as the final common pathway.

Damage to a lower motor neuron will cause motor impairment on the same (ipsilateral) side of the body, whereas damage to an upper motor neuron leads to motor impairment on the contralateral side. For example, the facial nerve (cranial nerve [CN] VII) is a lower motor neuron. Damage to the motor portion of the right facial nerve results in impaired movement of the right side of the face. However, if a stroke damages the right upper motor neuron that synapses with the right facial nerve, the result would be impaired motor function of the left side of the face, primarily its lower portion.

Lower motor neurons are either (1) alpha type, which when included with all muscle fibers supplied are called motor units, or (2) gamma type, which supply the muscle fibers of the neuromuscular spindle and control length and tension receptors for the stretch reflex and proprioception.

Extrapyramidal system. The extrapyramidal system is more complex than other motor pathways. It includes all the motor neurons originating in the motor cortex and the cerebellum outside the pyramidal tracts, in addition to the sensory (spinothalamic) tracts. The extrapyramidal tract integrates input from many sources and modifies the motor impulses of the pyramidal system, especially those needed to maintain posture, balance, and slow movement. Since the sensory tracts are located close to the corticospinal tracts in the spinal cord, it is common for both sensory and motor deficits to occur with spinal cord damage.

Peripheral Nervous System
Spinal nerves

Each spinal cord nerve segment communicates with specific parts of the body through 31 pairs of spinal nerves, both afferent and efferent, at that level (8 cervical, 12 thoracic, 5 lumbar, 5 sacral, and 1 coccygeal). Each nerve is designated by a letter and a number to indicate its location. For example, C8 is the eighth cervical nerve. Each spinal nerve has a dorsal root, which carries afferent (sensory) impulses to the cord, and a ventral root, which carries efferent (motor) impulses away from the cord. Sensory fibers (dorsal root) from a single spinal nerve that serve a particular skin surface are collectively called a dermatome (Figure 19.6). Because of considerable overlap between adjacent dermatome areas, sensory loss results only if a number of dermatomes are damaged.

Reflex arc

Reflexes are part of the motor system. They control automatic responses to stimuli at the level of the spinal cord (segmental response), freeing the cortex from involvement in most muscle movements that occur in the body. Reflexes provide rapid responses, such as withdrawal from painful stimuli. The simplest reflex arc is monosynaptic, in which the sensory fiber interacts directly with the motor neuron (Figure 19.7).

Skeletal muscles contract when they are stretched by contraction of the antagonistic muscle, the pull of gravity, or external manipulation. The muscles also contract when their tendons are stretched. Deep tendon reflexes, or muscle stretch reflexes, are segmental responses elicited by striking a tendon with a reflex hammer. This stimulus stretches the neuromuscular spindles of the muscle group.

Muscle spindles (gamma fibers), which are abundant in skeletal muscles, are capsules surrounding specialized muscle cells known as intrafusal fibers. Both ends of the intrafusal fiber consist of contractile tissue called the spindle pole, whereas the central portion, the nuclear bag, is expanded (nucleated). Primary afferent fibers are stimulated when the bag is stretched to carry impulses to the spinal cord, where alpha motor neurons are activated. The alpha motor neuron impulses terminate at the endplates of the skeletal muscle, and gamma efferent impulses terminate in the muscle spindle, stimulating both tendon and muscle contraction.

Figure 19.7 illustrates the deep tendon reflex, with the patellar tendon reflex used as an example. The patellar tendon of the quadriceps muscle is attached to the tibia. Tapping this tendon with a reflex hammer causes the muscle to be stretched, activating the muscle spindles and thereby the femoral (primary afferent) nerve, to the spinal cord. In the spinal cord the sensory neurons synapse with the alpha motor nerve in the cord segment (L3 and L4). The alpha efferent fibers carry impulses back to the muscle, resulting in contraction of the quadriceps muscle and extension of the leg. Dysfunction of the tendon reflex, therefore, could result from problems in the thigh muscle, the femoral nerve, or the segment of the spinal cord being tested.

Five Components of a Reflex Arc

1. Sensory (afferent) peripheral nerve
2. Intact interneuron (synapse) in the spinal cord
3. Motor (efferent) peripheral nerve
4. Intact neuromuscular junction (synapse in the muscle)
5. Competent muscle

figure **19.6**   Dermatomes of the body. Each dorsal (sensory) spinal root innervates one dermatome. The first cervical nerve usually has no cutaneous distribution. The trigeminal nerve (CN V) supplies most of the general somatic sensory innervation to the anterior part of the head. (*Modified from Rudy EB:* Advanced neurological and neurosurgical nursing, *St Louis, 1984, Mosby.*)

figure**19.7**   Deep tendon (stretch) reflex (knee-jerk or patellar tendon reflex). Inset shows afferent fibers from the muscle spindle and tendon organs, and efferent fibers to the muscle and spindle. Note that the patellar tendon of the extensor muscle attaches to the tibia below the knee.

Superficial reflexes. Superficial reflexes are reactions that can be elicited by stroking the skin or muscle. Examples of these reflexes include the abdominal reflex, which tests spinal cord levels T8 through T12 (see Figure 17.30); the cremasteric reflex, observed in males (T12-L2) when stroking of the skin of the inner upper thigh results in testicular movement on the same side; and the plantar reflex (L4-L5, S1-S2), elicited by firmly stroking the lateral surface of the sole of the foot to stimulate plantar flexion of the toes.

Cranial nerves

Twelve pairs of cranial nerves emerge from the brain or brainstem. Cranial nerves consist of fibers that have sensory (afferent) and motor (efferent) functions, as well as special sensory afferent functions such as vision, hearing, and equilibrium. Cranial nerves also contain special visceral efferent nerve fibers for voluntary motor function; special visceral afferent fibers carry visceral sensation, such as taste and smell (Figure 19.8).

CN I—olfactory nerve. The olfactory nerve is sensory for smell. The peripheral neurons of the olfactory nerve penetrate the nasal mucosa in the roof of the nose, the upper septum, and the medial wall of the superior nasal concha. Unless the individual sniffs or inspires deeply, most of the inspired air does not contact the olfactory epithelium; during normal respiration, inspired air does not rise that high in the nares (see Figure 13.5).

CN II—optic nerve. The optic nerve, sensory for sight, is described in Chapter 12 (see the discussions of examination of visual acuity, visual fields, retinal fields, and the optic disc).

CN III—oculomotor nerve; CN IV—trochlear nerve; CN VI—abducens nerve. The oculomotor, trochlear, and abducens nerves, which control movement of the eyeball, elevation of the eyelid, and pupillary constriction, are always tested together. These cranial nerves are also described in Chapter 12 (note the sections on neuromuscular and extraocular muscle function and tests of eye movement).

CN V—trigeminal nerve. The trigeminal nerve is motor to the muscles of mastication and sensory to the cornea, mucosa of the nose and mouth, and skin of the face and forehead in perceiving touch, temperature, and pain. The sensory fibers are contained in one of the

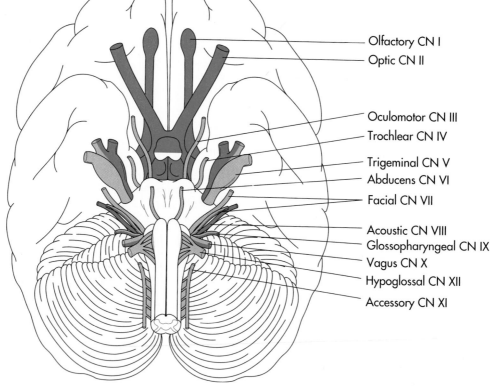

figure**19.8**   Diagram of the base of the brain showing the entrance or exit of the cranial nerves.

figure**19.9**   Cutaneous (sensory) fields of the head and upper part of the neck. The cutaneous fields of the three branches of the trigeminal nerve are identified as I, ophthalmic; II, maxillary; and III, mandibular.

three divisions of the nerve: ophthalmic, maxillary, or mandibular (Figure 19.9).

CN VII—facial nerve. The facial nerve is motor to the facial muscles and sensory to taste on the anterior two thirds of the tongue. Visceral sensation from the salivary glands and mucosa of the mouth and pharynx is also conducted by CN VII. In addition, the facial nerve carries parasympathetic fibers that stimulate secretion of the salivary glands, the lacrimal glands, and the mucosa of the nose, palate, and nasopharynx.

CN VIII—acoustic nerve. The acoustic nerve is composed of two divisions: the cochlear and the vestibular.

Cochlear division. The cochlear division is sensory for hearing. Tests for cochlear function are described in Chapter 13.

Vestibular division. Tests for vestibular functions, or equilibrium, are *not* routine in the physical examination. One method used to test vestibular function by producing changes in the flow of endolymph is the caloric test. In the caloric test, the examiner irrigates the client's ear with ice water; a normal reaction includes nausea, dizziness, and nystagmus.

Major Areas of Neurological Examination

1. Mental status (performed first during the interview, but in this chapter discussed after the other areas of examination)
2. Cranial nerves
3. Proprioception and cerebellar function
4. Motor function (see Chapter 18: Musculoskeletal System)
5. Sensory function
6. Deep tendon reflexes

CN IX—glossopharyngeal nerve; CN X—vagus nerve. The glossopharyngeal and vagus nerves are closely related both anatomically and physiologically, and they are tested as a unit. The glossopharyngeal nerve contains sensory and motor fibers. The sensory component is taste on the posterior third of the tongue and sensation from the tonsillar and pharyngeal mucosa. CN IX also has sensory fibers for the carotid sinus and body. The motor function of this nerve innervates the pharynx and parotid glands to control swallowing, gagging, and salivation.

The vagus nerve is sensory for the external ear and pharynx. It functions as a motor nerve to the soft palate, pharynx, larynx, and esophagus. CN X provides parasympathetic control to smooth and cardiac muscle and abdominal organs.

CN XI—spinal accessory nerve. The spinal accessory nerve supplies the sternocleidomastoid and trapezius muscles with motor innervation.

CN XII—hypoglossal nerve. The hypoglossal nerve provides motor fibers to the muscles of the tongue, making possible articulation of lingual speech sounds and swallowing.

Autonomic nervous system

The autonomic nervous system is made up of motor neurons called general visceral efferent neurons. The function of this system is to maintain a stable internal environment for the body. The sympathetic nervous system, also called the thoracolumbar division, is activated during stress and brings about widespread responses, such as increased heart rate, vasodilation in skeletal muscle, reduction in gastric secretions, and dilation of bronchioles. These "fight or flight" responses enable us to be physically prepared to handle potential danger. Sympathetic (thoracolumbar) preganglionic fibers emerge from T1 to L2 levels of the spinal column.

The parasympathetic system, also called the craniosacral division, is associated with conservation, restora-

tion, and maintenance of normal body functions, such as decreasing the heart rate and increasing gastrointestinal motility. Parasympathetic (craniosacral) preganglionic fibers emerge from the cranial nerves (III, VI, IX, X) and S1 through S4 segments of the spinal cord.

■ EXAMINATION OF THE NEUROLOGICAL SYSTEM

Health History

Clues to areas of abnormality may be evident during the client's history, such as orientation, speech, and ability to interact with the examiner. The presence of certain symptoms in a client who appears normal may indicate neurological problems. If any symptom is present, it is important to obtain further information about onset, duration, intensity, frequency, aggravating and alleviating factors, and effects on the client's activity (see Chapter 2 for interviewing techniques).

Present health status

1. Numbness, tingling, or loss of feeling
2. Difficulty with speaking, vision, or hearing
3. Any physical disability
4. Medications
5. Problems with coordination or balance
6. Change in ability to remember
7. Shakiness or tremors of the hands or legs
8. Presence of anxiety or depression
9. Recent changes in self, such as alterations in sleep habits, changes in sexual activity, unexplained weight gain or loss, difficulty in performing usual daily activities

Past health history

1. Seizures, fainting spells, or dizzy spells
2. Headaches
3. History of head injury or major trauma

Preparation for Examination: Client and Environment

The neurological examination begins as soon as you, the examiner, and the client are introduced. Begin to form an overall impression and continue to make general observations before focusing on problem areas. Conduct the interview and examination in a quiet, private room without interruption. Perform the mental status examination with both you and the client comfortably seated. Conduct the remainder of the neurological examination with the client seated on the edge of the examination table or standing. Ask the client to remove shoes, socks, and outer clothing that covers the extremities. Give the client a loose-fitting gown to wear.

PREPARATION FOR EXAMINATION

EQUIPMENT

Item	Purpose
Cottonball, disposable safety pin	Light touch, pain sensation, and localization
Tongue blade	Tongue strength, gag reflex
Tuning fork (512 cps)	Vibration sense
Ophthalmoscope	Optic nerve, pupil constriction
Reflex hammer	Deep tendon reflexes
Pencil and paper	Fine coordinated movements
Printed material	Reading and comprehension
Optional:	
Test tubes for cold and warm water	Temperature sensation
Aromatic substances	Olfaction
Sweet, sour substances	Taste
Calipers	Two-point discrimination

CLIENT AND ENVIRONMENT

Client clothed in loose-fitting gown over underwear
Quiet private room
Comfortable chairs
Examination table

HELPFUL HINT *Be cautious about interpreting results whenever a client does not do something you have instructed. It may be simply a misunderstanding of directions and not a neurological defect. An isolated abnormal finding is very difficult to interpret.*

Technique for Examination and Normal Findings
Cranial nerves

Table 19.1 summarizes the cranial nerves, including their functions, structures innervated, tests, and normal findings.

CN I (olfactory). Do not test CN I during a screening examination unless the history suggests a problem. Before testing the olfactory nerve, examine the nares for any signs of obstruction. Ask the client, with eyes

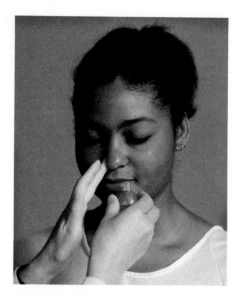

figure**19.10** Testing for the ability to smell. The examiner asks the client to sniff while placing a test tube containing the test substance beneath the nostril. The examiner holds the other nostril closed.

closed, to sniff familiar odors, such as coffee, vinegar, or chocolate. Test each side separately (Figure 19.10).

CN II (optic), III, IV, and VI (extraocular movements). See Chapter 12 for specific examination techniques.

CN V (trigeminal). With the client's eyes closed, test for the presence of several types of sensation, comparing both sides and testing areas innervated by the three branches of the trigeminal nerve (Figure 19.11). Check whether the client perceives sensation equally on both sides. Test the corneal reflex only on an unconscious client by touching a wisp of cotton lightly to the cornea and observing a blink response. Test for light touch by using a wisp of cotton and asking the client to localize where the sensation is perceived. By alternating the sharp and dull end of a safety pin, test for pain sensation; discard the safety pin after use. The sharp edge of a broken tongue blade can also be used. Test each branch on both sides of the face with a pain (sharp) stimulus. Testing for temperature sensation is not routine, since pain and temperature are both carried by the lateral spinothalamic tract.

Test muscles of mastication and the motor functions of the trigeminal nerve by palpating the masseter muscles (Figure 19.12) and the temporal muscles (Figure 19.13) while asking the client to bite down hard. Test jaw strength against resistance by applying downward pressure on the chin while asking the client to resist opening the mouth.

CN VII (facial). Inspect the client's face for symmetrical movement when he or she looks at the ceiling, wrin-

| table 19.1 | ***The Cranial Nerves*** |

Nerve	Function	Structure innervated	Test	Normal findings
I Olfactory	Sensory Smell	Olfactory epithelium in nasal cavity	Apply simple odors to one nostril at a time	Correct identification of odor
II Optic	Sensory Vision	Retina of eye	Visual acuity using Snellen chart Visual fields using a confrontation test Ophthalmoscopic examination	Correct identification of letters No visual fields defects Normal fundus
III Oculo motor	Motor Upward, downward, medial eye movement	Superior, medial, inferior rectus, inferior oblique, and levator palpebrae superior muscles	Flash light in one eye at a time EOM: Ask client to follow an object while you move it to left, then up and down left of midline; to right, then up and down right of midline	Direct and consensual light reflex Both eyes follow object in parallel
	Lid elevation Pupil constriction		Observe lids	Palpebral fissures equal Pupils constrict
IV Trochlear	Motor Downward, medial eye movement	Superior oblique muscle	EOM	Same as EOM of CN III

V Trigeminal	Sensory
	  Face
	  Scalp
	  Nasal mucosa
	  Buccal mucosa
	  Jaw muscles
	Motor
	  Masseter muscle
	  Temporal muscle
	  Digastric muscle
		Skin and mucosa of face and head via ophthalmic, maxillary, and mandibular divisions	Test tactile and pain sensation of all three divisions
			
			Feel two masseter muscles as client bites down
			Corneal reflex
				Normal sensory perception from entire face
				
				Equal contraction of masseters and no deviation of mandible
				Blinking of eye

VI Abducens	Motor Lateral eye movement	Lateral rectus muscle	EOM	Same as EOM of CN III

VII Facial	Sensory
	  External ear
	  Taste: anterior two thirds of tongue
	  Deep facial
		Taste buds of anterior two thirds of tongue
		Lacrimal, sublingual, and submandibular glands; other minor glands and mucosal surfaces
			Apply small amount of sugar or salt to anterior two thirds of tongue	Correct identification of substance

continued

table **19.1** **The Cranial Nerves—(cont'd)**

Nerve	Function	Structure innervated	Test	Normal findings

VII Facial— cont'd	Motor
	  Facial movement
	  Scalp muscle
	  Auricular muscle
	  Stylohyoid muscle
	  Digastric posterior belly
	Parasympathetic
	  Salivation: submax-illary glands, sublingual-glands
	  Lacrimation: lacrimal glands
	  Mucous membrane
	  Nasopharynx
	Sensory
		Facial, stapedius, stylo-hyoid, and posterior digastric muscles
		Middle ear
		External ear
			Ask client to wrinkle forehead, close eyes, show teeth, whistle	Normal execution of movements

VIII Acoustic	Cochlear: hearing	Spiral organ of cochlea	Hearing acuity using a watch or a whis-per Rinne test (tuning fork on mastoid process) Weber test (tuning fork on center of forehead) Otoscopic examina-tion	Normal and bilaterally symmetrical hearing Air conduction greater than bone conduc-tion Heard in both ears equally Normal tympanic membrane
	Vestibular: equilib-rium	Ampullae of semicircu-lar ducts and maculae of saccule and utricle	Romberg test* Caloric	Able to maintain bal-ance with eye closed Nystagmus

IX Glosso-pharyn-geal	Sensory
	  External ear
	  Taste: posterior third of tongue
	  Carotid: reflexes, baroreceptors and chemorecep-tors, sinus, body
		Taste buds of posterior third of tongue
		Parotid gland
		Pharynx (gag reflex), carotid sinus, posteri-or third of tongue, auditory tube, and middle ear
		Stylopharyngeus muscle
		External ear		

	Motor
	  Pharynx: gag re-flex, swallowing, pharyngeal mus-cles
	  Parotid gland: sali-vation
	Sensory
			Touch pharynx with cotton applicator	Gag reflex
				Able to swallow

X Vagus	External ear Pharynx	External ear Carotid and aortic bod-ies; muscles of soft palate, pharynx, lar-ynx, and esophagus	Listen to person talk	Lack of hoarseness

*Also a test of proprioception sense.

table 19.1   **The Cranial Nerves—(cont'd)**

Nerve	Function	Structure innervated	Test	Normal findings
X Vagus—cont'd	Motor Swallowing, gag reflex Pronation Cardiac slowing Bronchoconstriction Gastric secretion Peristalsis	Epiglottis	Ask person to say "ah"	Both sides of soft palate contract and uvula remains in midline
	Parasympathetic Thoracic and abdominal viscera Aortic arch Chemoreceptors Baroreceptors	Smooth and cardiac muscles and glands of thoracic and abdominal organs through transverse colon		
XI Accessory	Motor Swallowing pharyngeal muscles Turning of head: sternocleidomastoid muscles Elevation of shoulders: trapezius muscles	Larynx and pharynx (with CN X)	Ask client to turn head to each side and shrug shoulders while you resist the movements	Strong contractions of sternocleidomastoid and trapezius muscles
XII Hypoglossal	Motor Muscles that move tongue: hypoglossus, genioglossus, styloglossus	Extrinsic and intrinsic muscles of tongue	Ask client to protrude tongue fully Move client's tongue side to side against resistance with tongue blade	Tongue protrudes in midline Good tongue strength

A   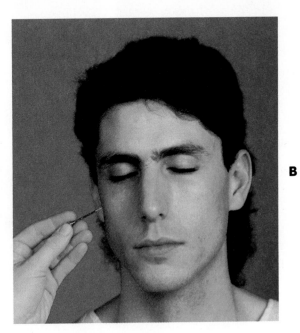 **B**

figure **19.11**   Testing for light touch (**A**) and pain (**B**) sensation. The examiner applies a wisp of cotton just firmly enough to stimulate the sensory nerve endings. To test for superficial pain, the examiner uses the sharp point of a safety pin, alternating with the dull end of the pin.

figure**19.12** Palpation of the masseter muscles for size, strength, and symmetry to test CN V (trigeminal nerve).

figure**19.13** Palpation of the temporal muscles for size, shape, and symmetry to test CN V (trigeminal nerve).

A   **B**   **C**

figure**19.14** Testing motor function of CN VII (facial nerve). The examiner inspects the client's ability to frown (**A**), smile (**B**), and puff out the cheeks (**C**).

kles the forehead, frowns, smiles, puffs out cheeks, and raises eyebrows (Figure 19.14). Ask the client to close the eyes, first lightly and then tightly, while you try to open them. In infants, evaluate the facial muscles during crying. Evaluate tone and note any atrophy and fasciculations, or twitching, of a muscle group.

Testing for taste, salivation, and lacrimation is generally not part of the routine physical examination. When it is appropriate to test taste sensation, use an applicator to apply salty or sweet solutions to the anterior of each side of the tongue. Use a different applicator for each substance, and allow the client a sip of water between tests to avoid mixing tastes. Have the client leave the tongue protruded until he or she identifies the taste. To avoid spreading the test substance over the tongue, give the client a card with the words salty, sweet, sour, and bitter (the vagus nerve innervates sour and bitter taste on the posterior tongue) and ask the client to point to the one that best describes the solution on the tongue (Figure 19.15). Record the number of correct responses.

CN VIII (acoustic). See Chapter 13: Ears, Nose, Mouth, and Throat.

CN IX (glossopharyngeal) and X (vagus). Testing of CN IX and CN X focuses on the musculature of the palate, pharynx, and larynx. Inspect the soft palate for symmetry. Identify the uvula and record any deviation from the midline. Test the gag reflex by touching the posterior wall of the pharynx with an applicator or a tongue blade; check for elevation of the palate and contraction of the pharyngeal muscles.

Note that the vagus nerve is functioning normally if the client can swallow and speak clearly without hoarseness. Ask the client to say "ah," and note whether the palate rises symmetrically. (See Chapter 13.)

CN XI (spinal accessory). To test the spinal accessory nerve, evaluate the symmetry, size, and strength of the muscles. Ask the client to turn the head to one side against the resistance of your hand while you palpate the opposite sternocleidomastoid muscle (Figure 19.16).

To assess the trapezius muscles, ask the client to shrug the shoulders while you exert downward pressure. Evaluate the muscles for strength and symmetry (Figure 19.17).

CN XII (hypoglossal). Inspect the tongue for size (atrophy), symmetry, and fasciculations. Ask the client to stick out the tongue as far as possible. Note the client's ability to stick the tongue straight out and the strength of the movement against lateral resistance produced with a tongue blade. Test the client's muscle strength by asking him or her to push out the cheek with the tongue while you push against it from the outside (Figure 19.18).

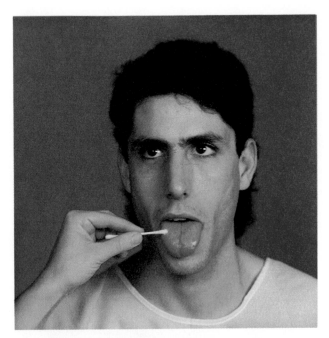

figure**19.15** Testing for taste sensation (CN VII [facial nerve] and CN IX [glossopharyngeal nerve]). The examiner applies salty or sweet solutions to the anterior two thirds of the tongue and sour or bitter solutions to the posterior one third of the tongue. The right and left sides of the tongue are tested while the client's tongue is projected.

figure**19.16** Assessing the symmetry, size, and strength of the sternocleidomastoid muscle in testing CN XI (spinal accessory nerve). The client is asked to turn the head to one side against the resistance of the examiner's hand. The contralateral sternocleidomastoid muscle will stand out as it contracts. The examiner palpates the visible muscle to assess tension.

figure**19.17** To test CN XI (spinal accessory nerve) and trapezius muscle strength, the client shrugs the shoulders against the resistance of the examiner's hands.

figure**19.18** Assessing the strength of the tongue. The examiner asks the client to push against the inner surface of the cheek with as much strength as possible. The examiner palpates the external surface of the cheek simultaneously.

Proprioception and cerebellar function

The proprioceptive system of the nervous system maintains posture, balance, and coordination. The neural structures involved in proprioception are the posterior columns of the spinal cord, the cerebellum, and the vestibular apparatus. The posterior columns of the spinal cord carry stimuli from the proprioceptors in tendons and joints in addition to fibers for touch and two-point discrimination. Lesions affecting the posterior column impair muscle and position sense. The cerebellum integrates muscle contractions to maintain posture. Lesions affecting the cerebellum impair balance and coordination.

The vestibular system is concerned with correcting movements. Vestibular disease is characterized by vertigo, nausea, and vomiting. Vertigo is the illusion of movement of the individual or the environment. Nausea and vomiting frequently accompany this condition. The following examination techniques are used to assess proprioception and cerebellar functions.

Finger-to-nose movements. Ask the client to touch his or her nose with the index finger of one hand and then the other, first with the eyes open and then with the eyes closed (Figure 19.19). A normal finding is the ability to accurately target the nose.

Finger-nose-finger movements. Ask the client, with the eyes open, to touch his or her nose and then your finger at a distance of approximately 45 cm. Have the

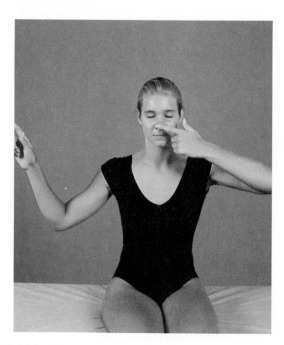

figure**19.19** Testing cerebellar function. The client attempts to alternately touch the nose with the index finger of each hand, repeating the motion with increasing speed.

client increase the speed as you move your finger (Figure 19.20). Test each hand separately. Note the speed and accuracy of movement.

Rapid alternating movements. Ask the client to pat his or her knees with the palms of the hands followed by the backs of the hands at an ever-increasing rate (Figure 19.21). Then have the client perform thumb-to-finger opposition by touching each finger of one hand to the thumb of the same hand as rapidly as possible (Figure 19.22).

Heel to shin. Ask the client to run the heel of each foot down the opposite shin (Figure 19.23).

Romberg test. Ask the client to stand with the feet together, first with the eyes open and then with the eyes

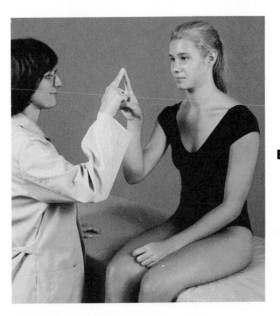

figure **19.20** Testing cerebellar function. The client attempts to move the finger from the nose (**A**) to the examiner's finger (**B**) rapidly. The examiner's index finger is about 18 inches from the client's eye and moves the position of the finger target.

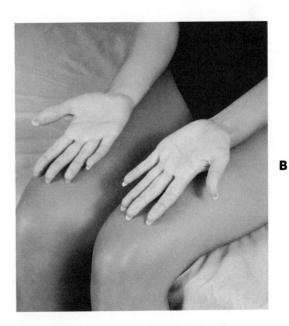

figure **19.21** Testing cerebellar function: pronation (**A**) and supination (**B**) of the hands with progressively more rapid movement.

figure**19.22** Testing cerebellar function. The examiner instructs the client to touch each finger to the thumb as rapidly as possible.

closed (Figure 19.24). Slight swaying is normal. Stand close enough to the client to prevent falling. The normal client is able to do this for about 15 seconds with the eyes closed.

Coordination. After the client opens the eyes, ask him or her to walk naturally, then in a heel-to-toe fashion (Figure 19.25), and then to stand on each foot (Figure 19.26). If the client does this without difficulty, ask him or her to hop on one foot and then the other (Figure 19.27), and to do a deep knee bend (Figure 19.28). Since shoes can interfere with balance, have the client perform these tests without shoes.

Sensory function

Although evaluating sensation over the entire skin surface is not necessary, stimuli should be applied strategically to test the dermatomes and the major peripheral nerves. A minimal number of test sites includes areas on the forehead, cheek, hand, and foot. In the screening examination, assume the nerve to be intact if sensation is normal at its most distal area. When there is evidence

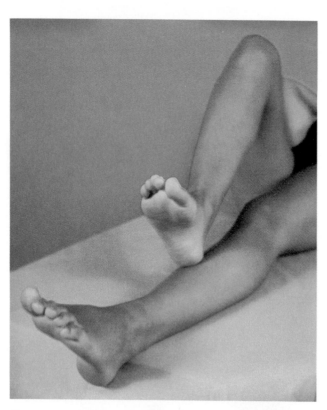

figure**19.23** Testing cerebellar function. The examiner asks the client to run the heel of each foot down the opposite shin.

figure**19.24** Testing the proprioceptive system. Romberg test: the client should be able to stand with the eyes closed and the feet together without swaying for approximately 5 seconds.

of dysfunction, localize the site of the dysfunction and map the boundaries. Sketch the region involved and describe the sensory change.

Variation in sensitivity of skin areas is normal. Use a stronger stimulus over the back, the buttocks, and areas where the skin is heavily cornified. Establish symmetry of sensation by checking first one spot and then the same area on the opposite side of the body.

Instruct the client to close the eyes during evaluation of sensory modalities. A client who is able to see the stimulus applied may be influenced by visual cues rather than responding to the specific sensory modality being tested.

> **HELPFUL HINT** *Ensure that both you and the client are rested, because fatigue may result in errors. Otherwise, you may interpret inattention or low motivation as a sensory loss. Also, to avoid predictability, vary the testing sites and the timing in applying the stimulus.*

The following terms are useful in describing and recording sensory dysfunction:

Anesthesia: Absence of normal sensation.

Hyperesthesia: Extreme sensitivity of one of the body's senses.

Hypoesthesia: Abnormal weakness of sensation in response to sensory stimulation.

Paresthesia: Any subjective sensation, experienced as numbness, tingling, or a "pins and needles" feeling.

Light touch sensation. Light touch and pain are mediated by different nerve endings. Sensory fibers for light touch enter the spinal cord and travel upward in the anterior spinothalamic tracts to the thalamus. Both anterior spinothalamic tracts must suffer destruction before transmission of light touch is lost.

Test light touch by contacting the skin with a wisp of cotton (see Figure 19.11, *A*). Does the client feel the touch of a wisp of cotton? Instruct the client to say "yes" or "now" when the touch is felt. If desired, combine this test with localization (a higher cortical func-

figure**19.25** Testing the proprioceptive system. The client attempts to walk a straight line, placing heel to toe.

figure**19.26** Testing the proprioceptive system. The client attempts to stand on one foot and then the other.

figure**19.27** Testing the proprioceptive system. The client attempts to hop in place on one foot and then the other.

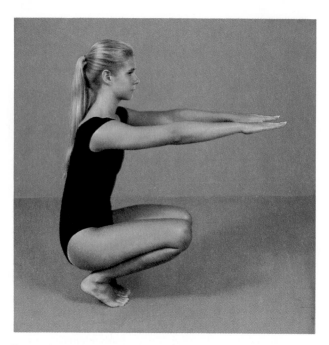

figure **19.28**   Testing the proprioceptive system. The client attempts a knee bend without support.

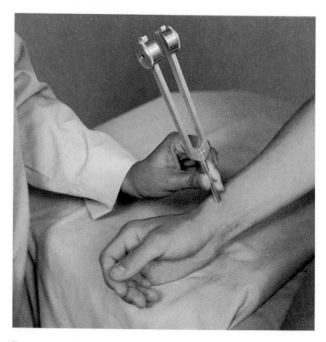

figure **19.29**   Testing sensitivity to vibration. The examiner applies the base of a vibrating tuning fork to a bony prominence, such as the wrist.

tion) by asking the client to state where he or she is touched. Compare each side of the body. Record areas of anesthesia or hyperesthesia.

Pain and temperature sensation. Pain and temperature fibers both travel in the lateral spinothalamic tract. A screening examination does not include temperature assessment unless pain sensation is abnormal. To test temperature sensation, roll tubes filled with warm and cold water against the client's skin over dermatome areas. (First test the stimuli on your own skin to avoid burning the client and to provide a comparison.) Ask the client to say "hot," "cold," or "can't tell."

Evaluate the sensory perception of superficial pain by using the sharp and dull points of a safety pin (see Figure 19.11, *B*). Compare each side of the body in the same locations as you test tactile sensation. To avoid any risk of infection, discard the safety pin after use. Instruct the client to say "sharp" or "dull" when touched. Remember that each area examined must be touched with a sharp stimulus because dull touch simply validates light touch perception.

Vibration sensation. The normal client can perceive vibration as a buzzing or tingling sensation when a bony prominence, such as the wrist, elbow, or ankle, touches the base of a vibrating tuning fork. With the client's eyes closed, test vibratory sensation by applying the vibrating tuning fork to the wrists, elbows, knees, and ankles (Figure 19.29). Ask the client to say "yes" or "now" (1) when first feeling the vibrations and (2) when the vibrations stop. Dampen the vibrations of the

tuning fork to move along more rapidly. Compare sensitivity from side to side and proximal to distal parts of the extremities. Apply the tuning fork to the most distal point of the extremity, since normal vibratory perception, or intactness of posterior columns, decreases from a proximal to a distal point.

A normal finding in the older client (older than 65 years) is diminished vibratory sensation, particularly in the extremities.

Tactile discrimination. Tactile discrimination requires interpretation by the cerebral cortex. Three types of tactile discrimination are tested: (1) stereognosis, (2) two-point discrimination, and (3) extinction.

Stereognosis is the ability to recognize objects by touching and manipulating them. Test stereognosis with universally familiar objects, such as a key, safety pin, or coin (Figure 19.30). Test graphesthesia by asking the client to identify letters or numbers written on each palm with a blunt point. The normal client can correctly identify the letters or numbers inscribed (Figure 19.31).

Two-point discrimination is the ability to sense whether one or two areas of the skin are being stimulated by pressure. There is considerable variability of perceptual ability over the different parts of the body. The following are minimal distances between the two points of the calipers at which the normal adult can sense simultaneous stimulation:

Tongue: 1 mm
Fingertips: 2.8 mm

figure**19.30** Testing for stereognosis. The normal client can identify a familiar object (coin, key) by touching and manipulating it.

figure**19.31** Testing for graphesthesia. The normal client can identify a number or letter written on the palm.

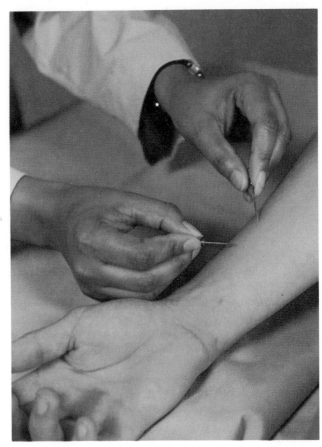

figure**19.32** Testing for two-point discrimination. Disposable pins or paper clips bent into a U shape can be used.

Palms of hands: 8 to 12 mm
Chest, forearms: 40 mm
Back: 40 to 70 mm
Upper arms, thighs: 75 mm

To test two-point discrimination, apply disposable pins or a paperclip bent into a U shape to the skin simultaneously. Ask the client if he or she feels one or two pinpricks (Figure 19.32).

To test for extinction, touch the skin on the same areas on both sides of the body. Failure to perceive touch on one side is called the extinction phenomenon. Normally, sensation is perceived on both sides.

Position sense. Position sense (kinesthetic sensation) is facilitated by proprioceptive receptors in the muscles, tendons, and joints. Perception of the position, orientation, and motion of limbs and body parts is obtained from kinesthetic sensations.

With the client's eyes closed and the joint in a neutral position, and with your fingers placed on each side of the client's digit (finger or toe), slightly move the position of the client's digit. Be careful not to touch other digits during this maneuver. Ask the client to describe how the position of the finger changes. Always move the digit to a neutral position before moving it again (Figure 19.33).

Reflexes

Deep tendon reflexes. Assess deep tendon reflexes to obtain information about the function of the reflex arcs and the spinal cord segments (Table 19.2). Elicit deep tendon reflexes by deforming (tapping) a tendon with a reflex hammer (Figure 19.34).

figure**19.33** Testing for position sense. With the client's eyes closed, the examiner slightly changes the position of a digit up or down. The client describes how the position was changed.

Record the symmetry of the reflex from one side of the body to the other. A succinct method of recording the reflex findings is the stick-figure representation (Figure 19.35). To obtain the best muscle contraction, test when the muscle is slightly stretched before the tendon is stretched (tapped with the reflex hammer).

Reinforcement is done to enhance a reflex. Ask the client to isometrically tense muscles not directly involved in the reflex arc being tested. For example, ask the client to clench the fists or to lock the fingers together and pull the hands apart (Figure 19.36) as you assess lower extremity reflexes. To reinforce the reflex arcs of the upper extremities, ask the client to clench the

figure**19.34** The examiner holds the reflex, or percussion, hammer in the dominant hand between the thumb and index finger and uses a striking motion to assess the deep tendon reflex.

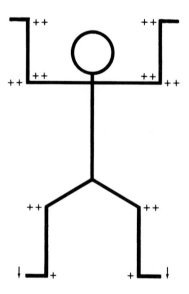

figure**19.35** Stick-figure drawing for recording reflexes usually tested in the screening examination. Responses are coded from zero to "++++," with "++" values considered normal.

table 19.2	Reflexes Commonly Tested in the Physical Examination and Segmental Levels of the Central Nervous System Involved		
Deep tendon reflexes	**Segmental level**	**Superficial reflexes**	**Segmental level**
Biceps	C5, 6	Pharyngeal (gag)	Medulla
Triceps	C6, 7, 8	Abdominal (upper)	T7, 8, 9
Brachioradialis	C5, 6	Abdominal (lower)	T12; L1
Patellar	L2, 3, 4	Cremasteric	L1, 2, 3
Ankle (Achilles)	S1, 2	Gluteal	L4, 5
		Plantar	L4, 5; S1, 2

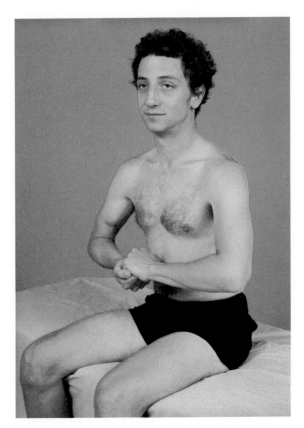

figure**19.36** Reinforcement maneuver for deep tendon reflexes.

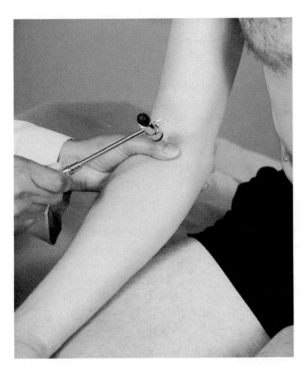

figure**19.37** Eliciting the biceps reflex. With the client's arm flexed, the examiner places the thumb over the biceps tendon and strikes the thumb with the reflex hammer.

Grading Deep Tendon Reflexes

0	No response
1+	Low normal, slightly diminished response
2+	Normal
3+	More brisk than normal, not necessarily indicative of disease
4+	Brisk, hyperactive, clonus of tendon associated with disease

jaw or to tense the quadriceps. Document that reinforcement was used to elicit the deep tendon reflex.

Biceps reflex (Figure 19.37). To check the biceps reflex, have the client flex the arm at the elbow. Place your thumb firmly over the biceps tendon to augment the tendon stretch. The thumb is struck with the reflex hammer. The normal response is flexion of the arm at the elbow.

> **HELPFUL HINT** *Compare reflexes bilaterally for symmetry, degree and speed of response, and recovery to original position. To accurately compare reflexes, make sure that each limb is in the same position.*

Triceps reflex (Figure 19.38). Tap the triceps tendon (above the olecranon process) with the reflex hammer. The normal response is extension of the elbow. Begin with the client's arm flexed at the elbow and resting in the client's lap. Alternatively, you can start with the client's arm flexed at the elbow and abducted while you hold it in position. The latter position sometimes allows for better viewing of the normal response of extension of the elbow.

Brachioradialis reflex (Figure 19.39). To test the brachioradialis reflex, begin with the client's arm in a relaxed position. Strike the styloid process of the radius with the hammer while palpating the tendon 3 to 5 cm above the wrist. The normal response is flexion of the elbow and pronation of the forearm. The fingers of the hand may also flex.

Patellar reflex (Figure 19.40). For this test, the client's legs should be hanging freely over the side of the bed or chair, or the client should be resting in a supine position. Palpate the muscle above the patella with one hand while striking the tendon with the reflex hammer directly below the patella. The normal response

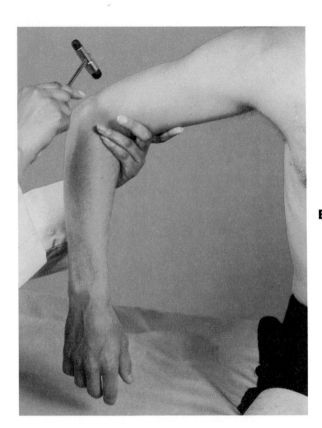

A

B

figure **19.38** Eliciting the triceps reflex. **A,** With the arm flexed at the elbow, the examiner taps the triceps tendon. **B,** The examiner holds the flexed arm in position. The normal response is straightening or extension of the arm.

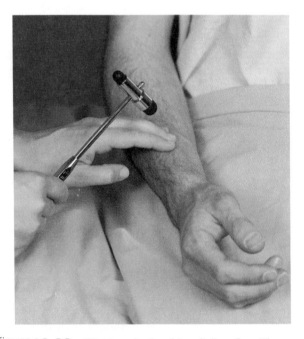

figure **19.39** Eliciting the brachioradialis reflex. The normal response is flexion of the arm at the elbow, pronation of the wrist, or slight flexion of the fingers.

is extension or kicking of the leg as the quadriceps muscle contracts.

Ankle (or Achilles) reflex (Figure 19.41). Hold the client's foot in a slightly dorsiflexed position with one hand and strike the Achilles tendon with the reflex hammer. The normal response is plantar flexion of the foot.

Superficial reflexes. Superficial, or cutaneous, reflexes are obtained by stimulating the skin.

Plantar reflexes (Figure 19.42). Plantar reflexes are superficial reactions. Use a pin, the sharp edge of a broken tongue blade, or the handle portion of the reflex hammer to elicit the reflex. Apply the stimulus to the lateral border of the client's sole, starting at the heel and continuing across the ball of the foot and ending beneath the great toe. The normal response is flexion of the toes (Figure 19.43). Extension or dorsiflexion of the great toe and fanning of the others, which is abnormal, is called the Babinski reflex. Before a child can walk, fanning and extension of the toes are the normal response.

Abdominal reflexes. The abdominal reflexes are described in Chapter 17.

Cremasteric reflex. Stimulate the male client's inner thigh with a sharp object, such as the stick end of an ap-

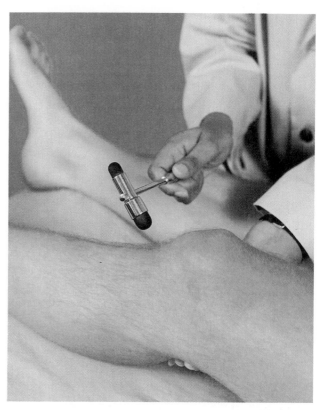

figure**19.40**   Eliciting the patellar reflex. With the client's legs hanging freely (**A**) or with the client in a supine position (**B**), the examiner strikes the tendon below the patella. The normal response is extension of the leg.

figure**19.41**   Eliciting the ankle reflex. **A,** Sitting. **B,** Lying down. The examiner strikes the Achilles tendon with the reflex hammer while holding the foot in a slightly dorsiflexed position. The normal response is plantar flexion of the foot.

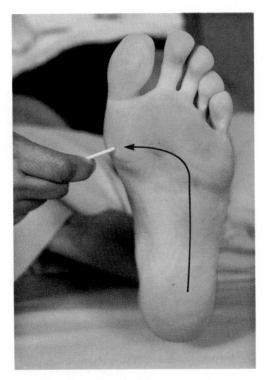

figure**19.42** Eliciting the plantar reflex. The examiner applies a hard object along the lateral surface of the sole, starting at the heel and moving along the ball of the foot, ending beneath the great toe.

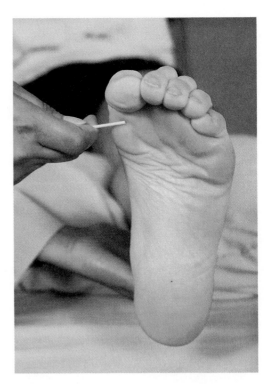

figure**19.43** The normal response to plantar stimulation: flexion of all the toes.

plicator. The expected response is retraction (elevation) of the scrotum on the same side that the cremaster muscle contracts.

Gluteal reflex. Spread the client's buttocks and stimulate the perianal area. The normal response is contraction of the anal sphincter.

■ ASSESSMENT OF MENTAL STATUS

Purpose of Examination

The purpose of the mental status examination is to assess the client's current emotional and mental capacity and functioning. The mental status examination provides a baseline for a client's psychological state and specific information that helps to establish a nursing diagnosis. The examination includes a description of the client's:

General appearance
Behavior
Mood or affect
Characteristics of speech
Orientation
Thought processes
Insight and judgment

Memory and learning
Perceptions and attitudes

The examiner focuses on assessing the client's ability to interact with the environment. Responses elicited during a single interview are only samples of the individual's thoughts and feelings. Fears regarding illness, family responsibilities, attitudes of others, and financial worries are some factors that can alter a client's feelings and behaviors. Considering the effects of prescription and illicit drugs on the client's mental processes and behaviors is important.

Examination of Mental Status
Health History

Assessment of mental status includes interviewing and inspection or observation. During the interview, make an overall assessment of whether the client is cooperative, friendly, or hostile. Obtain information about the client's educational and physical development; occupation; economic status; relationships; responsibilities felt toward family, work, or school; stressors (actual or perceived); goals (attainable and unrealistic); and support systems (individuals and affiliations).

Use therapeutic communication skills discussed in

Chapter 2. Focus on obtaining data about symptoms, including how the client views these symptoms and how disruptive they are to the client and others. Compare and contrast your observations with the client's perceptions. Document a client's behaviors and words accurately, succinctly, and in *measurable,* descriptive terms. Use short, direct quotes only when doing so enhances the client's meaning or clarifies the situation:

Incorrect: Client was very agitated during the interview.

Correct: During the 15-minute interview, client paced the room, bit fingernails, and stated 4 to 5 times, "I'm really nervous today."

Preparation for examination: client and environment

Equipment needed to conduct a mental status examination includes a pencil, paper, and reading material. The setting should be quiet and should provide privacy. Communication barriers related to age or culture can often be bridged through the use of qualified interpreters, friends, or family members. When information is obtained from sources other than the client, the examiner must understand the relationship of these individuals to the client.

General appearance

Carefully observe the client's general physical appearance, grooming, manner of dress, facial expression, and body posture as a measure of mental function. Do not focus too early on obvious abnormalities, since the subtle clues may be missed.

Grooming and manner of dress. Observe the client's clothing to determine its appropriateness to time, place, age, and lifestyle. Grooming of hair and nails and general cleanliness should be noted. A disheveled appearance in someone who was previously well groomed is especially significant.

Posture. Posture is important in providing clues to the client's feelings. The client who walks slowly into

---

table 19.3 *Levels of Consciousness (Responsiveness)*

Level	Behaviors
Consciousness	Appropriate response (rate and quality) to external stimuli; oriented to time, place, and person
Confusion	Inappropriate response to stimuli and decreased attention span and memory; reactions to simple commands
Lethargy (hypersomnia)	Drowsiness or increased sleep time; can be aroused; responds appropriately; may fall asleep again immediately
Delirium	Confusion, disorder perception, and decreased attention span; motor and sensory excitement; inappropriate reactions to stimuli; marked anxiety
Coma	Loss or lowering of consciousness
Stage I (stupor)	Arousable for short periods to verbal, visual, or painful stimuli; simple motor and verbal response to stimuli; slow responses; corneal and pupillary reflexes sluggish; deep tendon and superficial reflexes unaffected; pathological reflexes may be obtained
Stage II (light coma)	Simple motor and verbal (moaning) response to painful stimuli; mass motor movement or flexion (avoidance) response
Stage III (deep coma)	Decerebrate posturing to painful stimuli (extension of body and limbs and pronation of arms)
Stage IV	Flaccid muscles; pupillary reflex absent; apneic; on ventilator; superficial and some deep tendon reflexes present
Brain death	Two electroencephalographic (EEG) tracings 24 hours apart indicate absence of brain waves; cerebral function absent for 24 hours; failure of cerebral perfusion; expert opinion rules out hypothermia or drug toxicity (NOTE : All these behaviors must be present.)
Syncope	Temporary loss of consciousness (partial or complete) associated with increased rate of respiration, tachycardia, pallor, perspiration, and coolness of skin
Fugue state	Dysfunction of consciousness (hours or days) in which the individual carries on purposeful activity that he or she does not remember afterward
Amnesia	Memory loss over time or for specific subjects; individual affected responds appropriately to external stimuli

the room, barely lifting the feet, and who slumps in the chair while avoiding the examiner's glance may be showing a lack of affect or depression.

Coordination. Assess general coordination of movement by observing the client's gait (see Chapter 9: General Assessment, Including Vital Signs). To evaluate the complex coordination, give the client simple phrases to write and simple geometric figures to draw.

Behavior

Level of consciousness. Consciousness is awareness of one's thoughts and feelings and of the environment. The levels of consciousness (responsiveness) are generally described according to the behavior exhibited by the individual. Table 19.3 includes a useful categorization of the levels of consciousness. Response to pain may be the only indication of sensory stimulation. Stimuli used to assess response to pain include pinching of skin, pricking with a pin, pressure over supraorbital notches, or squeezing muscle masses or tendons, particularly the calf muscle. The client may respond by extension of limbs, facial grimacing, or withdrawal. Flexion responses are considered withdrawal responses and therefore purposeful. Nonpurposeful responses are mass reactions or extension of limbs.

Mood or affect. Affect is the observable manifestation of the internally experienced emotion or feeling state. In general, it is possible to estimate the client's emotional status or affective state from verbal and nonverbal behaviors. Affects may be described as labile if moods rapidly and abruptly shift. Observe the appropriateness and degree of affect to a given idea, as well as the range of affect.

Interview Protocol

How would you describe the problem that has brought you here?
What do you think is causing your problem?
Why do you think it happened to you?
Why do you think it started when it did?
How have your spirits been lately?
How do you feel life has been treating you?
Have you told anyone else about your feelings or problems?
Have you ever considered hurting yourself? If yes: Did you follow through and actually harm yourself? If yes: How did you do it?
Do you have any plans to harm yourself now? If yes: What are your plans?
Do you think about dying? If yes: How often?

To understand the client's perspective and to bring out the feelings of clients who resist offering information spontaneously, try the interview protocol described in the box below.

Characteristics of speech. Evaluate the client's comprehension of and ability to use the spoken language. The client's manner of speech may offer clues about his or her thought processes. The mentally healthy individual answers questions frankly. Responses to your questions and instructions give valuable information about the client's comprehension and willingness to cooperate. Note failure to answer a question, other evasive replies, and unwarranted criticism of you as the examiner.

Facial expression. Facial expression should be consistent with, and appropriate to the topic. In some Southeast Asian cultures, direct eye contact is avoided, especially by women, since the examiner is considered to hold a position of respect.

Cognitive functions

Assess the client's orientation, attention, memory, use of language, and intellectual skills. The Mini–Mental Status Examination (MMSE) is a practical 11-question instrument used to assess orientation, memory, concentration, calculation, and language abilities (see discussion of special screening tests).

Orientation. Assess orientation from the client's awareness of person, place, and time. The following questions can help in obtaining this information:

PERSON

What is your name? Address? Telephone number?
Who am I?
What is my job?

PLACE

Tell me where you are. What is the name of this place?
What is the name of the town you are in?
Who brought you here?

TIME

What day this is? Month? Year?

Record the degree of disorientation. Time is the orientation most frequently disordered in clients with mental disease. A disturbance of place orientation may ac-

---

🌐 CULTURAL CONSIDERATIONS

Behavior Variations
In many Asian cultures, an open display of one's distress is not considered appropriate behavior.

company organic mental disorders or schizophrenia. An individual may not be oriented to person in the aftermath of cerebral trauma or seizures.

Attention span. An appraisal of the individual's attention span includes the client's ability to maintain interest and to concentrate. Attention span is one of the first functions of the sensorium to become affected in individuals who are fatigued, anxious, or chemically impaired.

Memory. Memory is a function of general cerebral function. Impairment of memory occurs in both neurological and psychiatric disorders. Some general questions that may help to elicit a disorder in memory are as follows:

Have you noticed any loss of memory?

Do you remember those things that happened years ago best or those that happened today or yesterday?

Immediate memory. Immediate memory is verbalized remembering immediately after presentation. Test immediate memory by digit recall. Two sample tests follow.

To test your memory skills, I'd like you to repeat four series of numbers after me:

7, 4
9, 6, 5, 3
8, 9, 4, 1, 5
3, 8, 7, 4, 1, 6

I will say some numbers. You say them backward. For instance, I say *8, 2;* you say *2, 8:*

3, 8
7, 2, 0
5, 9, 2, 7

The average individual can generally repeat five to seven digits forward and four to six digits backward.

Recent memory. Recent memory is verbalized after several minutes to an hour. Examples of questions and exercises for assessing recent memory are as follows:

How long have you been here?

What were you doing before you came here?

What time did you get up today?

What did you eat for breakfast today?

Remote memory. Remote memory is verbalized after hours, days, or years. At the beginning of the interview, give the client three to five unrelated words to remember. Other examples of questions for assessing remote memory are as follows:

Where were you born?

Tell me the name of the high school you attended.

What was your mother's maiden name?

In testing for memory, do not ask questions for which the answers cannot be verified. Memory loss in organic dementia may involve disorders for immediate and recent events; however, affected individuals may be able to recall events from childhood with accuracy.

Intellectual functioning

Abstraction ability. To assess abstraction ability, ask the client to give the meaning of familiar proverbs:

A bird in the hand is worth two in the bush.

People who live in glass houses shouldn't throw stones.

Don't count your chickens before they hatch.

A rolling stone gathers no moss.

HELPFUL HINT *Interpretation of abstraction ability must take into consideration a client's cultural orientation, age, and educational level. Some proverbs may be culturally bound or more familiar to clients of a certain age group.*

Ability to learn (comprehension). The ability to learn includes abilities in perception, retention, association (interpretation), and recent memory. Give the client an address or a sentence that is not familiar and ask him or her to remember the content verbatim:

Listen to me carefully. I am going to give you an address that I want you to remember. Later on, I will ask you to repeat it for me: Apartment 13, Dover Hill Building.

Computation. The following exercise is useful in assessing the client's computational abilities:

Ask the client to subtract 7 from 100. Have the client continue subtracting 7 from the resulting remainder for several more calculations.

The normal client is able to complete the computation in 1½ minutes with fewer than four errors. Computation skills may be impaired by fatigue, depression, or anxiety.

Ability to read. Use a copy of a current newspaper to determine the client's reading skills. Be certain that the client is wearing corrective lenses if they are needed for reading. Impairment of the ability to read is called dyslexia.

General knowledge. Assessment of general knowledge may include an estimate of what the client has learned in school and his or her awareness of current events. Match inquiries to the educational, sociocultural, and life experiences of the client. Ask questions about presidents, capitals of countries, names of oceans, or current events in newspaper headlines.

Insight and judgment. Insight is the client's understanding of and beliefs about the cause and nature of his or her illness. Simple questions such as "Why did you decide to come here[name of health care facility] at this time?" allow clients to explain in their own words their comprehension of their health status. An example of an interview protocol designed to elicit information about

Mini–Mental Status Examination

MAXIMUM SCORE	SCORE	
		ORIENTATION
5	( )	What is the (year)(season)(date)(day)(month)?
5	( )	Where are we: (state)(country)(town)(hospital)(floor)?
		REGISTRATION
3	( )	Name three objects: 1 second to say each. Then ask the client to repeat them. Give 1 point for each correct answer. Then repeat them until all three are learned. Count trials and record.
		ATTENTION AND CALCULATION
5	( )	Serial 7's. 1 point for each correct. Stop after five answers. Alternatively spell "world" backward.
		RECALL
3	( )	Ask for three objects repeated above. Give 1 point for each correct.
		LANGUAGE
9	( )	Name a pencil and a watch (2 points)
		Repeat the following: "No ifs, ands, or buts" (1 point)
		Follow a three-stage command:
		"Take a paper in your right hand, fold it in half, and put it on the floor" (3 points)
		Read and obey the following:
		Close your eyes. (1 point)
		Write a sentence. (1 point)
		Copy design. (1 point)
30		Total score

ASSESS level of consciousness along a continuum

Alert	Drowsy	Stupor	Coma

INSTRUCTIONS FOR ADMINISTRATION OF MINI–MENTAL STATE EXAMINATION

ORIENTATION

(1) Ask for the date. Then ask specifically for parts omitted, for example, "Can you also tell me what season it is?" One point for each correct.

(2) Ask in turn "Can you tell me the name of this hospital (etc.)?" One point for each.

REGISTRATION

Ask the client if you may test memory. Then say the names of three unrelated objects, clearly and slowly, about 1 second for each. After you have said all three, ask the client to repeat them. This first repetition determines the score (0-3), but keep saying them until all three are repeated, up to six trials. If all three cannot be learned, recall cannot be meaningfully tested.

ATTENTION AND CALCULATION

Ask the client to begin with 100 and count backward by 7. Stop after five subtractions (93, 86, 79, 72, 65). Score the total number of correct answers. If the client cannot or will not perform this task, ask him or her to spell the word "world" backward. The score is the number of letters in correct order, e.g., dlrow = 5, dlorw = 3.

RECALL

Ask the client to recall the three words you previously asked him or her to remember. Score 0-3.

From Folstein MF, Folstein SE, McHugh PR: "Mini–mental state": a practical method for grading the cognitive state of patients for the clinician, *J Psychiatr Res* 12:189-198, 1975.

Mini–Mental Status Examination—cont'd

LANGUAGE

Naming: Show the client a wristwatch and ask what it is. Repeat for pencil. Score 0-2.

Repetition: Ask the patient to repeat the sentence after you. Allow only one trial. Score 0 or 1.

Three-stage command: Give the client a piece of plain blank paper, and repeat the command. Score 1 point for each part correctly executed.

Reading: On a blank piece of paper, print the sentence "Close your eyes" in letters large enough for the client to see clearly. Ask the client to read it and do what it says. Score 1 point only if the client actually closes his or her eyes.

Writing: Give the client a blank piece of paper, and ask him or her to write a sentence for you. Do not dictate a sentence; it is to be written spontaneously. It must contain a subject and verb and be sensible. Correct grammar and punctuation are not necessary.

Copying: On a clean piece of paper, draw intersecting pentagons, each side about 1 inch, and ask the client to copy it exactly as it is. All 10 angles must be present and 2 must intersect to score 1 point. Tremor and rotation are ignored.

Estimate the client's level of sensorium along a continuum, from alert on the left to coma on the right.

the client's mental representation or beliefs about his or her health or illness follows:

When did you first notice the problem?

What do you think this problem does to you?

How severe do you think this problem is?

What do you feel is causing the problem?

Have you noticed any troubling symptoms or feelings?

What do you think is the best treatment for this problem?

Judgment is a skill necessary for evaluation, assessment, and decision making, particularly in those situations in which two or more experiences are related to one another. The individual who is able to evaluate a situation and determine the appropriate reaction(s) is said to have good judgment or reasoning ability. Assess judgment through the client's expressed attitudes to his or her social, physical, occupational, and domestic status and plans for the future.

Judgment may be impaired in highly charged emotional states, mental retardation, organic mental disorder, schizophrenia, effects of drugs and alcohol, and anxiety. Two examples of questions that elicit judgment skills follow:

What would you do if you were in a theater when fire broke out?

What would you do if you found four stamped, addressed envelopes?

Thought processes. Verbal and nonverbal expressions are used to assess the client's ability to think logically and coherently and in a goal-directed sequence.

Screening Tests

Mini–Mental Status Examination

Using the Mini–Mental Status Examination (MMSE) (see box on p. 526 and above), ask the client the 11 questions. Score items so that a score of 30 indicates optimal function. The test takes about 10 minutes to administer to a client with normal mental status functioning.

Pain assessment scale

A systematic assessment of pain intensity and pain management uses a pain rating scale (Figure 19.44). The client is asked to rate pain from 0 (no pain) to 10 (worst pain). Ratings of 3 to 5 are considered mild pain; ratings of 5 to 7 are considered moderate pain; and ratings above 7 are considered severe pain. For children, happy and sad faces are used to make the pain rating.

Glasgow Coma Scale

The Glasgow Coma Scale is an assessment tool that rates level of consciousness by assigning a numerical score to three behavioral evaluations: eye opening, verbal response, and motor response. The score is the sum of these ratings (Table 19.4). A person with normal consciousness would obtain a score of 15. Common postures found in nonresponsive clients are decorticate, decerebrate, and flaccid.

Special Tests and Procedures

Data from standardized psychological tests to assess brain damage are more reliable than behavioral observations, although both examine the same functions, such

INITIAL PAIN ASSESSMENT TOOL

Date _____

Client's Name _____ Age _____

Diagnosis _____ Physician _____

Nurse _____

I. LOCATION: Client or nurse marks drawing.

II. INTENSITY: Client rates the pain. Scale* used _____

Present: _____

Worst pain gets: _____

Best pain gets: _____

Acceptable level of pain: _____

III. QUALITY: (Use client's own words, e.g., prick, ache, burn, throb, pull, sharp) _____

_____

IV. ONSET, DURATION VARIATIONS, RHYTHMS: _____

_____

V. MANNER OF EXPRESSING PAIN: _____

_____

VI. WHAT RELIEVES THE PAIN? _____

_____

VII. WHAT CAUSES OR INCREASES THE PAIN? _____

_____

VIII. EFFECTS OF PAIN: (Note decreased function, decreased quality of life) _____

Accompanying symptoms (e.g., nausea) _____

Sleep _____

Appetite _____

Physical activity _____

Relationship with others (e.g., irritability) _____

Emotions (e.g., anger, suicidal, crying) _____

Concentration _____

Other _____

IX. OTHER COMMENTS: _____

_____

*Pain rating scales: 0-10 Visual Analog Scale *(left)* and FACES Pain Rating Scale *(right).*

figure **19.44** Pain assessment form. *(Modified from McCaffery M, Beebe A: Pain: clinical manual for nursing practice,* St Louis, 1989, Mosby. *Wong-Baker FACES Pain Rating Scale is from Wong DL:* Whaley and Wong's nursing care of infants and children, *ed 5, St Louis, 1995, Mosby.)*

examination *step-by-step*

There is no one method for conducting the neurological examination. Each examiner may develop his or her own method. If abnormalities are found, a more complete examination of that area is necessary. The order below is a logical one for performing the complete mental status and neurological examination.

1. During the interview, assess cerebral function:
   a. Observe appearance and behavior for appropriateness to the situation.
   b. Assess mental status for orientation to person, place, and time; attention span; and calculation.
   c. Assess recent and remote memory and abstract reasoning.
   d. Assess emotional status, observing affect, mood, thought content, and expression of ideas.
   e. Assess communication skills; ability to express oneself and to listen; clarity of expression.
2. With the client standing:
   a. Observe gait.
   b. Assess Romberg's sign (standing with feet slightly apart, eyes closed).
   c. Observe heel-to-toe walking (tandem gait, toe-walking, heel-walking).
   d. Test standing on one foot, then the other; hopping on each foot.
   e. Assess deep knee bend (optional).
3. With the client sitting, examine the following regions in a head-to-toe direction.

Head and Face

1. Observe facial symmetry (CN VII).
2. Have the client frown, smile, puff cheeks, close eyes tightly, and resist the examiner opening eyes.
3. Ask the client, with eyes closed, to indicate when and where he or she is touched with a cotton wisp on three areas of the face innervated by CN V.
4. Ask the client, with eyes closed, to indicate "sharp" or "dull" sensation when touched with a pin on three areas of the face innervated by CN V.

Eyes

1. Observe symmetry of the lids, palpebral fissures (CN III).
2. Observe symmetry of the pupillary light reflex and pupil response (direct and consensual) to light and accommodation (CN III).
3. Test extraocular movements (CN III, IV, VI) for six fields of gaze.
4. Assess visual acuity using the Snellen chart (CN II).
5. Test visual fields by confrontation, having the client indicate when the examiner's fingers come into peripheral vision in eight visual fields (CN II).
6. Use an ophthalmoscope to examine CN II.

Ears

1. Test hearing acuity using Weber and Rinne tests (CN VIII).

Nose

1. Test smell (CN I) (not done in screening examination).

Mouth and Throat

1. Observe symmetrical rise of the soft palate with "ah" swallow (CN IX and X).
2. Assess jaw strength and symmetry (CN V).
3. Assess tongue strength (CN XII).
4. Test taste sensations (CN VII and IX) (not done in screening examination).

Neck

1. Test trapezius and sternocleidomastoid strength (CN XI).

Other

1. Assess cerebellar function and proprioception:
   a. Observe rapid alternating movements (upper and lower extremities).
   b. Perform finger-to-nose test.
   c. Perform finger-to-thumb test.
   d. Perform heel-down-shin test.
2. Test sensory function with the client's eyes closed:
   a. Assess light touch and pain on each extremity from distal to proximal.
   b. Test position sense.
   c. Check vibration sense.
   d. Test stereognosis.
   e. Test graphesthesia.
   f. Assess two-point discrimination.
3. Assess deep tendon reflexes:
   a. Test biceps reflex.
   b. Assess brachioradialis reflex.
   c. Test triceps reflex.
   d. Assess patellar reflex.
   e. Assess ankle jerk reflex.
   f. Assess plantar reflex.
4. Not tested in a screening examination:
   a. Extinction
   b. Reflexes: Corneal, abdominal, cremasteric, gluteal

table 19.4 *Glasgow Coma Scale*			
Best eye-opening response	Spontaneously	4	
	To verbal command	3	
	To pain	2	
	No response	1	
Best verbal response	Oriented, converses	5	**Decorticate:** Rigid flexion; upper arms held tightly to sides of body; elbows, wrists, and fingers flexed; feet are plantar flexed, legs extended and internally rotated; may have fine tremors or intense stiffness
	Disoriented, converses	4	
	Inappropriate words	3	
	Incomprehensible sounds	2	
	No response	1	
Best motor response	Obeys	6	
To verbal command	Localizes pain	5	
To painful stimulus	Flexion-withdrawal	4	
	Flexion-decorticate	3	
	Extension-decerebrate	2	**Decerebrate:** Rigid extension; arms fully extended; forearms pronated; wrists and fingers flexed; jaws clenched; neck extended; back may be arched; feet plantar flexed; may occur spontaneously, intermittently, or in response to a stimulus
	No response	1	
	TOTAL	(3-15)	

From Thompson JM, Wilson SF: *Health assessment for nursing practice,* St Louis, 1996, Mosby; modified from Chipps E, Clanin N, Campbell V: *Neurologic disorders,* St Louis, 1992, Mosby.

as the speed of response, level of comprehension, and use of language. Neuropsychological testing assesses visual memory and psychomotor skills in depth by using a wide range of standardized tests. Testing is performed by a skilled clinician specifically trained to administer and interpret these tests.

■ VARIATIONS FROM HEALTH

Variations in Sensory Function

Anosmia is the loss of the sense of smell. Hyposmia is an impaired sense of smell. In hyposmia, flavor perception is also impaired, since it is a synthesis of smell, taste, and perceptions from stimulation of end organs in the mouth and pharynx. The individual with CN I (olfactory) involvement may complain only of loss of the sense of taste.

Ageusia is the loss of taste or the lack of ability to discriminate sweet, sour, salty, and bitter tastes.

Shingles (herpes zoster) is caused by the herpes varicella-zoster virus, the same virus that causes chickenpox. The virus may remain dormant in the dorsal root ganglia of some spinal nerves. With increasing age, the immune system may not be as effective in keeping the virus inactive, and the reactivated virus causes shingles. Shingles appears on the skin as a painful papulovesicular rash that follows the course of peripheral, and sometimes cranial, nerves. No specific treatment is available, and these lesions may ulcerate and keratinize. Neuralgia or anesthesia may remain after the rash disappears.

Variations in Motor Function

Multiple sclerosis (MS) is a demyelinating disease that involves deterioration of myelin sheaths of neurons in the central nervous system. Without the myelin, nerve impulses become short-circuited and do not reach their intended destinations. Evidence exists that this is an autoimmune disease triggered by a virus.

Symptoms of MS first appear between the ages of 20 and 40 years. The disease may progress rapidly or slowly. Symptoms vary but may include muscle weakness or paralysis, partial loss of sensation, visual changes, loss of bowel and bladder control, and loss of spinal cord reflexes. Some individuals experience remissions, when symptoms disappear for an unpredictable period of time. No cure exists for MS at present.

Table 19.5 summarizes the causes and characteristics of upper and lower motor neuron lesions.

table 19.5	Deep Tendon Reflex and Muscle Changes in Upper and Lower Motor Neuron Lesions		
Lesion		**Common cause**	**Characteristics**
Upper motor neuron lesion (corticospinal tract)		Cerebral vascular occlusion Cerebral neoplasm	Hyperreflexia Paralysis of voluntary movement
Spasticity (usually includes damage to parallel pathways)		Trauma	Babinski's sign present Minimal muscle atrophy
Lower motor neuron lesion (anterior horn cell, somatic motor part of cranial nerves)		Poliomyelitis Neoplasm Trauma	Muscle weakness Paralysis Muscle atrophy Hyporeflexia or absent reflexes Fasciculations

Bell's palsy is a facial nerve palsy of acute onset and unknown cause. Evidence of this lower motor neuron disorder, which results in paralysis of an entire side of the face, is the closing of only one eye when the client attempts to close both eyes. When the client tries to raise the eyebrows, the eyebrow on the affected side does not rise and the forehead does not wrinkle. The client may exhibit overflow of tears or be unable to hold fluids orally because of a sagging mouth.

Neck trauma is the most frequent cause of dysfunction of the spinal accessory nerve (CN XI). Torticollis is a condition of intermittent or constant contraction of the sternocleidomastoid muscle in which the head is flexed forward and the chin is rotated away from the affected side.

A cerebrovascular accident (CVA), or stroke, is damage to a blood vessel in the brain that results in lack of oxygen to that part of the brain. Either a blood clot (thrombosis) or hemorrhage, often from the rupture of an aneurysm, causes the interruption in circulation. The symptoms depend on the part of the brain affected. The onset of symptoms may be slow if a clot formation decreases blood flow before complete occlusion occurs. In the case of a ruptured aneurysm, however, the onset may be sudden. Recovery from a CVA depends largely on its location and the extent of damage. In many individuals, especially those who begin rehabilitation early, the brain is able to establish new pathways to compensate for damaged areas.

Lesions of the Dominant Cerebral Hemisphere

Aphasia, the inability to comprehend or use language symbols, is caused by a lesion in the cerebral hemisphere dominant for speech. The most common cerebral pathological condition associated with aphasia is vascular disease. Data show that 95% of persons who are right-handed and have a language deficit have lesions of the left cerebral hemisphere, whereas 70% of left-handed individuals with language impairment also have a lesion of the left cerebral hemisphere.

If the motor cortex for speech is involved, the person can understand written and spoken words but cannot contract the muscles used for speech to form words properly. Damage to the interpretation area of the cortex for speech results in the inability to comprehend the meaning of spoken words. Aphasia often accompanies agnosia, the inability to recognize once-familiar objects.

Lesions of the Nondominant Cerebral Hemisphere

A disturbance in the ability to perform a purposeful act when comprehension is intact is termed apraxia. For example, if given a fork, the client may be unable to use it to eat; or the client may be unable to dress or button a shirt.

Variations in Cerebellar Function

The client with cerebellar disease has difficulty with rapid patting and supination-pronation alterations. The problem involves both smooth control of muscles and the starting and stopping of motion. Clumsiness of movement and irregular timing are characteristic of affected individuals.

Dyssynergia (impairment of muscle coordination or of the ability to perform movements smoothly) is loss of cerebellar function and results in intention tremor, or hypotonia.

Abnormalities of muscle tone, gait, speech, and nys-

Comparison of Disorders of the Cerebellum, Posterior Columns, and Vestibular Apparatus

CEREBELLAR DYSFUNCTION
Ataxia present with eyes opened or closed
Clumsiness
Poor coordination
Tremor
Hypotonia
Nystagmus

POSTERIOR COLUMN DYSFUNCTION
Ataxia made worse with eyes closed
Positive Romberg's sign (swaying with eyes closed)
Inability to recognize limb position
Loss of two-point discrimination
Astereognosis
Loss of vibratory sense

VESTIBULAR APPARATUS DYSFUNCTION
Nystagmus
Nausea
Vomiting
Ataxia present with eyes opened and closed

figure**19.45** Eliciting the grasp reflex. **A,** The examiner places the index and middle fingers in the client's palm and gently withdraws them. **B,** A positive response consists of the client's grasping the examiner's fingers.

tagmus in lateral gaze may also indicate cerebellar dysfunction. Disturbances in the timing of movements may also be evident.

Ataxia is the impairment of position sense.

The client with a cerebellar gait walks with a wide base; the trunk and head are held rigidly; the legs bend at the hips; arm movements are not coordinated with the stride; the client lurches and reels, frequently falling.

The client with cerebellar speech has slow, hesitant, or dysarthric verbalization.

Pathological Reflexes

Reflexes may be altered in pathophysiological changes involving the sensory pathways from the tendons and muscles or the motor component.

Babinski reflex

The Babinski reflex is dorsiflexion of the great toe and fanning of the other toes. Lesions of the pyramidal tract or motor nerves may be present in the client with a Babinski reflex.

Grasp reflex (Figure 19.45)

This reflex, while present in individuals with widespread brain damage, is normal in infants less than 4 months of age. To test the grasp reflex, place your index finger and middle finger in the client's palm, entering between the client's thumb and the index finger. Gently withdraw your fingers, pulling them across the skin of the client's palm. A positive response consists of the client's grasping of your fingers.

Lesions of the Corticospinal Tract

Clients with lesions of the corticospinal tract perform fine movements of the hands, such as picking up coins or pencils, slowly. Also, they are able to perform thumb-to-finger opposition less rapidly.

Signs of meningeal irritation

Meningeal irritation most commonly results from infection or intracranial hemorrhages. Nuchal rigidity

figure**19.46** Eliciting Brudzinski's sign. With meningeal irritation, pain is elicited when the head is flexed.

(stiff neck) is a common sign of meningitis and may be demonstrated by flexing the cervical spine, which produces discomfort in the posterior neck. In addition, the client cannot touch the chin to the chest.

Brudzinski's sign (Figure 19.46) is elicited with the client supine. Lift the client's head toward the sternum. The person with meningeal irritation will resist the movement and may flex the hips and knees. The movement is commonly accompanied by pain in the spine.

Variations in Mental Status

Confabulation is an attempt by the client to "fill in the gaps" with fabricated answers when he or she is unable to remember.

A client who rapidly skips from one complete idea to another without any relationship to the preceding idea may be manifesting flight of ideas.

It is important to carefully observe the client's affect to see whether it is congruent with the individual's verbal content. For example, a client who expresses little or no emotion while verbalizing the desire for self-harm or harm to others is demonstrating an incongruence between affect and verbal content.

Organic brain syndromes

Organic brain syndrome describes a symptom complex that causes an impairment of orientation, memory, or regulation of emotions. Affective symptoms, delusions, hallucinations, and obsessions may also be present. An acute brain syndrome (delirium) is one of short duration that is usually reversible. A chronic brain syndrome (dementia) is long-standing and often progressive in nature, with a less favorable prognosis.

Alzheimer's disease is a progressive, incurable form of mental deterioration that usually affects the elderly. Although the cause is not known, certain environmental factors bring out a genetic predisposition to this disease. Symptoms include confusion, forgetfulness, and loss of ability to execute simple tasks. As the disease progresses, a total loss of memory occurs. On autopsy the cerebral cortex shows structural changes, including increased fibrous tissue.

Affective (mood) disorders

The client with an affective disorder runs the gamut from depression to exaggerated euphoria, or mania. The highs and lows show little correlation with the person's life situation.

A bipolar disorder is diagnosed when mania is present or is indicated by the health history, whether or not depression occurs. Depression that occurs in the absence of mania is known as major unipolar depression.

Schizophrenic disorders

Hallucinations and delusions are the diagnostic signposts of schizophrenia. Delusions are false beliefs that are improbable in nature. Hallucinations are visual perceptions for which no external stimuli can be ascertained. Hallucinations may be suspected in the person who appears preoccupied.

Anxiety

The client who demonstrates symptoms of severe anxiety has recurrent periods of abrupt-onset anxiety that end without intervention. The client complains of fright without a known object. The autonomic nervous system is activated, possibly resulting in such signs and symptoms as palpitations, breathlessness, dizziness, feeling of impending doom, headache, fatigue, nausea and vomiting, and diarrhea.

Phobia

Phobia is a highly disturbing, recurring, and unrealistic fear that may relate to any situation or object.

■ FOCUSED HEALTH HISTORY *(SUBJECTIVE DATA)*

Mr. Z.'s chief complaint is that he feels too tired to get up in the morning. His wife died 3 months ago after a short illness. Since then, he reports feeling sad and lonely most of the time. Reports sleeping 2 to 3 hours per night and is tired all day. Reports a 10-lb weight gain in the past 2 months, which he attributes to increased intake of "junk" food, drinking 4 to 6 cans of beer per evening, and reduced physical activity. Says he sits home alone most of the time and has no close friends. Works on an assembly line and reports no job absences or injuries in the last 5 years but has been late for work 5 times in the past 2 weeks. Denies any history of mental illness, suicidal thoughts, or serious depression. Reports no sensory, motor, or coordination changes.

■ FOCUSED PHYSICAL EXAMINATION *(OBJECTIVE DATA)*

Mental status: Appears well-groomed; appropriate dress; slightly slumped posture. Gazed at the floor through most of the interview. Responds to questions appropriately. Oriented, alert, and cooperative throughout examination. Recent and remote memory intact.

Cranial nerves: Vision 20/30 both eyes with glasses (CN II); extraocular movement intact (CN III, IV, VI); jaw strength good (CN V); able to frown and smile (CN VII); correctly identifies whispered voice (CN VIII); swallows without difficulty (CN IX); palate rises symmetrically (CN X); able to turn head and shrug shoulders against resistance (CN XI); tongue midline (CN XII).

Cerebellar: Finger-to-nose, heel-to-shin, alternating movements done easily but slowly; Romberg negative; able to stand on each foot, hop, do knee bends, and heel-to-toe walk.

Face and extremities sensitive to light touch, localization, and pain; vibration and position sense intact.

DTRs: Bilaterally symmetrical, 1+, plantar reflex present.

diagnoses

HEALTH PROBLEM

Situational depression since death of spouse

NURSING DIAGNOSIS

Ineffective coping related to death of spouse

Defining Characteristics

- Presence of life stress
- Inability to meet role expectations
- Alteration in societal participation
- Excess food intake, alcohol consumption
- Digestive, bowel, appetite disturbance; chronic fatigue or sleep pattern disturbance

Male Genitalia

■ PURPOSE OF EXAMINATION

The purpose of the examination of the male genitalia is to assess the health of the male genital organs. The examination also provides an opportunity for teaching the client about genital area self-examination.

■ ANATOMY AND PHYSIOLOGY

The male genitalia (Figure 20.1) include the penis, scrotum, testes, epididymides, vas deferens, seminal vesicles, and prostate.

The shaft of the penis is formed by three columns of erectile tissue bound together by heavy fibrous tissue to form a cylinder. The dorsolateral columns are called the corpora cavernosa. The ventromedial column, which contains the urethra, is called the corpus spongiosum. Distally the penis terminates in a cone-shaped entity called the glans penis. The glans penis is formed by an extension and expansion of the corpus spongiosum penis, which fits over the blunt ends of the corpora cavernosa penis. The corona is the prominence formed where the glans joins the shaft. The urethra traverses the corpus spongiosum, and the external urethral orifice is a slitlike opening located slightly ventrally on the tip of the glans.

The skin of the penis is thin, hairless, darker than the other skin on a person's body, and only loosely connected to the internal parts of the organ. At the area of the corona, the skin forms a free fold, called the prepuce, or foreskin. When allowed to remain, this flap covers the glans to a variable extent. Often the prepuce is surgically removed through circumcision (Figure 20.2).

The penis serves as the terminal excretory organ for urine and, with erection, as the means of ejaculating sperm. The physiological process of erection occurs when the two corpora cavernosa become engorged with approximately 20 to 50 ml of blood through decreased venous outflow and increased arterial dilation. Orgasm is a major pleasurable sensation accompanying emission of secretions from the epididymides, vas deferens, seminal vesicles, prostate, and penis.

The scrotum is a deeply pigmented cutaneous pouch that contains the testes and parts of the spermatic cords (Figure 20.3). This sac is formed by an outer layer of

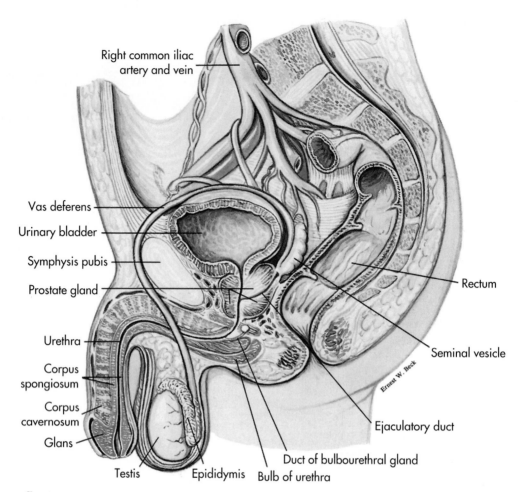

Right common iliac
artery and vein

Vas deferens

Urinary bladder

Symphysis pubis

Prostate gland

Urethra

Corpus
spongiosum

Corpus
cavernosum

Glans

Testis   Epididymis

Bulb of urethra

Duct of bulbourethral gland

Ejaculatory duct

Seminal vesicle

Rectum

Ernest W. Beck

figure**20.1**   Male genitalia. *(From Thibodeau GA:* Anatomy and physiology, *St Louis, 1987,*
Mosby.)

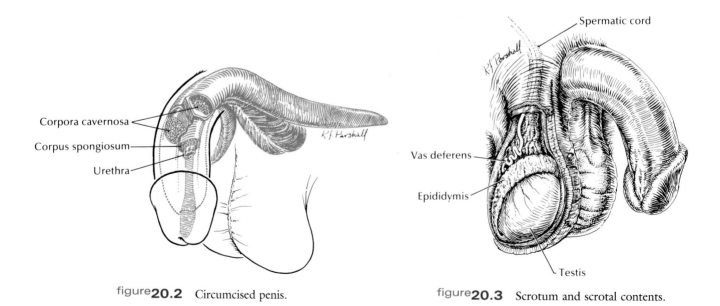

Corpora cavernosa

Corpus spongiosum

Urethra

figure**20.2**   Circumcised penis.

Spermatic cord

Vas deferens

Epididymis

Testis

figure**20.3**   Scrotum and scrotal contents.

thin, rugous skin overlying a tight muscle layer (cremaster muscle). The left side of the scrotum is often lower than the right side because the left spermatic cord is usually longer. Internally, the scrotum is divided into halves by a septum; each half contains a testis and its epididymis and part of the spermatic cord. The testes are ovoid and are suspended vertically, slightly forward; they lean slightly laterally in the scrotum. The mediolateral surfaces are flattened. Each testis is approximately 4 to 5 cm long, 3 cm wide, and 2 cm thick.

The testes produce both spermatozoa and testosterone. The epididymides serve as receptacles for storage, maturation, and transmission of sperm. The vas deferens serves as a mechanism of transit from each epididymis to the seminal vesicles. The prostate produces the bulk of ejaculatory fluid. The dartos muscle of the scrotum controls the temperature of the testes by adjusting the distance of the scrotum, and consequently the testes, from the body. Spermatogenesis requires temperatures below 37° C (98.6° F). Therefore the scrotum appears low in hot weather and high in cold weather.

The epididymis is a comma-shaped structure that is curved over the posterolateral surface and upper end of the testis. It creates a visual bulge on the posterolateral surface of the testis. The ductus deferens (vas deferens) begins at the tail of the epididymis, ascends the spermatic cord, travels through the inguinal canal, and eventually descends over the fundus of the bladder (see Figure 20.1).

The prostate, a slightly conical gland, lies under the bladder, surrounds the urethra, and measures approximately 4 cm at its base (or uppermost) part, 3 cm vertically, and 2 cm in its anteroposterior diameter. The prostate gland is roughly the size and shape of a chestnut. It has three lobes: left and right lateral lobes and a median lobe. These lobes are not well demarcated from one another. The median lobe is the part of the prostate that projects inward from the upper posterior area toward the urethra. Enlargement of this lobe causes urinary obstruction in benign prostatic hypertrophy.

The posterior surface of the prostate lies in close contact with the rectal wall and is the only portion of the gland that is accessible to examination. Its posterior sur-

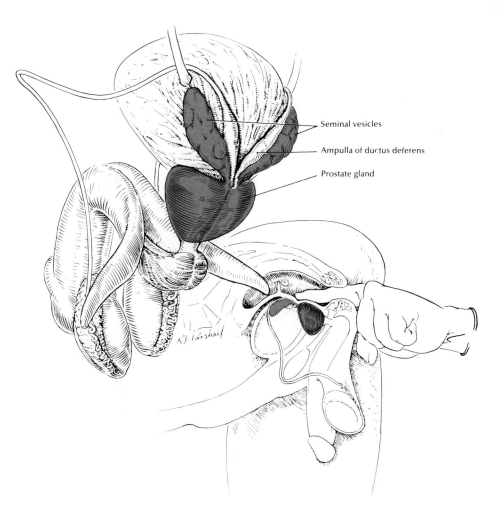

Seminal vesicles

Ampulla of ductus deferens

Prostate gland

figure**20.4** Prostate gland and seminal vesicles. Prostate examination.

figure**20.5** Inguinal lymph nodes. *(From Seidel HM et al: Mosby's guide to physical examination, ed 3, St Louis, 1995, Mosby.)*

face is slightly convex. A shallow median furrow divides all except the upper portions of the posterior surface into right and left lateral lobes.

The seminal vesicles are a pair of convoluted pouches, 5 to 10 cm long, that lie along the lower posterior surface of the bladder, anterior to the rectum (Figure 20.4).

The two groups of superficial nodes in the inguinal area are the superior and inferior inguinal nodes (Figure 20.5). These nodes receive most of the lymph drainage from the legs. The superior inguinal nodes lie somewhat horizontally along the inguinal ligament. They receive drainage from the abdominal wall below the umbilicus, the external genitalia (excluding the testes), the anal canal, the gluteal area, and the inferior inguinal nodes. The inferior group lies somewhat vertically below the junction of the saphenous and femoral veins. This is a group of large lymph nodes that receives lymph from the superficial regions of the leg and foot. Lymph from the penile and scrotal surfaces drains to the inguinal nodes, but lymphatic drainage from the testes is deep into the abdomen.

■ EXAMINATION

Health History

The health history of the male reproductive system is integrated with the urinary system history and the sexual history. The client may need some explanation about the reasons for the exploration of the sexual history and reassurance that such information is important in assessing overall health.

Throughout the health history, the following data about a symptom or problem should be recorded: (1) onset (specific date, sudden or gradual), (2) duration, (3) frequency, (4) precipitating factors, (5) aggravating or alleviating factors, (6) treatment received or self-care given, and (7) outcome. An outline for a regional history of the male genitourinary system follows.

Present health status

1. Changes in urination: Frequency, urgency, nocturia, dysuria, straining, difficulty in starting stream, incontinence (If present, describe frequency, amount of voidings, difficulty starting stream, changes in color or odor of urine, pain or burning with urination.)
2. Satisfaction with sexual functioning
3. Sexual partners: Sex, number, and their health
4. Use of contraceptives or safe sexual practices
5. Problems with sexual functioning: Pain, difficulty in obtaining or maintaining an erection, premature ejaculation (If present, investigate frequency, char-

---

RISK FACTORS	MALE CANCERS

TESTICULAR CANCER
Age 20 to 35
History of undescended testes, groin hernia, or testicular swelling with mumps
Family history of testicular cancer
White race
History of maternal use of oral contraceptives or diethylstilbestrol during pregnancy
Higher social class
Never married or married late

PROSTATE CANCER
Age over 50
Alcohol use
Diet high in animal fat
Family history of prostate cancer
Occupational exposure (e.g., cadmium, fertilizer, exhaust fumes)
Prostate specific antigen (PSA) level > 4 ng/ml
Residence in the United States

acteristics associated with intercourse, including partners, medications, and use of alcohol.)

6. Pattern of scrotal self-examination
7. Penile discharge (If present, determine color, amount, odor, associated symptoms, treatment, diagnoses.)
8. Penile lesions: Appearance, associated symptoms, treatment, diagnoses
9. Scrotal and groin masses, swelling, tenderness, pain, treatment, diagnoses
10. Enlargements or hernias in the inguinal area: Intermittent or constant; association with activity involving straining; groin pain; use of truss or similar device

Past health history

1. Urinary tract infections, kidney disease, kidney stones, flank pain, prostate problems
2. Reproductive history: Number of children and current health
3. Sexually transmitted diseases
4. Reproductive or hernia surgery
5. Trauma to genitourinary system

Associated conditions

1. Diabetes
2. Exposure to mumps after puberty

Family health history

1. Cancer of prostate or testes
2. Infertility problems
3. Mother's use of hormones during pregnancy or exposure to radiation during pregnancy

---

PREPARATION FOR EXAMINATION

EQUIPMENT

Item	Purpose
Disposable latex gloves	To protect examiner from infection
Flashlight	To transilluminate observed scrotal mass
Material to make slide or culture	To obtain specimen in case of abnormal discharge

CLIENT AND ENVIRONMENT

Client
Explain purpose and procedures
Uncovered from the waist down
Lying or standing

Environment
Warm
Private

Preparation for Examination: Client and Environment

Both the client and the practitioner usually perceive the examination of the genital organs as being different from the examination of other body parts. Characteristically, the genital and rectal examinations are the last portions of the physical assessment. The practitioner precedes the examination with a thorough history of the urinary system and a history of sexual functioning. The examiner should generally take the sexual history during the history-taking portion of the assessment while the client is dressed.

In preparation for the physical assessment, advise the client of its purpose and the procedures involved in the examination. Assemble the needed equipment.

The client may be lying down (with the examiner standing) or standing (with the examiner sitting or

---

HELPFUL HINT *For an effective examination, have the client void before the abdominal and pelvic area examination so that he will be more comfortable during palpation.*

Examination by a female practitioner

A female practitioner should feel emotionally comfortable with the examination. If she does not, she should routinely refer this part of the physical examination to a male practitioner. If she is comfortable with the examination, she must accept the fact that the male client may be reluctant to have a woman examine his genitalia. Cajoling a client into an uncomfortable procedure may destroy further rapport; the client's wishes in the situation should be respected. In most clinical settings, a male practitioner is available for a few minutes to examine the male genitalia. Our experience has been that most male clients are agreeable to examination by a woman; discomfort, if it exists, is usually on the examiner's part. It is therefore recommended that the beginning female examiner critically analyze her own feelings, fears, and beliefs; attempt male genital examination under supervision and with several cooperative clients; and then reexamine her feelings.

Conversation during examination

The client may perceive questioning about sexual activity or performance while the genitalia are being handled as evaluative or provocative.

Erection during examination

Erection can occur. If it does, reassure the client that an erection sometimes happens during the genital examination. Proceed with the examination without additional comment about the erection unless the client brings up the subject.

standing for various portions of the examination). Trousers and shorts should be removed. Put on rubber gloves before initiating the examination and wear them throughout the examination.

Technique for Examination and Normal Findings

Inspection of the genital area and penis

The techniques of inspection and palpation are used to examine the male genitalia. Inspection and palpation are done consecutively for each portion of the genitalia. After the inguinal and genital areas have been exposed, inspect the skin, hair, and gross appearance of the penis and scrotum (Figure 20.6). General examination of the skin and hair is discussed in Chapter 10. Assess the size of the penis and the secondary sex characteristics in relationship to the client's age and general development.

The onset of the appearance of adult sexual characteristics is extremely variable. Pubic hair appears and the testes enlarge between the ages of 12 and 16 years. Penile enlargement and the onset of seminal emission normally occur between the ages of 13 and 17 years. Table 20.1 contains a summary of developmental changes in the male genital system.

Genital hair is coarser than scalp hair. It is similar in color and appearance to axillary and chest hair. In the adult male, pubic hair will be abundant in the pubic region and will extend in a diamond pattern, narrowing upward toward the umbilicus. The penis is hairless, and the scrotum may have a sparse distribution of hairs.

An ambulatory, cooperative client can assist in the examination by handling the penis and scrotum during inspection. The examiner must do all the handling for the debilitated client. It is important to examine all the surfaces, including the posterior surfaces, of the male genitalia.

The color of the penis ranges from pink to light brown in whites and from light brown to dark brown in blacks. A prominent dorsal vein is often noted. Observe the entire penis for lesions, nodules, swelling, inflammation, and discharge. Then observe the glans and the urethral meatus for lesions and inflammation (Figure 20.7). If the client is uncircumcised, ask him to retract the prepuce from the glans, and carefully examine the glans and foreskin. If the uncircumcised client has retracted the foreskin for examination of the glans, remind him to return the foreskin to its usual position after the glans has been inspected.

If any discharge is present, obtain a smear and culture for gonorrhea and possibly chlamydial infection (see Chapter 21 for a discussion of procedures for obtaining smears and cultures). If the client has reported a discharge but none is present, request him to strip the penis from the base to the urethra. If a discharge is then

figure **20.6** Normal appearance of the male genitalia. **A,** Frontal view. **B,** Lateral view. (NOTE: The left testis is lower than the right because of the length of the spermatic cord.)

table 20.1 *Developmental Changes in Appearance of the Male Genital Organs*

Developmental time	Pubic hair	Appearance Penis	Testes and scrotum
Stage 1 Sexual maturity	None except for fine body hair such as on abdomen	Size proportional to body size as in childhood	Size proportional to body size as in childhood
Stage 2 Sexual maturity	Sparse, long, slightly pigmented, thin hair at base of penis	Slight enlargement	Enlargement of testes and scrotum; reddened pigmentation; texture more prominent
Stage 3 Sexual maturity	Darkens, becomes more coarse and curly; growth extends over symphysis	Elongation	Enlargement continues

Stage 1   Stage 2   Stage 3

Stage 4 Sexual maturity	Continues to darken, thicken, and become coarser and more curly; growth extends laterally, superiorly, and inferiorly	Breadth and length increase; glans develops	Enlargement continues; skin pigmentation darkens
Stage 5 Sexual maturity	Adult distribution and appearance; growth extends to inner thighs, umbilicus, and anus and is abundant	Adult appearance	Adult appearance
Elderly clients	Hair sparse and gray	Decrease in size	Testes hang low in scrotum; scrotum appears pendulous

Stage 4   Stage 5   Stage 6

Illustrations modified from Tanner JM: *Growth at adolescence,* ed 2, Oxford, 1962, Blackwell Scientific Publications.

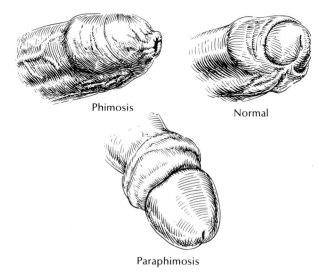

figure**20.7**   Usual position and appearance of the urethral meatus.

Penile epispadias

Penile hypospadias

figure**20.8**   Hypospadias, a malpositioning of the urethral meatus.

Phimosis

Normal

Paraphimosis

figure**20.9**   Phimosis, normal retraction of the prepuce, and paraphimosis.

present, make a culture. The procedure for stripping the penis is as follows:

1. Grasp the base of the penis with the thumb and fingers, with the thumb at the front and the fingers behind.
2. While applying a moderate amount of consistent pressure, move the thumb and the fingers slowly from the base to the tip of the penis.

The urethral meatus should appear pink and slitlike and should be positioned rather centrally on the glans. When the distal urethral ostium occurs on the ventral corona or at a more proximal and ventral site on the penis or perineum, the condition is called hypospadias (Figure 20.8). Epispadias is a similar malpositioning of the urethral meatus in the dorsal area.

When hypospadias or epispadias is noted, describe the location of the urethral meatus as precisely as possible. Hypospadias is classified as being glandular, penile, penoscrotal, or perineal. Epispadias is classified as being glandular, penile, or complete. *Glandular* refers to a location somewhere between the normal position and the junction of the glans with the body of the penis. *Penile* refers to a location on the penile shaft. *Penoscrotal* hypospadias indicates a positioning of the meatus along the anterior margin of the scrotum. *Perineal* hypospadias indicates a urethral orifice located on the perineum; in this condition, the scrotum is bifid. Epispadias is described as complete when the urethral orifice is located anterior to and off the penis.

The prepuce, if present, should be easily retractable from the glans and returnable to its original position. Phimosis exists when retraction cannot occur (Figure 20.9). This condition presents problems with cleanliness and prevents observation of the glans and interior surfaces of the prepuce. If the foreskin has been partially retracted but has impinged on the penis so that it cannot be returned to its usual position, the condition is called paraphimosis.

Palpation of the penis

Carefully palpate the penile shaft with the thumb and the first two fingers of the examining hand. The penis should feel smooth and semifirm. The overlying skin appears slightly wrinkled and feels somewhat movable over the underlying structures. Note any swelling, nodules, and induration as possibly abnormal findings. Occasionally, hard, nontender subcutaneous plaques are palpated on the dorsomedial surface. The client with this condition, called Peyronie's disease, may report penile bending with erection and painful intercourse.

Either compress the tip of the glans yourself or ask the client to compress the glans anteroposteriorly (Figure 20.10). This maneuver opens the distal end of the urethra for inspection. Observe for evidence of neoplastic lesions or inflammatory processes.

figure**20.10**   Compression of the glans to open the urethral meatus.

figure**20.11**   Normal appearance of the scrotum in the adult.

Inspection of the scrotum

Instruct the client to hold the penis out of the way, and observe the general size, superficial appearance, and symmetry of the scrotum (Figure 20.11). The scrotum normally appears asymmetrical because the left testis is generally lower than the right testis. Also, the tone of the dartos muscle determines the size of the scrotum; this muscle contracts when the area is cold and relaxes when the area is warm. In advanced age, the dartos muscle is somewhat atonic, and the scrotum may appear pendulous.

The scrotal skin is more darkly pigmented than that of the rest of the body. To observe the scrotal skin, spread its rugated surface. Also, remember to inspect the posterior and posterolateral and anterior and anterolateral skin areas. A common abnormality, occurring as a single lesion or as multiple lesions, is that of sebaceous cysts. These are firm, yellow to white, nontender cutaneous lesions measuring up to 1 cm in diameter.

Palpation of the scrotum

Before palpating the scrotum, assure the client that you will do this gently. The skin of the scrotum is not especially sensitive, but the contents are very sensitive. Palpate the contents of each half of the scrotal sac (Figure 20.12). Both testes should be present in the scrotum at birth. If they are not present, determine their location by retracing their course of descent back into the abdomen.

Palpate both testes with the first two fingers. Determine their consistency, size, shape, and response to pressure. The testes should be smooth, homogeneous in consistency, regular, equal in size, freely movable, and

figure**20.12**   Palpation of the scrotal contents.

slightly sensitive to compression. If possible, palpate both testes simultaneously to allow for comparison between them.

Next, palpate each epididymis. The epididymides are located in the posterolateral area of the testes in 93% of the male population. In approximately 7%, the epididymides lie in the anterolateral or anterior areas. Palpate them and note their size, shape, consistency, and tenderness. To palpate the epididymides, pick up the scrotum using the thumb, first finger, and middle finger of each hand just beneath the testes. Bring the fingers together under the testes. Next, move the fingers back several millimeters until the testes are felt. Just under and behind the testes, you should feel the epididymides as tubular structures that collapse when gently compressed. Become accustomed to differentiating the consistencies of the testes and the epididymides and where each begins and ends. The epididymides should feel smooth, discrete, larger cephalad, and nontender.

Then palpate each of the spermatic cords by bilaterally grasping each between the thumb and the forefinger, starting at the base of the epididymis and continuing to the inguinal canal. The vasa deferentia feel similar to smooth cords and are movable. The arteries, veins, lymph vessels, and nerves feel like indefinite threads along the side of the vas.

If swelling, irregularity, or nodularity is noted in the scrotum, an attempt should be made to transilluminate it by darkening the room and placing a lighted flashlight behind the scrotal contents. Transillumination is noted by a red glow. Serous fluid will transilluminate; tissue

and blood will not. On transillumination, the normal scrotum and epididymis will appear as dark masses with regular borders. Small areas of transilluminated space appear around the testes, with a larger transilluminated space appearing superior to the testes. The amount of transilluminated space superior to the testes is dependent on the amount of scrotal relaxation. Because of concern about the transmission of disease, a disposable flashlight or a flashlight with a disposable plastic cover should be used.

The scrotum can be edematous, and palpation may produce pitting. Edema of the scrotum can occur in any condition that causes edema in the lower trunk (e.g., cardiovascular disease).

Palpation of the regional lymph nodes

The lymph nodes of the inguinal areas may be assessed as part of the hernia examination or as part of the abdominal examination. Two sets of lymph nodes are assessed: superior inguinal and inferior inguinal (Figure 20.13).

The client must be lying down for examination of the inguinal nodes. Flex the client's leg at the knee to relax the muscles of the inguinal area. Abduct the leg slightly; you may see a shallow, hollow space. Begin your palpation here, lightly at first, and then more deeply. Palpate from the anterosuperior iliac spine to the pubic tubercle. Do not confuse Poupart's ligament with enlarged lymph nodes, which, if enlarged will be close to the surface and fairly easy to feel. See Figure 20.13 for an illustration of lymph node palpation areas.

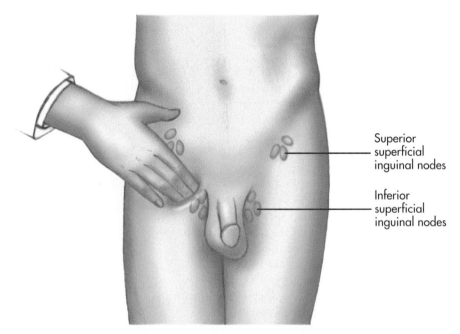

figure**20.13** Palpation of the inguinal lymph nodes.

Palpation of the prostate

With an ambulatory client, executing the rectal and prostate examination is done most satisfactorily with the client standing, hips flexed, toes pointed toward each other, and upper body resting on the examining table. This position flattens the buttocks, deters gluteal contraction, and makes the anus and rectum more accessible to evaluation. A debilitated client may be examined in the left lateral or lithotomy position. If the left lateral position is used, remind the client to flex his right knee and hip and to have his buttocks close to the edge of the examining table. The general procedure for the anal and rectal examination is described in Chapter 22. Perform the general rectal examination first. Then palpate the prostate gland and seminal vesicles with the pad of the index finger (Figure 20.14, *A*).

figure**20.14** Palpation of the prostate. **A,** Position of the examiner's finger. **B,** Prostatic massage. Arrows indicate the areas of the prostate that are massaged and the sequence and direction of the massage.

Visualize the prostate anatomy, its lobes, and its size in relationship to the bladder and the external anal sphincter. A common mistake of beginning practitioners is to palpate too deeply and mistake the base of the bladder for the prostate. Be sure to palpate the entire, accessible surface of the prostate. The prostate gland is located on the anterior rectal wall but should not be protruding into the rectal lumen. Prostatic enlargement, or protrusion of the prostate gland into the rectal lumen, is commonly described in grades:

Grade I: Encroaches less than 1 cm into the rectal lumen

Grade II: Encroaches 1 to 2 cm into the rectal lumen

Grade III: Encroaches 2 to 3 cm into the rectal lumen

Grade IV: Encroaches more than 3 cm into the rectal lumen

The gland should be approximately 3 cm long, approximately 4 cm across at its base, symmetrical, movable, and of a rubbery (like a pencil eraser) consistency. Its median sulcus normally can be felt. The lateral margins of the prostate gland should be discrete, and a moderate degree of mobility can be noted when the tip of the index finger is hooked over the upper border of the gland and the gland is pulled down gently.

The proximal portions of the seminal vesicles can sometimes be palpated as corrugated structures above the lateral to the midpoint of the gland. Normally, they are too soft to be palpated. Attempt to examine all available surfaces of the prostate gland and the entire area of the seminal vesicles. Significant abnormalities of the prostate gland or seminal vesicles include protrusion into the rectal lumen; hard, nodular areas; bogginess; tenderness; and asymmetry.

> **HELPFUL HINT** *In prostate examination, consider the following questions about the prostate:*
> - *Surface:* Smooth or nodular?
> - *Consistency:* Rubbery, hard, boggy, soft, or fluctuant?
> - *Shape:* Rounded or flat?
> - *Size:* Normal, enlarged, or atrophied?
> - *Sensitivity:* Tender or not?
> - *Movability:* Movable or fixed?

The prostate gland can be massaged centrally from its lateral edges to force secretions into the urethra (Figure 20.14, *B*). Stroke the prostate from its distal to proximal areas, with the order of strokes indicated in the figure. Secretions at the urethral opening can be examined and cultured. It is important that all areas of the prostate available for palpation be massaged.

Screening Tests and Procedures

The U.S. Preventive Services Task Force (1996) recommendation about screening for testicular cancer is as follows:

Periodic screening for testicular cancer by testicular examination is recommended for men with a history of cryptorchidism, orchiopexy, or testicular atrophy. There is insufficient evidence of clinical benefit or harm to recommend for or against routine screening of other asymptomatic men.

Because this recommendation is somewhat ambiguous and since the self-examination is easily and quickly done during a bath or a shower, consider teaching it to every client and recommending that it be done monthly on some target date.

---

examination *step-by-step*

1. Inspect the condition of the skin and hair in the pubic region.
2. Inspect the pubic hair distribution. Assess the consistency of findings with the client's age.
3. Inspect the penis:
   a. Ask the client to retract the foreskin (if present).
   b. Inspect the glans for inflammation.
   c. Check the condition and position of the urethral meatus.
   d. Assess the skin for color, lesions, and swelling.
4. Palpate the inguinal areas for nodes.
5. Palpate the penis:
   a. Compress the glans and check for inflammation or discharge.
   b. Examine the shaft of the penis for tenderness or induration (anterior and posterior surfaces).
   c. Strip the urethra for discharge (if symptomatic).
6. Inspect the scrotum:
   a. The client holds the penis out of the way.
   b. Inspect the skin and surface for color, symmetry, and swelling.
7. Palpate the scrotum:
   a. Spread the rugae to examine the surface for consistency, size, tenderness, and masses.
   b. Examine each spermatic cord for consistency, size, tenderness, and masses.
   c. Palpate the testes.
   d. Palpate the epididymides.
   e. Transilluminate any masses present.
8. Palpate the prostate gland (in conjunction with the rectal examination):
   a. Assess for extension into the lumen, size, contour, consistency, tenderness, and mobility.

The U.S. Preventive Services Task Force (1996) recommendation about screening for prostate cancer is as follows:

Routine screening for prostate cancer with digital examinations, serum tumor markers (e.g., prostate specific antigen), or transrectal ultrasound is not recommended.

■ VARIATIONS FROM HEALTH

Penis

Among the more common penile lesions are syphilitic chancre, condylomata acuminata, and cancer. The syphilitic chancre is the primary lesion of syphilis. It begins as a single papule that eventually erodes into an oval or round red ulcer with an indurated base that discharges serous material. It is usually painless.

Condylomata acuminata are wart-appearing growths. They are caused by human papillomavirus and may be seen occurring singly or in multiple cauliflower-like patches on the penis and throughout the genital area. They can be transmitted to a partner via sexual intercourse.

Carcinoma of the penis occurs most frequently on the glans and the inner lip of the prepuce. It may appear dry and scaly, ulcerated, or nodular. It is usually painless.

Scrotum

The common abnormalities of the scrotum are described and illustrated in Table 20.2. All scrotal masses should be described by their placement, size, shape, consistency, and tenderness and by whether they transilluminate.

Prostate

A hard single or multiple lesion on a firm and fixed prostate gland may indicate cancer. The initial lesion of carcinoma is frequently on the posterior lobe and can be easily identified during the rectal examination. A soft, symmetrical, boggy, nontender prostate gland may indicate benign prostatic hypertrophy, a condition very common in men over 50 years of age. In the later stages of this condition, the median sulcus may be obliterated. A boggy, fluctuant, or tender prostate gland may indicate acute or chronic prostatitis.

■ TEACHING SELF-ASSESSMENT

Genital self-examination is a means of early identification of scrotal cancer and sexually transmitted diseases. Individuals with malignant testicular tumors typically have the following characteristics:

Age 20 to 34
History of undescended testes
White race

table 20.2 **Description of Scrotal Abnormalities**

Abnormality	Definition/causation	Basis for diagnosis
Hydrocele	Accumulation of serous fluid between visceral and parietal layers of tunica vaginalis	Transilluminates; fingers can get above mass
Scrotal hernia	Hernia within scrotum	Bowel sounds auscultated; does not transilluminate; fingers cannot get above mass
Varicocele	Abnormal dilation and tortuosity of veins of pampiniform plexus; often described as "bag of worms" in scrotum*	Complaints of dragging sensation or dull pain in scrotal area; feels like soft bag of worms; collapses when scrotum is elevated and increases when scrotum is dependent; more commonly present on left side; usually appears at puberty
Spermatocele	Epididymal cyst resulting from partial obstruction of spermatic tubules*	Transilluminates; round mass, feels like a third testis; painless

Hydrocele   Scrotal hernia   Varicocele   Spermatocele

Epididymal mass   Epididymitis   Torsion of the spermatic cord   Testicular tumor

Abnormality	Definition/causation	Basis for diagnosis
Epididymal mass or nodularity	May be result of benign or malignant neoplasms, syphilis, or tuberculosis	Nodules are not tender; in tuberculosis lesions, vas deferens often feels beaded
Epididymitis	Inflammation of epididymis, usually resulting from *Escherichia coli, Neisseria gonorrhoeae,* or *Mycobacterium tuberculosis* organisms*	Spermatic cord often thickened and indurated; pain relieved by elevation
Torsion of spermatic cord	Axial rotation or volvulus of spermatic cord, resulting in infarction of testicle	Elevated mass; pain not relieved by further elevation; more common in childhood or adolescence; history of extreme pain and tenderness of testis, followed by hyperemic swelling and hydrocele
Testicular tumor	Multiple causes	Usually not painful; hydroceles may develop as result of a tumor; if testis cannot be palpated, fluid may need to be aspirated so that testis can be accurately evaluated

*From Betesh S, editor: *Diseases of the urinary tract and male genital organs,* Geneva, 1974, Council for Internal Organizations for Medical Sciences.

figure**20.15** Male genital self-examination. **A,** Examination of the urethral meatus. **B,** Scrotal assessment.

History of maternal use of oral contraceptives or diethylstilbestrol during early pregnancy

History of maternal abdominal or pelvic x-ray examination during pregnancy

Higher social class

Never married or late marriage

Clients with the following characteristics are at risk for sexually transmitted diseases: (1) more than one sexual partner and (2) intercourse with person(s) having multiple partners.

At the initiation of the teaching, assess the male client's level of knowledge about genital self-examination, reinforce the importance of a monthly self-examination, and provide instruction for the examination. The following outline can be used for the health teaching along with pictures of the anatomy of the male genitalia:

1. Cancer of the testes is one of the most curable forms of cancer when detected early. The cure rate is approximately 90%.
2. Cancer of the testes can affect males of any age but is most common between ages 15 and 35. It is much more likely in men whose testicles descended after infancy or never descended at all.
3. Men can have normal sexual relations after being treated for cancer of the testicle.
4. Examine the genitalia once a month.
5. Do the self-examination during or following a shower or warm bath, when the testes are relaxed, descended, and accessible for palpation.

6. Examine the penis for lesions and discharge:
   a. Inspect the head of the penis—retract the foreskin (if present).
   b. Examine the entire shaft.
   c. Inspect the urethral meatus for discharge (Figure 20.15, *A*).
7. Examine the skin and pubic hair for lesions and parasites.
8. Examine the scrotum:
   a. Use the thumbs and the index and middle fingers for examination, with the thumbs placed on the top and the fingers on the underside of the scrotum (Figure 20.15, *B*).
   b. Gently roll the contents of the scrotum between your thumbs and fingers. The normal testicle is about 1½ to 2 inches long. It feels smooth, rubbery, and firm but not hard. The epididymis is the storage tube found behind each testicle. Each should feel soft and spongy and sometimes slightly tender. The spermatic cords extend from the bottom of the epididymides and up into the pelvis. They should feel like smooth, firm tubes.
   c. The examination should be painless unless the pressure is too hard or some problem exists. A small amount of tenderness may be noticed during the palpation of the testes and the epididymides; this is normal.
   d. Any lump or change in texture, whether painful or not, should be reported to and as-

sessed by a health care provider as soon as possible.

■ ASSESSMENT OF THE INGUINAL AREA FOR HERNIAS

Purpose of Examination

The purpose of the inguinal area assessment for hernias is to determine the presence of inguinal and femoral hernias. This examination is addressed in conjunction with the male genital examination because most kinds of hernias are more common in males than in females. However, this discussion pertains to the physical examination of both sexes.

Anatomy and Physiology

The inguinal ligament (Poupart's ligament) extends from the anterosuperior spine of the ilium to the pubic tubercle. The inguinal canal is a flattened tunnel between two layers of abdominal muscle, measuring approximately 4 to 6 cm in the adult. Its internal ring is located 1 to 2 cm above the midpoint of the inguinal ligament. The spermatic cord traverses this internal ring, passes through the canal, exits the canal at its external (subcutaneous) ring, and then moves up and over the inguinal ligament and into the scrotum (Figure 20.16).

Hesselbach's triangle is the region superior to the inguinal canal, medial to the inferior epigastric artery, and lateral to the margin of the rectus muscle.

The femoral canal is a potential space just inferior to the inguinal ligament and 3 cm medial and parallel to the femoral artery. When the examiner's right hand is placed on the client's right anterior thigh with the index finger over the femoral artery, the femoral canal will be under the examiner's ring finger.

The three main types of pelvic area hernias are shown in Figure 20.17. In the indirect inguinal hernia, the hernial sac enters the internal inguinal canal, and its tip is located somewhere in the inguinal canal or beyond the canal. In men, indirect inguinal hernias may descend into the scrotum. The direct inguinal hernia emerges directly from behind and through the external inguinal ring. The femoral hernia emerges through the femoral ring, the femoral canal, and the fossa ovalis. The characteristics of the three main types of hernias are compared in Table 20.3.

Examination
Health history

Throughout the health history interview, the following data should be recorded about a symptom or problem: (1) onset (specific date, sudden or gradual), (2) duration, (3) frequency, (4) precipitating factors, (5) aggravating or alleviating factors, (6) treatment received or self-care given, and (7) outcome.

Present health status
1. Enlargement in the inguinal area
   a. Frequency: Intermittent or constant

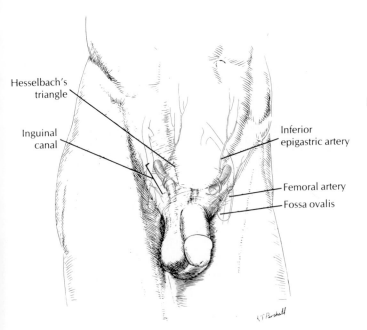

figure**20.16** Superficial anatomy of the anterior pelvic area.

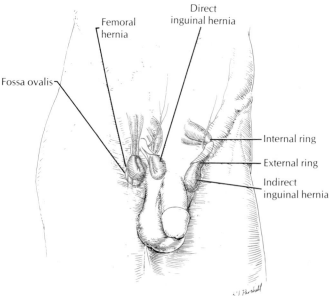

figure**20.17** Three common pelvic area hernias.

table 20.3 *Comparison of Inguinal and Femoral Hernias*

	Inguinal hernia		Femoral hernia
	Indirect	**Direct**	
Course	Sac emerges through internal inguinal ring, lateral to inferior epigastric artery; can remain in canal, exit external ring, or pass into scrotum	Sac emerges directly from behind and through external inguinal ring; located in region of Hesselbach's triangle	Sac emerges through femoral ring, femoral canal, and fossa ovalis; observed medial to femoral artery
Incidence	More common in infants under 1 year and in young men 16 to 20 years; more common in men than in women at a ratio of approximately 4:1; 60% of all hernias	Most often observed in men over 40 years of age; rarer than indirect hernia	Less common than inguinal hernias; seldom seen in children; more common in women; 4% of all hernias
Cause	Congenital or acquired	Congenital weakness exacerbated by (1) lifting, (2) atrophy of abdominal muscles, (3) ascites, (4) chronic cough, or (5) obesity	Acquired; may be caused by (1) stooping frequently, (2) increased abdominal pressure, (3) loss of muscle substance
Clinical symptoms and signs	Soft swelling in region of internal inguinal ring— swelling increases when client stands or strains, is sometimes reduced when client reclines; pain during straining	Abdominal bulge in area of Hesselbach's triangle, usually in area of internal ring; usually painless; easily reduced when client reclines; rarely enters scrotum	Right side more commonly affected; pain may be severe; strangulation frequent; sac may extend into scrotum, into labium, or along saphenous vein

b. Presence of pain: Character, location, association with lifting or straining
c. Association with lifting or straining
d. Change in size
e. Reducibility
f. Use of truss or other treatment
2. Swelling or lump in the inguinal area
Past health history
1. Surgery to the inguinal area
2. Infections in the legs or abdomen
Family health history
1. Hernias

Preparation for examination: client and environment

If a client has an inguinal or groin area hernia, he or she will probably complain of a swelling or bulging in that area, especially during abdominal straining. As part of the routine physical examination, all clients should be screened for inguinal and femoral hernias, even if they do not complain of groin swelling.

No special equipment is needed for the examination. The examiner should wear rubber gloves.

PREPARATION FOR EXAMINATION

EQUIPMENT

Item	**Purpose**
Rubber gloves	Protect examiner from infection

CLIENT AND ENVIRONMENT
Client
Uncovered from the waist
Preferably standing
Environment
Warm
Private

chapter
21

Female Genitalia

■ PURPOSE OF EXAMINATION

The purpose of the examination of the female genitalia is to assess the health of the female reproductive system and to screen for various sexually transmitted diseases and cervical cancer. The regional examination of the female genital system consists of (1) the abdominal examination, (2) inspection of the external genitalia, (3) palpation of the external genitalia, (4) the speculum examination, (5) specimen collection, (6) the bimanual vaginal examination, and (7) the rectovaginal examination. The examination of the inguinal area for hernias and nodes and the assessment of the anus and rectum are integrated into the examination of the genitalia.

■ ANATOMY AND PHYSIOLOGY

External Genitalia

The external female genitalia are termed the vulva or pudendum (Figure 21.1). The symphysis pubis is covered by a pad of fat called the mons pubis or mons veneris. In the postpubertal female, the mons is covered by a patch of coarse, curly hair that extends to the lower abdomen. The abdominal portion of the female escutcheon is flat and forms the base of an inverted triangle of hair.

The labia majora are two bilobate folds of adipose tissue extending from the mons to the perineum. After puberty, their outer surfaces are covered with hair and their inner surfaces are smooth and hairless. The labia minora are two folds of skin that are thinner and darker than the labia majora. The labia minora lie within the labia majora and extend from the clitoris to the fourchette. Anteriorly, each labium minus divides into a medial and a lateral part. The lateral parts join posteriorly to form the prepuce of the clitoris, and the medial parts join anterior to the clitoris to form the frenulum of the clitoris. The clitoris is composed of erectile tissue, homologous to the corpus cavernosum of the penis. Its body is normally about 2.5 cm long; the length of its visible portion is 2 cm or less.

The vestibule is the boat-shaped anatomic region between the labia minora. It contains the urethral and vaginal orifices. The urethral orifice is located approxi-

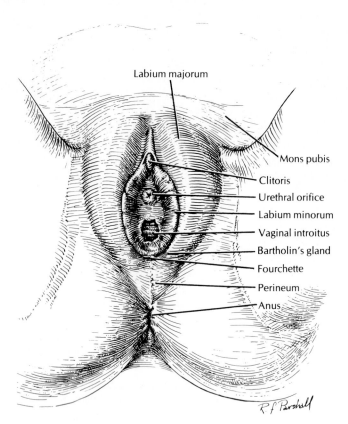

figure**21.1** Female external genitalia.

mately 2.5 cm posterior and inferior to the clitoris and is visualized as an irregular, vertical slit or an inverted V. The vaginal orifice, or introitus, lies immediately behind and inferior to the urethral orifice and can be observed as a thin vertical slit or as a large orifice with irregular skin edges, depending on the condition of the hymen. The hymen is a membranous, annular, or crescentic fold at the vaginal opening. When unperforated, it is usually a continuous membrane but on occasion may be cribiform. After perforation, small rounded fragments of hymen attach to the introital margins; these are called hymenal caruncles.

The ducts of two types of glands open on the vulva. Skene's glands are multiple, tiny organs located in the paraurethral area. They secrete a fluid that lubricates the vaginal vestibule during sexual intercourse. Their ducts, numbering approximately 6 to 31, lie inside and just outside of the urethral orifice and are usually not visible. These ducts open laterally and slightly posterior to the urethral orifice in approximately the 5 and 7 o'clock positions. The urethral orifice is the center of the clock. Bartholin's glands are small, ovoid organs located lateral and slightly posterior to the vaginal orifice, partially behind the bulb of the vestibule. During sexual excitement, these glands secrete mucus, which lubricates the introitus and promotes sperm motility and viability. Their ducts are approximately 2 cm long and open in

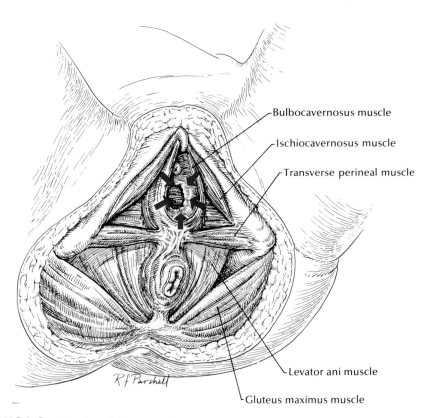

figure**21.2** Muscles of the pelvic floor. Arrows illustrate the direction of contraction of the bulbocavernosus muscle.

the groove between the labia minora and the hymen in approximately the 5 and 7 o'clock positions. These ducts are also usually not visible.

The perineum consists of the tissues between the introitus and the anus.

The pelvic floor consists of a group of muscles attached to points on the bony pelvis (Figure 21.2). These muscles form a suspended sling that assists in holding the pelvic contents in place. The muscles are pierced by the urethral, vaginal, and rectal orifices and function both passively as a pelvic support and actively in voluntary contraction of the vaginal and anal orifices.

Internal Genitalia

Figure 21.3 illustrates the internal genitalia. The vagina is a pink, transversely rugated, collapsed tube that in the adult is approximately 9 cm long posteriorly and 6 to 7 cm long anteriorly. It inclines posteriorly at approximately a 45-degree angle with the vertical plane of the body. The vagina is highly dilatable, especially in its superior portion and anteroposterior dimension. When collapsed, it is roughly H-shaped in transverse section. Superiorly and usually anteriorly, the vagina is pierced by the uterine cervix. The recess between the portion of the vagina adjacent to the cervix and the cervix is called the vaginal fornix. Although it is actually continuous, the fornix is anatomically divided into anterior, posterior, and lateral fornices.

The uterus is an inverted, pear-shaped, muscular organ that is flattened anteroposteriorly. It is usually found inclined forward 45 degrees from the vertical plane of the erect body and is approximately 5.5 to 8 cm long, 3.5 to 4 cm wide, and 2 to 2.5 cm thick. The uterus of the parous client may be normally enlarged an additional 2 to 3 cm in any of the three dimensions. The uterus is divided into two main parts: the body and the cervix. The body in turn is composed of three parts: the fundus, the prominence above the insertion of the fallopian tubes; the body, or main portion, of the uterus; and the isthmus, the constricted lower portion of the uterus, which is adjacent to the cervix. The cervix extends from the isthmus into the vagina.

The uterine cavity communicates with the vagina through an ostium, the cervical os. The os is a small, depressed, circular opening in the nulliparous client. In women who have borne children, the os is enlarged and irregularly shaped. The position of the uterus is not fixed; it is a relatively movable organ. The uterus may be anteverted, anteflexed, retroverted, or retroflexed in position; or it may be in midposition. (See Table 21.2 for illustrations of these positions.) In the normal adult with an empty bladder the uterus is usually anteverted and slightly anteflexed in position.

The ovaries are a pair of oval organs; each is approximately 3 cm long, 2 cm wide, and 1 cm thick. They are usually located near the lateral pelvic wall, at the level of the anterosuperior iliac spine. The two fallopian tubes insert in the upper portion of the uterus, are supported loosely by the broad ligament, and run laterally to the ovaries. Each tube is approximately 10 cm long.

The uterus, ovaries, and tubes are supported by four pairs of ligaments: the cardinal, uterosacral, round, and broad ligaments (Figure 21.4).

figure**21.3** Internal female genitalia.

figure**21.4** Ligaments of the internal female genitalia.

The rectouterine pouch, or Douglas' cul-de-sac, is a deep recess formed by the peritoneum as it passes over the intestinal surface of the rectum. It is the lowest point in the abdominal cavity.

The two groups of superficial nodes in the inguinal area are the superior and inferior inguinal nodes (see Figure 20.5). These nodes receive most of the lymph drainage from the legs. The superior inguinal nodes lie somewhat horizontally along the inguinal ligament. They receive drainage from the abdominal wall below the umbilicus, the external genitalia, the anal canal, the vulva and lower one third of the vagina, the gluteal area, and the inferior inguinal nodes. Lymph from around the internal female genitalia drains into deeper nodes, which are not accessible to palpation. The inferior group lies somewhat vertically below the junction of the saphenous and femoral veins. These large lymph nodes receive lymph from the superficial regions of the leg and foot.

■ EXAMINATION

Health History

The reproductive health history is fairly extensive. For a follow-up encounter in a health care system, much of the historical information will probably be on the record, and the focus of the interval history will be on the health need or problem. The gynecological and obstetrical regional history for a new adult client will be, out of necessity, somewhat lengthy (see below). Throughout the health history interview, record the following data about a symptom or problem: (1) onset (specific date, sudden or gradual); (2) duration; (3) frequency; (4) precipitating factors; (5) aggravating or alleviating factors; (6) treatment received or self-care given; and (7) outcome.

A. Menstrual history
   1. Age initiated (menarche)
   2. Date of last menstrual period [LMP = last menstrual period]
   3. Date of last normal menstrual period [LNMP] NOTE: This date may be the same as or different from the LMP. Discrepancies may be clinically significant.
   4. Pattern: Frequency (days), duration (days), and amount of bleeding (in total number of tampons and/or pads used); presence and size of clots (e.g., size of a quarter)
   5. Associated symptoms (dysmenorrhea): Pain, cramping, distention, weight gain, irritability, mood swings, breast engorgement
   6. Intermenstrual bleeding or spotting
   7. Changes in cycle: Metrorrhagia, oligomenorrhea

B. Self-care
   1. Pattern of douching (including solution used, strength of solution, and frequency)
   2. Use of feminine hygiene sprays
   3. Type of material in underpants and pantyhose worn
   4. Planning for pregnancy, if applicable
   5. Use of protection against sexually transmitted diseases
   6. Safe sexual practices
C. Gynecologic history
   1. Date and results of last Papanicolaou (Pap) smear
   2. Gynecological diagnoses, procedures, and surgeries
   3. Pregnancies: Dates, durations, complications, condition of infants if live births, and other relevant outcomes (include abortions [spontaneous, elective, therapeutic], and ectopic pregnancies)
   4. If postmenopausal: History of hot flashes, headaches, palpitations, sweats, mood swings, vaginal dryness and itching, other signs and symptoms
   5. Sexually transmitted diseases: Diagnoses and treatment
      a. Gonorrhea
      b. Herpes
      c. Vaginitis
      d. HIV
      e. Syphilis
   6. Infertility: Diagnosis and treatment
D. Medications: Contraceptive, hormonal, or other prescribed for management of reproductive system problems
   1. Name
   2. Dosage
   3. Purpose
   4. Frequency
   5. Duration
   6. Side effects
   7. Compliance
E. Sexual history
   1. Date of first intercourse
   2. Pattern and number of partners
   3. Health of partners
   4. Number and health of partners' partners
   5. Satisfaction with intercourse
   6. Current satisfaction with partner and opportunities for intercourse
   7. Dyspareunia
F. Present health/present illness (examples of history for common problems)
   1. *Abdominal/pelvic pain*
      a. Onset

b. Related factors

c. Character: Sharp, dull, aching, burning, knifelike

d. Location

e. Frequency

f. Intensity

g. Associated symptoms: Malaise, fever, nausea, vomiting, constipation

h. Relief measures

2. *Vaginal bleeding*

a. Onset

b. Related factors

c. Color: Pink, red, dark red, brown, other

d. Character: Thin, thick, watery, mixed with mucus; if clots, how many and how large

e. Amount: What size of saturation on underwear or saturation of how many pads or tampons in a specific time period

f. Frequency and relationship to menstrual cycle

g. Associated symptoms or events (e.g., cramping, injury)

3. *Vaginal discharge*

a. Onset

b. Color: White, yellow-green, gray, other

c. Character: Thin, curdlike, purulent, other

d. Odor: "Fishy," foul, other

e. Associated symptoms: Vulvar itching, vaginal itching, rash, pain with intercourse

f. Relief measures

g. Previous experiences with the same symptoms

4. *Urinary problems*

a. Character

b. Frequency

c. Previous diagnoses

d. Description of urine

e. Associated symptoms: Fever, chills, flank pain, urgency, frequency, dysuria, hematuria

f. Relationship of problems to changes in sexual intercourse frequency, technique, or partner

G. Associated conditions

1. Diabetes

2. Hypertension

3. Genitourinary problems

4. Cancer

H. Family history

1. Reproductive problems

2. Cancer

3. Diabetes

4. Mother's use of hormones during pregnancy

RISK FACTORS   FEMALE CANCERS

CERVICAL CANCER

Age: Between 40 and 50 years

History: Cervical dysplasias, condylomata acuminata lesions, herpes infection

First coitus: Early age

Sex partners: Multiple or partner with multiple partners

Pregnancies: Multiple

History: Exposure to diethylstilbestrol, smoking

ENDOMETRIAL CANCER

Age: Postmenopausal

Menarche: Early

Menopause: Late

Parity: Low or infertility

Body weight: Obese

History: Hypertension, diabetes, endometrial hyperplasia, liver disease

Estrogen: History of replacement

Family history: Endometrial, breast, or colon cancer

OVARIAN CANCER

Age: Between 40 and 60

History: Ovarian dysfunction, spontaneous abortions, cancer of breast or endometrium, irradiation of pelvic organs, endometriosis

Family history: Ovarian or breast cancer

Environment: Exposure to talc or asbestos

Preparation for Examination: Client and Environment

Most female clients perceive the examination of their reproductive organs as being different from the examination of other body parts. Past admonitions of "do not touch" and "keep it covered" have created a population of anatomically unaware and sometimes inappropriately "modest" women who are often unnecessarily difficult to examine. This is particularly true of older women and members of certain ethnic groups. Most practitioners believe that they can obtain a great amount of information about a female client by examining the genital area and performing screening tests. However, because of their experience with fearful and tense reactions of many clients, practitioners have sometimes routinely omitted the examination of the genital organs or have referred their clients to gynecological specialists for routine examinations.

One cause of the female client's tenseness during an examination of the genital area may be fear of discovery of sexual activity. During the history, investigate areas of anatomical and physiological function and dysfunction. The review of systems on all clients should include a

PREPARATION FOR EXAMINATION

EQUIPMENT

Item	Purpose
Disposable latex gloves	To protect examiner and client from transfer of infectious organisms
Speculums of various sizes	Inspection of internal genitalia
Sterile cotton swabs	To cleanse internal genitalia
	To obtain specimens for examination
Lubricant* (water soluble)	To facilitate insertion of speculum and fingers for examination
Cotton balls	To cleanse tissues
Sponge forceps	To insert cotton or gauze to cleanse tissues
Cytology fixative	To fix Papanicolaou (Pap) smear
Floor examination light	Visualization of internal structures
Ayre spatulas	To obtain cell samples for Pap smear
Cervical brushes	To obtain endocervical specimens for Pap smears
Culture media	Inoculation of specimens from cervical and vaginal areas
Glass slides	For Pap smears and for preparing a sample of vaginal discharge for examination
Hand mirror	To enable client to visualize internal genitalia
Normal saline	To prepare discharge on slides to assess for presence of specific organisms
Potassium hydroxide	To prepare discharge on slides to assess for presence of specific organisms
pH tape	To test pH of vagina

*An amount of lubricant, sufficient for the examination, should be placed on a piece of paper or gauze. The examiner should avoid handling the tube of lubricant during the examination, since it might become contaminated during handling and become a mechanism of infection transmission. Also, single-use tubes of lubricant are available.

CLIENT

Explain the procedure.

Have the client empty her bladder right before the examination.

Assist the client in assuming the lithotomy position.

1. Instruct the client to lie down on the examination table and help her to put her heels into the stirrups and to stabilize them. Some clients are more comfortable leaving their shoes and/or socks on. Also, padding the stirrups with a soft fabric is a helpful hint to increase comfort for the heels and feet.
2. Retract the end of the table if it is still extended.
3. Help the client to bring her buttocks to the very bottom edge of the table. Gently guide the client or advise her to feel and aim for the end of the table herself.
4. Redrape the client so that the knees and symphysis pubis are covered. Depress the drape between the knees so you can see the client's face for responses during the examination.
5. Reposition the upper torso so that the head and shoulders are slightly elevated to increase client comfort and assist relaxation of abdominal muscles.

ENVIRONMENT

Warm

Well lit with additional light available to assist the visualization of internal genitalia

Private

EXAMINER

Gloved throughout the examination

Standing and sitting (on a wheeled stool) between the client's legs during various parts of the examination

Monitoring the client's face throughout examination

sexual history. If you have skillfully accomplished this portion of the history and if the client has been cooperative, she should not be apprehensive about the possible discovery of sexual "secrets."

Other causes of tenseness during the pelvic examination include fear of discovery of disease and the memory of previous, uncomfortable pelvic examinations. Many clients are not knowledgeable regarding the anatomy of the pelvic area. Determine the client's need for basic information regarding the structure of the genital organs and provide this instruction before the pelvic examination, along with a demonstration of the instruments and an explanation of the procedure. Show the speculum to the client and demonstrate the mechanism used to open and close it. Advise the client about the clicking sounds normally made by a speculum as it is opened and closed. A relatively short amount of time taken to inform and orient all female clients at their first examinations provides long-term benefits in preventing anxiety and increasing cooperation.

HELPFUL HINT *Teaching the client a relaxation technique will often make an examination shorter in length and, in the case of a very tense client, possible at all.*

One successful relaxation technique is the following. Instruct the client to:
- *Place her hands on her chest at about the level of the diaphragm*
- *Breathe deeply and slowly through her mouth*
- *Concentrate on the rhythm of breathing*
- *Relax all body muscles with each exhalation*

The tense client is apt to hold her breath and tighten. Even the coached client may forget and hold her breath. A gentle reminder, advising her to keep breathing, usually enables the client to maintain relaxation. This technique is particularly helpful in the adolescent or virginal client, whose introitus may be especially small.

An additional relaxation, or, more specifically, distraction technique, is the placement of a sign or mobile above the examining table. Some clients appreciate having something to look at, and their attention is constructively diverted from the examiner's activities.

Most clients find it difficult to engage in lengthy conversations while in a lithotomy position. They do appreciate explanations and reassurances from examiners but prefer not to have to respond to questions until they are again upright and at eye level with the examiner. Questioning a client extensively during the pelvic examination is apt to make her tense.

Environmental conditions are also important in enhancing cooperation during examination of the genital area. The environment and the client should be warm. The examining area should be private and safe from unexpected intrusion. The room, the examiner's hands, and all materials touching the client should be warm.

Clients should be advised not to douche or use vaginal medications or other inserts during the 24 hours preceding the pelvic examination and reminded to empty their bladders immediately before the examination.

Materials needed for the examination should be assembled and readily available before the client is put in the lithotomy position (see Preparation for Examination box).

Some clients have difficulty assuming the lithotomy position, especially moving their buttocks sufficiently downward to the edge of the table. The practitioner can assist the client by asking the client to raise her buttocks (while the client is lying on the table with her heels in the stirrups) and by guiding the client's buttocks downward from a position at the client's side or from a position at the foot of the table. Clients usually feel more comfortable wearing shoes and/or socks when their feet are in the stirrups, rather than supporting their weight with their bare heels against the hard, cold metal of the stirrups.

The client and the examiner assume several positions for the examination. For the abdominal examination, the client is lying supine on the examination table and the examiner is facing the client's right side. For inspection and palpation of the external genitalia and the speculum examination, the client is in the lithotomy po-

figure**21.5** Lithotomy position for the female genital examination.

sition (Figure 21.5) and the examiner is seated on a stool, facing the client's genitalia. For the bimanual examination and the rectovaginal examination, the client remains in the lithotomy position, and the examiner is standing.

The abdominal examination is discussed in Chapter 17 on assessment of the abdomen. The examination of the female genital system should be preceded by a thorough examination of the abdomen.

Always wear gloves on both hands for the genital area examination. If infection is suspected, double gloves may provide additional protection for the examiner. Also, double gloving facilitates changing of gloves between the vaginal examination and the rectovaginal examination. The top pair can be shed right before the rectovaginal examination. However in the case of infection or suspected infection, the examiner may want to double glove throughout the examination.

Technique for Examination and Normal Findings
Palpation of regional lymph nodes

The lymph nodes of the inguinal areas are best assessed in the female client at the end of the abdominal examination. Two sets of lymph nodes are assessed: superior inguinal and inferior inguinal (see Figure 20.5).

The client must be lying down for the examination of the inguinal nodes. Flex the client's leg at the knee to relax the muscles of the inguinal area. Abduct the leg slightly; you may see a shallow, hollow space in the inguinal area. Begin your palpation here, lightly at first, and then more deeply. Palpate from the anterosuperior iliac spine to the pubic tubercle. Do not confuse Poupart's ligament with enlarged lymph nodes, which will be close to the surface and fairly easy to feel. See Figure 20.13 for an illustration of lymph node palpation areas.

Inspection of the external genitalia

With the client in the lithotomy position, sit on a stool, facing the external genitalia. Ask the client to relax and spread her legs. First, observe the skin and hair distribution. Adult female hair distribution should be approximately shaped as an inverse triangle. Some abdominal hair is normal and may be hereditary. Male (diamond-shaped) hair distribution patterns in women are abnormal.

In the adolescent client, assess sexual maturity by observing breast growth and pubic hair growth. Table 21.1 outlines and illustrates sexual maturity ratings for the appearance of the female genitalia. Along with changes in pubic hair, the following occur:
1. Increase in prominence in labia majora
2. Enlargement of the labia minora

3. Increase in size of the clitoris
4. Increase in elasticity of vaginal tissue
5. Enlargement of vagina and ovaries

Skin and hair. Although the client knows she will be touched, she may startle when the fingers are placed on the genitalia at the initiation of the palpation. To enable the client to accommodate to the touching, touch her first on the inner thigh with the back of a hand before touching any part of the genitalia. Tell the client you will be placing your hand against her thigh. Then place it gently, but firmly there. This helps relax the client and enables the examiner to assess the degree of relaxation.

Inspect the total skin area for lesions and parasites. Use the gloved fingers of one hand to spread the hair and labia so that all skin surfaces can be adequately visualized. The skin should be the same color as the remainder of the body or slightly darker. The hair is normally coarse in texture and somewhat curly to very curly. Sebaceous cysts are often seen on the labia.

Labia. The labia are flat in childhood, plump during adulthood, and atrophic in old age. Estrogen influences fat deposition, which causes a round, full appearance of the labia. The labia majora of the nulliparous client will be in close approximation, covering the labia minora and the vestibule area. After a vaginal delivery, the labia may appear slightly shriveled and gaping. Regardless of general appearance, the labia should appear reasonably symmetrical. The mucous membranes are normally dark pink in color and moist in appearance. The skin of the vulvar area is a slightly darker pigment than the skin of the rest of the body.

Clitoris. Examine the clitoris for size and examine the adjacent area for lesions. The visible portion of the clitoris should not exceed 2 cm in length and 1 cm in width. The area of the clitoris particularly is a common site for chancres of syphilis in the younger client and for cancerous lesions in the older client.

Urethral orifice. The urethral orifice appears slitlike, stellate, or as an inverted V and is of the same color as the membranes surrounding it. The openings of the paraurethral (Skene's) glands are not usually visible. Erythema or a polyp located in this area or a discharge from the urethra or gland ducts is abnormal.

Glandular areas. Observe the area of Bartholin's glands and their ducts for tenderness, swelling, erythema, duct enlargement, or discharge. The presence of any of these conditions is abnormal.

Perineum. Inspect the perineum for lesions and evidence of an episiotomy and its healing. Also inspect the anus at this time (see Chapter 22: Anus and Rectosigmoid Region).

Palpation of the external genitalia

Labia. Use one hand to spread the labia open while the other hand is used to palpate the labia majora and

table 21.1	*Developmental Changes in the General Appearance of Female Genitalia*		
Developmental stage	Description	Developmental stage	Description
Stage 1 sexual maturity (preadolescence)	No pubic hair, except for fine body hair	Stage 4 sexual maturity	Texture and curl of pubic hair as in adult but not as thick and not spread over thighs (usually seen between ages 13 and 14)
Stage 2 sexual maturity	Sparse growth of long, slightly pigmented, fine pubic hair, which is slightly curly and located along labia (usually seen between ages 11 and 12)	Stage 5 sexual maturity	Adult appearance in quality and quantity of pubic hair; growth is spread onto inner aspect of upper thighs
Stage 3 sexual maturity	Pubic hair becomes darker, curlier, and spreads over symphysis (usually seen between ages 12 and 13)	Elderly	Pubic hair is thin, sparse, brittle, and gray

labia minora. The labia should feel soft, and the texture should be homogeneous. Palpate any areas of observed abnormality below the skin surface to determine size, shape, consistency, movability, and tenderness.

Glands. Insert approximately half the index finger of the palpating hand into the vagina. First, gently milk the urethra and area of Skene's duct openings from about the level of 4 cm on the anterior vaginal wall down to the orifice (Figure 21.6). This procedure should not normally cause pain or discharge. If a discharge is present, a specimen is obtained with a swab and placed onto a Thayer-Martin culture plate. Then rotate the hand without removing the finger and palpate the area of Bartholin's glands and their ducts for swelling or tenderness (Figure 21.7). Palpate this area using the intra-

vaginal finger and the thumb of that same hand on the external surface. Normally, Bartholin's glands are not palpable.

Perineum and musculature of the vaginal introitus. While the finger is in the vagina, perform several maneuvers to assess the integrity of the pelvic musculature. Palpate the perineal area between the finger inside the vagina and the thumb of that same hand. In the nulliparous client, the perineum is felt as a firm, muscular body. After an episiotomy has healed, the perineum feels thinner and more rigid because of scarring. If this area is very thin and if the palpating fingers can almost approximate, the client may be experiencing bowel or sexual problems.

Ask the client to constrict her vaginal orifice around

figure **21.6** Palpation of Skene's glands.

figure **21.7** Palpation of Bartholin's glands.

the examiner's finger while placed in the vagina. A nulliparous client will demonstrate a high degree of tone; a multiparous client, less tone.

Presence of cystocele, rectocele, enterocele, and uterine prolapse. Place the index and middle fingers in the vagina, spread them laterally, and ask the client to push down against them. The presence of urinary stress incontinence, cystocele, rectocele, enterocele, or uterine prolapse can be observed if present. Cystocele is the prolapse into the vagina of the anterior vaginal wall and the bladder. Clinically, a pouching would be seen on the anterior wall as the client strains. Rectocele is the prolapse into the vagina of the posterior vaginal wall and the rectum. Clinically, a pouching would be seen on the posterior wall as the client strains. Enterocele is a hernia of the pouch of Douglas into the vagina. Clinically, a bulge would be seen emerging from the posterior fornix. If this is observed, the client should be additionally examined by assessing the effect of straining (1) during the speculum examination with the inserted speculum, half-opened, three fourths of its length into the vagina; and (2) during the bimanual examination with the intravaginal fingers in the posterior fornix.

There are three degrees of uterine prolapse. In first-degree prolapse, the cervix appears at the introitus when the client strains. In second-degree prolapse, the cervix is outside the introitus when the client strains. In third-degree prolapse, the whole uterus is outside the introitus, and the vagina is essentially turned inside out when the client strains.

Inspection of the internal genitalia— speculum examination

You will have obtained clues regarding the most appropriate type and size of speculum to use in the specu-

Tips for the Pelvic Examination

Elevation of the head of the examination table: Elevating the head of the examination table to about 30 degrees from the horizontal (1) allows eye contact and facilitates communication between the examiner and the client, (2) allows the practitioner to observe the client for responses to the examination, and (3) relaxes the abdominal muscles.

Examination lamp: The lamp is best positioned in front of the examiner's chest, a few inches below the chin, level with the perineum, but about 30 inches from it. This placement allows for maximum visibility for the examiner.

Pacing: Speed is important, but it is important not to be abrupt or too fast to obtain the needed information.

Speculum: Once inserted and locked into position, the speculum will generally stay in place without being held.

Failure to find the cervix on insertion of the speculum: This problem is usually caused by the speculum not being inserted far enough.

Bimanual examination: Pelvic structures are caught and palpated between the abdominal and vaginal examining hands. With the abdominal hand, apply pressure with the flat of the fingers.

lum examination through the history and inspection of the external genitalia. The two basic types of speculum shapes are the Graves speculum and the Pederson speculum (Figure 21.8). The Graves speculum is one of the most commonly used in examination of the adult female client. It is available in lengths varying from 3½ to 5 inches and in widths from ¾ to 1½ inches. The Pederson speculum is both narrower and flatter than the Graves speculum and is used with virgins, nulliparous clients, or clients whose vaginal orifices have contracted postmenopausally.

Warm metal speculums before insertion. An effective way to do this is to run warm water over it. The warm water also assists in lubricating both the metal and plastic speculums and should be used as the method of lubrication if cultures and smears are to be taken. Gel lubricant is bacteriostatic and also distorts cells on Pap smears. Therefore do not use lubricant if cultures or smears are to be obtained.

Use the following procedure for speculum insertion:

1. Place the index finger and middle finger of one hand about 2 cm into the vagina.

2. Spread the fingers and exert pressure toward the posterior vaginal wall. Advise the client that she will feel intravaginal pressure and ask her to relax the muscles you are pushing against.

3. Hold the speculum in the opposite hand with the blades between the index and middle fingers.

4. Ask the client to bear down. This maneuver helps to open the vaginal orifice and relax perineal muscles.

5. Insert the speculum blades obliquely along the top of the intravaginal fingers, taking advantage of the H configuration of the relaxed vagina (Figure 21.9, *A*).

6. Continue to insert the speculum at a plane parallel to the examining table until the end of the speculum has reached the tips of the fingers in the vagina. Then withdraw the intravaginal fingers (Figure 21.9, *B*).

7. Rotate the speculum to a transverse position, and alter the plane in adaptation to the plane of the vagina, approximately one of a 45-degree angle with the examining table (Figure 21.9, *C*). Insert

figure **21.8** Vaginal specula. From left to right: **A,** Short-billed pediatric, pediatric, small Pederson, Pederson, small Graves, large Graves, plastic Graves. **B,** Short-billed pediatric, pediatric, small Pederson, Pederson, small Graves, large Graves. *(From Seidel HM et al: Mosby's guide to physical examination, ed 3, St Louis, 1995, Mosby.)*

the speculum until it touches the end of the vagina.

8. Depress the lever of the speculum; this opens the blades and allows visualization. Ideally, the cervix is seen between the blades (Figure 21.9, *D*). Sometimes, however, especially for the beginning examiner, it is not. In such cases the speculum is either anterior (usually the situation) or posterior to the cervix. If this occurs, withdraw the speculum halfway and redirect it into a different plane. Be careful not to pinch the patient, because the blades can catch tissue between them as they are being closed and rotated.

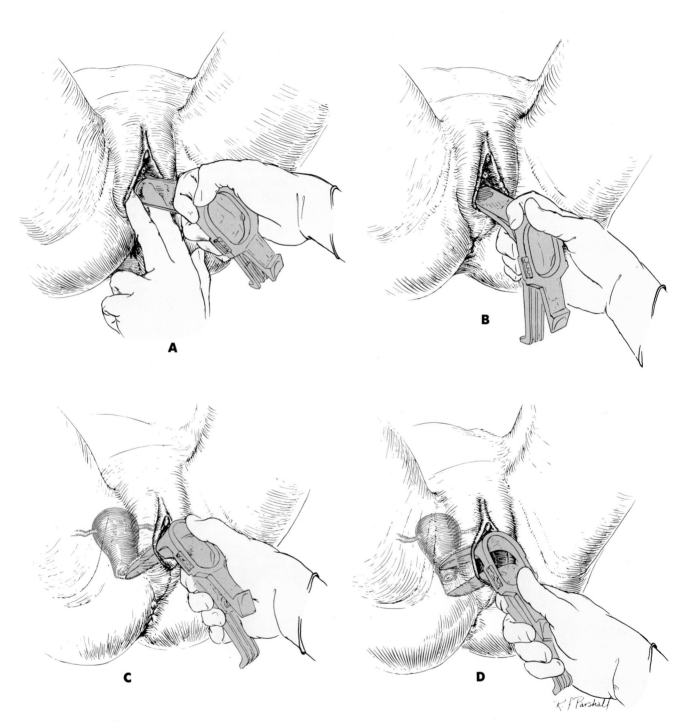

figure **21.9** Procedure for vaginal examination. **A,** Opening of the introitus. **B,** Oblique insertion of the speculum. **C,** Final insertion of the speculum. **D,** Opening of the speculum blades.

9. After the entire cervix is in view, fix the depressed lever in an open position.

If the client is tense and is resisting insertion of the speculum, do not withdraw the speculum but stop the insertion, leaving the speculum in its position. Remind the client to use relaxation techniques, and continue the examination when relaxation has occurred.

Cervix. Observe the cervix for color, position, size, projection into the vaginal vault, shape, general symmetry, surface characteristics, shape and patency of the os, and discharge:

Color. The normal color of the cervix is pink. The cervix is normally pale after menopause and cyanotic in pregnancy. Cyanosis can occur with any condition that causes systemic hypoxia or regional venous congestion. Hyperemia may indicate inflammation. An additional cause of pallor is anemia.

Position. The position of the cervix is related to the position of the uterus. The cervix is usually midline and extends approximately 2 cm into the vagina. A cervix projecting more deeply than 3 cm into the vaginal vault may indicate uterine prolapse. A cervix situated on a lateral vaginal wall may indicate tumor or adhesion of a superior structure.

Size. The cervix of women of childbearing age is usually 2 to 3 cm in diameter. A cervix larger than 4 cm in diameter is hypertrophied, and the presence of inflammation or tumor should be considered.

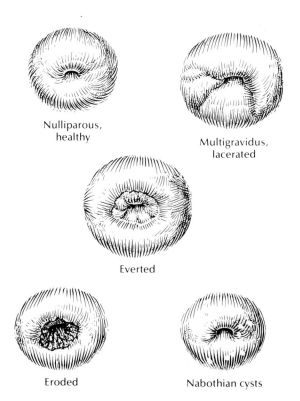

Nulliparous, healthy

Multigravidus, lacerated

Everted

Eroded

Nabothian cysts

figure**21.10** Common appearances and lesions of the cervix.

Surface characteristics. The cervix should look smooth and firm. Lesions and polyps are commonly seen on the cervix and require more than visual assessment to determine if a pathological condition exists. Any irregularity or nodularity of the cervical surface should be considered possibly abnormal (Figure 21.10). One relatively benign condition is the presence of nabothian cysts, which appear as smooth, round, small (less than 1 cm in diameter), yellow or grayish white lesions. Nabothian cysts are caused by obstruction of the cervical gland ducts.

When the squamocolumnar junction is on the ectocervix, the columnar epithelium will appear as a red, relatively symmetrical circle around the os. This condition is called eversion or ectropion. It may be a normal variation of the placement of the squamocolumnar junction, or it may be caused by the separation by speculum blades of a cervix whose external os has been altered and enlarged by childbirth. Erosions appear similar to eversions but are usually irregular, rough, and friable. Erosions frequently indicate pathological conditions and require further assessment and treatment. Because of the occasional presence of the squamocolumnar junction on the ectocervix and its visual similarity to erosions and other lesions, the differential assessment of a normal cervix from an abnormal cervix using inspection alone is impossible.

Diffuse punctuate hemorrhages, colloquially referred to as "strawberry spots," are occasionally observed in association with trichomonal infections.

Discharge. The character of the normal cervical mucus varies in the menstrual cycle. Normal discharge is always odorless and nonirritating. Its color and consistency may vary from clear to white and from thin to thick and stringy. Colored, malodorous, or purulent discharges exuding from the os or present in the area of the cervix are probably abnormal.

Shape of the os. The cervical os of the nulliparous client is small and evenly round. The cervical os of a parous client who has had a vaginal delivery shows the effects of the stretching and laceration of childbirth and is irregular in shape.

Many clients have not seen their cervices. The client should be asked if she wishes to see her cervix. This visualization can easily be accomplished through the use of a hand mirror.

After inspecting the cervix, obtain the Pap smear, culture for gonorrhea, and hanging drop specimen if indicated. The procedures for these are described at the end of this chapter.

Vagina. Next, inspect the vagina. This step is done during speculum insertion, while the speculum is open, and during its removal. Note the color and condition of the vaginal mucosa and the color, odor, consistency, and appearance of vaginal secretions. Pallor, cyanosis, and

hyperemia may be present for the same reasons as described for the cervix. Leukoplakia may also occur on vaginal mucosa.

As with cervical discharge, vaginal discharge is normally odorless, nonirritating, thin or mucoid, and clear or cloudy. Also, the presence of some whitish, creamy material (leukorrhea) is normal. Describe any other vaginal discharge according to its color, odor, consistency, amount, and appearance.

After the inspection of the vagina, slowly withdraw the speculum. As it is withdrawn, loosen the nut, or catch, and control the lever again with the thumb.

About Speculums

A vaginal speculum consists of two blades, a handle, and some mechanism to open the distal end of the blades. There are two basic types: reusable metal and disposable plastic.

Metal and plastic speculums operate somewhat differently, although both have (1) levers that, when depressed, open the distal ends of the blades; (2) mechanisms that allow for separation of the proximal ends of the blades; and (3) locking mechanisms. Metal speculums have two positioning devices: depression of the level opens the distal end of the blades, and fixing the screw on the lever locks the blades open at that point. In addition, the opening at the proximal end (and consequently the distal end) of the blades can be widened and locked wide by loosening and then lifting a plate attached to both the handle of the speculum and the upper blade.

The distal and proximal blade-opening mechanisms are connected in the plastic speculum. As the plastic lever is depressed in the plastic speculum, the distal end of the blades open. If the lever is fully depressed and then pushed upward on the handle, the proximal ends of the blades also widen. The lever fixes automatically into grooves on the handle of the speculum. The clicking sound of the plastic speculum is loud, sharp, and sometimes perceived as alarming to some clients, who think the speculum is breaking inside of them. Anticipatory warning about the sound of the plastic mechanism is advised. Plastic speculums also tend to get locked into position and are sometimes hard to release.

Because each type of speculum operates somewhat differently, the beginning examiner should practice with the mechanisms apart from examination and before use with clients.

Slowly close the blades as they are withdrawn, and carefully rotate the speculum so that all areas of vaginal tissue are inspected. As the blades are closed, be careful to prevent pinching of tissue or the catching of hairs between the blades.

Inspect the speculum for odors and either discard it (plastic) or place it in a soaking solution (metal). See box below, left, for more information about speculums.

Palpation of the internal genitalia—bimanual vaginal examination

The purpose of the bimanual examination is the palpation of the pelvic contents between the examiner's two hands (Figures 21.11 and 21.12): one in the vagina and the other on the lower abdomen. Examiners vary in their preference of the placement of the dominant, more sensitive hand. The beginning examiner should attempt alternating hands for examinations and then decide on a routine that is most workable individually.

The client remains in the lithotomy position. Stand between the client's legs. The vaginal examining hand assumes the obstetric position: index and middle fingers extended and together, thumb abducted, and fourth and little fingers folded on the palm of the hand. Lubricate the vaginal examining fingers. Spread the labia with the thumb and index finger of the opposite hand. Insert the lubricated fingers into the vagina with the palmar surface of the hand directed toward the anterior vaginal wall. Always palpate with the palmar surface of the fingers rather than with the less sensitive tips or backs. In the case of a young or old client with a small and narrow vagina, the examination may be performed with one intravaginal finger.

figure**21.11** Bimanual palpation of the uterus.

The other hand is placed on the abdomen and used to press the abdominal and pelvic contents toward the intravaginal hand. If the glove on this hand has been soiled by excessive discharge during the external genital inspection or speculum insertion, the glove on this hand should be changed.

Movement of both the intravaginal and abdominal hands should be slow and firm. To palpate adequately, the client must be relaxed. If the client becomes tense, stop the procedure and help the client relax; however, leave the examining hands in position.

Locate the cervix and assess it for size, contour, surface characteristics, consistency, position, patency of the os, and mobility. Use the palmar surfaces of both fingers to completely palpate the cervix and fornices. Gently place a fingertip into the external os to assess its patency. Determine on which vaginal wall the cervix is placed and if the cervix is approximately midline. Place the fingers in the lateral fornices, and move (wag) the cervix back and forth between the fingers for 1 to 2 cm in each direction to assess for CMT (cervical motion tenderness). The cervix and uterus should be freely movable and should move without tenderness. An immobile or tender cervix and uterus are abnormal.

The surface of the cervix normally feels smooth. Nabothian cysts, tumors, or lesions will make it feel nodular or irregular. The consistency of the cervix is firm and slightly resilient and feels analogous to the tip of the nose. The cervix softens in pregnancy and hardens with tumors. The cervix is normally located on the anterior wall in the midline or on the posterior wall. A laterally displaced cervix may indicate tumor or adhesion. The external os in the nonpregnant client should

admit a finger for about 0.5 cm. It should be open and firm. A stenosed external os is abnormal.

Assess the size, shape, surface characteristics, consistency, position, mobility, and tenderness of the uterine body and fundus. First, determine the position of the uterus because techniques used to assess the uterine body and fundus will vary with the uterine position in the client (Table 21.2). The uterus is in one of the three basic positions: anteversion, midposition, or retroversion. Version in this context indicates deflection, specifically the relationship of the long axis of the uterus to the long axis of the body. If the axis of the uterus is deflected anteriorly, the uterus is said to be anteverted; if the uterus is deflected posteriorly, the uterus is said to be retroverted; and if the long axis of the uterus is roughly parallel to that of the total body, the uterus is in midposition. When the long axis of the uterus is not straight but is bent on itself, the uterus is said to be flexed. Thus the anteverted or retroverted uterus can be flexed, or bent on itself, to produce two additional variations of position: anteflexion and retroflexion.

The position of the cervix provides clues of the uterine position. A cervix on the anterior wall may indicate an antepositioned or retroflexed uterus; a centrally located cervix probably indicates a uterus in midposition; and a cervix on the posterior vaginal wall suggests a retroverted uterus.

Because approximately 85% of uteri are in anteposition (i.e., anteverted or anteflexed), first attempt palpation of the uterus anteriorly. Place the intravaginal fingers in the anterior fornix. Place the hand on the abdomen flat on the midline and in a position approximately halfway between the symphysis pubis and the umbilicus. This hand acts as a resistance against which the intravaginal fingers palpate the pelvic organs. In thin women, the uterus is also palpated with the abdominal hand. With the fingers in the anterior fornix, gently lift the tissues against the hand on the abdomen. If the uterus is in anteposition, it will be palpated between the hands. If the uterus is not palpated anteriorly, place the fingers in the posterior fornix and again raise them forward toward the hand on the abdomen. If the uterus is in retroversion, only the isthmus will be felt between the hands, and the corpus may be felt with the backs of the intravaginal fingers.

Palpation of the body and fundus of the retroverted uterus is more difficult than palpation of the antepositioned uterus. In some cases the vaginal fingers can rotate the uterine fundus forward or upright by a combination of pressure in the posterior and lateral fornices combined with trapping of the fundus by the abdominal hand. If this cannot be done, palpate as much of the uterine surface as possible, and attempt a more thorough examination of the fundus during the rectovaginal examination.

figure**21.12** Bimanual palpation of the adnexa.

table 21.2   *Findings in Bimanual Vaginal and Rectovaginal Examination*

| | Bimanual | |
Position of uterus	Position of the cervix	Body and fundus
Anteverted	Anterior vaginal wall	Palpable by one hand on abdomen and fingers of other hand in vagina
Midposition	Apex of vagina	May not be palpable
Retroverted	Posterior vaginal wall	May not be palpable

Anterior and posterior portion of uterus	Rectovaginal	
	Cervix	Body and fundus
Palpable as uterus is rotated even more anteriorly	Palpable through rectovaginal septum	May not be palpable by fingers in rectum
May not be palpable	Posterior portion felt through rectovaginal septum	May not be palpable
Posterior portion may be palpable by fingers in posterior fornix	May not be palpable by fingers in rectum	Body easily palpable by fingers in rectum; fundus may not be palpable

continued

table 21.2   *Findings in Bimanual Vaginal and Rectovaginal Examination—cont'd*

Position of uterus	Bimanual	
	Position of the cervix	Body and fundus
Anteflexed	Anterior vaginal wall or apex	Easily palpable; angulation of isthmus may be felt in anterior fornix
Retroflexed	Anterior or posterior vaginal wall or apex	May not be palpable

Palpate the anterior, lateral, and posterior surfaces of the uterus by maneuvering its position and by "walking up" its surface with the intravaginal fingers.

After palpating the uterus, examine the adnexal areas. The adnexal areas are those structures and spaces surrounding the uterus, including the fallopian tubes and ovaries. The structures in these areas are of a size, consistency, and position that they may not be specifically palpated. If you have appropriately examined the area and no masses larger than the normal-size ovaries are identified, assume that no masses are present.

Palpate each of the adnexal areas, left and right. Place the index and middle finger of the intravaginal hand in one of the lateral fornices; place the hand on the ab-

domen on the ipsilateral iliac crest; and bring the hands together, moving in an inferior and medial direction, allowing the tissues lying between the two hands to slip between them (see Figure 21.12). The hand on the abdomen acts as resistance, and the intravaginal hand palpates the organs between the hands.

In premenopausal adult women, the ovaries are felt about half of the time. If normal ovaries are palpated, they are smooth, firm, slightly flattened, ovoid, and no larger than 4 to 6 cm in their largest dimension. Ovaries of prepubertal girls or postmenopausal women are normally smaller than 4 cm in their largest dimension. The ovaries are sensitive to touch but are not tender. They are highly movable and will easily slip between the pal-

Anterior and posterior portion of uterus	Rectovaginal	
	Cervix	Body and fundus
Easily palpable	Same as anteverted	Same as anteverted

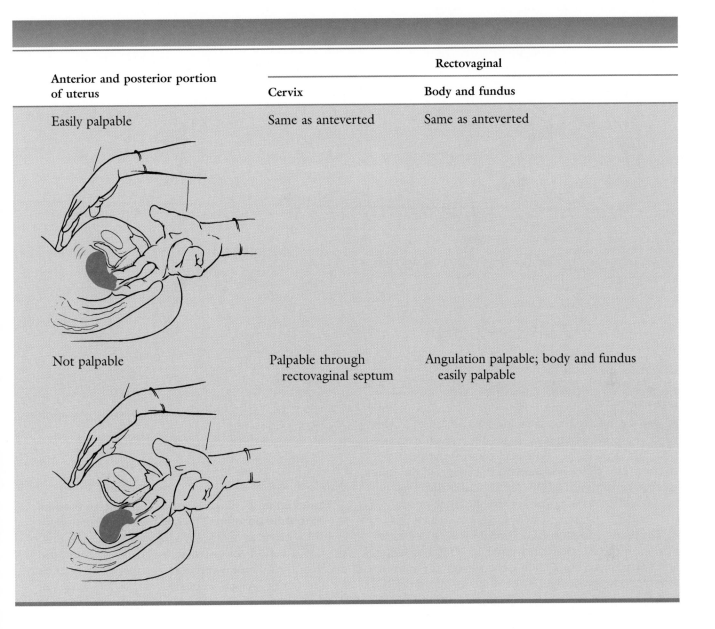

Not palpable	Palpable through rectovaginal septum	Angulation palpable; body and fundus easily palpable

pating hands. Normal fallopian tubes are not palpable. One clue to an ectopic pregnancy is the presence of arterial pulses in the adnexal areas.

Cordlike structures that are sometimes palpable are round ligaments.

Rectovaginal examination

The rectovaginal examination is uncomfortable for most women. However, because it enables examination not possible through the vaginal examination alone, it is recommended in all complete pelvic examinations. The rectovaginal examination allows for greater depth (approximately 2 cm higher) than the vaginal examination alone and enables assessment of the posterior portion of the uterus and pelvic cavity. Because the examination is uncomfortable, prepare the client for it by instruction regarding its purpose and anticipatory guidance about the possible feeling of urgency for bowel movement.

After completing the vaginal examination, withdraw the intravaginal hand, change the glove on the internal examining hand to prevent the possible transfer of infection from the vagina into the rectum, and lubricate the index and middle fingers. Advise the client that the next procedure is the last part of the pelvic examination and remind her to cooperate by relaxing the muscles. Next, ask the client to bear down. Then, place the index finger into the vagina in the posterior fornix of the cervix, and place the middle finger into the rectum. (See

figure**21.13** Rectovaginal palpation.

figure**21.14** Left lateral position for genital examination.

Chapter 22 for detailed explanation of the method for inserting the examining finger into the rectum.) Both fingers are inserted as far as possible. Place the other hand above the symphysis, as for the vaginal examination, and depress the abdominal hand. Bring the pelvic contents into closer proximity to the fingers in the vagina and the rectum. During this maneuver the rectal finger should be able to palpate the posterior portion of the uterus.

The uterine position is confirmed by the rectal examination. If the uterus is retroverted, its body and fundus are now palpated. In addition, the adnexal areas are reassessed. The procedure is the same as that described with the vaginal examination (Figure 21.13).

Palpate the areas of the rectovaginal septum and cul-de-sac. The rectovaginal septum should be palpated as a firm, thin, smooth, pliable structure. The posterior cul-de-sac is a potential space. The normal pelvic organs are palpated through it. Often, abnormal masses and normal ovaries are discovered in the cul-de-sac. Uterosacral ligaments may be palpable.

Complete the rectal examination (see Chapter 22), and help the client sit up when the examination is completed.

Because of the amount of lubricant used in the examination, the client will feel somewhat sticky. Provide her with disposable materials to clean herself and allow her to dress partially or completely (if the physical examination is completed). Often the pelvic and rectal examinations are the very last portions of the physical assessment, and complete dressing occurs before consultation about findings.

Special maneuvers

Examination of clients who are unable to assume the lithotomy position. The lithotomy position is optimal for a pelvic examination. However, it may be difficult for a very ill or debilitated client to assume and maintain the lithotomy position. An alternative position for the female genital examination is a left lateral or Sims' position (Figure 21.14). The client's buttocks should be as close to the edge of the examining table as safety allows. Position the right leg on top of or over the left leg and bend and abduct it. Stand behind the client. All the examination procedures described previously in this chapter can be performed with the client in this position.

Screening Tests and Procedures

The following recommendations are from the U.S. Preventive Services Task Force (1996).

Cervical cancer. Regular Pap tests are recommended for all women who are or have been sexually active. Testing should begin at the age when the woman initiates intercourse or around age 18 for women who are not sexually active. Pap tests are performed at an interval of 1 to 3 years, depending on the presence of risk factors, history, and clinical findings. Pap smears can be discontinued at age 65 *if the previous pattern of Pap*

RISK FACTORS	ABNORMAL PAP

Early onset of sexual activity (before age 18)
Multiple sexual partners
Sexual partner with multiple sex partners (>3)
Smoking
History of illicit drug use
History of genital condylomata
Sexual partner with genital condylomata
History of sexually transmitted diseases
History of abnormal Pap smears
Diethylstilbesterol (DES) exposure in utero

smear findings has been normal and no risk factors are present.

Chlamydial infection. Routine testing for *Chlamydia trachomatis* is recommended for the following groups of clients:

1. Asymptomatic persons who attend clinics for sexually transmitted diseases
2. Persons having specific risk factors for chlamydial infection: less than 20 years of age, multiple sexual partners, or sexual partner with multiple sexual contacts
3. Recent sexual partners of persons with positive cultures
4. Pregnant women in the high-risk group at the first prenatal visit and at later visits if the risk for infection is high

Gonorrhea. Routine cultures for gonorrhea are recommended for the following groups:

1. Asymptomatic persons in high-risk groups: prostitutes, persons with multiple sexual partners
2. Persons who have had sexual contact with a person diagnosed with gonorrhea
3. Persons with a history of repeated episodes of gonorrhea
4. Pregnant women at the first prenatal visit and at a later visit if the risk for infection is high

Cervical Papanicolaou smear

The Pap smear is taken to detect neoplastic cells in cervical and vaginal secretions. Normal and abnormal cervical and endometrial cells are shed onto the cervix and into the vagina and intermix with the normal secretions. The Pap smear is very accurate (95%) in detecting cervical cancer but only moderately effective in detecting endometrial cancer.

The client is in the lithotomy position, and the speculum has been inserted (only warm water should be used to lubricate the speculum). All materials listed ear-

figure**21.15** Endocervical specimen.

lier in the chapter are assembled. (Be sure the slides are clearly labeled with the client's identifying information.)

If a cervical mucus plug is present, remove it with a cotton ball held with forceps. There are many variations among laboratories regarding the areas from which cell samples are to be obtained, the mixing of cells from two or more areas, and the fixing of cells. One procedure is described here. However, variations are acceptable, and the practitioner should consult with the cytopathologist reading the smears for locally recommended procedures. The following paragraphs describe methods for obtaining samples from the endocervix, the cervix, and the vaginal pool.

Endocervical specimen. Figure 21.15 illustrates a procedure for obtaining a sample of cells from the endocervix:

1. Insert a sterile cotton-tipped applicator, moistened with normal saline, approximately 0.5 cm into the cervical os. Rotate it 360 degrees and leave it in 10 to 20 seconds to ensure saturation. The moistening with normal saline prevents the absorption of cells into the applicator and the shedding of cotton filaments onto the specimen collection slide.
2. Spread the endocervical smear on a slide labeled "endocervix." Rotate the swab so that all sampled areas are smeared on the slide. Avoid smearing thick areas on the slide, since the cells would be difficult to visualize microscopically. Fix the slide immediately by spraying it with a fixative or immersing it in a fixative solution.

An alternate procedure for obtaining an endocervical specimen is with a cytobrush. The brush is used in the same way the cotton swab is used, but it does not need to be moistened with saline. The procedure is:

1. Insert the brush into the cervical os until only the bristles closest to the handle are seen, and then rotate the brush 360 degrees in one direction (clockwise or counterclockwise).
2. Immediately rotate the entire surface of the brush onto a slide in the direction opposite to the one used to collect the specimen.
3. Avoid leaving a thick area of the specimen on the slide.
4. Fix the slide immediately by spraying it with a fixative or immersing it in a fixative solution.

Cervical specimen. Figure 21.16 illustrates the procedure for a cervical specimen:

1. Insert the larger humped end of the Ayre spatula into the cervical os so that the cervix fits comfortably into the groove created by the two humps. With moderate pressure, rotate the spatula 360 degrees, scraping the entire cervical surface and the squamocolumnar junction.
2. Spread the material from both sides of the spatula on a slide marked "cervix."
3. Fix the slide immediately by spraying it.

Vaginal pool smear

1. With the paddle or handle end of the Ayre spatula, scrape the area of the posterior cervical fornix.
2. Spread the material on the spatula in the area marked "vaginal pool."

figure**21.16** Cervical specimen taken using an Ayre spatula.

3. Fix the slide immediately by spraying it or immersing it in a fixative solution.

See box below for more information about Pap smears.

Gonorrheal culture

Cultures for gonorrheal infection are performed on men and women at risk for the infection. In addition, all pregnant women should be screened for gonorrhea because of possible fetal complications. Cervical cultures are done for women, urethral cultures for men, and rectal and throat cultures for persons engaged in rectal or

---

About Pap Smears

CLIENT PREPARATION

Advise the client to avoid douching, use of vaginal medications or other topical inserts, or tub baths for 48 hours before the procedure.

Defer if menstrual flow or infection.

Do not use lubricating jelly on the speculum.

Advise the client to avoid vaginal intercourse for 24 hours before the procedure.

Advise the client that a mild pinching may be momentarily felt as the endocervical sample and scrapings are taken.

Advise the client that a small amount of spotting may be noticed after the procedure.

FINDINGS

A report that indicates the presence of endocervical cells along with squamous cells or squamous metaplasia indicates an adequate sample.

Results are reported as labels, classes, or, in cervical intraepithelial neoplasia (CIN), levels:

Class 1, or normal: No abnormal cells are present.

Class 2, or atypia: Atypical cells are present, but there is no evidence of malignancy.

Class 3, or low-grade squamous intraepithelial lesion (SIL): Mild dysplasia. Cytological findings are suggestive of, but not conclusive of, malignancy. Requires immediate follow-up.

Class 4, or high-grade SIL: Carcinoma in situ. Cytological findings are strongly suggestive of malignancy.

Class 5, or invasive carcinoma: Cytological changes are conclusive of malignancy.

IMPORTANT

Secretions must be fixed before they dry. Drying will distort the cells and make interpretation difficult.

oral sex. Bacterial cultures use a special medium, such as Thayer-Martin, specifically designed for the cultivation of gonorrhea organisms.

The female client is in the lithotomy position with a speculum inserted. The male client is in a supine position to prevent possible falling if vasovagal syncope occurs with the introduction of the specimen-collecting swab into the urethra.

Endocervical culture

1. Obtain a specimen from the endocervical canal with a sterile cotton applicator. The technique is the same as that described for the Pap smear. Leave the applicator in the os for at least 30 seconds.

2. Inoculate a special culture plate or place the specimen in a special culture container as soon as possible.

3. If a Thayer-Martin culture plate is used, have the medium at room temperature; roll the swab in a large Z pattern on the culture plate; simultaneously rotate the swab as it is creating the Z so that all swab surfaces will be inoculated (Figure 21.17). Incubate the culture plate within 15 minutes of its inoculation in a warm, anaerobic environment. Place the culture plate, medium side up, in a candle jar, light the candle, tightly secure the cover of the jar, and leave the jar in a warm area until specimens can be placed in an incubator. In some clinics the inoculation is immediately cross-streaked with a sterile wire loop. Usually, however, this step is done in the laboratory, not in the examining room.

4. If another type of culture medium is used, follow instructions for specimen collection and handling.

Anal culture. Figure 21.18 illustrates the procedure for an anal culture:

1. Insert a sterile cotton-tipped applicator into the anal canal. Rotate the applicator 360 degrees and move it from side to side. Leave it in for 10 to 30 seconds to allow for absorption of secretion and organisms. If the swab contains feces, discard it and take another specimen.

2. Inoculate the culture plate and incubate it as described previously, using a separate culture plate labeled by source of specimen.

Oropharyngeal culture

1. Obtain a specimen of secretion from the oropharynx with a sterile swab.

2. Inoculate the medium and incubate as described for endocervical specimens.

See box below for more information about gonorrheal cultures.

About Gonorrhea Cultures

CLIENT PREPARATION—FEMALES
Advise the client to avoid douching, topical vaginal inserts, or tub baths for 24 hours.
Do not use a lubricant on the speculum.
Avoid taking specimens during menses—menses alter results.

CLIENT PREPARATION—MALES
Tell the client not to void within 1 hour of specimen collection—voiding washes out the organisms.

---

figure**21.17** Inoculation of the Thayer-Martin culture.

figure**21.18** Anal specimen.

Chlamydial culture

Chlamydia trachomatis is a common sexually transmitted disease. Detection is important because the organism causes trachoma, an eye disease resulting in the most common form of preventable blindness. Obtain vaginal and urethral specimens in the same manner described for the gonorrheal culture. Special culture material is inoculated with the specimen.

Testing for pH and wet mounts

The wet mount is a very commonly used, simple microscopic procedure that assists in the assessment of vaginal infections. It is indicated when there is vaginal discharge, vaginal or vulvar pruritis, vaginal or vulvar pain, or malodorous vaginal secretions.

Various vaginal conditions are associated with the pH status of the vagina. Normally, the vaginal pH is 4. Changes in pH are noted with the following conditions: candidiasis—pH 4 to 5; bacterial vaginitis—pH 5 to 6; and trichomoniasis—pH 6 to 7.

To test for vaginal pH, touch a piece of pH-testing tape to vaginal secretions collected in the speculum blade after it is removed. Compare the color changes with the color codes on the outside of the pH tape container.

The interpretation of wet mount preparations in the context of data obtained from the history and physical assessment is presented in Table 21.3. The following is the procedure for obtaining vaginal specimens for the testing of the presence of *Trichomonas vaginalis, Can-*

HELPFUL HINT *In preparing and examining wet mounts:*

- *If both saline and potassium hydroxide (KOH) slides are prepared, view the saline specimen first to allow time for the KOH to lyse cells.*
- *Tichomonads sometimes appear most mobile on a slide without a cover slip.*
- *Observe the slides with the ×10 objective and the light low.*
- *Start observing with the objective as close to the slide as possible.*
- *Use the coarse and fine focus knobs to improve visualization.*
- *First observe for squamous cells to estimate their number.*
- *Then switch to high power (×40) and increase the light if necessary.*
- *Look for bacteria, white blood cells, clue cells, trichomonads, and evidence of* Candida. *Vaginitis may have more than one cause, so do not stop examining the slide when one organism is found.*
- *When examining the KOH slide, start with low power. If hyphae are noted, confirm the impression under high power.*

Modified from Hawkins JW, Roberto-Nichols DM, Stanley-Haney JL: *Protocols for nurse practitioners in gynecologic settings,* ed 5, New York, 1995, Tiresias Press.

---

table 21.3 *Comparisons Among Commonly Observed Vaginal Conditions*

	Normal	*Candida*	*Gardnerella*	*Trichomonas*	Atrophic changes
Symptoms	None	Pruritis, burning	Pruritis, burning	Pruritis	Vaginal and vulvar dryness
Odor	None	Yeast smell	Fishy or musty	Variable	No characteristic
Erythema	None	Present	Variable	Present	Variable
pH	3.5-4.1	4.0-5.0	5.0-6.0	6.0-7.0	Up to 7.0
Saline smear	Rare WBCs, large gram-positive rods, squamous epithelial cells	Budding filaments, spores, pseudohyphae	Clue cells	Many WBCs, trichomonads	Many WBCs, parabasal and intermediate cells, scarce superficial cells
KOH preparation		Budding filaments, spores, pseudohyphae	Fishy odor with application of KOH		

WBCs, White blood cells; *KOH,* potassium hydroxide.

dida albicans, or *Gardnerella (Haemophilus) vaginalis:*

1. Obtain a specimen of vaginal secretions directly from the vagina or from material in the inferior speculum blade. For *Trichomonas vaginalis,* mix the secretions with a drop of normal saline solution on a glass slide. For *Candida albicans,* mix the secretions with a drop of 10% potassium hydroxide (KOH) solution on a slide. For *Gardnerella vaginalis* (also called *Hemophilus vaginalis*), the secretions are mixed with a 10% potassium hydroxide solution.

2. Place a glass cover slip on the slide.

3. If *G. vaginalis* is suspected, perform a "whiff" test as the slide is being prepared with the KOH. If *G. vaginalis* is present, an unpleasant, "fishy" odor will be noted after the drop of KOH is added. Immediately observe the slide under a microscope (Figure 21.19). If the specimen is positive for *T. vaginalis,* trichomonads will be seen on the saline slide. These are single-cell flagellates somewhat larger than a white blood cell (WBC), but smaller than a vaginal squamous epithelial cell. If the specimen is positive for *C. albicans,* hyphae and spores will be seen. If the specimen is positive for *G. vaginalis,* characteristic "clue cells" will be seen.

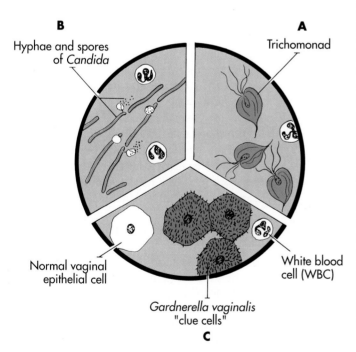

figure**21.19** Microscopic appearance of vaginal microorganisms. **A,** *Trichomonas.* **B,** Mycelia and spores. **C,** Epithelial cells stippled by *Gardnerella vaginalis.*

examination step-by-step

1. Palpate inguinal lymph nodes.
2. Inspect the external genitalia. Place your hand on the inner thigh to prepare the client for being touched.
   a. Skin color, condition, integrity
   b. Hair characteristics and distribution
   c. Labia majora: Symmetry, color, inflammation, lesions
   d. Clitoris: Size
   e. Labia minora
   f. Urethral opening: Discharge, inflammation
   g. Vaginal opening: Size, condition
   h. Perineum: Condition, inflammation, lesions
   i. Anus
3. Palpate the external genitalia.
   a. Labia
   b. Skene's glands
   c. Bartholin's glands
4. Assess support of the pelvic musculature.
   a. Palpate the perineum.
   b. Test the vaginal introitus musculature.
   c. Assess for rectocele, cystocele, enterocele, and uterine prolapse.
5. Perform the speculum examination.
   a. Insert the speculum.
   b. Inspect the cervix and os for color, position, size, surface characteristics, discharge, and shape.
   c. Obtain specimens for cervical and vaginal smears and cultures if needed.
   d. Inspect the vaginal wall for color, surface characteristics, and discharge.
6. Perform bimanual palpation.
   a. Vaginal wall: Smoothness, lesions
   b. Cervix and fornices: Size, shape, position, mobility, patency of os, surface characteristics, tenderness
   c. Uterus: Location, size, position, shape, mobility, tenderness
   d. Ovaries: Size, shape, consistency, tenderness
   e. Adnexal areas: Masses, tenderness
   f. Cul-de-sac: Masses, tenderness
7. Perform rectovaginal palpation.
   a. Anus
   b. Rectovaginal septum: Thickness, tone, nodules
   c. Rectum: Masses, tone
   d. Uterus and adnexae
   e. Cul-de-sac

> ### *Examination of a Client Who Has Had a Hysterectomy*
>
> Determine to the extent possible the details of the procedure, especially the extent of the procedure.
>
> On speculum examination the cervix will be absent. An identifiable suture line will be present. Take a Pap smear at the suture line with the blunt end of the spatula. Label the Pap smear requisition form with the fact of the hysterectomy.
>
> The vaginal walls may appear as they would after menopause without replacement therapy—decrease in rugae and secretions.
>
> In bimanual palpation, the uterus will obviously not be present, but the adnexal areas should be palpated as in the usual examination.

■ VARIATIONS FROM HEALTH

Skin and Labia

Common abnormalities of the skin and labia include parasites, skin lesions of all types, areas of leukoplakia, varicosities, hyperpigmentation, erythema, depigmentation, and swelling.

Parasites: Excoriations and erythematous areas are noted on the skin. Lice appear as dark spots on the skin, and their eggs (nits) are adherent to the pubic hair near the roots.

Skin lesions: Commonly seen skin lesions are those of herpes progenitalis, appearing as small, shallow vesicles with surrounding erythema; and condylomata acuminata, which appear in single or multiple cauliflower-like patches.

Leukoplakia: This appears as white, adherent patches on the skin; it may be likened to spots of dried white paint.

Vaginal Discharges

Vaginal discharges may result from various conditions of the uterus, cervix, and vagina. Causes include fungal, protozoal, viral, bacterial, spirochetal, and parasitic infections; benign and malignant neoplasms; chemical irritations; foreign bodies; fistulas; or poor hygiene. Full discussion of the various causes of discharges is beyond the scope of this text. However, clinical signs and symptoms accompanying common vaginal infections producing discharges are described (see Table 21.3) as follows:

Candida albicans: Candida albicans is a fungus that causes approximately 20% of vaginal infections. Common symptoms are vulvovaginal itching; vulvar redness and swelling; and thick, white, curdy (similar to cottage cheese) discharge. On examination the vulva and the vagina are frequently erythematous and edematous; curdy white discharge may be present in labial folds and in the vagina; and the vagina and cervix may appear edematous and covered with adherent, thrushlike patches.

Trichomonas vaginalis: This infection is caused by trichomonads, parasitic protozoans having motile flagella. Clients complain of watery, bubbly, profuse, yellowish green, malodorous discharge, which is generally most severe immediately after menses. On physical examination, the vulva may appear erythematous, and a yellow-green, foul-smelling discharge is present at the introitus and in the vagina. In addition, the vagina may be erythematous, and the vagina may have red, raised papules and petechiae.

Gardnerella vaginalis: This is a bacterial vaginosis that is thought to account for 50% to 60% of vaginal infections. Clients complain of increased, watery, gray, malodorous vaginal discharge. Findings characteristic of the physical examination include little to no vulvar edema, and a thin, creamy, gray-white, malodorous discharge covering the vagina and cervix.

■ TEACHING SELF-ASSESSMENT

The teaching of genital self-examination may be indicated for clients in the following situations:

1. Clients using barrier or intrauterine contraceptive devices. The clients need to check the placement of devices.
2. Clients who have recurring vaginal infections.
3. Clients at risk for sexually transmitted diseases.

The teaching session is initiated with a thorough presentation of the anatomy of the female genitalia and the normal appearance and feel of organs, structures, and discharge.

The following steps are recommended in teaching self-examination:

1. Find a comfortable position that will allow for viewing of the external genitalia with a mirror. A source of light from a nearby lamp is often necessary.
2. Inspect the condition of the hair and skin over the genitalia. Spread the hairs and inspect all the surfaces of the labia. Look for bumps, sores, warts, and blisters.
3. Spread the labia and look at the clitoris for bumps, blisters, sores, and warts.

4. Look at the urethral opening and the area of Bartholin's glands for swelling or redness.
5. Insert a finger into the vagina, feel the consistency of normal tissue, and get used to the plane of the vagina.
6. Insert a finger deep into the vagina and locate the cervix. Feel the os and then feel the entire surface by circling it with the finger.

7. Look carefully at the type of discharge that is on the finger when it is taken out.

Some women's self-help groups teach self-examination by vaginal speculum. This is not recommended because of the difficulty of this maneuver on oneself and because professional judgment is needed for adequate assessment.

---

sample documentation & diagnoses   CRITICAL THINKING

■ FOCUSED HEALTH HISTORY *(SUBJECTIVE DATA)*

Mrs. E., a 65-year-old female, is in for her annual gynecological examination. States that she has been feeling pressure "down there" all the time for the past 2 months. Feels as if she has to urinate all the time and dribbles urine frequently when she coughs, laughs, or sneezes. Has not had intercourse with her husband for 3 months because she is concerned she will urinate. Has been wearing pads to absorb urine leakage since about 6 months ago. Wears one pad during the day and one at night—they have been about half saturated when changed. Menarche was at age 14; cycle was regular every 30 days, with moderate to heavy flow for 5 days. Last menstrual period (LMP) was 15 years ago. Gravida 3/ para 3/ no abortions. Has had gynecological examinations yearly. Last Pap was 1 year ago, class I. No history of kidney disease. Had several bladder infections during her pregnancies and in early menopause, but no bladder infections for at least 10 years. Is not on hormone replacement therapy.

■ FOCUSED PHYSICAL EXAMINATION *(OBJECTIVE DATA)*

Female hair distribution. No masses, lesions, or swelling on labia, around clitoris, or perineum. Small amount of redness around urethral orifice. No discharge. No swelling or tenderness around Bartholin's glands. Old episeotomy scar on perineum.

Very weak vaginal musculature when asked to squeeze muscles around finger positioned in vagina. Anterior vaginal wall bulges and a drop of urine escapes from urethral orifice when asked to push down.

Vaginal mucosa and cervix pale. Few secretions in vagina. No lesions noted.

No pain or tenderness with vaginal examination. Uterus anteverted, small, and firm without masses. No pain on moving cervix. Ovaries not palpated. No adnexal masses.

No lesions, tenderness, or pain noted on rectovaginal examination. No hemorrhoids or masses in anus or lower rectum.

diagnoses

HEALTH PROBLEM
Urinary tract infection

NURSING DIAGNOSES

Stress incontinence related to prolapsed bladder
Defining Characteristics
- Dribbling with increased abdominal pressure
- Urinary frequency
- Urinary urgency
- Poor vaginal musculature
- Bladder prolapse on examination

Sexual dysfunction related to altered body structure and/or function
Defining Characteristics
- Verbalization of fear of sex due to incontinence
- Embarrassed about stress incontinence

Altered sexuality patterns related to altered body structure and/or function
Defining Characteristic
- Verbalization of fear due to incontinence

chapter

22

Anus and Rectosigmoid Region

■ PURPOSE OF EXAMINATION

The purposes of the rectal examination include assessment of anorectal status, the accessible pelvic viscera, the male prostate gland and seminal vesicles, and additional assessment of the female genitalia. The methods used to carry out this examination are inspection and palpation.

The rectal examination is an important component of every comprehensive physical examination. This type of examination is also indicated whenever the client is at risk for problems of the anorectal region or complains of symptoms that may indicate a problem or dysfunction of the region.

Because of the nature of the rectal examination, it is usually done at the end of the physical examination, which allows the client to clean himself or herself and dress on completion.

■ ANATOMY AND PHYSIOLOGY

The terminal gastrointestinal tract, which is called the rectosigmoid region, includes the anus, the rectum, and the caudal portion of the sigmoid colon.

The anal canal is the final segment of the colon. It is 2.5 to 4 cm long and opens into the perineum (Figure 22.1). The anal canal slants forward in a general line toward the umbilicus and forms a right angle with the rectum. The tract is surrounded by the external and internal sphincters, which keep it closed except when flatus and feces are passed. These sphincters are arranged in concentric layers. The striated external muscular ring is under voluntary control, whereas the internal smooth-muscle sphincter is under autonomic control. The internal sphincter is innervated from the pelvic plexus. Sympathetic stimulation contracts the sphincter; parasympathetic stimulation relaxes it. The anal canal, unlike the adjacent rectum, contains numerous somatic sensory nerves. Thus sensation in the canal is very keen. The distal portion of the external sphinc-

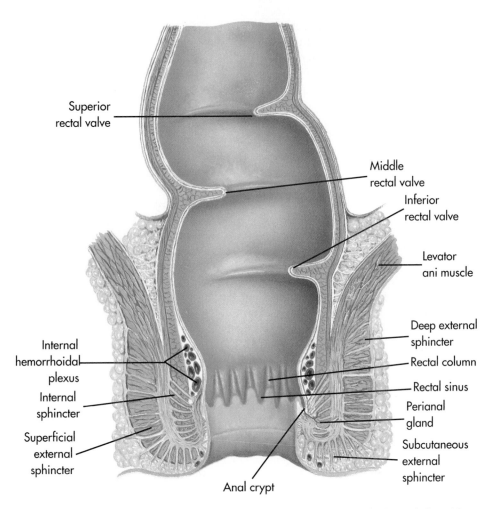

figure**22.1** Anatomy of the anus and rectum. *(From Seidel HM et al: Mosby's guide to physical examination, ed 3, St Louis, 1995, Mosby.)*

ter extends past the internal sphincter and may be palpated by the examining finger.

The stratified squamous epithelial lining of the anus is visible to inspection because it extends beyond the sphincters, where it merges with the skin. This junction is characterized by pigmentation and the presence of hair. Internally, the anal canal is lined by columns of mucosal tissue, which extend from the rectum and terminate in papillae. These anal columns, called the columns of Morgagni, fuse to form the anorectal junction, also called the pectinate, or dentate, line. The spaces between these columns are called crypts.

The anal columns are invested with cross channels of anastomosing veins, which form mucosal folds known as anal valves. These anastomosing veins form a ring termed the zona hemorrhoidalis. When dilated, these veins are called internal hemorrhoids. The lower section of the anal canal contains a venous plexus, which has only a minor connection with the zona hemorrhoidalis

and drains downward into the inferior rectal veins. Varicosed veins of this plexus are known as external hemorrhoids. Thus internal hemorrhoids occur superior to the pectinate line and are characterized by the moist, red epithelium of the rectum. External hemorrhoids are located inferior to the pectinate line and have the squamous epithelium of the anal canal or skin as their surface tissue.

The rectum is the portion of the gastrointestinal tract that is superior to the anal canal. Approximately 12 cm long, the rectum is lined with columnar epithelium. Superiorly, the rectum has its origin at the third sacral vertebra and is continuous with the sigmoid colon. Its distal end dilates to form the rectal ampulla, which contains flatus and feces. Four semilunar transverse folds, the valves of Houston, extend across half the circumference of the rectal lumen. The purpose of these valves is not clear. They may serve to support feces while allowing flatus to pass.

The sigmoid colon has its origin at the iliac flexure of the descending colon and terminates in the rectum. Approximately 40 cm long, it is accessible to examination with the sigmoidoscope. Flexible fiberoptic instruments have made possible inspection of the mucosal surfaces of the entire sigmoid colon and of the other portions of the colon.

■ EXAMINATION

Health History

In practice, the history of the anus and rectum is integrated into that of the gastrointestinal system. The regional history outlined here focuses on the distal portion of the gastrointestinal system. Throughout the health history interview, the following data are recorded about a symptom or problem: (1) onset (specific date, sudden or gradual), (2) duration, (3) frequency, (4) precipitating factors, (5) aggravating or alleviating factors, (6) treatment received or self-care given, and (7) outcome. A regional history of the entire abdominal area is required for an adequate history of the anus and rectum. (See Chapter 17 for a discussion of history taking of the abdominal area.)

Present health status

1. Diet
   a. Focus on fiber content and fluids
   b. Presence of lactose intolerance
2. Bowel habits
   a. Frequency
   b. Color
   c. Consistency
   d. Patterns of diarrhea and constipation
   e. Use of laxatives and enemas
3. Rest and activity patterns
4. Medications: Focus should be on medications intended to treat bowel problems and on those with intestinal tract side effects
5. Sexual practices involving anus and rectum

Present illness*

1. Bowel movement pattern changes
   a. Nature of change
   b. Type of stool: Color, consistency, presence of matter other than feces, odor
   c. Frequency of bowel movements
   d. Onset: Association with diet, illness, changes in daily pattern, stress, travel, other events
   e. Accompanying symptoms: Flatus, nausea, vomiting, distention, cramping, colic

*Current signs or symptoms of problems in region or in gastrointestinal tract.

f. Corrective measures taken and results
2. Anal region discomfort or pain
   a. Description of type of discomfort or pain: Character; duration; location; amount of itching, burning, discharge
   b. Association with body position: Sitting, standing, walking, lying down
   c. Timing with defecation or straining of stool
   d. Presence of blood, mucus, or other unusual substance in or on stool
   e. Corrective measures taken and results
3. Rectal bleeding
   a. Color of blood: Bright red, dark red, or red-black
   b. Amount: Blood on tissue, spotting in toilet, or active bleeding
   c. Location: Blood on stool or in stool
   d. Relationship to defecation and changes in stool and bowel habits
   e. Associated gastrointestinal and regional symptoms
   f. Duration
4. Discharge
   a. Type and character
   b. Pattern
   c. Relationship to bowel movements
   d. Amount
   e. History of trauma
   f. Pattern
5. Anal incontinence
   a. Amount
   b. Character
   c. Pattern
   d. Coping mechanisms
   e. History of previous anal surgery, obstetric injury, anorectal trauma, radiation-induced nerve or muscle injury, neurological disorders
6. Constipation (etiological factors)
   a. Deficient diet
   b. Poor bowel habits
   c. Medications
   d. Structural abnormalities of the large bowel or anus
   e. Motility disorders
   f. Psychiatric disorders
   g. Immobility
   h. Neurological disorders or injuries
   i. Endocrine disorders

Past health history and associated medical conditions

1. Past history of problems in region
2. Surgeries in region
3. Trauma to region
4. Recent travel to countries where exposure to parasitic diseases could have occurred
5. Diabetes
6. Low-flow cardiac conditions

RISK **FACTORS**	ANORECTAL PROBLEMS

Anal sexual practices
Travel to countries where parasitic and tropical
  diseases are common
Diabetes
Cardiac conditions
Malignancies
Family history of cancer, Crohn's disease, ulcera-
  tive colitis

PREPARATION FOR EXAMINATION

EQUIPMENT

Item	*Purpose*
Water-soluble lubricant	To enable more comfortable digital insertion and exami- nation
Disposable gloves	To protect examiner's hands from feces and infection
Penlight	To observe skin of anus
Material for testing stool	To determine presence of occult blood

CLIENT AND ENVIRONMENT

1. Provide a warm, private room with adequate lighting.
2. Explain examination.
3. Teach relaxation.
4. Reassure about sensations.
5. Position comfortably.
6. Drape adequately.

7. History of pelvic irradiation
8. Medications
9. Immobility

Family health history

1. Family history of cancer in region or in gastrointesti-
   nal tract
2. Crohn's disease
3. Ulcerative colitis
4. Bleeding disorders

Preparation for Examination: Client and Environment

Most clients experience a significant amount of em-
barrassment and apprehension about the rectal examina-
tion. They may be concerned about the cleanliness of
the area, the exploration of troubling symptoms, or
pain. These fears can cause spasms of the anal sphincters
and buttocks, which make the examination unnecessari-
ly uncomfortable. The following interventions can be
used to alleviate anxiety and facilitate client cooperation
so that a thorough and comfortable examination can be
performed:

1. Teach the client relaxation techniques. Remind
   the client to continue slow, deep breathing during
   the examination.
2. Advise the client that unusual sensations may
   occur during the examination, especially the feel-
   ing that defecation is imminent; reassure the
   client that defecation is unlikely. Tell the client
   that sometimes flatus is passed during the exami-
   nation and that this should not be a cause for em-
   barrassment. Remind clients that they may feel an
   urge to void when the prostate is palpated.
3. If the client has fecal incontinence, protect the
   client and the examination area with appropriate
   padding.
4. Proceed with the examination in a sympathetic
   but confident manner.
5. Maintain gentleness in approach, avoiding undue

force and allowing time for relaxation but not
withdrawing the examining hand until the exami-
nation has been completed. However, if the client
experiences extreme pain that persists, discontinue
the examination.
6. Drape the client to avoid unnecessary exposure of
   the genitalia.

Technique for Examination and Normal Findings

Examine the client in one of the following positions,
as shown in Figure 22.2:

1. *Left lateral or Sims' position.* The client lies on the
   left side with the superior thigh and knee flexed,
   bringing the knee close to the chest. The client's
   left hip should rest on a small, firm pillow or
   sandbag placed immediately adjacent to the side
   of the examination table, allowing the buttocks to
   be elevated and to project slightly over the edge
   of the table. The client's trunk should lie oblique-
   ly across the table top so that the head rests on a
   pillow near the opposite edge. The hips should be
   flexed to an angle slightly less than 90 degrees,
   with the lower leg placed close to the opposite
   side of the table and parallel to its edge. The right
   side of the body should be displaced slightly for-
   ward. In this position the rectal ampulla is pushed
   down and posteriorly and thus is advantageously

figure**22.2** Positions for rectal examination. **A,** Left lateral or Sims' position. **B,** Knee-chest position. **C,** Standing position. **D,** Lithotomy position. (Squatting position is not shown because it is infrequently used.)

aligned for the detection of rectal masses. However, the upper rectum and the pelvic structure tend to fall away in this position. This examination position is good for bed-bound clients, for males, and for females who are not receiving a pelvic examination during this assessment.

2. *Knee-chest position.* The client kneels on the examining table with the shoulders and head in contact with the examining table. The knees are positioned more widely apart than the hips. The angle at the hip is 75 to 80 degrees. The size of the prostate gland is best assessed with the client in this position. However, this position is uncomfortable and embarrassing for many clients.

3. *Standing position.* The client stands over the examining table with the hips flexed and the trunk resting on the table. This position is commonly used for examination of the prostate gland.

4. *Lithotomy position.* This position is used with female clients for a screening rectal examination following a pelvic examination. The client is supine with knees flexed and feet elevated and supported in stirrups.

5. *Squatting position.* The client squats on a firm, flat surface with the examiner behind the client. Rectal prolapse frequently can be noted when the client is in this position, and some lesions of the rectosigmoid region and pelvis can be felt especially well in this position.

For all rectal examinations, the examiner should wear gloves on both hands throughout the entire procedure. Thorough hand washing after degloving is recommended.

Inspection

The manner in which the client sits throughout the preceding portions of the assessment provides some evidence of discomfort in the anal region. A client who continuously changes position during the examination may be having some anal discomfort.

Inspect the sacrococcygeal area for a pilonidal cyst or sinus. Normally, this area appears smooth and the overlying skin is healthy. Inspect the pilonidal area (at the tip of the coccyx) for dimples, sinus openings, or signs of inflammation. Also, palpate the pilonidal area at this time for tenderness, induration, or swelling.

The skin over a pilonidal sinus may have abundant hair growth. The accumulation of secretions within the sinus often leads to infection, which is generally accompanied by foul-smelling discharge and local tenderness.

Next, examine the skin of the entire perineal area for lesions and inflammation.

Spread the buttocks carefully with both hands to examine the anus and the tissue immediately surrounding it. This skin is more pigmented and coarser than the rest of the perianal skin and is moist and hairless. Visually assess the perianal region for any lesions. Skin tags, scars, inflammation, perirectal abscesses, fissures, sentinel piles from rectal fissures, external hemorrhoids, fistula openings, condylomata acuminata (viral warts), tumors, and rectal prolapse may be observed through this inspection.

After the initial inspection, ask the client to strain downward, as though defecating, and inspect the anus during straining. With this maneuver, it is possible to identify rectal prolapse, polyps, or internal hemorrhoids. Describe any abnormal findings in terms of clock position, with the 12 o'clock position being the apex of the anus (point closest to the symphysis pubis).

Palpation

Spread the buttocks with the nondominant hand. If the sphincter tightens, instruct the client to relax and reassure the client. Then, when the sphincter has relaxed, continue the examination. Occasionally, painful lesions or bleeding may prevent completion of the examination unless a local analgesic agent is administered.

Lubricate the pad of the gloved index finger of the hand to be used for palpation. Instruct the client to strain downward against this finger. Then gently place the lubricated index finger of the examining hand against the anal verge. Exert firm pressure until the rectal sphincter begins to yield; then slowly insert the finger into the anal canal in the direction of the umbilicus as the sphincter relaxes (Figure 22.3). Ask the client to tighten the sphincter around the examining finger to provide a measurement of muscle strength of the anal sphincter. Hypertonicity of the external sphincter may occur with anxious voluntary or involuntary contraction or as a result of an anal fissure or other local pathological condition. A relaxed or hypotonic sphincter is seen occasionally after rectal surgery, or it may be caused by a neurological deficiency.

The anal canal is short. The distance from the anal verge to the anorectal junction is less than 3 cm, which is roughly equivalent to the distance from the fingertip to the interphalangeal joint. Palpate the subcutaneous portion of the external sphincter on the inner aspect of the anal verge. Rotate the palpating finger to examine the entire muscular ring. A palpable indentation marks the intersphincteric line. Palpate the deep external sphincter through the lower part of the internal sphincter, which it surrounds. Bidigital palpation of the sphincter area may yield more information than would be obtained by probing with the index finger alone. For bidigital palpation, press the thumb of the examining hand against the perianal tissue and move the examining index finger toward it. This technique is useful for detecting a perianal abscess and for palpating the bulbourethral (Cowper's) glands.

To assess the levator ani muscle, palpate laterally and

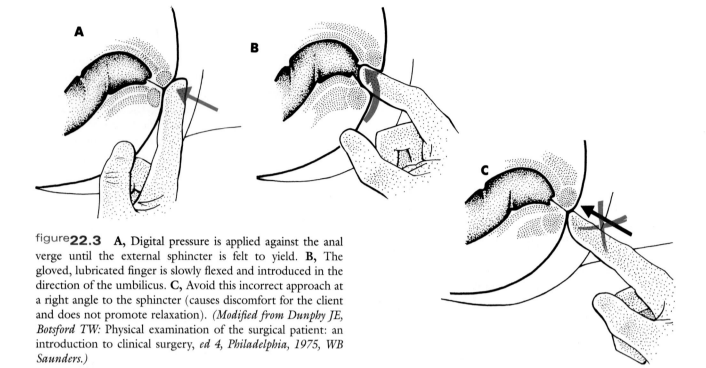

figure**22.3** **A,** Digital pressure is applied against the anal verge until the external sphincter is felt to yield. **B,** The gloved, lubricated finger is slowly flexed and introduced in the direction of the umbilicus. **C,** Avoid this incorrect approach at a right angle to the sphincter (causes discomfort for the client and does not promote relaxation). *(Modified from Dunphy JE, Botsford TW: Physical examination of the surgical patient: an introduction to clinical surgery, ed 4, Philadelphia, 1975, WB Saunders.)*

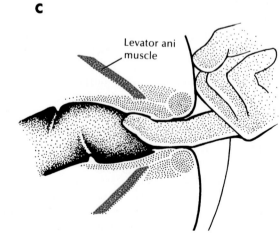

figure**22.4** The subcutaneous portion of the **external** sphincter is palpated **(A)**, followed by digital exploration **of** the deep external sphincter **(B)**. **C,** Palpation of the levator ani muscle. (NOTE: The techniques illustrated are for clients **in** the lithotomy position. Techniques need to be slightly modified for examination of clients in other positions. Examination principles and sequences remain the same.) *(Modified from Dunphy JE, Botsford TW: Physical examination of the surgical patient: an introduction to clinical surgery, ed 4, Philadelphia, 1975, WB Saunders.)*

posteriorly the area where the muscle is attached to the rectal wall on one side and then the other (Figure 22.4). Palpate the mucosa of the anal canal for tumors and polyps. Palpate the coccyx to determine its mobility and sensitivity. To assess muscular structures and the coccyx, perform bimanual examination with the index finger and the thumb.

The posterior wall of the rectum follows the curve of the coccyx and the sacrum and feels smooth to the palpating finger. The examining finger is able to palpate a distance of 6 to 10 cm of the rectal canal. To palpate the lateral walls of the rectum, rotate the index finger along the sides of the rectum. The ischial spines and the sacrotuberous ligaments can be identified through palpation. Rectal valves may be misinterpreted as protruding intrarectal masses, especially when they are well developed.

Because the prostate gland is situated anterior to the rectum, palpation through the mucosa of the anterior wall of the rectum allows for assessment of the size, shape, tenderness, surface characteristics, mobility, and consistency of the prostate gland. Ask the client to bear down so that an otherwise unreachable mass may be pushed downward into the range of the examining finger.

The prostate gland, a bilobed structure, has a normal diameter of approximately 4 cm at its widest part. The palpating finger is used to identify the smooth lateral lobes separated by a central groove. The prostate, which is approximately 3 cm long, should protrude about 1 cm into the rectum, should feel rubbery and smooth, and should be slightly movable. The prostate should be nontender to palpation. (Ask the client specifically to report any tenderness to touch.) Note the presence of nodules. (A complete discussion of the prostate examination is included in the discussion of the assessment of the male genitalia in Chapter 20.)

The normal cervix can be felt as a small round mass through the anterior wall of the rectum. In addition, a vaginal tampon or a retroverted uterus can be palpated through the rectal wall. (See Chapter 21 for a complete discussion of the assessment of the female genitalia.)

At the termination of the examination, assist the client to a more comfortable position and offer tissues to remove any lubricant remaining around the anal opening.

Examination of stool

After the examining finger has been withdrawn, examine the nature of any feces clinging to the glove (Table 22.1). Note the presence of pus or blood.

Next, test a small quantity of the feces for the presence of occult blood. This determination is made through a standard chemical test, as described later in this discussion. Small abrasions of the gastrointestinal tract are thought to be responsible for a blood loss of 1

table 22.1	Assessment of Stool Characteristics
Description of stool	**Possible explanation**
Yellow or green	Severe diarrhea, sterilization of bowel by antibiotics, diet high in chlorophyll-rich vegetables, and use of the drug calomel
Light tan, gray	Absence of bile pigments, as may be found in blockage of common bile duct, pancreatic insufficiency, obstructive jaundice, and diets high in milk or fat and low in meat
Black, tarry	Bleeding into upper gastrointestinal tract, ingestion of iron compounds or bismuth preparations, and high proportions of meat in diet
Red	Bleeding from lower gastrointestinal tract; some foods such as beets
Translucent mucus on stool	Spastic constipation, nucleus colitis, emotional disturbance, and excessive straining
Bloody mucus	Neoplasm or inflammation of rectal canal
Mucus with pus and blood	Ulcerative colitis, bacillary dysentery, ulcerating cancer of colon, and acute diverticulitis
Fat in stool	Malabsorption syndromes, enteritis and pancreatic diseases, surgical removal of a section of intestine, steatorrhea, and chronic pancreatic disease
Blood-stained mucus in liquid feces	Amebiasis
Intermittent pencil-like stools	Spasmodic contraction in rectum
Persistent pencil-like stools	Permanent stenosis from scarring or other obstruction
Pipe stem and ribbon stools	Lower rectal stricture

to 3 ml daily in the feces. The loss of more than 50 ml from the upper gastrointestinal tract will produce melena. To detect quantities of blood less than 50 ml or to determine whether black stools actually do contain blood, any of several reagents may be used.

Various factors other than bowel disease may contribute to occult blood in the stools. For example, the following factors might contribute to a positive test:

1. Bleeding gums following a dental procedure or resulting from another reason
2. Ingestion of red meat within 3 days of the test
3. Ingestion of fish, turnips, and horseradish
4. Drugs that cause gastrointestinal bleeding, such as anticoagulants, aspirin, colchicine, iron preparations, nonsteroidal antiarthritics, and steroids.
5. Other substances that might cause false-positive results for various reasons, such as oxidizing drugs, rauwolfia derivatives, and vitamin C

Tests for occult blood in the feces rely on substances that detect peroxidase as an indication of hemoglobin content demonstrated through color change in the stool specimen tested. Various reagent substances are used to detect occult blood. Their sensitivity varies as follows:

1. Orthotoluidine (Hematest, Occultest)—10 times more sensitive than benzidine
2. Benzidine—10 (or more) times more sensitive than guaiac
3. Guaiac (Hemoccult)—the least sensitive reagent

A single positive test result does not necessarily confirm the presence of gastrointestinal bleeding. A positive result is an indication to repeat the test at least three times while the client follows a meatless, high-residue diet.

The various commercially prepared screening tests for occult blood are packaged with complete instructions for use and are based on at least 3 days of specimens. Since the steps of the various tests are similar, the following instructions for the Hematest are presented as an example:

1. After the digital examination, wipe a bit of the feces on the glove of the examining finger on a square of filter paper supplied with the kit.
2. Place the filter paper with the stool smear on a glass slide.
3. Place a reagent tablet in the center of the smear on the filter paper.
4. Place one drop of water on the tablet, and allow the water to soak into the tablet for 5 to 10 seconds. Then add a second drop of water, which should run from the tablet onto the specimen and the filter paper.
5. After 2 minutes, the filter paper will turn blue if the test is positive. The color on the tablet itself or color appearing after 2 minutes is irrelevant.

If the screening test is positive, the client is retested after 48 to 72 hours. Instruct the client to refrain from eating meat, poultry, fish, turnips, and horseradish during the next testing period. In addition, the client may need to temporarily discontinue the use of the following substances: iron preparations, bromides, iodides, rauwolfia derivatives, indomethacin, colchicine, salicylates,

Other Investigative Techniques

ANOSCOPY

Use of an anoscope provides for a more complete examination of the anal canal and the internal hemorrhoidal zone.

PROCTOSCOPY

Use of a proctoscope provides visualization of the anus and the lower rectum. Approximately 9 to 15 cm of the lower intestinal tract can be visualized. The warmed and lubricated instrument is passed with the obturator for its full length. The obturator is removed, and the proctoscope is removed slowly while the examiner observes for ulcers, inflammation, strictures, or the cause of a palpable mass. Biopsy may be performed through the tube.

SIGMOIDOSCOPY

Visual examination of the upper portion of the rectum, an area that cannot be felt with the examining finger, is possible with a sigmoidoscope, which allows direct visualization of the lower 24 cm of the gastrointestinal tract. This examination is particularly important, since half of all carcinomas occur in the rectum and colon. The early detection of polyps and malignant lesions may result in early and successful treatment of an otherwise fatal disease.

MANOMETRY

This technique measures intraluminal pressure by a balloon probe attached to a catheter that is connected to a pressure transducer and a polygraph.

SPHINCTER ELECTROMYOGRAPHY

Needle or surface electrodes are used to detect the contractile activity of striated muscle and to obtain separate recordings from the external sphincter and from the puborectalis muscle.

DEFECOGRAPHY AND BALLOON PROCTOGRAPHY

These radiological investigations are designed to image the rectum and the pelvic floor at rest and during contraction and defecation.

phenylbutazone, oxyphenylbutazone, bismuth compounds, steroids, and ascorbic acid.

Screening Tests and Procedures

Screening for colorectal cancer is done through fecal occult blood testing and sigmoidoscopy. The U.S. Preventive Services Task Force (1996) recommends screening for colorectal cancer for all persons age 50 and older with fecal occult blood testing (FOBT) or sigmoidoscopy, or both. There is insufficient evidence to determine which of these screening methods is preferable or whether the combination produces greater benefits than either test alone. There is also insufficient evidence to recommend for or against routine screening with digital rectal examination. FOBT is recommended on an annual basis, but there is insufficient evidence to recommend a schedule for sigmoidoscopy screening, although a frequency of every 3 to 5 years is common.

For persons with a family history of hereditary syndromes associated with a very high risk of colon cancer and those previously diagnosed with ulcerative colitis, high-risk adenomatous polyps, or colon cancer, regular endoscopic screening should be a part of routine diagnosis and screening.

The presence of a pathological condition detected by digital examination may be further explored by one of the procedures shown in the box on p. 588.

■ VARIATIONS FROM HEALTH

Bright red blood, in small or large amounts, may originate in the large intestine, the sigmoid colon, the rectum, or the anus. The stool is likely to be red-black if the bleeding is coming from the ascending colon. Colonic bleeding should be suspected when blood is mixed with the feces. Rectal bleeding is probably occurring when blood is observed on the surface of the stool. The presence of a good deal of blood in the stool may be associated with marked malodor.

A black, tarry stool (melena) may result from bleeding in the stomach or the small intestine; the blood is partially digested during its passage to the rectum. On the other hand, the black color may result from ingested iron compounds and bismuth preparations.

Abscesses

Abscesses of the lower gastrointestinal tract that can be identified by physical examination (Figure 22.5) include the following types:

1. *Perirectal abscess:* May be palpated as a tender mass adjacent to the anal canal. The increased temperature of the mass may be helpful in identifying the inflammatory process.
2. *Ischiorectal abscess:* May be palpated as a tender mass protruding into the lateral wall of the anal canal.
3. *Supra–levator ani muscle abscess:* May be felt by the examining finger as a tender mass in the lateral rectal wall.

Anal Fissure

An anal fissure is a linear ulceration or laceration of the skin of the anus. A thin tear of the superficial anal mucosa, generally weeping, may be identified by asking the client to bear down as though straining to evacuate stool. The fissure is most commonly found in the posterior midline of the anal mucosa (in more than 90% of affected patients) and less frequently in the anterior midline (Figure 22.6). An anal fissure usually results from trauma, such as that associated with the passage of a large, hard stool or with anal intercourse. The client may complain of local pain, itching, or bleeding. Pain generally accompanies the passage of stool, and blood may be observed on the stool or on the toilet tissue. The inspection finding may include a sentinel skin tag or

---

examination *step-by-step*

Inspection
1. Spread the client's buttocks.
2. Observe the sacrococcygeal area.
3. Observe the perianal region for inflammation, lesions, hemorrhoids, and fissures.

Palpation
1. Lubricate the examining finger.
2. Insert the finger into the anus.
3. Place the pad of the finger gently along the anal verge.
4. Feel the sphincter tense and then relax. When the sphincter has relaxed, flex the tip of the finger and slowly insert it into the anal canal in the direction of the umbilicus.
5. Rotate the finger and palpate the entire muscular ring.
6. Assess tone by asking the client to contract the muscles.
7. Assess the perianal tissue and muscular structures through bidigital palpation.
8. Assess the remaining rectal wall.
9. *Men:* Palpate the prostate gland and the seminal vesicles on the anterior wall. *Women:* Perform the rectovaginal examination.

Assessment of stool
1. Withdraw the examining finger.
2. Examine the feces on the gloved finger.
3. Test the stool for occult blood.

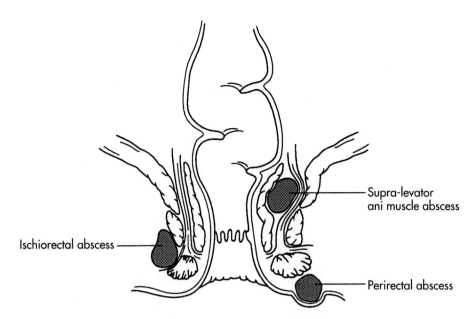

figure**22.5**   Common sites of abscess formation in the lower gastrointestinal tract.

figure**22.6**   Common problems of the anus and rectum.

ulcer through which the muscles of the internal sphincter may be visible at the base. Because the examination is painful to the client, which makes it difficult to relax the anal muscle, the use of a local anesthetic may be necessary.

Fecal Impaction

Fecal impaction is the accumulation and dehydration of fecal material in the rectum. When motility of the rectum is inhibited, the normal progression of feces does not occur and excessive amounts of water are reabsorbed through the bowel wall. The feces become hard and difficult to pass, and the accumulation may lead to complete obstruction. Fecal impaction is observed in individuals with chronic constipation and in those who have retained barium following gastrointestinal x-ray examination. The client complains of a sense of rectal fullness or urgency. Frequent small liquid-to-loose

table 22.2	Location of the Fistula Site Related to the External Opening	
	External opening	Location in anus
Goodsall's rule	Posterior to a line between ischial tuberosities	Posterior
	Radial from drainage site	Anterior
Salmon's law	Posterior to anus or more than 2.5 cm anterior or lateral	Posterior
	Anterior or less than 2.5 cm lateral	Anterior

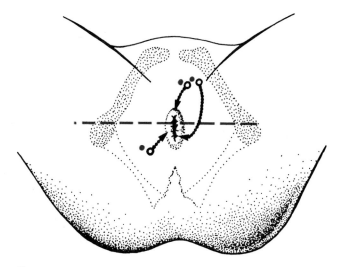

figure 22.7 Salmon's law. Fissure location related to the aperture of the fistula. (*Adapted from Dunphy JE, Botsford TW: Physical examination of the surgical patient: an introduction to clinical surgery, ed 4, Philadelphia, 1975, WB Saunders.*)

stools may occur in incomplete obstruction. The dehydrated fecal mass is easily felt on palpation.

Fistula-in-Ano

Fistula-in-ano is an abnormal opening on the cutaneous surface near the anus. It usually results from a local crypt abscess but is also common in Crohn's disease. A tract from an anal fissure or infection that terminates in the perianal skin or other tissue is termed an anorectal fistula. This type of fistula usually originates from local crypt abscesses. The fistula is a chronically inflamed tube, made up of fibrous tissue surrounding granulation tissue, that frequently can be palpated. The external opening is generally visible as a red elevation of granulation tissue. Local compression may result in the expression of serosanguineous or purulent drainage. Bidigital palpation is best accomplished with a finger in the anorectal cavity that compresses the tissue against the thumb on the skin surface. The fistulous tract feels like an indurated cord.

The site from which drainage from an anal infection occurs can be identified by relating the location of the external opening of the fissure to the anus (Table 22.2 and Figure 22.7).

Hemorrhoids

Hemorrhoids are dilated, congested veins. Hemorrhoidal swelling is associated with increased hydrostatic pressure in the portal venous system. The pressure associated with hemorrhoids correlates positively with pregnancy, straining at stool, chronic liver disease, and sudden increases in intraabdominal pressure. Bowel habits also play a role: for example, hemorrhoids frequently occur with diarrhea or incomplete bowel emptying.

Local factors such as abscess or tumor may also contribute to venous stasis.

Hemorrhoidal skin tags are ragged, flaccid skin sacs located around the anus. They cover connective tissue sacs and are the locus of resolved external hemorrhoids. Clients describe these tags as painless. Internal hemorrhoids occur proximal to the pectinate line (see Figure 22.6), whereas external hemorrhoids are those that are seen distal to this boundary. External hemorrhoids are covered by skin or anal squamous tissue.

External hemorrhoids are often painful, particularly if an increase in stool mass stretches the skin. Because the mass is located near the sphincter muscles, spasm is not uncommon. External hemorrhoids often cause itching and bleeding on defecation. These dilated veins may not be apparent at rest; however, they may appear as bluish, swollen areas at the anal verge when thrombosed. A thrombosed hemorroid is one in which blood has clotted, both within and outside the vein.

Internal hemorrhoids generally do not cause pain unless they are complicated by thrombosis, infection, or erosion of overlying mucosal surfaces. Discomfort is increased if the hemorrhoids prolapse through the anal opening. Bleeding may occur from the internal hemorrhoids with or without defecation. Proctoscopy is generally necessary for their identification.

Incontinence

Loss of the voluntary ability to control defecation is called incontinence. It may range from the involuntary passage of flatus to complete loss of sphincter tone. The

loss of fecal gases or liquids may also occur in the presence of a normal sphincter in hyperdynamic bowel states.

Masses

The presence of a mass in the rectum deserves special attention because nearly half of the rectal masses discovered are malignant. The client frequently denies pain or other symptoms. Early lesions are felt as small elevations or nodules with a firm base. Ulceration of the center of the lesion results in a crater that may be palpated. An ulcerated carcinoma may be identified through palpation by its firm, nodular, rolled edge. The lesion of carcinoma is described by including annular or tubular shape, degree of fixation, and distance from the anus. The consistency of the malignant mass is often stony and hard, and the contour is irregular. Extension of metastatic carcinoma from the peritoneum to the pelvic floor is described as a rectal shelf. It is palpated as a hard, nodular ridge.

Pilonidal Cyst and Sinus

A pilonidal cyst is a hairy sac that develops in the sacral region of the skin. A pilonidal sinus is an abnormal channel that contains a tuft of hair and is most frequently situated over or close to the tip of the coccyx. Even though it is thought to be a congenital lesion, a pilonidal sinus is commonly first diagnosed between the ages of 15 and 30 years. It is located superficial to the coccyx, or lower sacrum. The sinus opening may look like a dimple, with another very small opening found in the midline. In other cases of pilonidal sinus, a cyst can be observed and palpated. In more advanced conditions, a sinus tract can be palpated. The affected area may become edematous, erythematous, and tender, and a tuft of hair may be observed. The ingrowth of the hairs is probably the cause of infection, cyst, and fistula formation. These cysts and fistulas are generally removed surgically.

Pruritus Ani

Pruritus ani is a common chronic condition characterized by itching of the perianal skin. Excoriated, thickened, and pigmented skin may result from chronic inflammation associated with this condition. Itching and burning of the rectal area are most often traceable to pinworms in children and to fungal infections in adults. Clients with diabetes are particularly vulnerable to fun-

gal infections. A dull, grayish pink color of the perianal skin is characteristic of fungal infections. The radiating folds of skin may appear enlarged, and the skin may be cracked or fissured. Pruritus ani that is characterized by dry and brittle skin is thought to be related to psychosomatic disease.

Rectal Polyps

Rectal polyps, which feel like soft nodules, are encountered frequently. They may be pedunculated (on a stalk) or sessile (irregularly moundlike, growing from a relatively broad base, and closely adherent to the mucosal wall). Because of their soft consistency, rectal polyps may be difficult or impossible to identify by palpation. Proctoscopy is usually necessary for identification, and a biopsy is performed to identify malignant lesions. A pedunculated rectal polyp occasionally prolapses through the anal ring.

Rectal Prolapse

Internal hemorrhoids are the most common type of tissue protrusion through the anal ring. The pink-colored mucosa is described as appearing like a doughnut or rosette. In the older client, however, protruding mucosa may herald eversion or prolapse of the rectum. Incomplete prolapse involves only mucosa, whereas complete rectal prolapse is also associated with the sphincters.

The client describes the prolapse of tissue through the anal ring as occurring with exercise or while straining at stool. Frequently, the client is able to push the mass back in with digital pressure. Inspection reveals a red, bulging mucosal mass protruding through the anal ring.

Rectal Tenesmus

Rectal tenesmus is painful straining at stool associated with spasm of the anal and rectal muscles. The chief complaint is a distressing feeling of urgency. The client should be questioned concerning the nature of the stool. A hard, dry stool indicates constipation. A bloody, diarrheal stool might indicate ulcerative colitis. When the client's stools are normally constituted, a rectal fissure may be the cause of tenesmus. The client with a perirectal inflammation, such as prostatitis or proctitis, may also experience tenesmus.

The client who complains of constant rectal pain should be examined carefully for thrombosed rectal hemorrhoids.

sample documentation & diagnoses CRITICAL THINKING

▇ FOCUSED HEALTH HISTORY *(SUBJECTIVE DATA)*

Mrs. G., a 35-year-old married female, is complaining of burning and itching in the rectal area, especially after bowel movements, for about 2 months. Notes a small amount of blood on toilet tissue about once or twice a week after bowel movements. Over the past 2 months, bowel movements have not been regular (interval varies between 2× a day to once in 3 days). Stools are characteristically hard, and bowel movements are frequently painful. Has been taking a laxative (milk of magnesia) every 2 to 3 days for the past month. Denies abdominal pain, fecal incontinence, and a history of rectal infections, trauma, or surgeries. Has a history of hemorrhoids after her most recent pregnancy 3 years ago. Family history is negative for cancer and colon diseases. Three months ago started work outside of the home. Consequently, diet and activity patterns have changed. Eats fewer fruits and vegetables, drinks less water, and is less active.

▇ FOCUSED PHYSICAL EXAMINATION *(OBJECTIVE DATA)*

Abdomen: Flat; bowel sounds normal and heard in all four quadrants. No organomegaly or tenderness on palpation. No masses.

Perianal area: Clean, no fissures or lesions.

Rectum and anus: Small, 1 × 1 cm, reddish blue, shiny mass visible at 5 o'clock position at anal opening. Tender on palpation. Two small skin tags at 3 and 9 o'clock positions.

Sphincter tone: Good.

Rectal walls: Smooth and without tenderness.

Stool: Brown and formed.

Hemocult: Negative.

diagnoses

HEALTH PROBLEM

Constipation; external hemorrhoid

NURSING DIAGNOSIS

Constipation related to low-roughage diet, low fluid intake, and inadequate physical activity

Defining Characteristics

- Frequency less than normal pattern
- Hard, formed stools, decreased quality
- Straining at stool
- Painful defecation

chapter **23**

Integration of the Physical Assessment and Documentation

▌ PERFORMANCE OF THE INTEGRATED PHYSICAL EXAMINATION

This chapter includes three sections: description of and outline for the performance of a comprehensive, integrated physical examination; description of the documenting of the comprehensive physical examination; and a worksheet for documenting a physical examination.

After practicing and acquiring proficiency in the performance of regional examinations, it is important to develop a systematic pattern for performing an integrated physical examination. In practice, practitioners perform both regional examinations, such as in acute care settings, and comprehensive multisystem examinations, such as in health maintenance programs.

In developing a personal routine for a complete examination, consider factors of efficiency and client comfort. The examiner who performs procedures systematically and efficiently conserves time and is less likely to forget a procedure or a part of the body than is the examiner who performs examinations haphazardly.

Clients who are ill or debilitated lose energy quickly. A system of examination involving the fewest number of client position changes enhances acceptability and decreases the number of examinations and portions of examinations deferred because of client intolerance.

The manner in which the examiner conducts the physical examination can enhance or compromise rapport developed during the history-taking interview. A disorganized examiner who leaves the room to obtain missing equipment, who changes positions several times in a short time period, or who has the client change positions frequently may lose the client's confidence.

The outline presented in this chapter under Technique for Examination is a suggested format for performing the physical examination. It is intended as a guide for the beginning practitioner to use in practice sessions. In actual client care situations, this outline may require adapting because of the client's age or disability, examination protocols and priorities of the care agency, or examiner preference. The suggested format is designed to avoid excessive client and examiner movement. The approach integrates body systems into the examination of body regions.

PREPARATION FOR EXAMINATION

EQUIPMENT

The equipment needed for a complete physical examination includes the following (the purposes and uses of all the listed items have been explained in the preceding chapters):

Cotton balls
Cotton-tipped swabs or applicator sticks
Drapes
Flashlights—both large with transilluminator and penlight
Gauze squares
Glass of water
Gloves—latex, disposable examination
Marking pencil or pen
Materials for cover test
Materials to test pain and light touch sensation (pin, cotton ball)
Measuring tape
Nasal speculum (optional)
Odoriferous substances for cranial nerve examination
Ophthalmoscope
Otoscope with pneumatic bulb
Printed material for near visual acuity and comprehension examination
Reflex (percussion) hammer
Ruler
Scale with height measurement attachment
Sharp and dull testing materials
Snellen eye chart (far vision acuity)
Sphygmomanometer
Stethoscope with diaphragm and bell heads
Substances for taste sensation evaluation
Thermometer
Tongue blades
Tuning forks (one 500-1000 cycles per second [CPS] for testing auditory function and one 100-400 CPS for testing vibratory sense)

Watch that records seconds

If a pelvic or a rectal examination is to be done, add the following equipment and supplies:

Lubricant (water soluble)
Materials to collect and prepare vaginal secretions or specimens for laboratory examination
Materials to examine fecal material for occult blood
Mirror
Vaginal speculums

CLIENT AND ENVIRONMENT

The physical examination should occur in a comfortable room that provides privacy, adequate lighting, and a reasonable amount of space for client and examiner movement. The recommended equipment for an examination room includes the following:

Desk with two chairs
Examination lamp
Examining table
Scale
Sink
Stand or counter to hold supplies
Stool

In preparation for the examination, the following procedures are recommended:

1. Check for availability of needed materials within easy reach.
2. Review examination procedure with client.
3. Have client empty bladder.
4. Have client undress and put on gown.

Technique for Examination

The client enters the examination room, the examiner and the client greet each other, and the examiner observes the client (Figure 23.1).

Inspect general appearance

1. Skin color
2. Consistency of general appearance with age
3. General state of nutrition
4. Hygiene
5. Obvious physical deformities, limitations, use of assistive devices

Inspect stature and movement

1. Symmetry
2. Posture
3. Body build
4. Gait
5. Mobility

Inspect demeanor

1. Facial expression
2. Composure
3. Speech

figure**23.1**   Examiner greeting the client.

figure**23.2**   Interview for the health history.

4. Orientation and mental status
5. Disposition
6. Eye contact

Take health history

At this point in a comprehensive assessment, the examiner takes the health history (Figure 23.2). The comprehensive health history is discussed in Chapter 3. The student is referred to that chapter for review as needed. Allow the client to remain in street clothes for the history-taking interview. Just before starting the physical examination, have the client change from street clothes into the examination gown.

Take measurements

1. Measure weight.
2. Measure height.
3. Measure temperature.
4. Palpate pulses (radial and brachial).
5. Measure blood pressure (both arms).
6. Measure respiratory rate.

The client is sitting on the bed or examining table. The examiner is facing the client (Figure 23.3).

Inspect and palpate upper extremities

1. Examine skin (color, temperature, vascularity, lesions, hydration, turgor, texture, edema, masses), muscle mass, and skeletal configuration.
2. Examine nails (color and condition).

Examine head

1. Inspect configuration of skull.
2. Inspect condition of skin, scalp, and hair (masses, parasites, lesions).
3. Inspect hair distribution.
4. Inspect face—appearance, expression, symmetry of structure and features, movements.
5. Inspect head—size, shape, symmetry, extra movements.
6. Inspect movements of head and face.
7. Palpate skull, hair, and face (deformities, tenderness, lesions, texture, distribution, quantity).
8. Palpate and percuss paranasal sinus areas (tenderness).
9. Palpate temporomandibular joint (tenderness, crepitations).

Examine eyes

1. Inspect eyebrows, eyelids, eyelashes, conjunctiva, cornea, sclera, iris, pupil, and palpebral fissures.
2. Measure visual acuity (cranial nerve [CN] II).
3. Assess visual fields (CN II).
4. Determine alignment of eyes (perform cover test and corneal light reflex).
5. Test extraocular movements (CN III, CN IV, CN VI).
6. Palpate lacrimal sac.
7. Test pupillary responses (light and accommodation) (CN III).
8. Perform ophthalmoscopic examination of lens,

figure**23.3**   Client gowned and seated; examiner facing the client.

figure**23.4**   Client seated; examiner behind the client.

media, and retina (CN II). NOTE: The room should be darkened for the ophthalmoscopic examination.
9. Test corneal reflex (CN V, CN VII).

Examine ears

1. Inspect auricle (position, alignment, masses, lesions, tenderness).
2. Palpate auricle (masses, lesions, tenderness).
3. Perform otoscopic examination (inspect canals and tympanic membranes).
4. Determine auditory acuity (CN VIII).
5. Perform Weber and Rinne tests.

Examine nose

1. Inspect alignment of septum and surface characteristics.
2. Determine patency of each nostril.
3. Test for olfaction (CN I).
4. Inspect mucosa, septum, and turbinates (inflammation, allergy, lesions, epistaxis).

Examine mouth and pharynx

1. Inspect lips, total buccal mucosa, teeth, gums, tongue, sublingual area, roof of mouth, tonsillar area, and pharynx (as appropriate, for presence, condition, color, symmetry, surface characteristics, movement).
2. Palpate mouth with gloved hand if indicated.
3. Note mouth odor.
4. Test glossopharyngeal nerve (CN IX) and vagus nerve (CN X) ("ah" and gag reflex).
5. Test hypoglossal nerve (CN XII) (tongue movement).
6. Test taste (CN VII and CN IX).

Complete examination of cranial nerves

1. Test trigeminal nerve (CN V) (jaw clenching, lateral jaw movements, pain, and light touch to face).

2. Test facial nerve (CN VII). (Client smiles, raises eyebrows, shows teeth, puffs cheeks, keeps eyes closed against resistance.)
3. Test spinal accessory nerve (CN XI) (trapezius and sternocleidomastoid muscles).

Complete examination of head and examine neck

1. Inspect surface characteristics and range of motion of the head and neck.
2. Palpate nodes (preauricular, postauricular, occipital, parotid, sublingual, submandibular, submental, anterior cervical, posterior superficial cervical, posterior cervical, internal jugular, supraclavicular, and intraclavicular nodes).
3. Palpate carotid arteries.
4. Palpate for position of trachea.
5. Palpate thyroid gland.
6. Auscultate carotid arteries and thyroid gland for bruits.

The client is sitting on the bed or examining table, total chest uncovered if male, breasts covered if female (Figure 23.4). The examiner is standing behind the client.

Examine back

1. Inspect spine.
2. Palpate spine.
3. Inspect skin and thoracic configuration.
4. Palpate muscles and bones.

5. Palpate costovertebral area, asking client about tenderness.

Examine lungs (apices and lateral and posterior areas)

NOTE: Apical, posterior, and lateral lung regions can usually be examined from a position behind the client.
1. Inspect respiration (depth, rhythm, pattern) and posterior and lateral thorax.
2. Palpate for thoracic expansion and tactile fremitus.
3. Percuss systematically.
4. Determine diaphragmatic excursion.
5. Auscultate systematically (breath sounds and adventitious sounds).
6. Auscultate for vocal resonance.

The client is sitting on the bed or examining table, uncovered to the waist. The examiner is facing the client (Figure 23.5).

Examine lungs (anterior areas)

1. Inspect configuration and skin.
2. Palpate external thorax for skin temperature and consistency, tenderness, and thoracic configuration.
3. Palpate for general assessment and tactile fremitus.
4. Percuss systematically.
5. Auscultate lungs systematically.
6. Auscultate for vocal resonance.

figure**23.5**   Client seated and disrobed to the waist; examiner facing the client.

Examine heart

1. Inspect precordium (pulsations and heaving).
2. Palpate precordium (apical impulse, thrills, heaves, pulsations).
3. Auscultate precordium (aortic area, pulmonic area, left sternal border, apical area).
4. Inspect jugular venous pulses and pressure.

Examine breasts (female client and male client with gynecomastia)

NOTE: All men should have a breast examination in the supine position.
1. Inspect breasts with client's arms and hands at the sides, above the head, and pressed into the hips, eliciting pectoral contraction.
2. Inspect breasts with client leaning forward.
3. If lesions are suspected or client is at risk for other reasons, palpate breasts in all four quadrants.
4. If large breasts, perform a bimanual examination.

Complete palpation of nodes in upper body

1. Axillary nodes (lateral axillary, posterior axillary, central axillary, anterior axillary, and apical axillary)
2. Epitrochlear nodes

The client is supine. The examiner is at the right side of the client (Figure 23.6).

Examine breasts (male and female)

1. Palpate breasts systematically in all four quadrants and the tail of Spence.
2. Attempt to express secretion from the nipples.

Examine heart

1. Inspect precordium (pulsations and heaves).
2. Palpate precordium (apical impulse, thrills, heaves, pulsations).
3. Auscultate apical rate and rhythm.
4. Auscultate precordium (supine and on left side in all major sound areas).
5. Inspect jugular venous pulses and pressure.
6. Measure supine blood pressure (both arms).

Examine abdomen

1. Inspect abdomen at rest (skin characteristics, scars, contour, pulsations, movement).
2. Examine abdomen with head raised for integrity of abdominal musculature.
3. Auscultate bowel sounds, aorta, renal arteries, and femoral arteries.
4. Percuss abdomen.
5. Percuss and measure liver.
6. Percuss spleen.
7. Palpate all four quadrants lightly (tenderness, masses, organomegaly).

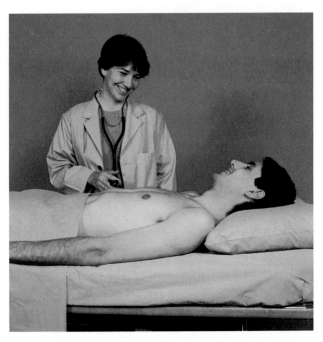

figure**23.6** Client supine; examiner standing at the right side of the client.

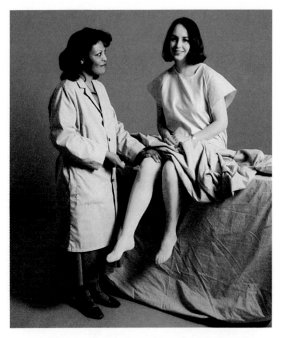

figure**23.7** Client seated; examiner facing the client.

8. Palpate all four quadrants deeply (tenderness, masses, organomegaly).
9. Palpate liver, spleen, inguinal and femoral node and hernia areas, and femoral pulses.
10. Test abdominal reflexes.
11. Palpate inguinal areas for pulses and nodes.

Examine lower extremities

1. Inspect skin, hair distribution, muscle mass, and skeletal configuration.
2. Palpate for temperature, texture, edema, popliteal pulses, posterior tibial pulses, and dorsal pedal pulses.
3. Test range of motion (toes, feet, ankles, knees, hips).
4. Test strength (toes, feet, ankles, knees, hips).
5. Test hips for stability.
6. Test sensation (pain, light touch, and vibration).
7. Test position sense.

The client is sitting on the bed or examining table. The examiner is standing in front of the client (Figure 23.7).

Assess neural system

1. Elicit deep tendon reflexes (biceps, triceps, brachioradialis, patellar, and Achilles reflexes).
2. Test for Babinski's reflex bilaterally.
3. Test for coordination of upper and lower extremities (cerebellar function).
   a. Touch nose with rapidly alternating index fingers.

b. Touch thumb with rapidly alternating fingers.
c. With index finger, alternately touch own nose and examiner's rapidly moving finger.
d. Run heel down tibia of opposite leg.
e. Alternately and rapidly cross leg over knee.
f. Perform figure-eight in air with leg.
4. Test sensory function (face and arms).
5. Test two-point discrimination—palms, thighs, back.
6. Test stereognosis, graphesthia.
7. Test position sense.

Assess upper extremities

1. Strength
2. Range of motion
3. Sensation
4. Vibration
5. Position sense

The client is standing. The examiner is standing next to and then behind the client (Figure 23.8).

Measure standing blood pressure in both arms
Examine spine and sacral area

1. Inspect with client bending over.
2. Test for range of motion—hyperextension, lateral bending, rotation of upper trunk.
3. Inspect sacrococcygeal and perianal areas.

figure**23.8** Client standing; examiner standing next to the client.

Assess neural system

1. Inspect gait (tandem, heel walking, toe walking, usual).
2. Test for proprioception and cerebellar function
   a. Perform Romberg test.
   b. With eyes closed, stand on one foot and then the other.
   c. Hop in place on one foot and then the other.
   d. Observe deep knee bends.

The male client is standing. The examiner is standing next to the client.

Examine external genitals

1. Inspect penis, urethral opening, pubic hair distribution, and scrotum.
2. Palpate penis.
3. Palpate scrotal contents.

Assess for presence of hernias

1. Observe for inguinal and femoral hernias at rest and with straining.
2. Palpate bilaterally for femoral hernias.
3. Palpate bilaterally for inguinal hernias.

Examination of the Bedridden Client

The regional and integrated examinations presented in this book are focused on clients who are able to sit and stand. For bedridden patients, the examination is adapted. A suggested sequence is (1) examination of the head, neck, anterior chest, and abdomen while the client is supine or supported in a sitting position on the bed; (2) examination of the back, posterior thorax, and skin while the client is rolled to the side; (3) completion of the examination with the client supine.

Rectal examination

NOTE: For this part of the examination, the client leans over the examination table.
1. Inspect perianal area.
2. Palpate rectum (sphincter tone and characteristics).
3. Palpate prostate and seminal vesicles.
4. Inspect characteristics of stool on gloved finger when removed.

The female client is in the lithotomy position, genital area uncovered. The examiner is sitting, facing the genital area.

Examine genitalia

1. Inspect genitalia (pubic hair condition and distribution, labia, clitoris, urethral opening, perineum, perianal area, and anus).
2. Palpate external genital area (labia, Bartholin's and Skene's glands).
3. Perform speculum examination (inspect vagina and cervix).
4. Obtain smears and cultures.
5. Perform bimanual vaginal examination (vagina, cervix, uterus, tubes, ovaries, muscle tone).

Examine rectum

1. Perform bimanual rectovaginal examination (sphincter tone, rectovaginal septum, ligaments, uterus, tubes, ovaries, cul-de-sac).
2. Inspect appearance of feces on gloved finger when removed.

Teaching Self-Assessment

While the client is still gowned, teach or review self-examinations appropriate to the situation. Generally, it is most effective to teach self-examinations during the cor-

Guidelines for Documenting the Physical Examination

1. Be specific.
2. Be concise.
3. Be complete.
4. Avoid using vague terms, such as "negative," "normal," or "good."
5. Specify portions of the examination omitted or deferred.
6. Use agreed-on and understood abbreviations.
7. Record exact size or placement of lesions—draw a picture or diagram.
8. Use illustrations when appropriate.

HELPFUL HINT *When performing the integrated physical examination:*
- *Warm hands and instruments.*
- *Keep fingernails short and smooth.*
- *Ensure a quiet, private setting.*
- *Adapt to the circumstances.*
- *Position the examining table away from a wall to enable maximum movement for yourself.*
- *Explain what you are doing and observing during the examination.*
- *Avoid vague or evaluative statements that the client may misunderstand.*
- *Advise the patient of specific, possible discomfort and unusual sensations.*
- *Ask the client to tell you about unusual sensations or pain elicited during the examination.*
- *Expose the area to be examined fully to ensure a complete assessment, but drape all areas not being examined appropriately.*

responding portion of the examiner's examination. However, there may be reasons to defer teaching until the end of the examination.

Completion of the Examination

When the examination and the teaching of self-examinations are completed, provide the client with disposable materials to clean areas where lubricant may remain. Then leave the examination room; allow the client privacy for dressing. Return to discuss findings and complete care.

▪ DOCUMENTING THE PHYSICAL EXAMINATION

The record should describe what the examiner saw, heard, palpated, and percussed. Whenever appropriate, write the exact description. Avoid evaluations such as "normal," "good," or "poor," or use them judiciously. Too frequently, examiners describe a major system, such as the cardiovascular system, in one word, "normal." This description is limited because it does not indicate what components of that system were assessed or the examiner's parameters of normal.

In documenting the physical examination, continuously attempt to achieve a balance between conciseness and comprehensiveness. To be concise, use outlines, phrases, and abbreviations. Sacrifice full sentences and write only essential words. Using a form for recording the physical examination is helpful. A form provides an

outline into which data can be entered. Forms also serve as reminders for completeness, and they save time. If all members of a health care system use the same forms systematically, they become extremely useful indexes for rapid information retrieval.

As recommended in the recording of the history (see Chapter 3: The Health History), the beginning practitioner should record as many details as possible, including all findings from the examination. With increased skill and discrimination regarding the significance of findings, the practitioner will be able to weed out irrelevant information and consolidate significant data.

Table 23.1 is a guideline designed to assist the beginning recorder (see also box above, left). The first column in Table 23.1 indicates the body systems or regions that are examined. The second column contains a list of the areas of recording. These areas should be described for most clients. The third column is a partial list of areas to be recorded if abnormalities are identified in the examination of that system. The fourth column contains examples of recording for each body system or area. The examples of recording do not relate to one client; therefore the fourth column should not be read as an example of the composite physical examination of one person. A sample worksheet for recording a physical examination can be found on pp. 609-613.

table 23.1 **Areas and Examples of Documentation for the Physical Examination**

Area of examination	Descriptions usually recorded	Descriptions recorded in detail if abnormalities are present (partial listing only)	Examples of documentation

Vital signs	Temperature: Oral, ear, axillary, or rectal
	Pulse
	Respiration
	Blood pressure; both arms in at least two positions (lying and sitting recommended)
	Weight (indicate if client is clothed or unclothed)
	Height (without shoes)
		Blood pressure in standing position and in both thighs	T: 37° C (98.6° F) (oral)
			P: 76/min—strong and regular
			R: 16/min
			BP:
			  Lying: R, 110/70/60; L, 112/68/60
			  Sitting: R, 116/74/67; L, 120/76/65
			Wt: 170 lb, unclothed
			Ht: 5 ft 3 in

General health	Appearance as relative to chronological age Apparent state of health Awareness Personal appearance Emotional status Nutritional status Affect Response Cooperation	Handshake Speech Respiratory difficulties Gross deformity Movements Unusual behavior	Slightly obese, alert, black male who looks younger than his stated age of 45; moves without difficulty; no gross abnormalities apparent; appears healthy and in no acute distress; is neatly dressed, responsive, and cooperative; responds appropriately; smiles frequently
Skin and mucous membranes	Color Edema Moisture Temperature Texture Turgor	Discharge Drainage Lesions: Distribution, type, configuration Superficial vascularity Mobility Thickness	Skin: Uniformly brown in color; soft, warm, moist, elastic, of normal thickness; no edema or lesions Mucous membranes: Pink, moist, slightly pale
Nails	Color of beds Texture	Lesions Abnormalities in size or shape Presence of clubbing	Nail beds pink; texture hard; no clubbing
Hair and scalp	Quantity Distribution Color Texture	Lesions Parasites	Hair: Normal male distribution; thick, curly; black color with graying at temples Scalp: Clean, no lesions
Cranium	Contour Tenderness	Lesions	Normocephalic, no tenderness

Area of examination	Descriptions usually recorded	Descriptions recorded in detail if abnormalities are present (partial listing only)	Examples of documentation
Face	Symmetry Movements Sinuses CN V CN VII	Tenderness Edema Lesions Parotid gland	Symmetrical at rest and with movement; jaw muscles strong, no crepitations or limitation in movement of temporomandibular joint; sinus areas not tender Sensory: Pain and light touch intact
Eyes	Visual acuity Visual fields Alignment of eyes Alignment of eyelids Movement of eyelids Conjunctiva Sclera Cornea Anterior chamber Iris Pupils: Size, shape, symmetry, reflexes (PERRLA may be used for "Pupils, equally round, react to light and accommodation") Lens Lacrimal apparatus Ophthalmological examination (disc, vessels, retina, macular areas)	Eyebrows Tonometry Lesions Exophthalmia	Vision (distant with glasses): R, 20/40; L, 20/30; can read newspaper at 18 in; visual fields full Alignment: No deviation with cover test; light reflex equal; palpebral fissure normal Extraocular movements: Bilaterally intact; no nystagmus, ptosis, lid lag Conjunctiva: Clear, slightly injected around area of R inner canthus Sclera: White Cornea: Clear, arcus senilis, R eye Anterior chamber: Not narrowed Iris: Blue, round Pupils: PERRLA Lens: Clear Funduscopic examination: Normal veins and arteries; disc round, margins well defined, color yellowish pink; macular areas visualized; no arteriolovenous (AV) nicking, hemorrhages, or exudates Lacrimal system: No swelling or discharge Corneal reflex: Present
Ears	Auricle Canal Otoscopic examination (color, presence of landmarks) Rinne and Weber tests	Position Discharge Pathological alterations present on otoscopic examination Lesions Mastoid tenderness General tenderness	Auricle: No lesions; canal free of cerumen and discharge Otoscopic examination: Drum intact; color pearly gray; landmarks and light reflex in proper positions Hearing: Finger rub heard in both ears at 3 ft Rinne and Weber tests heard equally in both ears, AC 2 × > BC or AC > BC 2:1

continued

Area of examination	Descriptions usually recorded	Descriptions recorded in detail if abnormalities are present (partial listing only)	Examples of documentation
Nose	Patency of each nostril Olfaction Turbinates and mucous membranes	External nose Vestibule Transillumination of sinuses	Nostrils patent: Odors identified Septum: Slightly deviated to R Turbinates and membranes: Pink, moist, no discharge
Oral cavity	Buccal mucosa Gums Teeth (decayed, missing, filled) Floor of mouth Hard and soft palate Tonsillar areas Posterior pharyngeal wall Taste Tongue position and movement	Breath odor Lips Lesions Laryngoscopic examination Palpation of mouth Parotid duct	Membranes: Pink and moist, no lesions Gums: No edema or inflammation Teeth: In good repair Palate: Intact; moves symmetrically with phonation; gag reflex present Tonsils: Present, not enlarged Pharynx: Pink and clean Tongue: Strong, midline; moves symmetrically Taste: Able to differentiate sweet and sour
Neck	Movements: Rotation and lateral bend Symmetry Thyroid gland Tracheal position Glands and nodes	Postural alignment Tenderness Tone of muscles Lesions Masses	Full ROM; strong symmetrically; thyroid not palpable; trachea midline; no enlargement of head and neck regional nodes
Breasts and axillae	Axillary nodes Supraclavicular nodes Infraclavicular nodes Breasts: Observation and palpation Nipples and areolar areas Discharge Masses	Retraction Dimpling	No nodes palpable—axillary, infraclavicular, or supraclavicular; no masses, retraction, or discharge Nipples symmetrically positioned No masses or tenderness palpated
Chest and respiratory system	Shape of thorax Symmetry of thorax Respiratory movements Respiratory excursion Palpation: Tactile fremitus, tenderness, masses Percussion notes Diaphragmatic excursion and level Auscultation: Breath sounds, adventitious sounds	Deformity Use of accessory muscles of respiration Vocal resonance Egophony, bronchophony, whispered pectoriloquy	Thorax oval; AP diameter < lateral diameter; symmetrical at rest and with movements; excursion equal bilaterally; tactile fremitus equal bilaterally; no masses or tenderness; percussion tones resonant; diaphragmatic excursion 5 cm bilaterally between T10 and T12; vesicular breath sounds bilaterally; no adventitious sounds

Area of examination	Descriptions usually recorded	Descriptions recorded in detail if abnormalities are present (partial listing only)	Examples of documentation
Central cardiovascular system	Position in which heart was examined; lying, sitting, left lateral, recumbent Inspection: Bulging, depression, pulsation (precordial and juxtaprecordial) Palpation: Thrusts, heaves, thrills, friction rubs Apical impulse Auscultation: Rate and rhythm, character of S_1, character of S_2, comparison of S_1 in aortic and pulmonic areas, comparison of S_1 and S_2 in major auscultatory areas, presence or absence of extra sounds—if present, description	Murmur or extra sound: whether systolic or diastolic; intensity; pitch; quality; site of maximum transmission; effect of position, respiration, and exercise; radiation	Examined in sitting and lying positions; no abnormal pulsations or lifts observed; PMI in 5th ICS, slightly medial to the LMCL; no abnormal pulsations palpated Apical pulse: 72, regular; heart sounds; S_1 single sound; S_2 splits with inspiration; S_1 heard loudest at apex; S_2 heard loudest at base; no murmurs or other sounds
Arterial pulses	Radial pulse: Rate, rhythm; consistency and tenderness of arterial wall Amplitude and character of peripheral pulses: Superficial temporal, brachial, femoral, popliteal, posterior tibial, dorsal pedal Carotid pulses: Equality, amplitude, thrills, bruits	Any abnormality (analysis of type)	Radial pulse: Bilaterally equal, regular, strong; no tenderness or thickening of vessels; 76/min Peripheral pulses: <table><tr><td></td><td>*Right*</td><td>*Left*</td></tr><tr><td>Temporal</td><td>2+</td><td>2+</td></tr><tr><td>Brachial</td><td>3+</td><td>3+</td></tr><tr><td>Femoral</td><td>2+</td><td>2+</td></tr><tr><td>Popliteal</td><td>0+</td><td>0+</td></tr><tr><td>Posterior tibial</td><td>2+</td><td>2+</td></tr><tr><td>Dorsal pedal</td><td>1+</td><td>1+</td></tr></table>Carotid pulses: Equal, strong, no bruits
Venous pulses and pressures	Jugular venous pulsations, presence of waves a, c, and v Venous pressure: Distention present at 45 degrees	Hepatojugular reflex Analysis of jugular venous waves	Jugular venous distention, 5 cm with client at 45 degrees

continued

table 23.1 **Areas and Examples of Documentation for the Physical Examination—cont'd**

Area of examination	Descriptions usually recorded	Descriptions recorded in detail if abnormalities are present (partial listing only)	Examples of documentation

Abdomen	Inspection: Scars, size, shape, symmetry, muscular development, bulging, movements
	Auscultation: Peristaltic sounds—present or absent; vascular bruits—present or absent
	Palpation
	  Masses
	  Tenderness (local, referred, rebound), tone of musculature
	  Liver: Size, contour, character of edge, consistency, tenderness
	  Kidney (indicate if palpable or not)
	  Costovertebral area: Tenderness
	Percussion: Liver size at MCL, spleen, masses
		Diastasis
		Distention
		Mass or bulging (specific description)
		Palpable spleen: Size, surface contour, splenic notch, consistency, tenderness, mobility
		Palpable kidney: Location, size, shape, consistency
		Distention of urinary bladder
		Fluid wave
		Flank dullness
		Shifting dullness
		Aorta
		Gallbladder
			Healed scar RLQ (appendectomy); slightly obese, protuberant; symmetrical, no bulging; bowel sounds present, no bruits; no abnormal movements; no masses; no tenderness; liver 11 cm in RMCL; no CVA tenderness; no organs palpated; muscle tone lax
			Area of midline diastasis: 6 cm × 2 cm inferior and superior to umbilicus
			
			3 cm

Neural system	Orientation Intellectual performance Emotional status Insight Memory Cranial nerves Coordination Sensory: Touch, pain, position, vibration Babinski's sign Romberg test Reflexes	Thought content Speech Sensory: Hot, cold, two-point discrimination Stereognosis Involuntary movements	Alert, oriented × 3; mood appropriate and stable; remote and recent memory intact; serial calculations by 6 accurate; insight normal; cranial nerves I-XII intact, examined and recorded in head and neck regions; all movement coordinated; able to perform rapid coordinated movements with upper and lower extremities.

table 23.1   Areas and Examples of Documentation for the Physical Examination—cont'd

Area of examination	Descriptions usually recorded	Descriptions recorded in detail if abnormalities are present (partial listing only)	Examples of documentation
			Deep tendon reflexes (0 to 4 +) 0 = absent + (or 1 +) = decreased + + (or 2 +) = normal + + + (or 3 +) = hyperactive + + + + (or 4 +) = clonus Sensory: Able to detect light touch, pain, and vibration to face, trunk, and extremities bilaterally and symmetrically; walks with coordination; able to maintain standing position with eyes closed
Extremities and musculoskeletal system	Both upper and lower extremities: General assessments—size, shape, mass, symmetry, hair distribution, color; temperature; edema; varicosities; tenderness; epitrochlear lymph nodes Bones and joints: Range of motion, tenderness, gait Muscles: Size, symmetry, strength, tone, tenderness, consistency Back: Posture; tenderness; movement—extension, lateral bend, rotation	Lesions Deformities Color and temperature: Changes on elevation and dependency Homans' sign Redness Heat Swelling Deformity Crepitations Contractures Muscle spasms Tenderness Atrophy Hypertrophy	Muscular development and mass normal for age; arms and legs symmetrical; skin warm, soft; male hair distribution on arms, legs, and feet; no edema, varicosities, or tenderness; no nodes palpated; joints nontender, not swollen; full ROM; good muscle tone, and strength equal bilaterally; back—full ROM; no tenderness or deformities

continued

table 23.1 **Areas and Examples of Documentation for the Physical Examination—cont'd**

Area of examination	Descriptions usually recorded	Descriptions recorded in detail if abnormalities are present (partial listing only)	Examples of documentation
Anus and rectum	Anal area Skin Hemorrhoids Sphincter tone Rectum Tumors Stool color Occult blood	Lesions Fissures Pilonidal sinus Condition of perineal body Tenderness Proctoscopic examination	Skin clean, no lesions; sphincter tone good; no hemorrhoids or masses noted; stools brown, guaiac negative
Inguinal area	Hernia: Inguinal, femoral Nodes	Size, shape, consistency, tenderness, reducibility of hernia or nodes	Hernias not present; no enlargement of nodes noted
Male genitalia	Penis: Condition of prepuce, skin Scrotum: Size, skin, testes, epididymides, spermatic cords Prostate gland: Size, shape, symmetry, consistency, tenderness Seminal vesicles: Size, shape, consistency	Scars Lesions Structural alterations Masses Swelling Nodules	Penis: Circumcised, clean, no lesions Scrotum and contents: Normal size, no masses or tumors noted Prostate and inferior portions of seminal vesicles: Palpated; normal consistency; nontender Prostate: Not enlarged; rubbery; nontender Seminal vesicles: Not palpable
Female genitalia	External: Hair distribution; labia; Bartholin's glands, urethral meatus, Skene's glands (BUS); hymen; introitus Vaginal observation: Presence or absence of rectocele, urethrocele, cystocele; tissue; discharge (smears or cultures taken); cervix Bimanual examination: Cervix, uterus, adnexa Rectovaginal examination: Uterus, cul-de-sac, septum	Lesions Tumors Prolapses	Normal female hair distribution; no lesions or masses BUS: No tenderness, redness, or discharge Hymen: Present in caruncles Labia: Pink, no lesions Introital tone: Good; no prolapses; no scars; perineum thick Vagina: Pink; discharge—small amount, thin, clean, nonodorous Cervix: Pink, nulliparous, firm, not tender, movable, midline Uterus: Pear shaped, movable, normal size, firm, no masses Tubes: Not palpable Ovaries: Palpable, movable, not tender, approximately $2 \times 3 \times 2$ cm; smooth surface, no lesions, firm consistency Rectovaginal septum: Thick and firm; no masses palpated in rectum or cul-de-sac

Worksheet for Documenting a Physical Examination

VITAL SIGNS

Temperature _____ Respiration _____ /min   BP (L) Arm (R)

_____ Supine _____

_____ Sitting _____

_____ Standing _____

Height _____ ft _____ in   Weight _____ lb (with or without clothes [circle])

GENERAL INSPECTION

SKIN, HAIR, NAILS, MUCOUS MEMBRANES

HEAD

Scalp _____

Face _____

(CNs V, VII) _____

_____

Sinus areas _____

Nodes _____

Cranium _____

EYES

Visual acuity _____

Visual fields _____

Ocular movements (CNs III, IV, VI) _____

Convergence _____

Lids, lacrimal organs _____

Conjunctiva, sclera _____

Cornea (CN V) _____

Lens and media _____

Pupils: Pupillary reflexes (CN III) _____

        Light, direct and consensual _____

        Accommodation _____

Fundi (CN II) _____

continued

Worksheet for Documenting a Physical Examination—cont'd

EARS

External structures _____

Canal _____

Tympanic membranes and landmarks _____

Hearing (CN VIII) _____

NOSE

External structure _____

Septum _____

Mucous membranes _____

Patency _____

Olfactory sense (CN I) _____

ORAL CAVITY

Lips _____

Buccal mucosa and ducts _____

Gums _____

Teeth _____

Palates and uvula (CNs IX, X) _____

Tonsillar areas _____

Tongue (CN XII) _____

Floor _____

Voice _____

Breath _____

Taste (CNs VII, IX) _____

NECK

General structure _____

Trachea _____

Thyroid _____

Nodes _____

Muscles (CN XI) _____

BREASTS AND AREA NODES (AXILLARY, SUPRACLAVICULAR, INFRACLAVICULAR)

Inspection _____

Palpation _____

CHEST, RESPIRATORY SYSTEM

Chest shape _____

Type of respiration _____

Expansion _____

Fremitus _____

General palpation _____

Worksheet for Documenting a Physical Examination—cont'd

Percussion _____

_____ Diaphragmatic excursion: (R) ___ cm (L) ___ cm

Breath sounds _____

_____

_____

Adventitious sounds _____

_____

CARDIOVASCULAR SYSTEM

Rate and rhythm: Radial (palpation) _____

Apical (auscultation) _____

Precordium: Inspection _____

Palpation _____

Auscultation _____

S_1 _____

S_2 _____

Other sounds _____

Murmur(s): Systolic _____

Distsolic _____

Carotid arteries _____

Jugular venous distention _____

_____

Description of peripheral pulses

Brachial	Radial	Femoral	Popliteal	Dorsal pedal	Post. tibial
R					
L					

ABDOMEN AND INGUINAL AREAS

Contour, tone _____

Scars, marks _____

Auscultation _____

_____

Liver _____ Span _____ cm at RMCL

Spleen _____

Kidneys _____ CVA tenderness _____

Bladder _____

Hernias _____

Masses _____

continued

Worksheet for Documenting a Physical Examination—cont'd

Palpation _____

_____

Percussion _____

_____

GENITALIA AND AREA NODES

_____

_____

_____

RECTAL EXAMINATION

MUSCULOSKELETAL SYSTEM
Gait _____

Upper extremities _____

Lower extremities _____

Deformities _____

Joint evaluation _____

_____

Muscle strength _____

_____

Muscle mass _____

Nodes _____

Range of motion _____
SPINE
Contour _____

Position _____

Motion _____

_____

NERVOUS SYSTEM
Mental status _____

Language _____

Cranial nerves (summarize) _____

Motor: Coordination: Upper extremities _____

Lower extremities _____

Involuntary movements _____

Worksheet for Documenting a Physical Examination—cont'd

DEEP TENDON REFLEXES:

NOTE: +s denote finger jerks, brachioradialis, biceps, triceps, reflexes, 4-quadrant abdominal scratch reflexes, patellar Achilles reflexes, and plantar reflexes. Abdominal reflexes are recorded as 0 or +. Scale: 0-4 (+ + + +); normal = 2 (+ +).

SENSORY

Light touch _____

Pain (pinprick) _____

Vibration _____

Position _____

chapter **24**

Pregnant Clients

■ PURPOSE OF EXAMINATION

This chapter focuses on the assessment of healthy pregnant women. It assumes and builds on knowledge of and skill in the physical examination of the adult client. The emphasis of this chapter is on the effects of the pregnant state on examination findings and the special techniques used to assess the health of the fetus and the woman's ability to deliver vaginally. To obtain complete information about the management of care for pregnant women, additional references are necessary.

■ PHYSICAL CHANGES IN PREGNANCY

A number of physical changes occur normally in pregnant women, many of which are noted in the physical assessment. All the physiological changes of pregnancy are directly or indirectly initiated by the hormones produced by the fetal chorionic tissues and the placenta. In early pregnancy the fetal trophoblast pro-

duces large amounts of human chorionic gonadotropic (HCG) hormone, which provides the basis for biological pregnancy testing. HCG is present in amounts detectable by immunological tests performed 8 to 10 days after conception.

Large amounts of estrogens and progesterone are produced during pregnancy. Estriol, an estrogen, is produced in large amounts during middle and late pregnancy. It is the basis for biological tests of placental and fetal well-being because a well-functioning placenta, a healthy fetus, and an intact fetal circulation are prerequisites for the continuous production of this hormone. The estrogens and progesterone maintain the decidua of pregnancy and cause the growth and hyperemia of the uterus, other pelvic organs, and the breasts.

In more than 50% of prenatal clients, the thyroid gland is symmetrically enlarged as a result of hyperplasia of glandular tissue, new follicle formation, and increased vascularity. The basal metabolic rate is increased, largely because of increased growth and oxygen consumption by the pregnant uterus, the fetus, and the placenta.

Reproductive System Changes

Changes in the uterus include the development of the decidua, hypertrophy of muscle cells, increased vascularity, formation of the lower uterine segment, and softening of the cervix. During pregnancy the overall size of the uterus increases five to six times, its weight increases about 20 times, and its capacity increases from approximately 2 to 5000 ml.

Hormones supply the initial stimulus for uterine hypertrophy. During the first 6 to 8 weeks of pregnancy, the uterus will increase in size whether the pregnancy is uterine or extrauterine. In early pregnancy the uterus is a pelvic organ and only internally palpable. At approximately 10 to 12 weeks' gestation, the growing uterus is double its nonpregnant size and reaches the top of the symphysis, where it is palpable abdominally. The uterine fundus lies approximately halfway between the symphysis and the umbilicus at about 16 weeks' gestation and reaches the umbilicus at about 20 to 22 weeks' gestation. After 20 weeks' gestation, the average upward growth of the uterus is about 3.75 cm per month (1 cm per week). At approximately 36 weeks' gestation, the uterus reaches the xiphisternum. In the last month of pregnancy, the fundus of the uterus may drop several centimeters if the fetal head descends deep into the pelvis.

The position of the uterus changes during gestation. In early gestation an exaggerated anteflexion is common. As the uterus ascends into the abdomen, a slight dextrorotation develops. In early pregnancy the uterus changes from a flattened pear shape to a globular shape. The globular shape continues until approximately 20 to 24 weeks, when a definite ovoid shape develops and continues until delivery.

At approximately 6 to 8 weeks' gestation, the uterine isthmus becomes softened and easily compressible, and the cervix, on palpation, seems almost detached from the uterine fundus. At about 8 weeks' gestation, the entire uterus softens.

During pregnancy the uterus contracts intermittently. Painless contractions, called Braxton-Hicks contractions, begin in early pregnancy and are first noted by the client and the examiner at about 24 weeks' gestation. These contractions can be stimulated by palpation of the uterus. If a contraction occurs during the abdominal examination, the examiner should wait until the contraction ends to continue palpation, and subsequently palpate more gently.

Three major changes occur in the cervix: (1) hypertrophy of the glands in the cervical canal, (2) softening of the cervix, and (3) bluish discoloration. These changes begin early in pregnancy—at about 6 weeks' gestation. Because of changes in the cervical epithelium, commonly a portion of the squamous epithelium is replaced by an outward extension of the columnar epithelium, producing an observable cervical ectropion or eversion of the cervical canal. This condition usually persists throughout pregnancy but disappears soon after the delivery.

The increase in pelvic vascularity causes a bluish discoloration of the cervix, vagina, and vulva at about 6 to 8 weeks' gestation. In addition, the vaginal mucosa thickens, the connective tissue becomes less dense, and the muscular areas hypertrophy. These changes are reflected in palpatory findings of softening and relaxation. The hypertrophied glands secrete more mucus. The total vaginal discharge is increased and more acidic than normal.

Breast Changes

Breast changes begin at about week 8 of pregnancy, with enlargement of the breasts. Shortly afterward the nipples become larger and more erectile, the areolae become more darkly pigmented, and the sebaceous glands (Montgomery's tubercles) in the areolae hypertrophy. Sometimes an irregular secondary areola develops, extending from the primary areola. Hypertrophy of the breasts often causes a slight tenderness. In women with well-developed axillary breast tissue, the hypertrophy may produce symptomatic lumps in the axillae. Colostrum can be expressed from the breast at about week 24 of pregnancy. The colostrum appears clear and yellowish at first but becomes cloudy later.

Stretching of the skin on the breast may produce striae gravidarum, and increased vascular supply may visibly engorge superficial breast veins.

Abdominal Area and Gastrointestinal System Changes

The muscles of the abdominal wall stretch to accommodate the growing uterus, and the umbilicus becomes flattened or protrudes. The rapid stretching of abdominal skin may cause the formation of striae gravidarum, which appear pink or red during pregnancy and become silvery white after delivery. In the third trimester of pregnancy, the rectus abdominis muscles are under considerable stress, and their tone is diminished. A wide permanent separation of these muscles, called diastasis recti abdominis, may occur. This condition allows the abdominal contents to protrude into the midline of the abdomen but requires no intervention.

In pregnancy, peristaltic activity is reduced, resulting in decreased bowel sounds. Smooth muscle relaxation, or atony, contributes to a variety of changes in gastrointestinal function. These changes include a high incidence of pregnancy-associated nausea and vomiting, heartburn, and constipation. In addition, the increased regional blood flow to the pelvis and venous pressure contribute to hemorrhoids, a source of discomfort in

late pregnancy. Nausea and vomiting usually do not persist beyond the third month, but heartburn, constipation, and hemorrhoids are more characteristic and troublesome in late pregnancy.

Less frequently noted gastrointestinal symptoms include ptyalism, or excessive salivation, and pica, a craving for substances of little or no food value. Pica is often an expression of the folkways of some cultural groups. It becomes a concern when it interferes with good nutrition.

The enlarging uterus displaces the colon laterally, upwardly, and posteriorly. Since this displacement changes the anatomical situation of the appendix, signs of appendicitis during pregnancy are not localized in McBurney's point of the right lower quadrant.

Skin, Mucous Membrane, and Hair Changes

The melanocytes in all portions of the skin are extremely active in pregnancy. There is a tendency toward generalized darkening of all skin, especially in skin that is hyperpigmented in the nonpregnant state. In some women a brownish-black pigmented streak may appear in the midline of the abdomen. This line of pigmentation is called the linea nigra. Some women develop a darkly pigmented configuration on the face that has been characteristically called the "mask of pregnancy," or chloasma. Scars and moles may also darken during pregnancy from the influence of melanocyte-stimulating hormone. Palmar erythema and spider nevi on the face and upper trunk also may accompany pregnancy.

Many pregnant women observe hypertrophy of the gums or epulis, resulting from hormonally induced, increased vascularity.

The hair of pregnant women may straighten and change in oiliness. Some women experience hair loss, especially in the frontal and parietal areas. Occasionally, increases in facial and abdominal hair, resulting from increased androgen and corticotropic hormone, are noted.

Cardiovascular System Changes

Many changes, too numerous to discuss adequately here, occur in the maternal circulatory system during pregnancy. However, several major changes that alter the physical examination findings are summarized as follows.

Blood volume is increased up to 45% and cardiac output is increased up to 30% in pregnancy, compared with the prepregnant state. Blood volume and cardiac output changes contribute to auscultatory changes that are common in pregnancy. Heart sounds are accentuated, and a low-grade systolic murmur (usually grade 2) is often noted.

As pregnancy advances, the heart is displaced upwardly and laterally. The apical impulse is displaced to a point 1 to 1.5 cm lateral to its location in the nonpregnant client. The pulse rate increases about 10 beats per minute from the prepregnancy rate, and palpitations may be noticed during pregnancy. The blood pressure is unchanged or may decrease in the second trimester.

A progesterone-induced generalized relaxation of the smooth muscle, arteriolar dilation, and increased capacity of the vascular compartment occur. The systolic blood pressure remains the same or is slightly lower during midpregnancy. There is no change in the venous pressure in the upper body, but the venous pressure increases in the lower extremities when the client is supine, sitting, or standing because of the pressure of the gravid uterus. This situation predisposes the woman to varicosities of the legs and the vulva, and to edema.

Respiratory System Changes

During pregnancy, the tidal volume increases and the respiratory rate increases slightly. Alveolar ventilation increases, and a more efficient exchange of lung gases occurs in the alveoli. Oxygen consumption rises by almost 20%, and plasma carbon dioxide content decreases.

As the uterus enlarges, it pushes the thoracic cage and diaphragm upward, and the thorax widens at the base. Physical assessment may reveal a change in respiration from abdominal to costal. In addition, dyspnea is a common complaint, especially in the last trimester, and deep respirations and sighing may be more frequent.

The tissue of the respiratory tract, sinuses, and nasopharynx manifests hyperemia and edema. This situation may contribute to engorgement of the turbinates, nasal stuffiness, and mouth breathing. Some women note increased nasal and sinus secretion and nosebleeds. Vocal cord edema may cause voice changes. Increased vascularity of the tympanic membranes and blockage of the eustachian tubes may contribute to decreased hearing, a sense of fullness in the ears, or earaches.

Musculoskeletal System Changes

The pelvic joints exhibit slight relaxation in pregnancy as a result of some unknown mechanism. This relaxation is maximal from about the seventh month onward. Because the gravid uterus has caused the pregnant client's weight to be thrust forward, the muscles of the spine are used to achieve a temporary new balance. The pregnant client throws her shoulders back and straightens her head and neck. The lower vertebral column is hyperextended (Figure 24.1).

The musculoskeletal changes are often reflected in postural and gait changes, lower backache, and fatigue. Often the pregnant woman's gait is described as waddling, and her balance is less stable from about week 24 onward.

figure**24.1** Posture of a pregnant woman.

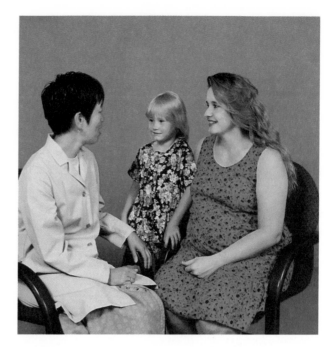

figure**24.2** Interview with a pregnant woman and another family member.

Urinary System Changes

A number of physiological changes occur during pregnancy, including a renal blood flow increased by as much as 50% and a glomerular filtration rate increased by up to 50% by the end of pregnancy. In addition, glucose reabsorption is decreased, resulting in glycosuria. The physical presence of the growing uterus causes displacement of the ureters and kidneys, especially on the right side. In the pelvis the growing uterus causes pressure on the bladder during the first and third trimesters, resulting in urinary frequency.

Neurological System Changes

Hypothalamic-pituitary neurohormonal changes occur during pregnancy. The interrelatedness of the body systems during pregnancy, combined with the major physical changes, makes it difficult to isolate exclusively neurological system changes. Alterations that may be primarily neurological in origin include headaches, and numbness and tingling of the hands. A complete summary of the physical changes that occur during pregnancy is provided in Table 24.1.

■ EXAMINATION

Prenatal Health History

A complete health history is an essential component of the initial visit for prenatal care (Figure 24.2). The structure of the health history is the same as that described for the adult client, with special attention given to the reproductive system and to the physical, social, and emotional readiness of the woman to incorporate a new child in her life.

The health history is important in pregnancy because information derived from it assists the practitioner in differentiating the client who is essentially normal and who will be expected to deliver a full-term, healthy baby from the high-risk expectant mother whose pregnancy is likely to affect her own or her fetus's health negatively. High-risk clients are given special care in most health care systems. The early identification of risk factors and their effective management enable the prenatal care to result in maximal benefit for the mother, family, and infant.

The health history for the obstetrical client follows the same basic protocol as that presented for all adults in Chapter 3. However, in prenatal care the following areas of history taking should receive special and complete attention:

Biographical information

1. Age
2. Race and/or ethnic background
3. Marital status and support network
4. Educational status

Sexual history

1. Pattern of sexual activity
2. Satisfaction with sexuality and sexual activity

table 24.1 *Summary of the Physical Changes of Pregnancy*

System or region	Summary of physiological and physical changes during pregnancy	System or region	Summary of physiological and physical changes during pregnancy
Skin and mucous membranes	Peripheral vascular vasodilation and increased numbers of capillaries result in increased blood flow, sweat, and sebaceous gland activity Increase in vascular spider veins and hemangiomas Thickening Fat is deposited in subdermal layers, especially on hips and buttocks Separations due to stretching Increased pigmentation of face, nipples, areolae, axillae, and vulva Palmar erythema Linea nigra Chloasma (mask of pregnancy) Gum hypertrophy		Increase in costal angle to about 100 degrees Increase in tidal volume Dyspnea
		Heart and blood vessels	Blood volume increases up to 45% Plasma volume increases 50% Splitting of S_1 and S_2 Loud S_1 S_3 may be heard Grade II systolic murmurs are commonly heard Diastolic murmurs are sometimes heard Increase in both thickness and mass of left ventricle Increase in stroke volume Cardiac output increases 30% Position of heart is shifted upward and to left Apex is rotated laterally—apex of heart is palpated more laterally than in nonpregnant state Vascular resistance decreases, and peripheral vasodilation occurs Varicose veins common in third trimester Increase in heart rate of 10 to 15 beats per minute Blood pressure may drop in second trimester
Thyroid	Slight enlargement—may be palpable Increased vascularity with possible bruit Increased T_4 and T_3 levels Decreased T_3 uptake Unchanged thyroid function		
Eyes	Mild corneal edema and thickening Fall in intraocular pressure Tears contain increase in lysozyme, resulting in blurred vision with contact lens wearing		
Ears, nose, and throat	Increased vascularity, resulting in symptoms of nasal stuffiness, decreased sense of smell, epistaxis, feeling of fullness in ears, and decreased hearing Increased vascularity and proliferation of gum tissue Laryngeal changes—hoarseness, voice changes, and cough	Breasts and axillae	Sensations of fullness, tingling, and tenderness Enlarge 2 to 3 times nonpregnancy size Expansion of ductal system and secretory alveoli; on palpation, breasts feel coarsely nodular Increase in glandular tissues displaces connective tissue; breasts become softer and looser Areolae become more deeply pigmented, and diameter increases Nipples become more prominent, darker, and more erectile Veins engorge and become more visible Colostrum is secreted Striae may appear
Respiratory system	Increase in thoracic transverse diameter of about 2 cm Rise in diaphragm up to 4 cm, compensated by increase in thoracic circumference of 5 to 7 cm		

table 24.1	*Summary of the Physical Changes of Pregnancy—cont'd*		
System or region	Summary of physiological and physical changes during pregnancy	System or region	Summary of physiological and physical changes during pregnancy
Abdomen	Loss of abdominal muscle tone Rectus abdominis muscles may separate (diastasis recti) Gastric motility decreases, resulting in delayed emptying time Esophageal reflux Bowel sounds are diminished Constipation, nausea, and vomiting are common Displacement of appendix Tendency to hemorrhoid formation Enlargement due to growing uterus and fetus Changes in bladder function and sensation	Anus and rectum	Decreased gastrointestinal tract tone and motility produce constipation Development of hemorrhoids is common
		Urinary system	Increased renal blood flow up to 50% in third trimester Increased glomerular filtration rate up to 50% Decreased reabsorption of glucose in renal tubules Displacement of ureters and kidneys Urinary frequency in first and third trimesters
Female genitalia	Uterine enlargement Softening of pelvic cartilage Strengthening of pelvic ligaments Pelvic congestion and edema Uterus, cervix, and isthmus soften, and cervix appears blue Thickening of mucosa of vaginal walls and connective tissue Smooth muscle cells hypertrophy Increased length of vaginal walls Vaginal secretions increase and have acidic pH	Musculoskeletal system	Increased mobility of sacroiliac, sacrococcygeal, and symphysis pubis joints Progressive lordosis in response to need to adjust to growing uterus
		Neurological system	Tension headaches Numbness and tingling of hands

3. Partners: Number and health
4. Contraception use

Past obstetrical history

1. Gravidity and parity: A five-number code with the abbreviation G-T-P-A-L is often used to summarize gravity and parity information.

   First digit = Total number of pregnancies, including current one (if applicable) (G)
   Second digit = Number of full-term births (T)
   Third digit = Number of preterm births (i.e., those between 21 and 37 weeks' gestation) (P)
   Fourth digit = Number of abortions (i.e., those terminated at or before 20 weeks' gestation (A)
   Fifth digit = Number of living children (L)
   Thus, for example, the gravidity/parity 5-2-1-1-3 indicates the following: the client is pregnant

for the fifth time; she has three living children, two of whom were delivered after full-term gestation and one of whom was premature; and she has had one abortion.

Alternate methods of indicating parity include two-digit, three-digit, and four-digit codes.

Two-digit codes: The first digit indicates gravidity, defined as the total number of pregnancies. The second digit represents parity, the number of live births (G-P). In the preceding example this code would be recorded as 5-3.
Three-digit codes: The first digit indicates gravidity, the second digit represents parity, and the third digit indicates abortions (G-P-A).
Four-digit codes: The first digit indicates gravidity, the second digit represents parity, the third digit indicates abortions, and the fourth digit

represents the number of living children (G-P-A-L).

NOTE: The term *nullipara* describes a woman who has not given birth to a viable offspring.

2. The following information is obtained for every past pregnancy:
   a. Date of delivery
   b. Duration of gestation
   c. Significant problems or complications
   d. Manner in which labor started, specifically whether labor was spontaneous or induced; if labor was induced, the reason for induction; if abortion, type (spontaneous [S], induced [I], or elective [E])
   e. Length of labor
   f. Complications of labor
   g. Presentation of infant at delivery
   h. Type of delivery: Vaginal or cesarean; if cesarean, the reason is noted
   i. Type of anesthesia used at delivery
   j. Condition of infant(s) at birth and birth weight
   k. Postpartum problems, especially infection, hemorrhage, and thrombophlebitis
   l. Problems such as jaundice, respiratory distress, infection, and congenital anomalies
   m. Type of infant feeding
   n. Current health of child

Present obstetrical history

1. Last normal menstrual period: An important task during the prenatal history is to estimate the expected date of confinement (EDC). Because the exact date of conception is unknown for the majority of prenatal clients, the EDC is calculated according to the first day of the last normal menstrual period (LNMP). The EDC is determined by counting backward 3 calendar months from the LNMP and adding 7 days (Nägele's rule). The year, of course, may change. For example, if the LNMP were 10-15-97, the EDC would be 7-22-98. If the client has a history of irregular menses, the EDC can be more accurately estimated by physical examination than by using the LNMP. Critical features that aid in determination or validation of the EDC are the date of quickening (when the mother first notices fetal movement, usually at about 18 weeks) and the time at which the fetal heart tones can be auscultated (at 10 to 12 weeks for a Doppler instrument and at 16 to 20 weeks for a fetoscope). Because of the variation that characterizes these events, ultrasonic measurement of fetal size and growth is being used more frequently to date pregnancy and assess fetal growth, along with measurement of the progressive enlargement of the uterus.

2. Symptoms of pregnancy
3. Feelings about pregnancy, especially determination of whether pregnancy was planned or unplanned
4. Bleeding since LNMP
5. Date when fetal movements were first felt
6. Fetal exposure to infections, radiation, and drugs (including oral contraceptives and spermacides)

Current and past medical gynecological history

1. Urinary tract infections
2. Sexually transmitted diseases
3. Bacterial and viral infections
4. Diabetes
5. Hypertension
6. Heart disease
7. Endocrine disorders
8. Anemia
9. Genital tract history, especially:
   a. Anomaly
   b. Cervical incompetence
   c. Myomas
   d. Contracted pelvis
   e. Ovarian mass
   f. Vaginal infections
   g. Surgery
   h. Abnormal Papanicolaou (Pap) test results
   i. Use of hormones (e.g., birth control pills)
   j. Menstrual history and functioning
   k. Endometriosis
10. Medication history: Over-the-counter and prescribed drugs
11. Current or past habitual use of alcohol, tobacco, mood-altering drugs or other nonprescribed drugs

Family and partner health history

Features of the family history that have special significance in pregnancy include diabetes, renal or hematological disorders, hypertension, multiple pregnancy, and congenital defects and retardation. It is important to know if the primigravida's mother had preeclampsia or high blood pressure during pregnancies, especially if she convulsed.

During pregnancy the health of the baby's father assumes special importance as a component of the health history. The following factors about the health and health history of the baby's father are especially important:

1. Current health and relationship
2. Blood type and Rh factor
3. History of potential inherited disorders
4. Use of tobacco, alcohol, and illicit drugs
5. Risk factors for sexually transmitted diseases

Emotional, psychological, and developmental status

Pregnancy is an important developmental event in a woman's life. The developmental tasks of pregnancy are incorporation of the fetus, differentiation of the fetus and mother, and, eventually, separation from the fetus. These tasks roughly coincide with the three trimesters of pregnancy.

During the first trimester of pregnancy, the gravida is involved with the process of accepting the fetus as a fact and a part of her body. Most women initially experience some ambivalence about their pregnancy and a resultant increase in anxiety. Many body changes occur that cause increased somatic awareness and inward focus. Relationships with key persons, especially the child's father and the gravida's mother, become especially important. Unresolved feelings and conflicts undergo reexamination. Feelings of dependency and vulnerability occur and can be additional causes of anxiety.

In the second trimester the fetus develops a separate identity. The gravida has had some time to become accustomed to her body changes and often feels better physically because the nausea has ceased. The fetus's movements are an important event, confirming the

RISK FACTORS / PRENATAL PROBLEMS

The following factors have been associated with increased morbidity and mortality of mothers and infants. The examiner should take special note of these factors during the health history interview and its recording.

HABITS
Smoking
Alcohol consumption
Drug addiction
Violent lifestyle

MATERNAL CHARACTERISTICS
Age—younger than 18 or older than 40
Poverty
Single status
Family disorganization
Conflict about pregnancy
Height less than 5 ft
Weight less than 100 lb
Inadequate diet
Low educational level

REPRODUCTIVE HISTORY
More than one previous abortion
Perinatal death
Infant weighing less than 2500 g
Infant weighing more than 4000 g
Infant with isoimmunization or ABO incompatibility
Infant with major congenital or perinatal disease
Uterine anomaly
Myomas
Ovarian masses
Sexually transmitted diseases

MEDICAL PROBLEMS
Hypertension
Renal disease
Diabetes mellitus

Heart disease
Sickle cell disease
Anemia
Pulmonary disease
Endocrine disorder

PRESENT PREGNANCY
Bleeding
Premature rupture of membranes
Anemia
No prenatal care
Preeclampsia or eclampsia
Hydramnios
Multiple pregnancy
Breech, transverse, or abnormal fetal position
Low or excessive weight gain
Hypertension (blood pressure greater than 140/90, a systolic increase of 30 mm Hg, or a diastolic increase of 15 mm Hg over baseline readings)
Abnormal fasting blood glucose level
Rh-negative sensitization
Exposure to teratogens
Viral infections
Sexually transmitted diseases
Bacterial infections
Protozoal infections
Postmaturity

A scoring system is useful in estimating the level or extent of risk for maternal or fetal illness or prematurity. Table 24.2 presents a tool for quantifying the risk of a prenatal client by using data collected through the history. Local populations may require adaptation of the content, the scoring mechanism, or the weighting of factors on this tool or any other tool selected. However, such a summarization of risk factors is usually helpful in the care of both individuals and a total clinic population.

table 24.2	*Rating Scale of Prenatal Risk Factors*

| | Factors | | | |
Score	Socioeconomic	Past history	Habits	Current pregnancy
1	Two children at home	First trimester abortion × 1 <1 year since last birth	Work outside home	Unusual fatigue
2	<20 years >40 years Single parent	First trimester abortion × 2	>10 cigarettes/day >6 cups coffee/day	<12 lb weight gain by 32 weeks Albuminuria Hypertension Bacteriuria
3	Low socioeconomic status Malnourished Less than 5 ft Less than 100 lb	First trimester abortion × 3	Unusual anxiety Heavy work Long, tiring trip Long commuting distance	Breech at 32 weeks Weight loss of 2 kg Head engaged before 34 weeks Febrile illness Leiomyomas
4	Less than 18 years	Pyelonephritis		Uterine bleeding after 12 weeks Effacement or dilation of cervix before 36 weeks Uterine irritability
5		Uterine anomaly Second trimester abortion Diethylstilbestrol (DES) exposure		Placenta previa Hydramnios
10		Premature delivery Repeated second trimester abortion		Twins Abdominal surgery

Modified from Zuspan FP, Quilligan EJ: *Practical manual of obstetric care,* St Louis, 1982, Mosby.
Total score is computed by adding the scores for the total set of factors present for given client. 0 to 5 points, minimal risk; 6 to 9 points, moderate risk; >10 points, high risk.

presence of the fetus and reminding the woman of the independence of the fetal movements from her control. The woman begins to think about the infant and their future. Worries about the possibility of producing an abnormal infant are common.

In the last trimester the gravida prepares for her separation from the fetus and her entrance into a new relationship with the newborn. This time is occupied with preparatory activities, such as attending parents' classes and buying clothing and equipment for the newborn. Concerns about labor and delivery and the physical discomforts of late pregnancy contribute to the woman's readiness for separation from the fetus and her movement toward the tasks of parenthood.

Social, economic, and cultural status

Because pregnancy and birth are important events in the development of any family and because the quality of the family affects the infant's health, the interviewer must assess the circumstances relating to the pregnancy and the family environment. The following are several important areas of exploration in the social history.

1. Client's desire for, and feelings about, this pregnancy
2. Feelings of significant others regarding this pregnancy
3. Client's personal and culturally derived health beliefs about pregnancy
4. Client's knowledge regarding pregnancy and parenting

5. Amount of support and assistance provided by family and significant others (including father of child and siblings)
6. Economic burdens imposed on client or family by pregnancy
7. Condition of the family's physical and emotional environment
8. Presence of physical abuse

General Physical Examination

A complete physical examination should be performed on the first prenatal visit because (1) the examination may reveal problems that need special or immediate attention, and (2) initial data provide the baseline against which changes that occur later in pregnancy can be compared. The initial general physical examination of the prenatal client is the same as for other clients, except for special emphasis on the diagnosis of pregnancy, the assessment of pelvic adequacy, and the assessment of fetal growth and well-being.

Several signs unrelated to the reproductive system may be normally altered in pregnancy. Such alterations of physical findings are listed in the box at right.

Diagnosis of Pregnancy

The diagnosis of pregnancy takes into account both the history of subjective symptoms noticed by the client and the objective signs noted by the examiner. In addition, laboratory tests are especially helpful in confirming early pregnancy.

Traditionally, the signs and symptoms of pregnancy have been categorized as (1) presumptive symptoms, (2) probable signs, and (3) positive signs. Presumptive symptoms are those concerns that the prenatal client identifies in the present illness and chief complaint portions of the history, as well as several additional general physical signs. They include the subjective data that may have led the client to seek confirmation of pregnancy. *Presumptive symptoms* include (1) absence of menses 10 or more days after the expected date of onset; (2) morning sickness, nausea, or appetite change; (3) frequent urination; (4) soreness or a tingling sensation in the breasts; (5) Braxton Hicks contractions; (6) quickening; (7) abdominal enlargement; and (8) bluish discoloration of the vagina.

The following are *probable signs* of pregnancy: (1) progressive enlargement of the uterus; (2) softening of the uterine isthmus (Hegar's sign); (3) asymmetrical, soft enlargement of one uterine cornu (Piskacek's sign); (4) bluish or cyanotic color of the cervix and upper vagina (Chadwick's sign); (5) softening of the cervix (Goodell's sign); (6) internal ballottement; (7) palpation of fetal parts; and (8) positive test results for HCG in urine or serum. These signs are termed "probable" because clinical conditions other than pregnancy can

---

Physical Findings Altered in Pregnancy

RESPIRATORY SYSTEM
Change in breathing from abdominal to costal
Shortening and widening at base of thoracic cage
Elevation of diaphragm
Increase in respiratory rate

CARDIOVASCULAR SYSTEM
Displacement of apical impulse laterally 1 to 1.5 cm
Grade 2 systolic murmur
Increase in pulse rate
Slight fall in blood pressure in second trimester

MUSCULOSKELETAL SYSTEM
Slight instability of pelvis
Alteration of standing posture and gait to compensate for gravid uterus

ABDOMINAL REGION
Contour changes because of gravid uterus
Striae gravidarum
Decrease in muscle tone
Linea nigra
Reduced peristaltic activity

SKIN AND MUCOUS MEMBRANES
Chloasma
Linea nigra
Hyperpigmentation of skin and bony prominences
Palmar erythema
Spider nevi on face and upper trunk
Striae gravidarum on breasts and abdomen
Gum hypertrophy

BREASTS
Enlargement
Large, erect nipples
Darkening of areolar pigment
Development of secondary areola
Hypertrophy of sebaceous glands in areola
Formation of colostrum
Tenderness on palpation
Striae gravidarum
Engorgement of superficial veins

OTHER ALTERATIONS
Straightening of hair
Loss of hair over frontal and parietal regions
Enlarged thyroid

---

cause any of them. However, if they occur together, a strong case can be made for pregnancy.

The *positive signs* of pregnancy are those that prove the presence of a fetus: (1) documentation of a fetal heartbeat by auscultation, electrocardiogram, or Doppler instrument; (2) palpation of active fetal movements; and

(3) radiological or ultrasonographic demonstration of fetal parts. Ultrasonographic techniques can demonstrate the presence of a gestational sac as early as 6 weeks' gestation. Doppler instruments can detect a fetal heartbeat as early as 10 to 12 weeks' gestation.

Currently, clinical diagnosis of pregnancy is made by using laboratory tests in conjunction with the probable signs of pregnancy. Technology and marketing have made available reliable, low-cost home and in-clinic pregnancy tests that, in conjunction with clinical findings, can confirm the diagnosis of pregnancy early in the first trimester. The commonly used immunological pregnancy tests are the hemagglutination inhibition test and the latex agglutination test. These tests depend on an antigen-antibody reaction between HCG and an antiserum obtained from rabbits immunized against this antigen. These tests are available for use by both health professionals and laypersons and are very sensitive. Most commercial tests use standardized anti-HCG rabbit serum and dead cells or standardized latex particles coated with HCG. Anti-HCG serum is mixed first with a sample of the client's urine; then HCG-coated red blood cells or particles are added. The lack of agglutination is a positive test because urine that contains HCG has neutralized the HCG antibodies. If the urine sample contains no HCG, agglutination occurs, indicating a negative test for pregnancy.

Pregnancy tests based on the presence of HCG in the urine can be reliably performed from 2 days after the first missed menses through 16 weeks' gestation. During this time the production of HCG is at its peak. Currently, home pregnancy testing is widely available to women and is becoming a common method of self-assessment. Home pregnancy tests vary in accuracy and instructions. Although the techniques are relatively simple and straightforward, mistakes are possible, and a

Laboratory Tests

In addition to the appropriate tests for relevant risk factors, the following laboratory tests are characteristically included in the initial prenatal assessment:

> Complete blood count
> Blood type and Rh identification
> General antibody screening test
> VDRL (Veneral Disease Research Laboratory) test
> Rubella titer
> Clean-catch urinalysis for glucose, albumin, and ketones and a microscopic examination
> Papanicolaou (Pap) smear
> Cervical smear for gonorrhea

The following additional tests are done as indicated for high-risk groups:

> Cervical smear for *Chlamydia trachomatis*
> Tine test for PPD (purified protein derivative) for tuberculosis
> Antibody screening for *Toxoplasma gondii,* cytomegalovirus, herpes simplex virus, human immunodeficiency virus (HIV), and hepatitis B surface antigen
> Hemoglobin electrophoresis for all black women

At 24 to 28 weeks' gestation, the following tests are often done:

> Repeat hemoglobin and hematocrit
> Repeat antibody screen
> Serum glucose screen and a mini–glucose tolerance test that consists of a fasting reading and a 1-hour glucose determination after a 50-g load

At 32 to 36 weeks' gestation, the following tests are often repeated:

> Hemoglobin and hematocrit
> VDRL
> Cervical smear for gonorrhea

PREPARATION FOR EXAMINATION

EQUIPMENT

In addition to all the equipment needed for a comprehensive physical examination that includes a pelvic examination, the following items are needed for the prenatal physical examination.

Item	Purpose
Long measuring tape	To assess growth of uterus
Doppler instrument or fetoscope	To auscultate fetal heart tones

CLIENT AND THE ENVIRONMENT

1. Provide a warm, private room.
2. Make sure that the client is adequately gowned and draped throughout the examination.
3. Help the client to assume various positions throughout the examination, as required by the assessment techniques.
4. Avoid allowing the client to lie on her back for extended periods because of the negative effects of the gravid uterus on the abdominal organs, the vessels, and the back. The most comfortable back-lying position is with the head elevated to about 45 degrees (Figure 24.3) and the knees slightly bent.

careful clinical assessment is always an important component of the diagnosis of pregnancy.

Several early clinical findings are used in conjunction with laboratory tests to diagnose pregnancy. In pregnancy, a pelvic examination done approximately 6 to 8 weeks after the last normal menses shows uterine enlargement. The uterus first enlarges in the pelvis. By 12 weeks' gestation, the examiner can palpate the uterus abdominally just above the symphysis pubis. In addition to enlarging, the uterus becomes globular and then ovoid.

The uterus softens during pregnancy because of its increased vascularity. The isthmus of the uterus is the first part to soften. At about 6 to 8 weeks' gestation, the softened isthmus produces a dramatic palpatory finding. On palpation, the enlarged globular uterus feels almost detached from the cervix, which is still not completely softened, because the isthmus feels so indistinct (Figure 24.4). This phenomenon is called Hegar's sign. By 7 or 8 weeks' gestation, the cervix and the uterus can be easily flexed at their junction (McDonald's sign). Speculum examination shows cyanosis of the cervix as early as 6 to 8 weeks' gestation, a change that results from the increased vascularity in the area.

Often, uterine enlargement does not progress symmetrically. Rather, the area of placental development enlarges more rapidly. This imbalance produces a palpatory asymmetrical enlargement of one uterine cornu, called Piskacek's sign (Figure 24.5).

The timetable for physical signs of pregnancy is presented in Table 24.3. This table also includes an outline of fetal development during pregnancy.

Technique for Examination and Normal Findings

Prenatal assessments include examination of both the mother and the developing fetus. After the initial assessment, examinations of the prenatal client are done at regular intervals. Reexamination schedules vary among clients. However, a common schedule includes examinations done approximately every 3 to 4 weeks during the first 28 weeks of pregnancy, then every 2 to 3 weeks until 36 weeks, and weekly thereafter.

figure**24.4** Hegar's sign: softening of the lower uterine segment.

figure**24.3** Elevation of the head and shoulders for a prenatal examination.

figure**24.5** Piskacek's sign: asymmetrical enlargement of the uterine fundus.

table 24.3 *Physical Signs of Pregnancy and Corresponding Stage of Fetal Development*

Sign	Approximate gestation (weeks since last menses)		Fetal development
Amenorrhea	2	0-4	Fertilization occurs Blastocyst implants Placental circulation established Organogenesis initiated Development of nervous system and vital organs initiated Anatomical structures and systems are in rudimentary form Size: 0.25 in by fourth week
Softening of cervix (Goodell's sign)	4-6		
Softening of cervicouterine junction (Ladin's sign)	5-6	5-8	All major organs in rudimentary form Fingers are present
Gestational sac may be noted by ultra-sonography	6		Ears and eyes are formed Heart complete and functioning
Compressibility of lower uterine segment (Hegar's sign)	6-8		Development of muscles is initiated Size: 1.25 in by eighth week
Dilation of breast veins			
Pulsation of uterine arteries in lateral fornices (Oslander's sign)			
Flexing of fundus of cervix (McDonald's sign)	7-8		
Asymmetrical softening and enlarging of uterus (Piskacek's sign)			
Uterus changes from pear to globular shape			
Bluish coloration of vagina and cervix (Chadwick's sign)	8-12	9-12	Organs forming and growing Swallowing and sucking reflexes present
Detection of fetal heartbeat with a Doppler instrument	10-12		Body movements increase Size: 3 in, 0.5 oz by 12th week
Uterus palpable just above symphysis pubis	12	13-16	Circulatory system established
Ballottement of fetus possible by abdominal and vaginal examination	16		Size: 6 in, 4 oz by 16th week
Uterus palpable halfway between symphysis and umbilicus			
Fetal movements noted by mother (quickening)	16-20	17-20	Rapid growth Size: 8 in, 8 ounces by 20th week
Pigment change may occur			
Uterine fundus at lower border of umbilicus	20	21-24	Meconium present in intestines
Fetal heartbeat auscultated with fetoscope			Size: 11 in, 1-1.5 lb by 24th week
Fetus palpable	24		
Mother begins to notice Braxton Hicks contractions	24-26	25-28	Nervous system can control breathing and temperature
Uterus changes from globular to ovoid shape			Size: 12 in, 2-3 lb by 28th week
Fetus easily palpable, very mobile, and may be found in any lie, presentation, or position	28	29-32	Fat deposits under skin Size: 13 in, 3-5 lb by 32nd week
Uterus is approximately half the distance from umbilicus to xiphoid			

table 24.3	*Physical Signs of Pregnancy and Corresponding Stage of Fetal Development—cont'd*		
Sign	Approximate gestation (weeks since last menses)		Fetal development
Fetus usually lies longitudinally with a vertex presentation	32	33-36	Primitive reflexes are present Size: 14 in, 5-6 lb by 36th week
Uterine fundus is approximately two thirds the distance between umbilicus and xiphoid			
Uterine fundus is just below xiphoid	34		
Vertex presentation may engage in pelvis	36-40	37-40	Less active because of crowding Size: 19-21 in, 6-8 lb by 40th week

At each prenatal revisit, the examiner usually assesses the following:

1. Interval history
2. Weight gain
3. Blood pressure
4. Urine for glucose, albumin, and ketones
5. Legs for edema
6. Abdomen
   a. Determination of uterine growth
   b. Determination of fetal presentation and position (beginning at 28 weeks and continuing to full term)
   c. Measurement of fetal heart rate

Interval history

At each visit, it is important to ask the client about new symptoms and signs and to update information about any health problems or issues noted in the initial history. Sometimes flow sheets with common signs and symptoms are used to facilitate documentation. Commonly reviewed areas include the presence and character of fetal movements, vaginal discharge or bleeding, cramps, pelvic pressure, and signs and symptoms of urinary tract infection.

Weight gain

At term, the infant, uterine contents, and other changes in the body account for approximately 20 pounds of weight. Optimal weight gain during pregnancy, based on the lowest rate of complications and optimal birth weight of infants, is 24 to 27.5 pounds (a wider range is 20 to 30 pounds). High prepregnancy weight correlates significantly with an increased risk of preeclampsia. Women with a low prepregnancy weight who gain little weight during pregnancy are more likely to have low-birth-weight infants (i.e., infants weighing 2500 g or less). Sudden weight gain, especially in the third trimester, usually indicates fluid retention, and this change should be evaluated in conjunction with maternal blood pressure. Apart from this transient cause of weight gain, many women tend to add to their body fat stores during pregnancy, and this weight gain may not be entirely lost after delivery. The gain in weight should occur gradually, averaging 1½ to 2 pounds per month during the first 24 weeks and ½ to 1 pound a week during the remainder of pregnancy.

Blood pressure

Mean systolic blood pressure and mean diastolic blood pressure are essentially unchanged during pregnancy, except for a mild and transient decrease during the middle trimester in a normal pregnancy. Hypertension, however, contributes significantly to prenatal morbidity and mortality, and pregnancy-induced hypertension is a disease peculiar to pregnancy. This disorder typically develops after week 24 of pregnancy and is characterized by some combination of the following factors:

1. Systolic blood pressure of at least 140 mm Hg or a rise of 30 mm Hg or more above the usual level in two readings done 6 hours apart
2. Diastolic pressure of 90 mm Hg or more or a rise of 15 mm Hg above the usual level in two readings done 6 hours apart
3. Proteinuria
4. Edema of the face or hands
5. Excessive weight gain (≥2.5 pounds per week)
6. Hyperreflexia

Assessment of edema and extremities

Ankle swelling and edema of the lower extremities occur in two thirds of women during late pregnancy. Women notice this swelling late in the day after they have been standing for some time. Sodium and water retention caused by steroid hormones, an increased hy-

drophilic property of intracellular connective tissue, and increased venous pressure in the lower extremities during pregnancy contribute to this edema. Assessment includes palpation of the ankles and pretibial areas to determine the extent of the edema and observation for hand, face, or generalized edema. Generalized edema may be manifested by pitting in the sacral area or by the appearance of a depression on the gravid abdomen from the rim of the fetoscope after it has been pressed against the abdomen to auscultate the fetal heart rate.

In addition to assessment for edema formation, examination of the legs includes inspection for varicose veins and dorsiflexion of the foot with the legs extended to check for Homans' sign and thrombophlebitis. In the presence of an elevated or a borderline elevated blood pressure, deep tendon reflexes should be assessed. Hyperreflexia and clonus, combined with other signs, may indicate preeclampsia.

Leg cramps during pregnancy may accompany extension of the foot and sudden shortening of leg muscles. This cramping may be caused by an elevation of serum phosphorus with a diet that includes a large quantity of milk.

Many discomforts and sensations in the legs result from compression of nerves caused by the pressure of the enlarging uterus. These include numbness in the lateral femoral area resulting from compression of that nerve beneath the inguinal ligament. Medial thigh sensation may result from the compression of the obturator nerve against the side walls of the pelvis. Periodic numbness of the fingers occurs in at least 5% of gravidas. This is apparently caused by a brachial plexus traction syndrome from drooping shoulders. Drooping is associated with the increased weight of the breasts as pregnancy advances. Finger movement may be impaired by compression of the median nerve in the arm and hand caused by physiological changes in the fascia, tendons, and connective tissue during pregnancy. This impairment, known as carpal tunnel syndrome, is characterized by a paroxysm of pain, numbness, tingling, or burning in the sides of the hands and fingers—particularly the thumb, second, and third fingers and the side of the fifth finger.

Abdominal examination

As pregnancy progresses, the uterus enlarges steadily. The height of the uterine fundus serves as a rough guide to fetal gestation and overall fetal growth. Figure 24.6 shows the expected fundal height at various gestational ages. At week 12 of pregnancy, the fundus is palpable just above the symphysis. At 16 weeks, the fundus is approximately halfway between the symphysis and the umbilicus. At week 20, the fundus usually reaches the lower border of the umbilicus. After week 20, the uterus increases in height by approximately 3.75 cm per month

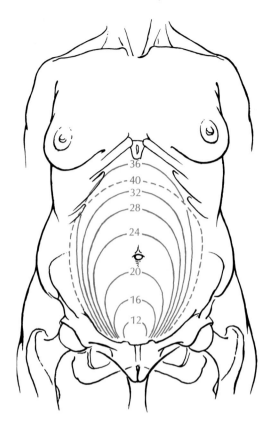

figure**24.6** Approximate levels of the uterine fundus at various gestational points. Numbers indicate weeks of gestation.

(or about 1 cm per week) until weeks 34 to 36, when the fundus almost reaches the xiphoid. Then, in approximately 65% of gravidas, the fetal head drops further into the pelvis with "lightening." If this occurs, the fundal measurement at 36 weeks may be greater than that noted later in pregnancy. These benchmarks are averages, and it should be noted that the length of the torso and the position of the umbilicus are highly variable among clients. In prenatal assessment, the client serves as her own control for assessment of adequate progress of fundal growth.

Unless the fetal head drops into the pelvis, the fundal height between weeks 37 and 40 will stay approximately the same. During this period, the fetus is growing, but the amount of amniotic fluid decreases.

The abdominal examination consists of the following components:

1. Inspection
2. Measurement of fundal height
3. Assessment of fetal position
   a. Fundal palpation
   b. Lateral palpation
   c. Pawlik's palpation
   d. Deep pelvic palpation
4. Auscultation

figure **24.7** Palpation to determine the height of the uterine fundus.

Inspection. In addition to the observations that are made during assessment of the abdomen (e.g., skin and scars), for the pregnant client the examiner observes the size and configuration of the enlarging uterus.

Normally, the uterine size should relate to the estimated gestational age. Any discrepancy between observed size and estimated gestational age requires further exploration. A uterus larger than expected may indicate incorrect gestational age estimation, multiple pregnancy, or polyhydramnios. A smaller uterus may indicate a poorly growing fetus or gestational miscalculation.

Observation of the abdomen may provide the first clue to fetal presentation and position. An asymmetrical appearance or distention in width versus longitudinal enlargement may suggest a transverse or oblique fetal lie that palpation can verify. After approximately week 28, fetal movements may be seen.

Measurement of fundal height. Measurement of the height of the fundus provides a general assessment of the development of the pregnancy. Therefore such measurements should be taken at each prenatal visit. Before the fundal measurement is done, calculate the estimated gestational age based on the last normal menstrual period, and use the estimate of age as a benchmark against which fundal growth is assessed. Between 20 and 31 weeks' gestation, the fundal height in centimeters is approximately equal to the gestational age in weeks. In general, a 1-cm increase per week is a normal pattern.

The procedure for measuring the fundal height is as follows:

1. Determine the top of the fundus (Figure 24.7).
   a. Stand at the right side of the supine client, facing her head.
   b. Place your hands on each lateral side of the uterus midway between the symphysis and the fundus.
   c. Move the uterus from side to side between your hands with gentle pressure.
   d. Palpate up the sides of the uterus to the fundus, being sure to stay on the sides of the uterus.
   e. As you come near the fundus, your hands will come together, meeting at the top of the fundus.
2. Measure the distance to the fundal edge from the upper border of the symphysis with a measuring tape. Place the zero point of the tape at the top of the symphysis and measure the distance to the top of the fundus (Figure 24.8).
3. When the fundus is below the umbilicus, record the measurement in centimeters above the symphysis (preferable) or below the umbilicus. When the measurement is above the umbilicus, record the measurement in centimeters above the symphysis.

The measurement of fundal height is approximate, and estimates of fundal height measurement may vary 1 to 2 cm among examiners. However, measurement, if done consistently by one examiner or a team of examiners within a clinical situation, should provide an excellent picture of fetal growth with each visit. If fundal height is <4 cm less than expected, additional assessments of menstrual history or fetal status are indicated.

figure**24.8**   Measurement of fundal height.

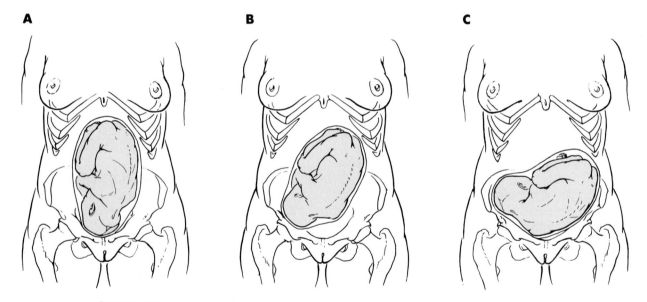

figure**24.9**   Examples of fetal lie. **A,** Longitudinal lie. **B,** Oblique lie. **C,** Transverse lie.

Assessment of fetal position. Next, palpate the abdomen to determine fetal lie, presentation, position, attitude, and size.

The lie is the relationship of the long axis of the fetus to the long axis of the uterus. The lie can be longitudinal, oblique, or transverse (Figure 24.9).

The presentation of the fetus is that fetal part that is most dependent. The presentation can be vertex, brow, face, shoulder, or breech (Figure 24.10).

The position is the relationship of a specified part of the fetal presentation, the denominator, to a particular part of the maternal pelvis (Figure 24.11). The denominator in a vertex presentation is the occiput (O); in a breech presentation, it is the sacrum (S); in a face presentation, it is the mentum (M), or chin; in a brow presentation, it is the frontum (F); and in a transverse lie presentation, it is the scapula (S). The position is standardly abbreviated according to the left or right of the

figure**24.10** Examples of fetal presentation. **A, Vertex. B,** Brow. **C,** Face. **D,** Shoulder. **E,** Breech.

LOA   LOT   LOP

figure**24.11** Examples of fetal position.

figure**24.12** Fetal attitude. **A,** Fully flexed. **B,** Poorly flexed. **C,** Extended.

figure**24.13** Engagement. Both the biparietal and suboccipitobregmatic diameters of the fetal head have passed into the inlet of the pelvis.

pelvis, the denominator, and the pelvic portion as follows:

Side of pelvis	Denominator	Pelvic portion
L = Left	O = Occiput	A = Anterior
R = Right	S = Sacrum	P = Posterior
	M = Mentum	T = Transverse
	F = Frontum	
	S = Scapula	

For example, if the occiput were presenting closest to the left anterior portion of the pelvis, the fetal position would be LOA.

The fetal attitude is the relationship of the fetal head and limbs to its body (Figure 24.12). The fetus may be fully flexed, poorly flexed, or extended. When the fetus is fully flexed, the spine is flexed, the head is flexed on the chest, and the arms and legs are crossed over the chest and abdomen.

Engagement occurs when both the biparietal diame-ter and the suboccipitobregmatic diameter of the fetal head (the smallest anteroposterior diameter of the head when it is well flexed during labor) pass into the inlet of the pelvis (Figure 24.13). When this occurs, the fetal head can be felt at the level of the ischial spines on vaginal palpation.

Abdominal palpation determines fetal lie, presentation, position, attitude, and size. Systematically palpate the abdomen using Leopold's maneuvers in the four sequential steps as follows:

1. Fundal palpation
2. Lateral palpation
3. Pawlik's palpation
4. Deep pelvic palpation

Leopold's maneuvers are usually not especially productive until 26 to 28 weeks' gestation, when the fetus is large enough for its parts to be differentiated through abdominal and uterine structures.

HELPFUL HINT	*In doing Leopold's maneuvers:*

In doing Leopold's maneuvers:
- *Use the palmar surface of the fingers for palpating.*
- *Keep the fingers of the hand together.*
- *Apply firm, smooth, steady pressure as necessary to determine needed information.*
- *Avoid jabbing or poking movements.*
- *If uterine contraction occurs, wait for it to pass and then palpate less strongly.*
- *Have the client bend the knees to facilitate her comfort.*
- *Review findings with the client and teach her to recognize the fetal parts.*

For this examination the client is supine. Elevating the client's head and shoulders and bending the knees may assist in decreasing tension of the abdominal muscles and in making the examination more comfortable for the client.

Fundal palpation

1. Stand at the client's right side, facing her head.
2. Place the palmar surface of both hands on the uterine fundus to determine what part of the fetus is occupying the fundus (Figure 24.14).

Usually the buttocks of the fetus are in the fundus; they are felt as a soft, irregular, and slightly movable mass. The lower limbs are felt adjacent to the buttocks. If the head is in the fundus, it is felt as smooth, round, hard, and ballottable. The groove of the neck is felt between the trunk and the upper limbs. The head is freely movable in contrast to the buttocks, which can move only sideways and with the trunk.

Lateral palpation (Figure 24.15)

1. While you are still facing the client's head, move both of your hands to either side of the uterus to determine the side on which the fetal back is located.
2. Support the fetus with one hand on one side while the other hand palpates the fetus on the other side.
3. Then reverse the procedure to palpate each side of the uterus.

The fetal back is felt as a continuous, smooth, firm object, whereas the fetal limbs, or small parts, are felt as small, irregular, sometimes moving objects. On each side, palpate the flank to the midline, making special note of the edge of the fetal back as a landmark in determining the fetal position.

figure**24.14** Palpation to determine the contents of the uterine fundus.

figure**24.15** Palpation of the lateral uterine fundus to determine the position of the back and extremities of the fetus.

Pawlik's palpation

1. Perform this procedure with the right hand only to determine what fetal part lies over the pelvic inlet. Place the right hand over the symphysis so that the fingers are on the left side of the uterus and the thumb is on the right side (Figure 24.16). The hand should be approximately around the fetal presenting part, usually the head.
2. Palpate the presenting part gently to determine its form and consistency.
3. Grasp and gently move the presenting part sideways back and forth between the thumb and fingers several times to determine its movability.

This palpation is done to confirm impressions about the presenting part and to determine if the presenting part (usually the fetal head) is engaged. If the fetal head is movable above the symphysis, it is not engaged. If the head is not movable, it may be engaged. The only method of confirming engagement is pelvic examination to determine if the biparietal diameter of the fetal head is level with the ischial spines.

Deep pelvic palpation

1. Change position (Figure 24.17). Remain on the client's right side but turn and face her feet.
2. Place a hand on each side of the uterus near the pelvic brim.
3. Ask the client to take a deep breath and to exhale slowly. As she does, allow your fingers to sink deeply above the pubic bones to palpate the presenting part and to determine the location of the cephalic prominence.

figure**24.16** Pawlik's palpation to determine the fetal presenting part.

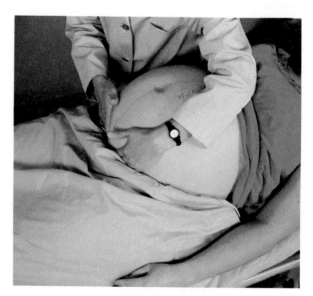

figure**24.17** Deep pelvic palpation to determine the fetal attitude and descent.

If the presenting part is the head, the location of the cephalic prominence (the forehead) helps determine the fetus's position and attitude. If the head is flexed, the occiput lies deeper in the pelvis, is flatter, and is less defined than the forehead, which is more prominent and on the same side as the small parts. If the head is not well flexed, the cephalic and occipital prominences are palpated at the same level, and the occipital portion, on the same side as the back, may be more prominent.

Throughout these maneuvers, assess the congruence of the size of the fetus with the gestational age.

Following is a series of questions that you, as the examiner, should mentally ask about each client during abdominal assessment and an indication of the procedures that assist in answering the questions.

Question	Source of evidence to answer question
What is the fetal lie?	Abdominal inspection
	Lateral abdominal palpation
What is the fetal presentation?	Fundal palpation
	Pawlik's palpation
	Deep pelvic palpation
What is the fetal position?	Lateral palpation
	Deep pelvic palpation
What is the fetal attitude?	Deep pelvic palpation
Is the fetal growth congruent with gestational age?	Fundal height measurement
	All Leopold's maneuvers

Auscultation The fetal heart rate is an indicator of fetal health status and requires monitoring throughout pregnancy. Auscultate the fetal heart rate with a special stethoscope called a fetoscope or a Doppler instrument. The Doppler instrument can be used to monitor the fetal heart rate after about 10 to 12 weeks' gestation as the fundus rises beyond the symphysis pubis. If you do not hear fetal heartbeats by Doppler monitoring after 12 to 14 weeks, reevaluate the gestational age estimate or fetal status. With a fetoscope, the fetal heart rate can first be heard between 16 and 20 weeks' gestation.

Use of the fetoscope is demonstrated in Figure 24.18. The fetal heart rate is rapid and soft. Use of a fetoscope avoids noises produced by fingers on the stethoscope and takes advantage of the benefits of both air and bone conduction. The bell of an ordinary stethoscope can be used to auscultate fetal heart tones, but it is less effective than a fetoscope in transmitting fetal heartbeats, especially around 20 weeks.

The fetal heart rate is normally between 120 and 160 beats per minute, and the heartbeats resemble the sound of a watch's ticking heard through a pillow. These sounds are best heard through the fetal back. When the fetus is large enough for its position to be determined, place the bell of the fetoscope or the Doppler head on the fetus's posterior thorax. When the fetus is

figure**24.18** Use of a fetoscope to auscultate the fetal heart. NOTE: The hand on the bell of the fetoscope is used to adjust it. When the fetal heartbeats are actually being measured, the hand should be removed.

less than 20 weeks' gestation, the heart rate is often best heard at the midline, just above the pubic hairline.

Count the fetal heart rate for at least 15 seconds, and record it in number of beats per minute according to the location of maximal intensity (by the abdominal quadrant in which it is most prominent). The fetal heart rate is normally much faster than the maternal heart rate, and therefore it can usually be well differentiated from it. Moreover, the fetal and maternal heart rates are not synchronous. Differentiate the maternal rate by palpating the mother's pulse while auscultating the abdomen.

Sounds other than the maternal and fetal heart tones can be heard in the uterus. Blood rushing through the placenta is called uterine souffle. The uterine souffle is a soft, blowing sound that is synchronous with the maternal pulse. The intensity of the souffle has been interpreted as an indicator of uterine blood flow and placental function. A loud uterine souffle has been associated with high levels of urinary estriol and a soft or absent souffle with lower estriol levels. Thus a soft or absent uterine souffle may indicate poor uterine blood flow and placental function, particularly in late pregnancy. Occasionally the blood flow in the umbilical artery can be auscultated. The sound is similar to a bruit and, as a rule, the rate is equal to the fetal heart tones. However, the sound does not have distinct heart sounds; rather it is similar to the uterine souffle. ■

The following steps outline interval abdominal assessment for the pregnant client:
1. Measure fundal height.
2. Palpate the abdomen to determine fetal position using Leopold's maneuvers:
   a. Fundal palpation
   b. Lateral palpation
   c. Pawlik's palpation
   d. Deep pelvic palpation
3. Auscultate fetal heart tones.

Examination of the Bony Pelvis

The purpose of the examination of the bony pelvis is to determine if the pelvic cavity is large enough to allow for passage of a full-term infant (term infant). Clinical pelvimetry is a gross estimate of the adequacy of the pelvis for delivery of a fetus. It is not uncommon for clients whose pelves have been assessed to be of borderline adequacy to deliver full-term infants vaginally. If the clinical assessment in early pregnancy indicates a possible inadequacy, the pelvis needs to be reassessed clinically and possibly by x-ray examination in late pregnancy and in relationship to the size of the infant at term. This examination is performed on the initial prenatal evaluation; it need not be repeated if the pelvis is of adequate size. However, if findings indicate that the pelvis is of borderline adequacy, or if you are unable to adequately perform the examination on the initial visit because of the client's tenseness and subsequent muscular contraction, repeat the examination at approximately 36 weeks' gestation. In the third trimester, the pelvic joints and ligaments relax, and the client is more accustomed to examination. Thus you can more thoroughly and accurately accomplish examination of the bony pelvis at that time.

The examination of the bony pelvis is done not so much to diagnose the type of pelvis but to determine its configuration and size. Because the examiner does not have direct access to the bony structures and because the bones are covered with variable amounts of soft tissue, estimates are approximate. X-ray examination can provide precise bony pelvis measurements. However, x-rays are not needed or indicated for the vast majority of prenatal clients.

The assessment of the bony pelvis must be put in the perspective of the capacity necessary to accommodate a full-term fetus. When the head of a full-term fetus is well flexed, the two largest presenting diameters are the biparietal and the suboccipitobregmatic, each measuring approximately 9.5 cm (Figure 24.19).

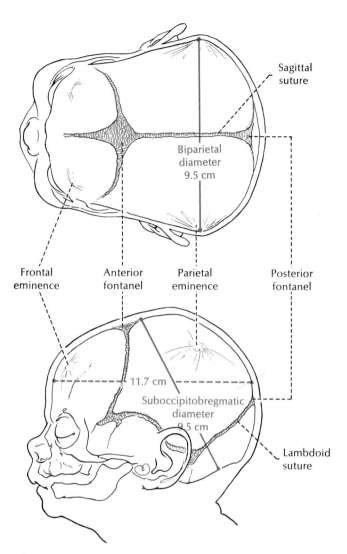

figure **24.19** Various diameters of the fetal head at term.

The pelvis consists of four bones: the two innominate bones, the sacrum, and the coccyx. Each innominate bone consists of three bones that fuse after puberty. These three bones are the ilium, the ischium, and the pubis (Figure 24.20). The innominate bones form the anterior and lateral portions of the pelvis.

The sacrum and the coccyx constitute the posterior portion of the pelvis. The sacrum is composed of five fused vertebrae. Its upper anterior portion is called the sacral promontory, which forms the posterior margin the pelvic brim. The coccyx is composed of three to five fused vertebrae and articulates with the sacrum.

The pelvis is divided by the brim into two parts: the false pelvis and the true pelvis. The false pelvis is that part above the brim and is of no obstetrical interest.

The brim and the area below it constitute the true pelvis. The true pelvis is divided into three parts: the inlet or brim, the midpelvis or cavity, and the outlet.

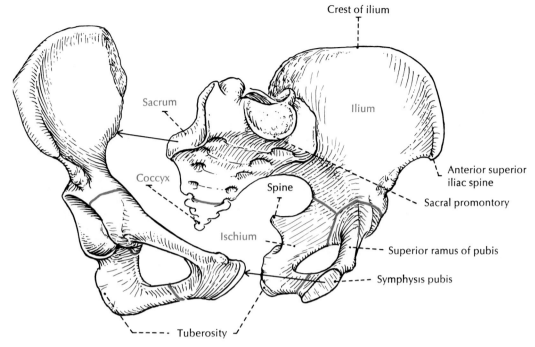

figure**24.20** Bones of the pelvis.

The inlet is formed anteriorly by the upper margins of the pubic bones, laterally by the iliopectineal lines, and posteriorly by the anterior upper margin of the sacrum, the sacral promontory. The cavity is formed anteriorly by the posterior aspect of the symphysis pubis, laterally by the inner surfaces of the ischial and iliac bones, and posteriorly by the anterior surface of the sacrum. The outlet, which is diamond shaped, is formed anteriorly by the inferior rami of the pubic and ischial bones, laterally by the ischial tuberosities, and posteriorly by the inferior edge of the sacrum (if the coccyx is movable).

Each of the pelvic portions can be imagined as a series of planes: the plane of the brim (or pelvic inlet), the planes of the midpelvis, and the plane of the outlet. These planes are illustrated in Figure 24.21.

The plane of the inlet in an average female pelvis measures approximately 11 to 13 cm in the anteroposterior diameter and 13 to 14 cm in the transverse diameter. The anteroposterior diameter of the inlet, measured from the middle of the sacral promontory to the superior posterior margin of the symphysis pubis, is called the true conjugate and is an important obstetrical measurement. However, only radiographic methods can be used to directly assess this measurement. The true conjugate can be estimated by measuring the diagonal conjugate, which is the distance between the inferior border of the symphysis pubis and the sacral promontory. The diagonal conjugate is approximately 1 to 2 cm longer than the true conjugate, depending on the

height and inclination of the symphysis. The clinical measurement of the diagonal conjugate, the most valuable single measurement of pelvic adequacy, is discussed later in this section.

The midpelvis contains the planes of greatest and least pelvic dimensions. The plane of least pelvic dimensions is bounded by the junction of the fourth and fifth sacral vertebrae, the symphysis, and the ischial spines. The average dimensions of this plane are 12 cm (anteroposterior diameter) and 10.5 cm (transverse diameter). The transverse diameter is the distance between the ischial spines.

The pelvic outlet is composed of two triangular planes, having a common base in the most inferior portion of the transverse diameter between the ischial tuberosities. The obstetrical anteroposterior diameter of the outlet is the distance between the inferior edge of the symphysis pubis and the edge of the sacrum (if the coccyx is movable). This measurement is usually 11.5 cm.

The transverse diameter of the outlet is the distance between the inner surfaces of the ischial tuberosities and usually measures approximately 11 cm (Figure 24.22).

Although there is a characteristic shape of the adult female pelvis that is different from the characteristically male pelvis, a female client may have any one of four types of human pelves, or a mixture of these types. In addition, the shape of the pelvis may have been distorted congenitally or by disease.

The four basic pelvic types, as originally classified by

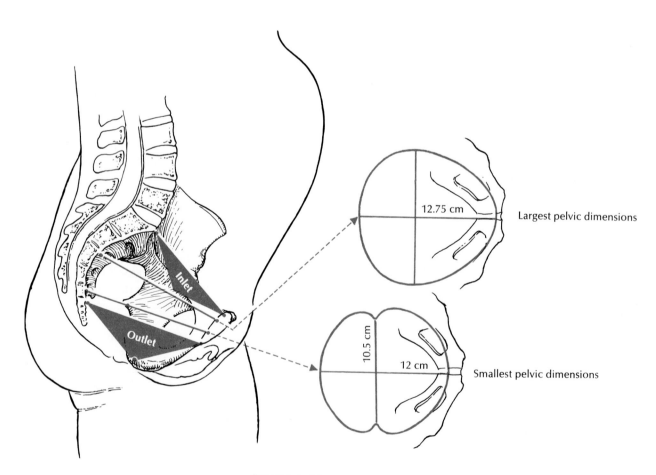

figure **24.21** Planes of the pelvic inlet and midpelvis. (Measurements are averages within normal limits.)

figure **24.22** Pelvic outlet.

Caldwell, Maloy, and Swenson (1939), are (1) gynecoid, (2) android, (3) anthropoid, and (4) platypelloid.

The typical female pelvis is the gynecoid pelvis, which is found in approximately 40% to 50% of adult women. This pelvis is characterized by a rounded inlet, except for a slight projection of the sacral promontory; a deep posterior half made possible by a wide sacrosciatic notch and concave sacrum; and a wide anterior half made possible by a wide, subpubic angle.

The android pelvis is found in approximately 15% to 20% of adult women. This pelvic type is roughly wedge- or heart-shaped, with the transverse diameter of the inlet approximately equal to the anteroposterior diameter but with the widest transverse diameter located closer to the sacrum. Other characteristics of the android pelvis include the following:

1. Narrow subpubic arch
2. Convergent side walls
3. Large, encroaching spines
4. Short sacrosciatic notch and sacrospinous ligament
5. Short interspinous diameter
6. Straight sacrum
7. Short intertuberous diameter

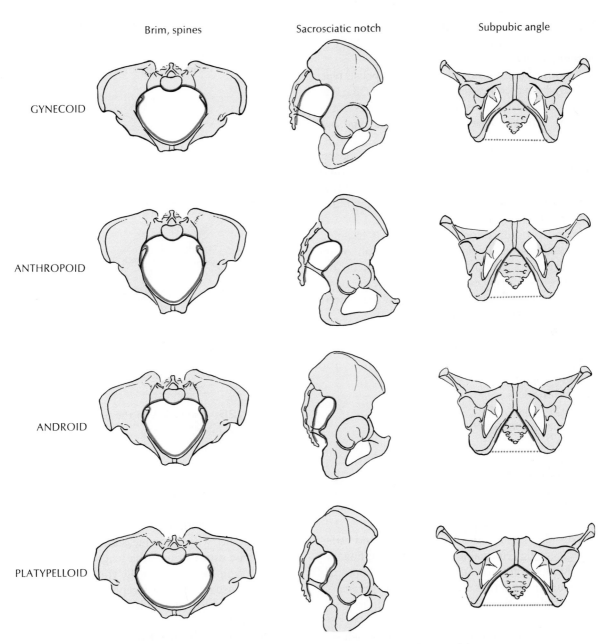

figure**24.23**   Comparisons of various portions of the four basic pelvic types.

The anthropoid pelvis has an elongated anteroposterior diameter and is found in approximately 25% to 35% of women. It is characterized by the following:

1. Narrow subpubic arch
2. Prominent ischial spines
3. Wide sacrosciatic notch and long sacrospinous ligaments
4. Deeply curved sacrum

The platypelloid pelvis has a flattened anteroposterior dimension with a relative widening of the transverse diameter. This pelvic type is seen in approximately 5% of women. The platypelloid pelvis is characterized by the following:

1. Wide subpubic arch
2. Flat ischial spines
3. Wide sacrosciatic notch and long sacrospinous ligaments
4. Straight sacrum

The various dimensions of the four basic pelvic types are compared and contrasted in Figure 24.23. Pure pelvic types are unusual; most pelves are mixtures of two pelvic types, with the characteristics of one type predominating.

Because examination of the bony pelvis can be uncomfortable, perform it after the internal examination of the soft pelvic organs. In preparing the client, include an explanation of the procedure, the client's emptying of her bladder, and instructions on relaxation.

A standard procedure for the bony pelvis examination is recommended. Begin with examination of the anterior pelvis, proceed to lateral examination on one side, compare the initially examined side with the opposite side, and conclude with examination of the posterior and inferior portions.

The following bony pelvis parts and landmarks are especially important in examining the pelvis:

1. Subpubic arch
2. Symphysis pubis
3. Side walls
4. Ischial spines
5. Sacrosciatic notch
6. Sacrum
7. Coccyx
8. Sacral promontory
9. Ischial tuberosities

The following is a recommended procedure for assessment of the bony pelvis:

1. Palpate the width of the subpubic arch, and estimate its angle. Normally, both examining fingers should fit comfortably in the arch, which optimally forms an angle that measures slightly greater than a right angle (90-degree angle) (Figure 24.24).
2. Estimate the length and inclination of the symphysis pubis by sweeping the examining fingers

figure**24.24** Method of estimating the angle of the subpubic arch.

figure**24.25** Estimation of the length and inclination of the symphysis pubis.

under the symphysis (Figure 24.25). Also, palpate the retropubic curve of the forepelvis and envision its configuration. Measurement difficulties created by a large amount of soft tissue in the area and reliability with slope measurements preclude a precise estimation of the length and inclination of the symphysis. Essentially, you are screening for an unusually long or steeply inclined symphysis pubis and for an angular rather than a rounded forepelvis.

3. Examine the right or the left lateral pelvic area. First, palpate the side walls to determine if they

figure**24.26** Measurement of the width of the sacrosciatic notch.

are straight, convergent, or divergent. Assess the splay of the side walls by following a line from the point of origin of the widest transverse diameter of the inlet downward to the inner aspect of the tuberosity. Another method for assessing the side walls is to place the examining fingers on the base of the ischial spine as a landmark and then to palpate above and below the landmark to determine the inclination.

4. Examine the ischial spine and the sacrospinous ligament on that same side. Assess the spines as being blunt, prominent, or encroaching. Outline the sacrosciatic notch with palpating fingers, if possible, and determine its width in centimeters or fingerbreadths. Often, tracing the entire notch is difficult, and the sacrospinous ligament is useful in estimating the width of the notch (Figure 24.26).

5. Examine the other side of the pelvis in the manner previously described to determine overall pelvic symmetry. Attempt to do this part of the examination with the palm of the hand up, rather than rotating the hand so that the palm is down.

6. Estimate the interspinous diameter by moving the examining fingers in a straight line from one spine across to the other (Figure 24.27). You may need to pronate the hand for this estimation. Calculate the estimate in centimeters. The usual measurement is 10.5 cm.

7. Next examine the sacrum and the coccyx. Sweep the fingers down the sacrum, noting whether it is straight, curved, or hollow and if its inclination is forward or backward. Examine the coccyx gently because it may be tender on movement. Gently

figure**24.27** Measurement of the interspinous diameter.

press the coccyx backward to determine if it is movable or fixed. Note its tilt as anterior or posterior.

8. Assess the diagonal conjugate last because this assessment can be uncomfortable for the client. A moderate amount of constant pressure is necessary to depress the perineum adequately. Exert pressure with your body rather than with the hand and forearm. Place your foot (the one on the same side as the examining hand) on a stool and the elbow of the examining arm on your thigh or hip. Then apply the needed pressure, controlling it with your body. For this examination, make sure that your fingers and wrist form a straight line with your forearm.

Locate the sacrum with the examining fingers,

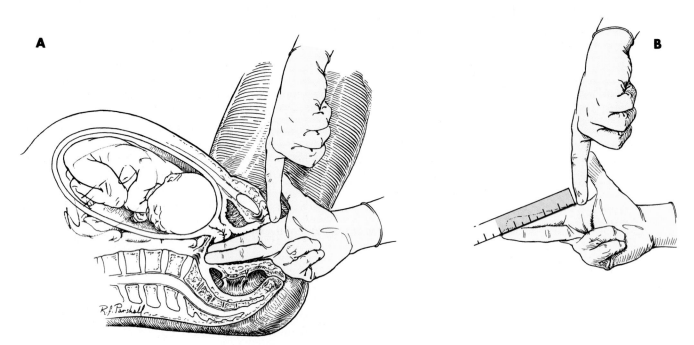

figure**24.28** Measurement of the diagonal conjugate. **A,** Internal palpation. **B,** Use of a ruler to specify the estimation in centimeters.

figure**24.29** Use of a fist to estimate the intertuberous diameter.

and with the middle finger "walk" up the sacrum until you reach the promontory or until you can no longer touch the sacrum. Mark the point where the client's symphysis touches your hand with the thumb of the opposite hand, and measure the distance in centimeters with a ruler (Figure 24.28). In obstetrical examining rooms, a ruler is often fixed to the wall for this measurement.

Often, you will not reach the sacral promontory. Become familiar with the "reach" of your examining fingers and record the findings as greater than (>) the centimeters of this reach. Normally, the diagonal conjugate is >12.5 cm.

9. Withdraw the examining hand from the vagina, and measure the intertuberous diameter. With both thumbs, externally trace the descending rami down to the tuberosities. Then make a fist and attempt to insert the fist between the tuberosities to measure the transverse diameter of an outlet (Figure 24.29). The intertuberous diameter is usually 10 to 11 cm. Again, know the span of your own fist and estimate the intertuberous diameter accordingly.

In summary, the areas of bony pelvic examination and the assessment descriptors for these areas follow:

Sequence of areas of bony pelvic examination	Assessment descriptors
1. Subpubic arch	*Inclination:* Less than 90 degrees, more than 90 degrees
2. Side walls	*Direction:* Parallel, convergent, divergent
3. Ischial spines	*Size:* Small, average, large *Prominence:* Blunt, prominent, encroaching
4. Sacrosciatic notch Sacrospinous ligament	*Length:* Estimated width or length in centimeters (usual length = 3 to 4 cm)
5. Opposite pelvic side	*Symmetry:* Symmetrical, asymmetrical
6. Interspinous diameter	*Length:* Estimated length in centimeters (usual length = 10.5 cm)
7. Sacrum	*Shape:* Concave, straight, convex
8. Coccyx	*Position:* Straight, projects anteriorly, projects posteriorly *Movability:* Movable, fixed
9. Diagonal conjugate	*Length:* Actual length or length greater than the measurement that the examiner can reach (usual length = 12.5 cm)
10. Intertuberous diameter	*Length:* Actual length in centimeters if Thom's pelvimeter is used, or an estimated length using a closed fist (usual length is 10 to 11 cm)

Screening Tests
General recommendations

The recommendations of the U.S. Preventive Services Task Force (1996) are provided in Tables 24.4 and 24.5.

Assessments near term

Two additional assessments of changes are done near the expected date of delivery: estimation of the length and dilation of the cervix and determination of the fetal station. Figure 24.30 illustrates a method of measuring the length of the cervix. Before 34 to 36 weeks' gestation, the cervix should maintain its usual length of 1.5 to 2 cm. During the last 4 weeks of gestation, the cervix shortens as the fetal head descends, and the internal cervical os softens and opens and is pulled upward and incorporated into the isthmus of the uterus. When the cervix shortens (effaces), it also begins to dilate. Cervical dilation is estimated by the diameter of the cervical os and is measured in centimeters—from 0 cm when closed to 10 cm when completely opened.

The degree of descent of the fetal presenting part, usually the head, is measured by the station. Station refers to the relationship of the presenting part to the plane of the ischial spines. If the lowest portion of the presenting part is at the level of the spines, it is at station 0. Other stations of the fetal presenting part are the following:

Minus 3	At the pelvic inlet
Minus 2	One third of the distance from the inlet to the spines
Minus 1	Two thirds of the distance from the inlet to the spines
Station 0	At the level of the ischial spines
Plus 1	One third of the distance between the spines and the pelvic floor
Plus 2	Two thirds of the distance between the spines and the pelvic floor
Plus 3	At the pelvic floor

figure**24.30** Measurement of cervical length.

table 24.4 Recommendations of the U.S. Preventive Services Task Force for All Pregnant Women

Screening recommendations	Other recommendations
FIRST VISIT SCREENING Blood pressure Hemoglobin/hematocrit Hepatitis B surface antigen RPR/VDRL *Chlamydia* screen (<25 yr) Rubella serology or vaccination history D(Rh) typing, antibody screen Offer CVS (<13 wk) or amniocentesis (15-18 wk) (age ≥35) Offer hemoglobinopathy screening Assess for problem or risk drinking Offer HIV screening Asymptomatic bacteriuria with urine culture (12-16 wk) **FOLLOW-UP VISIT SCREENING** Blood pressure Urine culture Offer multiple marker testing (15-18 wk) Offer serum α-fetoprotein (16-18 wk)	**COUNSELING** Tobacco cessation/effects of passive smoking Cease use of alcohol and other drugs Nutrition, including adequate calcium intake Encourage breast-feeding Use lap and shoulder belts Use infant safety car seats Sexually transmitted disease prevention **CHEMOPROPHYLAXIS** Multivitamin with folic acid

Data from US Preventive Services Task Force: *Guide to clinical preventive services: an assessment of the effectiveness of 169 interventions,* ed 2, Baltimore, 1996, Williams & Wilkins.
CVS, Chorionic villus sampling.

table 24.5 Recommendations of the U.S. Preventive Services Task Force for High-Risk Pregnant Women

Risk	Screening and counseling recommendations
High-risk sexual behavior	*Chlamydia* screening (first visit) Gonorrhea screening (first visit) HIV screening (first visit) HBsAg screening (third trimester) Repeat RPR/VDRL (third trimester)
Blood transfusion between 1978-1985	HIV screening (first visit)
Injection drug use	HIV screening (first visit) HBsAg (third trimester) Counseling to reduce infection risk
Unsensitized D-negative women	D(Rh) antibody testing (24-28 wk)
Risk factors for Down syndrome	Offer CVS (first trimester), amniocentesis (15-18 wk)
Prior pregnancy with neural tube defect	Folic acid 4.0 mg Offer amniocentesis (15-18 wk)

Data from US Preventive Services Task Force: *Guide to clinical preventive services: an assessment of the effectiveness of 169 interventions,* ed 2, Baltimore, 1996, Williams & Wilkins.
HBsAg, Hepatitis B surface antigen.

sample documentation & diagnoses CRITICAL THINKING

■ FOCUSED HEALTH HISTORY *(SUBJECTIVE DATA)*

Mrs. A., a 24-year-old primigravid client, is in for a routine prenatal visit (estimated gestation of 20 weeks). Has been feeling better since last visit, 1 month ago. Nausea and vomiting have ceased. Complains of mild pain in her breasts and a mild amount of lower abdominal and leg discomfort at night, which is alleviated by elevation in the evening. Less urinary frequency than in early pregnancy, but gets up to void about 2 times each night. She and her husband are becoming more enthusiastic about the baby. Husband is assisting more around the home. Plans to work until the baby is born and then take a 6- to 8-week postpartum leave. Fetal movements were first felt 3 weeks ago and are increasing in intensity. Occasional, mild Braxton Hicks contractions noted. No vaginal bleeding or discharge. No other problems.

■ FOCUSED PHYSICAL EXAMINATION *(OBJECTIVE DATA)*

BP: 118/76.
Weight: 165 lb (prepregnant = 140 lb); 8-lb weight gain since last visit.
Urine: Negative for glucose, albumin, and ketones.
Extremities: No edema.
Breasts: Full; consistently glandular in consistency; no lesions palpated. Small amount of watery fluid expressed from both nipples.
Abdominal assessment: Fundus at umbilicus (consistent with estimated 20-week gestation, measuring 19 cm. Fetal position uncertain because of small fetal size. Fetal heart tones heard in midline, regular at 158 beats/min.

diagnoses

NURSING DIAGNOSES

Altered nutrition: risk for more than body requirements
Defining Characteristics
- Weight 10% to 20% over ideal for height and frame
- Weight gain of 25 lbs in first 20 weeks of pregnancy

Pain related to physical body changes during pregnancy
Defining Characteristics
- Pain in breasts
- Pain in lower abdomen and legs

Sleep pattern disturbances related to frequent urination at night
Defining Characteristic
- Interrupted sleep 2 times each night to void

chapter 25

Pediatric Clients

■ PURPOSE OF EXAMINATION

Pediatric care is, to a large extent, health care aimed at promoting the health of the child and preventing illness and disability through early identification of problems, anticipatory guidance to help parents deal with physical and developmental issues before they become problems, and early and ongoing intervention for health care needs.

Ideally, the practitioner performs the examination of the child over an extended time in a planned sequential pattern. The dynamic changes that occur throughout the child's normal growth and development require that the practitioner assess certain aspects carefully: increments in growth; changes in physiological function; and development of cognitive, social, and motor skills of the child during each examination.

The health of the child is determined by comparing the individual child's current growth achievements and parameters of health with those found in his or her previous examinations, and with norms for children in the same age range. The practitioner should see the child frequently, usually every 2 to 3 months for well-child

care during infancy, when growth changes are most rapid and dramatic. The practitioner should assess the older child at regular, but less frequent, intervals for well-child care.

To provide holistic care to the child, it is also important to consider the needs and concerns of the child's primary caretaker(s), usually the parents. The adults responsible for the child's care often have questions and concerns about the child's development and about their own ability to manage care. The practitioner needs to encourage them to express their concerns and to discuss their needs in addition to the needs of the child. The examiner should have a sense of the parent as a person. What are the stresses and issues that the parents are dealing with? What impact do these factors have on their ability to parent? Parents who feel that their questions and concerns are being heard and that they are receiving support and respect will be better able to care for their children (Figure 25.1).

A part of each well-child assessment (and sick-child visit, if that is the only time that the family comes in for care, or if the potential for problems is apparent during

figure**25.1** Attention to the concerns of both the parent and the child is an important component of the assessment.

figure**25.2** The quality of the parent-child interaction needs to be assessed, and positive attitudes should be supported.

an acute care visit) should address anticipatory guidance. Anticipatory guidance involves teaching parents what to expect in terms of their child's physical, cognitive, emotional, and social development. The goal of anticipatory guidance is to promote positive parent-child relationships and prevent the development of emotional and behavioral disturbances related to difficulties in parent-child interactions. Frequently problems develop because parents or caregivers are unaware that "problem" behaviors are in fact normal stage-specific behaviors related to development. Examples include the "stranger anxiety" demonstrated when a 9-month-old is picked up by his grandmother whom he sees infrequently and the "negativism" of the 2-year-old. Helping the parent identify what is normal development versus abnormal or problem behavior can help parents feel more secure in their ability to respond to their children. For example, the 9-month-old will still cry when picked up by the "stranger," his grandmother, but his parents will be able to identify this reaction as a normal (although embarrassing) behavior rather than a reflection of being "spoiled" by the parents.

Anticipatory guidance also involves helping the parent identify and problem-solve around problematic areas. Examples include talking with a parent about how to deal with negativism or temper tantrums and anticipating what to do if the child has a tantrum in the grocery store, and helping parents who are planning to bring their 9-month-old child to a family reunion consider ways to introduce their child to relatives in a non-threatening manner. Anticipatory guidance can also be

used to help new parents address issues such as differences in attitudes toward discipline or the role each parent plays in child care activities before these differences become a source of family conflict.

Assessing the quality of the parent-child relationship is crucial. The practitioner should support positive interactions (Figure 25.2). Receiving recognition for their parenting skills is especially helpful for parents. The practitioner also should be alert to any signs of stress between the parent and the child. A mother who is concerned, anxious, or angry about a child's behavior or physical condition may be showing evidence of stress that can interfere with the mother-child relationship and ultimately with the child's development. The practitioner can identify difficulties in the parent-child interaction and initiate early interventions to promote better interactions. This issue emphasizes the importance of considering needs of the parent or other adults caring for the child in addition to those of the child.

The practitioner should always demonstrate respect for both the child and the parent, be willing to listen to problems, and help in finding adequate solutions. Both the child and the parent will be aware of the practitioner's attitudes and will respond according to their impressions. In essence, it is important to be sensitive to the child as a growing, developing human being who is always changing.

table 25.1   *Guidelines for Health Supervision*

	Infancy[3]								Early childhood[3]				
Age[4]	New-born[1]	2-4 days[2]	By 1 mo	2 mo	4 mo	6 mo	9 mo	12 mo	15 mo	18 mo	24 mo	3 yr	4 yr
History													
Initial/interval	•	•	•	•	•	•	•	•	•	•	•	•	•
Measurements													
Height and weight	•	•	•	•	•	•	•	•	•	•	•	•	•
Head circumference	•	•	•	•	•	•	•	•	•	•	•		
Blood pressure												•	•
Sensory screening													
Vision	S	S	S	S	S	S	S	S	S	S	S	O[5]	O
Hearing[6]	S/O	S	S	S	S	S	S	S	S	S	S	O	O
Developmental/ behavioral assessment[7]	•	•	•	•	•	•	•	•	•	•	•	•	•
Physical examination[8]	•	•	•	•	•	•	•	•	•	•	•	•	•
Procedures—general[9]													
Hereditary/metabolic screening[10]	←—————→												
Immunization[11]	•———————→			•	•	•		•	←—•—→				←
Lead screening[12]							•——→				•		
Hematocrit or hemoglobin						←——————→							
Urinalysis													
Procedures—patients at risk													
Tuberculin test[15]								★	★	★	★	★	★
Cholesterol screening[16]											★	★	★
STD screening[17]													
Pelvic exam[18]													
Anticipatory guidance[19]	•	•	•	•	•	•	•	•	•	•	•	•	•
Injury prevention[20]	•	•	•	•	•	•	•	•	•	•	•	•	•
Initial dental referral[21]									←———————→				

From Committee on Practice and Ambulatory Medicine, American Academy of Pediatrics, *Pediatrics* 96:373-374, 1995.

1. Breast-feeding encouraged and instruction and support offered.
2. For newborns discharged in less than 48 hours after delivery.
3. Developmental, psychosocial, and chronic disease issues for children and adolescents may require frequent counseling and treatment visits separate from preventive care visits.
4. If a child comes under care for the first time at any point on the schedule, or if any items are not accomplished at the suggested age, the schedule should be brought up to date at the earliest possible time.
5. If the patient is uncooperative, rescreen within 6 months.
6. Some experts recommend objective appraisal of hearing in the newborn period. The Joint Committee on Infant Hearing has identified patients at significant risk for hearing loss. All children meeting these criteria should be objectively screened. See the Joint Committee on Infant Hearing 1994 Position Statement.
7. By history and appropriate physical examination; if suspicious, by specific objective developmental testing.
8. At each visit, a complete physical examination is essential, with infant totally unclothed, older child undressed and suitably draped.
9. These may be modified, depending upon entry point into schedule and individual need.
10. Metabolic screening (e.g., thyroid, hemoglobinopathies, PKU, galactosemia) should be done according to state law.
11. Schedule(s) per the Committee on Infectious Diseases, published periodically in *Pediatrics*. Every visit should be an opportunity to update and complete a child's immunizations.

	Middle Childhood[3]				Adolescence[3]										
Age[4]	5 yr	6 yr	8 yr	10 yr	11 yr	12 yr	13 yr	14 yr	15 yr	16 yr	17 yr	18 yr	19 yr	20 yr	21 yr
History															
Initial/interval	•	•	•	•	•	•	•	•	•	•	•	•	•	•	•
Measurements															
Height and weight	•	•	•	•	•	•	•	•	•	•	•	•	•	•	•
Head circumference															
Blood pressure	•	•	•	•	•	•	•	•	•	•	•	•	•	•	•
Sensory screening															
Vision	O	S	S	O	S	O	S	S	O	S	S	O	S	S	S
Hearing[6]	O	S	S	O	S	O	S	S	O	S	S	O	S	S	S
Developmental/ behavioral assessment[7]	•	•	•	•	•	•	•	•	•	•	•	•	•	•	•
Physical examination[8]	•	•	•	•	•	•	•	•	•	•	•	•	•	•	•
Procedures—general[9]															
Hereditary/metabolic screening[10]															
Immunization[11]	•——→				•——————————————→										
Lead screening[12]															
Hematocrit or hemoglobin					←——————————————•[13]——————————————→										
Urinalysis	•				←——————————————•[14]——————————————→										
Procedures—patients at risk															
Tuberculin test[15]	★	★	★	★	★	★	★	★	★	★	★	★	★	★	★
Cholesterol screening[16]	★	★	★	★	★	★	★	★	★	★	★	★	★	★	★
STD screening[17]					★	★	★	★	★	★	★	★	★	★	★
Pelvic exam[18]					★	★	★	★	★	★	★←—★		★[18]	★	—★
Anticipatory guidance[19]	•	•	•	•	•	•	•	•	•	•	•	•	•	•	•
Injury prevention[20]	•	•	•	•	•	•	•	•	•	•	•	•	•	•	•
Initial dental referral[21]															

12. Blood lead screen per AAP statement "Lead Poisoning: From Screening to Primary Prevention" (1993).

13. All menstruating adolescents should be screened.

14. Conduct dipstick urinalysis for leukocytes for male and female adolescents.

15. TB testing per AAP statement "Screening for Tuberculosis in Infants and Children" (1994). Testing should be done upon recognition of high-risk factors. If results are negative but high-risk situation continues, testing should be repeated on an annual basis.

16. Cholesterol screening for high-risk patients per AAP "Statement on Cholesterol" (1992). If family history cannot be ascertained and other risk factors are present, screening should be at the discretion of the physician.

17. All sexually active patients should be screened for sexually transmitted diseases (STDs).

18. All sexually active females should have a pelvic examination. A pelvic examination and routine pap smear should be offered as part of preventive health maintenance between the ages of 18 and 21 years.

19. Appropriate discussion and counseling should be an integral part of each visit for care.

20. From birth to age 12, refer to AAP's injury prevention program (TIPP) as described in "A Guide to Safety Counseling in Office Practice" (1994).

21. Earlier initial dental evaluations may be appropriate for some children. Subsequent examinations as prescribed by dentist.

•, To be performed; ★, to be performed for patients at risk; S, subjective, by history; O, objective, by a standard testing method; ←•→, the range during which a service may be provided, with the dot indicating the preferred age.

NOTE : Special chemical, immunological, and endocrine testing is usually carried out upon specific indications. Testing other than newborn (e.g., inborn errors of metabolism, sickle disease, etc.) is discretionary with the physician.

This chapter discusses approaches to the child and the parent, as well as some techniques to obtain health information and to assess the child's health. In addition, it covers some of the physical differences between the child and the adult. Because it is not possible to include a survey of all the components of child development that are assessed, the reader is referred to the material on child developmental assessment in Chapter 4 and to standard pediatric texts for assistance in understanding the parameters of normal development and health of children.

■ GUIDELINES FOR HEALTH SUPERVISION

Much of the care given to children focuses on health promotion and the prevention of disease. The American Academy of Pediatrics (1995) suggests the schedule of well-child care shown in Table 25.1 for the care of children who (1) are receiving competent parenting, (2) have no manifestations of any important health problems, and (3) are growing and developing in a satisfactory fashion. The following situations may warrant additional visits:

1. Firstborn or adopted children or those not with natural parents
2. Parents with a particular need for education and guidance
3. Families from a disadvantaged social or economic environment
4. Presence or possibility of perinatal disorders (e.g., prematurity, low birth weight, congenital defects, or familial diseases)
5. Children with acquired illness or previously identified diseases or problems

■ EXAMINATION

Pediatric History

The pediatric history provides the opportunity to interview both the child and the parent to gather information about the child's health, development, relationships with others, and care. It also offers the opportunity for the child to become acquainted with the practitioner before being examined. The pediatric history is an adaptation of the model used for the adult history. It incorporates areas uniquely pertinent to the child, such as the history of the mother's health during the pregnancy, the history of birth and the neonatal period, and specific areas related to the child's psychosocial development (e.g., stage-related behaviors, school performance, peer relationships).

Cultural differences and individual parental beliefs about child-rearing and health influence the care of the infant and child and are revealed in the history of the child's care. The practitioner should respect these differences and make culturally sensitive decisions with regard to content and approaches in counseling.

The informant for the history may be a parent, a relative, a caretaker, and/or the child. Identify the informant and indicate the reliability of the information obtained. Commonly, the child, even the young child, participates in the interview and volunteers useful information. Indicate the information gained from the child as such in the history.

The comprehensive health history described in Chapter 3 is adapted for the pediatric client by making certain changes in format. The following developmental and nutritional data should be gathered before the review of systems, since these data are usually critical to the present health status of the infant or child:

1. Biographical information
2. Chief complaint or client's request for care
3. Present illness or present health status
4. Past health history
5. Developmental data
6. Nutritional data
7. Family health history
8. Review of systems
   a. Physical systems
   b. Sociological system
   c. Psychological system
9. Anticipatory guidance

Biographical information

The following information needs to be obtained in the biographical category. It is essentially the same as for the adult client with the addition of the parents' information.

1. Full name
2. Address
3. Birth date
4. Sex
5. Race
6. Religion
7. Birthplace
8. Parents' names
9. Parents' marital status
10. Parents' ages
11. Source of referral
12. Usual source of health care
13. Source and reliability of information
14. Date of interview

Chief complaint or client's request for care

The chief complaint statement gives the reason for making the visit and should be recorded in the words of the informant. The informant could be the parent or the child. Elicit this information with a neutral question ("How may I help you today?"), since the visit may be

for routine health care rather than for treatment of a health problem. The chief complaint statement for routine health care may be "It is time for his checkup" or "Well-baby check."

When the visit is for a well-child examination, you may want to ask: "Before we begin the examination, are there any particular questions or concerns that you would like to discuss?" This question encourages the client, parent, or child to raise issues that may not be addressed in the health history format and reinforces the idea that their questions and concerns are important.

Present illness or present health status

The present illness or present health status section incorporates the same categories of information obtained in the adult health history and includes a statement about the client's usual health; a description of the current concern, including the onset and chronological story; any relevant family history; any negative information; and a disability assessment. You may want to ask an open-ended question ("How has the baby been since you were last here?") to get a general picture of how things have been going (interval history). Also ask the parent the reason for seeking help at this time. Usually something significant has occurred that motivates the person to come for an evaluation. Physical changes in the child's condition, family stresses that make the problem more difficult to handle, or issues such as a similar problem in a friend or relative may have triggered the visit. Understanding these concerns will help in making your assessment of the situation and planning effective interventions.

Past health history

The past health history of infants, young children, and any child with a possible developmental deficiency should include the following information:
1. Prenatal history

a. Health of the mother while pregnant with this child
b. Mother's feelings about the pregnancy
c. Amount of prenatal care and when initiated
d. History of complications (excessive weight gain, hypertension, vaginal bleeding, nausea and vomiting, urinary problems, or infections such as rubella, cytomegalovirus, or venereal disease)
e. Medications or drugs prescribed or used during pregnancy
f. Use of alcohol, cigarettes, and other drugs (e.g., cocaine, heroin) during the pregnancy
2. Birth history
a. Date of birth
b. Hospital where child was born
c. Duration of the pregnancy
d. Parity of the mother
e. Nature and duration of the labor
f. Type of delivery
g. Use of sedation or anesthesia
h. Birth weight of the baby
i. State of the infant at birth and use of any *special* procedures
j. Apgar score, if known (Table 25.2)
3. Postnatal history
a. Any problems during the first days of life (including skin color, bleeding, seizures, respiratory distress, congenital anomalies or birth injuries, difficulty in sucking, rashes, or poor weight gain during the first days and weeks after birth)
b. Age of infant at discharge from hospital after birth

The past health history of *all* children includes the following information:
1. Past illnesses
a. Childhood illnesses (including communicable diseases such as chickenpox and rubeola)

table 25.2 *Apgar Scoring System for Newborns*

Clinical sign	Assigned score*		
	0	1	2
Heart rate	Absent	Slow (<100 beats per minute)	>100 beats per minute
Respiratory effort	Apnea	Slow and irregular	Immediate, strong
Muscle tone	Flaccid	Some flexion of arms and legs	Active movement
Reflex irritability†	No response	Grimace or cry	Crying vigorously
Color	Pale, blue	Body pink, extremities blue	Pink all over

*A score of 8 to 10 is excellent, 4 to 7 is guarded, and 0 to 3 is critical.
†Reaction when soft rubber catheter is inserted into the external nares.

Vaccine		Age									
	Birth	1 mo.	2 mos.	4 mos.	6 mos.	12 mos.	15 mos.	18 mos.	4-6 yrs.	11-12 yrs.	14-16 yrs.
Hepatitis B[1]		Hep B-1									
			Hep B-2			Hep B-3				Hep B[2]	
Diphtheria and Tetanus toxoids and Pertussis vaccine[3]			DTP	DTP	DTP	DTP (DTaP at ≥ 15 mo.)			DTP or DTaP	Td	
Haemophilus influenzae type B‡[4]			Hib	Hib	Hib	Hib					
Poliovirus[5]			OPV	OPV	OPV				OPV		
Measles-Mumps-Rubella[6]						MMR			MMR or MMR		
Varicella-Zoster Virus[7]						Var				Var	

■ Range of acceptable ages for vaccination   ▨ "Catch-up" vaccination[2]

figure **25.3** Recommended childhood vaccination schedule*—United States, July through December 1996. *(Modified from the Centers for Disease Control, Atlanta, Ga.; data from Advisory Committee on Immunization Practices, American Academy of Pediatrics, and American Academy of Family Physicians.)*

*Vaccines are listed under routinely recommended ages.

1. Infants born to hepatitis B surface antigen (HBsAg)–negative mothers should receive 2.5 μg of Recombivax HB* (Merck & Co.) or 10 μg of Engerix-B (SmithKline Beecham). The second dose should be administered 1 month after the first dose. Infants born to HBsAg-positive mothers should receive 0.5 ml hepatitis B immune globulin (HBIG) within 12 hours of birth, and either 5 μg of Recombivax HB or 10 μg of Engerix-B at a separate site. The second dose is recommended at age 1 to 2 months and the third dose at age 6 months. Infants born to mothers whose HBsAg status is unknown should receive either 5 μg of Recombivax HB or 10 μg of Engerix-B within 12 hours of birth. The second dose of vaccine is recommended at age 1 month and the third dose at age 6 months.

2. Adolescents who have not received 3 doses of hepatitis B vaccine should initiate or complete the series at age 11 to 12 years. The second dose should be administered at least 1 month after the first dose, and the third dose should be administered at least 4 months after the first dose and at least 2 months after the second dose.

3. The fourth dose of diphtheria and tetanus toxoids and pertussis vaccine (DTP) may be administered at age 12 months, if at least 6 months have elapsed since the third dose of DTP. Diphtheria and tetanus toxoids and acellular pertussis vaccine (DTaP) is licensed for the fourth and/or fifth vaccine dose(s) for children ≥15 months of age and may be preferred for these doses in this age group. Tetanus and diphtheria toxoids, absorbed, for adult use (Td) is recommended at age 11 to 12 years if at least 5 years have elapsed since the last dose of DTP, DTaP, or diphtheria and tetanus toxoids, absorbed, for pediatric use (DT).

4. Three *Haemophilus influenzae* type b (Hib) conjugate vaccines are licensed for infant use. If PedvaxHIB (Merck & Co.) *Haemophilus* b conjugate vaccine (meningococcal protein conjugate) (PRP-OMP) is administered at ages 2 and 4 months, a dose at 6 months is not required. After completing the primary series, any Hib conjugate vaccine may be used as a booster.

5. Oral poliovirus vaccine (OPV) is recommended for routine infant vaccination. Inactivated poliovirus vaccine (IPV) is recommended for persons—or household contacts of persons—with a congenital or acquired immune deficiency disease or an altered immune status resulting from disease or immunosuppressive therapy, and is an acceptable alternative for other persons. The primary 3-dose series for IPV should be given with a minimum interval of 4 weeks between the first and second doses and 6 months between the second and third doses.

6. The second dose of measles-mumps-rubella vaccine (MMR) is routinely recommended at age 4 to 6 years or at age 11 to 12 years but may be administered at any visit provided at least 1 month has elapsed since receipt of the first dose.

7. Varicella zoster virus vaccine (Var) can be administered to susceptible children any time after age 12 months. Unvaccinated children who lack a reliable history of chickenpox should be vaccinated by age 11 to 12 years. Use of trade names and commercial sources is for identification only and does not imply endorsement by the Public Health Service or the US Department of Health and Human Services.

b. Injuries
c. Hospitalizations
d. Operations
e. Other major illnesses
f. Frequency of infections
2. Allergies
a. Environmental
b. Food
c. Drug
d. Other
3. Immunizations, including booster inoculations (Figure 25.3) (NOTE: Immunization schedules are frequently updated by the American Academy of Pediatrics and the Centers for Disease Control [CDC] Advisory Committee on Immunization Practices. The most current schedule is reported in the journal *Pediatrics* and in the CDC's *Morbidity and Mortality Weekly Reports [MMWR]*.)
4. Habits
a. Sleep: Does child sleep through the night? Note naps, number of hours of sleep at night, bedtime routines
b. Elimination: Urination and bowel movements, toilet training, occurrence of accidents
c. Exercise: Types of activities, frequency, organized sports
d. Behavior patterns (e.g., fussiness, response to frustration, thumb sucking, nail biting): What is your child like? Does he or she have a particularly fussy time during the day?, etc.
e. Use of alcohol, tobacco, drugs, coffee, tea, colas
f. Discipline: Methods used, success, failure, concerns
g. Sexuality: Inquisitiveness about girl-boy differences and pregnancy; parental responses and sex education offered; concerns and questions parents/child may have about masturbation, menstruation, nocturnal emissions, development of secondary sex characteristics, dating, and sexual urges and activity
5. Medications taken regularly
a. By practitioner's prescription
b. By self-prescription (over-the-counter or use of prescription medications)

Developmental data

The assessment of the development of the child is discussed in detail in Chapter 4: Developmental Assessment Across the Life Span. The history of the child's development is a component of that assessment and should provide clues that indicate when a more formal assessment is indicated. The box on pp. 74–78 in Chapter 4 summarizes normal child developmental milestones from 1 month to 5 years. Table 25.3 describes developmental findings that indicate a need for referral.

The initial history should include the following information:
1. Age at which the child attained specific developmental achievements:
a. Held head erect
b. Rolled over
c. Sat alone
d. Walked alone
e. Said first words
f. Used sentences
g. Controlled feces
h. Learned urinary continence
2. Current developmental performance. Assess developmental performance by asking specific questions related to expected abilities for the child's age range (see pp. 74–78). You may want to ask a broad question ("What new things have you noticed your child doing since the last visit?") followed by a more specific question ("Has he rolled over yet?"). You may also determine development by use of a screening tool such as the Denver Developmental Screening Test II (see Figure 4.1).
3. Any periods of decreased or increased growth. Was this area evaluated? Were there any known or suspected causes for such growth (family stress, illness, etc.)? These questions can be asked either during the nutritional assessment or at this time.
4. Questions concerning developmentally appropriate activities (e.g., peer relationships, school achievement, dating) may be covered in the review of systems but are also appropriate to address here.

Nutritional data

Questions regarding nutrition vary according to the child's age. More detailed and specific information may be obtained for the infant, who is growing rapidly, than for the older child.

Early infancy (birth to 6 months)
1. Type of feeding (breast-feeding, brand of commercial formula, or home-prepared formula)
2. Frequency of feedings
3. Amount consumed with each feeding and during a 24-hour period. Be specific in terms of number of ounces per feeding, number and size of cans of formula used per day, type of formula and how formula is prepared (add water to concentrate versus ready to pour from can), and number of times and length of breast-feeding sessions per day
4. Any changes in feeding (e.g., from breast-feeding to bottle-feeding or addition of a supplementary bottle if breast-feeding, date of change, introduction of solids)
5. Any problems observed with feeding (e.g., colic or spitting up)

table 25.3 *Developmental Red Flags During the First Year*

Age	Rhythmicity and sleep/ autonomic stability	Social/ emotional skills	Cognitive and visual abilities	Language/ hearing	Fine motor (feeding/ self-care)	Gross motor (strength, coordination)
Newborn/ 1 mo	Apnea, poor suck/ swallow Tachypnea/ bradycardia with feeding Poor habitua- tion to external stimuli	Diffuse non- verbal cues Poor state transitions Irritable	Doll's eyes ?/ no RLR (red-light reflex) Poor alert state	No startle to sound/ sudden noises No quieting to voice High-pitched cry	Hands held fisted Absent or asymmetri- cal palmar grasp	Asymmetrical movements Hypotonia or hypertonia Asymmetrical primitive re- flexes
3 mo	Poor suck/ swallow/ breathing	Lack of social smile Withdrawn or depressed	No visual tracking Not fixing on face or object	Does not turn to voice, rattle, or bell No sounds, coos, squeals	Hands fisted with op- positional thumb No hand-to- mouth activity	Asymmetrical movements Hypotonia or hypertonia No attempt to raise head on stomach
6 mo	Continuation of any of above Poor feeding or sleep reg- ulation	No smiles No response to play Solemn ap- pearance	Not visually alert Does not reach for objects Does not look at caregiver	No babbles Does not respond to voice, bell, rattle, or loud noises even with startle	Does not hold rattle Does not hold hands to- gether Does not grasp at clothes	Does not at- tempt to sit with support Head lag with pull to sit Scissoring
8 mo	Control issues with feeding or sleep	Intense stranger anxiety	Lack of visual awareness Lack of reach- ing out for toys Lack of toy exploration visually or orally	Lack of single- or double- consonant sounds Lack of response to name or voice	No self- feeding No high- chair sit- ting No solids Does not pick up toy with one hand	Does not sit even in tri- pod position No lateral prop reflex Asymmetrical crawl, hand- edness, or other move- ments
12 mo	Poor sleep/ wake cycle persists Extreme inabil- ity to sepa- rate from parent	No response to game playing No response to reading or interac- tive activities Withdrawn or solemn	Not visually following activities in the environ- ment	Not imitating speech sounds Not using two to three words	Not attempt- ing to feed self or hold cup Not able to hold toy in each hand or transfer objects	Not pulling self to stand Not moving around the environment to explore

From Burns CE et al: *Pediatric primary care: a handbook for nurse practitioners*, Philadephia, 1996, WB Saunders; data from McMillan J: Watching for developmental lags and disabilities. In *The best of the whole pediatrician catalog I-III*, New York, 1983, McMillan; and Dixon S, Stein M: *Encounters with children*, St Louis, 1992, Mosby.

table 25.4 *Information on Drugs Affecting Breast-Feeding*

Drug	Effect
DRUGS THAT ARE CONTRAINDICATED DURING BREAST-FEEDING	
Bromocriptine	Suppresses lactation
Cocaine	Cocaine intoxication
Cyclophosphamide	Possible immune suppression; unknown effect on growth or association with carcinogenesis; neutropenia
Cyclosporine	Possible immune suppression; unknown effect on growth or association with carcinogenesis
Doxorubicin*	Possible immune suppression; unknown effect on growth or association with carcinogenesis
Ergotamine	Vomiting, diarrhea, convulsions (doses used in migraine medications)
Lithium	⅓ to ½ therapeutic blood concentration in infants
Methotrexate	Possible immune suppression; unknown effect on growth or association with carcinogenesis; neutropenia
Phencyclidine (PCP)	Potent hallucinogen
Phenindione	Anticoagulant; increased prothrombin and partial thromboplastin time in 1 infant (not used in United States)
DRUGS OF ABUSE THAT ARE CONTRAINDICATED DURING BREAST-FEEDING†	
Amphetamine	Irritability, poor sleep pattern
Cocaine	Cocaine intoxication
Heroin	
Marijuana	Only one report in literature; no effect mentioned
Nicotine (smoking)	Shock, vomiting, diarrhea, rapid heart rate, restlessness; decreased milk production
Phencyclidine	Potent hallucinogen
DRUGS THAT HAVE CAUSED SIGNIFICANT EFFECTS ON SOME NURSING INFANTS AND SHOULD BE GIVEN TO NURSING MOTHERS WITH CAUTION (MEASURE BLOOD CONCENTRATION IN THE INFANT WHEN POSSIBLE)	
Aspirin (salicylates)	Metabolic acidosis (dose related); may affect platelet function; rash
Clemastine	Drowsiness, irritability, refusal to feed, high-pitched cry, neck stiffness (1 case)
Phenobarbital	Sedation; infantile spasms after weaning from milk containing phenobarbital, methemoglobinemia (1 case)
Primidone	Sedation, feeding problems
Salicylazosulfapyridine (sulfasalazine)	Bloody diarrhea in 1 infant
DRUGS WHOSE EFFECTS ON NURSING INFANTS ARE UNKNOWN BUT MAY BE OF CONCERN	
Psychotropic drugs	Special concern when given to nursing mothers for long periods of time
Antianxiety drugs	
Diazepam	None
Lorazepam	None
Prazepam*	None
Quazepam	None
Antidepressants	
Amitriptyline	None
Amoxapine	None
Desipramine	None
Dothiepin	None
Doxepin	None
Imipramine	None
Trazodone	None
	None
Antipsychotic drugs	
Chlorpromazine	Galactorrhea in adult; drowsiness and lethargy in infant
Chlorprothixene	None
Haloperidol	None
Mesoridazine	None
Chloramphenicol	Possible idiosyncratic bone marrow suppression
Metoclopramide*	None described; potent central nervous system
Metronidazole	In vitro mutagen; may discontinue breast-feeding for 12-24 hours to allow excretion of dose when single-dose therapy is given to mother
Tinidazole	See Metronidazole

Modified from Committee on Drugs: The transfer of drugs and other chemicals into human milk, *Pediatrics* 93(1):137–150, 1994.

*Drug is concentrated in human milk.

†The Committee on Drugs believes strongly that nursing mothers should not ingest any of these compounds. Not only are they hazardous to the nursing infant, but they are detrimental to the physical and emotional health of the mother.

6. How long the mother plans to continue breast-feeding or bottle-feeding
7. Vitamin, iron, or fluoride supplements (including name of the preparation, when it was started, amount given, and method of administration)
8. Solid foods, including type (commercially prepared or home prepared), amount given, how they are given (by spoon or in bottle), and frequency
9. Water, including amount given, frequency offered, whether given plain or with a sweetener
10. Infant's appetite and reaction to eating

If the infant is breast-feeding, obtain the following information about the mother:

1. How the mother feels she is doing with breast-feeding
2. Any questions or concerns about herself or the baby
3. Any problems with her breasts (discomfort, blisters, chafing, tenderness, etc.)
4. How the mother cares for her breasts
5. Mother's program of daily exercise, rest, diet, and fluid intake
6. Medications being taken (specify name, frequency, purpose, and effectiveness) (see Table 25.4 for information on drugs known to be excreted in human milk and to have side effects in breast-fed infants)
7. Support mother receives from her spouse, family members, and/or friends
8. How long she plans to breast-feed and when (or if) she wants to introduce bottle-feeding
9. If using supplementary bottles, is she expressing breast milk or using formula? What kind of formula? How is she storing breast milk? Any problems with expressing milk?
10. Is there any other information that the mother would like (e.g., resources, support groups, lactation consultation)

To determine if the baby is getting enough breast milk, ask the mother:

1. How often the infant wets his or her diaper (should have at least eight wet diapers in a 24-hour period)
2. To describe the baby's bowel movements (should be large amount of yellow stool; may have bowel movements several times a day or every few days)

If the infant is receiving bottle-feedings, ask if he or she is held for all feedings or if the bottle is propped. The infant who receives a bottle of milk or juice at bedtime or naptime, to be used in much the same way as a pacifier, is at risk for dental caries and destruction of the anterior maxillary teeth (referred to as "baby bottle syndrome"[Figure 25.4]). This practice also puts the child at risk for aspiration of fluids and middle ear infections.

figure **25.4** Nursing-bottle caries in a 20-month-old child. Note extensive carious involvement of the maxillary primary incisors and first molars. *(Courtesy Drs. Abelson and Cameron, Lutherville, Md.)*

Later infancy (6 to 12 months). During this period the infant is beginning to vigorously manipulate his or her body and the environment. In addition to the questions outlined for the period of early infancy, ask questions regarding the infant's developing skills:

1. Has the infant started using a cup, finger-feeding, or using a spoon?
2. Does the infant receive coarser foods such as junior foods or table foods?
   a. What foods does he or she like?
   b. Has there been any problem (diarrhea, rash) after eating any particular food?
   c. How often does the infant eat solids (meals and snacks)?
3. How does the mother feel about the infant's developing independent feeding behaviors? What are her expectations of the child (e.g., child should not make a mess, should be able to use a spoon)?
4. Have there been any feeding problems?

Toddlerhood. During this stage the child's rapid growth rate slows. In addition, the child is experiencing an increased sense of independence and has the ability to feed himself or herself. This is a time when parents often become concerned about decreased food intake, and "battles" over feeding can develop. Therefore it is important to ask questions to determine the adequacy of food intake (recognizing that toddlers require smaller amounts of food than most parents realize) and the existence or signs of development of feeding problems.

1. What does the child eat during a typical day?
   a. What foods does he or she like?
   b. Has there been any problem (diarrhea, rash) after eating any particular food?
   c. How often does the child eat meals and snacks? What are the amounts (e.g., tablespoonfuls, number of crackers)
   d. How does the child feed himself or herself (fin-

gers, spoon, fork; holds cup; is still fed by parent)?

2. How do the parents feel about the toddler's feeding behaviors? What are their expectations of the child (should not make a mess, should be able to use a spoon, fork, etc.)?

3. Have there been any feeding problems?
   a. Have there been any "hunger strikes" (typical of an 18-month-old child)?
   b. Does the child go on "food jags" in which he or she will eat only one type of food?
   c. Is he or she a "picky eater"?
   d. Have there been many struggles for control (parent trying to make the child eat) over eating, and how do these resolve?

Preschool age, school age, and adolescence. The 24-hour recall method and the dietary history method are appropriate for obtaining information about the diet and eating habits of the child (see Chapter 5: Nutritional Assessment; sample forms for gathering nutritional data are included in Chapter 5). In addition to general nutrition patterns, find out about the parents' attitudes toward eating and their response to any eating problems that might exist. Pay special attention to preadolescents' and adolescents' concerns about being "overweight." Assess for possible eating disorders and crash dieting.

Family health history

The family medical history of the child is similar to the history obtained for the adult client (see Chapter 3: The Health History). It includes the health and age of the grandparents, maternal and paternal aunts and uncles, parents, and siblings and the age at death and cause of death for deceased relatives. In addition, the pediatric

family history should include information about miscarriages and stillbirths, congenital defects, and familial diseases.

Outline the family history information (or put it in the form of a family tree) to identify any illnesses or problems that may have implications for the child's future health and current health. The family tree, which is similar to the pedigree used in a genetic study, allows a study of the patterns of distribution of genetic traits in kindred people. When the information obtained in the family history reveals suspected genetic problems, refer the child and the parents to a specialist in genetics for diagnosis and counseling. Figure 25.5 illustrates a family tree for a pediatric client.

Review of systems

The review of systems is essentially the same as that for the adult history (see Chapter 3) except for age-appropriate modifications. The general format remains the same.

Physical systems

General (additional questions). Ask about recent and significant gain or loss of weight, failure to gain weight appropriate for age, or failure to increase in height.

Changes in behavior. Ask about behavior changes such as increased crying, irritability, nervousness, or withdrawal or changes in sleep patterns. These questions are usually found under the review of the central nervous system in the adult history. However, behavior changes in children may represent the first symptoms of a problem in any physical system or may indicate psychosocial problems, including abuse and neglect.

Skin (additional questions). Ask about birthmarks, rashes, and acne.

Head. Ask about injuries and headaches.

Eyes (additional questions). Ask about strabismus, discharge, vision disturbance (ask about behaviors that might be indicative of problems, such as sitting very close to the television, writing with the head near the desk, rubbing the eyes).

Ears (additional questions). Ask about ear infections, earaches, hearing loss (note loud speech, delayed speech, need to repeat questions), and previous hearing tests.

Nose (additional questions). Ask whether the child has a constant or frequent runny or stuffy nose (unilateral or bilateral); note the type of rhinorrhea.

Mouth and throat (additional questions). Ask about the age of eruption of teeth; whether the child was born with a cleft lip or cleft palate; the number of teeth at 1 year; whether the child had thrush.

Neck and nodes (additional questions). Ask about the limitation of movement or enlarged nodes.

Breasts (deletions and additional questions). In the newborn there may be breast enlargement secondary to

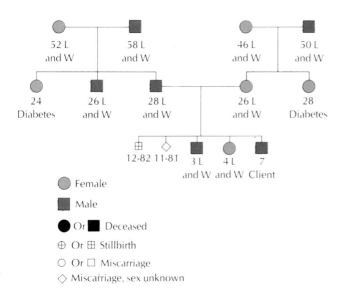

Female

Male

● Or ■ Deceased

⊕ Or ⊞ Stillbirth

○ Or □ Miscarriage

◇ Miscarriage, sex unknown

figure**25.5** Family tree used in a pediatric history.

maternal hormones that resolves spontaneously (but may be of concern to the parents).

Ask the preadolescent and the adolescent boy or girl if he or she has noticed changes in the breasts. (Figure 25.6 describes the normal stages of breast development in girls. Boys may experience some degree of transient gynecomastia during puberty.)

Ask about individual concerns regarding breast development, such as comparisons made with peers or the unequal development of the breasts. This subject may be approached by acknowledging that such concerns are common at this age and stating that you would be happy to answer any questions the adolescent may have. For girls, teach self-breast examination once breast buds have begun to develop.

Respiratory (additional questions). Ask about stridor, wheezing, episodes of croup, frequent colds, night-time coughing, and reduced exercise tolerance. Does the child play as actively as other children or curtail strenuous exercise?

Cardiovascular systems (additional questions). Ask about any history of heart murmur, and any evaluation and follow-up if a murmur is present; does the child experience fatigue on exertion?

Gastrointestinal system. Ask about abdominal pain, constipation, diarrhea, change in continence, toilet training, and "accidents."

Genital system (deletions and additional questions)

MALE. Ask the preadolescent and adolescent male questions about the development of the secondary sex characteristics. (Figure 25.7 describes normal changes.) This discussion also provides an opportunity to teach about the normal changes that have occurred or are going to occur and to reassure the client that what he is experiencing is normal. Characteristics to ask about include the following:

Appearance of hair on face and body
Appearance of axillary hair
Appearance of pubic hair
Increase in size of testes
Testicular self-examination (teach client)

Ask about individual concerns regarding sexual development. An effective approach is to universalize concerns. For example, say: "Many boys your age have questions about. . . . What questions would you like me to answer?" Delete the question about impotence until it is determined that the young man is sexually active.

FEMALE. Ask the preadolescent and adolescent female questions about the development of the secondary sex characteristics. (Figure 25.8 describes normal changes.) This discussion also offers the chance to teach about the normal changes that have occurred or are going to occur and to reassure the client that what she is experiencing is normal. Characteristics to ask about include the following:

Onset of menses (if menarche has occurred): determine if periods are painful
Appearance of axillary hair
Appearance of pubic hair

Ask about individual concerns regarding sexual development. Again, universalizing the question will make it more comfortable for the teenager to respond: "Many girls your age have questions about. . . . What questions would you like me to answer?"

Delete the questions about obstetrical history until you determine that the girl is sexually active.

Delete the question about Papanicolaou (Pap) tests until the girl is 15 years of age unless you determine that (1) the girl younger than 15 years is sexually active or (2) was exposed to diethylstilbestrol (DES) before birth and has begun to menstruate.

BOTH SEXES You should ask questions about sexual activity and sexually transmitted diseases once the child is about 10 years old. Explain the reason that the questions must be asked. Discuss "safer" sexual practices, contraception, and the option of abstinence, particularly if the client is sexually active.

Extremities and musculoskeletal system (additional questions). Ask about "growing pains," postural deformities or changes, changes in gait, and injuries to muscles or joints.

Central nervous system (additional questions). Ask about the ability to concentrate, hyperactivity, and headaches. Additional information about this system will be obtained in the developmental history and social history.

Sociological system

1. Relationship with family and significant others (can be done in the form of a family tree or genogram)
   a. Client's position in the family (birth order), natural child or adopted *(addition)*
   b. Person(s) with whom client lives
   c. Persons with whom client relates (Who is the primary caretaker? What are arrangements for baby-sitters? Does the child have special friends?)
   d. Recent family crises or changes (should include history of parental divorce, separation, or re-marriage and birth or adoption of siblings)
2. Environment
   a. Home (Heated? Adequate hot water? Well or city water? Number of rooms, toilets, cooking facilities? Where does child play?)
   b. Neighborhood (safety issues, play areas, sense of community)
   c. Recent changes in environment
   d. To what degree are cultural and religious practices observed?

Stage		Breast development

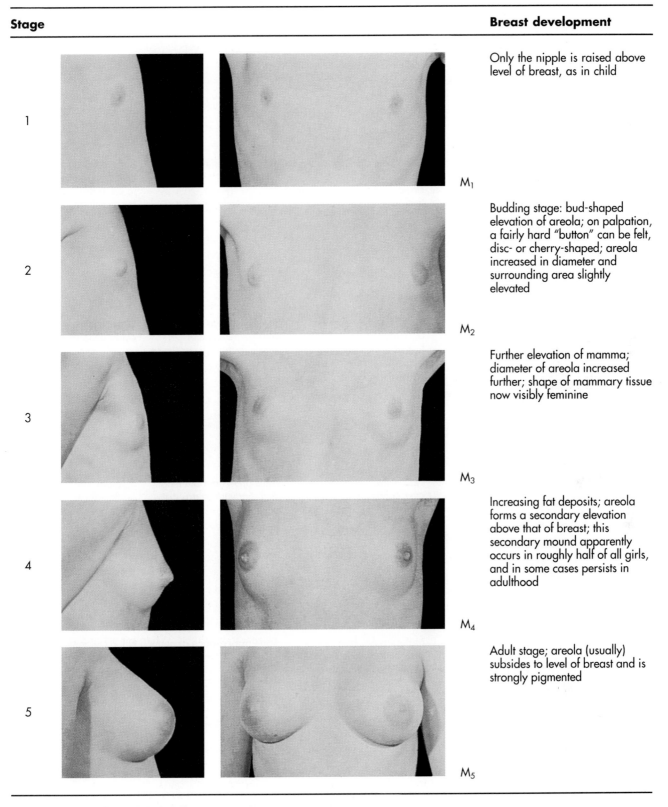

1 — M₁: Only the nipple is raised above level of breast, as in child

2 — M₂: Budding stage: bud-shaped elevation of areola; on palpation, a fairly hard "button" can be felt, disc- or cherry-shaped; areola increased in diameter and surrounding area slightly elevated

3 — M₃: Further elevation of mamma; diameter of areola increased further; shape of mammary tissue now visibly feminine

4 — M₄: Increasing fat deposits; areola forms a secondary elevation above that of breast; this secondary mound apparently occurs in roughly half of all girls, and in some cases persists in adulthood

5 — M₅: Adult stage; areola (usually) subsides to level of breast and is strongly pigmented

figure**25.6**   Five stages of breast development in females. (*Photographs from Van Wieringen JC: Growth diagrams 1965 Netherlands second national survey on 0-24-year-olds, Groningen, Netherlands, 1971, Wolters-Noordhoff; reprinted by permission of Kluwer Academic Publishers.*)

Stage		Pubic hair	Penis	Scrotum
1		No pubic hair	Appears like smaller child's penis	Testes begins to enlarge, but scrotum remains small and undeveloped
2		Pubic hair starting to develop; appears as straight, long, and downy texture	Little enlargement	Both testes and scrotum enlarge; scrotum begins to acquire darker skin tone and change in texture
3		Increasing hair growth over entire pubic region; hair is dark, curly, and beginning to become coarse	Penis begins to enlarge; enlargement is more in length than in general size	Growth and skin texture continue to develop
4		Hair is thick and coarse over entire pubic area	Penis grows in both length and diameter; glans also develops	Scrotum is like that of adult—darker tone and testes are almost adult size
5		Mature pubic hair distribution, including on upper medial thighs	Adult appearance of penis	Full development and adult-appearing testes

figure **25.7** Tanner's sex maturity development in males. *(Photographs from Van Wieringen JC: Growth diagrams 1965 Netherlands second national survey on 0-24-year-olds, Groningen, Netherlands, 1971, Wolters-Noordhoff; reprinted by permission of Kluwer Academic Publishers.)*

Stage		Pubic hair development
1		No growth of pubic hair
2		Initial, scarcely long, straight, downy and slightly pigmented pubic hair, especially along labia
3		Pubic hair is darker, coarser, and curly, and spread sparsely over entire pubis in typical female triangle
4		Pubic hair is denser, curly, and in an adult distribution, but less abundant and restricted to pubic area
5		Pubic hair is adult in quantity, type, and pattern, with lateral spreading to inner aspect of thighs
6		Further extension laterally, upward, or over the upper thighs (this stage may not occur in all women)

figure**25.8**   Tanner's sex maturity development in females. *(Photographs from Van Wieringen JC: Growth diagrams 1965 Netherlands second national survey on 0-24-year-olds, Groningen, Netherlands, 1971, Wolters-Noordhoff; reprinted by permission of Kluwer Academic Publishers.)*

3. Occupational history (if appropriate)
   a. Jobs held
   b. Satisfaction with present and past employment
   c. Current place of employment
   d. Future goals concerning occupation, career, etc.
4. Economic status and resources
   a. Parents' occupations and sources of income
   b. Parents' perception of adequacy or inadequacy of income
   c. Arrangements for child care while parent(s) are at work; type of care (baby-sitter, child care center, relatives, after-school program), satisfaction with care, concerns about child care
   d. Effect of child's illness on parents' economic status; plans for "sick child" care if both parents work outside the home
5. Educational level (this area may also be covered in the developmental assessment section)
   a. Name of child's school
   b. Current grade level (Has child ever been held back?)
   c. Judgment of intellect relative to age (parent may be asked to make this judgment by asking how this child performs compared with siblings or other children of the same age)
   d. Satisfaction with school, relationships with teacher, etc.
   e. Concerns about school performance
6. Daily profile
   a. Sleep, rest, activity patterns
   b. Social activities (play activities)
   c. Special weekend activities
   d. Recent changes in daily activities
   e. Parental concerns and management of any specific behavior, such as masturbation, thumb-sucking, nail-biting, temper tantrums, or bed-wetting
7. Patterns of health care
   a. Private and public primary care agencies
   b. Dental care
   c. Preventive care
   d. Emergency care

Psychological system. The outline for the psychological system review provided in Chapter 3 (and repeated here) is appropriate for use with the child and parent with the addition of information about the child's personality style. Include both the parent and the child because it will be the parent who is primarily responsible for the child's care during the childhood years. The adolescent child will be more responsible for self-care but will continue to need direction and support from an informed, understanding parent.

You can describe personality in general terms such as outgoing or shy. One way of describing personality that practitioners have found useful in working with families is to identify the child's behavioral or tem-

perament style. Temperament refers to the way an individual deals with new situations and life in general. Chess and Thomas (1986) have identified nine temperament categories (see box below) that can be combined to form three behavior profiles—the easy child, the difficult child, and the slow-to-warm-up child (see box on p. 663). These patterns appear to exist over long periods and may affect the child's adjustment to a variety of childhood situations. Chess and Thomas emphasize that the style itself is not problematic; it is the degree of "fit" between the child's style and his or her environment, in particular the parents, that determines the degree of difficulty experienced. Direct interventions at helping parents to understand their child's style and to work with that style rather than against it.

Attributes of Temperament

Activity: Level of physical motion during activity, such as sleep, eating, play, dressing, and bathing.

Rhythmicity: Regularity in the timing of physiological functions, such as hunger, sleep, and elimination.

Approach-withdrawal: Nature of initial responses to a new stimulus, such as people, situations, places, foods, toys, and procedures. *Approach* responses are positive, displayed by activity or expression; *withdrawal* responses are negative expressions or behaviors.

Adaptability: Ease or difficulty with which the child adapts or adjusts to new or altered situations.

Threshold of responsiveness (sensory threshold): Amount of stimulation, such as sounds or light, required to evoke a response in the child.

Intensity of reaction: Energy level of the child's reactions, regardless of quality or direction.

Mood: Amount of pleasant, happy, friendly behavior compared with unpleasant, unhappy, crying, unfriendly behavior exhibited by the child in various situations.

Distractibility: Ease with which a child's attention or direction of behavior can be diverted by external stimuli.

Attention span and persistence: Length of time a child pursues a given activity (*attention*) and the continuation of an activity in spite of obstacles (*persistence*).

Modified from Wong DL: *Whaley and Wong's nursing care of infants and children,* ed 5, St Louis, 1995, Mosby.

In assessment of the adolescent client (age 12 years and older), it is important to explore some additional areas, including depression and suicide potential, involvement with drugs and alcohol, and sexuality. The box below (right), the box on p. 664, and Table 25.5 give suggestions for what to cover and how to get the most information in the adolescent interview. Always inform teenage clients that the information that they share will be kept confidential unless they or someone else is in danger of physical harm. At the same time, encourage teens to talk with their parents about these issues.

1. Personality: How does the parent describe the child's general characteristics? What are his or her temperament characteristics (see box on p. 663)? How does this influence the child's interactions with family, friends, peers, etc.?
2. Cognitive abilities (for the child, this information may be included in the developmental assessment)
   a. Comprehension
   b. Learning patterns
   c. Memory
3. Response to illness and health
   a. Reaction to illness
   b. Coping patterns
   c. Value of health
   d. Use of well-child and health promotion services
4. Response to care
   a. Perceptions of the caregivers
   b. Compliance
5. Cultural implications for care
   a. Patterns of therapy
   b. Beliefs about child care and child-rearing
   c. Patterns of illness response

Anticipatory guidance

As noted earlier in the chapter, anticipatory guidance should be addressed at each visit. This area includes evaluating the parents' understanding of child development and education, upcoming developmental changes, and questions or issues of concern. The focus should be individualized to the family's needs. In addition, information about child safety (e.g., child-proofing the home, use of bicycle helmets, seat belts) (Figure 25.9) needs to be communicated. This information is most effective when it is offered just before a developmental

---

Behavior Profiles

EASY CHILD

Easygoing children are even tempered, regular, and predictable in their habits and have a positive approach to new stimuli. They are open and adaptable to change and display a mild to moderately intense mood that is typically positive.

DIFFICULT CHILD

Difficult children are highly active, irritable, and irregular in their habits. Negative withdrawal responses are typical, and they require a more structured environment. These children adapt slowly to new routines, people, or situations. Mood expressions are usually intense and primarily negative. They exhibit frequent periods of crying, and frustration often produces violent tantrums.

SLOW-TO-WARM-UP CHILD

Slow-to-warm-up children typically react negatively and with mild intensity to new stimuli and, unless pressured, adapt slowly with repeated contact. They respond with only mild but passive resistance to novelty or changes in routine. They are quite inactive and moody but show only moderate irregularity in functions.

Modified from Whaley LF, Wong DL : *Nursing care of infants and children,* ed 4, St Louis, 1991, Mosby.

Suicide Risk/Depression Screening

1. Sleep disorders (usually induction problems; also early/frequent waking or greatly increased sleep and complaints of increasing fatigue)
2. Appetite/eating behavior change
3. Feelings of "boredom"
4. Emotional outbursts and highly impulsive behavior
5. History of withdrawal/isolation
6. Hopeless/helpless feelings
7. History of past suicide attempts, depression, psychological counseling
8. History of suicide attempts, depression, or psychological problems in family or peers
9. History of drug/alcohol abuse, acting-out/crime, recent change in school performance
10. History of recurrent serious "accidents"
11. Psychosomatic symptomatology
12. Suicidal ideation (including significant current and past losses)
13. Decreased affect on interview, avoidance of eye contact—depression posturing
14. Preoccupation with death (clothing, music, media, art)

Modified from Goldenring JM, Cohen E: Getting into adolescent heads, *Contemp Pediatr* 5:75-86, 1988.

The HEADS Psychosocial Interview for Adolescents

HOME
Who lives with client? Where?
Own room?
What are relationships like at home?
What do parents and relatives do for a living?
Ever institutionalized? Incarcerated?
Recent moves? Running away?
New people in home environment?

EDUCATION AND EMPLOYMENT
School/grade performance—any recent changes? Any dramatic past changes?
Favorite subjects—worst subjects? (Include grades.)
Any years repeated/classes failed?
Suspension, termination, dropping out?
Future education/employment plans/goals?
Any current or past employment?
Relations with teachers, employers—school/work attendance?
Recent change of schools—number of schools in last 4 years?

ACTIVITIES
With peers (What do you do for fun? Where and when?)
With family or clubs?
Sports—regular exercise?
Church attendance, clubs, projects?

Hobbies—other home activities?
Reading for fun—what?
TV—how much weekly—favorite shows?
Favorite music?
Does patient have car, use seat belts?
History of arrests—acting-out—crime?

DRUGS
Use by peers? Use by patient? (Include alcohol/tobacco.)
Use by family members? (Include alcohol/tobacco.)
Amounts, frequency, patterns of use/abuse, and car use while intoxicated?
Source—how paid for?

SEXUALITY
Orientation?
Degree and types of sexual experience and acts?
Number of partners?
Masturbation? (Normalize.)
History of pregnancy/abortion?
Sexually transmitted diseases—knowledge and prevention?
Contraception? Frequency of use?
Comfort with sexual activity, enjoyment/pleasure obtained?
History of sexual/physical abuse

Modified from Goldenring JM, Cohen E: Getting into adolescent heads, *Contemp Pediatr* 5:75-86, 1988.

figure**25.9** Anticipatory guidance needs to be addressed at each visit and should be individualized to the family's needs.

change is about to occur. The boxes on pp. 666-667 and 668 provide guidelines for such information.

Anticipatory guidance information may be most easily integrated into other parts of the health history. For example, when you are getting information about the child's current developmental achievements, you can tell the parent what to look for over the next few months. For example, "Now that your baby has started to crawl, you can expect that he will start to explore new and potentially dangerous areas of your home." This approach can lead to a discussion of safety concerns that the parent will need to consider related to the child's mobility and ability to get into things (e.g., safety gates, plugs for electrical outlets, door/cupboard latches, need for syrup of ipecac).

Preparation for Examination: Client and Environment

How you conduct the interview and physical examination will vary according to the child's age, develop-

table 25.5 *Opening Lines—Good and Bad*

	Poor	Better	Reason
Home	Tell me about mom and dad.	Where do you live, and who lives there with you?	Parent(s) may have died or left the home. Open-ended question enables one to collect "environmental" as well as personal history.
Education	How are you doing in school?	What are you good at in school? What is hard for you? What grades do you get?	Poor questions can be answered "okay." Good questions ask for information about strengths and weaknesses and allow for quantification/objectification.
Activities	Do you have any activities outside of school?	What do you do for fun? What things do you do with friends? What do you do with your free time?	Good questions are open-ended and allow patient to express himself.
Drugs	Do you do drugs?	Many young people experiment with drugs, alcohol, or cigarettes. Have you or your friends ever tried them? What have you tried?	Good question is an expression of concern with specific follow-up. With younger teens, it is best to begin by asking about friends.
Sexuality	Have you ever had sex? Tell me about your boyfriend/girlfriend.	Have you ever had a sexual relationship with anyone? Most young people become interested in sexual relationships at your age. Have you had any with boys, girls, or both? Tell me about your sex life.	What does the term "have sex" really mean to teenagers? Asking only about heterosexual relationships closes doors at once.

From Goldenring JM, Cohen E: Getting into adolescent heads, *Contemp Pediatr* 5:75-86, 1988.

ment, and behavior and the type of setting in which the care is being provided. If you do not give consideration to the child's age and development, the examination likely will be incomplete. If the child is fearful or fatigued, you will need to be more creative, patient, and selective (if possible) in performing the examination.

In carrying out a pediatric examination, keep in mind that each visit for health care is a learning experience for the child and the parent(s). The experience may result in increased confidence in themselves and others, or it may produce feelings of failure and distrust toward the professionals who are caring for them. Thus it is important to provide opportunities to develop positive relationships during the visits for routine health care (Figure 25.10). Also, remember that any separation of the child from the parent may provoke anxiety in both parties and may increase their level of fear and distrust. Encourage parents to participate in the examination and support their young child. This participation may be done by holding the child during the examination or by

soothing the child in other ways. The older child may be able to participate more freely without the parent present. Most parents will recognize the older child's need to develop independence and encourage the child to participate alone. Finally, prepare the child and the parent for any new or painful procedures. An appreciation for the feelings of children and parents will make them more cooperative.

Developmental approach to examination

Conduct the physical examination of the child in an organized and systematic manner, taking into account differences between an adult and a pediatric examination. Perform distressing parts of the examination at the end if you believe that the child will be unable to cooperate. You can alter the order of the examination to accommodate the individual child's behavior (e.g., listening to the heart and lungs early in the examination before crying starts or becomes more vigorous). Similarly, you may begin the examination of a child with a body

Anticipatory Guidance Topics

PRENATAL AND NEWBORN

Prenatal Visit

Health: Pregnancy course, worries, tobacco, alcohol, drug use, hospital and pediatric office procedures

Safety: Infant car seat, crib safety

Nutrition: Planned feeding method

Child care: Help after birth, later arrangements

Family: Changes in relationships (spouse, siblings), supports, stresses, return to work

Newborn Visits

Health: Jaundice, umbilical cord care, circumcision, other common problems, when to call the physician's office

Safety: Infant car seat, smoke detector, choking, keeping tap water temperature below 120° F

Nutrition: Feeding, normal weight loss, spitting, vitamin and fluoride supplements

Development/behavior: Individuality, "consolability," visual and auditory responsiveness

Child care: Importance of interaction, parenting books, support for primary caregiver

Family: Postpartum adjustments, fatigue, "blues," special time for siblings

FIRST YEAR

0 to 6 Months

Health: Immunizations, exposure to infections

Safety: Falls, aspiration of small objects or powder, entanglement in mobiles with long strings, curtain cords

Nutrition: Supplementation of breast milk or formula, introduction of solids, iron

Development/behavior: Crying/colic, irregular schedules (eating, sleeping, eliminating), responding to infant cues, reciprocity, interactive games, beginning eye-hand coordination

Child care: Responsive and affectionate care, caregiving schedule

Family: Return to work, the nurturing of all family relationships (spouse and siblings)

12 MONTHS

Safety: Locks for household poisons and medications, gates for stairs, ipecac, poison center telephone number; outlet safety covers; avoidance of dangling cords or tablecloths; safety devices for windows/screens, toddler car seat at 20 pounds; avoidance of toys with small detachable pieces; supervision of child in tub or near water

Nutrition: Need to discourage use of bottle as a pacifier or while in bed; offer cup and soft finger foods (with supervision); introduce new foods one at a time

Development/behavior: Attachment, basic trust versus mistrust, stranger awareness, night waking, separation anxiety, bedtime routine, transitional object

Child care: Prohibitions few but firm and consistent across caregiving settings; discipline defined as "learning" (not punishment)

Family: Spacing of children

SECOND YEAR

2 Years

Health: Immunizations

Safety: Climbing and falls common; need to supervise outdoor play; ensure safety caps on medicine bottles; note dangers of plastic bags, pan handles hanging over stove, and space heaters

Nutrition: Avoidance of feeding conflicts (decreased appetite common); period of self-feeding, weaning from breast or bottle; need to avoid sweet or salty snacks

Development/behavior: Autonomy versus shame/doubt, ambivalence (independence/dependence), tantrums, negativism, getting into everything, night fears, readiness for toilet training, self-comforting behaviors (thumb-sucking, masturbation), speech, imaginative play, no sharing in play, positive reinforcement for desired behavior

Child care: Freedom to explore in safe place; day care; home a safer place to vent frustrations; needs show of affection, language stimulation through reading and conversation

Family: Sibling relationships

PRESCHOOL

2 to 5 Years

Health: Toothbrushing, first dental visit

Safety: Need for close supervision near water or street; home safety factors include padding of sharp furniture corners, fire escape plan for home, and locking up power tools; should have car lap belt at 40 pounds and bike helmet; should know (a) name, address, and telephone number; (b) not to provoke dogs; and (c) to say "no" to strangers

Nutrition: Balanced diet; need to avoid sweet or salty snacks; child should participate in conversation at meals

From Foye HR: Anticipatory guidance. In Hoekelman R et al: *Primary pediatric care,* ed 3, St Louis, 1997, Mosby.

Anticipatory Guidance Topics—cont'd

Development/behavior: Initiative versus guilt; difficulty with impulse control and sharing; developing interest in peers, high activity level; speaking in sentences by age 3; speech mostly intelligible to stranger by age 3; reading books; curiosity about body parts; magical thinking; egocentrism

Child care/preschool: Need for daily special time with parent(s), bedtime routine; need to talk about day in day care, limit TV and watch with child, reprimand privately, answer questions factually and simply; adjustment to preschool, kindergarten readiness

Family: Chores, responsibilities

MIDDLE CHILDHOOD

5 to 10 Years

Health: Appropriate weight; regular exercise; somatic complaints (limb and abdominal pain, headaches); alcohol, tobacco, and drug use; sexual development; physician and child dealings (more direct)

Safety: Bike helmets and street safety; car seat belts; swimming lessons; use of matches, firearms, and power tools; fire escape plan for home; saying "no" to strangers

Nutrition: Balanced diet, daily breakfast, limited sweet and salty snacks, moderate fatty foods

Development/behavior: Industry versus inferiority; need for successes, peer interactions, adequate sleep

School: School performance, homework, parent interest

Family: More time away but continuing need for family support, approval, affection, time together, and communication; family rules about bedtime, chores, and responsibilities; guidance in using money; parent(s) should encourage reading; limit TV watching and discuss programs seen together

Other activities: Organized sports, religious groups, other organizations, use of spare time

ADOLESCENCE

Discuss with Adolescent

Health: Alcohol, tobacco, and drug use; need for dental care, physical activity, immunizations

Safety: Bike and skateboard helmet and safety, car seat belts, driving while intoxicated, water safety, hitchhiking, risk-taking

Nutrition: Balanced diet, appropriate weight, avoidance of junk foods

Sexuality: Physical changes, sex education, peer pressure for sexual activity, sense of responsibility for self and partner, OK to say no, prevention of pregnancy and sexually transmitted diseases, breast and testes self-examination

Development/relationships: Identity versus role confusion, family, peers, dating, independence, trying different roles

School: Academics, homework

Other activities: Sports, hobbies, organizations, jobs

Future plans: School, work, relationships with others

Discuss with Parent

Communication: Let adolescent participate in discussion and development of family rules; needs frequent praise and affection, time together, interest in adolescent's activities

Independence: Parent and child ambivalence about independence; expect periods of estrangement; promote self-responsibility and independence; still needs supervision

Role model: Actions speak louder than words—parents provide model of responsible, reasonable, and compassionate behavior

---

part that is least likely to interfere with developing a sense of trust and confidence (e.g., the hands or the eyes). Table 25.6 presents a summary of the different approaches used for the physical examination at different developmental stages.

Infant. Usually, little difficulty is encountered in performing the physical examination of the infant in the first 6 months of life, since the infant has little fear of strangers. The parent or the examiner can distract the infant with repetitive vocal sounds and smiles. However, since the examination of the ears and mouth may cause distress, this area should be saved for the end of the examination. Take advantage of the opportunities that are

offered. If the infant is quiet or sleepy, start with the auscultation of the chest and do so while the caretaker is still holding the infant. If the infant is playful and active, start with the extremities and wait for a quieter moment to examine the chest.

During the last half of the first year of life, the infant experiences an increasing fear of strangers. In this situation, conduct the entire examination while the infant is held on the parent's lap (Figure 25.11). Even under the best of circumstances, creating an ideal situation may not be possible. The infant may remain resistant throughout the examination. If this happens, you need to be efficient in carrying out the examination in the least amount of

Pertinent Information for Anticipatory Guidance

A. Information about the *child*
1. Concerns—expressed by parent or child
2. Health current status and follow-up of past problems
3. Routine care—feeding, sleep, and elimination
4. Development—evaluated by school performance or with standardized tests (e.g., Denver Developmental Screening Test, Early Language Milestone Scale)
5. Behavior—temperament and interaction with family, peers, and others

B. Information about the *child's environment*
1. Family composition (at home)
2. Caregiving schedule—who and when
3. Family stresses—e.g., work, finances, illness, death, move, marital, and other relationships
4. Family supports—relatives, friends, organizations, material resources
5. Stimulation in the home
6. Stimulation/activities outside the home, e.g., preschool/school, peers, organizations
7. Safety

From Foye Jr HR: Anticipatory guidance. In Hoekelman R et al: *Primary pediatric care*, ed 3, St Louis, 1997, Mosby.

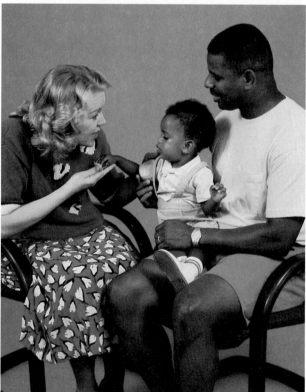

time and with minimal restraint of the infant. The parent often experiences discomfort or embarrassment because of the infant's behavior and will need reassurance that the infant is behaving normally. The situation is ideal for helping the parent to understand normal development and the needs of the infant at this age.

Toddler. The child from 1 to 3 years of age is a challenge to even the most experienced examiner. At this time the child is learning to use his or her body and to manipulate and experiment with all aspects of the environment. The child may see any restraint in the pursuit of desired activities as an interference, resulting in unhappiness or frustration for the child. At this age the child is experiencing a good deal of pleasure from recently acquired skills such as walking and talking and is enjoying the new ability to manipulate objects such as doors and wastebaskets. Yet the child is still unsure of strangers and needs the parent's presence to feel safe. The 2- or 3-year-old child may be charming and cooperative or difficult to examine. Whichever the case, you will be required to make many modifications in the organization of the ex-

figure**25.10** The physical examination can be a learning experience for both the parent and the child. It is important to listen to the parent's concerns and to assess the child's needs during the interview.

table 25.6	*Age-Specific Approaches to Physical Examination During Childhood*	
Position	**Sequence**	**Preparation**
INFANT		
Before sits alone: supine or prone, preferably in parent's lap; before 4 to 6 months: can place on examining table After sits alone: use sitting in parent's lap whenever possible If on table, place with parent in full view	If quiet, auscultate heart, lungs, abdomen Record heart and respiratory rates Palpate and percuss same areas Proceed in usual head-to-toe direction Perform traumatic procedures last (eyes, ears, mouth [while crying]) Elicit reflexes as body part examined Elicit Moro reflex last	Completely undress if room temperature permits Leave diaper on male Gain cooperation with distraction, bright objects, rattles, talking Have older infants hold a small block in each hand; until voluntary release develops toward end of the first year, infants will be unable to grasp other objects (e.g., stethoscope, otoscope) Smile at infant; use soft, gentle voice Pacify with bottle of sugar water or feeding Enlist parent's aid for restraining to examine ears, mouth Avoid abrupt, jerky movements
TODDLER		
Sitting or standing on/by parent Prone or supine in parent's lap	Inspect body area through play: "count fingers," "tickle toes" Use minimal physical contact initially Introduce equipment slowly Auscultate, percuss, palpate whenever quiet Perform traumatic procedures last (same as for infant)	Have parent remove outer clothing Remove underwear as body part examined Allow to inspect equipment; demonstrating use of equipment is usually ineffective If uncooperative, perform procedures quickly Use restraint when appropriate; request parent's assistance Talk about examination if cooperative; use short phrases Praise for cooperative behavior
PRESCHOOL CHILD		
Prefer standing or sitting Usually cooperative prone/supine Prefer parent's closeness	If cooperative, proceed in head-to-toe direction If uncooperative, proceed as with toddler	Request self-undressing Allow to wear underpants if shy Offer equipment for inspection; briefly demonstrate use Make up "story" about procedure: "I'm seeing how strong your muscles are" (blood pressure) Use paper-doll technique Give choices when possible Expect cooperation; use positive statements: "Open your mouth"
SCHOOL-AGE CHILD		
Prefer sitting Cooperative in most positions Younger child prefers parent's presence Older child may prefer privacy	Proceed in head-to-toe direction May examine genitalia last in older child Respect need for privacy	Request self-undressing Allow to wear underpants Give gown to wear Explain purpose of equipment and significance of procedure, such as otoscope to see eardrum, which is necessary for hearing Teach about body functioning and care
ADOLESCENT		
Same as for school-age child Offer option of parent's presence	Same as for older school-age child	Allow to undress in private Give gown Expose only area to be examined Respect need for privacy Explain findings during examination: "Your muscles are firm and strong" Matter-of-factly comment about sexual development: "Your breasts are developing as they should be" Emphasize normalcy of development Examine genitalia as any other body part; may leave to end

From Wong DL: *Whaley and Wong's nursing care of infants and children.* ed 5, St Louis, 1995, Mosby.

amination. You may examine the child in a standing position while you are seated or perform the examination with the child on the parent's lap. The child usually does not like to have all clothing removed at one time but will often cooperate if only one article of clothing is removed at a time while you carry out the examination. The child needs positive reinforcement for cooperative behaviors. He or she also needs the opportunity to handle and use the examining instruments (Figure 25.12). The child may enjoy doing so but may reject the offer if it is too fear-provoking. Despite the difficulties in examining the child of this age, the child's ability to relate more positively at each subsequent visit can be rewarding and profitable for the examiner.

Preschooler. At 3 or 4 years of age the child is usually able to understand and cooperate during the examination. He or she is anxious to please and is usually a delightful participant. At this stage the child has better control of feelings and behavior than the younger child does but may still lose control if fear is great. It is important to keep in mind the child's previous experiences with health care providers and the fears or problems associated with certain aspects of the examination (otoscopic examination in particular). The child should receive recognition for his or her efforts to participate so that the self-image will be enhanced. The child of this age especially enjoys trying out the examiner's equipment and will likely demonstrate new learning in future play activities; this experience is a way to incorporate the role of the examiner and to master fears (Figure 25.13). The child may prefer to try the equipment on a doll or a stuffed animal. Examination techniques or procedures can also be demonstrated first on a doll or stuffed animal. Again, for some children it may be helpful to permit the child to remain on the caregiver's lap.

School-age child. You can approach the school-age child in much the same way that you approach the adult. At this stage the child is usually curious and interested and benefits from explanations of what you are going to do. This child wants to perform well and will usually cooperate. However, the child may have concerns about his or her body and may feel threatened by the examination, particularly if he or she has had past negative experiences. Encourage the child to ask questions. Respect the child's sense of modesty, and attempt to conduct the examination with as little exposure as possible.

Adolescent. The adolescent period is a challenging one for parents, the adolescent, and health care providers. Many physical, developmental, and emotional changes

figure**25.11** The interview is a time for the child to become familiar with the examiner, as well as a time to gather information.

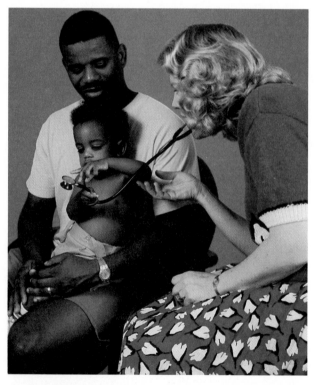

figure**25.12** The toddler needs the opportunity to handle and use the examining instruments from the safety of the parent's lap.

occur during this time (Table 25.7). Adolescents are not easy to anticipate, since behaviors are not predictable at this stage. They may be angry and hostile or charming and self-confident. Adolescents are primarily concerned about themselves and have the egocentric belief that others are as preoccupied with their own behavior and appearance as they are. They are likely to anticipate the responses of other people based on self-beliefs, self-criticism, and self-admiration. Adolescents self-consciously play to an audience because they believe that their behaviors, thoughts, and appearance are important to many people. Despite this egocentric view, adolescents will be responsive to a nonjudgmental examiner who encourages relevant conversation. This type of dialogue may not happen during the first visit, but if the experience is worthwhile to him or her, the adolescent may reveal more of these concerns at a later visit.

If possible, the adolescent should be the primary informant for the interview. The parent also provides significant data, particularly about the adolescent's past health history, the family health history, and the family situation, but the adolescent's perspective is also important. This approach supports the adolescent's sense of independence and can help in the development of rapport with the client.

Spend some time talking with the adolescent alone in addition to talking with the parents (Figure 25.14). This approach allows the adolescent to discuss private concerns. In general, the physical examination of the adolescent should be performed without the parent present. At the beginning of the visit, explain to the client and the parent that the policy is to meet with the parent and the child together for the history to make it as complete as possible and then to speak with and examine the child age 12 or older alone. Explain that after the examination, you will again meet with the parent and the child to discuss your findings and plans and to answer any questions that the parent and the child may have.

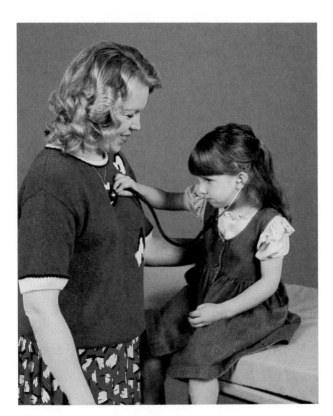

figure**25.13** The preschool-age child enjoys trying out the examiner's equipment.

figure**25.14** It is important to meet with the adolescent both alone and with the parent.

table 25.7 *Adolescent Psychosocial and Pubertal Development*		
Early adolescence (11 to 14 years)	**Middle adolescence (15 to 17 years)**	**Late adolescence (18 to 21 years)**
COGNITIVE DEVELOPMENT		
Concrete thinking: Present oriented; appreciate immediate reactions to behavior but little sense of later consequences	*Early abstract thinking:* Inductive/deductive reasoning; understands later consequences; very self-absorbed, introspective; lots of daydreaming and fantasies	*Abstract thinking:* Adult ability to think abstractly; philosophical; intense idealism about love, religion, social problems
SOCIAL/EMOTIONAL DEVELOPMENT		
Identity concerns:		
Concrete sense of morality and rule driven	More comfortable with sexual identity; gay youth at risk for depression and suicide ideation, also sadness	Focuses on vocational and personal options
Preoccupation with physical image		Uses life experience to generate options and temper decision making
Moody	Moodiness continues	
Friendship with same-sex peers	Identity centers on "Who am I?"	Capacity for moral reasoning
Experimentation is a common phenomenon	Strives toward autonomy	Able to formulate ethical principles
Peer values do not replace parents	Sensitive to social norms of peer group; conforms to perceived peer attitudes and behaviors	Capacity for mature emotional intimacy in relationships
May begin to experiment with mood or mind-altering substances	Identifies with group or clique	Adult sense of self
May experiment/explore homosexual behavior	May develop relationship with single romantic partner	
May experiment/explore heterosexual behavior	Limited capacity for emotional intimacy	

Most parents are not offended by this approach. If for cultural or individual reasons, it is not acceptable to the parent or the adolescent, conduct the history and examination with the family together.

Establishing a sense of confidentiality with the adolescent is important. Reassure the client that the information shared will remain between you and the client unless he or she gives you permission to share it with the parents or others or unless a problem becomes a threat to the client or to others. If you obtain information that cannot be kept confidential because of the laws of a particular state or the rules of health care practice, you must inform the client of this matter.

Since adolescent clients may be self-conscious and easily embarrassed, it is important to make sure that they wear a gown during the examination and that they are given complete privacy for dressing and undressing.

Technique for Examination and Normal Findings

The physical examination provides the opportunity to obtain objective information about the child. Al-

though, in general, most of the information comes from the history, physical examination findings assume greater importance when the parents are poor historians and the child is too young to communicate.

The physical examination of the infant or child varies according to the primary purpose of the visit. Three types of examinations might be performed. The first is the screening of a healthy child. Such an examination is usually complete but does not go into great depth in regard to a particular organ system. The second is the evaluation of a chief complaint, in which a more intensive examination of a particular area (and related regions) may be in order. The third is the follow-up examination of a complaint or disease that has been under treatment, in which the focus is usually one or two organ systems. Sometimes these three types of examinations are combined, particularly when it is the child's first visit and he or she is in need of a screening examination and a careful evaluation of the chief complaint.

Methods of restraint

On some occasions the physical examination involves an uncooperative child. You may need to use one or

table 25.7 *Adolescent Psychosocial and Pubertal Development—cont'd*

Early adolescence (11 to 14 years)	Middle adolescence (15 to 17 years)	Late adolescence (18 to 21 years)
SCHOOL-VOCATION		
Adjustment to middle school Need to be time efficient May see decrease in scholastic performance as demands increase Truancy may begin	Adjustment to senior high school Academic decisions Increased anxiety about academic performance, especially if college bound Safety in school; students carry weapons, may experience fear of physical harm	Decisions on whether to go to college, join workforce, or enter military Should be a time of choice and empowerment
FAMILY		
Heightened need for privacy Ambivalence about emotional independence Opinionated Challenges family rules, values, behaviors Still needs continued supervision and limit setting that promote increasing autonomy in decision making Family members are important role models Potential for sexual abuse increases as adolescent emerges sexually and begins to challenge behavior	Increased individuation and autonomy Extremely opinionated and challenging Increased family conflict, especially over issues of control Spends less time with family Peer groups take on greater importance Parents may be frustrated; continued communication is important	Relationships more accepting and harmonious More adult-to-adult interactions Family feels sense of loss as adolescent independence increases or can experience freedom

PHYSICAL

figure **25.15** Approximate timing of developmental changes in girls. Numbers indicate stages of development. The range of ages during which some of the changes occur is indicated by inclusive numbers below them. *(From Marshall WA, Tanner JM: Arch Dis Child 44:291, 1969).*

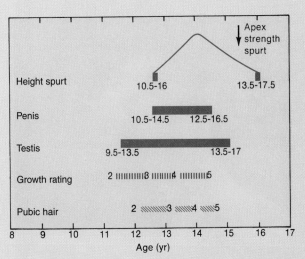

figure **25.16** Approximate timing of developmental changes in boys. Numbers indicate stages of development. The range of ages during which some of the changes occur is indicated by inclusive numbers below them. *(From Marshall WA, Tanner JM: Arch Dis Child 45:13, 1970.)*

Modified from Levenberg P, Elster A, editors: *Guidelines for adolescent preventive services (GAPS): clinical evaluation and management handbook,* Chicago, 1995, American Medical Association.

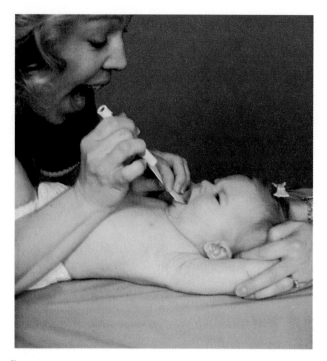

figure**25.17** Restraint of the young child with the parent assisting.

more of a variety of safe child-restraint methods. Clinical experience and knowledge of the child's behavior during previous visits will aid in choosing a safe restraint method. When restraint is necessary, carry out the procedure as quickly as possible and without criticism of the child.

One of the most common methods for restraining the infant or young child when examining the ears, nose, and mouth is done with the aid of the parent or another adult. Place the child in the supine position with the arms extended, and have the assisting adult hold the arms alongside the head (Figure 25.17). For an older child who cannot cooperate, use the same method with a second adult holding the child's legs.

Another method for the older child is sometimes called the "hug." Have the child sit on the parent's lap with the legs to the side and one arm tucked under the parent's arm while the parent holds the child's other arm securely (Figure 25.18). Obtain greater immobility of the child by having the parent place the child's legs between his or her own (Figure 25.19). If the parent is uncomfortable about assisting with restraint, you may ask another adult to help. However, the child usually feels less threatened if the parent does the holding.

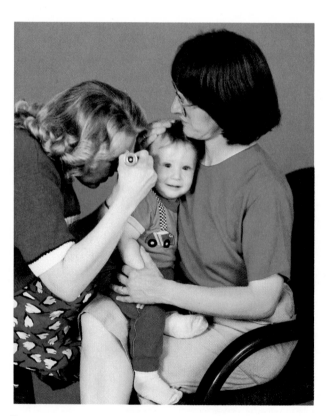

figure**25.18** Restraint using the "hug" restraint.

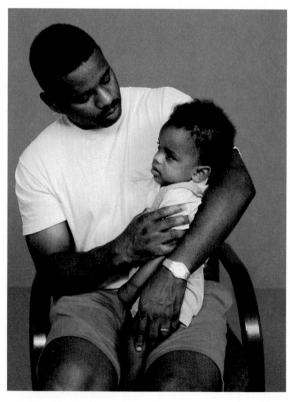

figure**25.19** Restraint of the older child using the leg restraint.

Measurements

Take measurements of the temperature, pulse rate, respiratory rate, blood pressure (for children over age 3 years), height, and weight as part of the physical examination of the child. In addition, note the measurements of the head circumference for the child who is less than 3 years of age. Comparing the physical measurements of a child with those of other healthy children over time makes it possible to determine if the child is progressing within normal parameters or if significant deviations exist.

Assessment of vital signs

Temperature. The body areas commonly used for obtaining temperature measurements—the mouth, the axilla, and the rectum, and a more recent approach, the ear canal and tympanic membrane—and types of thermometers are discussed in detail earlier in the book (see Chapter 9: General Assessment, Including Vital Signs) and are briefly reviewed here. The child's ability to cooperate and the health status determine the method selected.

Axillary temperature. You can obtain an axillary temperature on any child. This method reduces the risk of injury and is less intrusive than rectal or oral reading. Use the axillary route, whenever possible, to obtain the newborn infant's temperature. This approach may also be preferable for toddlers and preschoolers. Consider using an axillary temperature when the child objects to the rectal temperature and the oral temperature is not appropriate. Many practitioners recommend using the axillary method first and confirming an elevated temperature with a rectal or oral reading. Place the thermometer tip deep into the axilla and hold the arm close to the body for at least 5 minutes (a digital thermometer reading will be faster). Restrain the child by using the "hug" if necessary.

Rectal temperature. Obtaining a rectal temperature has been a common practice during the first few years of a child's life. However, many now recommend using this method only when no other route can be used. The main drawbacks are the danger of perforation of the rectum in the newborn and young infant and the increased discomfort for the young child, who experiences this as an intrusive procedure. Do not use this method with children who cannot tolerate this kind of stimulus to the central nervous system (CNS), as is the case with some children who have epilepsy, or with children who are receiving chemotherapy that affects the gastrointestinal mucosa.

A safe restraint method for taking a rectal temperature of a young infant is to lay the child face down on the parent's lap or on a padded table. Have the adult place the left forearm firmly across the child's hip area so that the child cannot raise the buttocks off the adult's lap or the table. Use the thumb and forefinger of the nondominant hand to separate the buttocks, and gently insert the lubricated thermometer with the dominant hand. Do not insert the thermometer any farther than 1 inch (2.5 cm). Deeper insertion increases the risk of perforation, since the colon curves posteriorly at a depth of 1¼ inches (3 cm). The temperature registers within 3 to 4 minutes on a glass thermometer (a digital thermometer reading is much quicker).

The infant's rectum is quite short; therefore insert the thermometer only a short distance. Three considerations help to determine sufficient entry: noting that the column of mercury is rising steadily, inserting no more than 1 inch (2.5 cm), and observing a decrease in the child's effort to push against the thermometer. It is normal for the child to push against the thermometer as the rectal sphincter muscles contract in response to the stimulus. Wait until the sphincter relaxes before continuing to insert. Hold the thermometer firmly enough to keep the child from pushing it out. Use care to hold the thermometer firmly but not to push it in further. Also, hold the child securely to prevent jerking and pushing the thermometer further into the rectum.

Oral temperature. Generally reserve oral temperature reading (with a glass thermometer) for children who are 5 to 6 years of age and older. Younger children may be able to use a digital thermometer. The child must be able to understand not to bite on the glass or digital thermometer and to keep the mouth closed during the procedure. Place the thermometer under the tongue for at least 5 minutes; it can take up to 7 minutes to reach the maximum temperature (for a glass thermometer, a digital thermometer will be much quicker). Sometimes the child's health condition (e.g., mouth breathing or limited intellectual functioning) interferes with being able to use this method.

Tympanic thermography. A more recent method for taking temperatures is tympanic thermography (see Chapter 9). The tympanic thermometer is placed in the ear canal and uses an infrared sensor to detect the temperature of blood flowing through the eardrum. It registers within 2 seconds. The ease and speed of this approach is making it the preferred method for use in many health care settings.

Temperature regulation is less exact in children than in adults. The rectal temperature is normally higher in infants and younger children, and the average temperature is above 37.2° C (99° F) until age 3 years. When a temperature is being recorded, it is important to indicate the route of measurement (rectal, oral, axillary, tympanic). However, do not add or subtract degrees based on route, since there is disagreement as to how much variability in temperature exists. The increase in temperature with even a minor infection is usually greater in infants and young children than in adults.

table 25.8	Normal Ranges of Heart Rates for Children		
	Rate (beats/min)		
Age	Resting (awake)	Resting (sleeping)	Exercise (fever)
Newborn	100-180	80-160	Up to 220
1 week to 3 months	100-220	80-180	Up to 220
3 months to 2 years	80-150	70-120	Up to 200
2 years to 10 years	70-110	60-100	Up to 180
10 years to adult	55-90	50-90	Up to 180

Modified from Gillette PC: Dysrhythmias. In Adams FH, Emmanouilides GC, Riemenschneider TA, editors: *Moss' heart disease in infants, children, and adolescents,* ed 4, Baltimore, 1989, Williams & Wilkins.

table 25.9	Amplitude, Quality of Heart Rate, and Site as They Relate to Differential Diagnosis of Heart Dysfunction in Young Infants and Children
Amplitude, quality, site	Cardiac dysfunction
Narrow, thready	Congestive heart failure Severe aortic stenosis
Bounding	Patent ductus arteriosus Aortic regurgitation
Pulsation in suprasternal notch	Aortic insufficiency Patent ductus arteriosus Coarctation of aorta
Palpable thrill in suprasternal notch	Aortic stenosis Valvular pulmonary stenosis Coarctation of aorta, occasionally patent ductus arteriosus

Data from Kempe CH et al: *Current pediatric diagnosis and treatment,* ed 9, Los Altos, Calif, 1987, Lange Medical Publications.

However, young infants with a severe infection may have a normal or subnormal temperature.

Pulse and respiration. Apprehension, crying, and physical activity, as well as the examination procedure itself, can alter a child's heart and respiratory rates. Thus, if possible, take these measurements while the child is at rest, either sleeping or lying quietly. If the child has been active, delay taking the measurement until the child has relaxed for about 5 to 10 minutes. If you must measure the respiratory rate and the heart rate while the child is crying or agitated, note this information next to your recording of the rate.

Examine the child's pulse for rate, rhythm, quality, and amplitude, just as for an adult. Auscultation of the heart—measuring the apical pulse—is the most easily obtained pulse in a young infant. The average heart rate of the infant at birth is 140 beats per minute. At 2 years of age the child's heart has adjusted downward to 110. At 10 years the rate is 85, and by the time the child reaches age 18, the pulse may have decreased to 82. A child, usually an adolescent, who engages in exercise regularly, such as swimming laps, may exhibit a much slower rate (i.e., in the 60s).

Table 25.8 lists the normal ranges of heart rates for children. Heart rhythm in children is not always regular. Often the rate will change in relation to the respiratory cycle. The heart rate accelerates during inspiration because of the increase in pressure in the thoracic cavity and decreases during expiration. This phenomenon, which is called sinus arrhythmia, is considered normal in children. Palpation of the brachial and femoral pulses is an essential step in the examination of the young infant. Irregularities often are the first signs of serious heart dysfunction. The amplitude and rhythm of the femoral pulse are expected to equal those of the brachial pulse. Absence or weakness of the femoral pulse indicates the possibility of coarctation of the aorta in the young infant. Table 25.9 compares some differences in amplitude, quality, and site and how they may relate to the differential diagnosis of heart disorders in children.

Obtain the respiratory rate by inspection or auscultation. In infants respiratory movements are primarily diaphragmatic and are observed by abdominal movement. Since these movements are frequently irregular, you need to count them for a full minute for accuracy. The average range of normal respirations is 30 to 80 per minute in the newborn period compared with 20 to 30 per minute in the 2-year-old. By 10 years of age the respiratory rate has adjusted to 17 to 22 per minute, and by age 20 it averages 15 to 20 per minute. Table 25.10 shows variations in respiration with age.

Blood pressure. The levels of systolic and diastolic blood pressure gradually increase during childhood, and normally a considerable variation exists in a child's pressure. The systolic pressure of the child may be raised by crying, vigorous exercise, or anxiety. Therefore choose a

table 25.10	Variations in Respiration with Age
Age	**Rate/min**
Premature	40-90
Newborn	30-80
1 yr	20-40
2 yr	20-30
3 yr	20-30
5 yr	20-25
10 yr	17-22
15 yr	15-20
20 yr	15-20

Data from Lowrey GH: *Growth and development of children*, ed 8, St Louis, 1986, Mosby.

time when the child is quiet and comfortable to obtain this measurement.

The National Task Force on Blood Pressure Control in Children recommends that children 3 years or older have their blood pressure measured annually as part of their regular health care. The child of this age is usually able to cooperate when you explain the procedure for obtaining a blood pressure measurement. Routinely measuring the blood pressure of the child less than 3 years of age is unnecessary unless there are indications of underlying problems such as renal or cardiac disease.

The most common method of measuring the blood pressure of the child is still auscultation with a mercury or aneroid sphygmomanometer. The selection of the cuff size and the method of measuring the blood pressure are described in detail in Figure 25.20. The size of the cuff is important because a cuff that is too small causes falsely elevated values. Pediatric cuffs are available in several sizes for newborns, infants, and children. A pediatric stethoscope with a small diaphragm is also essential when measuring the blood pressure of a young child. The systolic pressure is recorded as that point at which the Korotkoff sounds are initially heard. The diastolic pressure is recorded for the point at which the fourth-phase Korotkoff sound is heard, when the sound first becomes muffled. The fifth-phase Korotkoff sound is the disappearance of all sound. In young children the fourth and fifth sounds frequently occur simultaneously, and sometimes the Korotkoff sounds are heard all the way to zero.

The Doppler instrument, although relatively expensive, is useful with young infants and children. It mea-

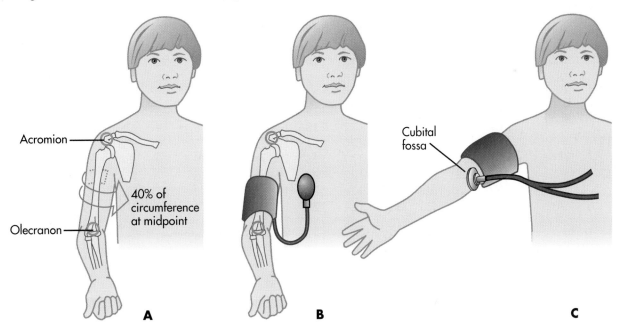

figure 25.20   Determination of proper cuff size and blood pressure measurement in children. **A,** The cuff bladder width should be approximately 40% of the circumference of the arm measured at a point midway between the olecranon and the acromion. **B,** The cuff bladder should cover 80% to 100% of the circumference of the arm. **C,** Blood pressure should be measured with the cubital fossa supported at the heart level. The stethoscope is placed over the brachial artery pulse, proximal and medial to the cubital fossa, below the bottom edge of the cuff. *(Modified from National High Blood Pressure Education Program Working Group on Hypertension Control in Children and Adolescents: Update on the 1987 Task Force Report on High Blood Pressure in Children and Adolescents, Pediatrics 98(4):649-658, 1996.)*

| table 25.11 | Blood Pressure Levels for the 90th and 95th Percentiles of Blood Pressure for Girls Ages 1 to 17 Years by Percentiles of Height | | | | | | | | | | | | | |

Age (yr)	Blood pressure percentile*	Systolic blood pressure by percentile of height (mm Hg)†							Diastolic blood pressure by percentile of height (mm Hg)†						
		5%	10%	25%	50%	75%	90%	95%	5%	10%	25%	50%	75%	90%	95%
1	90th	97	98	99	100	102	103	104	53	53	53	54	55	56	56
	95th	101	102	103	104	105	107	107	57	57	57	58	59	60	60
2	90th	99	99	100	102	103	104	105	57	57	58	58	59	60	61
	95th	102	103	104	105	107	108	109	61	61	62	62	63	64	65
3	90th	100	100	102	103	104	105	106	61	61	61	62	63	63	64
	95th	104	104	105	107	108	109	110	65	65	65	66	67	67	68
4	90th	101	102	103	104	106	107	108	63	63	64	65	65	66	67
	95th	105	106	107	108	109	111	111	67	67	68	69	69	70	71
5	90th	103	103	104	106	107	108	109	65	66	66	67	68	68	69
	95th	107	107	108	110	111	112	113	69	70	70	71	72	72	73
6	90th	104	105	106	107	109	110	111	67	67	68	69	69	70	71
	95th	108	109	110	111	112	114	114	71	71	72	73	73	74	75
7	90th	106	107	108	109	110	112	112	69	69	69	70	71	72	72
	95th	110	110	112	113	114	115	116	73	73	73	74	75	76	76
8	90th	108	109	110	111	112	113	114	70	70	71	71	72	73	74
	95th	112	112	113	115	116	117	118	74	74	75	75	76	77	78
9	90th	110	110	112	113	114	115	116	71	72	72	73	74	74	75
	95th	114	114	115	117	118	119	120	75	76	76	77	78	78	79
10	90th	112	112	114	115	116	117	118	73	73	73	74	75	76	76
	95th	116	116	117	119	120	121	122	77	77	77	78	79	80	80
11	90th	114	114	116	117	118	119	120	74	74	75	75	76	77	77
	95th	118	118	119	121	122	123	124	78	78	79	79	80	81	81
12	90th	116	116	118	119	120	121	122	75	75	76	76	77	78	78
	95th	120	120	121	123	124	125	126	79	79	80	80	81	82	82
13	90th	118	118	119	121	122	123	124	76	76	77	78	78	79	80
	95th	121	122	123	125	126	127	128	80	80	81	82	82	83	84
14	90th	119	120	121	122	124	125	126	77	77	78	79	79	80	81
	95th	123	124	125	126	128	129	130	81	81	82	83	83	84	85
15	90th	121	121	122	124	125	126	127	78	78	79	79	80	81	82
	95th	124	125	126	128	129	130	131	82	82	83	83	84	85	86
16	90th	122	122	123	125	126	127	128	79	79	79	80	81	82	82
	95th	125	126	127	128	130	131	132	83	83	83	84	85	86	86
17	90th	122	123	124	125	126	128	128	79	79	79	80	81	82	82
	95th	126	126	127	129	130	131	132	83	83	83	84	85	86	86

From National High Blood Pressure Education Program Working Group on Hypertension Control in Children and Adolescents: Update on the 1987 Task Force Report on High Blood Pressure in Children and Adolescents, *Pediatrics* 98(4):649-658, 1996.
*Blood pressure percentile was determined by a single reading.
†Height percentile was determined by standard growth curves.

table 25.12	**Blood Pressure Levels for the 90th and 95th Percentiles of Blood Pressure for Boys Ages 1 to 17 Years by Percentiles of Height**

Age (yr)	Blood pressure percentile*	Systolic blood pressure by percentile of height (mm Hg)†							Diastolic blood pressure by percentile of height (mm Hg)†						
		5%	10%	25%	50%	75%	90%	95%	5%	10%	25%	50%	75%	90%	95%
1	90th	94	95	97	98	100	102	102	50	51	52	53	54	54	55
	95th	98	99	101	102	104	106	106	55	55	56	57	58	59	59
2	90th	98	99	100	102	104	105	106	55	55	56	57	58	59	59
	95th	101	102	104	106	108	109	110	59	59	60	61	62	63	63
3	90th	100	101	103	105	107	108	109	59	59	60	61	62	63	63
	95th	104	105	107	109	111	112	113	63	63	64	65	66	67	67
4	90th	102	103	105	107	109	110	111	62	62	63	64	65	66	66
	95th	106	107	109	111	113	114	115	66	67	67	68	69	70	71
5	90th	104	105	106	108	110	112	112	65	65	66	67	68	69	69
	95th	108	109	110	112	114	115	116	69	70	70	71	72	73	74
6	90th	105	106	108	110	111	113	114	67	68	69	70	70	71	72
	95th	109	110	112	114	115	117	117	72	72	73	74	75	76	76
7	90th	106	107	109	111	113	114	115	69	70	71	72	72	73	74
	95th	110	111	113	115	116	118	119	74	74	75	76	77	78	78
8	90th	107	108	110	112	114	115	116	71	71	72	73	74	75	75
	95th	111	112	114	116	118	119	120	75	76	76	77	78	79	80
9	90th	109	110	112	113	115	117	117	72	73	73	74	75	76	77
	95th	113	114	116	117	119	121	121	76	77	78	79	80	80	81
10	90th	110	112	113	115	117	118	119	73	74	74	75	76	77	78
	95th	114	115	117	119	121	122	123	77	78	79	80	80	81	82
11	90th	112	113	115	117	119	120	121	74	74	75	76	77	78	78
	95th	116	117	119	121	123	124	125	78	79	79	80	81	82	83
12	90th	115	116	117	119	121	123	123	75	75	76	77	78	78	79
	95th	119	120	121	123	125	126	127	79	79	80	81	82	83	83
13	90th	117	118	120	122	124	125	126	75	76	77	78	79	80	
	95th	121	122	124	126	128	129	130	79	80	81	82	83	83	84
14	90th	120	121	123	125	126	128	128	76	76	77	78	79	80	80
	95th	124	125	127	128	130	132	132	80	81	81	82	83	84	85
15	90th	123	124	125	127	129	131	131	77	77	78	79	80	81	81
	95th	127	128	129	131	133	134	135	81	82	83	83	84	85	86
16	90th	125	126	128	130	132	133	134	79	79	80	81	82	82	83
	95th	129	130	132	134	136	137	138	83	83	84	85	86	87	87
17	90th	128	129	131	133	134	136	136	81	81	82	83	84	85	85
	95th	132	133	135	136	138	140	140	85	85	86	87	88	89	89

From National High Blood Pressure Education Program Working Group on Hypertension Control in Children and Adolescents: Update on the 1987 Task Force Report on High Blood Pressure in Children and Adolescents, *Pediatrics* 98(4):649-658, 1996.
*Blood pressure percentile was determined by a single measurement.
†Height percentile was determined by standard growth curves.

sures systolic blood pressure, which is the first sound heard. The Doppler device is useful for systolic measurement, but it has not been found to be reliable for diastolic pressure measurement.

If a Doppler instrument is unavailable, you can use the flush method to approximate the mean blood pressure. (This method is rarely used, but it is helpful to know it for situations in which advanced technology is unavailable.) Elevate the extremity, with the uninflated cuff in place. Stroke or milk the arm from the hand to the elbow. Inflate the cuff to a point above the estimated systolic blood pressure. Slowly release the pressure. A sudden reddening or "flush" of the extremity (as compared with the other extremity) will occur at a point about halfway between the systolic and diastolic pressures.

HELPFUL HINT *When taking a child's blood pressure:*

- *The child should be seated. Take the measurement routinely in the right arm held at heart level.*
- *Do not press too hard with the stethoscope.*
- *If no pediatric cuff is available, use an adult cuff around the child's thigh and place the stethoscope over the popliteal area (behind knee) to hear Korotkoff sounds. This measurement averages about 10 mm Hg higher than blood pressure taken in the arm.*
- *Refer the child with abnormally high serial readings to a physician.*
- *Blood pressure readings between the 90th and 95th percentiles are high-normal and require further evaluation for risk factors for hypertension.*
- *Significant hypertension is blood pressure persistently between the 95th and 99th percentiles for age, height, and sex.*

The 1996 American Academy of Pediatrics (AAP) Update on the 1987 Task Force Report on High Blood Pressure in Children and Adolescents found that body size, along with gender and age, must be considered to accurately assess blood pressure in children and adolescents. Frequently, very tall children have been misclassified as hypertensive. When height was factored in, their blood pressures were found to be normal. Conversely, very short children, judged to be normotensive, may in fact have high-normal or elevated blood pressures. Based on a detailed review of epidemiological samples, the AAP (1996) developed new blood pressure tables adjusted for height, as well as age and gender (Tables 25.11 and 25.12). To determine blood pressure status, obtain the height percentile from a standard growth chart (see example in Figure 25.21). Then compare the child's systolic and diastolic blood pressures with the

numbers provided in the boy's or girl's table (as appropriate) for age and height percentiles. If the child's systolic or diastolic blood pressure is at or above the 95th percentile, repeated measurements are indicated to rule out hypertension. Blood pressure measurements between the 90th and 95th percentiles are considered high-normal and require additional observation and evaluation for risk factors for hypertension. Although early essential hypertension is not a common problem in children, elevated blood pressure in children often correlates with hypertension in early adulthood (AAP, 1996). Monitoring blood pressure in children and promoting appropriate life style interventions in those at risk may help to avoid long-term problems.

Growth measurements

The routine measurement of growth is a screening procedure rather than a diagnostic procedure. Yet such measurement can provide clues to serious health problems. Growth is a continuous process that the practitioner must evaluate over time. Successive serial measurements plotted on a standardized growth chart provide objective information about the individual child's rate and pattern of growth in comparison with the general population. This information is useful in providing reassurance to parents and professionals regarding the child who is growing normally, in assessing the nutritional status of the child, and in identifying the child who may have abnormalities that are affecting the various growth parameters. Examples of abnormalities that could impair growth include growth-hormone deficiency, inflammatory bowel disease, and cardiac and renal disorders.

The three parameters of growth that are routinely measured during each examination of the child less than 3 years of age are recumbent length, body weight, and head circumference. For the child older than 3 years of age, it is sufficient to obtain standing height and weight measurements. Assessment of body segments, skinfold thickness, bone age, and dentition may be useful for further study of body growth, but it is not usually included in the routine physical examination.

Growth charts published by, or based on data from, the National Center for Health Statistics (NCHS) are most commonly used to record growth measurements (Figure 25.21). They are based on large, nationally representative samples of children. Two groups of charts were developed from the data: the first for the age interval from birth to 36 months and the second for the interval from 2 to 18 years. The charts for infants (birth to 36 months) were developed separately for boys and girls and include graphs for head circumference, recumbent length by age, weight by age, and weight by length. The charts for children ages 2 to 18 years are in separate versions for boys and girls and include graphs

BOYS: BIRTH TO 36 MONTHS
PHYSICAL GROWTH
NCHS PERCENTILES*

NAME_____ RECORD #_____

DATE	AGE	LENGTH	WEIGHT	HEAD CIRC.	COMMENT
	BIRTH				
	4 Mo	24"	13 lbs.		
	6½ Mo	26¾"	16.5 lbs.		
	8½ Mo	28¼"	18.5 lbs.		

MOTHER'S STATURE _____
FATHER'S STATURE _____
GESTATIONAL AGE _____ WEEKS

figure **25.21** Samples of physical growth charts for children. **A,** Boys: birth to 36 months, for length. *(Courtesy Ross Laboratories.)*

continued

figure**25.21, cont'd** **B,** Boys: birth to 36 months, for head circumference.

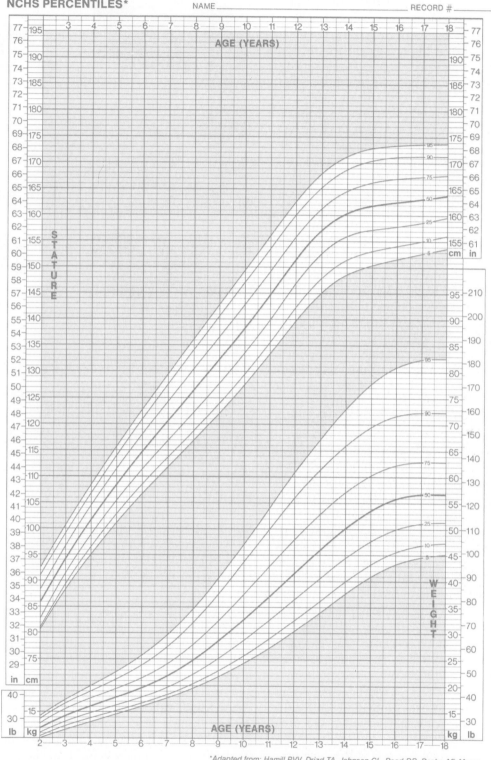

C

*Adapted from: Hamill PVV, Drizd TA, Johnson CL, Reed RB, Roche AF, Moore WM: Physical growth: National Center for Health Statistics percentiles. AM J CLIN NUTR 32:607-629,1979. Data from the National Center for Health Statistics (NCHS) Hyattsville, Maryland.

© 1980 ROSS LABORATORIES

figure**25.21, cont'd**   C, Girls: ages 2 through 18 years, for height and weight.

for stature (standing height) by age, weight by age, and weight by stature of prepubescent children.

The appropriate use of the charts requires that consistent measurement techniques be used at each point in time. For instance, do not record standing height or stature on the birth-to-36 months chart, since the infant will appear shorter than if the recumbent length were used. There can be a difference of up to 1 inch between recumbent and standing measures of the same child. Record standing height on the 2-to-18 year chart.

To interpret growth measurements, you need to take into account several factors. First, children whose weight and height fall between the 5th and 95th percentiles are likely to be growing normally. Evaluate and follow closely, however, those who fall below the 5th or above the 95th percentile. Consider the size of the parents and also the ethnic and racial background of the child. If both parents are small or large, their children's growth likely will be similar. Differences from the norm, which was determined for middle-class Caucasian children, have been noted for children of different ethnic groups. For example, based on standards from China, Chinese children's average weight and height fall in the 10th percentile on the NCHS charts rather than the 50th percentile. However, when investigators studied these children's growth patterns over time, their growth was normal (Wong, 1995). This example emphasizes that the overall pattern of growth is more important than any single measure.

The relationship between height and weight is also significant. Pay specific attention to children who have a disparity between these two measures. For example, a child whose height falls in the 75th percentile but whose weight falls in the 25th percentile needs more in-depth evaluation and monitoring. Other areas of concern are a child's failure to show expected increases in height and weight, particularly during peak growth periods such as infancy and adolescence, and sudden changes in height or weight from the child's growth curve (e.g., sudden increases or decreases).

Length or height. Measure recumbent length (birth to 3 years) with the child in the supine position with the legs extended. To measure length, facilitate the procedure by having two people participate. The parent is usually available and interested in providing this assistance. If you use a measuring board, place the infant's head against the fixed headboard, and have the parent hold it in the midline while you gently push on the infant's knees until the legs are fully extended and both heels are firmly touching the movable footboard. If a measuring device is not available, follow the same procedure, placing the child on a paper-covered flat surface and marking the paper at the top of the child's head and at the bottom of the heels (Figure 25.22, *A*). Measure the distance between the two points (Figure 25.22, *B*).

figure**25.22** **A,** Measuring recumbent length with the parent's assistance. The child is placed on a paper-covered flat surface, and marks are made at the head and feet. **B,** The distance between the two marks is measured while the child relaxes.

Measure standing height or stature (2 to 18 years) with the shoes off. Ask the child to stand as tall as possible and look straight ahead so that the top of the head is parallel with the ceiling. The feet should be together, and the shoulders, buttocks, and heels should be touching the wall without any flexion of the knees (Figure 25.23). Bring a block, squared at right angles against the wall, or a measuring board to the top of the child's head. When a measuring device is not available, you can make a mark on the wall at the top of the child's head and measure the distance from the floor.

Weight. To weigh the child, use an appropriately sized beam scale with nondetachable weights. Two

figure**25.23** Measurement of standing height.

scales are suggested: one for infants and small children, which measures weights to the nearest 0.5 ounce or 10 g, and one for older children and adults, which measures weights to the nearest 0.25 pound or 100 g. Before weighing the child, check the scale to determine if it is balanced. Return the weights to the zero setting and make sure that the balance is resting in the middle.

When infant growth charts (birth to 36 months) are used, weigh the child naked on the infant scale (Figure 25.24). With the charts for older children (2 to 18 years), use the upright adult scale, ideally with the child dressed only in underpants or a light gown (Figure 25.25).

Head circumference. Measure the head circumference during each examination between birth and 36 months of age and in any child whose head size is questionable. Pass a nonstretchable tape measure over the most prominent part of the occiput and just above the supraorbital ridges (Figure 25.26). The average head circumference at birth is 35 cm (14 inches) and by age 2 has increased to 49 cm (19.2 inches). The head circumference is an important measure to obtain because it is related to intracranial volume and allows an estimation of

figure**25.25** Weighing the older child. Ideally, the child would be dressed only in underwear or a light gown with shoes removed.

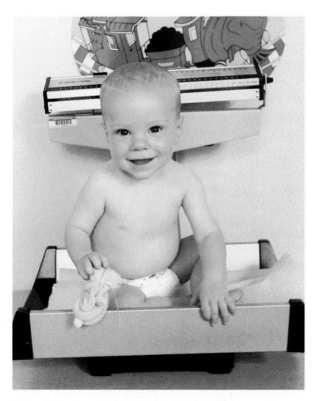

figure**25.24** Weighing the young infant.

figure**25.26** Appropriate placement of the measuring tape to obtain the head circumference. *(From Seidel HM et al: Mosby's guide to physical examination, ed 3, St Louis, 1995, Mosby.)*

the rate of growth of the brain. Plot sequential measurements on the appropriate NCHS growth chart. Check any discrepancy or deviation, with consideration given to the conditions of microcephaly and hydrocephaly.

Always measure the head circumference of the child who is suspected of having a neurological problem or a developmental delay, regardless of age.

Chest circumference. The measurement of the circumference of the chest at delivery and in early infancy has become significant in that it may indicate birth injury, congenital anomalies, or system dysfunction (e.g., cardiac enlargement). Otherwise, measuring the chest circumference on a regular basis beyond early infancy is unnecessary. Exceptions to this might include observed body disproportion or malformation of the thoracic cage. Measure the chest circumference of the child by placing a nonstretchable cloth tape measure at the level of the nipple, with the child in a supine position. Take the measurement midway between inspiration and expiration.

Growth curves of the body as a whole and of three types of tissue—lymphoid, neural, and genital—demonstrate the age ranges when children are expected to exhibit growth spurts (Figure 25.27).

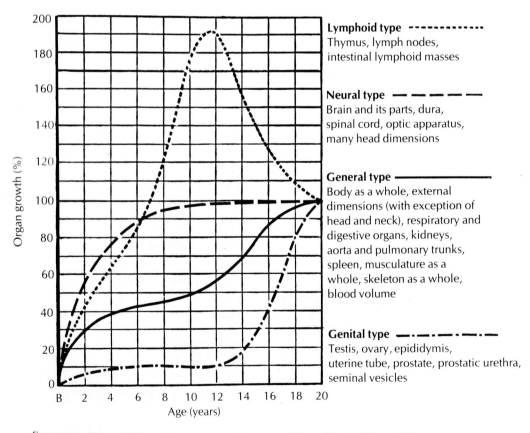

figure**25.27** Differential organ growth curves. *(From Harris JA et al: The measurement of man, Minneapolis, 1930, University of Minnesota Press.)*

HELPFUL HINT *Age- and sex-specific growth charts are readily available from the major formula manufacturers and from the makers of growth hormone. These charts have been standardized by using data from thousands of children so that comparisons can be made. Proper documentation of height and weight onto growth charts is as important as proper assessment. On the sample growth chart (see Figure 25.20), note that crossed lines are drawn with a straight edge to ensure that the child's age and measurements are recorded exactly. If the child is 9 years and 9 months old, the vertical line is drawn in a different place than if the child is 9 years and 2 months old. This distinction can make a big difference as to the percentile into which the child's height, weight, or head circumference falls.*

If a child is born prematurely, use the "corrected age" on growth charts and developmental assessments until the child is 2 ½ years old. To calculate "corrected age," subtract the number of weeks the child was born prematurely from the child's chronological age. Example: One would expect a 15-month-old child born 6 weeks prematurely to be in the same growth and developmental range of normal as a 13½-month-old.

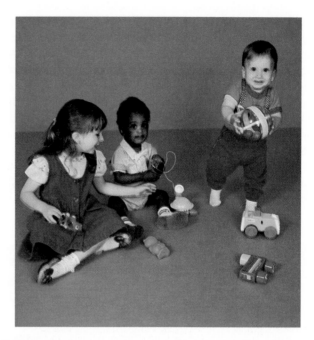

figure**25.28** Observations of children at play in the waiting area, as well as during the examination, can provide helpful information about their behavioral styles and development.

General inspection

The general inspection of the child includes observations similar to those of the adult examination (see Chapter 9). These include changes in facies, posture, and body contour; hygiene; and changes in gait. Also keep in mind those physical and behavioral characteristics that are expected for the individual child at the present chronological age (Figure 25.28). Chapter 4 describes the normal physical and behavioral changes that occur during the child's development. Observations made about the child's development during the interview and examination may indicate the need for a more formal assessment.

Observe and describe the child's behavior during the visit. Is this a quiet, shy child or an active, restless child? Is this child comfortable during the visit, or anxious and afraid? Does the child respond to the parent or other adults in an appropriate way?

Each child is a unique being, and it is a challenge to observe and record a description of any child's behavior. Keep in mind that behavior observed during a visit for health care may not be typical for that child.

Skin, hair, and nails

Assess the skin for color, texture, temperature, moisture, turgor, and any rashes or lesions. Observe the hair for color, texture, quality, and distribution. Assess the nails for color, shape, texture, and quality.

The examination of the skin provides valuable information about the general health of the child and evidence of specific skin problems. Inspect and palpate the skin of the entire body at each examination. Since the normal condition of the skin changes with age, it is important to become familiar with those changes seen in children, as described in the following sections.

Newborn and infant. The skin of the newborn is soft and smooth and appears almost transparent. The superficial vessels are prominent, giving the skin its red color. Use natural daylight to assess for jaundice. A mild degree of jaundice is frequently present after the second or third day in normal infants. If the jaundice is severe or occurs within the first 24 hours, however, you should consider the presence of a serious problem.

Small papular patches, called nevus flammeus, may be present over the occiput, forehead, and upper eyelids in the newborn period; these patches usually disappear by the end of the first year of life. The nose and cheeks are frequently covered by small white papules called milia (Figure 25.29), caused by plugging of the sebaceous glands during the neonatal period. Both sweat and sebaceous glands are present in the newborn, but they do not function until the second month of life. Some desquamation is common during the first weeks and varies in individual babies. Mongolian spots, which are blue or bluish brown, irregularly shaped, flat areas, occur in the

sacral and buttocks area of some infants, usually those who have darkly pigmented skin (Figure 25.30). These spots usually disappear by the end of the first or by the second year, but occasionally they persist for a longer time. A considerable amount of fine hair, called lanugo, covers the body of the newborn and is lost during the first weeks of life. The nails of the full-term newborn are well formed and firm in contrast to those of the premature infant, which are imperfectly formed.

During the first year of life, the proportion of subcutaneous fat continuously increases, and raw areas resulting from skin rubbing against skin are more prevalent in young, obese infants. This condition is called intertrigo (see Figure 10.29). During the second year of life, the proportion of subcutaneous fat decreases and intertrigo is less common. Skin turgor is a good indicator of hydration status. Check skin turgor by grasping the skin on the abdomen between your thumb and index finger, releasing it, and observing how quickly it returns to its normal shape (Figure 25.31).

Older child and adolescent. After the first year of life, the normal child shows little change in the skin until the onset of puberty, when considerable development of both sweat and sebaceous glands occurs. Asso-

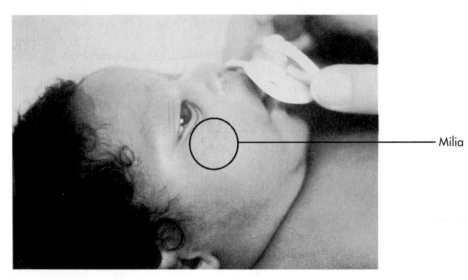

figure**25.29**   Milia in an infant. *(From Seidel HM et al: Mosby's guide to physical examination, ed 3, St Louis, 1995, Mosby.)*

figure**25.30**   Mongolian spots: extensive lesions over the back and buttocks. *(From Weston WL, Lane AT, Morelli JG: Color textbook of pediatric dermatology, ed 2, 1996, Mosby.)*

figure**25.31**   Checking skin turgor in an infant.

figure**25.32** Acne in an adolescent. *(From Habif TP: Clinical dermatology: a color guide to diagnosis and therapy, ed 3, St Louis, 1996, Mosby.)*

ciated with the development of the sebaceous glands is acne vulgaris, which is so common in its mildest forms that it is sometimes considered a normal physiological change. Early evidence of acne is the occasional comedo, or blackhead, on the nose and chin. At age 13 or 14 years, papules and small pustules may begin to appear (Figure 25.32). However, by age 16, many children will have recovered completely. Changes in the amount and distribution of hair also occur (see Figures 25.7 and 25.8). Hair growth becomes heavier; the appearance of pubic, axillary, and most of the more prominent body hair is influenced by sexual development during adolescence. (See Figures 10.17, *B* and *D,* 10.26, 10.28, 10.35, *B,* 10.38, *A,* 10.40, and 10.41 for common dermatological conditions in children and adolescents.)

Lymph nodes. Inspect and palpate the lymph nodes for size, mobility, temperature, and tenderness.

Lymph nodes in children have the same distribution as those in adults, but the nodes are usually more prominent until puberty (Figure 25.33). The amount of lymphoid tissue is considerable at birth and increases steadily, peaking between ages 8 and 10 and gradually decreasing during adolescence (see Figure 25.27). Shotty, discrete, movable, small, nontender nodes are common in the occipital, postauricular, anterior and posterior cervical, parotid, submaxillary, sublingual, axillary, epitrochlear, and in-

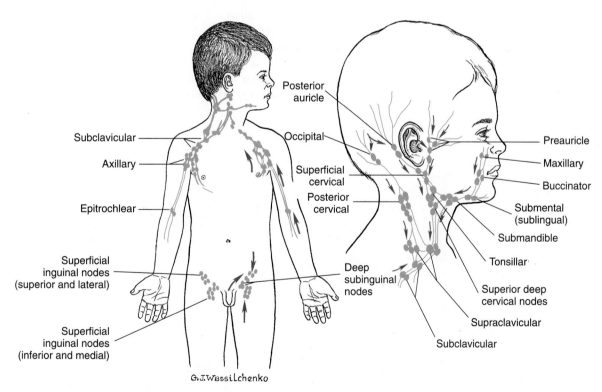

figure**25.33** Location of superficial lymph nodes. Arrows indicate directional flow of lymph. *(From Wong DL:* Whaley and Wong's nursing care of infants and children, *ed 5, St Louis, 1995, Mosby.)*

guinal areas in the normal healthy child. These are particularly notable in school-age children.

Examine lymph nodes during the examination of each part of the body.

Head and neck

Inspect the head for shape and symmetry. Palpate the fontanels in the infant and young child.

Newborn and infant. The shape of the newborn's head is often asymmetrical as a result of the molding that occurs during the passage through the birth canal. It may be a few days or weeks before the normal shape is restored. The newborn has a skull that molds easily because the bones of the cranium are not fused, which allows for some overlapping of the bones. Trauma may result in caput succedaneum or cephalhematoma. Caput succedaneum is an edematous swelling of the superficial tissues of the scalp manifested by a generalized soft swelling not bounded by suture lines. This condition is temporary and is usually resolved within the first few days of life. Cephalhematoma occurs as a result of bleeding into the periosteum and results in swelling that does not cross the suture line. Most cephalhematomas are absorbed within 2 weeks to 3 months. Flattening of the head often occurs in normal children, but it can also indicate problems such as mental retardation or rickets.

Palpate the sutures of the skull, which can usually be felt as ridges until the age of 6 months. Palpate the fontanels during each examination of the infant and young child to determine the size, shape, and presence of any tenseness or bulging. Normally, the posterior fontanel closes by 2 months of age and the anterior fontanel closes by the end of the second year (Figure 25.34). Tenseness or bulging of the fontanel is most

easily detected when the child is in a sitting position and should be assessed when the child is quiet. Bulging may occur with increased intercranial pressure (or when the child is crying). The fontanel may be depressed when the infant is dehydrated or malnourished. Note early closure or delayed closure of the fontanel. Early closure can result from microcephaly and delayed closure from prolonged intracranial pressure.

The importance of measuring the head circumference of the child up to 3 years of age has already been discussed.

Transillumination of the skull is a useful procedure in the initial examination of the infant and for any infant with an abnormal head size. Perform transillumination in a completely darkened room with an ordinary flashlight equipped with a rubber adaptor. Place the light against the infant's head. If the cerebrum is absent or greatly thinned, as from increased intracranial pressure, the entire cranium lights up. Often, defects transilluminate in a more limited way. Auscultation of the skull may reveal bruits, which are commonly found in normal children up to 4 years of age. After the age of 4 years, bruits are evidence of problems such as aneurysms or increased intracranial pressure.

Inspect the young infant's scalp for evidence of crusting, which often results from a seborrheic dermatitis commonly called "cradle cap" (Figure 25.35).

Inspect the shape of the face. A facial paralysis is most easily observed when the child cries or smiles and the asymmetry is increased. An abnormal or unusual facies may indicate a chromosomal abnormality such as Down syndrome.

Older child and adolescent. Percuss the frontal and maxillary sinuses by the direct method and palpate them

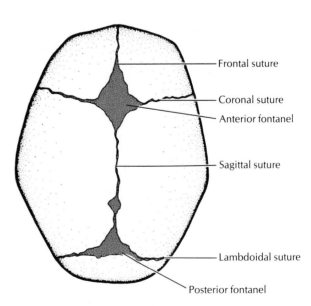

figure **25.34** Skull bones of the infant, showing fontanels and sutures.

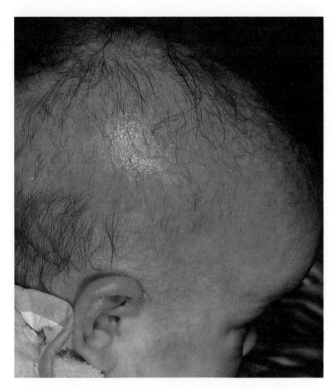

figure**25.35** Seborrheic dermatitis of the scalp in an infant. *(From Habif TP: Clinical dermatology: a color guide to diagnosis and therapy, ed 3, St Louis, 1996, Mosby.)*

in the child who is over 2 or 3 years of age. Until that age, the sinuses are too small and poorly developed for percussion or palpation (Figure 25.36).

Palpate the submaxillary and sublingual glands in the same way as in the adult examination. Check for local swelling of the parotid gland by observing the child in the sitting position with the head raised and the neck extended and by noting any swelling below the angle of the jaw. You can feel the swollen parotid gland by pal-

pating downward from the zygomatic arch. Unilateral or bilateral swelling of the parotid gland usually indicates mumps.

Examine the neck with the child lying flat on the back. Note the size of the neck. The neck of the infant normally is short. It lengthens at about 3 or 4 years of age. Palpate the lymph nodes, thyroid glands, and trachea. Carefully palpate the sternocleidomastoid muscle. A mass on the lower third of the muscle may indicate a congenital torticollis. Finally, determine the mobility of the neck by lifting the child's head and turning it from side to side or bringing the chin forward to touch the chest. Any resistance to flexion may indicate meningeal irritation.

Eyes

Examination of the eyes is most easily accomplished when the child is able to cooperate. The school-age child can participate in the adult format for the eye examination (see Chapter 12: Eyes). The infant and young child are much more of a challenge to the examiner.

Visual function at birth is limited, but it improves as the structures develop. Vision can be tested grossly in the very young infant by noting the pupillary response to light. This is one of the most primitive visual functions and is normally found in the newborn. The blink reflex is also present in normal newborns and young infants. The infant will blink the eyes when a bright light is introduced. It is important to make sure that the infant has a full red reflex in each eye. A white reflex could indicate a cataract or retinoblastoma.

At 5 or 6 weeks of age, the child should be able to fixate and give some evidence of following a bright toy or light. When 3 or 4 months old, the infant begins to reach for objects at different distances. At 6 to 7 months of age, the infant can have a funduscopic examination, although it is not routinely performed at this early an age. For children 3 to 6 years of age, a Snellen **E** chart

figure**25.36** Development of the frontal and maxillary sinuses. **A,** Early infancy. **B,** Early childhood. **C,** Adolescence. **D,** Adulthood.

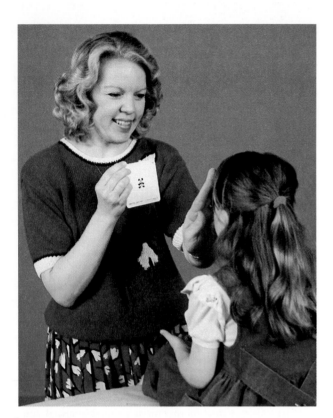

figure**25.37** Preparing the child for participation in testing of visual acuity.

can be used. Ask the child to hold the fingers in the same direction as the fingers of the E. You can also use Allen picture cards. The child identifies pictures, such as a tree, a telephone, a car, a house, and a teddy bear on an Allen card from a distance of 15 feet. Familiarizing the child with the procedure before testing may be helpful (Figure 25.37). The young child is normally farsighted and does not achieve visual acuity of 20/20 until the age of 7 years.

Tests for strabismus (squint, cross-eye), an imbalance of the extraocular muscles, are important because strabismus can lead to amblyopia, a type of blindness in the affected eye. Early recognition is essential to restore binocular vision, since the prognosis for a successful outcome for the child over 6 years of age is poor. An easy method for detecting strabismus is the corneal reflex test (or Hirschberg's test). Shine a bright light from a flashlight or ophthalmoscope directly into the eyes from about 16 inches (40.5 cm). In normal eyes the reflection of the light should fall symmetrically within each pupil. Any deviation warrants further evaluation. Another, more accurate, test to assess muscle imbalance is the cover-uncover test (see Chapter 11: Face, Head, Neck, and Regional Lymphatics). You can use this test in both younger and older children. Have the child focus on an object. Cover one eye with your hand, a card, or specially designed eyewear and observe the un-

covered eye for movement (Figure 25.38, *A*). Then uncover the eye and observe the recently covered eye for movement (Figure 25.38, *B*). If movement is noticed in either or both eyes, strabismus is present. The type of strabismus is determined by the combination of movements. Repeat the test to examine the other eye. Transient strabismus is common during the first months of life. If it persists beyond 6 months of age, however, or becomes fixed at an earlier age, the child should be referred to an ophthalmologist.

Test extraocular movements during the first weeks of life, as soon as the child is able to demonstrate following of movement. You can also at least partially examine the visual fields in infants and young children by having the child sit on the parent's lap with the head in the midline and one eye covered. As the light or bright object is brought into the visual field, the child will look at it or reach for it.

Inspect the outermost structures of the eyes in the same way as in the adult examination. The ophthalmoscopic examination depends on the child's ability to cooperate and the examiner's efficiency in observing as much as possible in a limited time. Attempts to restrain the child and force the eyes to remain open prove unsuccessful. If possible, direct the child's attention toward an object or light while you approach without touching the child. The appearance of the red reflex alone is important information for ruling out opacities of the cornea and lens and cataracts. Attempt to use the ophthalmoscope to observe the red reflex at each examination of the infant and child beginning in the first weeks of life.

Ears

Examination of the ears is often difficult; however, it is important because the immature structure of the young child's ears makes them more prone to infection. In the infant, the eustachian tube is shorter and wider than in the adult. It is also in a more horizontal position than in the adult, which makes it easier for pathogens to infect the middle ear.

> **HELPFUL HINT** *Pneumotoscopy is an important technique to learn, especially when working with children. It involves blowing air into the ear canal (either with a rubber squeeze bulb or gently blowing or sucking with the end of the rubber tube in the examiner's mouth). The normal tympanic membrane will move in and out as positive and negative pressures are applied. In the presence of infection, there is fluid behind the tympanic membrane and therefore a decrease in mobility when pressure is applied.*

A

B

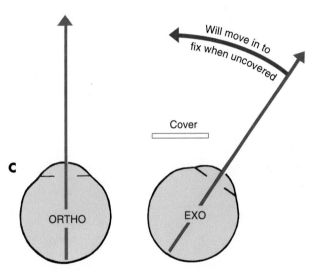

C

figure**25.38** Cover-uncover test for strabismus. **A,** Have the child look at an object (preferably a brightly colored toy) and cover one eye. Observe the uncovered eye for movement. **B,** While the child is still focused on the object, uncover the eye and observe it for movement. **C,** Exophoria: as the eye is uncovered, it shifts to fixate on the object. (**C** *from Prior JA, Silberstein JS, Stang JM:* Physical diagnosis: the history and examination of the patient, *ed 6, St Louis, 1981, Mosby.*)

figure**25.39** Ear alignment. **A,** Normal. **B,** Abnormal. *(From Whaley LF, Wong DL:* Nursing care of infants and children, *ed 4, St Louis, 1991, Mosby.)*

figure**25.40** It is helpful to let the child see the speculum and examine it in preparation for the otoscopic examination.

Inspect and palpate the external ear and the posterior mastoid areas for any obvious deformities. Note the position and size of the ears. Normally, the top of the ear is on a horizontal line with the inner and outer canthus of the eye (Figure 25.39).

Next, use the otoscope. This examination becomes more difficult as the infant grows older. It is usually helpful to spend some time preparing the child by letting him or her see the light and by inserting the speculum gently for only a few seconds and then removing it to assure the child that the procedure does not hurt (Figure 25.40). When restraint is necessary, have the parent firmly hold the child (Figure 25.41). Before inserting the otoscope, inspect the meatus for evidence of a foreign body or external otitis. In infancy and early childhood, the auditory canal is directed upward: pull the pinna of the ear down and back to aid in visualization (Figure 25.42). Hold the otoscope so that the hand holding it rests firmly on the head; the top of the speculum is inserted only ¼ or ½ inch into the canal to avoid any unnecessary discomfort. For the older child, pull the pinna up and back to visualize the tympanic membrane (Figure 25.43). Before you examine the tympanic membrane, carefully inspect the canal for evidence of furuncles or redness. Inspect the tympanic

A

B

figure**25.41** Positioning for restraining the child for an ear examination. **A,** Supine. **B,** Restraint using the hug.

A

Pull
pinna down
and back

B

Pull pinna
up and back

figure**25.42**   Straightening the ear canal in the infant **(A)** and in the child over 3 years of age **(B)**. *(From Whaley LF, Wong DL:* Nursing care of infants and children, *ed 4, St Louis, 1991, Mosby.)*

membrane for color, light reflex, and the usual landmarks of the bony prominences of the middle ear. If you suspect that fluid is present behind the tympanic membrane, you may want to use pneumotoscopy or a tympanogram. Figure 25.44 shows common middle ear findings. For additional examples of abnormal tympanic membranes, see Chapter 13: Ears, Nose, Mouth, and Throat.

If the canal is filled with cerumen, occasionally you may need to remove the cerumen by irrigation or curettage. The irrigation procedure is unpleasant, may cause vomiting, and is not done unless necessary. Never do this procedure if you suspect a perforation of the tympanic membrane. Avoid removing the cerumen with a curette unless you are skillful in doing so. The procedure may cause pain and bleeding and may result in increased crying, which only exacerbates the redness of the membrane. Flexible plastic curettes are now available and seem easier for many children to tolerate. Often cerumen that is not dry but fairly soft will move during the examination. Visualization of the membrane then becomes possible without the need for any special procedures to remove the cerumen. Avoid discomfort so that the child will not become conditioned to expect pain with future ear examinations.

In the infant, test hearing by asking an assistant to stand behind the child and make a noise, such as a hand slap, several inches away from the child's ear while you observe the child for an eye blink. This test is often inaccurate, since the child may be responding to air movement. In the young child, hearing can be grossly tested

figure**25.43**   Examination of the ear in an older child.

figure**25.44** Common conditions of the middle ear as assessed with the otoscope. *(Modified from Bluestone CD, Klein JO: Otitis media in infants and children, Philadelphia, 1988, WB Saunders.)*

NORMAL
Position–neutral
Color–normal
Translucency–translucent
Mobility–moves briskly with slight positive and negative pressure

NEGATIVE MIDDLE EAR PRESSURE
Position–retracted
Color–normal
Translucency–translucent
Mobility–moves only with applied negative pressure

ACUTE OTITIS MEDIA
Position–full to bulging
Color–red (can be pink, white, or yellow)
Translucency–opaque
Mobility–poor when both positive and negative pressures are applied

FLUID LEVEL
Position–retracted
Color–yellow or amber
Translucency–translucent
Mobility–same as with high negative pressure, but fluid level and bubbles change with applied pressure

OTITIS MEDIA WITH EFFUSION
Position–usually retracted
Color–white (or yellow or blue)
Translucency–opaque (may be translucent)
Mobility–poor when both positive and negative pressures are applied

PERFORATION (OR PATENT TYMPANOSTOMY)
Position–neutral or retracted
Color–white, pink, or normal
Translucency–translucent or opaque
Mobility–none

with the whispered voice. Stand behind the child, occlude one ear with your hand, and whisper the child's name. The child will usually turn when his or her name is heard. Repeat this step to test the other ear.

Nose

Purulent secretions are common with any nasal infection, including the common upper respiratory infection. Children with redness, discharge, and crusting on the outer edges of the alar may have a beta-hemolytic streptococcal infection. Watery nasal secretions may indicate foreign bodies, the common cold, or an allergy.

Note any unusual shape of the nose, flaring of the nostrils, and the character and amount of discharge.

Examine the septum, turbinates, and vestibule by pushing the tip of the nose upward with the thumb of the nondominant hand and shining a light into the naris. A speculum is usually not necessary for adequate visualization, and it might cause the child to be apprehensive.

Mouth and oropharynx

The mouth and oropharyngeal area can be examined last, since this examination often provokes fear in the child. However, it is helpful to some children to do this examination first. For example, the child who is anticipating discomfort may be relieved to have it accomplished and then can cooperate with the rest of the examination. Deciding on this approach requires knowledge about the individual child's behavior and responses. This information may be obtained during the history or in discussion with the parent.

The procedures are the same as in the adult examination. However, the young child will probably need to be restrained by the parent (Figure 25.45, *A*). The older child is usually able to cooperate (Figure 25.45, *B*). The examination findings are different from those of adults. The number of deciduous and permanent teeth and the pattern of eruption are determined by the child's age and development. There are 20 deciduous teeth, and their eruption is completed by the age of 2 ½ years. The first permanent molar and the lower incisor erupt at 6 years of age (Figure 25.46). The tonsils are normally larger in children than in adults, and they usually extend beyond the palatine arch until the age of 11 or 12 years (Figure 25.47). Figures 13.28 and 13.29 provide examples of enlarged tonsils. Inspect the palate for a cleft. A bifid uvula may indicate a submucous cleft palate (a cleft covered by membrane), which cannot be identified by inspection alone.

Chest

Begin the examination of the chest with an inspection of its general shape and circumference. In infancy the chest is almost round; the anteroposterior diameter equals the transverse diameter (i.e., barrel chest). This shape changes as the child grows from preschool to school age. The chest circumference is normally the same as, or slightly less than, the head circumference until age 2 years. Respiratory activity is abdominal and

A **B**

figure**25.45** Positioning the child for examination of the mouth. **A,** The young child often requires restraint by the parent and encouragement from both the parent and the examiner. **B,** The older child is usually cooperative.

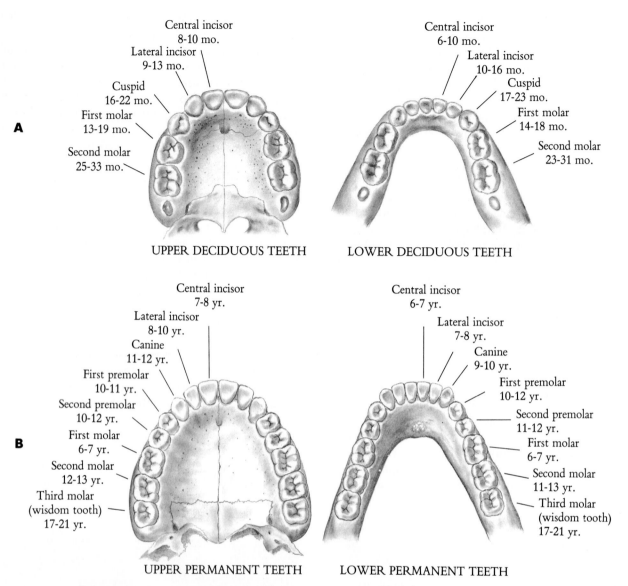

A

UPPER DECIDUOUS TEETH LOWER DECIDUOUS TEETH

Central incisor
8-10 mo.
Lateral incisor
9-13 mo.
Cuspid
16-22 mo.
First molar
13-19 mo.
Second molar
25-33 mo.

Central incisor
6-10 mo.
Lateral incisor
10-16 mo.
Cuspid
17-23 mo.
First molar
14-18 mo.
Second molar
23-31 mo.

B

UPPER PERMANENT TEETH LOWER PERMANENT TEETH

Central incisor
7-8 yr.
Lateral incisor
8-10 yr.
Canine
11-12 yr.
First premolar
10-11 yr.
Second premolar
10-12 yr.
First molar
6-7 yr.
Second molar
12-13 yr.
Third molar
(wisdom tooth)
17-21 yr.

Central incisor
6-7 yr.
Lateral incisor
7-8 yr.
Canine
9-10 yr.
First premolar
10-12 yr.
Second premolar
11-12 yr.
First molar
6-7 yr.
Second molar
11-13 yr.
Third molar
(wisdom tooth)
17-21 yr.

figure**25.46** **A,** Dentition of deciduous teeth and their sequence of eruption. **B,** Dentition of permanent teeth and their sequence of eruption. *(From Seidel HM et al:* Mosby's guide to physical examination, *ed 3, St Louis, 1995, Mosby.)*

does not become primarily thoracic until age 7 years. Little intercostal motion is seen in infants and young children. Therefore if you observe intercostal motion in the young child, suspect lung disease.

You can perform palpation and evaluate tactile fremitus while the child is crying. Perform percussion of the chest by using either the direct or the indirect method. The child's chest is normally more resonant than that of the adult. Breath sounds will seem much louder because of the thinness of the chest wall and are almost all bronchovesicular (Figure 25.48).

Heart

A quiet child and environment are necessary for accurate assessment of the heart (Figure 25.49). There-

fore making this the first part of the examination is a good idea. The examination of the cardiovascular system as discussed in Chapter 16 for the adult applies to the examination of the child; however, some cardiac findings of normal children are not considered normal in adults.

The pulse rate in children of different ages is discussed earlier in this chapter. The palpation of pulses in all the extremities is a part of the cardiovascular examination. The pulses in the lower extremities, especially the femoral pulses, are of special importance in children. Their absence or diminution may indicate coarctation of the aorta.

During infancy the position of the heart is more nearly horizontal and has a larger diameter in compari-

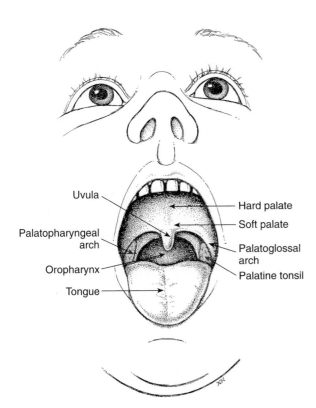

Uvula
Palatopharyngeal arch
Oropharynx
Tongue
Hard palate
Soft palate
Palatoglossal arch
Palatine tonsil

figure**25.47** Interior structures of the mouth. *(From Wong DL:* Whaley and Wong's nursing care of infants and children, *ed 5, St Louis, 1995, Mosby.)*

son with the total diameter of the chest than it does in the adult (Figure 25.50). The apex is one or two intercostal spaces above that considered normal for the adult. Therefore the apical impulse in young children is normally felt in the fourth intercostal space immediately to the left of the midclavicular line. This location changes gradually, and by 7 years of age the apical impulse is normally found in the fifth intercostal space at the midclavicular line.

Sinus arrhythmia is a normal finding in infants and children. The degree of arrhythmia is less in the young infant and greatest in the adolescent. The heart sounds are louder because of the thinness of the chest wall. They are also of a higher pitch and shorter duration than those of the normal adult. A splitting of the second heart sound can be heard in the second left intercostal space in most infants and children. The physiological split normally widens with inspiration. A third heart sound is present in approximately one third of all children and is best heard at the apex.

Many children have murmurs without heart disease. The significance of a murmur may be difficult to determine. Innocent murmurs are characteristically systolic in timing; are grade 1 or 2 in intensity; have a soft, blowing quality; and are not transmitted to other areas. It is not always possible to determine whether the murmur is innocent or pathological by auscultation alone, although

figure**25.48** Examination of the lungs. The young child is more comfortable and cooperative on the parent's lap.

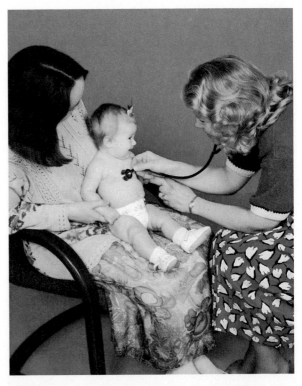

figure**25.49** Auscultation of the heart requires a quiet child. Doing the examination on the parent's lap increases the child's comfort and cooperation.

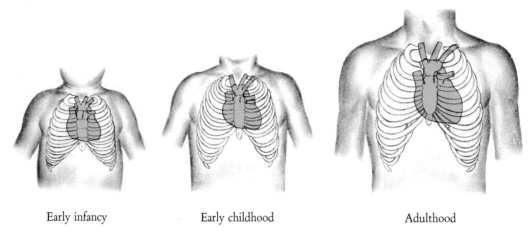

Early infancy   Early childhood   Adulthood

figure**25.50**   Position of the heart at various ages. *(From Seidel HM et al:* Mosby's guide to physical examination, *ed 2, St Louis, 1991, Mosby.)*

murmurs of grade 3 or louder usually indicate heart disease. A venous hum is commonly present in children. It is a continuous, low-pitched sound originating in the internal jugular vein that is heard either above or below the clavicles. It is accentuated in the upright position and disappears when the child is lying down. Because it is not pathologically significant, a venous hum should be differentiated from a murmur. Tables 16.9 and 16.10 provide a review of cardiac murmurs. Refer any murmur that is symptomatic (i.e., accompanied by chest pains or palpitations) to a physician.

figure**25.51**   Examination of the abdomen in an infant.

Abdomen

The abdomen is somewhat easier to examine in the child than in the adult because of the client's less well developed abdominal wall. To gain the child's cooperation, several approaches may be helpful. For example, a nursing bottle may calm the infant, or the young child may be more comfortable and relaxed if examined while sitting on the parent's lap. Find the approaches that are most productive in particular situations (Figure 25.51).

The order of the abdominal examination procedures for the young child should be inspection, auscultation, percussion, and then palpation. First, inspect the abdomen. The abdomen is larger than the chest in children less than 4 years of age and appears pot bellied in both supine and sitting positions. The child up to 13 years of age will have a pot belly in the standing position. This normal shape must be differentiated from true distention caused by enlargement of organs or the presence of tumors, cysts, or ascites. A depressed abdomen may result from dehydration or malnutrition. Respirations are largely abdominal in children up to 7 years of age. Any splinting or loss of movement may indicate peritonitis, appendicitis, or other acute problems. The umbilicus is normally closed, but umbilical hernias are common in Caucasian children up to 2 years of age and for longer periods in black children (Figure 25.52). Also, observe the abdomen for peristaltic waves (indicating pyloric stenosis) and dilated veins (indicating liver disease).

Carry out auscultation of the abdomen in the same manner as described in the examination of the adult—before percussion and palpation. Percussion may be useful in obtaining the boundaries of the liver, spleen, and any tumors. Children may be intrigued by the percussion sounds, especially the gastric bubble. Having the

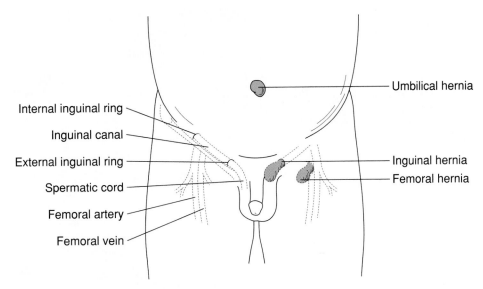

figure**25.52** Location of hernias.

Internal inguinal ring

Inguinal canal

External inguinal ring

Spermatic cord

Femoral artery

Femoral vein

Umbilical hernia

Inguinal hernia

Femoral hernia

HELPFUL HINT *In a relaxed child the abdomen is somewhat easier to examine than in the adult because the abdominal wall is less well developed and (usually) less adipose tissue is present. If a child's muscles become tense, however, the task becomes quite difficult.*

Many children become anxious or very ticklish during this part of the examination. To help the child relax, make sure he or she keeps the knees bent while lying on the back, and have the child keep a hand over yours as you palpate. You can also have the child's hand under your examining fingers during palpation.

child listen for the gastric bubble sound is one way to make the examination seem less threatening.

Perform palpation in the same way as in the examination of the adult except for the modifications in approach and in the positions of the child. Light palpation enables you to determine the tenseness of the abdominal muscles, the presence of superficial masses, and the presence of tenderness. The child is not able to pinpoint the area of tenderness, and only by watching the facial expressions can you determine the point of maximal tenderness. The liver is palpable 1 to 2 cm below the right costal margin in the first year of life. If it extends more than 2 cm below the costal margin, investigate further. The spleen is normally palpable 1 to 2 cm below the left costal margin in the first weeks of life. Note any increase in size. Any evidence of tenderness may indicate serious blood dyscrasias or other problems.

Determine tissue turgor by grasping a few inches of skin and subcutaneous tissue over the abdomen, pulling it up, and then quickly releasing it (see Figure 25.31). If the creases formed do not disappear immediately, dehydration is present. Do deep palpation in all four quadrants by single-hand or bimanual methods. Palpate the inguinal and femoral regions for hernias, lymph nodes, and femoral pulses (Figure 25.52).

Genitalia

The examination of the genitalia of both male and female children is usually carried out by inspection and palpation.

As part of the genital examination, you need to consider the child's or the adolescent's stage of pubertal development. The Sexual Maturity Rating (SMR) scale developed by Tanner (1962) is composed of five classes, which are based on pubic hair and breast development in females (see Figures 25.6 and 25.8) and pubic hair and genitalia in males (see Figure 25.7). This information is important for identifying abnormal puberty and also for reassuring the adolescent that he or she is normal. Record the SMR, or Tanner stage, at the initial visit and yearly thereafter.

Male genitalia. In the male child, two primary areas are examined: the penis and the scrotum. First examine the foreskin of the penis. The foreskin of the uncircumcised infant is normally tight for the first 2 or 3 months of life and does not retract easily. If the tightness persists beyond this period, it is called phimosis. Determine whether this condition causes any interference with urination. Do any retraction of the foreskin carefully, since the delicate membranes attached to the foreskin may be easily torn, resulting in adhesions. Next, examine the

figure**25.53**   **A,** Preventing the cremasteric reflex by having the child sit in the "tailor" position. **B,** Palpation of the scrotum to determine if the testes are descended, blocking the inguinal canal. (**A** *from Wong DL:* Whaley and Wong's nursing care of infants and children, *ed 5, St Louis, 1995, Mosby.*)

meatus to determine its position and the presence of any ulceration. The meatus is normally located at the tip of the shaft. An abnormal location of the meatus on the ventral surface is called hypospadias; an abnormal location on the dorsal surface is called epispadias.

Inspect the scrotum for evidence of enlargement. An enlarged scrotum may be indicative of a hernia or hydrocele. Palpate the scrotum to determine if the testes are descended (Figure 25.53). Use your index finger to block the inguinal canal and gently push toward the scrotum. Use the finger and thumb of the opposite hand to palpate the scrotum and grasp the testes as they are pushed downward into the scrotum. If you cannot easily palpate the testes in an older boy, have him sit in a chair with his legs apart, his heels on the seat of the chair, and his arms around his knees. This procedure interrupts the cremasteric reflex and creates pressure by flexing the abdomen and the thigh. You will feel the testes as a soft mass about 1 cm in diameter. They are normally descended if you can palpate them in the scrotum even if retraction into the inguinal canal occurs immediately. In an infant, block the inguinal canals with the nondominant hand and palpate the testes as soon as the diaper is removed before the cold room air causes retraction.

For the adolescent male, follow the same procedure as for the adult male (see Chapter 20: Male Genitalia).

Female genitalia. Inspect the genitalia of the female child by separating the labia majora with the thumb and the forefinger to expose the labia minora, urethral meatus, and vaginal orifice (Figure 25.54). Examine the young infant in a supine position on the mother's lap with the knees held in a flexed position and separated. Sit facing the mother and child. The older child can help by spreading back her labia with her hands (Figure 25.55). Urethral discharges are pathological and indicate infection somewhere in the urinary tract. A blood vaginal discharge during the first month of life (secondary to residual maternal hormones) is normal but not common. Purulent or mucoid vaginal discharges indicate infection or the presence of a foreign body. Inspect the labia and the clitoris for any abnormality in size or for evidence of adhesion or infection. Inspect the vaginal area; usually it is not palpated. An imperforate hymen may be apparent if there is fluid behind it.

The vaginal examination is usually omitted for the child. If concerns or symptoms require such an examination, an experienced clinician or a gynecologist should examine the child. Vaginal examinations should be done on the adolescent who is sexually active, has been sexu-

---

Orthopedic Disorders Common to Various Age Groups of Children

NEONATE

Oligohydramnios
  Compressed face
  Limb deformities
  Thoracic compression
  Lung hypoplasia
Prolonged breech position
Dislocation of hip
Deformations of knee
Hyperextension of knee
Dislocation of knee
Foot deformities
  Calcaneovalgus
  Metatarsus adductus
  Equinovarus
  Overlapping toes
Craniofacies
  Compressed face
    Molding of calvaria
    Mandibular asymmetry
  Torticollis
Dislocated hip(s)
Postural scoliosis

PRESCHOOLER

Postural-orthopedic abnormalities of foot
Abnormalities of toenail
Disorders of skin
Deviations in gait
Poor foot hygiene
Inadequate footgear

SCHOOL-AGE CHILD

Idiopathic adolescent scoliosis
Other types of scoliosis
Kyphosis
Lordosis
Alignment problems of lower extremity
Juvenile arthritis
Athletic injuries
  Unstable knee
  Upper extremity, elbow clean
  Epiphyseal injuries

YOUNG ADULT

Disabling low back pain
Osteoarthritis
Athletic injuries
  Jogging-related injuries

figure **25.56** Genu valgum (knock-knee) in the young child. *(From Seidel HM et al: Mosby's guide to physical examination, ed 3, St Louis, 1995, Mosby.)*

Infants generally have bowlegs until 12 to 18 months. When they begin walking, their gait is wide based. Some children tend to evert their feet so that they bear weight on the inner aspects of the feet, and this is normal. The young child also has a fat pad under the arch of the foot and may appear flat-footed until about 3 to 4 years of age. The child's bowlegged appearance changes as the gait improves, and then the child becomes mildly knock-kneed (Figure 25.56). The normal configuration of the legs develops by age 6 or 7 years.

Intoeing may result from metatarsus varus (forefoot turned in); medial tibial torsion, in which the entire foot turns in while the knee remains straight; or medial femoral torsion, in which the entire leg turns in with the foot and knee turned medially. A child who has intoeing as a result of a fixed deformity of the forefoot that cannot be corrected to neutral should be referred for orthopedic care. The problems of medial tibial torsion and

medial femoral torsion are more cosmetic than functional and usually disappear by age 4 or 5 years.

Examine the hips for congenital dislocation or subluxation at every routine visit during the first year of life. In congenital dislocation, the head of the femur is found outside the acetabulum, and relocation may or may not be possible. Subluxation means that the capsule is lax enough to allow the femoral head to be displaced but not dislocated. Clinical signs of an abnormal hip may be asymmetry of the skinfolds, creases on the dorsal surfaces, and an apparent leg length inequality (Figure 25.57). However, these signs may not be apparent in the young infant who has a hip that is susceptible to dislocation rather than a dislocated hip. The examination of the hips is done with the infant in the supine position. Flex the infant's hips and knees, and then abduct the hips fully. In the newborn, each thigh should abduct to almost 90 degrees (Figure 25.58). Any limitation in the abduction of either or both hips may indicate dislocation.

To check the stability of the individual hip, place your middle finger over the greater trochanter (Figure

figure**25.57** Examination of the hips. **A,** Normal gluteal folds. **B,** Abnormal gluteal folds.

figure**25.58** Examination of the hips for dislocation: abduction.

figure**25.59** Examination of the hips for dislocation: adduction.

25.59) with your thumb placed medially. Adduct the thigh while still in the flexed position and apply pressure along the long axis of the femur in the direction of the posterior lip of the acetabulum. As dislocation occurs, you will feel the click of exit (Barlow's test). You will feel a similar click or "clunk" when you reverse the maneuver by abducting the hip and the head of the femur slips back into the joint (Ortolani maneuver). When you feel lateral movement of the head of the femur without dislocation, the hip is subluxed. Most dislocated hips in

the newborn will relocate naturally. However, an unstable hip may become fixed in the dislocated position during the first weeks of life and the Ortolani maneuver cannot be done to replace the head. Dislocated hips can resolve spontaneously, but there is no way to be sure this will happen. Refer the infant suspected of having a dislocation to an orthopedist without delay, since treatment is far more effective at an early age.

All children should have a spinal examination during each health visit. In the young infant and child, a tuft of

figure**25.60** Defects of the spinal column. **A,** Normal spine. **B,** Kyphosis. **C,** Lordosis. **D,** Normal spine in balance. **E,** Mild scoliosis in balance. **F,** Severe scoliosis not in balance. **G,** Rib hump and flank asymmetry seen in flexion caused by rotary component.

hair or small dimple usually located toward the distal portion of the spine, but which may appear anywhere from the coccyx to the skull, may indicate underlying spina bifida or may be only a superficial anomaly. If a dimple is apparent, note its interior and depth. A dimple often indicates a dermoid cyst, which may become a site of infection. The young infant and child should be examined for congenital scoliosis, whereas the child of 10 years or older should be examined for idiopathic scoliosis. The method of examination is the same as for the adult (Figure 25.60). Observe the shoulders for symmetry in the standing position. Ask the child to bend the shoulders forward with the arms hanging freely and the head down. In this position you can observe any prominence of one side of the rib cage. Examine the young infant in a sitting position while bending the child forward on your hand. If a scoliosis is suspected, refer the child to an orthopedist.

Athletic injuries are becoming more common with the increase in organized sports activities for preadolescents and adolescents. The growing child is at risk for epiphyseal fractures where the least resistance to stress is found. Stress fractures of the tibia or the femur occur frequently, and the affected child complains of pain in the proximal region of the tibia or distal portion of the femur. A painful knee may be caused by a dislocation of the patella. The history of the child's recent activities will give some indication of the kind of injury sustained. The American Academy of Pediatrics has developed the 2-minute orthopedic examination, which tests for any loss of range of motion or function (Table 25.14).

Refer the child for evaluation by an orthopedist.

Neurological system

Although you must adapt the formal neurological examination of the infant or child to the age of the individual, at all times a complete examination consists of an assessment of the cranial nerves and special senses, the motor system, coordination and cerebellar function, sensation, and both superficial and deep reflexes. In children less than 2 years of age, the neurological assessment is closely related to the increasing myelinization and maturation of the neural system. In this age group you can only estimate the degree of maturation rather than quantify it.

In the newborn, infant, and child older than 2 years, the primary mode of examination is one of observation and inspection. This approach is usually reinforced by palpation and passive manipulation.

Observation of the child in the natural state and then

table 25.14	*The 2-Minute Orthopedic Examination*

Instructions	Observations
Stand facing examiner	Acromioclavicular joints, general habitus
Look at ceiling, floor, over both shoulders; touch ears to shoulders	Cervical spine motion
Shrug shoulders (examiner resists)	Trapezius strength
Abduct shoulders 90 degrees (examiner resists at 90 degrees)	Deltoid strength
Full external rotation of arms	Shoulder motion
Flex and extend elbows	Elbow motion
Arms at sides, elbows 90 degrees flexed; pronate and supinate wrists	Elbow and wrist motion
Spread fingers; make fist	Hand or finger motion and deformities
Tighten (contract) quadriceps; relax quadriceps	Symmetry and knee effusion; ankle effusion
"Duck walk" four steps (away from examiner with buttocks on heels)	Hip, knee, and ankle motion
Stand with back to examiner	Shoulder symmetry, scoliosis
Knees straight, touch toes	Scoliosis, hip motion, hamstring tightness
Raise up on toes, raise heels	Calf symmetry, leg strength

From *Sports medicine: health care for young athletes,* Elk Grove Village, Ill, 1991, American Academy of Pediatrics.

figure 25.61   Babinski reflex. *1,* Direction of stroke; *2,* dorsiflexion of big toe; *3,* fanning of toes. *(From Wong DL: Whaley and Wong's nursing care of infants and children, ed 5, St Louis, 1995, Mosby.)*

with purposeful stimulation is often the examiner's most valuable tool. Such observation is the best opportunity to determine how the child's overall function and behavior meet age-related norms. Seven assessment areas include symmetry of spontaneous movements, appearance, positioning, posture, movement of extremities, seizure activity, and responsiveness to the parents and the environment.

A good tool for assessing neurological status in an infant and young child is the Denver Developmental Screening Test II (see Figure 4.1). Gross and fine motor skills, language skills, and social skills provide clues to neurological status when the child is compared with other children of the same age. The Denver II is a major revision of the Denver Developmental Screening Test (DDST). It was developed to address criticisms of cultural and gender bias in the DDST.

Because the neurological system affects every other system, the neurological examination should be integrated with other parts of the physical examination. For example, changes in the pigmentation of the skin, lesions of the skin, masses in the abdomen, abnormal size and shape of the head, gaps and protrusions in the spinal column, and limited range of motion can all reflect a disease, lesion, or injury to the nervous system. In addition, because a child is going through an intense period of development that is in part related to the increasing myelinization and maturation of the neural system, meticulous observation of the child's developmental progress is important. The quality, pitch, loudness, and duration of a child's cry; drowsiness; irritability; and social, adaptive, language, and motor skills are all measures of how well the neurological system is functioning.

The automatic infant reflexes that are normal at birth disappear at approximately 4 to 6 months of age, as voluntary control begins to develop. They include the Moro reflex, palmar grasp reflex, plantar grasp reflex, placing reflex, stepping reflex, tonic neck reflex, and rooting reflex. Absence of these reflexes at birth may indicate a severe problem of the central nervous system. Persistence of these reflexes may be equally serious.

A positive Babinski reflex is normally present in the newborn and disappears by the age of 12 to 24 months or when the child begins to walk (Figure 25.61). Table 25.15 describes several reflexes found in full-term infants. Figure 25.62 illustrates these reflexes.

Examine the child who is 2 years of age or older with many of the same methods used for an adult. However, alter the conversation, directions, and developmental tasks to be more suitable to the child's interests and knowledge level. In a child of this age, more specific ex-

amination is possible, including auditory testing, funduscopic examination, and stereognosis testing. You can expand assessment to observe the quantity and quality of spontaneous voluntary motor activity, the ease in performing voluntary movements, lateral dominance, spontaneous drawing, articulation of sounds, and language acquisition. Also note the child's auditory discrimination, memory, reading, speech, and calculation skills. Last, test the child for awareness of body parts, spatial orientation, and emotional lability.

---

table 25.15 *Primitive Reflexes Routinely Evaluated: Procedure for Examination, Expected Findings, Time of Appearance and Disappearance*

Reflex (appearance)	Procedure and findings
Palmar grasp (birth)	Making sure the infant's head is in midline, touch the palm of the infant's hand from the ulnar side (opposite the thumb). Note the strong grasp of your finger. Sucking facilitates the grasp. It should be strongest between 1 and 2 months of age and disappear by 3 months (Figure 25.62, *A*).
Plantar grasp (birth)	Touch the plantar surface of the infant's feet at the base of the toes. The toes should curl downward. It should be strong up to 8 months of age (Figure 25.62, *B*).
Moro (birth)	With the infant supported in semisitting position, allow the head and trunk to drop back to a 30-degree angle. Observe symmetrical abduction and extension of the arms; fingers fan out and thumb and index finger form a **C**. The arms then adduct in an embracing motion followed by relaxed flexion. The legs may follow a similar pattern of response. The reflex diminishes in strength by 3 to 4 months and disappears by 6 months (Figure 25.62, *C*).
Placing (4 days of age)	Hold the infant upright under its arms next to the table or chair. Touch the dorsal side of the foot to the table or chair edge. Observe flexion of the hips and knees and lifting of the foot as if stepping up on the table. Age of disappearance varies (Figure 25.62, *D*).
Stepping (between birth and 8 weeks)	Hold the infant upright under the arms and allow the soles of the feet to touch the surface of the table. Observe for alternate flexion and extension of the legs, simulating walking. It disappears before voluntary walking (Figure 25.62, *E*).
Tonic neck or "fencing" (by 2 to 3 months)	With the infant lying supine and relaxed or sleeping, turn the head to one side so the jaw is over the shoulder. Observe for extension of the arm and leg on the side to which the head is turned and for flexion of the opposite arm and leg. Turn the infant's head to the other side, observing the reversal of the extremities' posture. This reflex diminishes at 3 to 4 months of age and disappears by 6 months. Be concerned if the infant never exhibits the reflex or seems locked in the fencing position. This reflex must disappear before the infant can roll over or bring its hand to its face (Figure 25.62, *F*).

Modified from Seidel HM et al: *Mosby's guide to physical examination,* ed 3, St Louis, 1995, Mosby.

figure **25.62** Elicitation of the primitive reflex. **A,** Palmar grasp. **B,** Plantar grasp. **C,** Moro reflex. **D,** Placing reflex. **E,** Stepping reflex. **F,** Tonic neck reflex. Proper positioning of the head and neck is shown, but this infant is too young for the reflex to be present. *(From Seidel HM et al:* Mosby's guide to physical examination, *ed 3, St Louis, 1995, Mosby.)*

Regardless of the child's age, if you suspect meningeal irritation during an illness episode, note the presence of paradoxical irritability, Kernig's sign, or Brudzinski's signs. In paradoxical irritability the child is not easily comforted when held by the parent, contrary to his or her usual behavior. To elicit Kernig's sign, have the child lie on the table, face up, with the leg bent at the knee. Attempt to extend the hip by raising the knee. If you encounter pain and resistance, the maneuver is positive for meningeal irritation. Obtain Brudzinski's sign by having the child lie supine on a table. Bend the neck gently. If the child's knees flex spontaneously, this sign is positive. Tables 25.16 and 25.17 give detailed information on techniques for evaluating cranial nerve function in infants and young children.

• • •

A thorough working knowledge of growth and development, combined with solid physical assessment skills and an appreciation of the need to include the family in the assessment process, will help the practitioner successfully assess pediatric clients and promote the health of children and their families (Figure 25.63).

table 25.16	*Testing Procedures and Expected Behaviors for Indirect Cranial Nerve Evaluation in Newborns and Infants*
Cranial nerves	**Procedures and observations**
CN II, III, IV, and VI	Optical blink reflex: shine a light at the infant's open eyes. Observe the quick closure of the eyes and dorsal flexion of the infant's head. No response may indicate poor light perception. Gazes intensely at close object or face. Focuses on and tracks an object with the eyes. Doll's eye maneuver: see CN VIII.
CN V	Rooting reflex: touch one corner of the infant's mouth. The infant should open the mouth and turn the head in the direction of stimulation. If the infant has been recently fed, minimal or no response is expected. Sucking reflex: place your finger in the infant's mouth, feeling the sucking action. The tongue should push up against your finger with a fairly good rate. Note the pressure, strength, and pattern of sucking.
CN VII	Observe the infant's facial expression when crying. Note the infant's ability to wrinkle the forehead and the symmetry of the smile.
CN VIII	Acoustic blink reflex: loudly clap your hands about 30 cm from the infant's head; avoid producing an air current. Note the blink in response to the sound. No response after 2-3 days of age may indicate hearing problems. Infant will habituate to repeated testing. Moves eyes in direction of sound. Freezes position with high-pitched sound. Doll's eye maneuver: hold the infant under the axilla in an upright position, head held steady, facing you. Rotate the infant first in one direction and then in the other. The infant's eyes should turn in the opposite direction of the head movement at exactly the same pace of the rotation. If the eyes do not move in the expected direction, suspect a vestibular problem or eye muscle paralysis.
CN IX and X	Swallowing and gag reflex.
CN XII	Coordinated sucking and swallowing ability. Pinch infant's nose: mouth will open and tip of tongue will rise in a midline position.

Modified from Seidel HM et al: *Mosby's guide to physical examination*, ed 3, St Louis, 1995, Mosby.

figure**25.63** Assessment of both the child and family is important for promoting health.

table**25.17** *Cranial Nerve Examination Procedures for Young Children*	
Cranial nerves	**Procedures and observations**
CN II	If the child cooperates, the Snellen **E** or Picture Chart may be used to test vision. Visual fields may be tested, but the child may need the head immobilized.
CN III, IV, and VI	Have the child follow an object with the eyes, immobilizing the head if necessary. Attempt to move the object through the cardinal points of gaze.
CN V	Observe the child chewing a cookie or cracker, noting bilateral jaw strength. Touch the child's forehead and cheeks with cotton and watch the child bat it away.
CN VII	Observe the child's face when smiling, frowning, and crying. Ask the child to show the teeth. Demonstrate puffed cheeks and ask the child to imitate.
CN VIII	Observe the child turn to sounds such as bell or whisper. Whisper a commonly used word behind the child's back and have the child repeat the word. Perform audiometric testing.
CN IX and X	Elicit gag reflex.
CN XI and XII	Instruct older child to stick out the tongue and shrug the shoulders or raise the arms.

From Seidel HM et al: *Mosby's guide to physical examination*, ed 3, St Louis, 1995, Mosby.

*sample*documentation&diagnoses   CRITICAL THINKING

■ FOCUSED HEALTH HISTORY *(SUBJECTIVE DATA)*

Debbie, a 7-year-old white female, has been brought to the clinic by her mother for a sore throat and fever for the past day. She has been in good health except for approximately 4 colds since her visit 1 year ago. She has no known allergies to any medications. Her mother states that Debbie has had a fever of up to 39.3° C (102.7° F; oral) since yesterday. The fever comes down with acetaminophen 320 mg. Her last dose of acetaminophen was about 3 hours ago. Debbie also complains of a sore throat. She has been drinking some liquids but eating little since she has had the fever and sore throat. Debbie denies any pain when bending her neck, abdominal pain, or pain with urination. Her mother states that Debbie is tired but alert and moderately active. She states that several of Debbie's classmates have strep throat and she is concerned that Debbie may also have strep throat. No one in her family is sick.

Debbie is in the second grade of the Urban elementary school. She states that she enjoys school but thinks her teacher "is too hard sometimes." Her mother says that all school reports are good and that Debbie has many friends in school and in the neighborhood and has recently started "sleeping over" with her girl friends. Her mother states that everyone in the family is fine—no major stresses or life changes.

■ FOCUSED PHYSICAL EXAMINATION *(OBJECTIVE DATA)*

General appearance: Cooperative, pleasant, 7-year-old white female who appears flushed and feverish.
Temperature: 38.8° C (101.8° F) (tympanic membrane).
Eyes: Clear, no discharge or redness.
Ears: Tympanic membranes pearly with landmarks visible.
Nose: Mucosa pink; slight, clear discharge.
Mouth: Pink, no lesions.
Throat: Tonsils red, swollen 3+ with yellow-white exudate.
Neck: Enlarged and tender tonsillar nodes bilaterally.
Chest: Lungs clear; breath sounds normal anteriorly and posteriorly, resonant to percussion, no adventitious sounds.

diagnoses

HEALTH PROBLEM

Pharyngitis; rule out group A streptoccal infection

NURSING DIAGNOSES

Pain related to inflammation of throat
Defining Characteristics

- Tonsils red, swollen, enlarged
- Verbal expression of sore throat
- Decreased intake related to sore throat

Altered nutrition: less than body requirements related to sore throat
Defining Characteristics

- Reported decreased food or drink intake
- Lack of interest in food
- Sore, inflamed throat

chapter 26

Aging Clients

■ PURPOSE OF EXAMINATION

This chapter highlights areas of the health history and physical examination that may differ in the older adult. The increased number of older adults who are living longer presents several challenges to health care professionals.

Demographics

The percentage of the American population over the age of 65 tripled between 1900 and 1990. Approximately 12.6% of the current population is over 65, and by 2030, when the baby boom generation has aged, about 22% of the population will be over 65. While the actual maximum life span has not increased (approximately 110 years), the number of older persons living into their 80s and 90s has increased. The fastest growing segment of the American population is the group of individuals 85 years and older.

The majority of older adults live active, independent lives in the community. Retired from one career, older adults may embark on a second career or pursue a life-long hobby on a full-time basis. Most older adults have

Major Chronic Conditions in Older Adults	
Arthritis	Orthopedic impairments
Hypertension	Sinusitis
Hearing impairments	Diabetes
Heart disease	Visual impairments
Cataracts	Varicose veins

at least one chronic health problem, and many have multiple chronic problems. The extent to which these chronic diseases cause illness and functional disability depends on the type and severity of the diseases, coexisting diseases, environmental factors such as financial and social resources, and the individual's perception of health and coping styles or coping strategies. The major chronic conditions in the older population are outlined by order of prevalence in the box above.

■ USE AND COST OF HEALTH CARE

Data reported by the American Association of Retired Persons and the Administration on Aging (1991) indicate that older individuals account for a disproportionate number of hospital stays and that, once in the hospital, the average length of stay is longer for older individuals than for younger ones, 8.9 days versus 5.3 days, respectively. Noninstitutionalized older adults also had more physician contacts than younger persons. About 1% of the population 65 to 74 years of age live in nursing homes, and by age 85, about 25% of older adults live in nursing homes. One third of the country's total personal health care dollars pay for health care for those over 65 years of age. Medicare and Medicaid cover about two thirds of these expenses. Medicare does not cover dental care. Many older adults must pay significant out-of-pocket health care expenses. This fact is important, since almost 20% of those over 65 are considered poor or near poor. Lack of financial resources can cause people to ration their medications and/or delay seeking care. This behavior may lead to worsening health conditions and lengthy, expensive hospital stays that might otherwise be controlled.

Nurses are likely to care for older clients in a variety of settings. And, since after age 65 there are 149 women for every 100 men, a majority of these clients are likely to be women.

■ EXAMINATION

Health History

Older adults are likely to have different types of problems than younger and middle-aged adults. This section discusses the presentation of conditions that are more likely to occur in an older population. These conditions are sometimes referred to as "geriatric syndromes" and include falls, incontinence, delirium, inappropriate medication use, mental status and mood impairment, functional impairment, and poor nutrition. While conditions are not diseases, these conditions place the client at risk for functional decline, morbidity, and mortality.

Altered clinical presentation

Diseases associated with "classic" symptoms in young and middle-aged adults may be associated with more general symptoms in later life. For example, a myocardial infarction may present with mental confusion, a fall, or nausea and vomiting, as opposed to crushing substernal pain radiating down the left arm. In addition, the presence of one condition may mask another. For example, a person with severe chronic obstructive lung disease may not be active enough to bring about the symptoms of angina despite the presence of severe ischemic heart disease.

Concomitant disease

Since multiple medical problems are common in older adults, an examination directed at one symptom may uncover more than one problem. When examining the client for a complaint of recurrent falls, the examiner may discover that the falls are related to hurrying to the bathroom to avoid an incontinent episode.

Accumulated life history

Intelligence does not decline with age. Treat older adults with respect for their intelligence, wisdom, and accumulated life experiences. Remember that the person has lived with his or her body a long time and may be able to detect subtle changes in health status better than the health professional. The older adult may have a long history of medical problems, and the interview may become lengthy. Whenever necessary, gently redirect the conversation to obtain the most pertinent history while at the same time avoiding giving the client the impression that offered information is not valued. To redirect the interview, say, "This is valuable information that I would like to hear about at some later point in time, but right now I need to focus on your problem of dizziness."

The following impairments are more frequently encountered in older adults. Awareness of these conditions will assist you in focusing questions on specific signs and symptoms.

Mental status and mood impairment

Dementia. Dementia is a clinical condition characterized by a decline in memory and intellectual functioning. Several different diseases may cause dementia. The most common cause of dementia is Alzheimer's disease, a disease in which neuron loss and a decrease in chemical transmitters occurs in certain areas of the brain. Other causes of dementia include multiple strokes, alcohol abuse, and Parkinson's disease, Huntington's disease, and acquired immunodeficiency disease. The box below lists the criteria from the revised third edition of the

DSM IV Dementia Criteria

A. Multiple cognitive deficits, including:
  1. Memory impairment
  2. One or more of the following:
    a. Aphasia
    b. Apraxia
    c. Agnosia
    d. Disturbance in executive function
B. No. 1 and No. 2 must significantly impair occupational or social functioning.

Diagnosis and Statistical Manual of Mental Disorders (DSM-IV) required to make a diagnosis of dementia.

Older clients are more likely to have symptoms of dementia, since the prevalence of dementia increases with age. At age 65, about 1.5% of the population has dementia; this percentage increases to about 50% at 90 years. If dementia is suspected, refer the client to a physician for a complete evaluation.

The answers to the following questions may provide information about the client's mental status:

Did the client come to the appointment alone or accompanied by someone?

Is the client appropriately dressed?

Is the client having difficulty answering questions?

Not all clients need a formal assessment of their mental status. If, however, the examiner suspects some impairment in mental status, he or she can use a number of standardized assessment instruments to evaluate mental status. The Mini-Mental Status Examination (MMSE) is a commonly used 30-item questionnaire that assesses orientation, registration, attention and calculation, recall, and language (see pp. 526–527). A score of 23 or less suggests some type of mental status impairment. The MMSE, however, is only a screening examination, and *no diagnosis is made or excluded solely on the basis of the examination score.* Dementia may be present with a score greater than 23.

Depression. Depression is the most common mood disorder in late life. The 1991 Consensus Development Conference on the Diagnosis and Treatment of Depression in Late Life defines depression as a syndrome that includes physiological, affective, and mental symptoms. The box below outlines the DSM-IV criteria for depression.

Depression is not more common in late life than in earlier life. About 3% of community-dwelling elderly suffer from major depression. In nursing homes, however, as many as 25% of residents may have depression. Some of the symptoms of depression, such as weight loss, sleep disturbances, and fatigue, may be associated

with other conditions, and the examiner may miss a diagnosis of depression in the older adult. Simply asking the client, "Do you feel sad, blue, or depressed much of the time?" provides insight into the client's mood. Assessing for depression is an important part of the health history for older adults, particularly for men, because older white men are at the highest risk for suicide of any age group.

A number of questionnaires are available to look for depressive symptoms. The Geriatric Depression Scale (GDS) is a 30-item questionnaire designed specifically to screen for depression in the elderly. Similar to the MMSE, the GDS score does not diagnose or exclude depression. Refer a client scoring high on the GDS to a physician or psychologist for further evaluation of a possible depression. Also, if the history suggests depression even in the absence of a high GDS score, refer the client for further evaluation.

Delirium. Delirium is an acute change in mental status with symptoms meeting the DSM-IV criteria outlined in the box below.

Delirium usually occurs during an acute medical illness, and studies have reported that 5% to 35% of hospitalized elderly develop delirium during their hospitalization. Delirium may develop in a few hours, and the client may have periods of clear thinking alternating with disorientation. Delirium is distinguished from dementia by its rapid onset. Delirium most often occurs in clients who had normal mental status before surgery or before developing an acute illness. Almost any acute disorder that affects brain function, such as hypoxia, fever, arrhythmias, and anemia, can cause delirium. One of the major causes of delirium in the older adult is medications. While delirium is most prevalent in hospitals, acutely ill older clients may be brought into a clinic accompanied by family members who report sudden and dramatic changes in the elderly person's mental status. These mental status changes may be the first sign of an acute illness.

Functional impairment

The older client's ability to maintain independence depends on his or her ability to meet basic physical and daily life management needs or to secure these needs

---

DSM IV Major Depression Criteria

Presence of five or more of the following:
1. Depressed mood
2. Diminished interest or pleasure
3. Weight loss or gain
4. Insomnia or hypersomnia
5. Psychomotor agitation or retardation
6. Fatigue or loss of energy
7. Feelings of worthlessness or guilt
8. Diminished energy to think or concentrate
9. Recurrent thoughts of death, suicidal ideation

DSM IV Delirium Criteria

Reduced attention
Impaired sensorium
Fluctuating course
Disorganized thinking
Subacute onset

through community resources. Basic physical needs are referred to as activities of daily living (ADLs), and life management needs are called instrumental activities of daily living (IADLs) (see boxes below). One or more physical and psychological impairments can greatly affect the client's ability to perform ADLs or IADLs. Assess ADL and IADL function in the older client.

The most accurate assessment of ADL and IADL function is direct observation of the client performing each specific task. This, however, is not practical in the clinic or hospital setting. Instead, ask clients whether they can perform the various ADL and IADL tasks alone or with assistance. If assistance is required, find out who provides the assistance and with what frequency. In addition, simply observe the client entering the room, sitting in a chair, and undressing for the examination for clues about several ADL functions. One quick and easy assessment of mobility is the timed get-up-and-go test. Time the client getting up from a chair, walking 10 feet, turning around, walking back to the chair, and sitting back down (Figure 26.1). Use a standard armchair with a seat height of about 46 cm. While the time required to perform this test varies with clients, highly mobile, independent older adults can perform this test in about 10 seconds. Detect changes over time by repeating this test at subsequent visits.

Standardized assessment questionnaires are also available for evaluating ADL and IADL tasks (see Chapter 27: Clients with Functional Limitations). The Katz Index of ADL and the Barthel Index are two examples of such questionnaires. The Barthel Index provides a score of 0 (total dependence) to 100 (total indepen-

dence), which is useful for following changes over time. The Assessment of Living Skills and Resources (ALSAR) is a form that assesses both the client's ability to perform IADLs and available resources.

Incontinence. Between 15% and 30% of older adults living at home and up to 50% of nursing home residents have incontinence. Incontinence is an involuntary loss of urine with or without warning. The incontinent older adult may experience physical, psychological, and financial burdens. For example, fear of an accident may lead to restriction of outside activities and contribute to social isolation.

Incontinence may be transient or established. Transient incontinence is acute in onset and is often related to a change in health status, such as a urinary tract infection, medications, stool impaction, delirium, polyuria, or restricted mobility. Often several of these factors are present during hospitalization, and it is not uncommon for older adults to develop incontinence when hospitalized.

Established incontinence occurs when leakage of urine persists after suspected causes (i.e., decreasing a

Activities of Daily Living	
Dressing	Bowel control
Transferring	Bladder control
Feeding	Walking
Bathing	Climbing stairs
Toileting	Grooming

Instrumental Activities of Daily Living	
Telephoning	Shopping
Reading	Meal preparation
Leisure	Laundering
Medication management	Housekeeping
Money management	Home maintenance

figure**26.1** The timed "get-up-and-go" test measures the time it takes the client to rise from a chair, walk 10 feet, turn around, return to the chair, and sit down.

table 26.1	*Common Causes of Incontinence*	
Urologic dysfunction	**Cause**	**Symptoms**
Detrusor muscle problem		
Overactivity	Stroke, dementia, Parkinson's disease	Urgency, little warning before voiding, usually large amounts of urine
Underactivity	Diabetes, bladder nerve injury	Bladder contracts reflexively without warning
Bladder outlet problem		
Incompetence	Relaxation of pelvic floor muscles	Involuntary loss of urine with increased abdominal pressure, such as coughing, sneezing, lifting, or standing
Obstruction	Prostatic hypertrophy	Overflow of urine from distended bladder

dose of diuretic) have been treated. Established incontinence is caused by a problem either with bladder muscle activity or with the bladder outlet. The bladder muscle, the detrusor, may be either overactive or underactive (Table 26.1). Detrusor overactivity is the most

figure 26.2 Many older clients use assistive devices, such as a Delta walker, to provide additional stability when ambulating.

common cause of incontinence in older adults and may result from stroke, Parkinson's disease, or Alzheimer's disease. This type of incontinence, also called urge incontinence, is characterized by little warning before voiding large amounts of urine. A client may state, "I just can't seem to get to the bathroom on time." Detrusor underactivity is less frequent and is caused by injury to the nerves of the bladder or to autonomic neuropathy, which may occur in diabetes. In this type of incontinence, the bladder contracts reflexively.

Stress incontinence is the second most common cause of incontinence in older women and is the result of bladder outlet incompetence. Relaxation of the pelvic floor muscles allows the proximal portion of the urethra and bladder neck to be displaced into the urogenital diaphragm with increased abdominal pressure. Stress incontinence causes involuntary loss of urine when abdominal pressure increases, such as when the woman coughs, laughs, lifts, or suddenly stands up. The amount of urine lost may vary from a few drops to a large quantity. Outlet obstruction, the second most common type of incontinence in older men, is due to prostatic enlargement, tumor, or urethral stricture. With outlet obstruction the bladder becomes distended with urine and eventually leaks urine from overflow.

Detrusor underactivity and overactivity, and outlet incompetence and obstruction are dysfunctions of the lower urinary tract that cause incontinence. Functional incontinence results from a variety of environmental and personal factors that impede getting to the bathroom before voiding occurs. Restricted mobility, bathroom location, and decreased manual dexterity or balance may cause incontinence in the absence of any urinary tract dysfunction or may exacerbate preexisting incontinence.

Clients are often reluctant to volunteer information about incontinence symptoms. Some individuals have the mistaken belief that incontinence is a normal part of aging that must be tolerated. State the following to help

the client relate incontinence symptoms, if present. "Some older people have a problem with leakage of urine at inappropriate times. This is not something that normally happens with aging and can often be treated. Do you ever have problems with leakage of urine?" Asking the question in this way informs the client that other people have a similar problem, it is not normal, and it may be treatable. If a client is experiencing symptoms, ask about the frequency and amount of the incontinence, associated activities, medications, eating and drinking habits, and current management of the problem by the client. Instruct the client on how to complete a voiding diary. The diary is an account of the frequency and amount voided, incontinent episodes, and associated activities.

Falls. Falls are a common occurrence in the older population. As many as one third of older adults living at home fall each year. This increases to about 50% by age 80. Accidents are the sixth leading cause of death for individuals over age 65; falls are the leading type of accident in this age group. About 5% of falls result in a fracture, with the most common fracture sites being the humerus, wrist, pelvis, ankle, and hip.

Risk factors for falls include sensory impairment such as visual changes and proprioceptive and vestibular dysfunction; neurological disorders resulting in gait impairment or mental status impairment; musculoskeletal disorders affecting strength and mobility; cardiovascular conditions, particularly orthostatic hypotension; and medications. Situational factors such as acute illness or an unfamiliar environment may precipitate a fall in individuals with or without predisposing risk factors. Falls are sometimes nonspecific signs of acute illness. For example, a nursing home resident falls, and in the course of the post-fall assessment the nurse measures a temperature of 38.9° C (102° F), and a subsequent diagnosis of pneumonia is made.

Ask clients whether they have fallen in the past 6 months. Obtain a detailed history about any reported falls, including risk factors for falls, frequency of falls, activity at the time of the fall, a description of the environment in which the fall occurred, and any injuries associated with the fall. For clients who live alone, always ask whether they were able to get up from the fall or whether they had to wait for help. The physical examination for clients who report a fall should include a neurological, musculoskeletal, and cardiovascular examination to assess for visual, balance, and gait impairment; muscle weakness; arrhythmias; and postural changes in blood pressure.

Inappropriate medication use

Older adults are the largest consumers of prescription drugs and also purchase many nonprescription medications. Several factors place the older client at risk for the ingestion of inappropriate medication, including multiple diseases, multiple health care providers, nonprescription medication use, sharing medications, and rationing medications. Older adults who see several different physicians for different problems may accumulate multiple medications, some of which may facilitate or impair the effect of others. Because of limited financial resources, the older adult may purchase only a portion of prescribed medications or may ration the medication, such as taking a pill once a day that is prescribed to be taken three times a day.

Medication dosage for some drugs may be altered for older clients because of age-related changes in the responsiveness of receptor cells to certain drugs, the distribution of drugs, and the metabolism and excretion of drugs. Since variability exists among older clients, consider medication dosages on an individual basis.

Instruct the client to bring all prescribed and non-prescribed medications to the examination, whether the client is currently taking them or not (people often stockpile unused medications at home). Using the last refill date on the bottle and the dose schedule, calculate the number of pills that should remain. Compare this number with the actual number of pills remaining to determine if the client is using the medication as ordered. Assess the number and type of medications in relation to the client's physical problems. Question the client about medications that do not seem to correspond with information obtained during the health history. For instance, a client might bring in a bottle of thyroid medication and fail to mention any thyroid problem. Conversely, the client may relate a diagnosis of hypertension and not have any antihypertensive medication. If you notice a discrepancy between the way in which a medication was prescribed and the way in which the client takes the medication, explore reasons for this discrepancy.

The greater the number of medications prescribed, the greater the likelihood that not all will be ingested. Clients may have difficulty opening the medication bottles, reading the labels, or remembering to take their medications. Advise clients that they can request easy-to-open pill bottles from their pharmacist. Suggest medication reminder boxes, which have compartments for both the days of the week and different times of the day. Medications can be sorted into these compartments either by the client, a family member, or a community nurse.

Poor nutrition

Nutritional status depends on the amount and type of food in the diet. Energy needs or caloric intake is based in part on the basal metabolic rate (BMR). The BMR depends on the amount of lean body mass. Since lean body mass declines with age, the BMR also declines. A declining BMR suggests that the older adult,

in general, needs fewer calories with increasing age. You must consider, however, the client's activity level and the presence of any acute or chronic illnesses when determining energy needs.

Since the client may need fewer calories with increasing age, the type of food the client eats becomes relatively more important to ensure adequate nutrient intake and to prevent poor nutritional status. The nutritional history should focus on both caloric needs and the types of food consumed.

Poor nutritional status, as defined by the 1991 Nutrition Screen Initiative Consensus Conference, includes nutritional deficiencies, as well as dehydration, undernutrition, nutritional imbalances, obesity, and excesses such as alcohol abuse. This consensus conference developed a plan for self-screening and professional nutritional screening for older adults. The client self-assessment screen is called the *Checklist to DETERMINE Nutritional Health*. This screening form asks the client to answer questions about the following nutritional risk factors:

Disease, chronic or acute
Eating habits
Tooth loss
Economic hardship
Reduced social contact
Multiple medications or drugs
Involuntary weight loss or gain
Needed assistance with self-care
Eighty years of age or greater

The purpose of this self-screening is to encourage clients to examine their nutritional intake and to seek professional help if they appear to be at risk.

The Nutrition Screen Initiative recommends two levels of professional nutritional screening. Level I screening identifies those individuals who either need preventive interventions, such as assistance with meals, or need a more in-depth nutritional assessment. Level I screening includes obtaining the client's height and weight history. Height may be difficult to obtain in some older clients because of kyphosis, inability to stand, or inability to maintain balance. When the client cannot stand, estimate height by measuring the length from the bottom of the foot to the anterior knee with the ankle and knee at a 90-degree angle.

Male height = 64.19 − (0.04 × Age in years) + (2.02 × Knee height [cm])

Female height = 84.88 − (0.24 × Age in years) + (1.83 × Knee height [cm])

The weight history includes questions about unintentional weight gain or loss in the past 6 months. Significant weight loss occurs if 5% or more of prior body weight is lost in 1 month, 7.5% in 3 months, or 10% or more in 6 months. Inquire about where the person eats, how often meals are skipped, the usual intake, the facilities available for food preparation, the resources available to purchase food, and the ability to perform ADLs. A 3-day diet record provides a good indication of food consumption, and many computer programs are available to calculate the energy and nutrient intake based on this 3-day record. You can mail this record, along with instructions for use, to clients before their appointment.

Perform level II screening, a more thorough nutritional assessment, when the client has an unintentional weight gain or loss in the past 6 months or appears underweight or overweight. Focus history questions on special dietary needs (i.e., is the client on a restricted sodium diet?); clinical symptoms such as sore mouth, difficulty chewing or swallowing; history of fractures; mood; mental status; and medications. Do laboratory screening for albumin level and serum cholesterol (see also Chapter 5: Nutritional Assessment).

Comprehensive geriatric assessment

It is apparent that the health assessment of the geriatric client may be complex and time-consuming. Older clients with multiple complex problems benefit from a comprehensive geriatric assessment (CGA). Such an assessment by team members from a variety of disciplines improves the accuracy of assessment, discharge planning and placement, and functional status. In addition, studies suggest that when geriatric teams provide care, prolonged survival, reduced medical care costs, reduced hospitalizations, decreased nursing home use, decreased medications, and increased use of home health services result.

In 1987 the National Institutes of Health convened a consensus conference on geriatric assessment. CGA was defined as the multidisciplinary evaluation in which the multiple problems of older persons are uncovered, described, and explained, if possible, and in which the resources and strengths of the person are catalogued, the need for services is assessed, and a coordinated care plan is developed to focus interventions for the person's problems. The various domains covered by CGA are physical, mental, social, economic, functional, and environmental status. In recent years more inpatient units and outpatient clinics offer comprehensive geriatric assessment. This type of thorough assessment generally takes several hours, during which time a core team—consisting of at least a physician, nurse, and social worker—sees and examines the client. Many teams also include physical and occupational therapists, a pharmacist, and a nutritionist. Often, the members of the various disciplines use standardized screening questionnaires, such as those mentioned previously, as they perform their assessment of the client. CGA is a time-consuming and costly evaluation, and not all older clients require

Questions to Target Potential Age-Related Impairments

1. Do you ever have a problem with urine leaking?
2. Have you fallen in the past 6 months?
3. Do you often feel sad, blue, down in the dumps, or depressed?
4. Do you often travel places away from home alone?
5. Do you have enough money to purchase your medications?
6. Do you sometimes skip your medications?
7. Do you skip meals often?

this type of extensive evaluation. Those clients likely to benefit most from CGA are over the age of 75 with potentially reversible functional disabilities.

Preparation for Examination: Client and Environment
Examiner-client interaction

Older adults may be accompanied by a spouse, adult child, or other relative or friend. Note whether the client is able to come into the examination room unaided. An inability to get to the examination room independently may indicate some type of sensory, functional, or mental status impairment. Sometimes relatives accompany independent and competent older adults into the examination room. Determine the client's wishes regarding the presence of others in the examination room. If the client requests that a relative or friend remain in the room, pay careful attention to who is answering questions and spontaneously providing information. A relative answering questions for the client may indicate that the client has some type of cognitive impairment and cannot answer. Politely but firmly inform the relative or friend that the client should be allowed to answer the questions first and that any additional information the relative or friend can supply will be welcomed after the client speaks.

Ask whether the client needs help in getting undressed for the examination or in getting dressed after the examination. Clients may need extra time and assistance in getting on and off the examining table. Some clients may tire quickly during the examination. If this occurs, adjust the sequence of the examination to include the most relevant assessments based on the presenting problem.

Sensory impairment

The loss of auditory acuity is the most common sensory loss among aging individuals and may impede history taking. Face the client directly, since many people with a hearing impairment rely to some extent on lipreading. Use simple, direct questions and avoid shouting. Shouting obscures the consonant sounds, sounds that are lost with hearing impairment in late life. Lowering the voice and speaking slightly louder may help. Amplification devices may assist in communication and are discussed later in this chapter.

Technique for Examination and Normal Findings
General inspection

The physical changes that highlight the aging process are graying hair and wrinkling of skin. Because of loss of connective tissue, body contours may appear sharper and hollows deeper, such as the orbits of the eyes and the axilla.

Skin

Age changes. Heredity, changes in the connective and epithelial tissues, endocrine alterations, and vascular changes all influence aging changes of the skin. Excessive exposure to sun accelerates these changes. The skin epidermis decreases in thickness. The melanocytes lose some of their ability to protect the skin from ultraviolet light. With chronic sun exposure, some melanocytes may be destroyed, resulting in hypopigmentation, or white spots, on the skin. Sun exposure can also stimulate melanocytes to produce hyperpigmented areas called lentigines. Lentigines are flat, tan to brown macules and are usually located on sun-exposed surfaces. They may be as large as 1 or 2 cm.

The dermis decreases in thickness, and as a result, the skin takes on a thin, translucent appearance. Sun exposure changes the structure of the dermal layer and contributes to sagging and wrinkling of the skin. With thinning of the dermis, less support exists for capillary walls, and blood vessel walls dilate. Visible dilated vessels are called telangiectasias or spider angiomas (see Figures 10.17, *C*, and 10.17, *E*). Skin capillaries are also more fragile. A bump to the skin can cause blood to leak through the capillaries into the dermis, resulting in bruising known as senile purpura. Ask the client how bruising occurred, since bruising may indicate a recent fall. A client unaware of bruising may have decreased sensory perception.

Subcutaneous fat decreases with age. While sebaceous glands may increase in size, their ability to function decreases. This decrease in function, together with water loss from the skin, contributes to dry skin or xerosis, a frequent complaint in older clients.

Lesions. Various skin lesions are common with increasing age. Seborrheic keratoses are benign, raised, warty-type lesions usually located on the face, shoulders, and trunk. The borders are irregular, and the surface scaly. These lesions have a "pasted-on," greasy appearance. Early lesions may be yellowish to tan, with the color changing to dark brown or black over time. Although benign, some people request their removal for cosmetic purposes (see Figure 10.21).

Skin tags are soft, flesh-colored lesions and are attached to the skin by a stalk. They vary in size from a pinhead to a pea and are most commonly found on the vertical and lateral surfaces of the neck and the axillary area. Like seborrhea keratoses, these lesions have little clinical importance but may be removed if they are irritated by clothing or for cosmetic reasons.

Cherry angiomas are another type of benign skin lesion occurring with increased frequency in older adults. These lesions are caused by proliferation and dilation of the superficial capillaries of the skin. They are bright red, soft, and dome shaped with a diameter of 1 mm or greater.

Actinic keratoses are pink to slightly red, dry lesions with indistinct borders. Rough adherent scales cover the lesions. These lesions occur over sun-exposed areas, such as the face, ears, and dorsal surfaces of the hands and arms. A small percentage of these actinic keratoses will transform into squamous cell skin cancers. Therefore these lesions are generally removed (see Figure 10.22).

Basal cell skin cancer is the most common of all cancers. Look for lesions that are nodular with rolled borders, translucent, and pearly in appearance. Telangiectasias are frequent inside the nodule. These lesions, which may be ulcerating, are most often located on sun-exposed body surfaces (Figure 26.3). Basal cell skin cancer is locally invasive and destructive but does not metastasize. Several techniques are available to remove these lesions, depending on the patient and the size and location of the cancer.

Hair and nails. Hair growth and nail growth change with age. Scalp, axillary, and pubic hair thins and decreases. Eyebrow, nostril, and ear hair becomes coarser, and some older women develop an increase in facial hair. A loss of hair pigment contributes to graying of hair. Nail growth slows and nails may yellow and lack luster. Some nails may become thin and split, whereas others, especially the toenails, may thicken.

Head and neck

Eyes. The cells responsible for lubricating the conjunctiva decrease, and "dry eye syndrome," characterized by a scratchy sensation with chronic irritation, may develop. Observe for an arcus senilis, the accumulation of calcium and cholesterol salts at the limbus of the eye

figure**26.3** Basal cell cancer on the nose.

(see Figure 12.33). This appears as a grayish to gray-white arc or halo and has no association with elevated serum cholesterol or other system illness. The cornea tends to become hazy. Pupils decrease in size, react more slowly to light, and dilate more slowly in the dark. As a result, the older adult requires more time adapting to a dark room. Restriction of upward movement of the pupil occurs with age, and the client may have to tip the head back further to look up.

Lids. Loss of fat from the orbit of the eye causes a sunken appearance. A decrease in strength of the muscles allowing the lids to shut tightly may result in an ectropion (see Figure 12.28). This is the turning out of the lower lid, exposing the punctum of the lower lid. If this occurs, tears do not drain properly and the client may complain of excess tearing. The opposite condition, entropion, is a turning inward of the lower lid caused by muscle spasm. The eyelashes of the lower lid contact the conjunctiva and cornea. If chronic irritation occurs, surgical correction may be necessary. The muscles that hold the upper lid open may weaken, causing lid droop or ptosis. The lid droop may hamper vision and can be corrected with surgery. Tear production may decrease and contribute to complaints of dry eyes.

Vision. The ability to accommodate decreases progressively with age. This condition is called presbyopia and increases with frequency after age 40. Assess for presbyopia by checking near vision with a hand-held reading card or newspaper. The ophthalmoscopic examination may be more difficult because of the smaller

pupil size. Look for mildly narrowed vessels, granular pigment in the macula, and a loss of bright macular and foveal reflexes. The fundus itself lacks luster and may appear more yellow.

Cataract, glaucoma, and age-related macular degeneration (AMD) are eye problems occurring more frequently in the older client. A cataract is an opacity in the lens, which gradually impairs vision (see Figure 12.35). A client who complains about glare from headlights when driving a car at night may have a cataract. The most common type of glaucoma in the older adult is open-angle glaucoma. Measuring intraocular pressures on a regular basis helps to detect glaucoma early. AMD, a loss of central vision, is one of the leading causes of blindness in the elderly. Laser therapy is one method of treatment for AMD. Clients with AMD may also be referred to low-vision specialists for assessment of magnification aids.

Ears

Outer ear. Aging changes begin to appear in the outer ear between ages 30 and 50. The skin becomes dry and less resilient, and connective tissue is lost. Pruritis may occur in the external auditory canal, leading to scratching. Remind clients not to use cotton tip applicators to relieve itching. Hair growth may be visible along the periphery of the helix, antihelix, and tragus of the pinna. The hairs are coarse and wirelike. The pinna increases in both length and width, and the earlobes are elongated. There is a decrease in cerumen production, and this reduction correlates with an increased dryness in cerumen. This may contribute to the increased tendency toward cerumen impactions.

Middle ear. Degenerative changes in the joints of the bones of the middle ear occur with increasing age. These changes, however, do not appear to have an appreciable effect on sound transmission.

Inner ear. The specialized cells of the auditory pathways have a limited ability to regenerate. Approximately 24% of individuals between ages 65 and 74 and 39% over age 75 have hearing loss. A variety of genetic and environmental factors contribute to this age-related hearing loss called presbycusis. Two common types of presbycusis are sensory and neural presbycusis. Sensory presbycusis is associated with degeneration of the organ of Corti and involves the inability to hear high-frequency sounds. Neural presbycusis is primarily a loss of speech discrimination. Neural presbycusis is associated with a decrease in the cochlear neurons while the organ of Corti remains functional.

A mild loss of speech frequency may pose little problem for the older person when listening to normal, clearly spoken conversation in a quiet room. In rooms with environmental noise such as churches, restaurants, or movie theaters, a mild hearing loss may present greater hearing problems.

figure**26.4**   In-the-ear hearing aid.

If you suspect hearing loss, check for and remove any cerumen impactions. If hearing problems persist, refer the client to an audiologist. Several aids are available for amplification of sound. The purpose of a hearing aid is to increase the intensity of the sound with as little distortion as possible. Several types of hearing aids are available: behind-the ear, eyeglass with aid, in-the-ear, in-the-canal, and body aids (Figure 26.4). The older adult may fear the social stigma associated with hearing aids. Successful adjustment to an aid depends largely on the client's motivation in wanting to use the aid.

Situation-specific assistive listening devices (ALDs) amplify speech for the hearing-impaired (Figure 26.5). An ALD is the size of a small transistor radio. A microphone is placed near the sound source while the listener places earphones in the ears. Sound travels to the earphones via infrared, audio loop, FM radio, or direct audio input. The sound is enhanced, and extraneous noise is reduced. Many theaters, churches, and lecture halls have such devices. They may also be used in examination rooms or hospital rooms.

Nose. Olfactory function decreases with age, and many older adults have a decreased ability to correctly identify odors. Although smell is not routinely assessed in the physical examination, question the client about altered smell, since failure to detect the smell of smoke or gas can be life-threatening. In addition, a decreased sense of smell may contribute to decreased food intake.

Mouth. The number of taste buds does not decline with aging. There is no age-related deterioration in the ability of healthy older adults to taste sweet, sour, salty, and bitter at usual concentrations. Older adults are re-

figure**26.5**   Assistive listening device.

taining more of their teeth longer. When tooth loss occurs, it is due to two major causes: dental caries and periodontal disease. Periodontal disease is the major cause of tooth loss in the older adult. Dental caries in older adults tends to develop at the root or bottom of the tooth along the gum where gingival recession or periodontal disease causes exposure of the root surface.

Healthy adults do not have diminished saliva production. Decreased salivary function does, however, occur commonly as a side effect of medications with anticholinergic effects. Decreased salivary function causes dry mouth or xerostomia (see box below). Xerostomia is also caused by irradiation of the salivary glands or salivary tumors. Observe for dry oral mucous membranes and dry tongue. Saliva has many functions, including antibacterial and antifungal activity, oral lubrication, buffering of bacteria-produced acids, mechanical cleansing, remineralization of teeth, and as an aid in mastication. Decreased saliva may contribute to caries formation. Instruct clients with xerostomia to brush their teeth after every meal and to avoid moistening their mouth with candy unless it is sugar-free. A variety of salivary lubricants are available to moisten the mouth in clients who have xerostomia.

The majority of oral cancers develop after age 40. Individuals with a history of tobacco and/or alcohol abuse are particularly at risk for developing an oral cancer. Carefully inspect the oral mucosa for red or white lesions. Remove any dentures during the examination, since poorly-fitting dentures can cause trauma to the oral mucosa. In addition, oral candidiasis may be present on areas of the mucosa where the dentures rest.

Breasts

With increasing age, the amount of fat in the breast increases as the glandular tissue atrophies. Breast consistency and shape change and are often described as pendulous (see Figure 14.5, *F*). The incidence of breast cancer in the United States increases with age; therefore the detection of a lump is significant and requires evaluation. Most recommendations suggest yearly mammo-

---

Classes of Medications Known to Cause Xerostomia

Anticholinergics	Decongestants
Antidepressants	Antiparkinsonians
Antihistamines	Antipsychotics
Antihypertensives	Diuretics
Antispasmodics	

grams for women between ages 50 and 59 and every 2 years after age 60.

Respiratory system

Calcification occurs in the costochondral joints of the ribs, and the chest wall becomes less compliant. Skeletal changes in the spine may cause an increase in the anteroposterior diameter of the chest. If this occurs, breath sounds may be more difficult to hear during auscultation.

Cardiovascular system

Age-related changes. Diseases of the cardiovascular system are common in the elderly and are the leading cause of death in this age group. Maximal heart rate decreases with age. Despite a decrease in heart rate, healthy older adults can maintain a normal cardiac output during exercise by increasing their stroke volume. While healthy older adults maintain normal cardiac output, many older clients do have cardiac disorders and do have decreased cardiac output and decreased activity tolerance.

Blood pressure. Isolated systolic hypertension and orthostatic hypotension are two problems commonly associated with changes in blood pressure in older adults.

Systolic blood pressure increases with age because of increased stiffness of the aorta and its branches. Isolated systolic hypertension occurs when the systolic blood pressure is greater than 160 mm Hg in the presence of a normal diastolic pressure. Isolated systolic hypertension occurs more frequently in older adults and is associated with an increased risk for strokes and fatal cardiovascular events. Research has shown that treating isolated systolic hypertension in older adults reduces the likelihood of strokes.

Postural or orthostatic hypotension occurs when the systolic blood pressure drops 20 mm Hg or more when the client goes from a lying or sitting position to a standing position. Baroreceptor sensitivity remains intact in healthy older adults and is not a likely cause of postural hypotension. One common cause of postural hypotension is medications, particularly antihypertensive medications, diuretics, and medications with anticholinergic effects.

In older clients, measure blood pressure in both arms with the client lying and standing, or sitting and standing. Have the client lying or sitting at rest at least 15 minutes before taking the initial blood pressure reading. Then have the client stand, and take the blood pressure immediately. If you record a drop in the standing blood pressure, retake the blood pressure again in 1 minute. A drop in blood pressure on rising places the older client at risk for light-headedness and falls. If these symptoms occur, refer the client to a physician for further evaluation. In addition, instruct the client to sit on the edge of the bed or chair for a couple of minutes before standing and have a firm object such as a heavy chair close by to use for support if needed.

Heart. Precordial palpation may be difficult in those elderly who have an increased anterorposterior diameter. Kyphosis, often occurring in the older client, may cause a downward dislocation of the cardiac apex (see Figure 18.57, *B*).

With age, there is an increase in fibrosis and calcification of the aortic valve cusps, a condition called aortic sclerosis. The thickening of these valves, together with dilation of the aorta, may cause a systolic murmur. Aortic sclerosis is of little clinical significance unless the sclerosed valve progresses to aortic stenosis. The aortic sclerosis murmur is best heard at the right base. It is low in intensity and short in duration, and it peaks early in systole. The differential diagnosis of aortic stenosis versus aortic sclerosis is difficult and best made by an echocardiogram. A fourth heart sound (S_4) is common with increased age and is often heard along with an aortic sclerotic murmur. An S_4 in the older client is most likely a result of decreased ventricular compliance.

Abdomen

In some older clients, the general loss of fibroconnective tissue and muscle wasting may make the abdominal wall slacker, thinner, and easier to palpate. In other clients, increased fat deposits around the abdomen may make palpation more difficult.

Reproductive system

Female client. Cells of the reproductive tract and the breasts are estrogen dependent for growth and function. The decline of estrogen production starting at menopause is responsible for many changes in the tissues of older female clients (see Table 21.1).

The ovaries, uterus, and cervix decrease in size. The ovaries may not be palpable. The vagina narrows and shortens. The vaginal epithelium atrophies; the surface is thin, pale, fragile, and easily traumatized; intercourse may be painful. The frequency of intercourse in older women depends on the availability of a partner, physical health, previous sexual activity, and desire. Table 26.2 lists changes in the phases of intercourse in the older woman. Vaginal estrogen creams often provide relief for painful symptoms associated with atrophic vaginitis. Observe for vaginal erosions, ulcerations, and adhesions.

Male client. Testosterone declines in older males. This decline occurs later than the decline in estrogen in the female. Testes decrease in size and are less firm on palpation. While sperm production either remains the same or decreases slightly, sperm motility decreases and size changes. The prostate gland is enlarged, and secretion is impaired. The seminal fluid is reduced in amount and viscosity.

These changes do not necessarily mean a decrease in libido or a loss in the sense of satisfaction from intercourse. Most men over 60 reported having intercourse one or two times a week. Table 26.3 notes changes in the phases of intercourse in the older man (see also Table 20.1).

Musculoskeletal system

With increasing age, thinning of the intervertebral disks and shortening or collapse of the intervertebral bodies result in loss of height. Changes in the spine also contribute to the development of kyphosis and an increase in anteroposterior diameter.

table 26.2	Changes in the Four Phases of Intercourse in the Aging Female Client
Phase	**Alteration**
Excitement	Delay in production of vaginal secretion and lubrication
Plateau	Reduction in vaginal length and width expansion
	Decreased uterine elevation
	Labia majora flaccid and do not elevate and flatten against perineum
	Labia minora do not undergo sex color change from pink to burgundy or become congested
	Clitoral size decreases after 60 years of age
Orgasm	Shorter than in younger persons
Resolution	Occurs more rapidly

table 26.3	Changes Observed in the Four Phases of Intercourse in the Aging Male Client
Phase	**Alteration**
Excitement	Slower increment in excitement
	Sex flush less in duration and intensity
	Diminished involuntary spasms
	Increased time to obtain erection
	Lessened testicular elevation and scrotal sac vasocongestion in erection
Plateau	Longer duration
	Increase in penile diameter due to less preejaculatory fluid emission
Orgasm	Shorter duration
	Fewer contractions in expulsion of semen bolus
Resolution	Lasts 12 to 24 hours
	Loss of erection may take only a few seconds

figure **26.6**   Heberden's and Bouchard's nodes.

Muscle mass and strength decrease with age. You can easily see atrophy of muscle by observing the back of the hands where grooves are present between the bones.

Osteoarthritis is a common age-related condition involving joints throughout the body, particularly the spine, knees, hips, and fingers. Most clients over 60 will have osteoarthritic changes in the spine. Accumulated injuries to the cartilage over time cause slow but progressive deterioration of the joint. With loss of cartilage, bony overgrowths protrude from the bone into the joint capsule. These overgrowths can cause angular deformities, pain, and limited mobility. In the spine, these overgrowths are called osteophytes. Bony enlargement of the dorsolateral and dorsomedial aspects of the distal and proximal joints of the fingers are called Heberden's nodes and Bouchard's nodes, respectively (Figure 26.6; see also Figure 18.63).

Nervous system

The assessment of mental status and cranial nerves has been discussed previously. Motor strength may decrease slightly with age. Investigate further any asymmetry of strength. Vibratory sensation decreases with age, especially in the feet and ankles. The posture may become stooped. Changes in gait, including a decreased stride length, anteroflexion of the upper torso, flexion of the arms and knees, and a diminished arm swing, may contribute to postural unsteadiness. Deep tendon reflexes remain intact in healthy elderly people, although they may be more difficult to elicit. In many older clients, ankle jerks may be diminished or absent.

■ SUMMARY

History taking is especially important in preparing for the physical examination of the older adult. Asking the following questions will help you to know if you need to seek additional information about potential problems that occur more frequently in older clients:

1. Do you ever have a problem with urine leaking?
2. Have you fallen in the past 6 months?
3. Do you often feel sad, blue, down in the dumps, or depressed?
4. Do you often travel places away from home alone?
5. Do you have enough money to purchase your medications?
6. Do you sometimes skip your medications?
7. Do you skip meals often?

Observe the client entering the examination room and note whether he or she walks slowly, uses a cane or walker, or is in a wheelchair. Watch how the client sits down in the chair. During the interview, determine if the client appears to have problems with memory, ambulation, and/or dressing. If the client has limitations in any of these areas, determine what assistance you will need to provide the client in undressing for the examination, getting on and off the examining table, and redressing. The procedure for performing the physical examination on the older adult is similar to that outlined in previous chapters for each body system. As with all clients, make sure the examination room is quiet and the temperature is comfortable.

sample documentation & diagnoses — CRITICAL THINKING

■ FOCUSED HEALTH HISTORY *(SUBJECTIVE DATA)*

Mrs. P., an 83-year-old female who lives alone, complains of dizziness when getting out of bed in the morning and occasionally later during the day when going from a sitting to a standing position. Describes the sensation as the room spinning around. Yesterday morning she lost her balance getting out of bed and fell. Reports no injuries. Denies unsteadiness when she walks. One week ago her doctor prescribed a diuretic for high blood pressure. She has been taking the tablet once daily in the morning as prescribed.

■ FOCUSED PHYSICAL EXAMINATION *(OBJECTIVE DATA)*

Vital signs: BP—lying: 160/70 right arm, 156/72 left arm; immediate standing: 130/64 right arm, 132/62 left arm; 1-minute standing: 140/80 right arm; 146/78 left arm. Temperature 37.1° C (98.8° F) (oral).

General appearance: Well-groomed, frail-looking woman, appropriately dressed and able to provide history without hesitation.

Lungs: Breath sounds vesicular without crackles or wheezes.

Heart: Rate and rhythm regular without murmurs or extra sounds.

Extremities: Pulses 2 +/4 in all extremities. Muscle strength 3/5 bilaterally. Skin thin, intact, no edema or lesions present.

Gait slow and slightly wide based. Romberg negative. Rising from a chair after sitting 15 minutes caused light-headedness and slight swaying on rising.

diagnoses

HEALTH PROBLEM
Orthostatic hypotension

NURSING DIAGNOSIS
Risk for injury related to vertigo secondary to orthostatic hypotension

Defining Characteristics
- Internal regulatory function—integrative dysfunction
- External—pharmaceutical agent (diuretic)

Clients with Functional Limitations

■ PURPOSE OF FUNCTIONAL ASSESSMENT

The various components of the physical examination and health history provide an indication of the health of a client's body systems and data about the relationship of the client with the environment, defined broadly. For most clients, the data also implicitly provide information about self-care and overall functional abilities. For special populations, however, including the elderly and handicapped, the usual components of the health assessment may be insufficient in providing adequate information regarding the client's capabilities and activities (i.e., a functional assessment). This chapter presents and discusses several approaches to measuring functional assessment and guidelines to incorporate a functional assessment into the routine health assessment.

In practice with a given client group, a practitioner may choose to use standardized tools for all clients or to integrate functional assessment questions and techniques into the routine health assessment as individual situations may indicate. Either method has advantages as well as disadvantages (see box on p. 729). Because

standardized tools are devised to yield comparable numerical scores, they are useful in situations where information must be summarized for communication across systems and providers, or when client, program, or other outcome evaluation is desired for general planning or discharge planning purposes. However, standardized tools often are not fully applicable across all groups and may include items not relevant for specific clients or client groups.

The examiner can integrate appropriate functional assessment parameters into the client's health assessment. Such integration can be effective if the examiner takes a highly individualized approach to the health history and physical examination and if sufficient time is available to add items. However, difficulty in obtaining reliable data in vulnerable populations may foster neglect in obtaining functional assessment information that could influence choice and scope of intervention.

Pinholt et al. (1987) compared the sensitivity and specificity of routine assessments and comprehensive functional assessment instruments. They found that physicians and nurses could identify severe impairments

Advantages and Disadvantages—Two Main Functional Assessment Approaches

APPROACH	EVALUATION
Integration into General Assessment	**Advantages**
	Flexible
	Individualized
	Focus on variables of interest
	Disadvantages
	Can be incomplete
	Lack of standardized terminology
	Generally unsuitable for statistical analyses
Standardized Tools	**Advantages**
	Objective
	Explicit
	Standardized
	Disadvantages
	May include irrelevant items
	Issues of validity and reliability

with routine approaches, but more prevalent and less prominent impairments were poorly recognized. The authors recommended the use of functional assessment instruments to detect moderate impairments, especially those remediable through early intervention.

■ INTRODUCTION TO KEY TERMS AND DEFINITIONS

Several conceptual definitions are useful for understanding the discussion in this chapter and other literature in the area of functional assessment. The World Health Organization (WHO) (1980) developed the following definitions to standardize terminology and facilitate communication in this area.

An *impairment* is any loss or abnormality of psychological, physiological, or anatomical structure or function. An impairment is independent of its etiology and does not necessarily mean that a disease is still present. An example of an impairment is loss of a limb.

A *disability* is any restriction or lack of ability to perform an activity in the manner or within the range considered normal for a person of the same age and similar circumstances. A disability may be temporary or perma-

nent and can occur in any component of human functioning. A disability is the functional consequence of an impairment. Different impairments may result in similar disabilities, and the same impairments do not necessarily result in similar disabilities. Not all impairments result in disability. An example of a disability is inability to climb stairs.

A *handicap* is a disadvantage for a given individual, resulting from an impairment or a disability, that limits or prevents the fulfillment of a role that is normal for that individual. A handicap is characterized by a difference between what an individual appears to be able to do and the expectations of the particular group of which he is a member. The state of being handicapped is strongly influenced by existing societal values. An example of a handicap is joblessness.

Functional status refers to the normal or characteristic performance of the individual. Functional status can be conceptualized into four categories:

1. *Physical function:* Sensory-motor performance.
2. *Mental function:* Intellectual, cognitive, or reasoning capabilities of the individual.
3. *Emotional function:* Affect and effectiveness in coping psychologically with life stresses.
4. *Social function:* Performance of social roles or obligations.

The following additional definitions are derived from legislative practice (NH Rev Stat Ann 464-A:2[VII], [XI] [1983]; cited in Nolan, 1984, p. 213).

Incapacity means a legal, not a medical, disability and shall be measured by functional limitations. It shall be construed to mean or refer to any person who has suffered, is suffering, or is likely to suffer substantial harm due to an inability to provide for his or her personal needs for food, clothing, shelter, health care, safety, or an inability to manage his or her property or financial affairs.

Functional limitations means behavior or conditions in an individual that impair his or her ability to participate in and perform minimal activities of daily living that secure and maintain proper food, clothing, shelter, health care, or safety for himself or herself.

The following models by Granger, Seltzer, and Fishbein (1987), based on the work of Nagi (1975) and Wood (1975), provide insight into the relationships among disease, impairment, and handicap.

Nagi Model

Pathologic → Impairment → Functional → Disability
condition   limitations

Wood Model

Disease or
disorder   → Impairment   → Disability   →   Handicap
(Intrinsic) → (Exteriorized) → (Objectified) → (Socialized)

■ INTEGRATING FUNCTIONAL ASSESSMENT INTO THE ROUTINE EXAMINATION

Functional Assessment Variables

Functional assessment can include a broad range of areas for examination. In practice, the examiner chooses those assessment areas relevant to a particular client or client group. For example, basic and instrumental activities of daily living would be important for assessment of a residential geriatric population, whereas the examiner would choose other assessment parameters for a rehabilitation unit accepting transfers from intensive care units. The following is a list of general categories of functional assessment topics:

BASIC ACTIVITIES OF DAILY LIVING (ADLs)

Grooming and personal hygiene
Skin care
Bathing
Dressing and undressing
Managing brace or prosthesis
Going to the toilet
Eating

INSTRUMENTAL ACTIVITIES OF DAILY LIVING (LADLs)

Managing personal finances
Managing business affairs
Shopping
Cooking
Preparing balanced meals
Using problem-solving skills
Managing medications

MOBILITY

Capability of upper and lower extremities
Body movement
Bed activities—turning, sitting, shifting
Transferring—between bed and wheelchair, wheelchair and chair, or chair and toilet
Operating a wheelchair
Walking on level surface
Ascending and descending stairs
Traveling

MEDICAL CONDITION

Amount of medical supervision needed
Continence—bowels and bladder
Speech

COMMUNICATION

Reading
Auditory comprehension
Language expression (verbal)
Language expression (gestural)
Writing (motor)
Written language expression

SENSES

Hearing
Vision

MENTAL CAPABILITY

Orientation
Understanding
Communication
Reading
Writing
Attention span
Memory
Judgment and reasoning
Ability to play games and work on hobbies
Awareness of current events
Ability to comprehend movies and books
Memory of appointments and commemorations
Ability to manage travel instructions

RESOURCES

Significant others
Amount of assistance received from others
Social support
Social interaction

BEHAVIOR PROBLEMS

Presence of emotional or psychiatric disorders
Amount of supervision required
Cooperation
Depression

General Assessment with Emphasis on Functional Status

You can perform the functional assessment at any time during the routine health assessment. If you are using a standardized tool, this assessment is probably most logical at the end of the history and before the examination. Findings may provide guidance for particular follow-up during the physical examination.

The functional assessment requires no equipment in addition to that used in a comprehensive examination; most of the approaches require only an interview and observation. Be prepared, however, to verify responses to various questions as needed. For example, you may want to ask the client to demonstrate operation of a wheelchair or ability to climb stairs. The best location for functional assessment is often the client's own surroundings, where environmental adaptations enable a full range of independent activities (Figures 27.1 through 27.3). Table 27.1 outlines the major components of the history and physical examination and iden-

figure**27.1** Assessing a client in his own surroundings allows for a full evaluation of the client's capabilities. This man with quadriplegia is able to work and manage a number of activities of daily living quite independently in his home. **A** and **B,** Using a computer to work at home. **C,** Adapting a telephone to enable full use of this resource. **D** and **E,** Using a board to transfer frozen meals into and out of a microwave oven for independent food preparation.

table 27.1	*Functional Assessment Emphases in the History and Physical Examination*
Areas of assessment	**Special emphases**
HISTORY	
Present illness	Determine how present illness interferes with client's ability to carry out self-care, work, and execute roles appropriate for age and social situation.
Past health history	Gain knowledge of abilities before incapacitating illness or situation in order to understand expectations and set rehabilitation goals.
Family health history	Note genetically transmitted disabling conditions.
Review of systems	Determine capabilities of the systems unaffected by the disability. These strengths will support rehabilitation. Complete a review of affected and likely-to-be-affected systems.
Social history	Describe in detail relationships and living arrangements and the adequacy of those relationships and living arrangements. For a hospitalized client after an unanticipated traumatic event, the accessibility of the living arrangements and the willingness of family and significant others to assist are important.
Employment history	Note the nature of the client's work and the client's ability to continue to manage that work or return to that work.
PHYSICAL EXAMINATION	

Neurological evaluation	Mental status
	Orientation to time, place, and person
	Memory
	Attention span
	Ability to perform calculations
	Abstract thinking
	Behavior
	Ability to follow commands
	Judgment
	Insight
	Mood
	Motor system
	    Atrophy
	    Spontaneous muscle activity
	    Tone
	    Increase in spasticity or rigidity
	    Hypotonia or flaccidity
	Sensory status—complete assessment
	Reflexes—complete assessment
	Vision
	Hearing
	Swallowing
	Speech and language
	Gait and mobility
	    Use of assistive devices
	    Ability to transfer
	    Demonstration of methods of mobility and transfer

table 27.1	*Functional Assessment Emphases in the History and Physical Examination—cont'd*
Areas of assessment	**Special emphases**
Musculoskeletal, soft tissue, and joint evaluation	Inspection—symmetry, postural attitudes, scars, edema, atrophy, masses, skin changes Palpation—muscles, bones, joints for local and general spasm, masses, swelling, or tenderness Measurement of active and passive range of motion with a goniometer Shoulder range of motion Finger flexion
Cardiac status	Complete assessment
Respiratory status	Adequacy of ventilation Ability to clear tracheobronchial secretions Physical endurance or capacity Psychological reaction to breathing difficulties
Skin	Condition of pressure areas—ischial, sacral, and trochanteric prominences
Bladder function	If incontinence or retention, extensive urological evaluation If intermittent self-catheterization or Foley used, review of technique
Bowel function	Review pattern and interventions used to achieve regular pattern
Pain	Quality, location, temporal characteristics, provocative factors, alleviating factors

A **B** **C**

figure **27.2**   The elderly enjoy being able to sit in familiar surroundings and engage in activities they have enjoyed all of their lives. **A,** This elderly man with a walking disability enjoys sitting at the kitchen table and reading the daily newspapers in several languages. **B,** He demonstrates his method of walking with the use of two canes. **C,** He demonstrates his method of lowering and lifting himself up from his chair.

figure**27.3** This man with paraplegia works outside his home each day and engages in a number of other outside activities. **A,** He demonstrates use of a mobile chair designed for his needs. **B,** He demonstrates his mobility in getting around his apartment building with a walker.

tifies the areas in which an assessment, focused on functional status, would require special emphasis.

■ FUNCTIONAL ASSESSMENT TOOLS

Choosing and Administering Functional Assessment Tools

If you choose to use standardized tools to measure functional assessment in a given population, first determine the variables of primary interest and then match those variables with items on extant tools. When examining potential screening and assessment tools, examine both the content of the items and the scope of measurement. For example, you may want to determine whether a certain functional disability exists, the extent to which the functions are enabled by human or mechanical assistance, or both.

Desirable characteristics of a functional assessment tool include the following:

1. *Applicability:* Appropriate for the client population.
2. *Continuity:* Applicable to the client population across phases of treatment.
3. *Ease in administration:* Can be administered by various health care professionals.
4. *Efficiency:* Balance between comprehensiveness and time required for administration.
5. *Reliability:* Demonstration of good test-retest and inter-rater reliability.
6. *Validity:* Findings consistent with other assessment data.
7. *Sensitivity:* Ability to differentiate among clients in general and a given client during various stages of treatment.

Although numerous tools have been developed to measure functional status, this chapter presents only some of the extant tools based on their perceived applicability to a health assessment framework. Criteria for selection include length of the tool, broad applicability to the elderly or the handicapped, ability to complement

the usual components of a history and physical examination, ease of administration, and published data about the tool's conceptual bases, validity, reliability, usability, and quality.

The functional assessment tools in this chapter generally are designed to be administered by health care professionals. Sometimes the care provider may wish the client or client caregiver to administer the tools (e.g., after hospital discharge and between clinic visits). However, findings from various studies comparing client self-report with professional and caregiver assessments indicate that the type of rater may influence scores. McGinnis et al. (1986) compared the use of a modified Barthel Index by clients and health care professionals. Findings indicated that assessments were significantly different between groups, with providers rating clients higher in abilities than they rated themselves at a time immediately before discharge.

Rubenstein et al. (1984) compared the ratings of hospitalized elderly by various groups using three instruments: the Lawton Personal Self-Maintenance Scale (PSMS), the Instrumental Activities of Daily Living (IADL) Scale, and the Katz Activities of Daily Living (ADL) Scale. Comparisons of ratings by the clients themselves, the clients' nurses, and the clients' significant others revealed that the PSMS scores by clients were significantly higher than those of significant others, that the clients' IADL scores were significantly higher than scores by the nurses and significant others, and that client scores for the ADLs were significantly higher than the nurses' scores. The authors concluded that clients may overestimate their abilities and that significant others may underestimate clients' functional abilities as compared with professional nursing assessments.

Another issue regarding functional assessment is the relative reliability of various forms of client self-report. Spiegel, Hirshfield, and Spiegel (1985) observed that clients with arthritis were more willing to admit difficulties with self-care activities in a self-administered questionnaire than in a personal interview.

Specific Functional Assessment Tools

This discussion presents a number of standardized functional assessment tools that may be useful with populations commonly seen in ambulatory and long-term care settings. Numerous other tools exist; see Frattali (1993), McDowell and Newell (1996), or Rothstein (1985) for additional information about the tools presented in this chapter and for information about tools designed for special populations and for research applications.

Katz ADL Index (Revised Version 1976)

The original Katz ADL tool was among the earliest tools to standardize functional assessment. Both the original and revised versions focus on several basic activities of daily living and are very easy to administer and score (Katz et al., 1963; Katz and Akpom, 1976). The revised version of the Katz ADL Index (Table 27.2) measures self-care and mobility, specifically the following activities:

Bathing
Dressing
Using the toilet
Transfer
Continence
Feeding

The examiner rates each activity as 1 or 0, 1 indicating performance of the activity without human help and 0 indicating performance of the activity with human assistance or that the activity is not performed at all. The scores form an ordinal or Gunman scale as noted on the top portion of Table 27.2.

The original Katz tool has been adapted for scoring by a Likert-type scale, using a scale range of 0 to 3 (0, complete independence; 1, use of a device; 2, use of human assistance; 3, complete dependence). No category exists for clients who use both a device and human assistance. The examiner adds the scores to obtain an overall score. A community-based version of the Katz tool adds items of walking and grooming but excludes continence. Brorsson and Asberg (1984) have judged the reliability and validity of the tool as good.

The Katz tool is a general measure of self-care and a very limited measure of mobility. It is probably most applicable with populations in which a level of disability is assumed or already established (e.g., individuals with chronic illness). The tool is short and very easy to administer; therefore the examiner could easily include a version on a printed history form. Its scoring approaches allow for comparison of a given individual over time or compilation across client groups.

PULSES Profile

The PULSES Profile was developed by Moskowitz and McCann (1957) to assess the functional independence of chronically ill, elderly persons. The PULSES instrument (Table 27.3) measures impairment, and the title of the tool is an acronym for its assessment components:

P = Physical condition
U = Upper limb functioning
L = Lower limb functioning
S = Sensory components
E = Excretory function
S = Support factors

The examiner scores each dimension using an ordinal scale from 1 to 4, with 1 representing essential intactness and 4 representing total dependence. The six categories are equally weighted, and the examiner sums the

table 27.2   *Index of Independence in Activities of Daily Living: Scoring and Definitions*

The index of Independence in Activities of Daily Living is based on an evaluation of the functional
independence or dependence of clients in bathing, dressing, going to toilet, transferring, continence, and
feeding. Specific definitions of functional independence and dependence appear below the index.

A—Independent in feeding, continence, transferring, going to toilet, dressing, and bathing

B—Independent in all but one of these functions

C—Independent in all but bathing and one additional function

D—Independent in all but bathing, dressing, and one additional function

E—Independent in all but bathing, dressing, going to toilet, and one additional function

F—Independent in all but bathing, dressing, going to toilet, transferring, and one additional function

G—Dependent in all six functions

Other—Dependent in at least two functions, but not classifiable as C, D, E, or F

Independence means without supervision, direction, or active personal assistance, except as specifically noted
below. This is based on actual status and not on ability. A client who refuses to perform a function is
considered as not performing the function, even though he or she is deemed able.

BATHING (SPONGE, SHOWER, OR TUB)

Independent: Assistance only in bathing a single part (such as back or disabled extremity) or bathes self
completely

Dependent: Assistance in bathing more than one part of body; assistance in getting in or out of tub or does
not bathe self

DRESSING

Independent: Gets clothes from closets and drawers; puts on clothes, outer garments, braces; manages
fasteners; act of tying shoes is excluded

Dependent: Does not dress self or remains partly undressed

GOING TO TOILET

Independent: Gets to toilet; gets on and off toilet; arranges clothes; cleans organs of excretion (may manage
own bedpan used at night only and may or may not be using mechanical supports)

Dependent: Uses bedpan or commode or receives assistance in getting to and using toilet

TRANSFER

Independent: Moves in and out of bed independently and moves in and out of chair independently (may or
may not be using mechanical supports)

Dependent: Assistance in moving in or out of bed and/or chair; does not perform one or more transfers

CONTINENCE

Independent: Urination and defecation entirely self-controlled

Dependent: Partial or total incontinence in urination or defecation; partial or total control by enemas,
catheters, or regulated use of urinals and/or bedpans

FEEDING

Independent: Gets food from plate or its equivalent into mouth (precutting of meat and preparation of food,
such as buttering bread, are excluded from evaluation)

Dependent: Assistance in act of feeding (see above); does not eat at all or parenteral feeding

Modified from Katz S et al: The index of independence in activities of daily living, progress in development of the index of ADL, *Gerontologist*
10:23, 1970.

table 27.3 PULSES Profile

	P Physical condition	U Upper extremities	L Lower extremities	S Sensory function	E Excretory functions	S Social and mental status
	Cardiovascular, pulmonary, and other visceral disorders	Shoulder girdles, cervical and upper dorsal spine	Pelvis, lower dorsal and lumbosacral spine	Vision, hearing, and speech	Bowel and bladder	Emotional and psychiatric disorders
Normal	1 Health maintenance	1 Complete function	1 Complete function	1 Complete function	1 Continent	1 Compatible with age
Mild	2 Occasional medical supervision	2 No assistance required	2 Fully ambulatory despite some loss of function	2 No appreciable functional impairment	2 Occasional stress incontinence or nocturia	2 No supervision required
Moderately severe	3 Frequent medical supervision	3 Some assistance necessary	3 Limited ambulation	3 Appreciable bilateral loss or complete unilateral loss of vision or hearing Incomplete aphasia	3 Periodic incontinence or retention	3 Some supervision necessary
Severe	4 Total care Bed or chair confined	4 Nursing care	4 Confined to wheelchair or bed	4 Total blindness Total deafness Global aphasia or aphonia	4 Total incontinence or retention (including catheter and colostomy)	4 Complete care in psychiatric facility

Modified from Moskowitz E: PULSES profile in retrospect, *Arch Phys Med Rehabil* 66:648, 1985; and Moskowitz E, McCann CB: Classification of disability in the chronically ill and aged, *J Chron Dis* 5:343, 1957.

P. *Physical* condition, including diseases of the viscera (cardiovascular, pulmonary, gastrointestinal, urologic, and endocrine) and cerebral disorders that are not enumerated in the lettered categories below.
  1. No gross abnormalities, considering the age of the individual.
  2. Minor abnormalities not requiring frequent medical or nursing supervision.
  3. Moderately severe abnormalities requiring frequent medical or nursing supervision yet still permitting ambulation.
  4. Severe abnormalities requiring constant medical or nursing supervision confining individual to bed or wheelchair.
U. *Upper* extremities, including shoulder girdle, cervical and upper dorsal spine.
  1. No gross abnormalities, considering the age of the individual.
  2. Minor abnormalities with fairly good range of motion and function.
  3. Moderately severe abnormalities but permitting the performance of daily needs to a limited extent.
  4. Severe abnormalities requiring constant nursing care.
L. *Lower* extremities, including the pelvis, lower dorsal and lumbosacral spine.
  1. No gross abnormalities, considering the age of the individual.
  2. Minor abnormalities with a fairly good range of motion and function.
  3. Moderately severe abnormalities permitting limited ambulation.
  4. Severe abnormalities confining the individual to bed or wheelchair.
S. *Sensory* components relating to speech, vision, and hearing.
  1. No gross abnormalities, considering the age of the individual.
  2. Minor deviations insufficient to cause any appreciable functional impairment.
  3. Moderate deviations sufficient to cause appreciable functional impairment.
  4. Severe deviations causing complete loss of hearing, vision, or speech.
E. *Excretory* function (i.e., bowel and bladder control).
  1. Complete control.
  2. Occasional stress incontinence or nocturia.
  3. Periodic bowel and bladder incontinence or retention alternating with control.
  4. Total incontinence, either bowel or bladder.
S. *Mental and emotional status.*
  1. No deviations, considering the age of the individual.
  2. Minor deviations in mood, temperament, and personality not impairing environmental adjustment.
  3. Moderately severe variations requiring some supervision.
  4. Severe variations requiring complete supervision.

	With help	Independent
1. Feeding (if food needs to be cut up = help)	5	10
2. Moving from wheelchair to bed and return (includes sitting up in bed)	5-10	15
3. Personal toilet (wash face, comb hair, shave, clean teeth)	0	5
4. Getting on and off toilet (handling clothes, wipe, flush)	5	10
5. Bathe self	0	5
6. Walking on level surface (or if unable to walk, propel a wheelchair)	10	15
	0*	5*
7. Ascend and descend stairs	5	10
8. Dressing (includes tying shoes, fastening fasteners)	5	10
9. Controlling bowels	5	10
10. Controlling bladder	5	10

From Mahoney FI, Barthel DW: Functional evaluation: the Barthel index, *Maryland State Med J* 14:61, 1965.
*Score only if unable to walk.
Instructions for scoring the Barthel Index (NOTE: A score of zero is given when the patient cannot meet the defined criterion):

1. Feeding
 10 = Independent. The patient can feed himself a meal from a tray or table when someone puts the food within his reach. He must put on an assistive device if this is needed, cut up the food, use salt and pepper, spread butter, etc. He must accomplish this in a reasonable time.
 5 = Some help is necessary (when cutting up food, etc., as listed above).
2. Moving from wheelchair to bed and return
 15 = Independent in all phases of this activity. Patient can safely approach the bed in his wheelchair, lock brakes, lift footrests, move safely to bed, lie down, come to a sitting position on the side of the bed, change the position of the wheelchair, if necessary, to transfer back into it safely, and return to the wheelchair.
 10 = Either some minimal help is needed in some step of this activity or the patient needs to be reminded or supervised for safety of one or more parts of this activity.
 5 = Patient can come to a sitting position without the help of a second person but needs to be lifted out of bed, or if he transfers with a great deal of help.
3. Doing personal toilet
 5 = Patient can wash hands and face, comb hair, clean teeth, and shave. He may use any kind of razor but must put in blade or plug in razor without help, as well as get it from drawer or cabinet. Female patients must put on own make-up, if used, but need not braid or style hair.
4. Getting on and off toilet
 10 = Patient is able to get on and off toilet, fasten and unfasten clothes, prevent soiling of clothes, and use toilet paper without help. He may use a wall bar or other stable object of support if needed. If it is necessary to use a bed pan instead of a toilet, he must be able to place it on a chair, empty it, and clean it.
 5 = Patient needs help because of imbalance or in handling clothes or in using toilet paper.
5. Bathing self
 5 = Patient may use a bathtub, a shower, or take a complete sponge bath. He must be able to do all the steps involved in whichever method is employed without another person being present.
6. Walking on a level surface
 15 = Patient can walk at least 50 yards without help or supervision. He may wear braces or prostheses and use crutches, canes, or a walkerette but not a rolling walker. He must be able to lock and unlock braces if used, assume the standing position and sit down, get the necessary mechanical aides into position for use, and dispose of them when he sits. (Putting on and taking off braces is scored under dressing.)
 10 = Patient needs help or supervision in any of the above but can walk at least 50 yards with a little help.
6a: Propelling a wheelchair
 5 = If a patient cannot ambulate but can propel a wheelchair independently. He must be able to go around corners, turn around, maneuver the chair to a table, bed, toilet, etc. He must be able to push a chair at least 50 yards. Do not score this item if the patient gets score for walking.
7. Ascending and descending stairs
 10 = Patient is able to go up and down a flight of stairs safely without help or supervision. He may and should use handrails, canes, or crutches when needed. He must be able to carry canes or crutches as he ascends or descends stairs.
 5 = Patient needs help with supervision of any one of the above items.
8. Dressing and undressing (Women need not be scored on use of a brassiere or girdle unless these are prescribed garments.)
 10 = Patient is able to put on and remove and fasten all clothing, and tie shoelaces (unless it is necessary to use adaptations for this). The activity includes putting on and removing and fastening corset or braces when these are prescribed. Such special clothing as suspenders, loafer shoes or dresses that open down the front may be used when necessary.
 5 = Patient needs help in putting on and removing or fastening any clothing. He must do at least half the work himself. He must accomplish this in a reasonable time.
9. Continence of bowels
 10 = Patient is able to control his bowels and have no accidents. He can use a suppository or take an enema when necessary (as for spinal cord injury patients who have had bowel training).
 5 = Patient needs help in using a suppository or taking an enema or has occasional accidents.
10. Controlling bladder
 10 = Patient is able to control his bladder day and night. Spinal cord injury patients who wear an external device and leg bag must put them on independently, clean and empty bag, and stay dry day and night.
 5 = Patient has occasional accidents or cannot wait for the bedpan or get to the toilet in time or needs help with an external device.

scores to produce a total score ranging from 6 to 24. Scores over 12 imply serious impairment, and scores over 16 usually reflect severe disability.

Several authors have reviewed the reliability and validity evidence for the scale (Jette, 1985; McDowell and Newell, 1996), and they have assessed it as acceptable.

The main limitations of the tool are the general focus on a broad array of categories and redundancy with items commonly measured in a routine history and physical examination. The instrument was designed for use in a rehabilitation setting and is probably most applicable in situations where changes in levels of impairment are anticipated.

Barthel Index

The Barthel Index (BI) (Mahoney and Barthel, 1965; Granger, 1982) (Table 27.4) is a weighted index for assessing dependence in various areas of self-care, mobility, and continence. The original scale contains 10 items that the examiner scores with a weighted rating of 15, 10, 5, or 0, depending on the amount of help the client needs to perform the function. Total scores range from 0 (total dependence) to 100 (total independence) and are intended to indicate the amount of assistance a client requires. A score of 60 indicates the threshold between independence and dependence; a score of 40 or below indicates severe dependence; and a score of 20 or below reflects total dependence in self-care and mobility. Granger, Albrecht, and Hamilton (1979) reported the test-retest reliability and inter-rater agreements as 89% and 95%, respectively.

Fortinsky, Granger, and Seltzer (1981) modified the original BI (Table 27.5). The modified BI contains 15 items and the following changes: two items of dressing (i.e., upper and lower body) rather than one general item; additional items for use of brace or prosthesis, transfer to toilet, transfer to tub or shower; and differentiation of items for walking and propelling a wheelchair.

Advantages of the BI include its widespread use, the clarity of scoring, and completeness of the set of items.

Instrumental ADL Scale

The Instrumental ADL Scale (Lawton, 1972) (Table 27.6) measures behaviors that are more cognitively and less directly physically oriented than the other self-care scales. The tool includes eight items measuring ability to use a telephone, shop, prepare food, keep house, do laundry, use public transportation, take responsibility for one's medications, and handle finances. The examiner scores each item on a 3-, 4-, or 5-point scale reflecting the amount of assistance used or limitation in performing the activity.

The Instrumental ADL Scale expands the concept of self-care beyond specific and basic physical ability by measuring performance in the usual household mainte-

table **27.5** *Modified Barthel Index Scoring*				
Independent		**Dependent**		
I Intact	**II** Limited	**III** Helper	**IV** Null	
10	5	0	0	Drink from cup/ feed from dish
5	5	3	0	Dress upper body
5	5	2	0	Dress lower body
0	0	−2	0	Don brace or prosthesis
5	5	0	0	Grooming
4	4	0	0	Wash or bathe
10	10	5	0	Bladder continence
10	10	5	0	Bowel continence
4	4	2	0	Care of perineum/ clothing at toilet
15	15	7	0	Transfer, chair
6	5	3	0	Transfer, toilet
1	1	0	0	Transfer, tub or shower
15	15	10	0	Walk on level 50 yards or more
10	10	5	0	Up and down stairs for one flight or more
15	5	0	0	Wheelchair/50 yards—only if not walking

Modified from the presentation of the Modified Barthel Index in Fortinsky RH, Granger CV, Seltzer GB: The use of functional assessment in understanding home care needs, *Med Care* 19:489, 1981.

nance activities. The examiner could use this scale with community-based populations and individuals whose mobility is compromised or who are at risk of progressive debilitation (e.g., the frail elderly).

Physical Self-Maintenance Scale

The Physical Self-Maintenance Scale (PSMS) (also known as the Lawton and Brody Scale, 1969) (Table 27.7) includes six items of self-care and mobility that the examiner rates using a unique Guttman-type scale for each item. The six items are toileting (including continence), feeding, dressing, grooming, physical ambulation, and bathing. The examiner may use either of two scoring methods: a count of the number of items for which disability is noted, or a severity scale summing the response codes for each item, resulting in a summary score ranging from 6 to 30.

table 27.6 *Instrumental Activities of Daily Living Scale*

A. Ability to use telephone
 1. Operates telephone on own initiative—looks up and dials numbers, etc.
 2. Dials well-known numbers.
 3. Answers telephone but does not dial.
 4. Does not use telephone at all.
B. Shopping
 1. Takes care of all shopping needs independently.
 2. Shops independently for small purchases.
 3. Must be accompanied on any shopping trip.
 4. Completely unable to shop.
C. Food preparation
 1. Plans, prepares, and serves adequate meals independently.
 2. Prepares adequate meals if supplied with ingredients.
 3. Heats and serves prepared meals, or prepares meals but does not maintain adequate diet.
 4. Needs to have meals prepared and served.
D. Housekeeping
 1. Maintains house alone or with occasional assistance.
 2. Performs light daily tasks such as dishwashing, bedmaking.
 3. Performs light daily tasks but cannot maintain acceptable level of cleanliness.
 4. Needs help with all home maintenance tasks.
 5. Does not participate in any housekeeping tasks.

E. Laundry
 1. Does personal laundry completely.
 2. Launders small items—rinses socks, stockings, etc.
 3. All laundry must be done by others.
F. Mode of transportation
 1. Travels independently on public transportation or drives own car.
 2. Arranges own travel by taxi but does not otherwise use public transportation.
 3. Travels on public transportation when assisted or accompanied by another.
 4. Travel limited to taxi or automobile with assistance of another.
 5. Does not travel at all.
G. Responsibility for own medications
 1. Is responsible for taking medications in correct dosages at correct time.
 2. Takes responsibility if medications are prepared in advance in separate dosages.
 3. Is not capable of dispensing own medications.
H. Ability to handle finances
 1. Manages financial matters independently (budgets, writes checks, pays rent, bills, goes to bank), collects and keeps track of income.
 2. Manages day-to-day purchases but needs help with banking, major purchases, etc.
 3. Incapable of handling money.

Modified from Brody E, Lawton MP: Philadelphia Geriatric Center, 5301 Old York Road, Philadelphia, PA 19141.

This tool demonstrates good reliability and validity (McDowell and Newell, 1996). The scale is probably most applicable to homebound or institutionalized populations. Administration is easy and rapid.

Functional Activities Questionnaire

The Functional Activities Questionnaire (FAQ) (Pfeffer et al., 1984) (Table 27.8) is a screening tool for assessing independence in daily activities. It is designed to measure universal skills among older adults and is completed by the client's significant other. The FAQ consists of 10 items relating to tasks necessary for independent living. For each activity, the respondent rates the client based on four levels, ranging from dependence (score = 3) to independence (score = 0). For activities the client does not usually perform, the respondent specifies whether the person would be unable to undertake the task if requested (score = 1). The total score is the sum of individual items, with higher scores reflecting greater dependency.

The authors of the FAQ are in the process of revising and testing a new version of this tool that includes the addition of four items on activities of daily living and one item on initiative.

McDowell and Newell (1996) have reviewed the evidence regarding validity and reliability of the original tool and concluded that the initial findings were very promising.

Rapid Disability Rating Scale

The Rapid Disability Rating Scale–2 (Linn and Linn, 1982) (Table 27.9) is an 18-item global disability scale measuring assistance needed with activities of daily living, disability, and special problems according to the assistance required, degree of disability, or degree of special problems. Each item is briefly defined and has options of four scale points. The total scores range from 18 to 72, with higher values indicating greater disability.

The scale demonstrates high reliability in use (McDowell and Newell, 1996; Rothstein, 1985), and the initial results of validity examination are positive.

This tool contains several items that the examiner

table 27.7 *Physical Self-Maintenance Scale*

A. Toilet
1. Cares for self at toilet completely, no incontinence.
2. Needs to be reminded, or needs help in cleaning self, or has rare (weekly at most) accidents.
3. Soiling or wetting while asleep more than once a week.
4. Soiling or wetting while awake more than once a week.
5. No control of bowels or bladder.

B. Feeding
1. Eats without assistance.
2. Eats with minor assistance at mealtimes and/or with special preparation of food, or help in cleaning up after meals.
3. Feeds self with moderate assistance and is untidy.
4. Requires extensive assistance for all meals.
5. Does not feed self at all and resists efforts of others to feed him.

C. Dressing
1. Dresses, undresses, and selects clothes from own wardrobe.
2. Dresses and undresses self, with minor assistance.
3. Needs moderate assistance in dressing or selection of clothes.
4. Needs major assistance in dressing but cooperates with efforts of others to help.
5. Completely unable to dress self and resists efforts of others to help.

D. Grooming (neatness, hair, nails, hands, face, clothing)
1. Always neatly dressed, well-groomed, without assistance.
2. Grooms self adequately with occasional minor assistance, (e.g., shaving).
3. Needs moderate and regular assistance or supervision in grooming.
4. Needs total grooming care, but can remain well-groomed after help from others.
5. Actively negates all efforts of others to maintain grooming.

E. Physical ambulation
1. Goes about grounds or city.
2. Ambulates within residence or about one block distant.
3. Ambulates with assistance of (check one)
   a ( ) another person, b ( ) railing,
   c ( ) cane, d ( ) walker, e ( ) wheelchair.
   1 _____ Gets in and out without help.
   2 _____ Needs help in getting in and out.
4. Sits unsupported in chair or wheelchair, but cannot propel self without help.
5. Bedridden more than half the time.

F. Bathing
1. Bathes self (tub, shower, sponge bath) without help.
2. Bathes self with help in getting in and out of tub.
3. Washes face and hands only, but cannot bathe rest of body.
4. Does not wash self but is cooperative with those who bathe him.
5. Does not try to wash self and resists efforts to keep him clean.

Modified from the Physical Self-Maintenance scale in Lawton MP, Brody EM: Assessment of older people: self-maintaining and instrumental activities of daily living, *Gerontologist* 9:180, 1969.

would include in the routine health assessment (e.g., hearing, sight, diet, medication), and it may be most appropriate for screening situations.

Functional Status Rating System

The Functional Status Rating System (Forer, 1981) (Table 27.10) measures the amount of assistance needed in self-care and mobility and the amount of impairment in communication, psychosocial adjustment, and cognitive function. It is unusually comprehensive for a functional assessment tool, covering 30 items under five topics. Although the tool may in small part duplicate portions of the health assessment, most of the items measure new assessment factors.

The amount of currently available psychometric information about the tool is limited.

Functional Independence Measure (tool) and Functional Assessment Measures Tool

A recent innovation in the field of rehabilitation medicine is the proposal of a uniform, national data system for functional assessment. This standardized database would establish a uniform language and set of definitions for communicating disability and rehabilitation

Text continued on p. 747

table 27.8 *Functional Activities Questionnaire*

Activities questionnaire to be completed by spouse, child, close friend, or relative of the participant.

Instructions: The following pages list 10 common activities. *For each activity,* please read all choices, then choose the *one* statement that best describes the *current* ability of the participant. Answers should apply to *that person's* abilities, not your own. Please check off a choice for *each* activity; do not skip any.

1. Writing checks, paying bills, balancing checkbook, keeping financial records
   _____ A. Someone has recently taken over this activity completely or almost completely.
   _____ B. Requires frequent advice or assistance from others (e.g., relatives, friends, business associates, banker), which was *not previously necessary.*
   _____ C. Does without any advice or assistance, but finds it more difficult than used to or does less good job.
   _____ D. Does without any difficulty or advice.
   _____ E. Never did and would find it quite difficult to start now.
   _____ F. Didn't do regularly but can do normally now with a little practice if he or she has to.

2. Making out insurance or Social Security forms, handling business affairs or papers, assembling tax records
   _____ A. Someone has recently taken over this activity completely or almost completely, and that someone did not used to do any or as much.
   _____ B. Requires more frequent advice or more assistance from others than in the past.
   _____ C. Does without any more advice or assistance than used to, but finds it more difficult or does less good job than in the past.
   _____ D. Does without any difficulty or advice.
   _____ E. Never did and would find it quite difficult to start now, even with practice.
   _____ F. Didn't do routinely, but can do normally now should he or she have to.

3. Shopping alone for clothes, household necessities, and groceries.
   _____ A. Someone has recently taken over this activity completely or almost completely.
   _____ B. Requires frequent advice or assistance from others.
   _____ C. Does without advice or assistance, but finds it more difficult than used to or does less good job.
   _____ D. Does without any difficulty or advice.
   _____ E. Never did and would find it quite difficult to start now.
   _____ F. Didn't do routinely but can do normally now should he or she have to.

4. Playing a game of skill, such as bridge, other card games, or chess, or working on a hobby, such as painting, photography, woodwork, or stamp collecting
   _____ A. Hardly ever does now or has great difficulty.
   _____ B. Requires advice, or others have to make allowances.
   _____ C. Does without advice, or assistance, but finds it more difficult or is less skillful than used to be.
   _____ D. Does without any difficulty or advice.
   _____ E. Never did and would find it quite difficult to start now.
   _____ F. Didn't do regularly, but can do normally now should he or she have to.

5. Heat the water, make a cup of coffee or tea, and turn off the stove
   _____ A. Someone else has recently taken over this activity completely or almost completely.
   _____ B. Requires advice or has frequent problems (e.g., burns pots, forgets to turn off stove).
   _____ C. Does without advice or assistance but occasional problems.
   _____ D. Does without any difficulty or advice.
   _____ E. Never did and would find it quite difficult to start now.
   _____ F. Didn't usually, but can do normally now, should he or she have to.

Modified from R.I. Pfeffer, MD.

table 27.8 *Functional Activities Questionnaire—cont'd*

6. Prepare a balanced meal (e.g., meat, chicken, or fish; vegetables; dessert)
   _____ A. Someone else has recently taken over this activity completely or almost completely.
   _____ B. Requires frequent advice or has frequent problems (e.g., burns pots, forgets how to make a given dish).
   _____ C. Does without much advice or assistance, but finds it more difficult (e.g., switched to TV dinners most of the time because of difficulty).
   _____ D. Does without any difficulty or advice.
   _____ E. Never did and would find it quite difficult to do now even after a little practice.
   _____ F. Didn't do regularly, but can do normally now should he or she have to.

7. Keep track of current events, either in the neighborhood or nationally
   _____ A. Pays no attention to, or doesn't remember outside happenings.
   _____ B. Some idea about *major* events (e.g., comments on presidential election, major events in the news, or major sporting events).
   _____ C. Somewhat less attention to, or knowledge of, current events than formerly.
   _____ D. As aware of current events as ever was.
   _____ E. Never paid much attention to current events, and would find it quite difficult to start now.
   _____ F. Never paid much attention, but can do as well as anyone now when he or she tries.

8. Pay attention to, understand, and discuss the plot or theme of a 1-hour television program; get something out of a book or magazine
   _____ A. Doesn't remember, or seems confused by, what he or she has watched or read.
   _____ B. Aware of the *general idea,* characters, or nature while he or she watches or reads, but may *not recall* later; may *not grasp theme* or have opinion about what he or she saw.
   _____ C. Less attention, or less memory than before; less likely to catch humor, points that are made quickly, or subtle points.
   _____ D. Grasps as quickly as ever.
   _____ E. Never paid much attention to or commented on T.V., never read much and would probably find it very difficult to start now.
   _____ F. Never read or watched T.V. much, but reads or watches as much as ever and gets as much out of it as ever.

9. Remember appointments, plans, household tasks, car repairs, family occasions (such as birthdays or anniversaries), holidays, medications
   _____ A. Someone else has recently taken this over.
   _____ B. Has to be reminded some of the time (more than in the past or more than most people).
   _____ C. Manages without reminders but has to rely heavily on notes, calendars, schemes.
   _____ D. Remembers appointments, plans, occasions, etc., as well as he or she ever did.
   _____ E. Never had to keep track of appointments, medications, or family occasions, and would probably find it very difficult to start now.
   _____ F. Didn't have to keep track of these things in the past, but can do as well as anyone when he or she tries.

10. Travel out of neighborhood: driving, walking, arranging to take or change buses and trains, planes
   _____ A. Someone else has taken this over completely or almost completely.
   _____ B. Can get around in own neighborhood but gets lost out of neighborhood.
   _____ C. Has more problems getting around than used to (e.g., occasionally lost, loss of confidence, can't find car, etc.) but usually OK.
   _____ D. Gets around as well as ever.
   _____ E. Rarely did much driving or had to get around alone and would find quite difficult to learn bus routes or make similar arrangements now.
   _____ F. Didn't have to get around alone much in past, but can do as well as ever when he or she has to.

table 27.9 *Rapid Disability Rating Scale–2*

Directions: Rate what the person *does* to reflect current behavior. Circle one of the four choices for each item. Consider rating with any aids or prostheses normally used.

ASSISTANCE WITH ACTIVITIES OF DAILY LIVING

Eating	None	A little	A lot	Spoon-feed: intra-venous tube
Walking (with cane or walker if used)	None	A little	A lot	Does not walk
Mobility (going outside and getting about with wheelchair, etc., if used)	None	A little	A lot	Is housebound
Bathing (include getting supplies, supervising)	None	A little	A lot	Must be bathed
Dressing (include help in selecting clothes)	None	A little	A lot	Must be dressed
Toileting (include help with clothes, cleaning, or help with ostomy, catheter)	None	A little	A lot	Uses bedpan or unable to care for ostomy/catheter
Grooming (shaving for men, hairdressing for women, nails, teeth)	None	A little	A lot	Must be groomed
Adaptive tasks (managing money/possessions; telephoning; buying newspaper, toilet articles, snacks)	None	A little	A lot	Cannot manage

DEGREE OF DISABILITY

Communication (expressing self)	None	A little	A lot	Does not communicate
Hearing (with aid if used)	None	A little	A lot	Does not seem to hear
Sight (with glasses, if used)	None	A little	A lot	Does not see
Diet (deviation from normal)	None	A little	A lot	Fed by intravenous tube
In bed during day (ordered or self-initiated)	None	A little (<3 hr)	A lot	Most/all of time
Incontinence (urine/feces, with catheter or prosthesis, if used)	None	Sometimes	Frequently (weekly +)	Does not control
Medication	None	Sometimes	Daily, taken orally	Daily: injection (+ oral if used)

DEGREE OF SPECIAL PROBLEMS

Mental confusion	None	A little	A lot	Extreme
Uncooperativeness (combats efforts to help with care)	None	A little	A lot	Extreme
Depression	None	A little	A lot	Extreme

Modified from the presentation of the Rapid Disability Rating Scale–2 as published in Linn MW, Linn BS: The rapid disability rating scale–2, *J Am Geriatr Soc* 30:380, 1982.

table 27.10 **Functional Status Rating System**

FUNCTIONAL STATUS IN SELF-CARE

A. *Eating/feeding:* Management of all aspects of setting up and eating food (including cutting of meat) with or without adaptive equipment.

B. *Personal hygiene:* Includes setup, oral care, washing face and hands with a washcloth, hair grooming, shaving, and makeup.

C. *Toileting:* Includes management of clothing and cleanliness.

D. *Bathing:* Includes entire body bathing (tub, shower, or bed bath).

E. *Bowel management:* Able to insert suppository and/or perform manual evacuation, aware of need to defecate, has sphincter muscle control.

F. *Bladder management:* Able to manage equipment necessary for bladder evacuation (may include intermittent catheterization).

G. *Skin management:* Performance of skin care program, regular inspection, prevention of pressure sores, rashes, or irritations.

H. *Bed activities:* Includes turning, coming to a sitting position, scooting, and maintenance of balance.

I. *Dressing:* Includes performance of total body dressing except tying shoes, with or without adaptive equipment (also includes application of orthosis and prosthesis).

FUNCTIONAL STATUS IN MOBILITY

A. *Transfers:* Includes the management of all aspects of transfers to and from bed, mat, toilet, tub/shower, wheelchair, with or without adaptive equipment.

B. *Wheelchair skills:* Includes management of brakes, leg rests, maneuvering and propelling through and over doorway thresholds.

C. *Ambulation:* Includes coming to a standing position and walking short to moderate distances on level surfaces with or without equipment.

D. *Stairs and environmental surfaces:* Includes climbing stairs, curbs, ramps or environmental terrain.

E. *Community mobility:* Ability to manage transportation.

FUNCTIONAL STATUS IN COMMUNICATION

A. *Understanding spoken language*

B. *Reading comprehension*

C. *Language expression (non-speech/alternative methods):* Includes pointing, gestures, manual communication boards, electronic systems.

D. *Language expression (verbal):* Includes grammar, syntax, and appropriateness of language.

E. *Speech intelligibility*

F. *Written communication (motor)*

G. *Written language expression:* Includes spelling, vocabulary, punctuation, syntax, grammar, and completeness of written response.

FUNCTIONAL STATUS IN PSYCHOSOCIAL ADJUSTMENT

A. *Emotional adjustment:* Includes frequency and severity of depression, anxiety, frustration, lability, unresponsiveness, agitation, interference with progress in therapies, motivation, ability to cope with and take responsibility for emotional behavior.

B. *Family/significant others/environment:* Includes frequency of chronic problems or conflicts in client's relationships, interference with progress in therapies, ability and willingness to provide for client's specific needs after discharge, and to promote client's recovery and independence.

C. *Adjustment to limitations:* Includes denial/awareness, acceptance of limitations, willingness to learn new ways of functioning, compensating, taking appropriate safety precautions, and realistic expectations for long-term recovery.

D. *Social adjustment:* Includes frequency and limitation of social contacts, responsiveness in one-to-one and group situations, appropriateness of behavior in relationships, and spontaneity of interactions.

FUNCTIONAL STATUS IN COGNITIVE FUNCTION

A. *Attention span:* Includes distractability, level of alertness and responsiveness, ability to concentrate on a task, ability to follow directions, immediate recall as the structure, difficulty, and length of the task vary.

B. *Orientation*

C. *Judgment reasoning*

D. *Memory:* Includes short- and long-term.

E. *Problem-solving*

SUMMARY OF RATING SCALES

Self-Care and Mobility Items

1.0 = Unable—totally dependent
1.5 = Maximum assistance of 1 or 2 people
2.0 = Moderate assistance
2.5 = Minimal assistance
3.0 = Standby assistance
3.5 = Supervised
4.0 = Independent

Communication, Psychosocial, and Cognitive Function Items

1.0 = Extremely severe
1.5 = Severe
2.0 = Moderately severe
2.5 = Moderate impairment
3.0 = Mild impairment
3.5 = Minimal impairment
4.0 = No impairment

Modified from S.K. Forer.

table 27.11 *Functional Assessment Measures Summary Worksheet*

Rating Scale: 7 Complete independence (timely, safely)
6 Modified independence (extra time, device)
5 Supervision
4 Minimal assist (subject 75% of task)
3 Moderate assist (50%-74% of task)
2 Maximal assist (25%-49% of task)
1 Total assist (subject 25% of task)

SELF-CARE ITEMS

1. Feeding   Adm _____ Goal _____ D/C _____ F/U _____
2. Grooming   Adm _____ Goal _____ D/C _____ F/U _____
3. Bathing technique _____   Adm _____ Goal _____ D/C _____ F/U _____
4. Dressing upper body   Adm _____ Goal _____ D/C _____ F/U _____
5. Dressing lower body   Adm _____ Goal _____ D/C _____ F/U _____
6. Toileting   Adm _____ Goal _____ D/C _____ F/U _____
7. Swallowing*   Adm _____ Goal _____ D/C _____ F/U _____

SPHINCTER CONTROL

8. Bladder management   Adm _____ Goal _____ D/C _____ F/U _____
9. Bowel management   Adm _____ Goal _____ D/C _____ F/U _____

MOBILITY ITEMS

Transfers Technique _____

10. Bed, chair, wheelchair   Adm _____ Goal _____ D/C _____ F/U _____
11. Toilet   Adm _____ Goal _____ D/C _____ F/U _____
12. Tub or shower   Adm _____ Goal _____ D/C _____ F/U _____
13. Car transfers*   Adm _____ Goal _____ D/C _____ F/U _____

Locomotion

14. Walking/wheelchair   Adm _____ Goal _____ D/C _____ F/U _____
15. Stairs   Adm _____ Goal _____ D/C _____ F/U _____
16. Community mobility*   Adm _____ Goal _____ D/C _____ F/U _____

COMMUNICATION ITEMS

17. Comprehension   Adm _____ Goal _____ D/C _____ F/U _____
18. Expression   Adm _____ Goal _____ D/C _____ F/U _____
19. Reading*   Adm _____ Goal _____ D/C _____ F/U _____
20. Writing*   Adm _____ Goal _____ D/C _____ F/U _____
21. Speech intelligibility*   Adm _____ Goal _____ D/C _____ F/U _____

PSYCHOSOCIAL ADJUSTMENT ITEMS

22. Social interaction   Adm _____ Goal _____ D/C _____ F/U _____
23. Emotional adjustment*   Adm _____ Goal _____ D/C _____ F/U _____
24. Adjustment to limitations*   Adm _____ Goal _____ D/C _____ F/U _____
25. Vocational reentry*   D/C _____ F/U _____

COGNITIVE FUNCTION

26. Problem solving   Adm _____ Goal _____ D/C _____ F/U _____
27. Memory   Adm _____ Goal _____ D/C _____ F/U _____
28. Orientation*   Adm _____ Goal _____ D/C _____ F/U _____
29. Attention*   Adm _____ Goal _____ D/C _____ F/U _____

The Functional Assessment Measures tool was developed by the staff of the Santa Clara Medical Center, Santa Clara, Calif.
D/C, At discharge; *F/U*, at follow-up.
*Items added to the original FIM assessment tool. The FIM was developed by the Task Force for the Development of a Uniform Data System for Medical Rehabilitation, Department of Rehabilitative Medicine, Buffalo General Hospital, Buffalo, N.Y.

information. Toward this end, the major researchers in the field have developed the minimum data set for the field, the Functional Independence Measure (FIM) tool. The FIM tool measures 18 items in the categories of self-care, mobility, locomotion, communication, and social cognition. The seven-point rating scale is designed to assess the patient's level or degree of independence, the amount of assistance required, use of adaptive or assistive devices, and the percentage of a given task completed successfully. The FIM requires 15 to 20 minutes for administration and can be performed by a variety of health care professionals.

The staff of the Santa Clara Medical Center has expanded the FIM to a 29-item scale, titled the Functional Assessment Measures (FAM). The expanded tool uses the same rating scheme and requires 20 to 25 minutes for administration. The summary rating scale for the FAM is in Table 27.11. Comprehensive tools like the FIM and FAM are likely to be used in long-term care rehabilitation programs.

■ SUMMARY

Use of an organized functional assessment is recommended for all clients whose daily activities may be affected by impairments or disabilities; the elderly and the handicapped are the more obvious examples of such groups. The literature has shown that health care providers often do superficial assessments of this assessment area and may not appreciate the client's capabilities or limitations. This lack of appreciation may cause inappropriate or insufficient treatment, lack of support, and neglect of problems that may be treatable.

The approaches and tools presented in this chapter have applicability across the range of settings and circumstances in which practitioners perform health assessments. Because the functional assessment is not a routine component of the health assessment, an approach standardized across practitioners does not exist for general populations. The practitioner is advised to explore the assessment options and to select and use, as indicated, the most applicable and useful approaches and tools.

sample documentation & diagnoses — CRITICAL THINKING

■ FOCUSED HEALTH HISTORY (SUBJECTIVE DATA)

Mr. K., a 59-year-old plumber who owns his own business, has just been transferred from the neurological intensive care unit onto the medical floor to stabilize his condition before transfer to the rehabilitation center. Six days after he suffered a cerebrovascular accident, he has a diagnosis of left hemiplegia and aphasia. Because of Mr. K.'s speech dysfunction, his history was provided by his wife. Mr. K. was admitted 6 days ago, unconscious after he did not awaken to the alarm clock. He was noted to respond only to deep pain; his left arm and leg were limp. Two days later, he regained consciousness, was unable to move his left arm or leg, and was unable to speak clearly, swallow, or perform any activities of daily living (ADLs). Wife states client is unable to move his left arm or leg, speak clearly, swallow, or do his own ADLs.

■ FOCUSED PHYSICAL EXAMINATION (OBJECTIVE DATA)

Mental status: Client is lying in bed; body slumps slightly to left; appears alert but has difficulty maintaining eye contact. Speech slow, requires much effort, and is garbled. Hard to determine if appropriate. Seems to understand words spoken to him. Follows requests slowly but appropriately within limits of motor weakness.

Cranial nerves:
  I: Not tested.
  II: Acuity normal, fields by confrontation—left homonymous hemianopia, fundi normal.
  III, IV, VI: Extraocular movements (EOMs) intact; slight left-sided ptosis; no nystagmus; pupils equal, round, react to light and accommodation (PERRLA).
  V: Sensation intact to pinprick and light touch. Jaw strength weak on left.
  VII: Flat nasolabial fold on left; motor weakness on left lower face. Unable to wrinkle forehead bilaterally; unable to smile on left side.
  VIII: Hearing intact.
  IX, X: No swallowing or gag reflex present; uvula rises slightly to right on phonation.
  XI: Shoulder shrug; head movement weaker on left.
  XII: Tongue protrudes slightly to right; no tremors.

Cerebellar: Unable to move left hand or leg, unable to support weight. Spasticity in left arm and leg. Unable to stand and walk unassisted. Unable to perform finger-to-nose or heel-to-shin maneuver on left side. Right side intact but slow.

Sensory: Pinprick and light touch present but decreased on left arm and leg. Vibration intact. Position sense decreased on left, intact on right. Stereognosis intact.

Deep tendon reflexes (DTRs): Right side intact 1+; left side 0; Babinski present left side. Plantar reflex absent left side, intact on right side.

continued

diagnoses

NURSING DIAGNOSES

Impaired swallowing related to neuromuscular impairment (absent gag reflex)
Defining Characteristics
- Observed evidence of difficulty swallowing
- Observed coughing/choking when swallowing
- Assessed no gag or swallowing ability

Altered nutrition: less than body requirements related to muscle weakness (mastication and swallowing)
Defining Characteristics
- Inability to swallow
- No gag reflex
- Observed inadequate food intake

Risk for impaired skin integrity related to prolonged immobility
Defining Characteristics
- Physical immobility—cannot move left side
- Incontinence of both bladder and bowel—excretion on skin

Bowel incontinence related to cognitive/perceptual impairment
Defining Characteristics
- Involuntary passage of stool
- Inability to communicate need (aphasia)

Total incontinence related to cognitive/perceptual impairment
Defining Characteristics
- Lack of perineal or bladder filling awareness
- Unawareness of incontinence
- Inability to communicate need (aphasia)

Impaired physical mobility related to neuromuscular impairment
Defining Characteristics
- Inability to purposefully move within the physical environment
- Decreased muscle strength
- Impaired coordination
- Level IV—is dependent and at this time does not participate in movement

diagnoses—cont'd

Total self-care deficit related to neuromuscular impairment
Defining Characteristics
- Inability to wash body or body parts
- Inability to obtain or get to water source
- Inability to regulate temperature or flow of water
- Impaired ability to put on or take off necessary items of clothing
- Impaired ability to obtain or replace articles of clothes, fasten clothing, and maintain appearance at a satisfactory level
- Level IV—is dependent and does not participate in self-care at this time

Sensory-perceptual alterations (kinesthetic) related to neuromuscular impairment
Defining Characteristics
- Measured change in sensory acuity
- Altered communication patterns
- Inability to sit or stand
- Motor incoordination

Unilateral neglect related to neuromuscular impairment, inability to move left side
Defining Characteristics
- Consistent inattention to stimuli on affected side
- Lack of positioning and/or safety precautions regarding left side
- Does not look toward affected side

Body image disturbance related to nonintegration to change in body function and limitations
Defining Characteristics
- Verbalized fear of rejection or reaction by others
- Verbalized feelings of powerlessness in relation to body
- Depersonalization of part or loss by impersonal pronoun
- Refusal to verify actual change in body
- Change in ability to estimate spatial relationship of body to environment

Impaired verbal communication related to neuromuscular impairment
Defining Characteristics
- Speaks or verbalizes with difficulty
- Difficulty forming words
- Difficulty expressing thoughts verbally

Impaired social interaction related to communication barrier and limited physical mobility
Defining Characteristics
- Observed discomfort in social situations
- Observed inability to communicate a satisfactory sense of belonging

abatement Decrease in intensity of a pain or other symptom.

abduction Movement away from the axial line (for a limb) or the median plane (for the digits).

acceptance Recognition of what is said without necessarily agreeing.

accommodation Process by which the refractive power of the lens of the eye is increased through contraction of the ciliary muscle, which causes increased thickness and curvature of the lens. The accommodation response of the pupils consists of convergence of the eyes and constriction of the pupils as the gaze shifts from a distant to a near point.

acculturation Process of adapting to a culture different from the one in which a person was encultured.

acini Small, saclike dilations found in various glands.

acoustic stethoscope Instrument used in mediate auscultation, consisting of two earpieces connected by means of flexible tubing to a diaphragm, which is placed on the client's skin.

actinic keratoses Pink to slightly red, dry, scaly lesions with indistinct borders and a malignant potential.

active listening Communication technique that involves concentration on what is said by blocking out environmental noise, distractions, and intrusive thoughts. Active listening conveys a nonverbal message to the speaker that what is being said is valued.

active range of motion Purposeful joint movement performed by the client without assistance from the examiner.

activities of daily living Basic physical needs of dressing, transferring, feeding, bathing, toileting, bowel and bladder control, walking, climbing stairs, and grooming.

acute Characterized by sharpness and severity; usually involves rapid onset and short duration.

adaptation Process by which the eye becomes more sensitive to either reduced or increased illumination.

adduction Movement toward the axial line (for a limb) or the median plane (for the digits).

adnexal Being next to or near another, related structure—the ovaries in the case of female genitalia.

adolescence The stage of life beginning at puberty and extending to adulthood.

affect Outwardly manifested emotional range attached to ideas. *Appropriate affect:* emotional tone in harmony with the accompanying idea, thought, or verbalization. *Blunted affect:* disturbance manifested by a severe reduction in the intensity of affect. *Flat affect:* absence or near absence of any signs of affective expression. *Inappropriate affect:* incongruence between the emotional feeling tone and the idea, thought, or speech accompanying it. *Labile affect:* rapid changes in the emotional feeling tone that are unrelated to external stimuli.

afferent neuron Any neuron that transmits nerve impulses from the periphery toward the central nervous system (sensory).

age-related macular degeneration Degeneration of the macula leading to decreased central vision.

ageusia Loss of the sensation of taste or of the ability to discriminate sweet, sour, salty, and bitter tastes.

agnosia Inability to discriminate sensory stimuli. *Acoustic or auditory agnosia:* impaired ability to recognize familiar sounds. *Tactile agnosia:* impaired ability to recognize familiar objects by touch or feel. *Visual agnosia:* impaired ability to recognize familiar objects by sight. *Somatagnosia:* disturbance in recognition of body parts.

alopecia Partial or complete lack of hair resulting from normal aging, endocrine disorder, drug reactions, skin disease, and other causes.

alveoli Small, thin-walled sacs through which gas exchange takes place between alveolar air and pulmonary capillary blood.

amblyopia Reduced vision in an eye that appears structurally normal on ophthalmoscopic examination.

amenorrhea Absence of menstruation.

ampulla Rounded, saclike dilation of a duct, canal, or any tubular structure.

anastomosing Joining.

anesthesia Absence of normal sensation, especially sensitivity to pain, such as induced by an anesthetic substance or hypnosis or as occurs with traumatic or pathophysiological damage to nerve tissue.

aneurysm Localized dilation of an artery. Most prominent and significant in the aorta but also occurs in peripheral vessels.

angina pectoris Pain that is substernal and/or radiating to the left arm, neck, or jaw; frequently correlated with myocardial ischemia. May be accompanied by a feeling of suffocation or impending death. Attacks are often related to exertion, emotional stress, or exposure to intense cold.

anisocoria Condition in which the pupils of the two eyes are of unequal size.

ankylosis Rigidity and consolidation of a joint.

annulus Dense, fibrous ring surrounding the tympanic membrane.

anonychia Complete absence of the nail.

anorexia Loss of appetite.

anosmia Inability to smell.

anterior triangle Landmark on the neck formed by the edge of the mandible (superiorly), the sternocleidomastoid muscle (laterally), and the midline of the trachea (medially). Used to describe the location of physical findings.

anuria Absence of excretion of urine.

anxiety Motor tension, autonomic hyperactivity, apprehension, or hyperattentiveness.

aortic valve Heart valve separating the left ventricle from the aorta.

aphasia Dysfunction or loss of the ability to express thoughts by speech, writing, symbols, or signs. *Fluent aphasia:* ability to produce words but with frequent errors in the choice of appropriate words or in the creation of words. *Nonfluent aphasia:* inability to produce words, either in spoken or written form.

apical impulse Pulsation of the apex of the heart against the chest wall, normally at the fifth left intercostal space in the midclavicular line.

Apley's sign Pain, locking of the knee, or clicking evoked with rotation of a flexed knee. Positive sign is indicative of a loose object in the knee (cartilage) that occurs with a torn meniscus.

apnea Cessation of breathing in the end-expiratory position.

apraxia Impairment of the ability to carry out purposeful skilled acts despite an intact sensory and motor system, such as an inability to draw or construct forms of two or three dimensions.

aqueous humor Fluid secreted in the ciliary body, which is found in the anterior chamber of the eye.

arcus senilis Grayish to gray-white, opaque arc or halo surrounding the cornea; generally occurs in individuals older than 50 years.

areolae Pigmented areas surrounding the nipples. Their color varies from pink to brown.

arrhythmia Any deviation from the normal pace of the heart. Kinds of arrhythmias include atrial fibrillation, atrial flutter, heart block, premature atrial contraction, and sinus arrhythmia.

arterial insufficiency Inadequate supply of blood by way of the arteries to peripheral areas.

arterial pressure Force exerted by the blood against the arterial walls.

arteriosclerosis Common arterial disorder characterized by hardening, thickening, loss of elasticity, and calcification of arterial walls, resulting in a decreased blood supply, especially to the cerebrum and the lower extremities.

arteritis Inflammatory condition of the inner layers or the outer coat of one or more arteries.

arthralgia Any pain that affects a joint.

arthritis Inflammation of a joint.

ascites Abnormal accumulation of fluid containing large amounts of protein and electrolytes within the abdominal cavity.

asthma Paroxysmal dyspnea (wheezing) resulting from obstruction of the bronchi or spasm of smooth muscle.

astigmatism Condition involving irregularity of the spherical curve of the cornea in which light rays cannot be focused in a point on the retina.

ataxia Impairment of coordination of muscular activity.

atelectasis Incomplete expansion of a lung compromised since birth; collapse of the adult lung.

atherosclerosis Type of arteriosclerosis characterized by deposits (atheromas) of cholesterol, lipoid material, and lipophages in the walls of large arteries and arterioles. This condition usually occurs with aging and is often associated with obesity, hypertension, and diabetes.

atony (atonic) Weak; lacking normal tone.

atrioventricular (AV) block Impairment of impulse conduction from the atria to the ventricles that occurs at the AV node or the bundle of His (or its branches).

atrioventricular (AV) valves Valves in the heart through which blood flows from the atria to the ventricles. The left AV valve is the mitral valve. The right AV valve is the tricuspid valve.

atrium (*pl*, atria) One of the two upper chambers of the heart. The right atrium receives deoxygenated blood from the superior and inferior vena cavae. The left atrium receives oxygenated blood from the pulmonary veins.

atrophy Wasting; decrease in the size of a cell, tissue, organ, or body part.

auditory ossicles Series of three small bones (malleus, incus, stapes) that extend across the middle ear.

augmentation Technique used to reinforce expression of deep tendon reflexes. The individual isometrically tenses muscles not directly involved in the reflex arc.

auricle External ear; also called pinna.

auscultation Examination technique done by listening, usually through a stethoscope.

autonomic nervous system Part of the peripheral nervous system that regulates involuntary vital function, including the activity of the cardiac muscle, the smooth muscle, and the glands. It has two divisions: (1) the sympathetic nervous system accelerates heart rate, constricts blood vessels, and raises blood pressure; (2) the parasympathetic nervous system slows heart rate, increases intestinal peristalsis and gland activity, and relaxes sphincters.

axillary tail of Spence Anatomical projection of breast tissue into the axilla.

axon Cylindrical extension of a nerve cell that conducts impulses away from the neuron cell body.

Baker's cyst Swelling in the popliteal space resulting from herniation of the synovial membrane of the knee.

ballottement Palpation technique used to assess a floating object. Fluid-filled tissue is pushed toward the examiner's hand so that the object will float against the examiner's fingers.

basal cell skin cancer Nodular, translucent lesions with small blood vessels often seen inside the nodule.

behavior Any observable, recordable, and measurable move, response, or act (verbal or nonverbal) of an individual.

bigeminal, bigeminy Pattern of arrhythmia consisting of coupled or paired ventricular beats; alternating QRS complexes are ventricular premature depolarizations.

bigeminal pulse Abnormal pulse in which two beats in close succession are followed by a pause during which no pulse is felt.

bipolar disorder Affective or mood disorder characterized by periods of mania alternating with periods of depression, with normal mood intervals occurring between the two.

bitemporal hemianopsia Loss of vision in both temporal fields of vision.

blepharitis Inflammation of the eyelid margins.

body image A person's subjective concept of his or her physical appearance.

body language The conveyance of messages by movements or gestures of the body or limbs, facial expressions, and eye contact. Body posture may convey a variety of emotions, including anger, anxiety, boredom, attention, or indifference.

borborygmi Audible bowel sounds, generally caused by gas propulsion through the intestine.

bounding pulse Pulse that, on palpation, feels full and spring-like because of an increased thrust of cardiac contraction or an increased volume of circulating blood within the elastic structures of the vascular system.

bradycardia Circulatory condition in which the myocardium contracts steadily but at a rate of less than 50 beats per minute.

bradypnea Abnormally slow rate of breathing.

brainstem Portion of the brain that comprises the medulla oblongata, the pons, and the mesencephalon. It performs motor, sensory, and reflex functions and contains the corticospinal and the reticulospinal tracts. The 12 pairs of cranial nerves arise mainly from the brainstem.

Braxton Hicks contraction Irregular tightening of the uterus that begins in the first trimester and increases in frequency, duration, and intensity as the pregnancy advances.

bronchiectasis Chronic dilation of one or more bronchi.

bronchioles Small airways of the respiratory system extending from the bronchi into the lobes of the lungs.

bronchitis Inflammation of one or more bronchi; condition may be chronic or acute.

bronchophony Sound of the voice as heard with abnormally increased clarity and intensity through the stethoscope over the lung parenchyma in an area of consolidation.

bronchovesicular Related to breath sounds from bronchial tubes and alveoli.

bruit Murmur or blowing sound heard over the peripheral vessels, indicating increased flow or stenosis of the vessel.

bruxism Compulsive, unconscious grinding of the teeth, especially during sleep.

buccal Pertaining to the cheek.

buffalo hump Accumulation of fat on the back of the neck associated with the prolonged use of large doses of glucocorticoids or the hypersecretion of cortisol caused by Cushing's syndrome.

bursa Sac or saclike cavity filled with fluid and located in sites where friction would otherwise develop, such as in a joint or over a bony prominence.

bursitis Inflammation of a bursa.

caput succedaneum Localized pitting edema in the scalp of a newborn that may overlie the sutures of the skull.

caries Decay of the calcified protein of teeth.

carpal tunnel syndrome Entrapment of the median nerve in the carpal tunnel, resulting in paresthesia, pain, and muscle weakness.

caruncle Small, fleshy projection located at the inner canthus of the eye.

cataplexy Condition characterized by sudden muscular weakness and hypotonia, caused by emotions, such as anger, fear, or surprise; often associated with narcolepsy.

cataract Opacity in the lens that gradually impairs vision over time.

caudad Toward the tail or end of the body; away from the head.

central sleep apnea Form of sleep apnea resulting from a decreased respiratory center output. Characterized by cessation of both airflow and respiratory movements.

cephalad Toward the head; away from the tail or end.

cephalhematoma Swelling caused by subcutaneous bleeding and accumulation of blood in the scalp of a newborn; usually the result of birth trauma.

cerebellum Part of the brain located in the posterior cranial fossa behind the brainstem. Its functions are concerned with coordinating voluntary muscular activity.

cerebrum Largest part of the brain, consisting of the right and left cerebral hemispheres. Its many functions include movement, sensation, learning, and memory.

cerumen Earwax produced by the apocrine and sebaceous glands within the ear canal.

chalazion Sebaceous cyst on the eyelid that is formed by distention of a meibomian gland.

cherry angiomas Benign, bright red, small, dome-shaped skin lesion.

chief complaint The major reason for seeking care stated in the client's own words.

chloasma Tan or brown pigmentation, particularly of the forehead, cheeks, and nose.

choana Funnel-shaped channel.

cholesterol Fat-soluble crystalline steroid alcohol found in animal fat, oil, and egg yolk. Increased levels of serum cholesterol may be associated with the pathogenesis of atherosclerosis.

chordae tendineae Strands of tendon attaching the atrioventricular valves to the papillary muscles at the heart.

chorionic Pertaining to the chorion, a fetal membrane composed of trophoblast that forms the fetal portion of the placenta.

choroid Thin, highly vascular membrane covering the posterior five sixths of the eye, located between the retina and the sclera.

chronic obstructive pulmonary disease General term for disease involving airway obstruction, such as chronic bronchitis, emphysema, or asthma.

Chvostek's sign Spasm of the facial muscle evoked by tapping branches of the facial nerve; may be caused by hypocalcemia or hypomagnesemia.

ciliary body Thickened part of the vascular tunic of the eye that joins the iris with the anterior portion of the choroid; produces aqueous humor and regulates its outflow.

ciliary movement Waving motion of the hairlike processes projecting from the epithelium of the respiratory tract.

circadian pattern (circadian rhythm) Cyclical pattern or period based on a 24-hour cycle, especially the repetition of certain physiological phenomena, such as sleeping and waking.

circumduction Circular movement.

cirrhosis Disease characterized by destruction of liver parenchyma. The affected liver is characterized by fibrous tissue and yellow-tan nodules.

claudication Weakness of the legs accompanied by cramplike pains in the calves, caused by poor circulation of the blood to the leg muscles. This condition is exacerbated by walking.

clubbing Proliferation of soft tissue of the terminal phalanges, generally associated with relative hypoxia of peripheral tissues, loss of the angle between the skin and the nail base, and sponginess of the nail base.

coarctation Tightening or compression of the walls of a vessel, producing a narrowed lumen.

cochlea Conical bony structure of the inner ear, perforated by numerous apertures for passage of the chochlear division of the acoustic nerve.

cognitive Pertaining to the mental processes of knowing, thinking, learning, and judging.

colic Acute abdominal pain associated with smooth muscle contraction of the gastrointestinal tract.

colitis Inflammation of the colon.

concha Body structure that is shell shaped, such as the cavity in the external ear that surrounds the external auditory meatus.

conduction Process in which heat is transferred from one substance to another because of a difference in temperature.

conductive hearing loss Diminished ability to hear caused by the inability of vibrations to travel to or through the inner ear to an intact auditory nerve.

condyloma (condylomata acuminata) Hyperkeratotic exophytic lesions of stratified squamous epithelium; these develop as small, elevated, soft nodules that enlarge and coalesce to become cauliflower-like excrescences.

confabulation Fabrication of facts or events in response to questions about situations that are not recalled because of memory impairment.

congenital Present at birth.

conjunctiva Mucous membrane that lines the inner surfaces of the eyelids and the anterior part of the sclera.

conjunctivitis Inflammation of the conjunctiva.

consensual reaction Constriction of the pupil of one eye when the other eye is being stimulated by light.

consolidation Process in which liquid or solid replacement of lung parenchyma as exudate from an inflammatory condition is amassed.

constipation Infrequent or difficult evacuation of feces; often associated with drying and hardening of the stool.

contour Surface outline or shape of the part being described.

contracting A contract is an oral or written agreement between the provider and client that makes explicit the expectations of each party.

contractures Abnormal, usually permanent condition of a joint, characterized by flexion and fixation and caused by atrophy and shortening of muscle fibers or loss of the normal elasticity of the skin.

convection Transfer of heat through a gas or liquid by the circulation of heated particles.

convergence Coordinated medial movement of the eyes in fixing on a near object.

Cooper's ligaments Suspensory ligaments of the breast.

cor pulmonale Right-sided heart hypertrophy and right ventricular failure resulting from pulmonary hypertension.

cornea Convex, transparent anterior part of the eye that makes up one sixth of the outermost tunic of the eye bulb.

cornu Any horn-shaped structure.

coronary artery disease Any one of the abnormal conditions that may affect the arteries of the heart and produce various pathological effects, especially the reduced flow of oxygen and nutrients to the myocardium.

corticotropic Of or pertaining to stimulation of the adrenal cortex.

crackles Discrete, noncontinuous sound resembling fine crackling, radio static, or hairs being rubbed together as heard through a stethoscope; generally produced by air bubbling through an exudate.

cramp Involuntary, painful skeletal muscle contraction.

crepitus (crepitation) Dry, crackling sound in (1) the lung, when air passes through abnormally accumulated moisture; (2) the joints, when dry synovial surfaces rub together; and (3) the skin, when air is present subdermally.

cretinism Disease caused by congenital lack of thyroid hormone; characterized by retarded physical and mental development, deafness, dystrophy of bones and soft tissue, and abnormally low concentrations of thyroid hormones.

cribriform Perforated, like a sieve.

crisis Sudden change in the course of a disease.

cryptorchidism Failure of one or both of the testicles to descend into the scrotum.

cue Something that is noted by using the five senses (taste, touch, smell, sight, and hearing). A cue can be either subjective data or objective data.

culture Complex, integrated system that includes knowledge, beliefs, skills, art, morals, law, customs, and any other acquired habits and capabilities of a group of people.

cupping Increased posterior curvature of the optic disc caused by the increased intraocular pressure of glaucoma, which gradually exerts pressure posteriorly against the optic disc.

cyanosis Dusky blue color of the skin and mucous membranes, seen especially in the lips and nail beds, caused by an excess of deoxygenated hemoglobin in the blood (saturation less than 75% to 85% or PaO_2 less than 50 mm Hg), or a structural defect in the hemoglobin molecule.

cystocele Herniation of the urinary bladder into the anterior vaginal wall.

dacryoadenitis Inflammation of the lacrimal gland.

dacryocystitis Inflammation of the lacrimal sac.

decidua Endometrium during pregnancy that is shed in the postpartum period.

defervescence The diminishing or disappearance of a fever.

defining characteristics Signs and symptoms that help to confirm a diagnosis.

delirium Clouded state of consciousness; reduction in clarity of awareness of the environment accompanied by a reduced capacity to shift, focus, and sustain attention to environmental stimuli.

delusion False belief that is improbable in nature; not influenced by contrary experience or related to the client's cultural and educational background.

dementia Loss of cognitive abilities of sufficient magnitude to interfere with social or occupational functioning. It involves impairment of memory, abstract thinking, or judgment or other disturbance of high cortical function.

dendrite Branching process that extends from the cell body of a neuron. Each neuron usually possesses several dendrites, which receive impulses that are conducted to the cell body.

depression Term used to define (1) a mood, (2) a syndrome, and (3) an illness. The mood of depression is described as dejection and lowering of functional activity; it is a normal experience that may be incurred in response to frustration and loss. The syndrome of depression includes a depressed mood in combination with one or more of the following symptoms: inability to concentrate, anorexia, weight loss, and suicidal ideas. The illness of depression is characterized by the syndrome of depression but lasts longer. Related functional impairment may include the inability to carry on daily activities, particularly work.

dermatome Area on the surface of a body innervated by afferent fibers from one spinal root.

detrusor Bladder muscle.

dextrocardia Rare condition in which the position of the heart is reversed and lies on the right side of the chest.

diagnostic Pertaining to the identification of a disease or condition by a scientific evaluation of physical signs, symptoms, history, laboratory tests, and procedures.

diarrhea Increased frequency and liquid content of fecal evacuation.

diastasis recti abdominis Separation of the two rectus muscles along the median line of the abdominal wall. May occur as a result of pregnancy or obesity.

diastolic (diastole) The force of blood against the arterial wall during the filling phase of the cardiac cycle, and the time between contractions of the atria or the ventricles during which the blood enters the relaxed chambers.

dicrotic notch Interval between the two peaks of a dicrotic pulse.

dicrotic pulse Presence of two sphygmographic waves to one beat of the pulse.

diplopia Double vision; simultaneous perception of two images for a single object.

disease Abnormality of structure or function that has a single pathogenic mechanism and a predictable course.

disorientation Lack of awareness as to time, place, or person.

dorsiflexion Backward bending.

dullness Decreased resonance on percussion, such as percussion sound produced over the liver.

dysarthria Difficult, poorly articulated speech.

dyschezia Painful defecation.

dyscoria Abnormality in the shape of the pupil.

dyslexia Disturbance in understanding the written word; difficulty in reading.

dysmenorrhea Painful menstruation.

dyspareunia Difficult or painful sexual intercourse in women.

dyspepsia Impairment of the ability to digest food, especially discomfort after eating a meal.

dysphagia Difficult or painful swallowing.

dysplasia Disorder in the size, shape, or organization of adult cells; any abnormal development of tissues or organs.

dyspnea Difficult or labored respiration; shortness of breath.

dyssynergia Inability to perform movements smoothly or an impairment in muscle coordination.

dysuria Difficult or painful urination.

ecchymosis Discoloration of an area of the skin or mucous membranes caused by the extravasation of blood into the subcutaneous tissues as a result of trauma to the underlying blood vessels or fragility of the vessel walls.

ecogram Diagram that maps the network of significant others, including friends, neighbors, peers, and associates.

ectocervix The outside portion of the cervix.

ectomorph A person whose physique is characterized by slenderness, fragility, and predominance of structures derived from the ectoderm.

ectopic pregnancy Abnormal pregnancy in which the conceptus implants outside the uterine cavity.

ectropion Turning outward of the lower lid of the eye.

edema Abnormal increase in the quantity of interstitial fluid.

efferent neuron Any neuron that transmits nerve impulses from the central nervous system toward the periphery (motor).

egophony Voice sound of a nasal or bleating quality, as heard through a stethoscope; often defined by asking the client to say "ee," which sounds like "ay" in an area of consolidation.

ejection click High-pitched clicking sound produced by the forceful opening of a diseased aortic or pulmonic valve, heard soon after the first heart sound.

embolism Sudden obstruction of an artery by a clot or other foreign substance. Symptoms vary with the degree of occlusion that the embolism causes, the character of the embolus, and the size, nature, and location of the occluded vessel.

embolus Foreign object, quantity of air or gas, bit of tissue or tumor, or piece of thrombus that circulates in the bloodstream until it becomes lodged in a vessel.

emphysema Condition involving entrapment of air within tissue, either interstitial or pulmonary. *Pulmonary emphysema*, or chronic obstructive pulmonary disease, results from permanent dilation or enlargement of the passages peripheral to the terminal bronchiole, which causes increased resistance to airflow. *Interstitial emphysema* is the presence of air in the subcutaneous tissue mediastinum or connective tissue of the lung resulting from air leakage through a damaged portion of the respiratory passages or alveoli; may result in swelling of tissue or a distinctive crackling sound called crepitation.

enculturation Process of acquiring one's cultural identity as it is transmitted by the previous generation.

endocardium Lining of the heart chambers.

endocervical Pertaining to the inside of the cervix.

endocervix Membrane lining the canal of the uterine cervix.

endolymph Fluid found in the membranous labyrinth of the internal ear.

endometriosis Presence of endometrial stroma and glands in ectopic locations, such as the ovaries, pelvic peritoneum, or colon.

endomorph A person whose body build is characterized by a soft, round physique with a large trunk and thighs, tapering extremities, an accumulation of fat throughout the body, and a predominance of structures derived from the endoderm.

enophthalmos Recession of the globe of the eye within the orbit.

enterocele Herniation of the intestine into the vagina.

entropion Turning inward of the lower lid of the eye.

enuresis Involuntary urination.

epiphora Tearing that results from faulty drainage of the eyes.

episiotomy Surgical procedure in which an incision is made in a woman's perineum to enlarge her vaginal opening for delivery.

epispadias Congenital anomaly in which the urethra opens on the dorsum of the penis.

epistaxis Bleeding or hemorrhage from the nose.

epulis Any tumor or growth on the gingiva.

equilibrium Ongoing process of maintaining the orientation and position of the body in relationship to the ground and in space.

erythema Dilation of capillaries, resulting in redness of the skin.

esophoria Deviation of the visual axis of one eye toward that of the other eye that occurs in the absence of visual stimuli for fusion.

esotropia Strabismus characterized by an inward deviation of one eye relative to the other eye.

essential hypertension Elevated arterial pressure for which no cause can be found and that is often the only significant clinical finding.

ethnic group Group of persons with shared traits, such as common national or regional origin and linguistic, ancestral, and physical characteristics.

ethnocentrism Tendency to view people unconsciously by using one's group and one's own customs as the standard for all judgments.

euphoria False sense of elation or well-being; pathological elevation of mood. This condition is most notable in clients who are experiencing the manic phase of bipolar disorder.

eustachian tube Cartilaginous and bony passage between the nasopharynx and the middle ear that allows equalization of air pressure between the middle ear and the external environment.

evaporation The change of a substance from a solid or liquid state to a gaseous state. The process of evaporation is hastened by an increase in temperature and a decrease in atmospheric pressure.

eversion Turning outward or inside out, as of the eyelid.

exophoria Deviation of the visual axis of one eye away from that of the other eye that occurs in the absence of visual stimuli for fusion.

exophthalmos Abnormal condition characterized by a marked protrusion of the eyeballs.

exostosis Abnormal benign growth on the surface of a bone.

exotropia Strabismus characterized by the outward deviation of one eye relative to the other.

extension Straightening of a limb so that the joint angle is increased.

external rotation Turning of a body part away from the central axis or midline of the body.

extinction Loss of touch perception on one side of the body.

extrapyramidal system Tract of motor nerves from the brain to the anterior horns of the spinal cord, except for the fibers of the pyramidal tract. It controls and coordinates the postural, static, supporting, and locomotor mechanisms and causes contractions of muscle groups in sequence or simultaneously.

extrasystole Cardiac contraction that is abnormal in timing or in origin of impulse; premature contraction of the heart.

facial nerve (CN VII) Cranial nerve that innervates the scalp, forehead, eyelids, muscles of facial expression, cheeks, and jaw.

fasciculation Observable, localized, uncoordinated, uncontrollable twitching movements resulting from contraction of a fasciculus (bundle of muscle fibers) served by one anterior horn cell; usually does not cause movement of a joint.

fever Pyrexia; elevation of the body temperature above normal for a given individual.

fibrillation Fine, continuous twitching caused by irregular, random contraction of a single muscle or group of fibers. Fibrillation of a chamber of the heart results in inefficient random contraction of that chamber and disruption of the normal sinus rhythm of the heart. This condition is usually described by the part that is contracting abnormally (e.g., atrial fibrillation or ventricular fibrillation). Atrial fibrillation is usually benign; ventricular fibrillation can be life-threatening.

fibroadenoma Benign tumor composed of dense epithelial and fibroblastic tissue. A fibroadenoma of the breast is nontender, encapsulated, round, movable, and firm.

fibromyositis Any one of a large number of disorders in which the common element is stiffness and joint or muscle pain accompanied by localized inflammation of the muscle tissues and of the fibrous connective tissues.

field of vision Area simultaneously visible to a motionless eye.

fist percussion Striking the body with the lateral aspect of the hand to elicit pain or tenderness.

flatulence Presence of an excessive amount of gas in the gastrointestinal tract.

flexion Bending of a joint so that the joint angle is decreased.

flight of ideas Nearly continuous flow of rapid speech with abrupt changes from topic to topic. This condition is noted most frequently in organic mental disorders, schizophrenia, and psychotic disorders and as a reaction to stress.

floaters Spots that appear to drift in front of the eye and are caused by a shadow cast on the retina by vitreous debris.

fornix Archlike structure of space.

fourchette Tense band of membranes connecting the posterior angle of the vagina to the posterior ends of the labia minora.

fovea centralis Central spot of color vision on the retina that contains only cones and no rods.

fremitus Palpable vibration.

frenulum Restraining portion or structure. An example is the sublingual frenulum.

friction rub Crackling, grating sound as heard through a stethoscope when two inflamed, roughened surfaces rub together.

fundus The base or deepest part of any organ.

gait Manner of progression in walking. In *ataxic gait* the foot is raised high and the sole strikes down suddenly.

gallop rhythm Heart rate characterized by three sounds.

ganglia Type of nerve cell, chiefly collected in groups outside the central nervous system. Individual cells and very small groups abound in association with alimentary organs.

genogram Diagram that depicts family relationships over at least three generations.

gigantism Excessive growth of the body or its parts; may be a result of hypersecretion of growth hormone in childhood.

gingivitis Inflammation of the papillary and marginal gingiva.

glans Small, rounded mass. *Glans penis:* caplike, conical tip of the penis that covers the end of the corpora cavernosa penis and the corpus spongiosum.

glaucoma Ocular disease in which increased intraocular pressure causes atrophy and excavation of the optic nerve, producing visual field defects.

goiter Increase in size of the thyroid gland.

goniometer Instrument used to measure joint angles.

gout Disease caused by deposition of crystals of monosodium urate; characterized by a disorder in purine metabolism and associated with exacerbations of arthritis of a single joint.

graphesthesia Ability to identify letters or numbers inscribed with a blunt object on the palm of the hand, back, or other areas. Higher cortical integration is required to perform this function.

grasp reflex Normal reflex in young infants elicited by stroking the infant's palms; the examiner's fingers are grasped so firmly that the child can be lifted into the air. (In older individuals the tonic grasp reflex is pathological, occurring in diseases of the premotor cortex.)

Grey Turner's sign Bruising of the flank skin.

gynecomastia Hypertrophy of breast tissue in a male subject.

health history Comprehensive body of information obtained from the client and other select sources. Includes information on the client as a whole, the health/illness status (past and present), the social and physical environment, and past interactions with health care systems.

Heberden's nodes (nodules) Small, hard nodules of the terminal interphalangeal joints, associated with osteoarthritis.

helix Superior and posterior free margin of the ear.

hematemesis Vomiting of blood.

hematopoietic Relating to the formation and development of blood cells in the bone marrow.

hematuria Presence of blood in the urine.

hemianopsia Defective vision or blindness in one half of the visual field.

hemoptysis Spitting or coughing up of blood from the respiratory tract.

hemorrhoid Dilation of a part of the venous hemorrhoidal plexus in the mucosal membrane of the rectum. A hemorrhoid may occur as a result of increased hydrostatic pressure in the venous system, such as in pregnancy, or from disease that causes portal hypertension and straining at stool. *Internal hemorrhoids:* varicosity of superior or middle hemorrhoidal veins below the anal mucosa; may result in bleeding. *External hemorrhoids:* varicosity of the inferior hemorrhoidal vein under the anal skin; may cause pain and swelling around the anal sphincter and itching and bleeding.

hepatomegaly Abnormal enlargement of the liver, usually a sign of liver disease.

hernia Abnormal protrusion of an organ or tissue through an opening. *Incarcerated hernia:* protrusion of abdominal contents through a weakness in the abdominal wall so that the contents cannot be returned to the abdominal cavity. *Direct inguinal hernia:* protrusion of abdominal contents through a weakness in the abdominal musculature in the region of Hesselbach's triangle. *Indirect inguinal hernia:* protrusion (generally indirect) of abdominal contents into the scrotal sac. *Strangulated hernia:* hernia in which the blood supply to the protruded tissue is obstructed.

herpes zoster Acute infection caused by the varicella-zoster virus, affecting primarily adults and characterized by the development of painful vesicular skin eruptions that follow the underlying route of cranial or spinal nerves inflamed by the virus.

hertz (Hz) Unit of frequency of a periodic process equal to 1 cycle per second.

high-density lipoprotein (HDL) Plasma protein containing about 50% protein with cholesterol and triglycerides. It may serve to stabilize very low-density lipoprotein. Called "good" cholesterol, it is involved in transporting cholesterol and other lipids from the plasma to the tissues.

hirsutism Excessive hairiness, especially in females.

homeostasis Relative constancy in the internal environment of the body, naturally maintained by adaptive responses that promote healthy survival.

homonymous Having the same name.

homonymous hemianopsia Blindness or defective vision in the right or left half of the visual field of both eyes.

hordeolum Inflammation of a sebaceous gland of the eyelid; sty.

horn Projection or protuberance of a body structure. Examples include the gray horns of the spinal cord, horn of the hyoid bone, and iliac horn.

hydrocele Circumscribed collection of fluid, particularly in the scrotum.

hypercholesterolemia Condition in which greater than normal amounts of cholesterol are present in the blood. High levels of cholesterol and other lipids may lead to the development of atherosclerosis.

hyperesthesia Abnormally increased sensitivity of one of the body's sense organs, such as pain or touch receptors in the skin.

hyperlipidemia Excess of lipids in the plasma.

hyperopia Farsightedness.

hyperplasia Increase in the number of cells in a body part.

hyperpnea Increased depth of respiration with or without an increase in rate.

hypersomnia (1) Sleep of excessive depth or abnormal duration; (2) extreme drowsiness, often associated with lethargy; (3) a condition characterized by periods of deep, long sleep.

hypertension Common, often asymptomatic disorder characterized by elevated blood pressure that persistently exceeds 140/90 mm Hg.

hyperventilation Increase in rate and depth of respiration.

hyphema Blood in the anterior chamber of the eye.

hypoesthesia Abnormal weakness of sensation in response to stimulation of the sensory nerves.

hypopyon Purulent material in the anterior chamber of the eye.

hyposmia Diminished sense of smell.

hypospadias Developmental anomaly in which the urethra opens on the underside of the penis.

hypotension Abnormal condition in which the blood pressure is not adequate for normal perfusion and oxygenation of the tissues.

hypotonia Decrease in body tonus.

idiopathic Without a known cause.

immediate (direct) percussion Use of the finger or hand to strike the body to evaluate the sound waves produced.

incontinence Failure of control of excretory functions.

incus One of the three ossicles of the inner ear, resembling an anvil. It communicates sound vibrations from the malleus to the stapes.

infarction Obstruction of circulation followed by ischemic necrosis.

inference How one perceives or interprets a cue.

insomnia Chronic inability to sleep or to remain asleep throughout the night; wakefulness; sleeplessness.

inspection Visual evaluation of the body that incorporates the senses of sight, smell, and hearing.

instrumental activities of daily living Life management skills of telephoning, reading, leisure, medication management, money management, transportation, shopping, meal preparation, laundering, housekeeping, home maintenance, etc.

insufficiency Inadequate closure of a heart valve, resulting in backflow of blood into the ventricles or atria.

intensity Loudness of sound.

intercostal space Space between two ribs.

intermittent claudication *Claudication* is a weakness of the legs accompanied by cramplike pains in the calves caused by poor circulation to the leg muscles. *Intermittent claudication* is a form of this disorder that is manifested only at certain times, usually after an extended period of walking, and is relieved by a period of rest.

internal rotation Turning of the body part toward the central axis or midline of the body.

interpersonal distance Distance between two individuals interacting that will vary by the nature of the relationship or cultural practices.

interpretation Sharing the meaning of the facts provided so that the client has an opportunity to confirm, deny, or offer an alternative explanation.

intertrigo (intertriginous) Erythematous irritation in areas where two skin surfaces come together, such as the groin area or the folds between large, pendulous breasts.

intraepithelian Within the epithelium.

introitus Entrance or orifice to a cavity or a hollow tubular structure of the body.

inversion (1) Turning inward. (2) Invagination or depression of the nipple's central portion. Can occur congenitally or as a response to an invasive process.

ipsilateral Pertaining to the same side of the body.

iridescent vision Perception of halos around lights, particularly with corneal edema.

iritis Inflammation of the iris.

ischial spines The two relatively sharp bony projections into the pelvic outlet from the ischial bones that form the lower border of the pelvis.

isolated systolic hypertension Systolic blood pressure greater than 160 mm Hg and normal diastolic blood pressure.

jaundice Accumulation of bilirubin-to-serum concentration greater than 2 mg/dl; produces yellow-green to bronze color of skin and itching.

jugular venous pulse Pulse wave in the jugular veins reflecting cardiac activity on the right side of the heart.

keloid Scar formation caused by a dense overgrowth of fibrous tissue, usually raised and thickened.

keratinization Process by which epithelial cells exposed to the external environment lose their moisture and are replaced by horny tissue.

kinesthetic sensation Feeling facilitated by the proprioceptive receptors in the muscles, tendons, and joints.

Korotkoff sounds Turbulent sounds heard when auscultating the blood pressure.

Kussmaul respiration Rapid and deep respiratory cycles resulting from stimulation of the medullary respiratory center in metabolic acidosis; associated with a pH less than 7.2 in diabetic ketoacidosis.

kyphosis Increased posterior convexity of the spine (humpback).

labile Readily altered, unstable.

labyrinth Intricate communicating passageway, such as the bony and membranous labyrinths of the inner ear.

lacrimation Production of tears, especially in excess.

laminar flow Airflow that is concentrated into a narrow pathway.

lens Transparent biconvex structure located behind the pupil and in front of the vitreous body.

lentigines Flat, tan to brown macules located in sun-exposed surfaces.

leukorrhea White discharge from the vagina.

lichen planus Nonmalignant, chronic, pruritic skin condition characterized by small, flat, purplish papules or plaques. The cause is unknown.

lid lag Condition in which the eyelid margin is above the limbus and some sclera is visible; it may indicate thyroid disease.

limbus Edge of the cornea at the point where it meets the sclera.

linea nigra Pigmentation of the linea alba, the tendinous median line on the anterior abdominal wall, during pregnancy.

lineae albicantes (striae) Atrophic lines or streaks that differ in texture and color from the surrounding skin and are caused by disrupted elastic fibers of the reticular layer of the skin.

lithotomy position Position assumed by the patient lying supine with the hips and the knees flexed and the thighs abducted and rotated externally.

lobes Glandular tissue units in the breast situated in a circular, spokelike fashion.

lobule Small lobe, such as the soft, pendulous lower part of the external ear.

lordosis Anterior concavity of the lumbar spine (swayback, saddleback).

low-density lipoprotein (LDL) Plasma protein containing relatively more cholesterol and triglycerides than protein. Called "bad" cholesterol, it is involved with the formation of atherosclerotic plaques.

lower motor neuron Peripheral neuron with a motor (efferent) function. Its cell body is located in the anterior horns of the spinal cord or brainstem nuclei, and it terminates in skeletal muscles.

lumpectomy Surgical excision of a tumor without removal of large amounts of surrounding tissue or adjacent lymph nodes.

luxation Dislocation.

lymphadenopathy Any disorder of the lymph nodes or lymph vessels.

macula Area of the retina where the receptors for color vision are most concentrated; located temporal to the optic disc.

malaise Feeling of general discomfort or uneasiness.

malleus One of the three ossicles of the middle ear; resembles a hammer; connected to the tympanic membrane.

mammary folds Crescent-shaped ridges of breast tissue found at the inferior portions of very large or pendulous breasts. May be confused with breast masses but are nonpathological.

mammography Radiography of the soft tissues of the breast to allow identification of various benign and malignant neoplastic processes.

mastication Chewing, tearing, or grinding food with the teeth while it becomes mixed with saliva.

mastitis Inflammation of breast tissue.

mastoid process Bony prominence of the posterior portion of the temporal bone, located posterior to the lower part of the auricle, serving as the attachment for various muscles, including the sternocleidomastoid.

McBurney's point Anatomical landmark located approximately 2 inches above the right anterosuperior iliac spine on a line between the umbilicus and the spine.

McMurray's sign Inability to extend the flexed knee may indicate a loose object in the knee (cartilage) due to a torn meniscus.

meatus Passage or opening, especially at the external portion of a canal.

mediastinum Portion of the thoracic cavity in the middle of the thorax, between the pleural sacs that contain the two lungs.

mediate (indirect) percussion Technique in which the middle finger of one hand strikes the middle finger of the other hand to emit a sound or vibration.

meibomian gland One of several sebaceous glands that secrete sebum from the ducts on the posterior margin of each eyelid. The glands are embedded in the tarsal plate of each eyelid.

melanocyte Body cell capable of producing melanin.

menarche First menstruation and commencement of cyclic menstrual function.

menopause Gradual cessation of the menses, usually occurring between 45 and 60 years of age.

menorrhagia Abnormally heavy or long menstrual periods.

mental status examination Record of current findings that includes a description of a client's appearance, behavior, motor activity, speech, alertness, mood, cognition, intelligence, reactions, views, and attitudes.

mesomorph A person whose physique is characterized by a predominance of muscle, bone, and connective tissue, structures that develop from the mesodermal layer of the embryo.

metrorrhagia Irregular and/or dysfunctional uterine bleeding.

microaneurysm Outpouching in the wall of a capillary that appears as a red dot on the retina.

middlescence Term for the years of middle adulthood.

migraine Recurring vascular headache characterized by a prodromal aura, unilateral onset, severe pain, photophobia, and autonomic disturbances during the acute phase, which may last for hours or days.

minority group Any group that receives different and unequal treatment from others in the larger group or society and whose members see themselves as victims of discrimination.

miosis Constriction of the pupil.

mitral regurgitation Backward flow of blood from the left ventricle to the left atrium associated with an incompetent mitral valve.

mitral valve Left atrioventricular valve.

mitral valve stenosis Fibrosis and thickening of the cusps of the mitral valve with narrowing of the aperture between the left atrium and the left ventricle.

mixed hearing loss Combination of conductive and sensorineural loss in the same ear.

mixed sleep apnea Condition marked by signs and symptoms of both central sleep apnea and obstructive sleep apnea.

Montgomery's glands Small sebaceous glands located on the areola.

morning sickness Nausea and vomiting occurring from the fifth or sixth week through the fourteenth to sixteenth week of pregnancy.

Moro reflex Normal mass reflex in a young infant elicited by a sudden loud noise resulting in flexion of the legs, an embracing posture of the arms, and usually a brief cry. Also called startle reflex.

morphology Study of the physical shape and size of a specimen, plant, or animal.

multiparous Having delivered one or more viable infants.

murmur Blowing sound caused by turbulence of blood flow; heard through the stethoscope over the heart; when heard in the great vessels, the sound is called a bruit.

Murphy's sign Sign noted by a maneuver done during deep palpation in the approximate location of the gallbladder. On deep inspiration, the liver descends, bringing the gallbladder in contact with the examiner's hand. Pain is elicited in the presence of cholecystitis.

mycelia Masses of interwoven, branched, threadlike filaments that make up most fungi.

mydriasis Dilation of the pupil.

myelination Development of the myelin sheath around a nerve fiber.

myocardial infarction Occlusion of a coronary artery caused by atherosclerosis or thrombosis, resulting in damage to the myocardium.

myocardium Thick, contractile middle layer of the heart; composed of muscle tissue that forms the bulk of this organ.

myopia Nearsightedness; condition in which parallel rays of light come to focus in front of the retina.

myxedema Hypothyroidism. Hypometabolism is present, and nonpitting edema results from the presence of hydrated mucopolysaccharides in connective tissue.

nabothian cysts Cystlike formations of the mucosa of the uterine cervix resulting from an accumulation of retained secretion in occluded glands.

narcolepsy Syndrome characterized by sudden sleep attacks, cataplexy, sleep paralysis, and visual or auditory hallucination at the onset of sleep.

nasolabial fold Crease in the skin extending from the angle of the nose to the corner of the mouth.

nausea Feeling that vomiting is impending.

neoplasia New and abnormal development of cells that may be benign or malignant.

neuromuscular spindle Any one of a number of small bundles of delicate muscular fibers, enclosed by a capsule, in which sensory nerve fibers terminate. Spindles vary in length from 0.8 to 5 mm, accommodating as many as four large myelinated nerve fibers that pierce the capsule and lose their myelin sheaths.

nevus Well-demarcated, pigmented, congenital skin blemish that is usually benign but may become cancerous.

nicking Appearance of indentation of an optic vein where an arteriole crosses it.

night blindness Slow adjustment from bright to dim light.

nocturia Excessive urination at night.

nocturnal enuresis Urinary voiding during sleep.

nodularity Lumpiness.

nuchal Pertaining to the nape of the neck.

nuchal rigidity Pertaining to limited range of motion of the cervical spine, usually associated with pain.

nullipara (nulliparous) Woman who has not given birth to a viable offspring.

nursing diagnosis Statement that describes a client's health state, or response to illness, treatable by a nurse.

nystagmus Involuntary rhythmic motion of the eye; may be horizontal, vertical, rotary, or mixed.

obesity Condition in which the amount of fat in the body is excessive in relation to total body weight; exceeding 20% of ideal body weight.

obstipation Severe constipation.

obstructive sleep apnea Form of sleep apnea involving a physical obstruction of the upper airway.

oligomenorrhea Decreased frequency of menstruation with an interval of 38 to 90 days.

oliguria Abnormally decreased urine secretion (less than 400 ml/24 hr).

opening snap Snapping sound produced by the opening of a diseased mitral or tricuspid valve. It is an early diastolic sound heard soon after the second heart sound.

orchiopexy Operation in which an undescended testis is mobilized, brought into the scrotum, and attached so that it will not retract.

orientation Conscious awareness of person, place, and time.

orifice An opening.

oropharynx One of the three anatomical divisions of the pharynx. It extends behind the mouth from the soft palate (above) to the level of the hyoid bone (below) and contains the palatine tonsils and the lingual tonsils.

orthopnea Dyspnea that begins or increases when the client lies down, and is relieved by sitting upright.

orthostatic (postural) hypotension Lower blood pressure of greater than 30 mm Hg that occurs on rising from a lying or sitting to an erect position.

osteoporosis Disorder characterized by loss of bone density, occurring most frequently in postmenopausal women, in sedentary or immobilized individuals, and in persons on long-term steroid therapy.

ostium Orifice.

otalgia Earache.

palpation Examination technique that involves feeling or touching the object to be evaluated.

palpebra Eyelid.

palpebral fissure Opening between the margins of the upper and lower eyelids when the eye is open.

palpitation Pulsations of the heart and arteries that are perceptible to the client and are associated with normal emotional responses or with certain heart disorders.

papilledema Edema of the optic disc.

paranasal sinus One of the air cavities in various bones around the nose. Examples are the frontal sinus in the frontal bone lying deep to the medial part of the superciliary ridge and the maxillary sinus within the maxilla between the orbit, the nasal cavity, and the upper teeth.

paraphimosis Condition characterized by an inability to replace the foreskin in its normal position after it has been retracted behind the glans penis.

parenchyma Tissue of an organ as distinguished from supporting or connective tissue.

paresis Slight or incomplete paralysis; weakness.

paresthesia Abnormal or perverted sensation; may include burning, itching, pain, or a feeling of electric shock.

Parkinson's disease Progressive disorder of the basal ganglia, characterized by tremor, difficulty in initiating voluntary movements, muscle weakness and rigidity, and a peculiar gait.

paronychia Inflammation and infection of the folds of tissue surrounding a fingernail.

parous Having borne one or more viable offspring.

paroxysmal nocturnal dyspnea Sudden onset of dyspnea after a period of lying down. Sitting upright helps relieve the dyspnea.

pars flaccida Less taut portion of the tympanic membrane.

pars tensa Taut portion of the tympanic membrane.

passive range of motion Joint movement of the client that is produced by the examiner.

peau d'orange Orange-peel appearance of the breast caused by edema of the breast and resultant blocked lymph drainage.

pectus carinatum Structural deformity of the thoracic cage where the sternum is displaced anteriorly, increasing the anteroposterior diameter. The costal cartilages adjacent to the sternum are depressed.

pectus excavatum Structural deformity of the thoracic cage where the lower sternum is depressed. Compression of the heart and great vessels may cause murmurs.

perception Awareness of objects and relations that follows stimulation of the peripheral sense organs.

percussion Examination technique used to evaluate the size, borders, and consistency of certain internal organs and to determine the presence of and evaluate the amount of air and fluid in a body cavity. It involves listening to reverberation of tissue after striking the surface with short, sharp blows.

pericardium Fibrous sac that surrounds the heart and the roots of the great vessels.

periorbital edema Accumulation of fluid in the eyelids and other tissues surrounding the eye.

peritonitis Inflammation of the peritoneum.

petechiae Tiny purple or red spots that appear on the skin as a result of minute hemorrhages within the dermal or submucosal layers.

Peyronie's disease Disease of unknown cause resulting in fibrous induration of the corpora cavernosa of the penis. The chief symptom is painful erection.

phimosis Narrowness of the opening of the prepuce that causes difficulty in retraction of the foreskin of the penis.

phobia Persistent and exaggerated fear of a particular object or situation.

phoria Mild weakness of the extraocular muscle(s); appears as a deviation of the eye when fusion is suspended.

photophobia Abnormal sensitivity to light.

physiologic cup (physiologic depression) Small depression just temporal to the center of the optic disc.

pincer grasp The index finger in apposition to the thumb.

pinguecula Small, yellowish white subconjunctival elevation located between the corneoscleral limbus and the canthus.

pinna Projecting part of the external ear; the auricle.

pitch Quality of a tone or sound that is dependent on the relative rapidity of the vibrations by which it is produced.

pituitary dwarfism Condition of being abnormally small, especially small of stature due to a deficiency of growth hormone.

plantar flexion Bending of the foot toward the floor.

platypnea Respiratory distress that increases when a person is upright.

plethora Pertaining to a red, florid complexion.

pleural effusion Fluid of any kind in the pleural cavity.

pleurisy Pleural inflammation accompanied by pain.

polydipsia Excessive thirst.

polymenorrhea Abnormally frequent menstruation.

polyphagia Excessive ingestion of food.

polysomnography Multicomponent sleep study that monitors arterial oxygen saturation, brain waves (electroencephalogram [EEG]), eye movements (electrooculogram [EOG]), muscle tone and movements (electromyelogram [EMG]), intraesophageal pressure, inspiratory flow, and rib cage and abdominal circumference changes. The length of time slept, the total number of apneic periods, the number of apneic periods per hour, the percentage of apneic time, the mean duration of apneas, and the cumulative SaO_2 are calculated for each individual.

polyuria Excessive urinary excretion.

posterior triangle Landmark on the neck formed by the sternocleidomastoid muscle (laterally), the trapezius muscle (posteriorly), and the clavicle (inferiorly), used to describe the location of physical findings.

Poupart's ligament Inguinal ligament; the fibrous band that runs from the anterosuperior iliac spine to the pubic spine.

precordium Area of the anterior chest wall overlying the heart and the great vessels.

prepuce Foreskin.

presbycusis Age-related hearing loss.

presbyopia Decreased ability of the optic lens to accommodate to near vision with increasing age.

preterm infant Infant born before 37 weeks of gestation.

proctitis Inflammation of the rectal mucosa.

proctoscopy Examination of the rectum with a short cylindrical instrument called a proctoscope.

pronation (1) Assumption of the prone (face down) position; (2) turning the forearm so that the palm is posterior; or (3) eversion and abduction of the foot.

prostatitis Acute or chronic inflammation of the prostate gland, generally in conjunction with cystitis and urethritis. Symptoms include low back and perineal pain, fever, urinary frequency, and dysuria.

pruritus Itching.

pterygium Abnormal triangular thickening of the bulbar conjunctiva on the cornea, with the apex directed toward the pupil.

ptosis Drooping of the upper eyelid, often interfering with vision.

puberty The period of life at which the ability to reproduce begins.

pulmonic valve Heart valve separating the right ventricle from the pulmonary artery.

pulse Palpable, rhythmic expansion of an artery caused by ejection of blood from the left ventricle during systole.

pulse deficit Condition that exists when the peripheral pulse count is less than the ventricular rate taken at the apex of the heart. It indicates a lack of peripheral perfusion for some of the heart contractions.

pulse pressure The difference between the systolic and diastolic blood pressure.

pulsus alternans (alternating pulse) Pulse characterized by a regular alternation of weak and strong beats without changes in the length of the cycle.

pulsus bisferiens Arterial pulse that has two palpable peaks, the second of which is slightly stronger than the first.

pulsus paradoxus (paradoxical pulse) Abnormal decrease in systolic pressure and pulse-wave amplitude during inspiration. The normal fall in pressure is less than 10 mm Hg. An excessive decline may be a sign of precordial tamponade, adhesive pericarditis, severe lung disease, advanced heart failure, or other conditions.

puncta Tiny apertures in the margins of each eyelid that open into the lacrimal ducts.

pupil Aperture in the iris that allows for the passage of light.

pyogenic Substance that tends to cause a rise in body temperature.

pyorrhea Purulent inflammation of the gums.

pyramidal tract Pathway composed of groups of nerve fibers in the white matter of the spinal cord through which motor impulses are conducted to the anterior horn cells from the opposite side of the brain. These descending fibers regulate the voluntary and reflex activity of the muscles through the anterior horn cells.

pyrexia Fever; elevation of the body temperature above normal for a given individual.

pyrosis Heartburn.

pyuria Presence of pus in the urine.

race Classification of human beings on the basis of physical characteristics, such as skin pigmentation, head form, or stature, that are transmitted through generations.

radiation Emission of energy, rays, or waves.

Raynaud's phenomenon Intermittent attacks of ischemia of the extremities, especially the fingers, toes, ears, and nose.

rectocele Herniation of the rectum into the posterior vaginal wall.

reflection Repeating a phrase or sentence the client has said. Allow a period of silence lasting at least 5 to 10 seconds to allow the client to think before answering a question or responding to a suggestion; after 10 seconds without a response, the interviewer will need to initiate another question or suggestion.

reflex Involuntary functioning or movement of any organ or part of the body in response to a particular stimulus. The function or action occurs immediately, without the involvement of the will or consciousness.

regurgitation Backward flow of blood through a defective heart valve.

REM sleep Rapid eye movement sleep characterized by episodic bursts of rapid eye movements on the electrooculogram and by low-voltage, high-frequency waves on the electroencephalogram.

resonance Low-pitched, hollow sound produced over normal lung tissue when the chest is percussed.

reticular activating system Functional system in the brain that is essential for wakefulness, attention, concentration, and introspection. A network of nerve fibers in the thalamus, hypothalamus, brainstem, and cerebral cortex contribute to the system.

retina Delicate nervous tissue membrane of the eye that is continuous with the optic nerve; receives images of external objects and transmits visual impulses through the optic nerve to the brain.

retinal exudates White or yellow infiltrates that develop on the retina.

retraction (1) Condition of being drawn back. (2) Appears as a depression or pucker on the skin (also called dimpling). It usually is caused by the fibrotic shortening and immobilization of Cooper's ligament by an invasive process.

rhonchus Wheezing or snoring sound produced by airflow across a partially constricted air passage. *Sibilant rhonchus:* high-pitched wheeze produced in a small air passage. *Sonorous rhonchus:* low-pitched wheeze produced in a large air passage.

rigor Common term for shivering accompanying a chill or for muscle rigidity accompanying depletion of adenosine triphosphate, such as in death (rigor mortis).

Rinne test Test comparing air conduction and bone conduction through the use of a tuning fork. In normal hearing, air conduction sounds are heard longer than bone conduction sounds (positive Rinne).

rugated Having ridges or folds.

S_1 First heart sound in the cardiac cycle. It is associated with closure of the mitral and tricuspid valves and is synchronous with the apical pulse. Auscultated at the apex, it is louder, longer, and lower than the second sound (S_2), which follows it.

S_2 Second heart sound in the cardiac cycle. It is associated with closure of the aortic and pulmonary valves immediately before ventricular diastole. Auscultated at the base of the heart, the second sound is louder than the first.

S_3 Third heart sound; related to early ventricular filling. Normally, this sound is audible only in children and physically active young adults. In older people it is an abnormal finding and usually indicates myocardial failure.

S_4 Fourth heart sound; related to late ventricular filling. This sound occurs late in diastole on contraction of the atria.

Rarely heard in normal clients, it indicates an abnormally increased resistance to ventricular filling, such as in hypertensive cardiovascular disease, coronary artery disease, myocardiopathy, and aortic stenosis.

salpingitis Inflammation of the fallopian tubes as a result of infection. Leukorrhea, adnexal tenderness, abdominal pain, and fever may be present.

sciatica Pain, weakness, or paresthesias associated with the course of the sciatic nerve; may affect the posterior aspect of the thigh and the posterolateral and anterolateral aspects of the leg into the foot.

sclera Tough, inelastic opaque membrane that covers the posterior five sixths of the eye bulb; maintains the size and form of the bulb and attaches to muscles that move the bulb.

scoliosis Lateral deviation of the spine.

scotoma Islandlike area of blindness in the field of vision.

screening Preliminary procedure, such as a test or examination, to detect the most characteristic sign or signs of a disorder that may require further investigation.

sebaceous Pertaining to or secreting sebum, an oily secretion composed of fat and epithelial debris.

sebaceous cyst Retention of the fatty secretion of the sebaceous gland.

seborrheic keratoses Benign, raised, wartlike skin lesions appearing with increasing age.

self-esteem The degree of worth and competence one attributes to oneself.

semilunar valves Valves with half-moon–shaped cusps located between the ventricles and the great vessels. The left semilunar valve is the aortic valve. The right semilunar valve is the pulmonic valve.

senile purpura Skin bruising caused by leakage of blood through fragile skin capillaries.

sensorineural hearing loss Diminished ability to hear caused by the inability of the acoustic nerve to transmit nervous impulses from the middle ear to the brain. Also called perceptive hearing loss.

sequela Any abnormal condition that follows and results from a disease, treatment, or injury.

sign Objective evidence of disease that is perceptible to the examiner.

sinus Hollow cavity in a bone or other tissue.

skin tags Benign, soft, flesh-colored skin lesions.

sleep State marked by reduced consciousness, diminished activity of the skeletal muscles, and depressed metabolism. People normally experience sleep in patterns that follow four observable, progressive stages.

sleep apnea Periodic cessation of breathing during sleep.

sleep apnea syndrome (SAS) Sleep disorder characterized by multiple episodes of cessation of breathing during sleep.

sleep terror disorder Condition occurring during stage 3 or 4 of nonrapid eye movement (nonREM) sleep that is characterized by repeated episodes of abrupt awakening, usually with a panicky scream, accompanied by intense anxiety, confusion, agitation, disorientation, unresponsiveness, marked motor movements, and amnesia concerning the event.

somnambulism Sleepwalking; a condition occurring during stage 3 or 4 of nonrapid eye movement (nonREM) sleep that is characterized by complex motor activity, usually culminating in leaving the bed and walking about, with no recall of the episode on awakening.

spasm Involuntary sudden contraction of a muscle or group of muscles accompanied by pain and interference with function.

speculum Device made of two narrow blades or a hollow tube, used to assist in opening a body cavity.

spermatogenesis Process of development of spermatozoa, the male germ cells.

spinal accessory nerve (CN XI) Function of this nerve is essential for speech, swallowing, and certain movements of the head and shoulders.

squamocolumnar junction Area of the cervix where the membranes covered by squamous cells of the vaginal portion of the cervix meet the membranes of the columnar portion of the cervix.

standard precautions Constellation of safeguards for handling materials, tissues, and fluids that may contain human pathogens; exposure to blood and body fluids is minimized by using removable and disposable barriers (e.g., latex and vinyl gloves, protective eyewear, masks and gowns, and "sharps" containers).

stapes One of the three ossicles of the middle ear, resembling a tiny stirrup. It transmits sound vibrations from the incus to the internal ear.

steatorrhea Abnormal increase of fat in the feces.

stereognosis Faculty of perceiving and understanding the form and nature of objects by the sense of touch. Higher cortical integration is required to perform this function.

sternocleidomastoid muscles Symmetrical muscles of the neck extending from the upper sternum and proximal portion of the clavicle to the mastoid process of the temporal bone behind the ear.

strabismus Disparity in the anteroposterior axes of the eyes; the optic axes cannot be directed to the same object because of lack of muscular coordination.

stress incontinence Involuntary urination incurred by straining, coughing, or lifting.

stressor Stimulus perceived by the individual or the organism as challenging, threatening, or damaging.

stria (*pl.,* striae) (lineae albicantes) Atrophic line or streak that differs in texture and color from the surrounding skin because of disrupted elastic fibers of the reticular layer of the cutis.

striae gravidarum Atrophic, pinkish or purplish scarlike lesions observed on the breasts, thighs, abdomen, and buttocks during pregnancy; lesions later become silvery white.

stridor Abnormal, high-pitched respiratory sound caused by an obstruction in the trachea or larynx.

sty Inflammation of a sebaceous gland of the eyelid; also called hordeolum.

subculture Group of persons within a culture with one or more shared traits.

subluxation Partial discoloration.

sulcus Shallow groove, depression, or furrow on the surface of an organ, such as one that separates the convolutions of the cerebral hemisphere.

supination Assumption of the supine (lying down) position.

symmetry Similarity in size, shape, and position to the body part on the opposite side.

symptom Client's subjective perception of an alteration of bodily or mental function from basal conditions; change perceived by the individual.

synapse Joining; point of contact between two neurons or between a neuron and an effector organ, across which nerve impulses are transmitted through the action of a neurotransmitter, such as acetylcholine or norepinephrine.

syncope Fainting; temporary unconsciousness.

systolic (systole) The force of blood against the arterial wall during the ejection phase of the cardiac cycle, or contraction of the heart.

tachycardia Rapid heart rate (≥100 beats per minute). *Atrial flutter:* rapid, regular, uniform atrial contraction caused by AV block; ventricular rhythm varies with the degree of AV block. *Atrial tachycardia:* arrhythmia caused by the atria; rapid, regular beat of the entire heart. *Ventricular tachycardia:* arrhythmia caused by the ventricles; rapid, relatively regular heartbeat.

tachypnea Rapid respiratory rate.

tangential lighting Use of light shining from the side to create shadows over the area being examined; accentuates subtle differences in contour and movement.

taxonomy Framework for classifying and organizing information according to hierarchical categories.

telangiectasias Visible dilated capillaries located in skin.

temporal Of or limited by time.

temporal artery Artery on the head that runs anterior to the ear over the temporal bone and onto the forehead.

temporomandibular joint One of two joints connecting the mandible of the jaw to the temporal bone of the skull.

tenesmus Persistent, ineffectual spasms of the rectum accompanied by the desire to empty the bowel.

term infant Infant born between 37 and 41 weeks of gestation.

therapeutic relationship Relationship in which the focus of exchange is on the client and the client's needs.

therapeutic use of self Communication technique in which the use of personal qualities of the interviewer supports the client's perspective or feelings by finding a common connection. This technique can be especially helpful when the client's ethnicity, race, or socioeconomic status appear to be very different from that of the interviewer.

thrill Fine vibration accompanying turbulent blood flow in the heart or the great vessels. It is palpable when the examiner's fingers are placed over the site of the altered blood flow.

thrombophlebitis Inflammation of a vein, often accompanied by formation of a clot.

thrombus Aggregation of platelets, fibrin, clotting factors, and the cellular elements of the blood attached to the interior wall of a vein or artery that sometimes occludes the lumen of the vessel.

thyroid gland Endocrine gland at the front of the neck, consisting of bilateral lobes connected in the middle by a narrow isthmus. Secretes thyroxine, which is essential for growth and metabolic stability.

timbre The quality of a sound that distinguishes it from other sounds of the same pitch and volume.

tinnitus Sensation of noise in the ear caused by abnormal stimulation of the auditory apparatus or its afferent pathways; may be described as ringing, buzzing, swishing, roaring, blowing, or whistling.

tonic neck reflex Normal response in newborns to extend the arm and the leg on the side of the body to which the head is quickly turned while the infant is supine and to flex the

limbs of the opposite side. The reflex prevents the infant from rolling over until adequate neurological and motor development occurs and disappears by 3 to 4 months of age. At this time the reflex is replaced by symmetrical positioning of both sides of the body.

tophi Deposits of monosodium urate, associated with gout.

torticollis Abnormal condition in which the contraction of neck muscles causes the head to be inclined to one side. This condition may be congenital or acquired.

tragus Projection of the cartilage of the auricle at the opening of the external auditory meatus.

transient ischemic attack Occlusion of a central nervous system vessel that results in a focal neurological disturbance.

transillumination Passage of light through a solid or liquid substance.

trapezius muscles Symmetrical, large, flat triangular muscles of the shoulder and upper back. These muscles extend from the occipital bone, the ligamentum nuchae, and the spinous processes of the seventh cervical and all the thoracic vertebrae. They act to rotate the scapula, raise the shoulder, and abduct and flex the arm.

tremor Involuntary, somewhat rhythmic, oscillatory quivering of muscles caused by alternating contraction of opposing groups of muscles. *Cerebellar tremor:* occurs during intentional movement, becoming more pronounced near the end of the movement; associated with lesions of the dentate nucleus. *Coarse tremor:* slow and large-amplitude movements. *Essential (familial) tremor:* usually initially appears around age 50 with fine tremors of the hands; aggravated by intentional movement; commonly affects the head, jaws, lips, or voice. *Fine tremor:* rapid (10 to 20 oscillations/sec) and low-amplitude movements, usually in the fingers and hands. *Moderate tremor:* medium-rate and medium-amplitude movements. *Passive tremor:* present at rest; may improve during intentional movement (e.g., pill-rolling tremor or Parkinson's disease.) *Physiological tremor:* experienced by healthy people in fatigue, cold, and stress. *Toxic tremor:* caused by endogenous (thyrotoxicosis, uremia) or exogenous toxins (alcohol, drugs).

tricuspid valve Right atrioventricular valve.

trigeminal nerve (CN V) Cranial nerve that mediates sensation of the face. It has three branches: ophthalmic, maxillary, and mandibular.

trimester Period of 13 weeks.

trochanteric Pertaining to the two bony projections on the proximal end of the femur that serve as the attachment of various muscles.

trophoblast Peripheral cell layer of the blastocyst that attaches the fertilized ovum to the uterine wall and becomes the placenta and the membranes.

tropia Permanent deviation of the axis of an eye; strabismus.

tuberosity Elevation or protuberance, especially of a bone.

two-point discrimination Ability to sense the simultaneous stimulation of two areas of skin. Higher cortical integration is required to perform this function.

tympanic membrane Eardrum; membranous structure separating the external ear from the middle ear.

tympany Resonant sound produced over an air-filled region obtained by percussion.

ulnar deviation Turning the wrist away from the midline of the body.

umbo Landmark on the tympanic membrane created by the attachment of the membrane to the malleus.

upper motor neuron Long neurons with cell bodies in the motor portion of the cerebral cortex and axons that extend down the spinal cord, terminating at segmental levels of the spinal cord. They transmit impulses to lower motor neurons.

uvula Small cone-shaped process, suspended in the mouth from the middle of the posterior border of the soft palate.

valgus Deviation of an extremity outward, away from the midline. *Genu valgum:* condition in which the knees are abnormally close together; knock-knee.

validation Process of making sure the information or data collected is factual or true.

varicocele Distention of the veins of the spermatic cord.

varicose Dilated, distended, or bulging. This term is used particularly to describe a vein.

varus Deviation of an extremity toward the midline. *Genu varum:* condition in which the knees are abnormally separated; bowleg.

ventricle One of two muscular pumping chambers of the heart. The left ventricle pumps blood into the pulmonary artery.

ventricular fibrillation Cardiac arrhythmia marked by rapid, disorganized depolarizations of the ventricular myocardium.

ventricular tachycardia Tachycardia that usually originates in the ventricular Purkinje system.

vertigo Illusion of movement, with imagined rotation of oneself (*subjective vertigo*) or one's surrounding (*objective vertigo*).

vestibule Space or cavity that serves as the entrance to a passageway.

vital or cardinal signs Indicators of bodily function such as blood pressure, temperature, pulse, and respiration.

vitreous humor Transparent substance contained in the posterior chamber of the eye.

von Recklinghausen's disease Also known as neurofibromatosis, this congenital condition is characterized by fibrous tumors of the nerve tissue (neurofibromas), café-au-lait spots on the skin, and, in some cases, developmental anomalies of the muscles, bones, and viscera.

Weber test Test of bone conduction through the use of a tuning fork placed on the top of the skull or middle forehead. A normal result occurs when the client reports that the sound is heard equally in both ears. The sound lateralizes when hearing loss is present.

wheeze Form of rhonchus characterized by a high-pitched musical quality. Caused by a high-velocity flow of air through a narrowed airway, it is heard during both inspiration and expiration.

whispered pectoriloquy Increased resonance of the whispered voice as heard through a stethoscope in an area of consolidation.

xanthelasma Soft yellow spot or plaque that usually occurs in groups on the eyelids.

xeromammography Done with a xerographic plate instead of film.

xerostomia Dry mouth, usually caused by medications or radiation therapy.

xiphoid Lowest portion of the sternum; composed of bone and cartilage.

bibliography

Chapter 1

Alfaro R: *Application of nursing process: a step-by-step guide,* Philadelphia, 1986, JB Lippincott.

Engle GL: The need for a new medical model: a challenge for biomedicine, *Science* 196:129-196, 1970.

Gordon M: *Nursing diagnoses: process and application,* ed 3, St Louis, 1994, Mosby.

Gordon M: *Manual of nursing diagnosis 1997-1998,* St Louis, 1997, Mosby.

Maslow A: *Motivation and personality,* New York, 1970, Harper & Row.

Orem D: *Nursing: concepts of practice,* ed 5, St Louis, 1995, Mosby.

Rantz MJ, LeMone P: *Classification of nursing diagnoses: proceedings of the eleventh conference,* NANDA, Glendale, Calif, 1995, CINAHL Information Systems.

Sparks SM, Taylor SM: *Nursing diagnosis reference manual,* Springhouse, Pa, 1991, Springhouse.

Yura H, Walsh MB: *The nursing process: assessing, planning, implementing, and evaluating,* ed 5, New York, 1988, Appleton-Century-Crofts.

Chapter 2

Berlin EA, Fowkes WC: A teaching framework for cross-cultural health care, *West J Med* 139:934-938, 1983.

Long L: *Understanding/responding: a communication manual for nurses,* ed 2, Boston, 1992, Jones & Bartlett.

Kleinman A, Eisenberg L, Good B: Culture, illness, and care, *Ann Intern Med* 88:251-258, 1978.

Molde S: Understanding patient agendas, *Image J Nurs Sch* 18:145-147, 1986.

Putsch RW: Cross-cultural communication, *JAMA* 254:3344-3348, 1985.

Stuart GW, Sundeen SJ: *Principles and practice of psychiatric nursing,* ed 5, St Louis, 1995, Mosby.

Sundeen SJ et al: *Nurse-client interaction: implementing the nursing process,* ed 5, St Louis, 1994, Mosby.

Chapter 3

Bernstein L, Bernstein RS: *Interviewing: a guide for health professionals,* ed 4, Norwalk, Conn, 1985, Appleton-Century-Crofts.

Billings JA, Stoeckel JD: *The clinical encounter: a guide to the medical interview and case presentation,* St Louis, 1989, Mosby.

Cohen-Cole SA: *The medical interview: the three function approach,* St Louis, 1991, Mosby.

Crouch MA, Thiedke CC: Documentation of family health history in the outpatient medical record, *J Fam Pract* 22:169-174, 1986.

Fuller J, Schaller-Ayers J: *Health assessment: a nursing approach,* ed 2, Philadelphia, 1994, JB Lippincott.

Gordon M: *Nursing diagnosis: process and application,* ed 3, St Louis, 1994, Mosby.

Kraytman M: *The complete patient history,* ed 2, New York, 1991, McGraw-Hill.

Lipson LG, Dibble SL, Minarik PA: *Culture and nursing care: a pocket guide,* San Francisco, 1996, UCSF Nursing Press.

Mosby's medical, nursing, and allied health dictionary, ed 4, St Louis, 1994, Mosby.

Pagana KD, Pagana TJ: *Mosby's diagnostic and laboratory test reference,* ed 3, St Louis, 1997, Mosby.

Roter DL, Hall JA: Physicians' interviewing styles and medical information obtained from patients, *J Gen Intern Med* 2:325-329, 1987.

Sherwood MJ et al: *Determining nursing diagnosis through assessment,* Baltimore, 1988, Williams & Wilkins.

Smith RC: *The patient's story: integrated patient-doctor interviewing,* Boston, 1996, Little, Brown.

US Preventive Services Task Force: *Guide to clinical preventive services,* ed 2, Alexandria, Va, 1996, International Medical Publishing.

Wasson J et al: *The common symptom guide,* ed 4, New York, 1996, McGraw-Hill.

Wong DL: *Whaley and Wong's nursing care of infants and children,* ed 5, St Louis, 1995, Mosby.

Chapter 4

Berk LE: *Child development,* ed 2, Boston, 1991, Allyn & Bacon.

Blair KA: Aging: physiological aspects and clinical implications, *Nurse Pract* 15(2):14-28, 1990.

Comfort A: *A good old age,* New York, 1976, Crown.

Duvall E, Miller B: *Marriage and family development,* ed 6, New York, 1984, Harper & Row.

Erikson EH: *Childhood and society,* ed 2, New York, 1963, WW Norton.

Erikson EH: *Identity: youth and crisis,* New York, 1968, WW Norton.

Erikson EH: *Adulthood,* New York, 1978, WW Norton.

Foster RLR et al: *Family-centered nursing care of children,* Philadelphia, 1989, WB Saunders.

Frankenburg WK, Camp BW, editors: *Pediatric screening tests,* Springfield, Ill, 1975, Charles C Thomas.

Frankenburg WK, Dodds JB: The Denver Developmental Screening Test, *J Pediatr* 71:181-191, 1967.

Gilligan C: *In a different voice, psychological theory and women's development,* Cambridge, Mass, 1982, Harvard University Press.

Hall CS, Nordby VJ: *A primer Jungian psychology,* New York, 1973, New American Library.

Havinghurst R: *Human development and education,* St Louis, 1953, Warren H Green.

Holmes TH, Rahe RH: The social readjustment rating scale, *J Psychosom Res* 11:213-218, 1967.

Jones DA et al: *Health assessment across the life span,* New York, 1984, McGraw-Hill.

Kimmel DC: *Adulthood and aging: an interdisciplinary development view,* ed 3, New York, 1989, John Wiley & Sons.

Levinson DJ et al: *The seasons of a man's life,* New York, 1979, Ballantine.

Marlow DR, Redding BA: *Textbook of pediatric nursing,* ed 6, Philadelphia, 1988, WB Saunders.

Murray RB, Zentner JP: *Nursing assessment and health promotion strategies through the life span,* ed 4, Norwalk, Conn, 1989, Appleton & Lange.

Piaget J: *The construction of reality in the child,* New York, 1975, Ballantine.

Rahe RH: Epidemiological studies of life changes and illness, *Int J Psychiatry Med* 6(1-2):133-146, 1975.

Sarason IG, Johnson JH, Siegel JM: Assessing the impact of life changes: development of the life experiences survey, *J Consult Clin Psychol* 46:932-946, 1978.

Schuster CS, Ashburn SS: *The process of human development: a holistic life span approach,* ed 3, Philadelphia, 1992, JB Lippincott.

Sheehy G: *The silent passage: menopause,* New York, 1991, Random House.

Sheehy G: *New passages,* New York, 1995, EP Dutton.

Stein M: *In midlife: a Jungian perspective,* Dallas, 1983, Spring Publications.

Stevenson JS: *Issues and crises during middlescence,* New York, 1977, Appleton-Century-Crofts.

Wadsworth B: *Piaget's theory of cognitive and affective development,* ed 3, White Plains, NY, 1988, Longman.

Wong DL: *Whaley and Wong's nursing care of infants and children,* ed 5, St Louis, 1995, Mosby.

Chapter 5

American Dietetic Association: Position of the American Dietetic Association: nutrition, aging, and the continuum of health care, *J Am Diet Assoc* 93:80-82, 1993.

Charuhas PM: Nutrition support of the cancer patient, *RD* 10:1-12, 1990.

Chumlea WMC, Guo SS, Steinbaugh ML: Prediction of stature from knee height for black and white adults and children with application to mobility-impaired or handicapped persons, *J Am Diet Assoc* 94:1385-1391, 1994.

Council on Practice Quality Management Committee, American Dietetic Association: Identifying patients at risk: ADA's definitions for nutrition screening and nutrition assessment, *J Am Diet Assoc* 94:838-839, 1994.

Daly LE, et al: Folate levels and neural tube defects, *JAMA* 274:1698-1702, 1995.

Detsky AS, Smalley PS, Chang J: Is this patient malnourished? *JAMA* 271:54-58, 1994.

Dwyer JT: Health aspects of vegetarian diets, *Am J Clin Nutr* 48(3 suppl):712-738, 1988.

Elmore MF et al: Developing an effective adult nutrition screening tool for a community hospital, *J Am Diet Assoc* 94:1113-1118, 1121, 1994.

Ernst ND, Obarzanek E: Child health and nutrition: obesity and high blood cholesterol, *Prev Med* 23:427-436, 1994.

Expert Panel: Summary of the second report of the National Cholesterol Education (NCEP) Expert Panel on detection, evaluation, and treatment of high blood cholesterol in adults (Adult Treatment Panel II), *JAMA* 269:3015-3023, 1993.

Foltz NO, Schiller MR, Ryan AS: Nutrition screening and assessment: current practices and dietitians' leadership roles, *J Am Diet Assoc* 93:1388-1395, 1993.

Gregory RP, Davis DL: Use of carbohydrate counting for meal planning in type I diabetes, *Diabetes Educ* 20:406-409, 1994.

Heitmann BL, Lissner L: Dietary underreporting by obese individuals—is it specific or nonspecific? *BMJ* 311:986-989, 1995.

Heymsfield SB, Tighe A, Wang ZM: Nutritional assessment by anthropometric and biochemical methods. In Shils ME, Olson JA, Shike M: *Modern nutrition in health and disease,* ed 8, Philadelphia, 1994, Lea & Febiger.

Jenkins DJA et al: Glycemic index of foods: a physiological basis for carbohydrate exchange, *Am J Clin Nutr* 34:362-366, 1981.

Joy EA, Donnell C, Husu K: Outpatient management of disordered eating, *Your Patient and Fitness* 9(2):21-24, 1995.

Kouba J: Nutritional care of the individual with cancer, *Nutr Clin Pract* 3:175-182, 1988.

Kushner RF et al: National Coordinating Committee clinical indicators of nutrition care, *J Am Diet Assoc* 94:1168-1177, 1994.

Lissner L, Nelson Steen S, Brownell K: Weight reduction diets and health promotion, *Am J Prev Med* 8:154-158, 1992.

Nutrition recommendations and principles for people with diabetes mellitus, *Diabetes Care* 17:519-522, 1994 (position statement).

The Nutrition Screening Initiative: *Report of nutrition screening,* vol 1, *Toward a common view,* Washington, DC, 1991, The Nutrition Screening Initiative.

Nutritionist IV Diet Analysis and Nutrition Evaluation: N-Squared Computing, 3040 Commercial Street SE, Salem, Ore, 1993.

Pennington JAT: *Bowes and Church's food values of portions commonly used,* ed 15, New York, 1989, HarperCollins.

Scandanavian Simvastatin Survival Study Group: Randomised trial of cholesterol lowering in 4444 patients with coronary heart disease: the Scandanavian Simvastatin Survival Study (4S), *Lancet* 344:1383-1389, 1994.

Tarnopolsky MA: Protein, caffeine, and sports, *Physician Sportsmed* 21:137-149, 1993.

Underbakke G: Computer applications in clinical nutrition. In Kaud FA, editor: *Effective computer management in food and nutrition services,* Gaithersburg, Md, 1989, Aspen.

US Preventive Services Task Force: *Guide to clinical preventive services,* ed 2, Alexandria, Va, 1996, International Medical Publishing.

Wright HS et al: The 1987-88 Nationwide Food Consumption Survey: an update on the nutrient intake of respondents, *Nutr Today* 26:21-27, 1991.

Chapter 6

Bliwise DL, Benkert RE, Ingham RH: Factors associated with nightly variability in sleep-disordered breathing in the elderly, *Chest* 100(4):973-976, 1991.

Feinsilver SH: Recognizing and treating the sleep apnea syndromes, *Emerg Med* 19(11):147-159, 1987.

Goothe B: Recognizing sleep apnea syndrome, *Respir Manage* 17(1):27-30, 1987.

Gordon M: *Manual of nursing diagnosis,* 1997-1998, St Louis, 1997, Mosby.

Guilleminault C: *Sleep and its disorders in children,* New York, 1987, Raven Press.

Jaquis J: Obstructive sleep apnea syndrome, *Nurse Pract* 12(6):50-56, 1987.

Kryger MH, Roth T, Dement WC: *Principles and practice of sleep medicine,* ed 2, Philadelphia, 1994, WB Saunders.

Martin RJ: *Cardiorespiratory disorders during sleep,* ed 2, Mount Kisco, NY, 1990, Futura Publishing.

Mendelson WB: *Human sleep: research and clinical care,* New York, 1987, Plenum Publishing.

Reite ML, Nagel KE, Ruddy JR: *Concise guide to the evaluation and management of sleep disorders,* Washington, DC, 1990, American Psychiatric Press.

Williams RL, editor: *Sleep disorders: diagnosis and treatment,* ed 2, New York, 1988, John Wiley & Sons.

Chapter 7

AAN Expert Panel on Culturally Competent Nursing Care: AAN expert panel report: culturally competent health care, *Nurs Outlook* 40:277-283, 1992.

American Nurses Association: *Cultural diversity in the nursing curriculum: a guide for implementation* (ANA No G-171:11), Kansas City, Mo, 1986, American Nurses Association.

Andrews MM, Bouyle JS: *Transcultural concepts in nursing care,* ed 2, Boston, 1995, Little, Brown.

Barker JC: Cultural diversity—changing the context of medical practice in cross-cultural medicine—a decade later, *East J Med* 157 (special issue): 248-254, 1992.

Buchwald D et al: Caring for patients in a multicultural society, *Patient Care* 28(11):105-120, 1994.

DeSantis L, Thomas JT: Health education and the immigrant Haitian mother: cultural insights for community health nurses, *Public Health Nurs* 9:87-96, 1992.

Fuchs VR, Hahn JS: How does Canada do it? A comparison of expenditures for physicians' services in the United States and Canada, *N Engl J Med* 323:884-890, 1990.

Giger JN, Davidhizar RE: *Transcultural nursing: assessment and intervention,* ed 2, St Louis, 1995, Mosby.

Hartog J, Hartog EA: Cultural aspects of health and illness behavior in hospitals, *West J Med* 139:911-916, 1983.

Hautman MA: Folk health and illness beliefs, *Nurse Pract* 4:4, 1979.

Health Resources and Service Administration: *Health status of minorities and low income groups,* DHHS Pub No HRS-P-DV 85-1, Washington, DC, 1985, US Government Printing Office.

Helman C: *Culture, health and illness,* ed 2, London, 1990, John Wright & Sons.

Henderson G, Primeaux M: *Transcultural health care,* Menlo Park, Calif, 1981, Addison-Wesley.

Kleinman A, Eisenberg L, Good B: Culture, illness and care: clinical lessons from anthropologic and cross-cultural research, *Ann Intern Med* 88:251-258, 1978.

Kluckhohn F: Dominant and variant value orientations. In Brink PJ, editor: *Transcultural nursing: a book of readings,* Englewood Cliffs, NJ, 1976, Prentice Hall.

Krause N, Goldenhar LM: Acculturation and psychological distress in three groups of elderly Hispanics, *J Gerontol* 47:S279-S288, 1992.

Leininger MM: *Transcultural nursing: concepts, theories and practices,* New York, 1978, John Wiley & Sons.

Lipson JG, Dibble SL, Minarik PA: *Culture and nursing care: a pocket guide,* San Francisco, 1996, USCF Nursing Press.

Martin MM, Henry M: Cultural relativity and poverty, *Public Health Nurs* 6:28-34, 1989.

Morse JM, Young DE, Swartz L: Cree Indian healing practices and Western health care: a comparative analysis. *Soc Sci Med* 32:1361-1366, 1991.

National Center for Health Statistics, *Prevention profile, Health United States,* 1991, Hyattsville, Md, 1992, Public Health Service.

Olness K: Cultural issues in primary pediatric care. In Hoekelman RA et al: *Primary pediatric care,* ed 2, St Louis, 1992, Mosby.

Overfield T: Biological variation: concepts from physical anthropology. In Henderson G, Primeaux M, editors: *Transcultural health care,* Menlo Park, Calif, 1981, Addison-Wesley.

Rauh VA, Wasserman GA, Brunelli SA: Determinants of maternal child-rearing attitudes, *J Am Acad Child Adolesc Psychiatry* 29:375-381, 1990.

Rogler LH, Cortes DE, Malgady RG: Acculturation and mental health status among Hispanics, *Am Psychol* 46:585-605, 1991.

Smith LS: Ethnic differences in knowledge of sexually transmitted diseases in North American Black and Mexican-American migrant farmworkers, *Res Nurs Health* 11:51-58, 1988.

Snow LF: Folk medical beliefs and their implications for the care of patients: a review based on studies of black Americans. In Henderson G, Primeaux M, editors: *Transcultural health care,* Menlo Park, Calif, 1981, Addison-Wesley.

Snow LF, Johnson SM: Folklore, food, female reproductive cycle, *Ecol Food Nutr* 7:41-49, 1978.

Spector R: *Cultural diversity in health and illness,* ed 4, Norwalk, Conn, 1996, Appleton & Lange.

Starn JR: Family culture and chronic conditions. In Jackson PL, Vessey JA: *Primary care of the child with a chronic condition,* ed 2, St Louis, 1996, Mosby.

Stulc DM: The family as bearer of culture. In Cookfair JN, editor: *Nursing process and practice in the community,* St Louis, 1991, Mosby.

Syme SL: Social determinants of disease, *Ann Clin Res* 19:44-52, 1987.

Thierderman SB: Ethnocentrism: a barrier to effective health care, *Nurse Pract* 11:53-59, 1986.

Tripp-Reimer T: Cultural assessment. In Bellack J, Edlund B, editors: *Nursing assessment and diagnosis,* Boston, 1992, Jones & Bartlett.

Tripp-Reimer T, Brink PJ, Saunders JM: Cultural assessment: content and process, *Nurs Outlook* 32:78-82, 1984.

US Bureau of the Census: *Statistical abstract of the United States: 1992,* ed 112, Washington, DC, 1992, US Government Printing Office.

US Department of Health and Human Services, Public Health Service: *Healthy people 2000: national health promotion and disease prevention objectives,* 1990, DHHS Pub No 91-50213, Washington, DC.

Villarruel AM, Ortiz de Montellano B: Culture and pain: a Meso-American perspective, *Adv Nurs Sci* 15:21-32, 1992.

Wong DL: *Whaley and Wong's nursing care of infants and children,* ed 5, St Louis, 1995, Mosby.

Zborowski M: Cultural components in response to pain, *Soc Issues* 8:16-30, 1952.

Zborowski M: *People in pain,* San Francisco, 1969, Jossey-Bass.

Zola IK: Culture and symptoms: an analysis of patients presenting complaints, *Am Soc Rev* 31:615-630, 1966.

Chapter 8

Breslow L, Somers AR: The lifetime health monitoring program: a practical approach to preventive medicine, *N Engl J Med* 296:601, 1977.

King C: Refining your assessment techniques, *RN* 46:42-47, 1983.

Kozier B, Erb G, Blais K: *Fundamentals of nursing: concepts, process and practice,* ed 5, Menlo Park, Calif, 1995, Addison-Wesley.

Leavell HR, Clark EG: *Preventive medicine for the doctor in his community,* ed 3, New York, 1965, McGraw-Hill.

Talbot L, Marquardt M: *Pocket guide to critical care assessment,* ed 3, St Louis, 1997, Mosby.

US Preventive Services Task Force: *Guide to clinical preventive services,* ed 2, Alexandria, Va, 1996, International Medical Publishing.

Chapter 9

American Heart Association: *Heart and stroke facts,* 1996 statistical supplement, Dallas, 1995, The Association.

American Heart Association of Wisconsin: *Blood pressure education program instructor's manual,* Milwaukee, 1996, The Association.

Carnoni-Huntley, LaCroix AZ, Havlik RJ: Race and sex differentials in the impact of hypertension in the United States, *Arch Intern Med* 149:780, 1989.

Centers for Disease Control: Recommendations for prevention of HIV transmission in health-care settings, *MMWR* (suppl 36):SS, Aug 1987.

Fever and tympanic thermometry: a symposium, *Clin Pediatr* (suppl):30, 1991.

Gelfand JA, Dinarello CA, Wolff SM: Alteration in body temperature. In Isselbacher KJ et al, editors: *Harrison's principles of internal medicine,* vol 1, ed 13, New York, 1994, McGraw-Hill.

Gordon M: *Manual of nursing diagnosis 1997-1998,* St Louis, 1997, Mosby.

Guyton AC: *Textbook of medical physiology,* ed 9, Philadelphia, 1995, WB Saunders.

Hill MN, Grim CM: How to take a precise blood pressure, *Am J Nurs* 91:38, 1991.

Joint National Committee on Detection, Evaluation, and Treatment of High Blood Pressure: *The fifth report of the Joint National Committee on detection, evaluation, and treatment of high blood pressure,* NIH Pub No 93-1088, Bethesda, Md, 1993, National Institutes of Health.

Magee DJ: *Orthopedic physical assessment,* ed 2, Philadelphia, 1992, WB Saunders.

Mountcastle VB: *Medical physiology,* vol 2, ed 14, St Louis, 1980, Mosby.

National High Blood Pressure Education Program Working Group on Hypertension Control in Children and Adolescents: Update on the 1987 Task Force Report on High Blood Pressure in Children and Adolescents, *Pediatrics* 98(4):649-658, 1996.

Summers S: Axillary, tympanic and esophageal temperature measurement: descriptive comparisons in postanesthesia patients, *J Post Anesth Nurs* 6:420, 1991.

Thibodeau GA, Patton KT: *Anatomy and physiology,* ed 3, St Louis, 1996, Mosby.

Timby BK, Lewis LW: *Fundamental skills and concepts in patient care,* ed 6, New York, 1996, JB Lippincott.

Wong DL: *Whaley and Wong's nursing care of infants and children,* ed 5, St Louis, 1995, Mosby.

Chapter 10

Archer CB, Robertson SJ: *Black and white skin diseases,* Cambridge, Mass, 1995, Blackwell Science.

Daniel CR et al: Don't overlook skin surveillance, *Patient Care* 30(11):90-107, 1996.

Fitzpatrick TB et al: *Dermatology in general medicine,* ed 4, New York, 1993, McGraw-Hill.

Gaskin F: Detection of cyanosis in the person with dark skin, *J Natl Black Nurses Assoc* 1(1):52-60, 1986.

Gordon M: *Nursing diagnosis: process and application,* ed 3, St Louis, 1994, Mosby.

Habif TP: *Clinical dermatology: a color guide to diagnosis and therapy,* ed 3, St Louis, 1996, Mosby.

Kopf AW et al: Techniques of cutaneous examination for detection of skin cancer, *Cancer* 75(suppl 2):684-690, 1995.

Lawrence CM, Cox NH: *Physical signs in dermatology,* London, 1993, Mosby-Wolfe.

The NIH Consensus Development Panel on Melanoma: Diagnosis and treatment of early melanoma, *JAMA* 268:1314-1319, 1992.

Pariser RJ, editor: Diagnostic and therapeutic techniques for evaluation and treatment of skin disorders, *Primary Care* 16(3):823-846, 1989.

Samman PD: *The nails in disease,* ed 4, London, 1986, William Heinemann Medical Books.

Sauer GC: *Manual of skin diseases,* ed 7, Philadelphia, 1996, JB Lippincott.

Sawaya ME, Stough DB: Untangling misconceptions about hair, *Patient Care,* pp 193-213, May 15, 1992.

US Preventive Services Task Force: *Guide to clinical preventive services,* ed 2, Alexandria, Va, 1996, International Medical Publishing.

Chapter 11

Abrams DI, Foon KA, Gold JWM: Lymphadenopathy: a diagnostic plan, *Patient Care* 4(30):94-112, 1988.

Carpenter DR, Hudacek S: Polymyalgia rheumatica: a comprehensive review of this debilitating disease, *Nurse Pract* 19(6):50-58, 1994.

Cummings C et al: Age: a clue in neck mass diagnosis, *Patient Care* 24(1):38-47, 1990.

DeGroot LJ et al: *The thyroid and its diseases,* ed 5, New York, 1994, John Wiley & Sons.

Derman H: Migraine headache: precision in diagnosis and improved therapeutic prospects, *Consultant* 31(5):57-63, 1991.

Diamond S, Dalessio DJ, editors: *The practicing physician's approach to headache,* ed 4, Baltimore, 1986, Williams & Wilkins.

Giger JN, Davidhizar RE: *Transcultural nursing,* ed 2, St Louis, 1995, Mosby.

Gilbert R, Warfield C: Evaluating and treating the patient with neck pain, *Hosp Pract* 22(8):223-232, 1987.

Gordon M: *Manual of nursing diagnosis 1997-1998,* St Louis, 1997, Mosby.

Haase GR et al: When facial pain is the problem, *Patient Care* 24(12):119-124, 1990.

Heitman R, Irizarry A: Hypothyroidism: common complaints, perplexing diagnosis, *Nurse Pract* 20(3):54-60, 1995.

Peatfield R: *Headache,* Berlin, 1986, Springer-Verlag.

Purath J: Assessing headache pain, *RN* 54(10):26-31, 1991.

Schleper J: Prevention, detection and diagnosis of head and neck cancers, *Semin Oncol Nurs* 5(3):139-149, 1989.

Schneiderman H, Garibaldi RA: Physical examination of HIV-infected patients: head and neck, eyes, mouth and throat, and lymph nodes, *Consultant* 30(1):45-51, 1990.

Smith LS: Evaluation and management of the muscle contraction headache, *Nurse Pract* 13(1):20-27, 1988.

Thompson JM et al: *Mosby's clinical nursing,* ed 4, St Louis, 1997, Mosby.

US Preventive Services Task Force: *Guide to clinical preventive services,* ed 2, Alexandria, Va, 1996, International Medical Publishing.

Weiss J: Assessment and management of the client with headaches, *Nurse Pract* 18(4):44-57, 1993.

Whitney CM: New headache classification: implications for neuroscience nurses, *Neurosci Nurs* 22(6):385-388, 1990.

Wollenberg SP: Primary care diagnosis and management of Bell's palsy, *Nurse Pract* 14(12):14-18, 1989.

Yeomans AC: Assessment and management of hypothyroidism, *Nurse Pract* 15(1):8-15, 1990.

Chapter 12

Apple DJ, Rabb MF: *Ocular pathology: clinical applications and self-assessment,* ed 4, St Louis, 1991, Mosby.

Arffa RC: *Grayson's diseases of the cornea,* ed 3, St Louis, 1991, Mosby.

Boyd-Monk H: Assessing acquired ocular diseases, *Nurs Clin North Am* 25(4):811-822, 1990.

Gordon M: *Manual of nursing diagnosis 1997-1998,* St Louis, 1997, Mosby.

Harrington DO, Drake MV: *The visual fields: text and atlas of clinical perimetry,* ed 6, St Louis, 1990, Mosby.

Hoskins HD, Kass MA: *Becker-Shaffer's diagnosis and therapy of the glaucomas,* ed 6, St Louis, 1989, Mosby.

Jones M, Tippett T: Assessment of the red eye, *Nurse Pract* 5: 10-15, Jan-Feb 1980.

Lawlor MC: Common ocular injuries and disorders. 2. Red eye, *J Emerg Nurs* 15(1):36-41, 1989.

Newell FW: *Ophthalmology: principles and concepts,* ed 8, St Louis, 1996, Mosby.

Sapira JD, Schneiderman H: The funduscopic examination: how to make the most of it, *Consultant* 30(6):22-27, 1990.

Schneiderman H, Garibaldi RA: Physical examination of HIV-infected patients: head and neck, eyes, mouth and throat, and lymph nodes, *Consultant* 30(1):42-51, 1990.

Small RG: Red eye: five steps toward a differential diagnosis, *Consultant* 31(7):29-32, 1991.

Chapter 13

Bates B: *A guide to physical examination and history taking,* ed 6, Philadelphia, 1995, JB Lippincott.

Gordon M: *Manual of nursing diagnosis 1997-1998,* St Louis, 1997, Mosby.

Koufman JA: *Core otolaryngology,* Philadelphia, 1990, JB Lippincott.

Lee KJ: *Textbook of otolaryngology and head and neck surgery,* New York, 1989, Elsevier.

Netter FH: *CIBA collection of medical illustrations,* vol 3, *Digestive system,* part I, *Upper digestive tract,* Summit, NJ, CIBA Medical Education Div. 1983.

Potter PA, Perry AG: *Basic nursing: theory and practice,* ed 3, St Louis, 1995, Mosby.

Riley MAK: *Nursing care of the client with ear, nose and throat disorders,* New York, 1987, Springer.

Schuller DE: *DeWeese and Saunders' otolaryngology—head and neck surgery,* ed 8, St Louis, 1994, Mosby.

Seidel HM et al: *Mosby's guide to physical examination,* ed 3, St Louis, 1995, Mosby.

Serra AM: *Ear, nose and throat nursing,* Cambridge, Mass, 1986, Blackwell Science.

Chapter 14

Annonier C: *Female breast examination,* Berlin, 1986, Springer-Verlag.

Baines CJ: Breast self-examination, *Cancer Suppl* 69:1942, 1992.

Baines CJ, Miller AB, Bassett AA: Physical examination: its role as a single screening modality in the Canadian National Breast Screening Study, *Cancer Suppl* 63:1816, 1992.

Barth V, Prechtel K, Heywang SH: *Atlas of breast diseases,* Philadelphia, 1991, BC Decker.

Blackwell RE, Grotting JC: *Diagnosis and management of breast disease,* Cambridge, Mass, 1996, Blackwell Science.

Bland KI, Copeland EM: *The breast: comprehensive management of benign and malignant diseases,* Philadelphia, 1991, WB Saunders.

Bondy ML et al: Validation of a breast cancer risk assessment model in women with a positive family history, *J Natl Cancer Inst* 86(8):620-625, 1994.

Champion V: Role of breast self-examination in breast cancer screening, *Cancer Suppl* 69:1985, 1992.

Denton S, editor: *Breast cancer nursing,* San Diego, 1995, Singular Publishing.

Dodd GD: American Cancer Society guidelines on screening for breast cancer, *Cancer Suppl* 69:1885, 1992.

Donegan WL, Spratt JS, editors: *Cancer of the breast,* ed 4, Philadelphia, 1995, WB Saunders.

Foster RS et al: Clinical breast examination and breast self examination, *Cancer Suppl* 69, 1992.

Gordon M: *Nursing diagnosis: process and application,* ed 3, St Louis, 1994, Mosby.

Hindle WH: *Breast disease for gynecologists,* Norwalk, Conn, 1990, Appleton & Lange.

Hughes LE, Mansel RE, Webster DJT: *Benign disorders and diseases of the breast,* London, 1989, Baillière Tindall.

Isaacs JH: *Textbook of breast disease,* St Louis, 1992, Mosby.

Johnson ET: *Breast cancer, black women,* Montgomery, Ala, 1993, Van Slyke & Bray.

Judkins AF, Boutwell WB: A model program for teaching nurses breast examination and cancer screening, *J Contin Educ Nurs* 22(6):233-236, 1991.

Leucht W: *Teaching atlas of breast ultrasound,* ed 2, Stuttgart, 1992, Georg Thieme Verlag.

Love SM: *Dr. Susan Love's breast book,* ed 2, Reading, Mass, 1995, Addison-Wesley.

Mettlin C: Breast cancer risk factors, *Cancer Suppl* 69:1904, 1992.

Mitchell GW, Bassett LW: *The female breast and its disorders,* Baltimore, 1990, Williams & Wilkins.

Pagana KD, Pagana TJ: *Mosby's diagnostic and laboratory test reference,* ed 3, St Louis, 1997, Mosby.

Smallwood JA, Taylor I: *Benign breast diseases,* Baltimore, 1990, Urban & Schwarzenberg.

Stoll BA, editor: *Reducing breast cancer risk in women,* Boston, 1995, Kluwer Academic Publishers.

US Department of Health and Human Services: *Healthy people 2000,* Washington, DC, 1991, DHHS.

US Preventive Services Task Force: *Guide to clinical preventive services,* ed 2, Alexandria, Va, 1996, International Medical Publishing.

Chapter 15

Burton GG, Hodgkin JE, Ward JJ: *Respiratory care: a guide to clinical practice,* ed 4, Philadelphia, 1997, JB Lippincott.

Cotes JE: *Lung function: assessment and application in medicine,* ed 5, Oxford, 1993, Blackwell Science.

Dettenmeier PA: *Pulmonary nursing care,* St Louis, 1992, Mosby.

George RB et al: *Chest medicine: essentials of pulmonary and critical care medicine,* ed 3, Baltimore, 1995, Williams & Wilkins.

Gordon M: *Nursing diagnosis: process and application,* ed 3, St Louis, 1994, Mosby.

Loudon RG: The lung exam, *Clin Chest Med* 8:265-272, 1987.

Martin L: *Pulmonary physiology in clinical practice: the essentials for patient care and evaluation,* St Louis, 1987, Mosby.

Mitchell RS, Petty TL, Schwarz MI: *Synopsis of clinical pulmonary disease,* ed 4, St Louis, 1989, Mosby.

Mosby's medical, nursing, and allied health dictionary, ed 4, St Louis, 1994, Mosby.

Nunn JF: *Applied respiratory physiology,* ed 3, Oxford, 1993, Butterworth-Heineman.

Op't Holt TB: *Assessment-based respiratory care,* New York, 1986, John Wiley & Sons.

Pagana KD, Pagana TJ: *Mosby's diagnostic and laboratory test reference,* ed 3, St Louis, 1997, Mosby.

Providing respiratory care, Springhouse, Pa, 1996, Springhouse.

Ruppel GE: *Manual of pulmonary function testing,* ed 6, St Louis, 1995, Mosby.

US Preventive Services Task Force: *Guide to clinical preventive services,* ed 2, Alexandria, Va, International Medical Publishing.

Weinberger SE: *Principles of pulmonary medicine,* ed 2, Philadelphia, 1992, WB Saunders.

Wilby ML: *Delmar's instant nursing assessment: respiratory,* Albany, NY, 1996, Delmar.

Wilkins RL, Hodgkin JE, Lopez B: *Lung sounds: practical guide,* ed 2, St Louis, 1996, Mosby.

Wilkins RL, Krider SJ, Sheldon RL: *Clinical assessment in respiratory care,* ed 3, St Louis, 1994, Mosby.

Witkowski AS: *Pulmonary assessment: a clinical guideline,* Philadelphia, 1985, JB Lippincott.

Chapter 16

Adolph RJ: The value of bedside examination in an era of high technology, part 1, *Heart Dis Stroke* 3(3):128-131, 1994.

Baker JD: Assessment of peripheral arterial occlusive disease, *Crit Care Nurs Clin North Am* 3(3):493-498, 1991.

Blank CA, Irwin GH: Peripheral vascular disorders: assessment and intervention, *Nurs Clin North Am* 25(4):777-793, 1990.

Braunwald E, editor: *Heart disease: a textbook of cardiovascular medicine,* ed 5, Philadelphia, 1996, WB Saunders.

Bright LD, Georgi S: Peripheral vascular disease: is it arterial or venous? *Am J Nurs* 92(9):34-43, 1992.

Butman SM et al: Bedside cardiovascular examination in patients with severe chronic heart failure: importance of rest or inducible jugular venous distension, *J Am College Cardiol* 22(4):968-974, 1993.

Davis E: The diagnostic puzzle and management challenge of Raynaud's syndrome, *Nurse Pract* 18(3):18-20, 1993.

DeLeon AC: Fine-tuning the examination of the heart, *Consultant* 29(4):51-61, 1989.

Epstein DE: Changing interpretations of angina pectoris associated with transient myocardial ischemia, *J Cardiovasc Nurs* 7(1):1-13, 1992.

Erickson B: *Heart sounds and murmurs: a practical guide,* ed 3, St Louis, 1997, Mosby.

Fabius DB: Solving the mystery of heart murmurs, *Nursing 94* 24(7):39-44, 1994.

Fabius DB: Uncovering the secrets of snaps, rubs, & clicks, *Nursing 94* 24(7):45-50, 1994.

Fellows E, Jocz AM: Getting the upper hand on lower extremity arterial disease, *Nursing 91* 21(8):34-41, 1991.

Gehring P: Vascular assessment, *RN* 55(1):40-47, 1992.

Gersony WM: Coarctation of the aorta, *Hosp Med* 27(5):53-63, 1991.

Herr KA: Night leg pain in the elderly, *Geriatr Nurs* 13(1):13-16, 1992.

Jessup M et al: CHF in the elderly: is it different? *Patient Care* 26(14):40-61, 1992.

Meyers DG: Review of cardiac auscultation, (part 1), *Hosp Med* 29(10):25-52, 1993.

Notowitz LB: Normal venous anatomy and physiology of the lower extremity, *J Vasc Nurs* 11(2):39-42, 1993.

Recognizing valvular heart disease, *Emerg Med* 22(7):56-71, 1990.

Thompson JM, Wilson SF: *Health assessment for nursing practice,* St Louis, 1996, Mosby.

Tilkian AG, Conover MB: *Understanding heart sounds and murmurs,* ed 3, Philadelphia, 1993, WB Saunders.

US Preventive Services Task Force: *Guide to clinical preventive services,* ed 2, Alexandria, Va, 1996, International Medical Publishing.

Whitaker L, Kelleher A: Raynaud's syndrome: diagnosis and treatment, *J Vasc Nurs* 12(1):10-13, 1994.

Wong DL: *Whaley and Wong's nursing care of infants and children,* ed 5, St Louis, 1995, Mosby.

Yacone-Morton L: Cardiac assessment, *RN* 54(12):28-35, 1991.

Chapter 17

Bowers AC, Thompson JM: *Clinical manual of health assessment,* ed 4, St Louis, 1992, Mosby.

Centers for Disease Control: Hepatitis B virus: a comprehensive strategy for eliminating transmission in the United States through universal childhood vaccination—recommendations of the Immunization Practices Advisory Committee (ACIP), *MMWR* 40 (No RR-13), 1991.

Christensen J: *Bedside logic in diagnostic gastroenterology,* New York, 1987, Churchill Livingstone.

Gordon M: *Nursing diagnosis: process and application,* ed 3, St Louis, 1994, Mosby.

Johnson LR: *Gastrointestinal physiology,* ed 5, St Louis, 1997, Mosby.

Reece SM: Immunization strategies for the elimination of hepatitis B, *Nurse Pract* 18:42-50, 1993.

Seidel HM et al: *Mosby's guide to physical examination,* ed 3, St Louis, 1995, Mosby.

Thompson JM et al: *Mosby's clinical nursing,* ed 4, St Louis, 1997, Mosby.

US Preventive Services Task Force: *Guide to clinical preventive services,* ed 2, Alexandria, Va, 1996, International Medical Publishing.

Chapter 18

American Academy of Orthopaedic Surgeons: *Joint motion: method of measuring and recording,* Chicago, 1965, The Academy.

Ausenhus MK: Osteoporosis: prevention during the adolescent and young adult years, *Nurse Pract* 13:19-24, 1988.

Beetham W, Polley H: *Rheumatologic interviewing and physical examination of the joints,* ed 2, Philadelphia, 1978, WB Saunders.

Collo MC et al: Evaluating arthritic complaints, *Nurse Pract* 16:9-20, 1991.

Daniels L, Worthingham C: *Muscle testing: techniques of manual examination,* ed 5, Philadelphia, 1986, WB Saunders.

Gordon M: *Nursing diagnosis: process and application,* ed 3, St Louis, 1994, Mosby.

Hoppenfeld S: *Physical examination of the spine and extremities,* New York, 1976, Appleton-Century-Crofts.

Magee DJ: *Orthopedic physical assessment,* ed 2, Philadelphia, 1992, WB Saunders.

Mann RA, editor: *DuVries' surgery of the foot,* ed 5, St Louis, 1986, Mosby.

McCarty DJ, Koopman WJ, editors: *Arthritis and allied conditions,* ed 12, Philadelphia, 1993, Lea & Febiger.

Mendelsohn, BA, Paiement GD: Physical examination of the knee, *Primary Care* 23:321-328, 1996.

Mercier LR: *Practical orthopedics,* ed 4, St Louis, 1995, Mosby.

Mourad LA: *Orthopedic disorders,* St Louis, 1991, Mosby.

US Preventive Services Task Force: *Guide to clinical preventive services,* ed 2, Alexandria, Va, 1996, International Medical Publishing.

Chapter 19

Alspach JG: *Core curriculum for critical care nursing,* ed 4, Philadelphia, 1991, WB Saunders.

Bates B: *A guide to physical examination and history taking,* ed 6, Philadelphia, 1995, JB Lippincott.

Bowers AC, Thompson JM: *Clinical manual of health assessment,* ed 4, St Louis, 1992, Mosby.

Chipps E, Clanin N, Campbell V: *Neurologic disorders,* St Louis, 1992, Mosby.

DeJong RN et al: *Essentials of the neurological examination,* Philadelphia, 1978, SmithKline.

Hickey JV: *The clinical practice of neurological and neurosurgical nursing,* ed 4, Philadelphia, 1996, JB Lippincott.

Jones D: *Health assessment manual,* New York, 1986, McGraw-Hill.

Lewis SM, Collier IC, Heitkemper MM: *Medical-surgical nursing: assessment and management of clinical problems,* ed 4, St Louis, 1996, Mosby.

Matthews PJ, Carlson CE: *Spinal cord injury: a guide to rehabilitation nursing,* Rockville, Md, 1987, Aspen.

Potter P: *Pocket guide to health assessment,* ed 3, St Louis, 1994, Mosby.

Rudy EB, Gray VR: *Handbook of health assessment,* ed 3, Norwalk, Conn, 1991, Appleton & Lange.

Scanlon VC, Sanders T: *Essentials of anatomy and physiology,* Philadelphia, 1991, FA Davis.

Seidel HM et al: *Mosby's guide to physical examination,* ed 3, St Louis, 1995, Mosby.

Snyder M: *A guide to neurological and neurosurgical nursing,* ed 2, Albany, NY, 1991, Delmar.

Sparks SM, Taylor CM: *Nursing diagnosis reference manual,* Springhouse, Pa, 1991, Springhouse.

Stuart GW, Sundeen SJ: *Principles and practice of psychiatric nursing,* ed 5, St Louis, 1995, Mosby.

Thompson J, Wilson S: *Health assessment for nursing practice,* St Louis, 1996, Mosby.

Thompson JM et al: *Mosby's clinical nursing,* ed 4, St Louis, 1997, Mosby.

Watson C: *Basic human neuroanatomy: an introductory atlas,* ed 5, Boston, 1995, Little, Brown.

Chapter 20

Blandy JP, Lytton B: *The prostate,* London, 1986, Butterworth.

Blesch KS: Health beliefs about testicular cancer and self-examination among professional men, *Oncol Nurs Forum* 13:29-33, 1986.

Edmunds MW, Mayhew MS: *Procedures for the primary care practitioner,* St Louis, 1996, Mosby.

Gillenwater JY et al: *Adult and pediatric urology,* ed 3, St Louis, 1996, Mosby.

Gordon M: *Nursing diagnosis: process and application,* ed 3, St Louis, 1994, Mosby.

Mayhew HE, Selman SH: Genitourinary problems in the male patient, *Prim Care* 16:857-1068, 1989.

Nyhus LM, Condon RE: *Hernia,* ed 3, Philadelphia, 1989, JB Lippincott.

Pagana KD, Pagana TJ: *Mosby's diagnostic and laboratory test reference,* ed 3, St Louis, 1997, Mosby.

Rous SN: *Urology: a core textbook,* ed 2, Cambridge, Mass, 1996, Blackwell Science.

Sherwood MJ et al: *Determining nursing diagnosis through assessment,* Baltimore, 1988, Williams & Wilkins.

Smith LE, editor: *Practical guide to anorectal testing,* ed 2, New York, 1994, Igaku-Shoin Medical Publishers.

Stanford J: Testicular self-examination, *Prof Nurse* 1:132-133, 1986.

Stanford J: Testicular self-examination: teaching, learning and practice by nurses, *J Adv Nurs* 12:13-19, 1986.

US Preventive Services Task Force: *Guide to clinical preventive services,* ed 2, Alexandria, Va, 1996, International Medical Publishing.

Vogt HB, McHale MS: Testicular cancer, *Postgrad Med* 93:93-96, 1992.

Chapter 21

Barber HRK, Fields DH, Kaufman SA: *Quick reference to OB GYN procedures,* ed 3, Philadelphia, 1990, JB Lippincott.

Beckmann CRB: *Obstetrics and gynecology,* ed 2, Baltimore, 1995, Williams & Wilkins.

Clarke-Pearson DL, Dawood MY: *Green's gynecology,* ed 4, Boston, 1990, Little, Brown.

Firth PA, Watanabe SJ: *Women's health,* Albany, NY, 1996, Delmar Publishers.

Gordon M: *Nursing diagnosis: process and application,* ed 3, St Louis, 1994, Mosby.

Gulanick M, Gradishar D, Puzas MK: *Obstetric and gynecologic nursing,* Albany, NY, 1994, Delmar Publishers.

Hawkins JW, Roberto-Nichols DM, Stanley-Haney JL: *Protocols for nurse practitioners in gynecologic settings,* ed 5, New York, 1995, Tiresias Press.

Herbst AL et al: *Comprehensive gynecology,* ed 2, St Louis, 1992, Mosby.

Knaus JV, Isaacs JH, editors: *Office gynecology,* New York, 1993, Springer-Verlag.

Lichtman R, Papera S: *Gynecology: well-woman care,* Norwalk, Conn, 1990, Appleton & Lange.

Mackay EV et al: *Illustrated textbook of gynaecology,* ed 2, Sydney, 1992, Harcourt Brace Jovanovich.

Mosby's medical, nursing, and allied health dictionary, ed 4, St Louis, 1994, Mosby.

Olsson HM, Gullberg MT: Role of the woman patient and fear of the pelvic examination, *West J Nurs Res* 9:357-367, 1987.

Pagana KD, Pagana TJ: *Mosby's diagnostic and laboratory test reference,* ed 3, St Louis, 1997, Mosby.

Ryan KJ, Berkowitz RS, Barbieri RL: *Kistner's gynecology: principles and practice,* ed 6, St Louis, 1995, Mosby.

Seidel HM et al: *Mosby's guide to physical examination,* ed 3, St Louis, 1995, Mosby.

Sherwood MJ et al: *Determining nursing diagnosis through assessment,* Baltimore, 1988, Williams & Wilkins.

Stenchever MA: *Office gynecology,* ed 2, St Louis, 1996, Mosby.

Symonds EM, Macpherson MBA: *Color atlas of obstetrics and gynecology,* London, 1995, Mosby-Wolfe.

US Preventive Services Task Force: *Guide to clinical preventive services,* ed 2, Alexandria, Va, 1996, International Medical Publishing.

Willson JR, Carrington, ER: *Obstetrics and gynecology,* ed 9, St Louis, 1991, Mosby.

Chapter 22

Beahrs OH, Higgins GA, Weinstein JJ: *Colorectal tumors,* Philadelphia, 1986, JB Lippincott.

Cherry DA, Rothenberger DA: Pelvic floor physiology, *Surg Clin North Am* 68:1217-1230, 1988.

Ger R: Surgical anatomy of the pelvis, *Surg Clin North Am* 68:1202-1216, 1988.

Gordon M: *Nursing diagnosis: process and application,* ed 3, St Louis, 1994, Mosby.

Gordon PH: The anorectum: anatomic and physiologic considerations in health and disease, *Gastroenterol Clin North Am* 16(1):1-15, 1987.

Kirsner JB, Shorter RG, editors: *Diseases of the colon, rectum, and anal canal,* Baltimore, 1988, Williams & Wilkins.

Localio SA, Eng K, Coppa GF: *Anorectal, presacral, and sacral tumors: anatomy, physiology, pathogenesis, and management,* Philadelphia, 1987, WB Saunders.

Marti MC, Givel JC: *Surgery of anorectal diseases,* Berlin, 1990, Springer-Verlag.

Pagana KD, Pagana TJ: *Mosby's diagnostic and laboratory test reference,* ed 3, St Louis, 1997, Mosby.

Payne JE: Symptoms and the diagnosis of bowel cancer: a critical view, *Med J Aust* 148:505-507, 1988.

Raufmann JP, Straus EW: Endoscopic procedures in the AIDS patient: risks, precautions, indications, and obligations, *Gastroenterol Clin North Am* 17:495-506, 1988.

Schrock TR: Diseases of the anorectum. In Sleisenger MH, Fordtran JS: *Gastrointestinal disease,* ed 4, Philadelphia, 1986, WB Saunders.

Sherwood MJ et al: *Determining nursing diagnosis through assessment,* Baltimore, 1988, Williams & Wilkins.

Smith LE, editor: *Practical guide to anorectal testing,* ed 2, New York, 1994, Igaku-Shoin Medical Publishers.

US Preventive Services Task Force: *Guide to clinical preventive services,* ed 2, Alexandria, Va, 1996, International Medical Publishing.

Chapter 24

Andolsek KM: *Obstetric care: standards of prenatal, intrapartum, and postpartum management,* Philadelphia, 1990, Lea & Febiger.

Barber HRK, Fields DH, Kaufman SA: *Quick reference to OB-GYN procedures,* ed 3, Philadelphia, 1990, JB Lippincott.

Beckmann CRB: *Obstetrics and gynecology,* ed 2, Baltimore, 1995, Williams & Wilkins.

Caldwell WE, Maloy HC, Swenson PC: The use of the roentgen ray in obstetrics: anatomical variations in the female pelvis and their classification according to morphology, *Am J Roentgenol* 41:505, 1939.

DeCherney AH, Pernoll ML: *Current obstetric and gynecologic diagnosis and treatment,* ed 8, Norwalk, Conn, 1994, Appleton & Lange.

Firth PA, Watanabe SJ: *Women's health,* Albany, NY, 1996, Delmar Publishers.

Gabbe SG, Niebyl JR, Simpson JL: *Obstetrics: normal and problem pregnancies,* ed 2, New York, 1991, Churchill Livingstone.

Gordon M: *Nursing diagnosis: process and application,* ed 3, St Louis, 1994, Mosby.

Gulanick M, Gradishar D, Puzas MK: *Obstetric and gynecologic nursing,* Albany, NY, 1994, Delmar Publishers.

James DK, Stirrat GM, editors: *Pregnancy and risk: the basis for rational management,* Chichester, NY, 1988, John Wiley & Sons.

Lichtman R, Papera S: *Gynecology: well-woman care,* Norwalk, Conn, 1990, Appleton & Lange.

Merkatz IR, Thompson JE, *New perspectives on prenatal care,* New York, 1990, Elsevier.

Mosby's medical, nursing, and allied health dictionary, ed 4, St Louis, 1994, Mosby.

Nagey DA: The content of prenatal care, *Obstet Gynecol* 74:516, 1989.

Oxorn H: *Oxorn-Foote human labor and birth,* Norwalk, Conn, 1986, Appleton-Century-Crofts.

Pagana KD, Pagana TJ: *Mosby's diagnostic and laboratory test reference,* ed 3, St Louis, 1997, Mosby.

Sherwood MJ et al: *Determining nursing diagnosis through assessment,* Baltimore, 1988, Williams & Wilkins.

Symonds EM, Macpherson MBA: *Color atlas of obstetrics and gynecology,* London, 1995, Mosby-Wolfe.

Tucker S: *Pocket guide to fetal monitoring,* ed 3, St Louis, 1996, Mosby.

US Preventive Services Task Force: *Guide to clinical preventive services,* ed 2, Alexandria, Va, 1996, International Medical Publishing.

Varney H: *Nurse-midwifery,* ed 2, Boston, 1987, Blackwell Scientific Publications.

Willson JR et al: *Obstetrics and gynecology,* ed 9, St Louis, 1991, Mosby.

Chapter 25

American Academy of Pediatrics: *Guidelines for health supervision II,* ed 2, Elk Grove Village, Ill, 1988, The Academy.

American Academy of Pediatrics: *Report of the committee on infectious diseases,* ed 22, Elk Grove Village, Ill, 1991, The Academy.

American Academy of Pediatrics: Committee on Practice and Ambulatory Medicine Recommendation for Preventive Pediatric Health Care, *Pediatrics* 96:373-374, 1995.

American Academy of Pediatrics: Committee on Immunization Practice Recommended Childhood Immunization Schedules, *Pediatrics* 98(1):751, 1996.

Burns C et al: *Pediatric primary care: a handbook for nurse practitioners,* Philadelphia, 1996, WB Saunders.

Chess S, Thomas A: *Temperament in clinical practice,* New York, 1986, Guilford Press.

Daniels SR: Primary hypertension in childhood and adolescence, *Pediatr Ann* 21:224-234, 1992.

Dixon SD, Stein MT: *Encounters with children: pediatric behavior and development,* ed 2, St Louis, 1992, Mosby.

Gemberling C: Preparticipation sports evaluation: an overview, *Nurse Pract Forum* 7(3):125-135, 1996.

Goidenring JM, Cohen E: Getting into adolescent heads, *Contemp Pediatr* 5:75-86, 1988.

Hoekelman RA et al: *Primary pediatric care,* ed 3, St Louis, 1997, Mosby.

Levenberg P, Elster A, editors: *1995 guidelines for adolescent preventive services (GAPS): clinical evaluation and management handbook,* Chicago, American Medical Association.

Lichtman R, Papera S: *Gynecology: well woman care,* Norwalk, Conn, 1990, Appleton & Lange.

Lowrey GH: *Growth and development of children,* ed 8, St Louis, 1986, Mosby.

National Heart, Lung and Blood Institute: Report of Second Task Force on Blood Pressure Control in Children—1987, *Pediatrics* 79:1-25, 1987.

National High Blood Pressure Education Program Working Group on Hypertension Control in Children and Adolescents: Update on the 1987 Task Force Report on High Blood Pressure in Children and Adolescents, *Pediatrics* 98(4):649-658, 1996.

Satter E: *Child of mine: feeding with love and good sense,* Palo Alto, Calif, 1991, Bull Publishing.

Schwartz MW et al: *Pediatric primary care: a problem-oriented approach,* ed 3, St Louis, 1996, Mosby.

Seidel HM et al: *Mosby's guide to physical examination,* ed 3, St Louis, 1995, Mosby.

Strassburger V, Brown R: *Adolescent medicine: a practical guide,* Boston, 1991, Little, Brown.

Tanner JM: *Growth at adolescence,* ed 2, Oxford, 1962, Blackwell Scientific Publications.

US Department of Health, Education and Welfare: *NCHS growth curves for children birth to 18 years,* Hyattsville, Md, 1977, National Center for Health Statistics.

US Department of Health and Human Services, Public Health Service: *Healthy people 2000: national health promotion and disease prevention objectives,* DHHS No 91-50213, Washington, DC, 1990.

Wong DL: *Whaley and Wong's nursing care of infants and children,* ed 5, St Louis, 1995, Mosby.

Zimmerman R, Giebink G: Childhood immunizations: a practical approach for clinicians, *Am Fam Physician* 45:1759-1776, 1992.

Zitelli B, Davis H: *Atlas of pediatric physical diagnosis,* ed 3, New York, 1996, Gower Medical Publishing.

Chapter 26

American Association of Retired Persons and the Administration of Aging, Program Resources Department: *A profile of older Americans,* Washington, DC, 1991, US Department of Health and Human Services.

American Psychiatric Association: *Diagnosis and statistical manual of mental disorders,* ed 4, Washington, DC, 1994, The Association.

Cassel CK et al: *Geriatric medicine,* ed 2, New York, 1990, Springer-Verlag.

Consensus conference differential diagnosis of dementing diseases, *JAMA* 258:3411-3416, 1987.

Dwyer J: *Screening older Americans' nutritional health: current practices and future possibilities,* Washington, DC, 1992, Nutritional Screening Initiative.

Folstein M, Folstein SE, McHugh PR: Mini-mental state: a practical method for grading the cognitive state of patients for the clinician, *J Psychiatr Res* 12:189-198, 1975.

Gordon M: *Manual of nursing diagnosis 1997-1998,* St Louis, 1993, Mosby.

Hirsch CH et al: The natural history of functional morbidity in hospitalized older patients, *Am Geriatr Soc* 38:1296-1303, 1990.

Katz S et al: Studies of illness in the aged: the index of ADL: a standard measure of biologic and psychosocial function, *JAMA* 185:914-919, 1963.

Levkoff SE et al: Delirium: the occurrence and persistence of symptoms among elderly hospitalized patients, *Arch Intern Med* 152:334-340, 1992.

Mahoney Fl, Barthel DW: Functional evaluation: the Barthel Index, *Maryland State Med J* 14:61-65, 1965.

Podsiadlo D, Richardson S: The timed "up & go": a test of basic functional mobility for frail elderly persons, *J Am Geriatr Soc* 39:142-148, 1991.

Schor JD et al: Risk factors for delirium in hospitalized elderly, *JAMA* 267:827-831, 1992.

Williams JH et al: Development and testing of the assessment of living skills and resources (ALSAR) in elderly community-dwelling veterans, *Gerontologist* 31:76-83, 1991.

Yesavage JA et al: Development and validation of a geriatric depression screening scale: preliminary report, *J Psychiatr Res* 17:37-49, 1983.

Chapter 27

Brorsson B, Asberg KH: Katz index of independence in ADL: reliability and validity in short-term care, *Scand J Rehabil Med* 16:125-132, 1984.

Buchanan B: Functional assessment: measurement with the Barthel Index and PULSES profile, *Home Health Nurse* 4:11-17, 1986.

Forer SK: *Revised functional status rating instrument,* Glendale, Calif, 1981, Rehabilitation Institute, Glendale Adventist Medical Center.

Fortinsky RH, Granger CV, Seltzer GB: The use of functional assessment in understanding home care needs, *Med Care* 19:489-497, 1981.

Frattali CM: Perspectives on functional assessment: its use for policy making. *Disabil Rehabil* 15:1-9, 1993.

Fuhrer MJ, editor: *Rehabilitation outcomes: analysis and measurement,* Baltimore, 1987, Brookes.

Golden RR, Teresi JA, Gurland BJ: Development of indicator scales for the comprehensive assessment and referral evaluation (CARE) interview schedule, *J Gerontol* 39:138-146, 1984.

Goodgold J: *Rehabilitation medicine,* St Louis, 1988, Mosby.

Gordon M: *Nursing diagnosis: process and application,* ed 3, St Louis, 1994, Mosby.

Gotland B et al: The SHORT-CARE: an efficient instrument for the assessment of depression, dementia, and disability, *J Gerontol* 39:166-169, 1984.

Granger CV: Health accounting—functional assessment of the long-term patient. In Kottke FJ, Stillwell GK, Lehmann JF, editors: *Krusen's handbook of physical medicine and rehabilitation,* ed 3, Philadelphia, 1982, WB Saunders.

Granger CV, Albrecht GL, Hamilton BB: Outcome of comprehensive medical rehabilitation: measurement by PULSES profile and the Barthel index, *Arch Phys Med Rehabil* 60:145-154, 1979.

Granger CV, Gresham G, editors: *Functional assessment in rehabilitation medicine,* Baltimore, 1984, Williams & Wilkins.

Granger CV, Seltzer GB, Fishbein CF: *Primary care of the functionally disabled: assessment and management,* Philadelphia, 1987, JB Lippincott.

Granger CV et al: Advances in functional assessment for medical rehabilitation, *Top Clin Rehabil* 1:59-74, 1986.

Gulick EE: The self-assessment of health among the chronically ill, *Top Clin Nurs* 8:74-82, 1986.

Gurland B et al: The comprehensive assessment and referral evaluation (CARE)—rationale, development and reliability, *Int J Aging Human Develop* 8:9-42, 1977.

Hamilton GG et al: A uniform national data system for medical rehabilitation. In Fuhrer J, editor: *Rehabilitation outcomes: analysis and measurement,* Baltimore, 1987, Brookes.

Hertanu JS et al: Stroke rehabilitation: correlation and prognostic value of computerized tomography and sequential functional assessments, *Arch Phys Med Rehabil* 65:505-508, 1984.

Hoeman S: *Rehabilitation nursing: process and application,* ed 2, St Louis, 1996, Mosby.

Jacelon CS: The Barthel index and other indices of functional ability, *Rehabil Nurs* 11:9-11, 1986.

Jette AM: State of the art in functional status assessment. In Rothstein JM: *Measurement in physical therapy,* New York, 1985, Churchill Livingstone.

Katz S, Akpom CA: Index of ADL, *Med Care* 14:116-118, 1976.

Katz S et al: Studies of illness in the aged: the index of ADL: a standardized measure of biological and psychosocial function, *JAMA* 185:914-919, 1963.

Keith RA: Functional assessment measures in medical rehabilitation: current status, *Arch Phys Med Rehabil* 65:74-78, 1984.

Keith RA et al: The functional independence measure: a new tool for rehabilitation. In Eisenberg MG, Grzesiak RC, editors: *Advances in clinical rehabilitation,* New York, 1987, Spring.

Lawton MP: Assessing the competence of older people. In Kent D, Kastenbaum R, Sherwood S, editors: *Research, planning and action for the elderly,* New York, 1972, Behavioral Publications.

Lawton MP, Brody EM: Assessment of older people: self-maintaining and instrumental activities of daily living, *Gerontologist* 9:180, 1969.

Linn MW, Linn BS: The rapid disability rating scale–2, *J Am Geriatr Soc* 30:378-382, 1982.

Mahoney FI, Barthel DW: Functional evaluation: the Barthel index, *Maryland State Med J* 14:61, 1965.

McDowell I, Newell C: *Measuring health: a guide to rating scales questionnaires,* ed 2, New York, 1996, Oxford University Press.

McGinnis GE et al: Program evaluation of physical medicine and rehabilitation departments using self-report Barthel, *Arch Phys Med Rehabil* 67:123-135, 1986.

Mosby's medical, nursing, and allied health dictionary, ed 4, St Louis, 1994, Mosby.

Moskowitz E: PULSES Profile in retrospect, *Arch Phys Med Rehabil* 66:647-648, 1985.

Moskowitz E, McCann CB: Classification of disability in the chronically ill and aging, *J Chron Dis* 5:342-346, 1957.

Nagi S: *Disability, concepts and prevalence.* Unpublished paper presented at the First Mary Switzer Memorial Seminar, Cleveland, Ohio, May 1975.

Ninos M, Makohon R: Functional assessment of the patient, *Geriatr Nurs* 6:139-142, 1985.

Nolan BS: Functional evaluation of the elderly in guardianship proceedings, *Law, Med Healthcare* 12(2):10-12, 18, 1984.

O'Toole DM, Goldberg RT, Ryan B: Functional changes in vascular amputee patients: evaluation by Barthel, PULSES profile and ESCROW scale, *Arch Phys Med Rehabil* 66:508-511, 1985.

Pfeffer RI et al: Index in older adults: reliability, validity, and measurement of change over time, *Am J Epidemiol* 120:922-935, 1984.

Pinholt EM et al: Functional assessment of the elderly: a comparison of standard instruments with clinical judgment, *Arch Intern med* 147:484-488, 1987.

Rothstein JM: *Measurement in physical therapy,* New York, 1985, Churchill Livingstone.

Rubenstein LZ et al: Systematic biases in functional status assessment of elderly adults: effects of different data sources, *J Gerontol* 39:686-691, 1984.

Sheikh K et al: Repeatability and validity of a modified activities of daily living (ADL) index in studies of chronic disability, *Int Rehab Med* 1:51, 1979.

Special issue—Critical issues in functional assessment, *Am J Occup Ther* 47:199-259, 1993.

Spiegel JS, Hirshfield MS, Spiegel TM: Evaluation of self-care activities: comparison of a self-reported questionnaire with an occupational therapist interview, *Br J Rheumatol* 24:357-361, 1985.

Teresi JA, Golden RR, Gurland BJ: Concurrent and predictive validity of indicator scales developed for the comprehensive assessment and referral evaluation interview schedule, *J Gerontol* 39:158-165, 1984.

Teresi JA et al: Construct validity of indicator scales developed from the comprehensive assessment and referral evaluation interview schedule, *J Gerontol* 39:147-157, 1984.

Wood P: *Classification of impairments and handicaps,* Geneva, 1975, World Health Organization.

World Health Organization: *International classification of impairments, disabilities, and handicaps,* Geneva, 1980, The Organization.

Page numbers in *italics* indicate illustrations. Page numbers followed by a *t* indicate tables.

NURSING DIAGNOSES GROUPED BY FUNCTIONAL HEALTH PATTERNS

Health Perception–Health Management Pattern

Altered Health Maintenance
Altered Protection
Effective Management of Therapeutic Regimen: Individuals
Energy Field Disturbance
Health-Seeking Behaviors (Specify)
Ineffective Management of Therapeutic Regimen: Community
Ineffective Management of Therapeutic Regimen: Families
Ineffective Management of Therapeutic Regimen: Individuals
Noncompliance (Specify)
Risk for Infection
Risk for Injury
Risk for Perioperative Positioning Injury
Risk for Poisoning
Risk for Suffocation
Risk for Trauma

Nutritional-Metabolic Pattern

Altered Nutrition: Less Than Body Requirements
Altered Nutrition: More Than Body Requirements
Altered Nutrition: Risk for More Than Body Requirements
Altered Oral Mucous Membrane
Effective Breastfeeding
Fluid Volume Deficit
Fluid Volume Excess
Hyperthermia
Hypothermia
Impaired Skin Integrity
Impaired Swallowing
Impaired Tissue Integrity
Ineffective Breastfeeding
Ineffective Infant Feeding Pattern
Ineffective Thermoregulation
Interrupted Breastfeeding
Risk for Altered Body Temperature
Risk for Aspiration
Risk for Fluid Volume Deficit
Risk for Impaired Skin Integrity

Elimination Pattern

Altered Urinary Elimination
Bowel Incontinence
Colonic Constipation
Constipation
Diarrhea
Functional Incontinence

Perceived Constipation
Reflex Incontinence
Stress Incontinence
Total Incontinence
Urge Incontinence
Urinary Retention

Activity-Exercise Pattern

Activity Intolerance
Altered Growth and Development
Altered Tissue Perfusion (Specify Type)
Bathing/Hygiene Self-Care Deficit
Decreased Cardiac Output
Disorganized Infant Behavior
Diversional Activity Deficit
Dressing/Grooming Self-Care Deficit
Dysfunctional Ventilatory Weaning Response (DVWR)
Dysreflexia
Feeding Self-Care Deficit
Fatigue
Impaired Gas Exchange
Impaired Home Maintenance Management
Impaired Physical Mobility
Inability to Sustain Spontaneous Ventilation
Ineffective Airway Clearance
Ineffective Breathing Pattern
Potential for Enhanced Organized Infant Behavior
Risk for Activity Intolerance
Risk for Disorganized Infant Behavior
Risk for Disuse Syndrome
Risk for Peripheral Neurovascular Dysfunction
Toileting Self-Care Deficit

Sleep-Rest Pattern

Sleep Pattern Disturbance

Cognitive-Perceptual Pattern

Acute Confusion
Altered Thought Processes
Chronic Confusion
Chronic Pain
Decisional Conflict (Specify)
Decreased Adaptive Capacity: Intracranial
Impaired Environmental Interpretation Syndrome
Impaired Memory
Knowledge Deficit (Specify)
Pain
Sensory-Perceptual Alterations (Specify)
Unilateral Neglect

Self-Perception–Self-Concept Pattern

Anxiety
Body Image Disturbance
Chronic Low Self-Esteem

Fear
Hopelessness
Personal Identity Disturbance
Powerlessness
Risk for Loneliness
Risk for Self-Mutilation
Self-Esteem Disturbance
Situational Low Self-Esteem

Role-Relationship Pattern

Altered Family Processes
Altered Family Processes: Alcoholism
Altered Parenting
Altered Role Performance
Anticipatory Grieving
Caregiver Role Strain
Dysfunctional Grieving
Impaired Social Interaction
Impaired Verbal Communication
Parental Role Conflict
Relocation Stress Syndrome
Risk for Altered Parent/Infant/Child Attachment
Risk for Altered Parenting
Risk for Caregiver Role Strain
Risk for Violence: Directed at Others
Risk for Violence: Self-Directed
Social Isolation
Social Isolation or Social Rejection

Sexuality-Reproductive Pattern

Altered Sexuality Patterns
Rape-Trauma Syndrome
Rape-Trauma Syndrome: Compound Reaction
Rape-Trauma Syndrome: Silent Reaction
Sexual Dysfunction

Coping–Stress Tolerance Pattern

Defensive Coping
Family Coping: Potential for Growth
Impaired Adjustment
Ineffective Community Coping
Ineffective Denial
Ineffective Individual Coping
Ineffective Family Coping: Compromised
Ineffective Family Coping: Disabling
Posttrauma Response
Potential for Enhanced Community Coping

Value-Belief Pattern

Potential for Enhanced Spiritual Well-Being
Spiritual Distress (Distress of Human Spirit)

Modified from *NANDA nursing diagnosis: definitions and classifications 1997–1998*, North American Nursing Diagnosis Association; and Gordon M: *Manual of nursing diagnosis 1997–1998*, St Louis, 1997, Mosby.